Patrick C. Walsh, M.D.

Urologist-in-Chief, James Buchanan Brady
  Urological Institute
The Johns Hopkins Hospital
Professor and Director
  Department of Urology
The Johns Hopkins University
  School of Medicine
Baltimore, Maryland

Ruben F. Gittes, M.D.

Urologist-in-Chief
Brighman and Women's Hospital
Professor of Urological Surgery
Harvard Medical School
Boston, Massachusetts

Alan D. Perlmutter, M.D.

Chief, Department of Pediatric Urology
Children's Hospital of Michigan
Professor of Urology
Wayne State University School of Medicine
Detroit, Michigan

Thomas A. Stamey, M.D.

Professor of Surgery and
Chairman, Division of Urology
Stanford University School of Medicine
Stanford, California

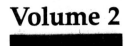

Volume 2

Campbell's

UROLOGY

FIFTH EDITION

1986

W.B. SAUNDERS COMPANY

Philadelphia • London • Toronto • Mexico City • Rio de Janeiro • Sydney • Tokyo • Hong Kong

W. B. Saunders Company: West Washington Square
Philadelphia, PA   19105

Library of Congress Cataloging in Publication Data
Urology.
Campbell's Urology.
1. Urology.   I. Campbell, Meredith Fairfax, 1894-1968.   II. Walsh, Patrick C.   III. Title. [DNLM: 1. Urologic diseases. WJ 100 C192]
RC871.U758 1986   616.6   83-20427
ISBN 0-7216-9088-2 (set)

Listed here is the latest translated edition of this book together with the language of the translation and the publisher.

Italian (3rd Edition)—   Casa Editrice Universo,
                          Rome, Italy

Portuguese (1st Edition)—Editora Guanabara Koogan,
                          Rio de Janeiro, Brazil

Editor: Carroll Cann
Cover Designer: Terri Siegel
Production Manager: Bob Butler
Manuscript Editor: Connie Burton
Illustration Coordinator: Walt Verbitski

Volume 1 ISBN   0-7216-9085-8
Volume 2 ISBN   0-7216-9086-6
Volume 3 ISBN   0-7216-9087-4
Set ISBN   0-7216-9088-2

Campbell's Urology

Last digit is the print number: 9   8   7   6   5   4   3   2   1

CONTRIBUTORS

HERBERT L. ABRAMS, M.D.

Philip H. Cook Professor of Radiology, Harvard Medical School; Senior Radiologist, Brigham and Women's Hospital, Boston, Massachusetts.

Computed Tomography of the Kidney; Renal and Adrenal Angiography; Renal Venography

DOUGLASS E. ADAMS, M.D.

Professor of Radiology, Harvard Medical School; Director, NMR Division, Department of Radiology, Brigham and Women's Hospital, Boston, Massachusetts.

Renal and Adrenal Angiography

S. JAMES ADELSTEIN, M.D., Ph.D.

Professor of Radiology, Harvard Medical School; Director, Joint Program in Nuclear Medicine, Brigham and Women's Hospital, Beth Israel Hospital, The Children's Hospital, Dana Farber Cancer Institute, Boston, Massachusetts.

Radionuclides in Genitourinary Disorders

ERNEST H. AGATSTEIN, M.D.

Senior Resident, Division of Urology, University of California, Los Angeles, School of Medicine; Staff, UCLA Medical Center, Los Angeles, California.

Imperforate Anus, Persistent Cloaca, and Urogenital Sinus Outlet Obstruction

RODNEY U. ANDERSON, M.D.

Associate Professor of Surgery (Urology), Stanford University School of Medicine; Chief of Urology, Santa Clara Valley Medical Center, San Jose, California.

Urinary Tract Infections in Spinal Cord Injury Patients

STUART B. BAUER, M.D.

Assistant Professor of Urology (Surgery), Harvard Medical School; Associate in Surgery (Urology), The Children's Hospital Medical Center, Boston, Massachusetts.

Anomalies of the Upper Urinary Tract

RICHARD E. BERGER, M.D.

Associate Professor, Department of Urology, University of Washington School of Medicine; Chief, Department of Urology, Harborview Medical Center, Seattle, Washington.

Sexually Transmitted Diseases

JAY BERNSTEIN, M.D.

Clinical Professor of Pathology, Wayne State University School of Medicine; Director, Department of Anatomic Pathology, William Beaumont Hospital, Royal Oak, Michigan.

Renal Cystic Disease and Renal Dysplasia

WILLIAM E. BRADLEY, M.D.

Professor, Department of Neurology, University of California, Irvine, School of Medicine; Neurology Service, Veterans Administration Medical Center, Long Beach, California.

Physiology of the Urinary Bladder

CHARLES B. BRENDLER, M.D.

Assistant Professor of Urology, The Johns Hopkins University School of Medicine, Baltimore, Maryland.

Perioperative Care

v

C. EUGENE CARLTON, Jr., M.D.

Russell and Mary Hugh Scott Professor and Chairman, Department of Urology, Baylor College of Medicine; Chief, Urology Service, Methodist Hospital; Active Staff, Ben Taub General Hospital, St. Luke's Episcopal Hospital, Texas Children's Hospital; Consulting Staff, Veterans Administration Hospital, Houston, Texas.

Initial Evaluation, Including History, Physical Examination, and Urinalysis.

WILLIAM J. CATALONA, M.D.

Professor and Chief, Division of Urologic Surgery, Washington University Medical Center; Attending Urologist, Barnes Hospital, Jewish Hospital, St. Louis Children's Hospital, St. Louis County Hospital, Veterans Administration Hospital, St. Louis, Missouri.

Carcinoma of the Prostate

THOMAS S. K. CHANG, Ph.D.

Assistant Professor, James Buchanan Brady Urological Institute, The Johns Hopkins University School of Medicine, Baltimore, Maryland.

The Testis, Epididymis, and Ductus Deferens

DONALD S. COFFEY, Ph.D.

Professor of Urology, Professor of Oncology, and Professor of Pharmacology and Experimental Therapeutics, The Johns Hopkins University School of Medicine; Director of the Research Laboratories of the Department of Urology, The Johns Hopkins Hospital, Baltimore, Maryland.

Biochemistry and Physiology of the Prostate and Seminal Vesicles.

GIULIO J. D'ANGIO, M.D.

Professor of Radiology, Radiation Therapy, and Pediatric Oncology, University of Pennsylvania School of Medicine; Director, Children's Cancer Research Center, Children's Hospital of Philadelphia, Philadelphia, Pennsylvania.

Pediatric Oncology

JEAN B. DE KERNION, M.D.

Professor of Surgery/Urology, and Head of Urologic Oncology, University of California, Los Angeles, School of Medicine; Director for Clinical Programs, Jonsson Cancer Center; Attending Physician, UCLA Hospital, Wadsworth Veterans Administration Hospital, Los Angeles, California.

Renal Tumors

FRANCESCO DEL GRECO, M.D.

Chief, Section of Nephrology-Hypertension, and Professor of Medicine, Northwestern University Medical School, Chicago, Illinois.

Other Renal Diseases of Urologic Significance

CHARLES J. DEVINE, Jr., M.D., F.A.C.S., F.A.A.P.

Professor and Chairman, Department of Urology, Eastern Virginia Medical School; Staff, Medical Center Hospitals, Norfolk General Hospital, De Paul Hospital, Leigh Memorial Hospital; Consultant in Urology, U.S. Naval Regional Medical Center, Portsmouth; Chief of Urology, Children's Hospital of the King's Daughters, Norfolk, Virginia.

Surgery of the Urethra

ROBERT G. DLUHY, M.D.

Associate Professor of Medicine, Harvard Medical School; Physician, Brigham and Women's Hospital, Boston, Massachusetts.

The Adrenals.

GEORGE W. DRACH, M.D.

Professor of Surgery and Chief of Urology, University of Arizona College of Medicine, Tucson, Arizona.

Urinary Lithiasis.

MICHAEL J. DROLLER, M.D.

Professor and Chairman, Department of Urology, Mount Sinai Medical School; Consultant, Bronx Veterans Administration Medical Center, Elmhurst General Hospital; Director of Urology, Mount Sinai Medical Center, New York, New York.

Transitional Cell Cancer: Upper Tracts and Bladder

JOHN W. DUCKETT, M.D.

Professor of Urology, University of Pennsylvania School of Medicine; Director, Division of Urology, Children's Hospital of Philadelphia, Philadelphia, Pennsylvania.

Hypospadias; Disorders of the Urethra and Penis

RICHARD M. EHRLICH, M.D., F.A.C.S., F.A.A.P.

Professor of Surgery/Urology, University of California, Los Angeles, School of Medicine; Staff, UCLA Medical Center, Los Angeles, California.

Imperforate Anus, Persistent Cloaca, and Urogenital Sinus Outlet Obstruction

AUDREY E. EVANS, M.D.

Professor of Pediatrics, University of Pennsylvania School of Medicine; Director, Division of Oncology, Children's Hospital of Philadelphia, Philadelphia, Pennsylvania.

Pediatric Oncology

LARRY L. EWING, Ph.D.

Professor, The Johns Hopkins University School of Hygiene and Public Health, Baltimore, Maryland.

The Testis, Epididymis, and Ductus Deferens

STEWART FELDMAN, M.D.

Formerly, Resident in Urology, Case Western Reserve University School of Medicine, Cleveland, Ohio.

Extrinsic Obstruction of the Ureter

JOHN F. GAETA, M.D.

Professor of Pathology and Associate Professor of Urology, State University of New York at Buffalo School of Medicine; Director, Tissue Pathology, Buffalo General Hospital, Buffalo, New York.

Tumors of Testicular Adnexal Structures and Seminal Vesicles

KENNETH D. GARDNER, Jr., M.D.

Professor of Medicine, University of New Mexico School of Medicine; Chief of Renal Diseases, Department of Medicine, University of New Mexico Hospital, Albuquerque, New Mexico.

Renal Cystic Disease and Renal Dysplasia

FREDRICK W. GEORGE, Ph.D.

Assistant Professor of Cell Biology, University of Texas Health Science Center at Dallas, Southwestern Medical School, Dallas, Texas.

Embryology of the Genital Tract

JAY Y. GILLENWATER, M.D.

Professor and Chairman, Department of Urology, University of Virginia School of Medicine; Chief of Urology, University of Virginia Hospital, Charlottesville, Virginia.

The Pathophysiology of Urinary Obstruction

RUBEN F. GITTES, M.D.

Elliot C. Cutler Professor of Urological Surgery, Harvard Medical School; Chief of Urology, Brigham and Women's Hospital, Boston, Massachusetts.

Partial Nephrectomy: In Situ or Extracorporeal; The Adrenals

JAMES G. GOW, M.D., Ch.M., F.R.C.S.

Formerly, Clinical Lecturer, University of Liverpool; Lourdes Private Hospital, Liverpool, England.

Genitourinary Tuberculosis

HARRY GRABSTALD, M.D., F.A.C.S.

Professor of Urology, Mount Sinai School of Medicine; Acting Director, Department of Urology, Beth Israel Medical Center, New York, New York.

Benign and Malignant Tumors of the Male and Female Urethra; Surgery of Penile and Urethral Carcinoma

JOHN T. GRAYHACK, M.D.

Professor and Chairman, Department of Urology, Northwestern University Medical School; Chief, Northwestern Memorial Hospital; Consultant, Veterans Administration Lakeside Hospital, Chicago, Illinois.

Surgical Management of Ureteropelvic Junction Obstruction.

LAWRENCE F. GREENE, M.D., Ph.D.*

Formerly, Clinical Professor of Surgery/Urology, University of California, San Diego, School of Medicine; Chief of Urology, Veterans Administration Hospital, San Diego, California.

Transurethral Surgery

JAMES E. GRIFFIN, M.D.

Associate Professor of Internal Medicine, University of Texas Health Science Center at Dallas, Southwestern Medical School; Attending Physician, Parkland Memorial Hospital, Dallas, Texas.

Disorders of Sexual Differentiation

H. ROGER HADLEY, M.D.

Assistant Professor, Loma Linda University School of Medicine; Consultant, Riverside General Hospital; Staff, Jerry Pettis Veterans Hospital, San Bernardino County Hospital, Loma Linda University Medical Center, Loma Linda, California.

The Treatment of Male Urinary Incontinence

W. HARDY HENDREN, M.D.

Professor of Surgery, Harvard Medical School; Chief of Surgery, The Children's Hospital; Visiting Surgeon, Massachusetts General Hospital, Boston, Massachusetts.

Urinary Undiversion: Refunctionalization of the Previously Diverted Urinary Tract

STANLEY C. HOPKINS, M.D., C.M., F.R.C.S.(C)

Assistant Professor of Surgery, Division of Urology, University of South Florida College of Medicine; Acting Chief, Urology Section, James A. Haley Veterans Administration Hospital, Tampa, Florida.

Benign and Malignant Tumors of the Male and Female Urethra

---

*Deceased.

STUART S. HOWARDS, M.D.

Professor of Urology and Physiology, University of Virginia School of Medicine; Urologist, University of Virginia Medical Center, Charlottesville, Virginia.

Male Infertility; Surgery of the Scrotum and Its Contents

DOMINIK J. HUBER, M.D.

Radiologist, Long Island Jewish Medical Center, New Hyde Park, New York.

Computed Tomography of the Kidney

PERRY B. HUDSON, M.D.

Professor of Surgery, University of South Florida College of Medicine; Chief, Urology Section, Veterans Administration Medical Center, Bay Pines, Florida

Perineal Prostatectomy

SARWAT HUSSAIN, M.B.B.S.

Department of Radiology, Aga Khan University Medical College, Islamabad, Pakistan.

Computed Tomography of the Adrenal Gland

ROBERT D. JEFFS, M.D., F.R.C.S.(C).

Professor of Pediatric Urology, The Johns Hopkins University School of Medicine; Director of Pediatric Urology, The Johns Hopkins Hospital; Consultant in Pediatric Urology, Francis Scott Key Medical Center, University of Maryland Hospital, John F. Kennedy Institute, Baltimore, Maryland.

Management of the Exstrophy-Epispadias Complex and Urachal Anomalies

JOSEPH J. KAUFMAN, M.D.

Professor of Surgery/Urology, and Chief, Division of Urology, University of California, Los Angeles, School of Medicine; Chief, UCLA Urology Hospital; Director, Clark UCLA Urological Center; Consultant, Wadsworth Veterans Administration Hospital, Sepulveda Veterans Administration Hospital, Cedars/Sinai Hospital, Los Angeles, California.

Surgical Treatment of Renovascular Hypertension

ROBERT W. KINDRACHUK, M.D.

Chief Resident in Urology, Stanford University Medical School; Staff, Stanford University Medical Center, Stanford, California.

Urinalysis

LOWELL R. KING, M.D.

Professor of Urology and Associate Professor of Pediatrics; Head, Section on Pediatric Urology, Duke University School of Medicine; Division of Urology, Duke University Medical Center, Durham, North Carolina.

Vesicoureteral Reflux, Megaureter, and Ureteral Reimplantation

FREDERICK A. KLEIN, M.D.

Assistant Professor of Urology, Virginia Commonwealth University Medical College of Virginia School of Medicine; Staff, Medical College of Virginia Hospitals, Richmond, Virginia.

Surgery of the Ureter

STEPHEN A. KOFF, M.D.

Associate Professor of Surgery; Head, Section of Pediatric Urology, Ohio State University Medical College, Columbus, Ohio.

Enuresis

WARREN W. KOONTZ, Jr., M.D.

Professor and Chairman, Division of Urology, Associate Dean for Clinical Affairs, Virginia Commonwealth University Medical College of Virginia School of Medicine; Staff, Medical College of Virginia Hospitals, Richmond, Virginia.

Surgery of the Ureter

ROBERT J. KRANE, M.D.

Professor and Chairman, Department of Urology, Boston University School of Medicine; Urologist-in-Chief, University Hospital, Boston, Massachusetts.

Sexual Function and Dysfunction.

R. LAWRENCE KROOVAND, M.D.

Associate Professor of Surgery (Pediatric Urology) and Pediatrics, and Director of Pediatric and Reconstructive Urology, Bowman Gray School of Medicine of Wake Forest University; Director of Pediatric and Reconstructive Urology, North Carolina Baptist Hospital, Winston-Salem, North Carolina.

Myelomeningocele

ELROY D. KURSH, M.D.

Associate Professor of Urology, Case Western Reserve University School of Medicine; Staff, University Hospitals of Cleveland, Cleveland, Ohio.

Extrinsic Obstruction of the Ureter

PAUL H. LANGE, M.D.

Professor of Urologic Surgery, University of Minnesota Medical School; Chief, Urology Section, Veterans Administration Medical Center, Minneapolis, Minnesota.

Diagnostic and Therapeutic Urologic Instrumentation

JAY STAUFFER LEHMAN, M.D.*

Formerly, Assistant Director, The Edna McConnell Clark Foundation, New York, New York.

Parasitic Diseases of the Genitourinary System

---

*Deceased.

HERBERT LEPOR, M.D.

Postdoctoral Fellow, Department of Urology, The Johns Hopkins University School of Medicine; Chief Resident, Department of Urology, The Johns Hopkins Hospital, Baltimore, Maryland.

Management of the Exstrophy-Epispadias Complex and Urachal Anomalies

BRUCE R. LESLIE, M.D.

Staff Physician, Division of Hypertensive Diseases, Ochsner Medical Institutions, New Orleans, Lousiana.

Normal Renal Physiology

SELWYN B. LEVITT, M.D.

Adjunct Clinical Professor of Urology, New York Medical College; Attending Pediatric Urologist, Albert Einstein College Hospital; Co-Director, Section of Pediatric Urology, Westchester County Medical Center; Attending Pediatric Urologist, Montefiore Hospital and Medical Center and Bronx Municipal Hospital Center, New York, New York.

Vesicoureteral Reflux, Megaureter, and Ureteral Reimplantation

MICHAEL M. LIEBER, M.D.

Associate Professor of Urology, Mayo Medical School, Consultant in Urology, Mayo Clinic; Staff, Methodist Hospital, St. Mary's Hospital, Rochester, Minnesota.

Open Bladder Surgery

GARY LIESKOVSKY, M.D.

Assistant Professor of Surgery/Urology, University of Southern California School of Medicine, Los Angeles, California.

Use of Intestinal Segments in the Urinary Tract

BERNARD LYTTON, M.B., F.R.C.S.

Professor of Surgery/Urology, Yale University School of Medicine; Chief of Urology, Yale–New Haven Medical Center, New Haven, Connecticut.

Surgery of the Kidney

MAX MAIZELS, M.D.

Assistant Professor of Urology, Northwestern University Medical School; Staff, Children's Memorial Hospital, Northwestern Memorial Hospital, Chicago, Illinois.

Normal Development of the Urinary Tract

TERRENCE R. MALLOY, M.D.

Professor of Urology, University of Pennsylvania School of Medicine; Chief, Section of Urology, Pennsylvania Hospital, Philadelphia, Pennsylvania.

Surgery of the Penis

FRAY F. MARSHALL, M.D.

Associate Professor of Urology, The Johns Hopkins University School of Medicine; Active Staff, The Johns Hopkins Hospital, Baltimore, Maryland.

Anatomy of the Retroperitoneum and Adrenal

VICTOR F. MARSHALL, M.D., D.Sc.

Emeritus Professor of Surgery (Urology), Cornell University Medical College; Professor of Urology, University of Virginia; Emeritus Attending Surgeon, Memorial Hospital for Cancer and Allied Diseases; Consultant in Urology, University of Virginia Hospital, Charlottesville, Virginia.

Suprapubic Vesicourethral Suspension (Marshall-Marchetti-Krantz) for Stress Incontinence.

EDWARD J. McGUIRE, M.D.

Professor of Surgery and Head, Section of Urology, University of Michigan Medical School, Ann Arbor, Michigan.

Neuromuscular Dysfunction of the Lower Urinary Tract

EDWIN M. MEARES, Jr., M.D.

Charles M. Whitney Professor of Urology, and Chairman, Division of Urology, Tufts University School of Medicine; Chairman, Department of Urology, and Urologist-in-Chief, New England Medical Center Hospitals, Boston, Massachusetts.

Prostatitis and Related Disorders

HARRY Z. MELLINS, M.D.

Professor of Radiology, Harvard Medical School; Director, Diagnostic Radiology, Brigham and Women's Hospital, Boston, Massachusetts.

Urography and Cystourethrography

EDWARD M. MESSING, M.D.

Assistant Professor of Surgery and Human Oncology, Division of Urology, University of Wisconsin School of Medicine; Attending Surgeon, University of Wisconsin Hospital and Clinics; Consulting Surgeon, Middleton Veterans Administration Hospital, Madison, Wisconsin.

Interstitial Cystitis and Related Syndromes

BRUCE A. MOLITORIS, M.D.

Assistant Professor of Medicine, Division of Renal Diseases, University of Colorado School of Medicine; Staff, University Hospital, Denver Veterans Administration Medical Center, Denver, Colorado.

Etiology, Pathogenesis, and Management of Renal Failure

MICHAEL J. MORSE, M.D.

Assistant Professor of Surgery (Urology), Cornell University Medical College; Clinical Assistant Attending, Urologic Service, Memorial Sloan-Kettering Cancer Center, New York, New York.

Neoplasms of the Testis; Surgery of Testicular Neoplasms

EDWARD C. MUECKE, M.D.

Clinical Professor of Surgery (Urology), Cornell University Medical College; Attending Surgeon (Urology), The New York Hospital; Associate Attending Surgeon (Urology), Lenox Hill Hospital, New York, New York.

Exstrophy, Epispadias, and Other Anomalies of the Bladder

GERALD P. MURPHY, M.D.

Professor of Surgery, State University of New York at Buffalo School of Medicine; Director, Roswell Park Memorial Institute, Buffalo, New York.

Tumors of Testicular Adnexal Structures and Seminal Vesicles

JOHN B. NANNINGA, M.D.

Associate Professor of Urology, Northwestern University Medical School; Attending Urologist, Northwestern Memorial Hospital; Consultant in Urology, Veterans Administration Lakeside Hospital; Chief, Division of Surgery, Rehabilitation Institute of Chicago, Chicago, Illinois.

Suprapubic and Retropubic Prostatectomy

WALTER R. NICKEL, M.D.

Clinical Professor of Dermatology and Pathology, University of California, San Diego, School of Medicine; Civilian Consultant, U.S. Naval Regional Medical Center, San Diego, California.

Visible Lesions of the Male Genitalia; Cutaneous Diseases of External Genitalia

VINCENT J. O'CONOR, Jr., M.D.

Professor of Urology, Northwestern University Medical School; Chief of Urology, Northwestern Memorial Hospital; Attending Urologist, Veterans Administration Lakeside Hospital, Chicago, Illinois.

Suprapubic and Retropubic Prostatectomy

CARL A. OLSSON, M.D.

Lattimer Professor and Chairman, Department of Urology, College of Physicians and Surgeons, Columbia University; Chief of Urology and Director, Squier Urologic Clinic, Presbyterian Hospital, New York, New York.

Anatomy of the Upper Urinary Tract

JOHN M. PALMER, M.D.

Professor of Urology, University of California, Davis, School of Medicine; Consultant, Veterans Administration Medical Center, Kaiser Permanente Medical Center, Sutter Community Hospitals Cancer Center, Sacramento, California.

Surgery of The Seminal Vesicles

JEROME P. PARNELL, II, M.D.

Clinical Assistant Professor of Surgery-Urology, University of North Carolina at Chapel Hill School of Medicine, Chapel Hill, North Carolina.

Suprapubic Vesicourethral Suspension (Marshall-Marchetti-Krantz) for Stress Incontinence

DAVID F. PAULSON, M.D.

Professor and Chief, Division of Urology, Department of Surgery, Duke University Medical Center, Durham, North Carolina.

Principles of Oncology

ALAN D. PERLMUTTER, M.D.

Professor of Urology, Wayne State University School of Medicine; Chief, Department of Pediatric Urology, Children's Hospital of Michigan, Detroit, Michigan.

Anomalies of the Upper Urinary Tract; Management of Intersexuality; Temporary Urinary Diversion in Infants and Young Children

LESTER PERSKY, M.D.

Clinical Professor of Urology, Case Western Reserve University School of Medicine; Staff, University Hospitals of Cleveland, St. Luke's Hospital, Cleveland, Ohio.

Extrinsic Obstruction of the Ureter

PAUL C. PETERS, M.D.

Professor and Chairman, Division of Urology, The University of Texas Health Science Center at Dallas, Southwestern Medical School; Chief of Urology, Parkland Memorial Hospital, Children's Medical Center; Attending Staff, Baylor University Medical Center, Presbyterian Hospital, Medical Arts Hospital, John Peter Smith Hospital (Ft. Worth), Dallas Veterans Administration Hospital, Dallas, Texas.

Genitourinary Trauma

ROBERT T. PLUMB, M.D.

Clinical Professor of Surgery (Urology), University of California, San Diego, School of Medicine; Senior Staff, Mercy Hospital, Donald N. Sharp Memorial Community Hospital, Coronado Hospital, San Diego, California.

Visible Lesions of the Male Genitalia; Cutaneous Diseases of External Genitalia

JACOB RAJFER, M.D.

Associate Professor of Surgery/Urology, University of California, Los Angeles; School of Medicine; Chief, Division of Urology, Harbor/UCLA Medical Center, Los Angeles, California.

Congenital Anomalies of the Testis

R. BEVERLY RANEY, Jr., M.D.

Associate Professor of Pediatrics, The University of Pennsylvania School of Medicine; Associate Director for Education and Training, and Senior Physician, Division of Oncology, Department of Pediatrics, Children's Hospital of Philadelphia, Philadelphia, Pennsylvania.

Pediatric Oncology

VASSILIOS RAPTOPOULOS, M.D.

University of Massachusetts Medical School; University of Massachusetts Medical Center, Worcester, Massachusetts.

Ultrasound

SHLOMO RAZ, M.D.

Associate Professor of Surgery/Urology, University of California, Los Angeles, School of Medicine; UCLA Center for the Health Sciences, Los Angeles, California.

The Treatment of Male Urinary Incontinence

MARTIN I. RESNICK, M.D.

Professor and Chairman, Division of Urology, Case Western Reserve University School of Medicine; Staff, University Hospitals of Cleveland, Cleveland, Ohio.

Extrinsic Obstruction of the Ureter

ALAN B. RETIK, M.D.

Professor of Surgery (Urology), Harvard Medical School; Chief, Division of Urology, The Children's Hospital, Boston, Massachusetts.

Anomalies of the Upper Urinary Tract; Ectopic Ureter and Ureterocele; Temporary Urinary Diversion in Infants and Young Children

JEROME P. RICHIE, M.D.

Associate Professor of Urological Surgery, Harvard Medical School; Chief, Urologic Oncology, Brigham and Women's Hospital, Boston, Massachusetts.

Ureterointestinal Diversion

ARTHUR I. SAGALOWSKY, M.D.

Associate Professor, Division of Urology, and Surgical Director, Renal Transplant, The University of Texas Health Science Center at Dallas, Southwestern Medical School; Attending Staff, Dallas Veterans Administration Hospital, Children's Medical Center, St. Paul Hospital, Baylor University Medical Center Hospital, Parkland Memorial Hospital, Dallas, Texas.

Genitourinary Trauma

OSCAR SALVATIERRA, Jr., M.D.

Professor of Surgery and Urology, and Chief, Transplant Service, University of California, San Francisco, School of Medicine, San Francisco, California.

Renal Transplantation

PETER T. SCARDINO, M.D.

Associate Professor of Urology, Baylor College of Medicine; Active Staff, The Methodist Hospital, Ben Taub General Hospital; Assistant Staff, St. Luke's Episcopal Hospital; Courtesy Staff, Veterans Administration Hospital, Texas Children's Hospital, Houston, Texas.

Initial Evaluation, Including History, Physical Examination, and Urinalysis

ANTHONY J. SCHAEFFER, M.D.

Associate Professor, Northwestern University Medical School; Attending, Northwestern Memorial Hospital; Associate Attending, Children's Memorial Hospital; Consultant in Urology, Veterans Administration Lakeside Hospital, Chicago, Illinois.

Other Renal Diseases of Urologic Significance; Surgical Management of Ureteropelvic Junction Obstruction

PAUL F. SCHELLHAMMER, M.D.

Professor of Urology, Eastern Virginia Medical School; Director, Urology Training Program, Eastern Virginia Graduate School of Medicine; Active Staff, General Hospital of Virginia Beach, Norfolk General Hospital, Leigh Memorial Hospital, Children's Hospital of the King's Daughters, DePaul Hospital, Norfolk, Virginia.

Tumors of the Penis

JAN SCHÖNEBECK, M.D.

Associate Professor of Urology, University of Linköping, Sweden; Head of Urology, Department of Surgery, Central Hospital, Norrköping, Sweden.

Fungal Infections of the Urinary Tract

ROBERT W. SCHRIER, M.D.

Professor and Chairman, Department of Medicine, University of Colorado School of Medicine; Head, Division of Renal Diseases; Staff, University Hospital, Denver Veterans Administration Medical Center, Denver General Hospital, Rose Medical Center, Denver, Colorado

Etiology, Pathogenesis, and Management of Renal Failure

WILLIAM W. SCOTT, Ph.D., M.D., D.Sc.

Professor of Urology, Emeritus, The Johns Hopkins University School of Medicine; The Johns Hopkins Hospital, Baltimore, Maryland.

Carcinoma of the Prostate

STEVEN E. SELTZER, M.D.

Associate Professor of Radiology, Harvard Medical School; Radiologist and Director, Computed Tomography, Brigham and Women's Hospital, Boston, Massachusetts.

Computed Tomography of the Kidney

RICHARD J. SHERINS, M.D.

Chief, Section on Reproductive Endocrinology, Developmental Endocrinology Branch, National Institute of Child Health and Human Development, Bethesda, Maryland.

Male Infertility

LINDA M. DAIRIKI SHORTLIFFE, M.D.

Assistant Professor of Surgery (Urology), Stanford University School of Medicine; Chief, Urology Section, Veterans Administration Medical Center, Palo Alto, California.

Infections of the Urinary Tract: Introduction and General Principles; Urinary Infections in Adult Women; Urinary Incontinence in the Female: Stress Urinary Incontinence

DONALD G. SKINNER, M.D.

Professor and Chairman, Division of Urology (Surgery), University of Southern California School of Medicine; Chief of Staff, Kenneth Norris, Jr., Cancer Hospital and Research Institute, Los Angeles, California.

Ureterointestinal Diversion; Use of Intestinal Segments in the Urinary Tract

EDWARD H. SMITH, M.D.

Professor and Chairman, Department of Radiology, University of Massachusetts Medical School, Worcester, Massachusetts.

Ultrasound

BRENT W. SNOW, M.D.

Assistant Professor, University of Utah School of Medicine, Salt Lake City, Utah.

Disorders of the Urethra and Penis

HOWARD McC. SNYDER, III, M.D.

Assistant Professor of Urology in Surgery, University of Pennsylvania School of Medicine; Assistant Surgeon, Division of Urology, Children's Hospital of Philadelphia, Philadelphia, Pennsylvania.

Pediatric Oncology

JOSEPH T. SPAULDING, M.D.

Assistant Clinical Professor of Urology, University of California, San Francisco, School of Medicine; Active Staff, St. Francis Memorial Hospital, St. Mary's Medical Center, Pacific Presbyterian Medical Center, San Francisco, California.

Surgery of Penile and Urethral Carcinoma

THOMAS A. STAMEY, M.D.

Professor of Surgery and Chairman, Division of Urology, Stanford University School of Medicine, Stanford, California.

Urinalysis; Infections of the Urinary Tract: Introduction and General Principles; Urinary Infections in Adult Women; Urinary Incontinence in the Female: Stress Urinary Incontinence

RALPH A. STRAFFON, M.D.

Chairman, Division of Surgery; Member, Department of Urology, Cleveland Clinic Foundation, Cleveland, Ohio.

Surgery for Calculus Disease of the Urinary Tract

RONALD S. SWERDLOFF, M.D.

Professor of Medicine, University of California, Los Angeles, School of Medicine; Chief, Division of Endocrinology, Harbor-UCLA Medical Center, Los Angeles, California.

Physiology of Male Reproduction: Hypothalamic-Pituitary Function

EMIL A. TANAGHO, M.D.

Professor and Chairman, Department of Urology, University of California, San Francisco, School of Medicine, San Francisco, California.

Anatomy of the Lower Urinary Tract

SALVATOR TREVES, M.D.

Associate Professor of Radiology, Harvard Medical School; Chief, Division of Nuclear Medicine, The Children's Hospital Medical Center, Boston, Massachusetts.

Radionuclides in Genitourinary Disorders

TIMOTHY S. TRULOCK, M.D.

Fellow in Pediatric Urology, Emory University School of Medicine, Atlanta, Georgia.

Prune-Belly Syndrome

SABAH S. TUMEH, M.D.

Assistant Professor of Radiology, Harvard Medical School; Radiologist, Brigham and Women's Hospital; Consultant in Oncodiagnostic Radiology and Nuclear Medicine; Dana Farber Cancer Institute, Boston, Massachusetts.

Radionuclides in Genitourinary Disorders

RICHARD TURNER-WARWICK, B.Sc., D.M. (Oxon.), M.Ch., F.R.C.S., F.R.C.P., F.A.C.S.

Consultant Urological Surgeon, The London University Institute of Urology, Middlesex Hospital, St. Peter's Group Hospitals, Royal National Orthopaedic Hospital, London, England.

Urinary Fistulae in the Female

DAVID C. UTZ, M.D.

Anson L. Clark Professor of Urology, Mayo Clinic and Mayo Medical School; Staff, Methodist Hospital, Saint Mary's Hospital, Rochester, Minnesota.

Open Bladder Surgery

E. DARRACOTT VAUGHAN, Jr., M.D.

James J. Colt Professor of Urology in Surgery, Cornell University Medical College; Attending Surgeon, The New York Hospital, Memorial Sloan-Kettering Cancer Center; Visiting Physician, The Rockefeller University Hospital, New York, New York

Normal Renal Physiology; Renovascular Hypertension; Suprapubic Vesicourethral Suspension (Marshall-Marchetti-Krantz) for Stress Incontinence

M. J. VERNON SMITH, M.D., Ph.D.

Professor of Urology, Virginia Commonwealth University Medical College of Virginia School of Medicine; Staff, Medical College of Virginia Hospitals, Richmond, Virginia.

Surgery of the Ureter

FRANZ VON LICHTENBERG, M.D.

Professor of Pathology, Harvard Medical School; Pathologist, Brigham and Women's Hospital, Boston, Massachusetts.

Parasitic Diseases of the Genitourinary System

PATRICK C. WALSH, M.D.

David Hall McConnell Professor and Director, Department of Urology, The Johns Hopkins University School of Medicine; Urologist-In-Chief, The James Buchanan Brady Urological Institute, the Johns Hopkins Hospital, Baltimore, Maryland.

Benign Prostatic Hyperplasia; Radical Retropubic Prostatectomy

ALAN J. WEIN, M.D.

Professor of Urology and Chairman, Section of Urology, University of Pennsylvania School of Medicine, Philadelphia, Pennsylvania.

Surgery of the Penis

LESTER WEISS, M.D.

Clinical Professor of Pediatrics, University of Michigan, Medical School; Director, Medical Genetics and Birth Defects Center, Henry Ford Hospital, Detroit, Michigan.

Genetic Determinants of Urologic Disease

ROBERT M. WEISS, M.D.

Professor, Department of Surgery/Urology, Yale University School of Medicine; Adjunct Professor, Department of Pharmacology, Columbia University, College of Physicians and Surgeons, New York, New York; Medical Staff, Gaylord Hospital, Wallingford; Attending, Yale–New Haven Hospital; Consulting, West Haven Veterans Administration Hospital, Waterbury Hospital, Sharon Hospital, William Backus Hospital, Norwalk Hospital, St. Raphael's Hospital, New Haven, Connecticut.

Physiology and Pharmacology of the Renal Pelvis and Ureter

WILLET F. WHITMORE, Jr., M.D.

Professor of Surgery (Urology), Cornell University Medical College; Attending Surgeon, Urologic Service, Memorial Sloan-Kettering Cancer Center, New York, New York.

Neoplasms of the Testis; Surgery of Testicular Neoplasms

JEAN D. WILSON, M.D.

Professor of Internal Medicine, University of Texas Health Science Center at Dallas, Southwestern Medical School; Attending Physician, Parkland Memorial Hospital, Dallas, Texas.

Embryology of the Genital Tract; Disorders of Sexual Differentiation

JAN WINBERG, M.D.

Professor of Pediatrics, Karolinska Institute; Chairman, Department of Pediatrics, Karolinska Hospital, Stockholm, Sweden.

Urinary Tract Infections in Infants and Children

JOHN R. WOODARD, M.D.

Professor of Surgery (Urology) and Director of Pediatric Urology, Emory University School of Medicine; Chief, Urology Service, Henrietta Egleston Hospital for Children, Atlanta, Georgia.

Prune-Belly Syndrome; Neonatal and Perinatal Emergencies

PHILIPPE E. ZIMMERN, M.D.

Resident in Urology, University of California, Los Angeles, School of Medicine, Los Angeles, California.

The Treatment of Male Urinary Incontinence

PREFACE

Urology has undergone remarkable growth and change since the Fourth Edition of this textbook was published. In creating this edition we recognized the need for an authoritative textbook incorporating the new advances in basic science, clinical medicine, instrumentation, and surgical technique. At the outset we knew we had the opportunity to create the best textbook of urology ever written and, in doing so, to improve the quality of care provided by all urologists for their patients.

We began by re-evaluating every chapter in the Fourth Edition with the help of our residents. No one is more critical or frank than the resident in training, and these evaluations were helpful in focusing new goals. We recognized that it was possible to consolidate the pathophysiologic material contained in the early chapters into a smaller space while providing more information. This enabled us to expand the clinical and surgical sections.

In keeping with past tradition there has been a significant turnover of participants in the book in order to ensure fresh approaches to specific topics. In this edition, for example, there are 26 new authors and 9 new chapters. The anatomy chapter has been subdivided into three sections: the retroperitoneum and adrenal, the upper urinary tract, and the lower urinary tract and genitalia. All three sections are now under new authorship and have new illustrations, new depth, and new emphasis on surgical considerations. The sections on normal renal function; renovascular hypertension; the etiology, pathogenesis, and management of renal failure; and renal diseases of urologic significance have new authorship. They have been completely updated and modernized and contain succinct, factual, specific applications for the urologist. A new chapter on diagnostic and therapeutic urologic instrumentation has been provided. This excellent chapter on endourology incorporates all the new information in this rapidly developing field. The section on sexual function and dysfunction, which also has new authorship, contains the newer concepts of physiology of penile erection along with extensive recommendations regarding the evaluation and management of patients with sexual dysfunction. In the recognition that a major portion of the urologist's practice involves the management of patients with cancer, a new chapter, "Principles of Oncology," has been included. Urologists have been called upon to provide an ever increasing level of sophisticated care for cancer patients. This chapter will enable the urologist to have a more informed understanding of the principles of oncology and their applications to clinical care. A new chapter on pre- and postoperative care of the urologic patient is also included. This chapter amounts to a "mini-textbook" of medicine and is an excellent synopsis of the modern concepts of pre- and postoperative care that the urologic surgeon should know.

Over 50 per cent of the chapters on urologic surgery have new authors and new illustrations. Examples from this section of the book include new chapters on urinary undiversion and the surgery of calculus disease. In addition, new approaches are presented to the management of extracorporeal renal surgery and partial nephrectomy, the surgical management of ureteropelvic junction obstruction, the surgical management of the ureter, open bladder surgery, transurethral prostatectomy, surgery of the penis, and surgery of the scrotum and its contents. The chapter on the use of intestinal segments provides an excellent description of the Kock pouch, a technique that has received widespread attention from urologists because it provides a form of urinary diversion that does not require an external appliance. In addition, the chapter on radical retropubic prostatectomy emphasizes the new "nerve-sparing" modifications that preserve postoperative potency following radical prostatectomy and cystoprostatectomy.

We wish to thank the authors of prior editions, since this new edition has been built upon the solid foundation they laid. Our gratitude is greatest for the contingent of contributing authors who collectively represent the finest scientists and clinicians associated with the field of urology. We wish to pay tribute to the late J. Hartwell Harrison, who coedited the Third Edition with the late Meredith Campbell and who led all of us through the major transition incorporated in the Fourth Edition. His untimely death prevents his witnessing our present efforts.

A work of this scope and magnitude cannot be accomplished without the assistance of a great number of persons whose efforts may not be specifically attributed within this book. Finally, we wish to express our thanks to Carroll C. Cann, Robert Butler, Constance Burton, Carolyn Naylor, and the staff of the W. B. Saunders Company for their patience and help in bringing this ambitious undertaking to publication.

PATRICK C. WALSH, M.D.
For the Editors

CONTENTS

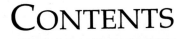

VOLUME 1

SECTION I. ANATOMY AND PHYSIOLOGY

SECTION II. THE UROLOGIC EXAMINATION AND DIAGNOSTIC TECHNIQUES

6
INITIAL EVALUATION, INCLUDING HISTORY, PHYSICAL EXAMINATION, AND URINALYSIS

7
RADIOLOGY OF THE URINARY TRACT

SECTION III. THE PATHOPHYSIOLOGY OF URINARY OBSTRUCTION

9

10

SECTION VIII. URINARY LITHIASIS

SECTION IX. GENITOURINARY TRAUMA

26
GENITOURINARY TRAUMA 1192
Paul C. Peters, M.D., and Arthur I. Sagalowsky, M.D.

VOLUME 2

SECTION X. BENIGN PROSTATIC HYPERPLASIA

27
BENIGN PROSTATIC HYPERPLASIA 1248
Patrick C. Walsh, M.D.

SECTION XI. TUMORS OF THE GENITOURINARY
TRACT IN THE ADULT

28
PRINCIPLES OF ONCOLOGY 1268
David F. Paulson, M.D.

SECTION XII. EMBRYOLOGY AND ANOMALIES OF THE GENITOURINARY TRACT

SECTION XIII. PEDIATRIC UROLOGIC SURGERY

VOLUME III

SECTION XIV. RENAL DISEASES OF UROLOGIC SIGNIFICANCE

SECTION XV. UROLOGIC SURGERY

BENIGN PROSTATIC HYPERPLASIA

CHAPTER 27

Benign Prostatic Hyperplasia

PATRICK C. WALSH, M.D.

Benign prostatic hyperplasia (BPH) is probably the most common neoplastic growth that occurs in men. Beginning with the early observations of Morgagni (1760), it was recognized that benign hyperplasia arose from the inner periurethral glands of the prostate, and a century later surgical techniques were developed for the removal of this tissue. Although over the ensuing years these advances have provided a logical and satisfactory form of treatment for this disorder, much remains to be learned about the causes, pathogenesis, and possible medical management of prostatic hyperplasia. It is hoped that with the recent development of radioimmunoassays for the measurement of both steroidal and polypeptide hormones in the serum, and with improved insight into the target-organ mechanisms underlying the action of androgens and estrogens in the prostate, a greater understanding can be obtained about the factors that regulate normal and abnormal growth of the prostate. This chapter reviews the most recent information available on the incidence, pathology, causes, and clinical manifestations of this common disorder.

INCIDENCE

As demonstrated by Swyer many years ago (1944), there is a very slow increase in the size of the prostate from the time of birth until puberty (Berry et al., 1984) (Fig. 27–1). At that time, a rapid increase in size occurs that continues until after the third decade is reached. The size of the prostate then remains constant until about the age of 45 years. Beginning at this time, either the prostate may undergo benign hyperplasia, in which case its volume commences to increase at a rapid pace and continues to do so until death, or it may not show this pathologic change, in which case it commences to atrophy and progressively decreases in size. Consequently, benign prostatic hyperplasia is characteristically a disease of men older than the age of 40 years. Few, if any, patients with true nodular hyperplasia have been observed before this age. In Moore's series (1944) of more than 700 prostates, the youngest individual with a true nodule within the prostate was 39 years of age, and the nodules in this case were microscopic in size.

Histologically, BPH is also rarely identified in men under the age of 40 years (Moore, 1944; Swyer, 1944; Franks, 1954; Haugen and Harbitz, 1972; Pradhan and Chandra, 1975). However, beginning in the 40's, the incidence of BPH increases from an average of 23 to 88 per cent by the ninth decade (Berry et al., 1984) (Fig. 27–2). Although this reflects the incidence of BPH as determined in histologic sections by the pathologist, it does not indicate the sizes of the prostates associated with this disease. Figure 27–2 illustrates the average prostatic weight at autopsy of 740 men and the average prostatic weight at the time of simple perineal prostatectomy performed for BPH in the early part of the century at the Brady Urological Institute (Gover, 1923).

These data indicate that with age there is a gradual increase in average prostatic weight beginning at approximately the fifth decade. This finding is accompanied by an increase in the incidence of BPH identified histologically by the pathologist. In addition, the amount of tissue removed at the time of simple prostatec-

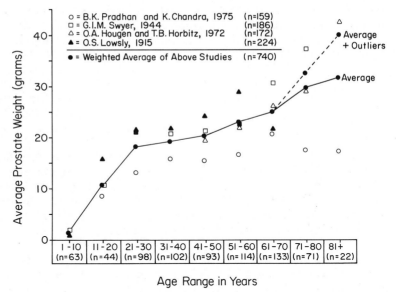

Figure 27–1. Age-related changes in the size of the human prostate. Data summarized from four published autopsy series from a total of 740 human subjects (Lowsly, 1915; Swyer, 1944; Haugen and Harbitz, 1972; Pradhan and Chandra, 1975). The solid line connecting the dark circles denotes the weighted average obtained from the four studies. Two of the four studies contained a few specimens that were extremely large and could be shown to be outliers from the general average. When they are included they raise the overall average, as shown by the broken line. (From Berry, S. J., et al.: J. Urol., *132*:474, 1984.)

tomy also appears to increase with advancing age. These data support the progressive nature of this disease in the aging male.

Although most patients over the age of 50 will have histological evidence of benign prostatic hyperplasia and many patients will suffer symptoms resulting from urethral compression, not all patients require a prostatectomy for relief of these symptoms. In 1968 Lytton et al. suggested that the probability of a 40-year-old man requiring an operation for BPH, if he lives to 80 years of age, is approximately 10 per cent. Recently, Birkhoff (1983) suggested that because the rate of prostatectomy has doubled since that study was performed, the chance now

of a 50-year-old man requiring a prostatectomy during his lifetime is 20 to 25 per cent.

Although the development of BPH is almost a universal phenomenon in aging men, the cause and pathogenesis of this disorder are poorly understood. Attempts at identifying risk factors based on epidemiologic studies have not been very helpful. Recently, Rotkin (1983) summarized these data and suggested that "there are no confirmable data to suggest relationships of sociocultural variables, celibacy, specific blood groups, use of tobacco and/or alcohol, gerontologic conditions, such as coronary heart disease, cerebral vascular disease, hypertension, diabetes mellitus, and cirrhosis of the liver, to

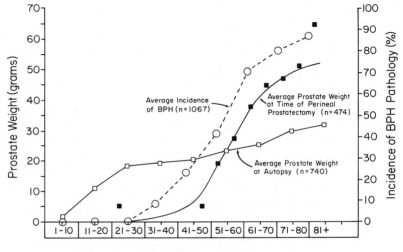

Figure 27–2. Age-related alterations in human prostatic pathology: incidence of BPH at autopsy in 1067 men based on histologic criteria (open circles); average prostatic weight at autopsy in 740 men (open boxes); average prostatic weight at time of simple perineal prostatectomy for BPH in 474 men (closed boxes). (From Berry, S. J., et al.: J. Urol., *132*:474, 1984.)

the onset of BPH." Furthermore, he concluded that there was no further information to support the claimed association of BPH as a precursor developing into prostatic cancer.

PATHOLOGY

The adult prostate is a compact organ lying at the neck of the bladder and surrounding the urethra. In young men, distinct lobes cannot be identified. Yet, McNeal (1981) identified four distinct zones within the prostate having morphologic, functional, and pathologic significance: (1) the anterior fibromuscular stroma, (2) the peripheral zone, (3) the central zone, and (4) preprostatic tissue (see Chapter 5). The last zone, which is the smallest and most complex in its arrangement of both glandular and nonglandular elements, is the exclusive site of origin of BPH. The main component of the preprostatic zone is a cylindrical smooth muscle sphincter that surrounds the urethra. This sphincter prevents the reflux of semen into the bladder at the time of ejaculation. Inside this cylinder of smooth muscle are tiny periurethral glands. Although the lateral expansion (away from the urethra) of most of these glands is limited by the smooth muscle cylinder, at the distal margins some ducts escape the most distal rings of smooth muscle, thus enabling them to develop outside its confines. This group of ducts, arising at a single point at the junction of the proximal and distal urethral segments, is the transition zone (Fig. 27–3). The transition zone

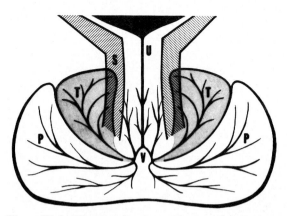

Figure 27–3. Diagram of gross appearance of the prostate sectioned in the oblique coronal plane parallel to the urethra. Ducts of the transition zone (T) leave urethra lateral to verumontanum (V) and just proximal to highest ducts of peripheral zone (P). These ducts spread laterally around distal border of preprostatic sphincter (S) and follow it proximally toward bladder neck. (From McNeal, J. E.: Invest. Urol., *15*:340, 1978.)

and other periurethral glands are the exclusive site of origin of BPH.

According to McNeal (1978, 1981, 1983), as early as the fourth decade, nodules begin to develop in the transition zone and periurethral tissue of the prostate. The nodules in the periurethral tissue are of pure stromal composition and usually remain small throughout life. In contrast, almost all nodules in the transition zone are glandular from their inception, and later in life these nodules enlarge to form the main mass of BPH tissue. The formation of these nodules involves the budding of new small glands from pre-existing ducts with the creation of new glandular architecture. The formation of new ductal and acinar architecture (McNeal, 1983) is generally a forbidden process in adult organs. For this reason, he suggested (1978) that BPH results from a reawakening of embryonic inductive interactions between incompletely developed prostatic glands and inappropriate nonprostatic stroma, which arises from the smooth muscle sphincter.

The growth of BPH appears to involve three independent processes: (1) nodule formation; (2) diffuse enlargement of the transition zone; and (3) enlargement of nodules (McNeal, 1978). McNeal found that in men ages 50 to 70 years, although the volume of the transition zone doubled, nodules accounted for only 14 per cent of the mass of the transition zone. Thus, diffuse enlargement of the transition zone was the major reason for size increase in most men younger than age 70. Beginning in the seventh decade and increasing abruptly in the eighth, there was a dramatic increase in nodule mass that accounted for the major increase in prostatic size after that time. In most cases, McNeal found that clinically significant BPH was almost entirely the result of bilateral expansion of nodules in the transition zone. The nodules in the periurethral zone usually increased at a much slower rate and only if the stromal nodules were incorporated by gland buds from nearby periurethral ducts. The degree of expansion of the periurethral nodules tends to be greatest proximally and gives rise to the so-called middle lobe, which projects into the bladder posterior to the urethral lumen.

On microscopic examination, the hyperplasia is characteristically nodular, and both epithelium and stroma are involved in varying degrees (Fig. 27–4). Based on the histologic pattern, Franks (1976) recognized five types: (1) stromal, (2) fibromuscular, (3) muscular, (4) fibroadenomatous, and (5) fibromyoadenomatous. The last, which is most common, is made

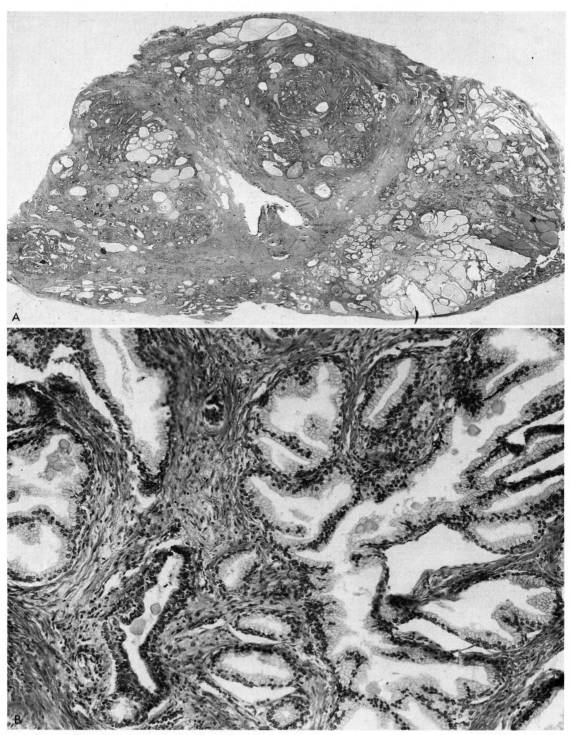

Figure 27–4. Photomicrograph of a cross section of a human prostate with early benign hyperplasia. *A,* Whole mount, low power, *B,* High power ×160.

up of a stromal component composed of interlacing strands of smooth muscle and collagen, arranged in much the same way as in the normal prostate, and glandular elements of differing types. Commonly, there are groups of small or large acini, some of which may be cystic, in which there are often many papillary infoldings. The epithelium is generally made up of tall columnar cells with pale-staining granular cytoplasm, basal vesicular nuclei, and rather indefinite luminal margins (see Fig. 27–4). In addition, there is often an inconspicuous basal layer of flattened cells beneath the cell surface resembling that in the normal prostate (Franks, 1976). In other areas, the hyperplasia may involve small acini lined with two or more layers of darker cuboidal cells. The absence of mitotic figures in the hyperplastic prostate is puzzling and suggests one of these possibilities:

1. That the mitotic cycle is either very fast or very slow.

2. That the process is hypertrophy and not hyperplasia.

3. That it represents remnants of a previous stimulus with little growth.

4. That the growth is amitotic (Mostofi, 1970).

Hyperplastic glands are further differentiated from normal glands on the basis of secondary changes in the hyperplastic areas that result from the mechanical effects of nodules expanding within the relatively confined prostatic area. Evidence of recent or healed infarction is observed in approximately 25 per cent of hyperplastic glands (Mostofi, 1970). Cellulitis from ascending duct infection, dilatation of acini, retention of secretion due to ductile obstruction, focal atypical hyperplasia, and metaplasia of the epithelium are other changes that are of significance in the diagnosis of prostatic hyperplasia (Mostofi, 1970). Finally, areas of prostatic cancer, usually extending from the posterior portion of the gland, are found in approximately 10 per cent of all patients (Franks, 1976). Prostatic infarction, inflammation, or carcinoma may be additional factors that are responsible for the urinary outflow obstructive symptoms that we commonly attribute to benign nodular hyperplasia alone.

ETIOLOGY

Based upon all available information, it appears clear that the two major factors necessary for the onset of BPH in men are the presence of the testes and aging. Consequently, much research has been directed at identifying a hormonal cause. Although there is conflicting information, there are several factors that strongly support the possibility that BPH in men is under endocrine control:

1. Benign prostatic hyperplasia does not occur in men who are castrated prior to puberty.

2. Regression of established BPH has been reported to occur following castration.

3. In an animal model, BPH can be reproduced by hormones.

What is the nature of these hormonal influences?

Over the past decade, the factors that interact to cause the development of BPH have come under intense scrutiny. The various theories and approaches to this problem can be distilled down to three possibilities (Grayhack, 1983):

1. BPH reflects merely a reaction of normal prostatic cells to an abnormal endocrine environment.

2. BPH reflects a stimulated growth of substantially altered prostatic cells by a minimally altered hormonal environment.

3. BPH reflects a variable mixture of these factors.

The remainder of this section details the various etiologic factors that have been considered to be important in the pathogenesis of BPH.

Role of the Testis

It is generally believed that BPH does not occur in patients who are castrated prior to puberty and that it is rare in males who are castrated prior to the age of 40. Only one documented exception has been reported: Scott (1953) performed a prostatectomy on a 60-year-old man with urinary retention who had been castrated at the age of 28 years.

Whether the testes play a permissive or active role in the development of BPH is uncertain. Theoretically, the most convincing way to demonstrate a direct effect of the testes on BPH would be the demonstration of regression following castration of patients with established BPH. As stated by Huggins and Stevens in 1940: *Whether benign hypertrophy of the prostate is under endocrine control or not is a problem of immediate interest since not all workers are agreed on this point. Determination of the effect of castration on this disease is one of the most critical ways to settle this problem, but contradiction of opinion exists at the present time as to the effect of removal of the gonads on enlargement of the prostate.*

Unfortunately, this statement is as true today as it was in 1940. In a classic study by White in 1895, 111 men were castrated for the treatment of bladder outlet obstruction. Approximately 87 per cent of these men showed rapid atrophy of the prostatic enlargement after orchiectomy. The following year Cabot presented a longer follow-up of 61 cases (Cabot, 1896). Substantial improvement was demonstrated in 84 per cent of men undergoing orchiectomy for BPH. These reports were followed quickly by other publications reporting failure of relief of prostatic enlargement following castration, and 30 to 40 years elapsed before Deming et al. (1935) revived the subject. They reported no effect of castration on prostatic enlargement in one patient whom they followed for 3 months. In 1940, Huggins and Stevens castrated three men for treatment of BPH. Atrophy was not present 29 days after castration in one patient, but appeared in the other two at 86 and 91 days respectively, after the operation. They concluded that "the prostatic epithelium, at least, is under the control of the testes."

Believing that more data were necessary to prove a relationship between established BPH and the testes and recognizing that purposeful castration of a large number of men with the condition was not feasible, Wendel et al. (1972) compared the histologic findings of BPH in patients with prostatic carcinoma who had been treated with castration and estrogen therapy with the histologic findings in patients with prostatic cancer who were not treated. They concluded that the BPH present in patients with carcinoma of the prostate treated with orchiectomy and estrogen is a lower grade than that found in those patients not receiving this treatment. Infolding of the acinar epithelium and the secretory phase were virtually absent in the group receiving orchiectomy and estrogen compared with their presence in patients not having this treatment. This finding in patients with occult or untreated prostatic cancer suggests that the differences are correlated with orchiectomy and estrogen and not with the presence of carcinoma itself. They believe that their observations support the theory that the cells of BPH are subject to continuing stimulation by the testes. Summarizing all of these findings, one returns to the conclusion of Huggins and Stevens (1940) concerning the influence of the testes upon the prostatic epithelium.

In all of these studies, there has been no accurate quantitation of the stromal component of the disease. It is well recognized that in experimental animals following castration, there is more rapid and complete regression of epithelial components than their stromal counterparts (Neubauer et al., 1981). Consequently, it is possible that castration may have its most powerful influence in those cases of BPH characterized by epithelial overgrowth and the least influence in those cases in which the disease is mainly stromal. In the future, further attempts should be made to clarify the influence of the testes on BPH.

The "Dihydrotestosterone Thesis"

It is well recognized that dihydrotestosterone (DHT) is the major intracellular androgenic metabolite within the prostate (Bruchovsky and Wilson, 1968; Anderson and Liao, 1968) (see Chapter 5). Recognizing the central regulatory role of DHT in growth of the prostate, Wilson et al. (1970) first suggested that DHT accumulation might be implicated in the etiology of BPH. This suggestion was based initially on an investigation of several different animal species to determine whether the capacity of the prostate to form DHT could be correlated with prostatic growth (Wilson and Gloyna, 1970). Their study demonstrated that in most animals the prostate loses its ability to form DHT with age. However, in two animal species, the dog and man, high rates of DHT formation persist throughout life. Because these are the two animal species that spontaneously develop prostatic hyperplasia, it was proposed that BPH might be the result of the unregulated production of DHT over many years. To explore this possibility further, Siiteri and Wilson (1970) measured the androgen content in normal and hyperplastic human prostates. Although they found no significant difference in the content of testosterone in the two types of tissue, the content of DHT was three- to four-fold greater in hyperplastic tissue than in normal glands. Subsequently, this observation has been confirmed by other investigators. For the past dozen years, research into the etiology of BPH has focused on factors that may be responsible for the accumulation of supranormal levels of DHT and the mechanism by which this induces prostatic hyperplasia (Geller et al., 1976; Hammond, 1978; Meikle et al., 1978; Krieg et al., 1979).

While investigating the value of using measurements of DHT content as a marker for the hormonal responsiveness of prostatic cancer, our laboratory recently noted that the content of DHT in normal and benign hyperplastic tissues obtained at open surgical procedures was similar (Walsh et al., 1983). We measured DHT content in normal peripheral and benign hyperplastic prostatic tissue obtained at open surgical procedures on 29 men ages 36 to 82 years. The DHT content in normal prostates (mean ± SE, 5.1 ± 0.4 ng/gm tissue) and in BPH (5.0 ± 0.4) was similar. In 11 patients in whom both normal and hyperplastic prostatic tissue was harvested simultaneously at the same operation, there was no significant difference in the content of DHT in the two types of tissue. These findings failed to confirm the widespread belief that DHT content is elevated in BPH. Our data differ from the reported literature in one major respect: The DHT content of normal peripheral prostate in this study is three to four times higher than previously reported (Table 27–1). In reviewing the literature to determine why we were unable to confirm the findings of others, we learned that the "elevated" levels of DHT in BPH reported by others were based upon measurements performed on surgically removed specimens, whereas the "low levels" of DHT in normal tissue were based upon measurements performed on tissues obtained at autopsy. This observation suggested that the conditions of tissue harvesting may have significantly influenced the endogenous levels of androgen within the prostate. To explore this possibility further, DHT content was measured in seven cadavers ranging in age from 19 to 82 years. The results of this experiment suggested that the DHT content of prostatic tissue removed at autopsy is facticiously low (0.7 to 1.0 ng/gm tissue) (Table 27–1).

Several investigators have justified the use of prostatic tissue procured at autopsy for the measurement of DHT content by demonstrating that when prostatic tissue was incubated at 20°C,

there was no fall in DHT content. However, the unclothed body of an adult in an environmental temperature of 60°F only cools at 1°F per hour during the first 3 hours after death and then 2°F per hour during the next 3 hours. If the body is clothed, the rate of cooling is 66 per cent slower (Marshall and Hoare, 1962). These facts encouraged us to determine the influence of incubations performed at 37°C on DHT content. When in vitro incubations of fresh prostatic tissue were performed at 37°C, DHT content was reduced to low levels within 2 hours.

The finding that DHT content in BPH is identical to levels in normal tissue questions the role of DHT accumulation as a causative factor in the etiology of BPH. The speculative role of DHT as a causative factor in BPH has been supported experimentally by studies in the dog that demonstrated these two phenomena:

1. Canine BPH is characterized by increased prostatic DHT concentration (Gloyna et al., 1970).

2. Steroid treatment regimens that increase prostatic growth in the dog increase prostatic DHT concentrations (Moore et al., 1979).

However, recent studies from our laboratories have questioned these findings. In age-matched dogs, we could demonstrate no difference in DHT content between dogs with histologically normal prostates and those with spontaneous BPH (Ewing et al., in press). Second, although a positive correlation was observed between prostatic weight and DHT content in castrated or intact beagles treated with 11 of 15 different steroid regimens, there were four additional treatment regimens (intact or castrated beagles treated with either DHT or 3α-androstanediol alone) that resulted in high concentrations of prostatic DHT but that failed to evoke equivalent increases in prostatic weight (Ewing et al., in press). Finally, there was a dramatic

TABLE 27–1. SUMMARY OF PUBLISHED DATA ON DIHYDROTESTOSTERONE (DHT) CONTENT IN NORMAL AND HYPERPLASTIC PROSTATIC TISSUE

| | Source of Tissue | | DHT ng/gm tissue + SE | |
Authors	NORMAL	BPH	NORMAL	BPH
Siiteri and Wilson (1970)	Autopsy	Surgery	1.3 ± 0.5	6.0 ± 1.0
Geller et al. (1976)	Autopsy	Surgery	2.1 ± 0.3	5.6 ± 0.9
Hammond (1978)	Autopsy	Surgery	1.3 ± 0.3	5.5 ± 0.5
Meikle et al. (1978)	Autopsy	Surgery	1.3 ± 0.6	4.0 ± 1.9
Kreig et al. (1979)	Autopsy	Surgery	1.6 ± 1.0	4.5 ± 1.4
Walsh et al. (1983)	Surgery	Surgery	5.1 ± 0.4	5.0 ± 0.4
	Autopsy	Autopsy	0.7 ± 0.1	1.0 ± 0.2

Abbreviation: BPH = Benign prostatic hyperplasia.

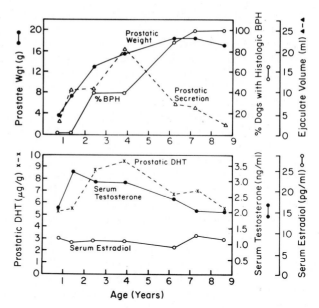

Figure 27–5. The relationships between prostatic weight, histology, volume of prostatic secretion, tissue dihydrotestosterone content, and serum levels of testosterone and estradiol in the beagle with age.

biphasic change in prostatic DHT concentrations with advancing age in the beagle (Fig. 27–5). After age 4 years, although DHT content in the prostate fell, the incidence of BPH continued to increase (Ewing et al., 1983).

In another study, we observed that the prostatic secretory function in the beagle peaks at approximately 4 years of age and then declines dramatically (Brendler et al., 1983). However, as the secretory capacity of the prostate diminishes, the gland continues to grow and histologic changes of BPH become more evident (Fig. 27–5).

These data suggest that the factors regulating growth of the canine prostate and at least one differentiated function (i.e., secretion) may be controlled separately and the fact that abnormal growth continues in the face of declining DHT levels suggests that regulatory factors other than DHT may be involved in the etiology of the hyperplastic growth of the dog prostate. Recognizing that human BPH occurs in the presence of normal tissue levels of DHT should focus research efforts to identify other factors that may sensitize this tissue and accelerate growth.

The Role of Estrogen/Androgen Synergism

The role of estrogens in the physiologic regulation of prostatic growth in man is one of great speculation. For years it has been assumed that estrogen may be responsible in some way for the spontaneous development of prostatic hyperplasia in man. This speculation was strengthened by the observation that in the dog, estrogen acts synergistically with androgen in the experimental induction of BPH.

Using the dog as a model, Wilson et al. (1975) demonstrated previously that young castrated dogs that were treated for 2 years with either testosterone or DHT failed to develop BPH while intact control dogs over a similar interval spontaneously developed the disease. Based upon this observation, they speculated that one or more testicular hormones, other than testosterone or DHT, were required for the development of prostatic hyperplasia.

Based on these findings, Walsh and Wilson (1976) subsequently examined the possible role of estradiol and androstanediol in this process. In this series of experiments, dogs received treatment with androstanediol or DHT with or without estradiol. In the animals treated with androstanediol, the average weight of the prostate increased 10 gm in 1 year and two of the five animals developed BPH. Even more striking results were produced by the combination of androstanediol plus estradiol; the average increase in gland size was 31.2 gm and all five animals had massively enlarged prostates. These results were in striking contrast to previous studies in which prostatic weights of similar animals treated with identical doses of testosterone and DHT averaged only 3.6 and 6.0 gm, respectively. Thus, for the first time, enlargement of the prostate, comparable with that seen in prostatic hyperplasia, was produced by hormonal treatment subsequent to early castration in the dog.

These results have been confirmed by others since. In addition, it has been demonstrated that when DHT is administered in combination with estradiol, prostatic hyperplasia is induced (DeKlerk et al., 1979).

To gain insight into the mechanism by which estrogen produces this synergistic effect, the androgen and estrogen receptors in the canine prostate have been characterized. The canine prostate contains high concentrations of an estrogen receptor (Chaisiri et al., 1978; Trachtenberg et al., 1980, Hawkins et al., 1980). Furthermore, when castrated dogs are treated with estradiol, there is a two-fold increase in cytosolic androgen receptor (Moore et al., 1979). This observation led Moore et al. (1979) to propose that the mechanism of estrogen/androgen synergism in the experimental induction of canine BPH may be explained by estradiol-mediated increases in the androgen receptor. Our laboratory subsequently demonstrated that spontaneously arising canine hyperplasia in young dogs was characterized by increases in nuclear androgen receptor content and that the administration of estradiol plus androstanediol to castrated dogs significantly increased the prostatic nuclear androgen receptor content over that found in dogs treated with androstanediol alone (Trachtenberg et al., 1980). From this observation, we concluded that an increase in nuclear androgen receptor content appeared to be an important event in the development of spontaneously arising and experimentally induced canine prostatic hyperplasia and that the mechanism of androgen/estrogen synergism in the experimental induction of canine BPH may be explained by estradiol-mediated increases in nuclear androgen receptor content (Trachtenberg et al., 1980). Although this is an attractive hypothesis to explain the experimental induction of canine prostatic hyperplasia, it is not known whether or not estrogen synergism is responsible as well for spontaneous BPH in the dog.

In man, a number of investigators have explored the possibility of estrogen/androgen synergism by measuring steroid hormone levels in the plasma of men as they age. Although some investigators have suggested that there is no alteration in plasma testosterone levels with aging (Harman and Tsitouras, 1980), most laboratories agree that with aging there is a gradual fall in plasma testosterone levels. The reason for the disagreement on this important subject was recently explained by the observation that in old age there is attenuation of the early morning rise in testosterone levels that are characteristic of young men (Bremner et al., 1983). To correct for this, Zumoff et al. (1982) measured 24-hour mean plasma concentrations of androgens and estrogens in healthy men over a wide range of ages. They found that plasma testosterone concentrations showed a slow continuous decline with age, decreasing about 35 per cent between 21 and 85 years of age (Fig. 27–6). However, there was no alteration with age in plasma estrone or estradiol. These findings are in agreement with those of Harman and Tsitouras (1980), but are in contrast to other findings that demonstrated an increase in plasma estradiol with age (Rubens et al., 1974; Pirke and Doerr, 1975). Regardless, whether estradiol concentrations increase or remain stable with aging, because plasma testosterone levels fall there is an alteration in the ratio of estrogen to androgen. As emphasized by Wilson (1980), because these endocrine changes probably do not commence until after the initiation of the pathologic process it is unlikely that these alterations in plasma hormones are causally linked to the initiation of the hyperplasia. However, it is clear that the continued growth of the hyperplastic process during the fifth and sixth decades takes place on the background of decreased levels of plasma androgen relative to normal or increased levels of plasma estrogen. This is the major evidence that suggests a possible pathogenic role for estrogen in the induction of BPH.

Recognizing that the characterization of steroid hormones in the canine prostate has helped to clarify the estrogen/androgen synergism responsible for the experimental induction of BPH in the dog, similar studies have been carried out in man. The canine prostate contains abundant quantities of a high-affinity estrogen receptor. However, reports on estrogen binding in the human prostate have been conflicting. (For review, see Ekman et al., 1983.) The percentage of specimens classified as estrogen receptor–positive from numerous laboratories is highly variable, and the estrogen receptor content differs from one report to another and within the same studies. To explore this subject further, we recently characterized the estrogen receptor in the human prostate and determined that the human prostate contains multiple sites for estrogen binding in cytosol as well as nuclear preparations (Ekman et al., 1983). One class of binding sites (Type I) corresponds to the classical, high-affinity estrogen receptor (K_d for [^{3}H] estradiol 0.10 nM). This receptor has been characterized in normal and BPH tissues. In both

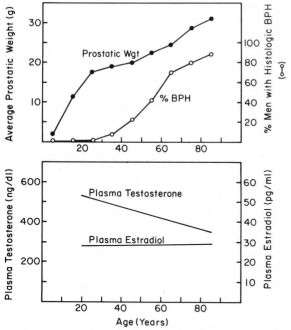

Figure 27–6. The relationships between prostatic weight and histology and plasma testosterone and estradiol in man with age. The data on prostatic weight and histology are repeated from Figure 27–2. The data on plasma testosterone and estradiol represent regression lines calculated from 24 hour mean plasma concentrations measured on 35 healthy male volunteers aged 21 to 85 years. (From Zumoff, B., et al.: J. Clin. Endocrinol. Metab., *54*:534, 1982.)

the cytosol, nuclear salt–extractable, and nuclear salt–resistant compartments, the level of the classical estrogen receptor in BPH is significantly lower than in normal tissue. In addition to the estrogen receptor, progesterone and androgen receptors have also been characterized. With the recognition that estrogens are known to induce the progesterone receptor in breast and uterine target tissues, the existence of a progesterone receptor in human BPH suggests the possibility that this tissue may be under estrogenic stimulation. To investigate this possibility, progesterone receptor content was measured in normal and hyperplastic tissues (Ekman et al., 1982). Cytosolic progesterone receptor content in normal and BPH tissue were similar; nuclear salt–extractable and nuclear salt–resistant receptors were undetectable. These findings failed to provide evidence for preferential estrogenic stimulation of human BPH. When androgen receptor content was measured in the three subcellular compartments, elevated levels of receptor were identified in both the nuclear salt–extractable and nuclear salt–resistant compartments in BPH tissue (54 and 41 per cent, respectively) (Barrack et al., 1983).

In summary, studies on the role of estrogen in the pathogenesis of BPH have been reviewed. Evidence in favor of a role for estrogen includes:

1. *Experimental* induction of BPH in the dog in which estrogen synergizes with 5α-reduced androgens.

2. Estrogen induction of the androgen receptor in the canine prostate, a proposed mechanism for estrogen/androgen synergism.

3. Alteration in estrogen/androgen production with aging in man favoring a possible role for estrogen in the maintenance, but not induction of BPH.

4. The presence of the classical estrogen receptor in human BPH.

5. Increased nuclear androgen receptor levels in human BPH, similar to findings in spontaneous and experimentally induced canine BPH (Barrack et al., 1983).

On the other hand, there are also factors that fail to support a role for estrogen in the pathogenesis of BPH:

1. The alterations in estrogen/androgen production that occur with aging appear rather minor and occur after the apparent onset of the disease.

2. Cytoplasmic and nuclear estrogen receptor levels in human BPH are significantly lower than in the normal prostate and considerably lower than estrogen receptor content in the canine prostate.

3. The similar levels of cytosolic progesterone receptor content in normal and BPH tissues fail to provide evidence for preferential estrogenic stimulation of human BPH (Ekman et al., 1982).

Thus, although estrogen synergism is an attractive hypothesis as a mechanism for the induction of BPH, further evidence is necessary before this thesis can be accepted. Documentation of definite increases in estrogen stimulation with age is necessary. Furthermore, more information is necessary to document the fact that human BPH is actually a target organ for estrogenic stimulation. In many species, treatment of castrated animals with estrogen produces a marked change in the morphologic organization of the prostate from a predominantly atrophic epithelium to one characterized by squamous metaplasia and fibromuscular stroma. When estrogen is administered to humans, although squamous metaplasia occurs in the urethra and ducts of the prostate, the acini are rarely involved (Moore and McLellan, 1938; Mostofi, 1970). This is further evidence against a primary role for estrogens in the stimulation of BPH.

The Role of Stromal-Epithelial Interactions

Reawakening of the inductive potential of the prostatic stroma during adulthood is a rather recent and particularly attractive hypothesis in the unending search for an answer to the etiology of BPH (McNeal, 1978). In the embryo, *androgenic hormone* is the inducer that triggers the budding of the prostatic ducts from the urethral lining into the adjacent stroma. Cunha (1980) has shown that the *mesenchyme* is the actual target organ for androgenic steroids that mediates the morphogenetic effects of hormones upon the epithelium. The mesenchyme induces the urogenital epithelium to express its normal program of morphogenesis and cytodifferentiation.

McNeal (1983) observed that in BPH, *gland budding* and *branching* toward a central focus is considered most often a primary event. He cites the formation of new ductal and acinar architecture, which he states is a forbidden process in adult organs, as evidence for embryonic capacity for this tissue. He believes that some humoral-inducing agent from the stroma may be the inciting agent for gland proliferation. The earliest changes of BPH have been noted to occur in a very small area of the prostate termed by McNeal as the *transition zone*. According to McNeal, the early formation of nodules may represent an entirely local event having no endocrine determinants. In contrast, the growth of nodules, which McNeal found occurring in men older than age 70, appears synchronized and occurs simultaneously in many nodules of the same gland. This could well represent an endocrine change. Thus, the induction of BPH could be viewed as a multifactorial event.

At present, there is no solid evidence that "embryonic reawakening" occurs in adult tissues. However, the hypothesis as set forth by McNeal is most attractive and deserves serious consideration and investigation.

Summary of Etiologic Findings

The etiology of benign prostatic hyperplasia has been examined, and various hypotheses have been reviewed. There is still much to be learned. It remains to be determined whether or not human BPH is under the regulation of the testes. It should be possible to evaluate the role of the testes using various pharmacologic manipulations that selectively and reversibly block testicular secretions, e.g., luteinizing hormone releasing hormone LHRH agonists, antiestrogens, antiandrogens, or inhibitors of steroidogenesis. If indeed it is possible to demonstrate an effect of testicular secretions on the growth of BPH, it will remain to be determined whether or not this effect is direct or merely permissive.

Based upon experimental studies in the dog, it appears that the factors regulating growth of the prostate and at least one differentiated function (i.e., secretion) may be controlled separately and, furthermore, that abnormal growth continues in the face of declining levels of serum testosterone and tissue DHT. These data suggest that regulatory factors other than serum testosterone and tissue levels of DHT may be involved in the etiology of the hyperplastic growth of the dog prostate. Recognizing that human BPH occurs in the presence of normal tissue levels of DHT should focus research efforts to identify other factors that may sensitize this tissue and accelerate growth. In the dog, estrogen serves this function in the experimental induction of the disease. However, it remains to be determined whether estrogenic synergism plays a role in the induction of BPH in man. Additional studies are necessary to determine the relationship between estrogen secretion, aging, and the development of BPH in man. In addition, further evidence needs to be accumulated to document the fact that human BPH is indeed a target organ for estrogenic stimulation.

A recent and attractive area for research involves epithelial-stromal interactions and "embryonic reawakening" in the pathogenesis of BPH. This appears to be an ideal mechanism to explain the early induction of the disease relegating an abnormal endocrine environment to a secondary role involved in the maintenance and proliferation of the disease once it has been induced. This attractive hypothesis needs further work.

DIAGNOSIS

Clinical Manifestations

Enlargement of the prostate per se causes no obvious physiologic manifestations. The disturbances that result are secondary to the effects on the urethra, the bladder, the kidneys, and, less frequently, the prostate itself. Urethral obstruction results from the elongation, tortuosity, and compression of the posterior urethra. When only the lateral lobes are involved in the process, the urethral lumen is compressed into an elongated, narrow but broad, ribbon-like channel (Culp, 1975). Enlargement of the median lobe may be in one of two directions. It may be confined by the internal urethral sphincter and expand in a subtrigonal direction, elevating the bladder base and displacing or angulating the internal urethral orifice forward. Less frequently, the median lobe enlargement expands into the bladder lumen through the internal urethral sphincter. Such a median lobe is called a subcervical lobe, since it extends into the bladder on a relatively small stalk whose base is located distal to the bladder neck. Because of its mobility, it tends to fall over the internal urethral orifice, producing a ball-valve obstruction. Consequently, one or more of these mechanisms are responsible for the urinary tract obstruction produced by hyperplasia.

In an effort to overcome the obstruction, the detrusor musculature undergoes compensatory hypertrophy, resulting in the characteristic ribbed appearance of the muscle bands. Muscular activity that increases the intravesical pressure for the purpose of overcoming the obstruction at the bladder neck leads to the herniation of the mucosa through the thinner parts of the bladder wall, forming diverticula. Untreated, the process progresses to decompensation with dilatation of the bladder and thinning of the wall, resulting in weakening of the vesical musculature that supports the intramural portion of the ureter. Dilatation of the ureter and pelvis and secondary infection may eventually lead to renal insufficiency and hypertension.

Symptoms

In early cases, the patient usually has minimal symptoms, because the detrusor musculature is capable of compensating for the increased outlet resistance to urine flow. With increasing encroachment on the urethra as a result of growth of the adenoma, however, the patient eventually develops a constellation of symptoms called "prostatism":

1. Diminution in the caliber and force of the urinary stream.

2. Hesitancy in initiating voiding.

3. Inability to terminate micturition abruptly, with postvoiding dribbling.

4. A sensation of incomplete emptying of the bladder.

5. Occasionally, urinary retention.

These are *obstructive* symptoms, and they must be carefully distinguished from irritative lower urinary tract symptoms such as dysuria, frequency, and urgency. Disastrous results can follow a prostatectomy performed on a patient whose symptoms stemmed from irritation, such as inflammatory or infectious processes, rather than from obstruction. As prostatic obstruction progresses, about 50 to 80 per cent of them will develop unstable bladders with secondary symptoms of frequency, urgency, and urgency incontinence (Bates et al., 1979). As the amount of residual urine increases, the patient may note nocturia, diurnal frequency, a mass in the lower abdomen, and overflow urinary incontinence. Residual urine also predisposes to recurrent urinary tract infections.

Some patients with "silent" prostatism present with symptoms that represent the secondary effects of the bladder neck obstruction. Slowly progressive obstruction may permit a gradual adjustment to the symptoms. Thus, the patient presents for examination without complaints. The examination, however, may show the secondary anemia of renal insufficiency, a lower abdominal midline mass representing an incompletely emptied bladder, an elevated blood urea nitrogen (BUN) or creatinine level, or other findings associated with renal insufficiency. Hematuria may be another symptom of obstruction, especially if it is terminal. Hematuria is more common in early benign hyperplasia than in carcinoma of the prostate. As urinary tract obstructive symptoms increase in severity, the patient may develop urinary retention. Acute urinary retention is frequently precipitated by chilling; ingestion of alcohol; a prolonged delay in voiding; infection; or the ingestion of anticholinergics, antidepressants, tranquilizers, or decongestants.

Physical Examination

Prior to examination, the physician should observe the patient voiding to completion to document the decrease in size and force of the urinary stream. These findings on the general physical examination may suggest the presence of severe obstruction:

1. Evidence of loss of weight or edema of the hands and face.

2. Pallor or other evidence of secondary anemia.

3. Cardiomegaly or pulmonary edema.

4. Tenderness in the renal areas.

5. A mass in the lower abdomen.

The rectal examination is performed with a well-lubricated glove index finger, and a 360-degree digital exploration is carried out. The prostate is palpated with attention to size, consistency, and shape. Hyperplasia usually produces a smooth, firm, elastic enlargement of the prostate. The size of the prostate on rectal examination, however, does not permit one to estimate the degree of bladder neck obstruction. Patients with marked enlargement of the prostate may have no urinary tract obstruction, whereas if there is median lobe hypertrophy, the patient may have marked outflow obstructive symptoms without palpable enlargement of the gland. In addition to revealing the individual characteristics of the prostate, the rectal examination also affords the physician an opportunity to evaluate the intactness of the rectal sphincter, which indirectly reflects the state of vesical innervation (Culp, 1975). The symptoms of neurogenic bladder may simulate bladder neck obstruction secondary to BPH.

Further Investigations

Many men with BPH present to the urologist early in the disease process because of concern about the cause for their new symptom complex and about the possible presence of cancer. In these men, a careful history, physical examination, and urinalysis (if normal) are usually all that are necessary. The patient should be reassured about the benign nature of his condition, the long and uncertain natural history of the disease, and the advisability of yearly follow-up evaluations.

In men who present with a more advanced disease process (e.g., marked outlet obstructive symptoms, obstructive and irritative symptoms, or recurrent infection), I usually catheterize the patient with a No. 16 Coude catheter following completion of the physical examination. This simple maneuver rules out the presence of a narrow urethral stricture and quantitates the amount of residual urine. In addition to a routine urinalysis, a urine culture is obtained to exclude infection, blood urea nitrogen and serum creatinine levels are determined to estimate the degree of renal function, and an acid phosphatase sample is drawn (preferably prior to prostatic examination). In the past, at this point patients were often asked to return for an intravenous pyelogram and cystourethroscopy.

Cystourethroscopy

To evaluate vescial neck obstruction properly, there is no adequate substitute for cystourethroscopy. When the diagnosis is uncertain, cystoscopy may be carried out in the office. In the patient who is markedly symptomatic, however, this examination is best performed immediately prior to prostatectomy to guide the surgeon in choosing an operative approach. This examination should include a complete evaluation of the interior of the bladder, with special reference to the presence of trabeculation, cellules, or diverticula. The vesical neck is examined for the presence of contracture, bar formation, or intravesical intrusion of the prostate. The length of the posterior urethra is measured from the bladder neck to the verumontanum to aid in estimating the size of the prostate. Once the contours of the lobes, their number, and their depth have been estimated, the bladder is filled with water, and with the sidearm of the cystourethroscope open, the instrument is withdrawn to determine whether the lobes are occlusive. When interpreting the significance of these findings, the urologist should recognize that most men over 50 years of age will have some degree of outlet obstruction that can be detected by cystourethroscopy. Thus, this finding alone is not a sufficient indication for surgical treatment.

Intravenous Urography

An intravenous pyelogram with postvoiding film will document the degree of upper urinary tract obstruction, identify the presence of bladder calculi, and estimate the degree of bladder emptying. In addition, the presence of a filling defect in the bladder, especially when the lower end of the ureters pursue a hooked course in entering the bladder, suggests the presence of marked intravesical prostatic enlargement. However, the value of routine intravenous urography in the evaluation of men with BPH has been questioned (Marshall et al., 1974; Abrams et al., 1976; Anderson et al., 1977). These studies demonstrated a low incidence (approximately 15 per cent) of coexisting pathology detected by urography. This finding, coupled with the risk of a contrast medium reaction and the cost of the investigation, suggests that routine urography in the evaluation of the uncomplicated patient with BPH is unnecessary. For this reason, unless other indications are present, e.g. hematuria, it is probably wise to delay excretory urograms until patients are scheduled for prostatectomy. I find that the information provided by an intravenous pyelogram is most valuable in planning and executing a safe surgical procedure.

Urodynamic Evaluation

The measurement of urinary flow rate, although not mandatory, can provide useful information in the evaluation of patients who present with obstructive symptoms. The flow curve reflects the net result of bladder function and outlet resistance. If the maximum flow rate is greater than 15 ml/sec, patients rarely have infravesical obstruction (Abrams and Griffiths, 1979). Conversely, in the absence of primary bladder dysfunction, patients with flow rates less than 10 ml/sec almost always prove to be obstructed. In patients who have flow rates between these two extremes, repeat testing is necessary. Cystometry is indicated in those patients with a clinical suspicion of bladder dysfunction unrelated to obstruction, e.g., patients who present primarily with urgency and frequency. In addition, it is useful in documenting the presence of detrusor instability in those patients with advanced outlet obstruction (Bates et al., 1979). In patients who deny significant outflow obstructive symptoms but who are found to have marked trabeculation and a large quantity of residual urine, a more formal urodynamic evaluation may be necessary. This should include, in addition to urinary flow measurements, simultaneous measurements of intravesical and intraurethral pressure profiles.

DIFFERENTIAL DIAGNOSIS

Usually there is no difficulty in establishing the diagnosis of benign prostatic hyperplasia. Carcinoma of the prostate, bladder neck contracture, urethral stricture, bladder calculus, carcinoma of the bladder, chronic prostatitis, and neurogenic bladder may simulate the clinical picture of BPH, however, because they also may produce bladder outlet obstructive symptoms. The presence of irritative lower urinary tract symptoms, such as dysuria, urgency, and frequency, should alert the physician to consider conditions other than obstruction as the cause of the patient's symptoms. In the absence of a large amount of residual urine, frequency and nocturia are not caused by benign prostatic hyperplasia. Bladder neck contractures, urethral strictures, bladder calculi, and bladder neoplasms are best evaluated with endoscopy. In some patients with diffuse carcinoma of the bladder in situ (a condition in which patients frequently present with lower urinary tract symptoms) the lesion may be difficult to recognize on cystoscopy, and urinary cytology and random bladder biopsies may be necessary to confirm its presence. Likewise, young men with diffuse infiltrating carcinoma of the prostate often present with lower urinary tract obstructive symptoms.

TREATMENT

Because there is no effective medical management for the treatment of benign prostatic hyperplasia at present, all comments in this section are predicated on the fact that the only effective treatment available is surgery. Consequently, because the vast majority of men older than the age of 60 years have some evidence of benign prostatic hyperplasia, the mere presence of this disorder is not an indication for its treatment. The general indications for the relief of prostatic obstruction are:

1. Acute urinary retention.
2. Hydronephrosis.
3. Recurrent urinary tract infection aggravated by residual urine.
4. Severe hematuria from a congested prostate.
5. Outflow obstructive symptoms that are of sufficient concern to the patient to cause him to desire treatment.
6. Obstructive symptoms associated with the development of bladder instability (urgency and urgency incontinence).

When following patients with obstructive symptoms conservatively, one should consider the development of bladder instability as an absolute indication for the surgical relief of obstruction. In these patients, conservative measures have failed. In patients with this finding, detrusor instability will improve in 75 per cent of patients following prostatectomy, but in 25 per cent it will remain unchanged (Turner-Warwick, 1979). Thus, every effort should be made to detect this condition early in its onset and to relieve obstruction as soon as possible thereafter.

When the patient is seen relatively early following the onset of obstructive symptoms—before any of these relative indications are present—he frequently wishes to know what the natural history of the disease will be. This question is difficult to answer, because many patients who receive no therapy whatsoever will have no change in their symptoms over many years (Birkhoff, 1983). In the classic study of Clarke (1937), in which 93 patients were followed more than 4 years, many patients showed a sustained improvement after instrumentation alone. Consequently, in the group of patients who lack definite indications for prostatectomy, it appears advisable to examine the patient periodically to observe the natural history of the disease rather than to anticipate its development by advising prophylactic prostatectomy.

In subsequent chapters (see Chapters 75, 77 and 78), the surgical approaches to the prostate are reviewed, and the indications, technique, and complications are discussed. Although surgery is the only modality known to be effective for the treatment of obstructive BPH, the current status of medical therapy is reviewed next.

Stimulated by the early studies of White (1895), which demonstrated a beneficial effect of castration in patients with symptomatic benign prostatic hyperplasia, many investigators have sought a "pill" for treatment of the benign prostate. Treatment with estrogens (Peirson, 1946) or estrogen-androgen combinations (Kaufman and Goodwin, 1959) has been used in the past to ameliorate the symptoms of outflow obstruction. The results with these two forms of therapy, however, are too inconsistent to warrant absolute conclusions.

Beginning in the 1960's, when antiandrogens became available, a number of clinical studies were initiated. Because spontaneous remission of symptoms frequently occurs in untreated patients, these studies have often been difficult to interpret. The earliest antiandrogens that were used were progestational agents. Geller et al. (1965) first reported good results with 17 α-hydroxyprogesterone and later with chlormadinone acetate. A careful review of both reports, however, fails to demonstrate a significant effect. Wolf and Madsen (1968) tested two other progestational agents that they found ineffective. In a later report on progestational agents, Rangno et al. (1971) reported encouraging results with medrogestone. Urinary flow rates were not determined, however, and there was no significant improvement in residual urine. The factors that did improve (symptoms, rectal estimations of prostatic size, and cystoscopy) are the least reliable, thus making the interpretation of the results open to debate. Subsequently, Paulson and Kane (1975) engaged in a study quite similar to that of Rangno et al. (1971), except that the dose of medrogestone was reduced. Although the authors reported a significant increase in peak urine flow, mean urine flow, and total volume and urine voided during micturition in patients treated with 15 mg of this agent twice a day, subsequent analysis of these data suggested no difference in

these measurements (Scott and Coffey, 1975). Megestrol acetate is another potent progestational agent that has been tested by several investigators. In a recent summary of this experience, Donkervoort (1983) concluded that although megestrol acetate had a slight positive effect on voiding patterns of patients with BPH, the optimal dosage and duration of treatment were unclear and loss of libido was a significant side effect.

Using cyproterone acetate in low doses (50 mg/day), Soctt and Wade (1969) treated 13 patients with symptomatic BPH. Urinary flow rates improved in 9 patients, the amount of residual urine decreased in 8, plasma testosterone levels decreased in 11, and histologic examination of the prostate demonstrated regression in 8.

More recently, Ekman et al. (1981) evaluated cyproterone acetate, 50 mg/day in combination with bromocriptine, 2.5 mg/day (to block the influence of prolactin), in a randomized study including a placebo control. The hormonally treated patients experienced a 75 per cent improvement in symptoms, a 23 per cent reduction in prostatic size, as estimated by computed tomography, and a 60 per cent improvement in urinary flow rate compared with the placebo control group, in which the response was 25, 2, and 5 per cent, respectively. The authors concluded that although these results were encouraging, two patients who experienced a marked reduction in prostatic size continued to suffer from outlet symptoms and, furthermore, that the side effects of the combination treatment seemed to limit its usefulness.

Gestonorone caproate is an agent that has received considerable attention. Although early reports were encouraging, they generally lacked a control group. Two other studies have had appropriate placebo groups that have permitted a critical appraisal to be done. Gingell et al. (1972) studied 21 patients in a double-blind cross-over protocol, administering placebo or hormone intramuscularly once a week for 24 weeks. They failed to demonstrate improvement in flow rates and residual urine, although treated patients did appear to have less diurnal frequency.

Aubrey and Khosla (1971), also using gestonorone caproate, studied 24 men. Eleven patients received the placebo first and then the hormone; there was a 50 per cent improvement in symptoms after administration of the placebo, and no further improvement following the hormone therapy. Thirteen patients received the hormone first and then the placebo; there was a 60 per cent improvement after the hormone was administered, increasing to 73 per cent after administration of the placebo. Although the authors were encouraged by these results, it still appears uncertain whether predictable benefit can be derived from this agent.

Flutamide (Sch 13521), a potent nonsteroidal antiandrogen, was tested by Caine et al. (1975a). In a placebo-controlled, randomized study of 30 patients with significant BPH and residual urine, they found no difference in residual urine, gross prostatic size, or histologic findings in prostatic biopsies. The only observable improvement was a significant increase in urinary flow rates in patients treated with flutamide. A large number of patients receiving the active compound did develop nipple tenderness or gynecomastia.

Caine addressed the medical management of BPH from a different approach. In 1975 he demonstrated the presence of alpha-adrenergic receptors in prostatic tissue (Caine et al., 1975b) and a year later reported on the beneficial effects of alpha-adrenergic blockers in the management of BPH (Caine et al., 1976). More recently, he reported on the results of treatment utilizing phenoxybenzamine in 200 cases of BPH (Caine et al., 1981). He found that 80 per cent of patients achieved improvement in obstructive symptoms; furthermore, the treatment was useful in aiding catheter removal after an attack of acute retention. Side effects were reported in 30 per cent of patients. In contrast to these encouraging results, Brooks et al. (1983) reported on their experience utilizing phenoxybenzamine (10 mg/day) in the treatment of men with BPH. They found no statistically significant benefit on flow rate, residual urine, or urethral pressure profile. They concluded that phenoxybenzamine in low doses was ineffective in reducing the physical obstruction of the enlarged prostate gland. Thus, the ultimate role of alpha-adrenergic blocking agents in the management of obstructive BPH remains to be clarified.

In summary, there has been no controlled study of any drug that has demonstrated a meaningful improvement in patients with obstructive BPH. It is hoped that future studies of more potent agents, or possibly combinations of agents, may provide convincing evidence. For many elderly men who are not candidates for surgery, such a drug would be most welcome. One study has suggested a potential problem with their use, however. Neri (1972) noted that in the dog, prostatic hyperplasia that receded following treatment with flutamide returned to its enlarged size 8 weeks after the antiandrogen was discontinued. If this proves to be true in future studies in man, patients who elect "the male pill" may look forward to a lifetime of medication.

References

Abrams, P. H., and Griffiths, D. J.: The assessment of prostatic obstruction from urodynamic measurements and from residual urine. Br. J. Urol., 51:129, 1979.

Abrams, P. H., Roylance, J., and Feneley, R. C. L.: Excretion urography in the investigation of prostatism. Br. J. Urol., 48:681, 1976.

Andersen, J. T., Jacobsen, O., and Standgaard, L.: The diagnostic value of intravenous pyelography in infravesicle obstruction in males. Scand. J. Urol. Nephrol., 11:225, 1977.

Anderson, K. M., and Liao, S.: Selective retention of dihydrotestosterone by prostatic nuclei. Nature, 219:277, 1968.

Aubrey, D. A., and Khosla, T.: The effect of 17-alpha-hydroxy-19-norprogesterone caproate (SH 582) on benign prostatic hypertrophy. Br. J. Surg., 58:648, 1971.

Barrack, E. R., Bujnovszky, P., and Walsh, P. C.: Subcellular distribution of androgen receptors in human normal, benign hyperplastic, and malignant prostatic tissues: Characterization of nuclear salt–resistant receptors. Cancer Res., 43:1107, 1983.

Bates, C. P., Whiteside, C. G., and Turner-Warwick, R.: Synchronous cine pressure-flow cystourethrography. Br. J. Urol., 42:714, 1979.

Berry, S. J., Coffey, D. S., Walsh, P. C., and Ewing, L. L.: The development of human benign prostatic hyperplasia with age. J. Urol., 132:474, 1984.

Birkhoff, J. D.: Natural history of benign prostatic hypertrophy. In Hinman, F. (Ed.): Benign Prostatic Hypertrophy. New York, Springer-Verlag, 1983, p. 5.

Bremner, W. J., Vitiello, M. V., and Prinz, P. N.: Loss of circadian rhythmicity in blood testosterone levels with aging in normal men. J. Clin. Endocrinol. Metab., 56:1278, 1983.

Brendler, C. B., Berry, S. J., Ewing, L. L., McCullough, A. R., Cochran, R. C., Strandberg, J. D., Zirkin, B. R., Coffey, D. S., Wheaton, L. G., Hiler, M. L., Bordy, M. C., Scott, W. W., and Walsh, P. C.: Spontaneous benign prostatic hyperplasia in the beagle: Age-associated changes in serum hormone levels and the morphology and secretory function of the canine prostate. J. Clin. Invest., 71:1114, 1983.

Brooks, M. E., Sidi, A. A., Hanani, Y., and Braf, Z. F.: Ineffectiveness of phenoxybenzamine in treatment of benign prostatic hypertrophy: A controlled study. Urology, 21:474, 1983.

Bruchovsky, N., and Wilson, J. D.: The conversion of testosterone to 5α-androstane-17β-ol-one by rat prostate in vivo and in vitro. J. Biol. Chem., 243:2012, 1968.

Cabot, A. T.: The question of castration for enlarged prostate. Ann. Surg. 24:265, 1896.

Caine, M., Perlberg, S., and Gordon, R.: The treatment of benign prostatic hypertrophy with flutamide (SCH 13521): A placebo-controlled study. J. Urol., 114:564, 1975a.

Caine, M., Perlberg, S., and Shapiro, A.: Phenoxybenzamine for benign prostatic obstruction: Review of 200 cases. Urology, 17:542, 1981.

Caine, M., Pfau, A., and Perlberg, S.: The use of alpha adrenergic blockers in benign prostatic hypertrophy. Urology, 48:255, 1976.

Caine, M., Raz, S., and Zeigler, M.: Adrenergic and cholinergic receptors in the human prostate, prostatic capsule, and bladder neck. Br. J. Urol., *47*:193, 1975*b*.

Chaisiri, N., Volataire, Y., Evans, B. A. J., and Pierrepoint, C. G.: Demonstration of a cytoplasmic receptor protein for estrogen in the canine prostate gland. J. Endocrinol., *78*:131, 1978.

Clarke, R.: The prostate and the endocrines: A control series. J. Urol., *9*:254, 1937.

Culp, D. A.: Benign prostatic hyperplasia. Early recognition and management. Urol. Clin. North Am., *2*:29, 1975.

Cunha, G. R., Chung, L. W. K., Shannon, J. M., and Reese, B. A.: Stromal-epithelial interactions in sex differentiation. Biol. Reprod., *22*:19, 1980.

DeKlerk, D. P., Coffey, D. S., Ewing, L. L., McDermott, I. R., Reiner, W. G., Robinson, C. H., Scott, W. W., Strandberg, J. D., Talalay, P., Walsh, P. C., Wheaton, L. G., and Zirkin, B. R.: Comparison of spontaneous and experimentally induced canine prostatic hyperplasia. J. Clin. Invest., *64*:842, 1979.

Deming, C. L.: The effect of castration on benign hypertrophy of the prostate in man. J. Urol., *33*:388, 1935.

Deming, C. L., Jenkins, R. H., and van Wagenen, G.: Further studies in the endocrinological relationships of prostatic hypertrophy. The effect of castration of the sub-urethral glands in the posterior urethra of the rat. J. Urol., *34*:678, 1935.

Donkervoort, A. K.: Megesterol acetate in treatment. *In* Hinman, F. (Ed.): Benign Prostatic Hypertrophy. New York, Springer-Verlag, 1983, p. 277.

Ekman, P., Barrack, E. R., Greene, G. L., Jensen, E. V., and Walsh, P. C.: Estrogen receptors in human prostate: Evidence for multiple binding sites. J. Clin. Endocrinol. Metab., *57*:166, 1983.

Ekman, P., Barrack, E. R., and Walsh, P. C.: Simultaneous measurement of progesterone and androgen receptors in human prostate: A microassay. J. Clin. Endocrinol. Metab., *55*:1089, 1982.

Ekman, P., Johansson, B., Ohlsen, H., and Ringertz, H.: Drug therapy in benign prostatic hyperplasia. Scand. J. Urol. Nephrol. Suppl., *60*:77, 1981.

Ewing, L. L., Berry, S. J., and Higginbottom, E. G.: Dihydrotestosterone content of beagle prostatic tissue: Effect of age and hyperplasia. Endocrinology, *113*:2004, 1983.

Franks, L. M.: Benign prostatic hyperplasia: Gross and microscopic anatomy. *In* Grayhack, J. T., Wilson, J. D., and Scherbenske, M. J. (Eds.): Benign Prostatic Hyperplasia. NIAMDD Workshop Proceedings, Feb. 20-21, 1975. DHEW Publication Number (NIH) 76-1113, p. 63. Washington, D. C., U. S. Government Printing Office, 1976.

Franks, L. M.: Benign nodular hyperplasia of the prostate: A review. Ann. R. Coll. Surg., *14*:92, 1954.

Geller, J., Albert, J., Lopez, D., Geller, A., and Niwayama, G.: Comparison of androgen metabolites in benign prostatic hypertrophy (BPH) and normal prostate. J. Clin. Endocrinol., *43*:686, 1976.

Geller, J., Angrist, A., Nakao, K., and Newman, H.: Therapy with progestational agents in advanced benign prostatic hypertrophy. J.A.M.A., *210*:1421, 1969.

Geller, J., Bora, R., Roberts, T., Newman, H., Lin, A., and Silva, R.: Treatment of benign prostatic hypertrophy with hydroxyprogesterone caproate. J.A.M.A., *193*:121, 1965.

Gingell, J. C., Miller, I. M., and Roberts, B. M.: Clinical trial of gestronol hexanoate (SH 582) in benign prostatic hypertrophy. Proc. R. Soc. Med., *65*:12, 1972.

Gloyna, R. E., Siiteri, P. K., and Wilson, J. D.: Dihydrotestosterone in prostatic hypertrophy. II. The formation and content of dihydrotestosterone in the hypertrophic canine prostate and the effect of dihydrotestosterone on prostate growth in the dog. J. Clin. Invest., *49*:1746, 1970.

Gover, M.: A statistical study of the etiology of benign hypertrophy of the prostate gland. Johns Hopkins Hospital Rep., *21*:2131, 1923.

Grayhack, J. T.: Directions for future research. *In* Hinman, F. (Ed.): Benign Prostatic Hypertrophy. New York, Springer-Verlag, 1983, p. 313.

Hammond, G. L.: Endogenous steroid levels in the human prostate from birth to old age: A comparison of normal and diseased states. J. Endocrinol., *78*:7, 1978.

Harbitz, T. B., and Haugen, O. A.: Histology of the prostate in elderly men. Acta. Pathol. Microbiol. Scand. [A], *80*:756, 1972.

Harman, S. M., and Tsitouras, P. D.: Reproductive hormones in aging men. I. Measurement of sex steroids, basal luteinizing hormone, and Leydig cell responses to human chorionic gonadotropin. J. Clin. Endocrinol. Metab., *51*:35, 1980.

Haugen, O. A., and Harbitz, T. B.: Prostatic weight in elderly men. Acta Path. Microbiol. Scand. Section A, *80*:769, 1972.

Hawkins, E. F., Trachtenberg, J., Hicks, L. L., and Walsh, P. C.: Androgen and estrogen receptors in the canine prostate. J. Androl., *1*:234, 1980.

Huggins, C.: The etiology of benign prostatic hypertrophy. Bull. N.Y. Acad. Med., *23*:696, 1947.

Huggins, C., and Stevens, R.: The effect of castration on benign hypertrophy of the prostate in man. J. Urol., *43*:705, 1940.

Huggins, C., and Stevens, R.: The effect of castration on benign hypertrophy of the prostate in man. J. Urol., *43*:705, 1940.

Kaufman, J. J., and Goodwin, W. E.: Hormonal management of the benign obstructing prostate: Use of combined androgen-estrogen therapy. J. Urol., *81*:165, 1959.

Krieg, M., Bartsch, W., Janssen, W., and Voigt, K. D.: A comparative study of binding metabolism and endogenous levels of androgens in normal, hyperplastic, and carcinomatous human prostate. J. Steroid Biochem., *11*:615, 1979.

Lytton, B., Emery, J. M., and Harvard, B. M.: The incidence of benign prostatic hyperplasia. J. Urol., *99*:639, 1968.

Marshall, T. K, and Hoare, F. E.: The rectal cooling after death and its mathematical expression. J. Forensic Sci., *7*:56, 1962.

Marshall, V., Singh, M., and Blandy, J. P.: Is urography necessary for patients with acute retention of urine before prostatectomy? Br. J. Urol., *46*:73, 1974.

McNeal, J. E.: Origin and evolution of benign prostatic enlargement. Invest. Urol., *15*:340, 1978.

McNeal, J. E.: The zonal anatomy of the prostate. Prostate, *2*:35, 1981.

McNeal, J. E.: The prostate gland. Morphology and pathobiology. 1983 Monographs in Urology, *4*:1, 1983.

Meikle, A. W., Stringham, J. D., and Olsen, D. C.: Subnormal tissue 3α-androstanediol and androsterone in prostatic hyperplasia. J. Clin. Endocrinol., *47*:909, 1978.

Moore, R. A.: Benign hypertrophy and carcinoma of the prostate. Surgery, *16*:152, 1944.

Moore, R. J., Gazak, J. M., Quebbeman, J. F., and Wilson, J. D.: Concentration of dihydrotestosterone and 3-androstanediol in naturally occurring and androgen-induced prostatic hyperplasia in the dog. J. Clin. Invest., *64*:1003, 1979.

Moore, R. J., Gazak, J. M., Wilson, J. D.: Regulation of cytoplasmic dihydrotestosterone binding in dog prostate. J. Clin. Invest., *63*:351, 1979.

Morgagni, G. B.: The Seats and Causes of Disease Investigated by Anatomy. Book 3, p. 460. London, Johnson and Payne, 1760.

Mostofi, F. K.: Benign hyperplasia of the prostate gland. *In* Campbell, M. F., and Harrison, J. H., (Eds.): Urology. 3rd ed., p. 1065. Philadelphia, W. B. Saunders Co., 1970.

Neri, R. O., and Monahan, M.: Effects of a novel nonsteroidal antiandrogen on canine prostatic hyperplasia. Invest. Urol., *10*:123, 1972.

Neubauer, B. L., and Mawhinney, M. G.: Actions of androgen and estrogen on guinea pig seminal vesicle epithelium and muscle. Endocrinol., *108*:680, 1981.

Paulson, D. F., and Kane, R. D.: A prospective study in the pharmaceutical management of benign prostatic hyperplasia. J. Urol., *113*:811, 1975.

Peirson, E. L.: A study of the effect of stilbestrol therapy on the size of the benignly hypertrophied prostate gland. J. Urol., *55*:73, 1946.

Pirke, K. M., and Doerr, P.: Age related changes in free plasma testosterone, dihydrotestosterone, and oestradiol. Acta Endocrinol., *80*:171, 1975.

Pradhan, B. K., and Chandra, K.: Morphogenesis of nodular hyperplasia-prostate. J. Urol., *113*:210, 1975.

Rangno, R. E., McLeod, P. J., and Ruedy, J.: Treatment of benign prostatic hypertrophy with medrogestone. Clin. Pharmacol. Ther., *12*:658, 1971.

Rotkin, I. D.: Origins, distribution, and risk of benign prostatic hypertrophy. *In* Hinman, F. (Ed.): Benign Prostatic Hypertrophy. New York, Springer-Verlag, 1983, p. 10.

Rubens, R., Dhont, M., and Vermeulen, A.: Further studies on Leydig cell function in old age. J. Clin. Endocrinol., *39*:40, 1974.

Scott, W. W.: What makes the prostate grow? J. Urol., *70*:477, 1953.

Scott, W. W., and Coffey, D. S.: Nonsurgical treatment of human benign prostatic hyperplasia. Vitam. Horm., *33*:439, 1975.

Scott, W. W., and Wade, J. C.: Medical treatment of benign nodular hyperplasia with cyproterone acetate. J. Urol., *101*:81, 1969.

Siiteri, P. K., and Wilson, J. D.: Dihydrotestosterone in prostatic hypertrophy. I. The formation and content of dihydrotestosterone in the hypertrophic prostate of man. J. Clin. Invest., *49*:1737, 1970.

Swyer, G. I. M.: Post-natal growth changes in the human prostate. J. Anat., *78*:130, 1944.

Trachtenberg, J., Hicks, L. L., and Walsh, P. C.: Androgen- and estrogen-receptor content in spontaneous and experimentally induced canine prostatic hyperplasia. J. Clin. Invest., *65*:1051, 1980.

Turner-Warwick, R.: Clinical urodynamics. Urol. Clin. North Am., *6*:13, 171, 1979.

Walsh, P. C., Hutchins, G. M., and Ewing, L. L.: The tissue content of dihydrotestosterone in human prostatic hyperplasia is not supranormal. J. Clin. Invest., *72*:1772, 1983.

Walsh, P. C., and Wilson, J. D.: The induction of prostatic hypertrophy in the dog with androstanediol. J. Clin. Invest., *57*:1093, 1976.

Wendel, E. F., Brannen, G. E., Putong, P. B., and Grayhack, J. T.: The effect of orchiectomy and estrogens on benign prostatic hyperplasia. J. Urol., *108*:116, 1972.

White, J. W.: The results of double castration in hypertrophy of the prostate. Ann. Surg., *22*:1, 1895.

Wilson, J. D.: The pathogenesis of benign prostatic hyperplasia. Am. J. Med., *68*:745, 1980.

Wilson, J. D., and Gloyna, R. E.: The intranuclear metabolism of testosterone in the accessory organs of reproduction. Recent Prog. Horm. Res., *26*:309, 1970.

Wilson, J. D., Gloyna, R. E., and Siiteri, P. K.: Androgen metabolism in the hypertrophic prostate. J. Steroid Biochem., *6*:443, 1975.

Wolf, H., and Madsen, P. O.: Treatment of benign prostatic hypertrophy with progestational agents: A preliminary report. J. Urol., *99*:780, 1968.

Zumoff, B., Strain, G. W., Kream, J., O'Connor, J., Rosenfeld, R. S., Levin, J., and Fukushima, D. K.: Age variation of the 24-hour mean plasma concentrations of androgens, estrogens, and gonadotropins in normal adult men. J. Clin. Endocrinol. Metab., *54*:534, 1982.

TUMORS OF THE GENITOURINARY TRACT IN THE ADULT

CHAPTER 28

Principles of Oncology

DAVID F. PAULSON, M.D.

The current philosophy that prompts selection of surgery, radiotherapy, or chemotherapy, either singly or in combination, for control of malignant genitourinary neoplasms requires an understanding of the biology of the malignant cell. The discussion that follows will focus on the principles of solid tumor oncology as applied to genitourinary malignancy. This focus does not imply that the other solid or liquid tumors are unimportant, nor does it imply that the study of these tumors has not provided preliminary information that has subsequently been translated into the area of the urologic neoplasms. This focus simply reflects the necessary limitations placed on this discussion by constraints of space.

THEORIES OF CARCINOGENESIS

Many postulates have been advanced to explain the phenomenon of carcinogenesis. No single theory has successfully embraced in a unifying concept the multiple observations made. The current theories of carcinogenesis can be grouped in four general categories segregated by proposed mechanism. These are (1) somatic mutation, (2) aberrant differentiation, (3) virus activation, and (4) cell selection.

THE THEORY OF SOMATIC MUTATION

Somatic mutation relates the initiation of neoplastic growth to abnormalities in one or several of the genes that regulate cell growth and differentiation. These abnormalities may occur at any time during the life of the cell. One or several of the mutations necessary for the development of neoplastic growth may be vertically transmitted. Thus, the affected indi-

vidual may have an increased susceptibility to neoplasia, as fewer mutational steps must then occur in the affected cell to complete the carcinogenic process. Ionizing radiation and the alkylating chemicals produce their mutagenic effects by altering the genetic structure of the cell. There is much biologic evidence to support the theory of somatic mutation: (1) The genetic constitution of the organism may influence the susceptibility to cancer; (2) there seems to be a direct relationship between mutagenicity and carcinogenicity; and (3) there is a frequent documented occurrence of chromosomal abnormalities in the neoplastic cell.

What evidence is there to indicate that the genetic constitution of the organism may influence susceptibility to malignant disease? Certain chromosomal disorders are associated with the appearance of specific neoplastic diseases (Harnden, 1977; Knudson, 1973, 1975; Mulvihill, 1975; Hecht and McCaw, 1977). The most familiar ones are the trisomies, such as Down's syndrome (trisomy 21), Klinefelter's syndrome (XXY), and trisomy D, all of which predispose to the development of leukemia. Trisomy 18, which is thought to increase susceptibility to neoplasia and dysplasia, is associated with an elevated incidence of Wilms' tumor (Knudson, 1973, 1975). Twenty-five to 30 per cent of phenotypically female males who have gonadal dysgenesis with an X-Y chromosomal pattern may demonstrate gonadoblastomas. It is postulated that the presence of the Y chromosome may be responsible even when the cells containing the Y chromosome reside only within the gonad (Mulvihill, 1975). It also has been postulated that the carcinogenic impact of the Y chromosome results from its presence in an abnormal environment, such as occurs in the heterotopic transplantation of embryo cells beneath the testicular capsule in mice (Stevens, 1970; Pierce and Cox, 1978).

Susceptibility to specific neoplastic disorders may be inherited either as a mendelian recessive or a mendelian dominant trait. The phakomatoses are inherited as a mendelian dominant trait and are characterized by congenital defects and tumor syndromes of various types, with neurofibromatosis being the most common (Knudson, 1973). The von Hippel–Lindau syndrome is a rare phakomatosis associated with renal tumors. Wilms' tumor and neuroblastoma demonstrate a distribution consistent with dominant mendelian inheritance. Tumors tend to occur earlier and are more frequently bilateral in members of affected families than they are in the general population (Knudson, 1975; Knudson and Strong, 1972). It has been estimated that about 38 per cent of all Wilms' tumors and 20 to 25 per cent of all neuroblastomas are hereditary (Knudson, 1973). Further evidence of the potential contribution of genetic abnormalities to the development of human solid tumors is based upon the identification of chromosomal abnormalities within these solid tumors. Further, the degree of malignant degeneration or tumor aggressiveness seems to be related to the degree of chromosomal abnormality. This is most evident in the field of urologic malignant disease when one examines the association of marker chromosomes or abnormal chromosome number and recurrent malignant disease within the bladder. A considerable body of evidence supports the current concepts that the karyotype of the malignant cell is unstable and variable (Nowell, 1976).

Finally, there seems to be a correlation between carcinogenicity and mutagenicity. Many of the known carcinogenic agents, such as ionizing radiation, nitrogen mustard, and certain of the polycyclic aromatic hydrocarbons, are both carcinogenic and mutagenic (Miller and Miller, 1971, 1977; Magee, 1977; Rinkus and Legator, 1979).

THE THEORY OF ABERRANT DIFFERENTIATION

The theory of aberrant differentiation proposes that abnormalities of genes or chromosomes need not occur to prompt a neoplastic change. Rather, disturbances in gene regulation, either through faulty repression or through derepression, may cause alterations of growth with loss of cellular differentiation, which is subsequently interpreted as the neoplastic change. Because this defect involves only changes in gene regulation, not changes in gene structure, it is considered to be epigenetic rather than genetic (Weinstein et al., 1975). This theory is supported by observations that have demonstrated the totipotentiality of the cancer cell genome. A unique study, in which the nuclei from Lucke frog renal carcinoma cells were transplanted into enucleate frog eggs, did not produce new Lucke frog renal carcinoma cells but gave rise to normal embryos, and subsequently to normal tadpoles (McKinnell et al., 1969). This experiment argues that the genes responsible for normal differentiation and regulation of cells are intact and capable of normal function when provided with the proper environment and stimulus.

The importance of the local environment on the expression of the gene is further illustrated by the observation that heterotopic transplantation of mouse embryo tissue beneath the capsule of the testis results in murine teratocarcinoma (Stevens, 1970; Pierce and Cox, 1978). Tumors that are dedifferentiated may, under the influence of the normal events of aging or either radiation or chemotherapy, undergo differentiation to a more benign state. This is best recognized when one examines the clinical course of those malignant neuroblastomas that, with progressive maturation, become benign ganglioneuromas; similarly, some malignant teratocarcinomas, under the influence of chemotherapy, undergo progressive differentiation to benign teratomas. In each instance, the malignant cell has expressed those characteristics that are associated with benignity (Everson and Cole, 1966).

THE THEORY OF VIRAL CARCINOGENESIS

Current dogma holds that the oncogenic virus produces its effect by integrating the genetic information contained within its own nucleic acid into the genetic material of the host cell (Baltimore, 1975; Tooze, 1973; Temin, 1975). It is believed that this viral information, having been integrated into the genetic material of the host cell, constitutes part of the normal inheritance of the cell and is subject to regulation by repression or derepression, which occurs with the original genetic material of the cell. The two hypotheses proposed to encompass this philosophy, the "oncogene" hypothesis and the "protovirus" hypothesis, merge the viral theory of carcinogenesis and the genetic theory of carcinogenesis into a unifying concept.

The "oncogene" hypothesis proposes that the genetic material of the C-type RNA viruses consists of "virogenes," which code for viral replication, and "oncogenes," which code for neoplastic transformation of the host cell. These viral genomes are transmitted vertically within the host and may play a functional role in the normal growth of the cell. Cancer results from derepression of the viral oncogenes, either because of the impact of external carcinogens or through spontaneous occurrence of mutational events. The derepression of the virogenes, which leads to virus production, does not produce neoplastic transformation (Tooze, 1973; Todaro, 1977).

The "protovirus" hypothesis proposes that the genetic information is transmitted among the somatic cells from the "protovirus" region of the genetic material (DNA) into RNA intermediates. This genetic information is then encoded into DNA sequences by the activities of RNA-dependent DNA transcriptase, with these new DNA sequences being reinserted into the genetic material. Thus, existing genes are thought to be amplified with new DNA sequences involved in the process of differentiation without affecting the stability of the germ line. The phenomenon of "misevolution" of the protoviruses, either by alteration in their base sequences or by faulty integration of the subsequent DNA genomic material into the wrong area of the host genome, is proposed to produce the neoplastic transformation seen in the affected cell (Binns and Meins, 1973; Temin, 1975).

THE THEORY OF CELL SELECTION

Neoplastic stimuli that enhance the probability of malignancy are, according to this philosophy, thought to do so by promoting the proliferation of malignant cells that otherwise might remain dormant. The stimulus required to promote this evolution may involve cytotoxic effects, which tend to select for cells that have already passed through the preliminary stages of neoplastic transformation. Thus, the progression of the tumor cells toward malignancy may occur as the sequential appearance and selected outgrowth of increasingly autonomous subpopulations that evolve through stepwise mutation-like changes and proliferate under the influence of sustained selection pressures (Foulds, 1975; Farber, 1973).

THE INFLUENCE OF CHEMICAL CARCINOGENS

The first documented environmental malignancy was described by Sir Percival Pott in a series of letters in *Lancet*, in which he identified the high incidence of scrotal cancer among the chimney sweeps of London. The development of this malignancy was related to the constant exposure of the scrotal skin to soot (Weisburger, 1973; Weinstein, 1978). However, over 100 years passed before any concerted effort was made to identify the impact of environmental carcinogens. It is now known, however, that there are a large number of environmental carcinogens, many of which impact directly upon the genitourinary system (Table 28–1). The mechanism of chemical carcinogenesis is thought to be the impact of the carcinogenic agent on molecular structure and subsequently on biologic activity. The process of chemical carcinogenesis can be segregated into two steps: initiation and promotion (Berenblum, 1979). Initiation involves a permanent mutation-like alteration in the genetic material, whereas promotion is dependent on reversible alterations in epigenetic regulation (Weinstein, 1978). Mutagens tend to behave as initiators, whereas hormones and other growth-stimulating factors seem to function as promoters. Both initiating agents and promoting agents are important in the production of malignancy in humans. Most of the environmental carcinogens require metabolic activation within the host in order to effect carcinogenesis (Miller and Miller, 1977; Miller, 1979). Although the metabolic sequence of events may be necessary to allow the parent compound to achieve its malignant potential, it is recognized that the metabolism of the parent compounds to form the "proximate" carcinogens is necessary before these agents can react with their macromolecular targets (Miller, 1979). The majority of the carcinogens that have been tested under conditions allowing their activation to the proximate form function as mutagens (Rinkus and Legator, 1979). These proximate carcinogens ultimately achieve their impact by covalently binding to the informational macromolecules within the cell.

Although the mechanisms of radiation carcinogenesis are unknown, it is currently felt that radiation induces changes at the cellular level by producing alterations in the chromosomal structure.

TUMOR FORMATION

Once the malignant change has occurred, there are additional external factors that determine a cell's pattern of growth, such as the adjacent substratum, adjacent cells, or growth-stimulating compounds that must impinge on the cell surface. The three components of the

TABLE 28-1. CHEMICALS OR INDUSTRIAL PROCESSES ASSOCIATED WITH CANCER INDUCTION IN HUMANS: COMPARISON OF TARGET ORGANS AND MAIN ROUTES OF EXPOSURE IN ANIMALS AND HUMANS

	Humans			Animals		
CHEMICAL OR INDUSTRIAL PROCESS	MAIN TYPE OF EXPOSURE*	TARGET ORGAN	MAIN ROUTE OF EXPOSURE†	ANIMAL	TARGET ORGAN	ROUTE OF EXPOSURE
4-Aminobiphenyl	Occupational	Bladder	Inhalation, skin, PO	Mouse, rabbit, dog Newborn mouse Rat	Bladder Liver Mammary gland, intestine	PO SC injection SC injection
Auramine	Occupational	Bladder	Inhalation, skin, PO	Mouse, rat Rabbit, dog Rat	Liver Negative Local, liver, intestine	PO PO SC injection
Benzidine	Occupational	Bladder	Inhalation, skin, PO	Mouse Rat Rat Hamster Dog	Liver Liver Zymbal gland, liver, colon Liver Bladder	SC injection PO SC injection PO PO
Cadmium-using industries (possibly cadmium oxide)	Occupational	Prostate, lung‡	Inhalation, PO	Rat	Local, testis	SC or IM injection
Cyclophosphamide	Medicinal	Bladder	PO, injection	Mouse Rat 	Hematopoietic system, lung Various sites Bladder‡ Mammary gland Various sites	IP, SC injection PO IP IP IV
2-Naphthylamine	Occupational	Bladder	Inhalation, skin, PO	Hamster, dog, monkey Mouse Rat, rabbit	Bladder Liver, lung Inadequate	PO SC injection PO
N,N-Bis (2-chloroethyl)-2-naphthylamine	Medicinal	Bladder	PO	Mouse Rat	Lung Local	IP SC injection
Phenacetin	Medicinal	Kidney	PO		No adequate tests	
Soot, tars, oils	Occupational, environmental	Lung, skin (scrotum)	Inhalation, skin	Mouse, rabbit	Skin	Topical

*The main types of exposures mentioned are those by which association has been demonstrated; exposures other than those mentioned may also occur.

†The main routes of exposure given may not be the only ones by which such effects could occur.

‡Indicative evidence.

From Tomatis, L., Agtha, C., Bartsch, H., et al.: Cancer Res., 38:877, 1978.

cell surface are extracellular matrix, cytoplasmic or plasma membrane, and intracellular matrix. Each of these components seems to be involved in growth regulation, and each is altered in transformed cells. The ability to metastasize is also felt to be dependent upon cell surface properties (Pardee, 1964). Extensive study has been done on a large extracellular protein called fibronectin. It does not occur in some neoplastic cells, possibly being removed by a proteolytic system, plasminogen activator, which is secreted by these malignant cells (Reich et al., 1975). Although fibronectin does not seem to be related to the neoplastic event, it may be related to membrane activity. The plasma membrane holds the cells together and provides a barrier between intracellular and extracellular processes. It functions as a selective transport of molecules into and out of the cell and binds growth factors and other proteins to its surface. What occurs within the cell membrane with malignant change is unknown. Some of the transport mechanisms increase in activity after malignant transformation (Hatanaka, 1974). Functional properties of the cell membrane are most probably changed after transformation in response to the altered metabolic rate of the cell.

Recent studies have demonstrated that tumor cells within a primary malignant tumor have differing metastatic potential (Hart and Fidler, 1980, 1981; Poste, 1982; Nicolson, in press). The rate of appearance of metastatic lesions seems to be statistically related to the size of the primary tumor, the incidence increasing as the tumor size increases. However, the same histologic type of cancer may produce quite diverse survival patterns among individual patients (Sugarbaker, 1981). This marked variation in the metastatic potential of human malignancies, even those of the same histologic type, indicates that there may be no simple relationship between the size of the primary tumor and the expected incidence of metastases. Current thinking holds that metastases may result either from random arrest and survival of tumor cells in distant organs or from nonrandom, preferential implantation, survival, and growth of tumor cells in specific sites.

Recent studies also demonstrate that phenotypic instability and clonal stabilization occur in vivo at metastatic sites (Poste et al., 1982). Using isolated clones from individual lung tumor colonies produced by the B16 melanoma, Poste and coworkers demonstrated that "early" metastases excised after 18 days were composed primarily of clones that showed indistinguisha-

ble metastatic phenotypes (intralesional clonal homogeneity) in over 80 per cent of the individual early metastases that were tested. However, the metastatic phenotypes of clones isolated from different metastases in the same animal differed significantly (intralesional clonal heterogeneity). When "late metastases" were excised after 40 days of growth, intralesional clonal homogeneity was found in only 30 per cent of the metastases, the remainder containing two or more clonal subpopulations of tumor cells with differing metastatic properties (intralesional clonal heterogeneity). Thus, with the passage of time, the inherent genetic instability of the tumor cell is demonstrated and intralesional clonal heterogeneity is regenerated.

In metastatic deposits, as in primary deposits, tumor evolution and progression are determined by the properties of those cells that constitute that deposit. In both the primary and the metastatic lesion formed by the occurrence, survival, and proliferation of a single cell, diversity is eventually achieved by phenotypic variability of that initial cell. The rate of tumor cell release from the primary tumor is believed to be quite high. Cells released from the primary tumor may enter either the lymphatic or the venous circulation. Using a model system of a murine mammary tumor implanted into the ovary, Butler and Gullino (1975) isolated arterial inflow and venous efflux to count the number of tumor cells released from the implanted tumor with time. They demonstrated that 1 gm of "primary" or implanted tumor would release several million viable cells per 24 hours. Not only are single cells released from a primary tumor but also multicellular clumps are released.

The interaction of circulating tumor cells with blood components, such as fibrin, is thought to be important in the isolation and initiation of metastatic deposits within the microvasculature (Chew et al., 1976; Warren, 1973; Gershon et al., 1967). Formation of a fibrin thrombus or fibrin coating around the arrested malignant cell occurs in many of the tumor systems and appears to be related to the thromboplastic and procoagulation activity (Day et al., 1959; Mootse et al., 1965). When malignant tumor cell arrest on the endothelium has occurred, the metastatic cell usually escapes from the vascular component by invasion of the vessel wall rather than by expansive growth with subsequent rupture of the vessel (Nakamura et al., 1977). Extravasation of the tumor cell from the vascular compartment may occur through an endothelial defect, but more commonly the mechanism of extravasation involves tumor cell separation with invasion of the intercellular junction between adjacent endothelial cells (Wood, 1958; Winkelhake and Nicholson, 1976) or penetration of the endothelial cell cytoplasm by tumor cell pseudopodia (Dingemans, 1974). These events are followed by adhesion to and subsequent destruction of the underlying endothelial basal lamina or basement membrane (Fig. 28–1).

One of the more important host responses that occur during metastasis involves the formation of new blood vessels. This response is called neovascularization or angiogenesis (Folkman, 1974, 1975). All tumor colonies do not require additional blood flow from the host; however, once these colonies achieve a diameter of approximately 2 mm, ingrowth of new vessels must occur or continued growth will be limited (Folkman, 1975; Folkman and Cotran, 1976).

Algire and Chalkey were among the first to establish that tumor cells will alter the host environment by inducing angiogenesis. The factor (or factors) that prompts new vessel formation is called tumor angiogenesis factor(s) (TAF) (Folkman, 1974, 1975; Folkman and Cotran, 1976). Angiogenesis involves several processes: endothelial cell mitogenesis, endothelial cell chemotaxis, and endothelial cell invasion. Angiogenesis is not a tumor-specific process. It is a normal response that occurs during physiologic repair after tissue wounding, inflammation, or other cellular rearrangements. Tumor angiogenesis factor may not be a tumor-specific molecule but may be a normal molecule or molecules released by tumor cells that are capable of stimulating normal host responses.

PRINCIPLES FOR DETERMINING THE EXTENT OF DISEASE IN THE UNTREATED OR PREVIOUSLY TREATED PATIENT

Following the histologic confirmation of the presence of malignant disease, the physician must institute an orderly assessment of the anatomic extent of disease in the individual patient, as this will determine treatment selection. Failure to accurately identify the extent and site of disease will cause the physician to select a treatment that may be inappropriate and that may not be of long-term benefit to the patient. Failure to determine the extent of disease spread in the previously treated patient may cause the physician to select inappropriate rescue therapy and worsen the subsequent clinical course of the patient.

GLOBAL (SYSTEMIC) EVALUATION

Serum marker proteins, when produced by a specific genitourinary tumor, may be the most global indicator of disease spread. Prostatic acid phosphatase has long been known to be an indicator of the presence of widespread prostatic malignancy. Normally, the acid phosphatase produced by the cells that line the acini of the prostatic ducts is released into a ductal system that effectively excludes it from contact with the interstitial fluids and the lymphatic and venous systems. However, when neoplastic growth occurs, the malignant prostate epithelial cells may lose contact with this ductal system. Consequently, acid phosphatase, when released from the surface of the malignant epithelial cells, is released directly into interstitial fluids and gains

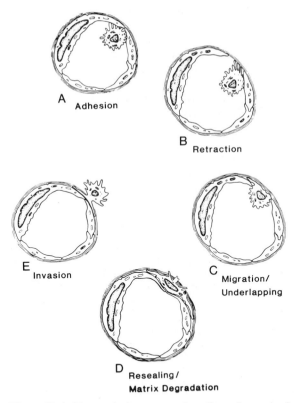

Figure 28–1. Events during metastatic cell attachment and invasion of vascular endothelial cell monolayers and their underlying extracellular matrix. *A*, The tumor cell attaches to the endothelial cell. *B*, The endothelial cell retracts. *C*, The tumor cell migrates and attaches to the underlying extracellular matrix and works beneath adjacent endothelial cells. *D*, There is destruction of the endothelial basal matrix with re-formation of endothelial cell junctions. *E*, There is invasion of the malignant cell into surrounding tissue parenchyma. (After Nicolson, G. L., and Poste, G.: Curr. Probl. Cancer, 7(6):54, 1982.)

A   Adhesion

B   Retraction

C   Migration/ Underlapping

D   Resealing/ Matrix Degradation

E   Invasion

access to the systemic circulation, where it appears as an elevation above normal of the serum prostatic acid phosphatase. This normal biologic protein becomes abnormal only when it is detected in increased amounts in the systemic circulation. It is released from the prostatic epithelium with a diurnal variation that is unpredictable, and serum levels of prostatic acid phosphatase may fluctuate as much as 50 per cent above or below the mean level within a 6-hour period (Brenckman et al., 1981) (Fig. 28–2). Thus, in the evaluation of a patient with an elevated serum acid phosphatase value, a single observation that is increased or decreased may be an indicator of nothing more than the normal biologic variation of this marker protein. Further, any event that breaks down the blood-prostate barrier in the nontumor may produce transient elevations of the serum prostatic acid phosphatase. Two common events are instrumentation and manipulation. Urethral dilation and prostatic massage may both produce a transient increase in the serum acid phosphatase. Thus, detection of an elevated serum acid phosphatase value after manipulation of the prostate may not be an indicator of systemic disease in a patient who is not thought to have disseminated malignancy. Likewise, any event within the prostate that breaks down this barrier, such as inflammation or infarction, may produce transient elevation of the serum prostatic acid phosphatase.

Alpha fetoprotein and beta subunit HCG, which are associated with testicular malignancy, may reflect either disseminated disease or production of these marker proteins by the testicular primary tumor when the primary tumor continues in situ. However, when the diagnosis of testicular malignancy has been established by removal of the testis, persistence of the elevated serum marker protein beta subunit HCG or alpha fetoprotein indicates that the disease is disseminated. The identification of alpha fetoprotein or beta subunit HCG provides a biologic marker by which the presence of testicular malignancy can be determined (Lange et al., 1976; Maier and Sulak, 1974; McIntire et al., 1975; Mizejewski et al., 1975; Moore et al., 1976).

The beta subunit molecule is made up of two polypeptide chains, alpha and beta. The beta chain is responsible for the biologic activity of the hormone and is not present in normal adult males (Vaitukaitis and Ross, 1973; Vaitukaitis et al., 1972; Braunstein et al., 1973). Thus, the elevation of this marker protein after the primary tumor has been removed should indicate metastatic disease. Radioimmunoassay techniques have been developed for the detection of serum beta subunit HCG in the presence of high levels of luteinizing hormones. Alpha fetoprotein, an alpha-1-globulin, occurs in adults only in pathologic states (Bracken et al., 1975; Shepheard, 1974). It can be found in patients with both hepatocellular and testicular malignancy. When elevated levels of alpha fetoprotein are found in the serum of patients with testicular malignancy, embryonal elements are usually identified with malignancy. Persis-

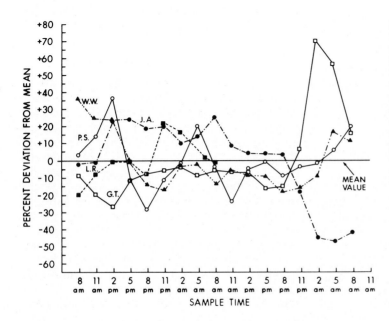

Figure 28–2. Percentage deviation of serum tartrate–labile ("prostatic") acid phosphatase activity from sample mean values during 24 hours (patient 1) and 48 hours (patients 2,3,4, and 5) of observation. Samples were obtained every 3 hours. Substrate was alphanaphthyl phosphate. Horizontal line indicates mean value; closed squares, patient 1; open squares, patient 2; closed circles, patient 3; open circles, patient 4; closed triangles, patient 5. (From Brenckman, W. D., Lastinger, L. B., and Sedor, F.: JAMA, 245:2501, 1981. Used by permission.)

tent marker elevation after orchiectomy may indicate the presence of residual disease at distant sites. The clinician must have a knowledge of the half-life of the marker proteins in order to correctly interpret the meaning of elevated levels in the detection of persistent disease. Alpha fetoprotein has a half-life of approximately 5 days, whereas beta subunit HCG has a half-life of approximately 16 hours. The clinician may wish to establish half-life curves in order to ensure that the marker substance that is being detected is not from tumor previously removed. Elevated marker proteins after orchiectomy indicate disease in other than the primary site. Should marker proteins remain elevated after lymphadenectomy, the clinician must assume that the patient has residual postoperative disease.

When the patient whose tumor produces marker proteins is being monitored, delayed appearance of marker proteins indicates the recurrence of disease. However, not all prostatic and testicular tumors release marker proteins, and tumors may lose their ability to produce marker proteins with time. Therefore, the disappearance of marker proteins, or the absence of elevation, does not necessarily indicate that the patient is tumor-free or that the disease has not become active. The presence of serum marker protein elevation, whether acid phosphatase, alpha fetoprotein, or beta subunit, in the presence of either prostatic or testicular malignancy, should alert the physician to the possibility of disseminated disease.

Once the clinician has performed the most global assessment of metastatic disease, he should focus on distant parenchymal and bony sites. Most metastatic deposits in the lung, when originating from genitourinary sites, present as a nodular density within the lung parenchyma. Thus, a screening chest film is appropriate as the focus turns more sharply to the primary tumor site.

The clinician should first study the axial and appendicular skeleton. Each of the primary genitourinary tumors may produce either a blastic or a lytic lesion. These often are easily detected by plain radiographs. Long bone films are unnecessary in patients who are undergoing assessment of skeletal extension. Patients who have normal bone on both chest and KUB studies should undergo radioisotopic bone scanning. The radioisotopic bone scan is not specific, indicating increased uptake of the radioisotope in areas of increased bony metabolism. However, the isotopic bone scan is much more sensitive than routine bone films in detecting

metastatic disease. Depending on the site of the primary lesion, the isotopic bone scan is estimated to detect disease in up to 20 per cent of patients considered to be without bony extension by routine bone films. This has been well demonstrated in patients with prostatic malignancy; in these cases, metastatic disease is detected in about 22 per cent of individuals with normal bone films, with the incidence of metastatic disease increasing as the volume of local disease increases (Fig. 28–3).

At this point in the evaluation, the clinician should determine whether extension to the liver has occurred. The likelihood of hepatic extension increases when the liver function studies are abnormal. Hepatic spread can be detected by either isotopic scanning or computerized imaging. Neither modality is foolproof, and one must be aware of the possibility of both false positive and false negative determinations. Following evaluation of metastatic disease in distant parenchymal or bony sites, the extent of regional disease should be determined. Malignant disease of genitourinary origins metastasizes to regional nodes. Early involvement of these regional nodes occurs frequently. Thus, the urologic surgeon, recognizing that simple surgical management of the malignancy may be inadequate in the face of systemic disease, must take care to establish that there is no regional or distal nodal involvement.

Metastatic disease in regional lymph nodes can be detected by computerized axial tomography, by bipedal lymphangiography, or by surgical removal. Large-volume nodal disease is accurately detected by computerized axial tomography or bipedal lymphangiography; selection of one of these two noninvasive staging modalities is based upon the institutional expe-

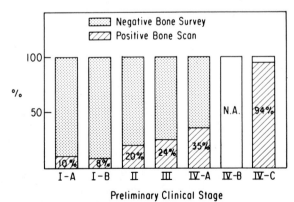

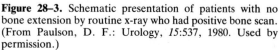

Figure 28–3. Schematic presentation of patients with no bone extension by routine x-ray who had positive bone scan. (From Paulson, D. F.: Urology, *15*:537, 1980. Used by permission.)

rience of the practitioner. The presence of malignant disease in abnormally large nodes may be confirmed by skinny-needle aspiration, thus sparing the patient a surgical procedure. However, the clinician must be aware that microscopic deposits of disease within lymph nodes are poorly detected by these methods, and therefore, he must rely on a surgical dissection with pathologic examination of the removed nodes in order to determine the presence of metastatic disease. This problem has been carefully defined in the area of prostatic malignancy, wherein it has been found that abnormal lymphangiograms are pathologically positive 88 to 90 per cent of the time. On the other hand, negative lymphangiograms may be pathologically incorrect in 20 to 30 per cent of all patients (Paulson, 1980*a, b*). Finally, the local extent of the tumor, whether there is involvement of adjacent structures or not, may be determined by a combination of careful physical examination and computerized axial tomography.

When evaluating the patient with genitourinary malignancy, one should initiate a systematic evaluation of disease extent, moving from the most global assessment to focus on the primary tumor deposits. Failure to accurately assess the distribution of disease will result in inadequate information at the time of treatment selection. The necessity for careful and sequential assessment has been demonstrated in a series of patients with prostatic carcinoma who were initially classified as to anatomic extent on the basis of serum acid phosphatase, routine bone films, and rectal examination. Patients then underwent isotopic bone scanning and, when no bone disease was detected, bipedal lymphangiography, followed by a staging pelvic lymphadenectomy. As can be seen in Figure 28–4, approximately 40 per cent of all patients

believed to have localized prostatic malignancy were upgraded to a higher disease category by this sequential approach. Failure to define the extent of disease would have produced inadequate information, hampering treatment selection and causing inaccuracies in assessing of treatment results.

Current thinking suggests that the anatomic distribution of disease is the single most important factor in treatment selection and disease course. The pathologic grade or cell type of the tumor seems to be important only as a visual predictor of the statistical probability of disease spread. Sufficient data have been derived from studies of carcinoma of the kidney, bladder, and prostate to support this thesis. With renal carcinoma, it seems clear that the relative value of the anatomic extent of disease in predicting treatment response is well established and that pathologic grade and cell type merely predict the biologic aggressiveness of the individual tumor. The data of Selli and coworkers (1983) indicate that patients with organ-confined renal adenocarcinoma $(T_1T_2N_0M_0)$ experience virtually a 90+ per cent survival at 10 years as opposed to a 65 per cent survival in $T_3N_0M_0$ patients at 5 years. This clearly demonstrates that the survival of patients without metastatic disease is related to the local extent of the tumor (Fig. 28–5).

When one examines the survival of nonmetastatic patients with regard to grade of the primary tumor $(T_{any}M_0N_0)$, one sees that as the grade of the primary tumor increases, the survival decreases. The survival advantage in M_0N_0 patients, which was noted with Grade 1 and Grade 2 tumors versus Grade 3 and Grade 4

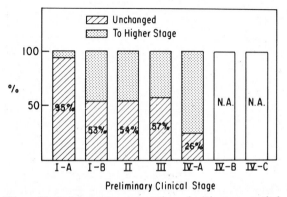

Figure 28–4. Schematic presentation of patients upgraded after careful staging. (From Paulson, D. F.: Urology, *15*:537, 1980. Used by permission.)

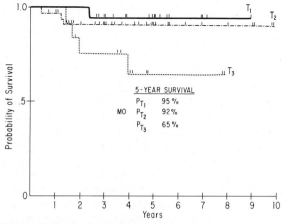

Figure 28–5. Survival of patients with Stage N_0M_0 renal adenocarcinoma after nephrectomy. (From Selli, C., Hinshaw, W., Woodard, B. H., and Paulson, D. F.: Cancer, *52*(5):899, 1983. Used by permission.)

tumors, most probably reflects the enhanced probability of undetected metastatic disease among patients with high-grade tumors (P > 0.001) (Fig. 28–6). Nephrectomy in patients with metastatic disease does not alter the subsequent disease course. This is not expected, as survival of these patients is dependent not on the local tumor but on the distant disease process and the biologic aggressiveness of the individual tumor cells. In addition, the similar mortality rate among patients with bony as opposed to soft tissue metastases supports the hypothesis that the risk of death is related to the biologic aggressiveness of the individual tumor and not to the site of the lesion (Swanson et al., 1981).

The impact of the anatomic extent of disease on the prognosis of patients with solid genitourinary tumors is even more apparent when one examines transitional cell carcinoma of the bladder. Once the malignant transitional cell has demonstrated the ability to penetrate the lamina propria, the host is at greater risk for death (Anderstrom et al., 1980) (Table 28–2). Patients who have a conservatively treated Grade 2 or Grade 3, Stage 0 transitional cell carcinoma can expect a 98 per cent survival at 5 years and a 94 per cent survival at 10 years. The accumulated experience indicates that only 4 to 6 per cent of all patients who have transitional cell tumors that do not penetrate the lamina propria will succumb secondary to widespread transitional cell malignancy. However, once the disease has penetrated the lamina propria, the survival at 5 years drops. Eighty-eight per cent of patients who have a Grade 2 transitional cell malignancy that penetrates the lamina propria will survive 5 years with conser-

TABLE 28–2. TRANSITIONAL CELL CARCINOMA (TCC) WITH AND WITHOUT LAMINA PROPRIA INVASION

	5-Year Survival (%)	10-Year Survival (%)
NO INVASION		
Grade 2	98	94
Grade 3	98	94
LP INVASION		
Grade 2	83	83
Grade 3	63	56
Grade 4	50	

From Anderstrom, C., et al.: J. Urol., *124*:23, 1980.

vative treatment only. However, 66 per cent of conservatively treated patients with a Grade 3 transitional cell malignancy that penetrates the lamina propria will survive 5 years; only 50 per cent of patients who have a Grade 4 tumor of similar stage will be expected to survive 5 years.

In similarly treated patient populations, penetration of the lamina propria indicates a tumor with enhanced biologic aggressiveness. Thirty per cent of all tumors that penetrate the lamina propria will recur with either muscle invasion or distant metastases, the majority within 2 years (Heney et al., 1983). Thus, in considering the treatment of superficial transitional cell carcinoma, one must accurately determine whether the disease has penetrated the lamina propria, as there seems to be a marked difference in survival dependent upon the depth of penetration. Whether the high disease-control failure in conservatively treated lamina propria–invasive disease occurs because therapy has not eradicated the disease or because the disease is systemic at the initiation of treatment is unknown. Since only 10 per cent of patients with clinical Stage 0 or Stage A disease show muscle invasion or regional lymph node involvement on pathologic study, the failure rates associated with conservative treatment may very well be due to failure of local treatment to control the tumor within the bladder.

The notion that node-positive transitional cell malignancy is a disease that is uncontrollable by surgical intervention alone is supported by the data of Whitmore and associates. One hundred and thirty-four patients with node-positive disease underwent pelvic lymphadenectomy and radical cystectomy. The authors categorized the extent of nodal disease as seen in Table 28–3 (Smith, 1981). When one examines the time to failure and the survival in patients with node-positive disease, it becomes apparent that survival is dependent primarily on the volume of nodal disease (Table 28–4) (Smith,

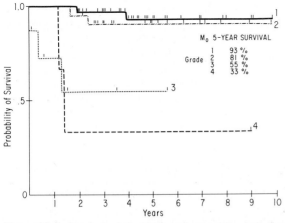

Figure 28–6. Survival of the N_0M_0 patients with renal adenocarcinoma after radical nephrectomy, as a function of tumor grade. (From Selli, C., Hinshaw, W., Woodard, B. H., and Paulson, D. F.: Cancer, *52*(5):899, 1983. Used by permission.)

TABLE 28–3. STRATIFICATION OF NODAL DISEASE

N_1—Single node distal to common iliac bifurcation (30 pts.)
N_2—Unilateral involvement of > 1 node distal to C.I. bifurcation (41 pts.)
N_3—Bilateral node involvement, ≥ 1 distal to the C.I. bifurcation (38 pts.)
N_4—Any node above the C.I. bifurcation (25 pts.)

From Smith, J. A., Jr., and Whitmore, W. F., Jr.: J. Urol., *126*:591, 1981.

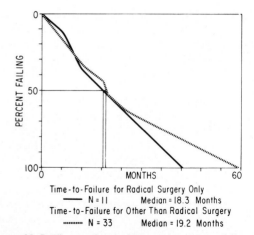

Time-to-Failure for Radical Surgery Only
—— N = 11   Median = 18.3 Months
Time-to-Failure for Other Than Radical Surgery
·········· N = 33   Median = 19.2 Months

Figure 28–7. Time to first incidence of treatment failure for patients with node-positive disease treated by radical surgery, radiation therapy, or delayed endocrine therapy. (From Paulson, D. F., Cline, W. A., et al.: J. Urol., *127*:935, 1982. Used by permission.)

1981). Thus, the conclusion can be drawn that the short survival of patients with large-volume nodal disease, as opposed to the lengthened survival of patients with small-volume nodal disease, merely reflects the enhanced survival potential of patients with low-volume systemic disease as opposed to the decreased survival potential of patients with high-volume systemic disease. The accumulated experience with prostatic malignancy similarly supports the concept of the anatomic extent of disease as the predictor of treatment response.

Kramer and coworkers (1981) examined the impact of radical prostatectomy and pelvic lymphadenectomy in patients with and without histologically proven pelvic nodal extension. Using time to first evidence of distant disease as the end point of this study, they demonstrated a considerable difference in the time to failure between the two pathologic groups, with 50 per cent of patients who demonstrated node-positive disease showing evidence of distant spread within 19.5 months (Kramer et al., 1981; Paulson, 1980*b*). In a follow-up study, all patients who had node-positive prostatic extension were assigned (on the basis of physician preference) to radical prostatectomy; to external-beam radiation therapy employing 5000 rad to the full pelvis and the periaortic lymph nodes to the upper level of L1, with a 2000 rad boost to the prostate; or to delayed androgen-deprivation therapy (Kramer et al., 1981; Paulson, 1980*b*). Patients who had histologically proven pelvic lymph node extension showed no disease control advantage when treated with radical prostatec-

tomy, external-beam radiation therapy, or delayed androgen deprivation (Fig. 28–7). These results strongly support the premise that pelvic lymph node extension identifies a tumor that not only has the potential for systemic spread but also has already initiated systemic dissemination in the host and thus can no longer be controlled by treatment with only local or regional effects.

The single-institution experience of Whitmore and coworkers demonstrated that after pelvic lymphadenectomy and 125-I implantation, 40 per cent of patients who had pelvic lymph node extension showed bony spread within 24 months and 75 per cent had treatment failure within 60 months (Grossman et al., in press). Although one might argue that an occasional patient with a single microscopic nodal focus could conceivably benefit from lymphadenectomy, the accumulated data strongly support the concept that pelvic lymphadenectomy is not therapeutic but that the identification of node-positive disease identifies tumors that are systemic in nature. This concept is substantiated

TABLE 28–4. FIVE-YEAR STATUS OF PATIENTS BY N-GROUPS

	N_1	N_2	N_3	N_4	**Total**
Total Cases	*30*	*41*	*38*	*25*	*134*
Alive, no evidence of disease	5 (17%)	2 (5%)	2 (5%)	0	9 (7%)
Dead of TCC	23 (77%)	34 (83%)	31 (82%)	21 (84%)	109 (82%)
Median survival	22 mo.	13 mo.	11 mo.	7 mo.	
Median time to recurrence	135 mo.	10 mo.	7 mo.	5 mo.	

From Smith, J. A., Jr., and Whitmore, W. F., Jr.: J. Urol., *126*:591, 1981.

by the observation that only an incremental enhancement of disease control is observed in patients with just one positive node versus those with more than one positive node, irrespective of the treatment employed (Paulson et al., 1982) (Fig. 28–8).

Even with a treatment that is regional rather than local, the volume of local disease and the extent of disease spread markedly influence the ability of that treatment to establish control. An examination of the Uro-Oncology Group data is interesting. In this study, patients with normal serum prostatic acid phosphatase, negative isotopic bone scans, and absence of pelvic nodal extension, whose disease was digitally confined to the prostate, were randomly assigned to either external-beam radiation therapy or radical prostatectomy. Patients who showed no evidence of distant disease but whose disease was outside the anatomic limits of the prostate by rectal examination were assigned either to radiation therapy or to delayed androgen deprivation; patients who had histologically confirmed node-positive disease were assigned to extended-field radiation therapy or to delayed androgen deprivation. In these three treatment groups, the end point of the study was first evidence of distant disease, as identified by the appearance of a positive bone scan, and/or elevation of serum prostatic acid phosphatase, and/or the appearance of parenchymal or soft tissue extension. If one examines the relative impact of external-beam radiation therapy to control organ-confined disease versus regional disease versus node-positive disease, one can see that as the extent and volume of disease

increase, the ability of equivalently applied radiation therapy to control the disease decreases (Fig. 28–9). One may question whether this differential in disease-control impact reflects the inability of radiation therapy to control the tumor as volume increases or whether it is due to an increase of systemic disease as a function of the size of the primary tumor.

Use of histologic grading to predict the probability of extended disease is well demonstrated when one uses the histologic appearance of the prostatic primary lesion to predict the presence of pelvic lymph node extension. Gleason and coworkers proposed a system of histopathologic grading based upon the glandular pattern of tumor growth identified at relatively low magnification ($\times$ 40 to 100) (Gleason and Mellinger, 1974). The Gleason sum, as assigned to the primary tumor, is a reasonable predictor of nodal extension (Table 28–5). The incidence of node-positive disease increases with the loss of differentiation within the cells that make up the primary tumor. This observation has been supported by many other investigators using both the Gleason method and alternative criteria for grading prostatic primaries. The accu-

TABLE 28–5. COMPARISON OF GLEASON SUM WITH NODE BIOPSY

	Node Biopsy			
Gleason Sum	POSITIVE (%)	NEGATIVE (%)	N/GROUP	
2–5	13.9	86.1	36	
6	32.4	67.6	34	
7	49.9	50.1	21	$X^2 = 28.2$
8	75.0	25.0	12	$p < 0.0005$
9–10	100.0	0	7	
No Diagnosis	33.3	66.7	12	

From Uro-Oncology Research Group: Report. American Urological Association, 1979. Used by permission.

TABLE 28–6. COMPARISON OF THE TWO CLASSIFICATION SYSTEMS FOR STAGING OF RENAL CELL CARCINOMA

	TNM (1978)	Robson
Small tumor, no enlargement of kidney	T_1	A
Large tumor, cortex not broken	T_2	A
Perinephric or hilar extension	T_3	B
Extension to neighboring organs	T_4	D
Nodal invasion	N_+	C
Renal vein involved	V_1	C
Vena cava involved	V_2	C
Distant metastases	M_+	D

From Selli, C., Hinshaw, W. M., Woodard, B. H., and Paulson, D. F.: Cancer, 52:899, 1983.

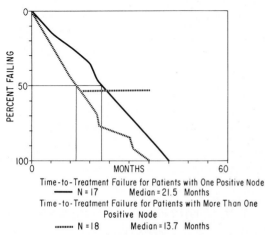

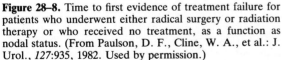

Time-to-Treatment Failure for Patients with One Positive Node
—— N = 17   Median = 21.5 Months
Time-to-Treatment Failure for Patients with More Than One Positive Node
········ N = 18   Median = 13.7 Months

Figure 28–8. Time to first evidence of treatment failure for patients who underwent either radical surgery or radiation therapy or who received no treatment, as a function as nodal status. (From Paulson, D. F., Cline, W. A., et al.: J. Urol., *127*:935, 1982. Used by permission.)

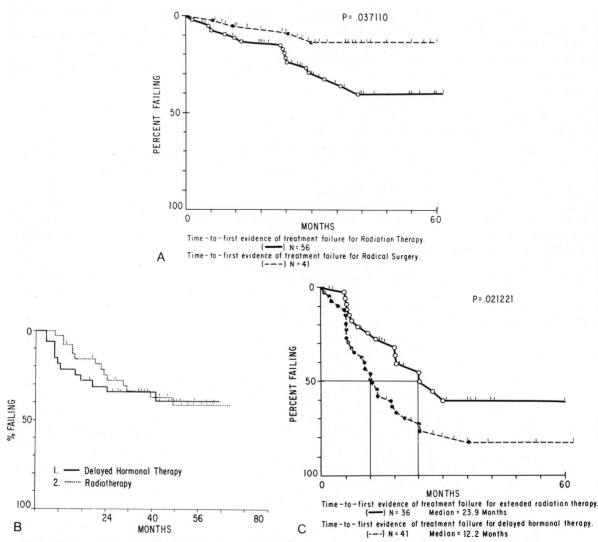

Figure 28–9. *A,* Time to treatment failure for patients randomized to radiation therapy or radical surgery, whose disease is confined to the prostate. *B,* Failure rate among patients with node-negative Stage C disease randomized to either radiation therapy or delayed hormonal therapy. *C,* Time to first evidence of treatment failure for patients with node-positive disease randomized either to extended field radiation therapy or to delayed hormonal therapy. (*A* from Paulson, D. F., Lin, G. H., et al.: J. Urol. *128*:502, 1982; *B* from Hodge, G. B., Paulson, D. F., et al.: J. Urol., in press; *C* from Paulson, D. F., Cline, W. A., et al.: J. Urol., *127*:935, 1982. Used by permission.)

mulated data indicate that the histologic grade of the primary tumor is a visual indicator of the statistical probability of metastatic disease. However, in patients who are accurately staged by the most current staging modalities, the anatomic extent of disease seems to be the most important prognosticator of treatment impact. Thus, the clinician should employ the staging system that most accurately determines the anatomic extent of disease and that can best be used for communication between treating physicians. The TNM system, as devised by the American Joint Committee for Cancer Treat-

ment Results Reporting of the American College of Surgeons, is strongly recommended. The TNM system and the classic staging systems currently employed in the United States are compared in Tables 28–6 to 28–9.

TREATMENT OF MALIGNANT DISEASE

Malignant genitourinary disease is treated with surgery, radiation therapy, and chemotherapy, either singly or in combination. Certain

TABLE 28–7. STAGING SYSTEMS OF BLADDER CANCER

Jewett (1946)	Jewett (1952)	Marshall (1952)	Bladder Cancer Staging (Clinical-Pathologic)	American Joint Committee UICC—1974 CLINICAL	PATHOLOGIC
		No tumor-definitive specimen		T_0	P_0
		0	Carcinoma in situ	TIS	PIS
A	A		Papillary tumor—no invasion	T_A	P_A
		A	Papillary tumor—lamina propria invasion	T_1	P_1
B	B_1	B_1	Superficial ⎱ muscle invasion	T_2	P_2
	B_2	B_2	Deep ⎰	T_{3A} ⎱	P_3
C	C	C	Invasion of perivesical fat	T_{3B} ⎰	
		D_1	Invasion of contiguous viscera	T_4	P_4
			Involvement of pelvic nodes		N_{1-3}
		D_2	Involvement of juxtaregional nodes		N_4
			Distant metastases		M_1

From Droller, M. J.: Curr. Probl. Surg., *18*:205, 1981.

TABLE 28–8. TNM CLASSIFICATION

Primary Tumor (T)
TX   Minimum requirements cannot be met.
T0   No tumor palpable; includes incidental findings of cancer in a biopsy or operative specimen. Assign all such cases a G, N, or M category.
T1   Tumor intracapsular surrounded by normal gland.
T2   Tumor confined to gland, deforming contour, and invading capsule, but lateral sulci and seminal vesicles are not involved.
T3   Tumor extends beyond capsule with or without involvement of lateral sulci and/or seminal vesicles.
T4   Tumor fixed or involving neighboring structures. Add suffix (m) after "T" to indicate multiple tumors (e.g., T2m).

Nodal Involvement (N)
NX   Minimum requirements cannot be met.
N0   No involvement of regional lymph nodes.
N1   Involvement of a single regional lymph node.
N2   Involvement of multiple regional lymph nodes.
N3   Free space between tumor and fixed pelvic wall mass.
N4   Involvement of juxtaregional nodes.
Note: If N category is determined by lymphangiography or isotope scans, insert "l" or "i" between "N" and appropriate number (e.g., Nl2 or Ni2). If nodes are histologically positive after surgery, add " + ," if negative, add " − ."

Distant Metastasis (M)
MX   Not assessed
M0   No (known) distant metastasis
M1   Distant metastasis present
Specify _____
Specify sites according to the following notations:

Pulmonary—PUL	Bone Marrow—MAR
Osseous—OSS	Pleura—PLE
Hepatic—HEP	Skin—SKI
Bain—BRA	Eye—EYE
Lymph Nodes—LYM	Other—OTH

Note: Add " + " to the abbreviated notation to indicate that the pathology (p) is proved.

From Paulson, D. F.: *In* DeVita, V. T., Hellman, S., and Rosenberg, S. A. (Eds.): Cancer: Principles and Practice of Oncology. Philadelphia, J. B. Lippincott Co., 1982, p. 756.

TABLE 28–9. STAGING OF TESTICULAR MALIGNANCY

Clinical Stage	History, Physical, Chest X-Ray	Lymphangiogram, IVP	Serum Markers	Laparotomy	Surgical Pathology Stage
I	Negative	Negative	Negative	Negative	I—Negative nodes
	Negative	Negative	Negative	Microscopic nodes positive	IIa—Microscopic nodes positive
II	Negative	Negative	Elevated	Microscopic nodes positive	
	Negative	Positive	Negative or elevated	Macroscopic nodes positive	IIb—Macroscopic nodes clearly resected
					IIc—Macroscopic nodes not clearly resected
					IId—Macroscopic nodes not resected
IIIa IIIb	Positive	Positive/negative	Positive/ negative	Positive/negative	Any of the above possibilities

From Paulson, D. F.: Curr. Probl. Cancer, 6(11):20, 1982.

principles apply in the selection of these treatments. Current concepts indicate that surgery is appropriate only when disease is confined to a single organ site and inappropriate for controlling regional or distant metastatic disease. The survival of patients with distant metastatic disease, who have surgery for control of both a primary lesion and the metastatic site, probably results from the biology of the tumor rather than from the treatment alone. Radiation therapy can be considered a regional treatment—one that is applicable both to malignant disease in a single organ site and to local extension of the disease from that site. Chemotherapy is the best choice when the disease is systemic. Combinations of these three treatments may be used to gain control of disease that is other than organ-confined.

Surgical Oncology

Of major importance in the selection of patients for surgical treatment is a consideration of the potential benefit of surgery versus the risk of surgical intervention. There are a series of identified determinants of operative risk. These are (1) the general health status of the patient, (2) the severity of the underlying disease process, (3) the degree to which the form of surgical intervention selected will alter normal physiologic function, (4) the technical complexity of the surgical procedure chosen, (5) the type of anesthesia selected and the potential impact of that anesthetic on physiologic function, and (6) the experience of the surgical personnel involved. In patients with malignant urologic disease, the disease process is a major determinant of operative mortality, which is defined as death within 30 days of a major procedure. It should be recognized that patients who undergo palliative surgery for metastatic disease have a higher operative mortality than those who undergo a similar procedure in the absence of metastatic disease. The surgical death rate due to the anesthetic alone appears to be related linearly to the physical status of the patient. The current anesthetic mortality in patients undergoing elective cancer surgery is approximately 0.1 per cent.

Surgical intervention plays a major role in the diagnosis, anatomic staging, treatment, rehabilitation, and palliation of the patient with malignant disease. Nowhere is this more evident than in the management of prostatic carcinoma. The diagnosis of prostatic carcinoma may be strongly suspected on the basis of physical examination, radiographic findings, or serum biochemical abnormalities. However, the diagnosis is established only by obtaining tissue. The presence of prostatic malignancy is most frequently confirmed by needle biopsy of the area defined as suspicious by rectal examination. As stated earlier, it is important to identify the anatomic extent of disease in order that treatment selection can be made with precision. The failure to obtain proper staging information will lead to poor treatment planning and will compromise the ability to control malignant disease. Surgery seems to be the optimal treatment for patients with solid tumor malignancy when that tumor is confined to the anatomic site of origin.

The surgeon's role is to identify the best procedure for the primary cancer, select the appropriate mode of therapy, and, when appropriate, integrate surgery with other treatment modalities. Surgery may be useful in reducing the bulk of residual disease in tumors other than genitourinary tumors, but this does not appear to be appropriate for patients with urologic disease.

Principles of Radiation Therapy

CHARACTERISTICS

Ionizing radiation causes the ejection of an orbital electron. It may be electromagnetic or particulate. Electromagnetic radiation may be divided into roentgen and gamma radiation, which are produced by different mechanisms. Gamma rays are produced intranuclearly by the decay of radioactive isotopes, whereas roentgen radiation is electrical (except when it is produced by orbital electron rearrangement during the decay of 125-I).

Electromagnetic radiation dissipates as the inverse square of the distance from the source, the dose of radiation 2 cm from a point source being 25 per cent of the dose for 1 cm. Absorption of electromagnetic radiation occurs by three mechanisms, the energy of the radiation being the determining factor. Photoelectric absorption predominates at lower energies. Photon interaction produces ejection of a tightly bound orbital electron. The vacancy in the atomic shell then is filled by an electron falling from an outer shell of the same atom or from outside the atom. The photon energy is lost in this process. Photoelectric absorption varies with the cube of the atomic number. This is important, as it is the reason why materials with high atomic numbers, such as lead, are effective shielding materials.

Compton absorption is a second form of radiation absorption. The interaction is with a distal electron that has a very low binding energy. In this absorptive process, the photon gives up a portion of its energy to a single electron. A portion of the residual energy reappears as a secondary photon. Compton absorption does not depend on atomic number but on electron density.

Pair production is the final type of absorption. This requires an incident photon energy greater than 1.02 MeV. In pair production, a positive and a negative electron are simultaneously produced. The interaction of radiation with matter is described as the amount of energy absorbed per unit mass. The absorbed dose is measured in joules per kilogram. One joule/kg equals one gray (Gy) (1 gray = 100 rad). The roentgen (R) is a unit of roentgen or gamma radiation based upon the ability of radiation to ionize air. One R of roentgen or gamma radiation results in a dose of somewhat less than 1 rad (0.01 Gy) in soft tissue. The range of electromagnetic radiation used in clinical practice is defined as (1) superficial radiation or roentgen radiation from approximately 10 to 125 KeV; (2) orthovoltage radiation consisting of electromagnetic radiation between 125 and 400 KeV; and (3) supervoltage radiation for all energies above 400 KeV. It is important to recognize the various ranges for electromagnetic radiation because (1) as the energy of radiation increases, the penetration of the roentgen rays increases; and (2) with supervoltage energies, the absorption of bone is not higher than that of surrounding soft tissues. Supervoltage radiation also is "skin-sparing," meaning that the maximum dose is not reached at the skin level but occurs at a depth below the surface.

Two general types of technique are used in the delivery of radiation therapy—brachytherapy and teletherapy. In brachytherapy, the radiation source is placed either within or close to the target volume as an interstitial or intercavitary radiation. Teletherapy uses a device distant from the patient. In brachytherapy the radiation source is usually close to the target volume; therefore, the dose is largely determined by inverse square considerations, indicating that the geometry of the implant is important. In teletherapy, dose depends on inverse square considerations and tissue absorption, with the distribution of radiation related to the characteristics of the machine and the patient. The isotope curve for any specific therapy program is dependent upon the energy of radiation, the distance from the source of radiation, and the density and atomic number of the absorbing material. The goal of each treatment plan in radiotherapy is to maximize the dose to the tumor volume while minimizing the dose to normal surrounding tissues. Thus, it is important that the tumor dose be homogeneous, since the maximum dose in the tumor tissue or target volume frequently is the cause of complications, and the minimum dose in this same volume determines the potential for tumor recurrence.

BIOLOGIC IMPACT OF RADIATION THERAPY

There are two possible mechanisms for production of cell kill by radiation therapy; these result from the impact of energy transfer to biologically important molecules. The mechanisms for interaction with these biologically important molecules that control cell life are the direct effect of radiation on the target molecule and the indirect effect produced by intermediate radiation products. Deoxyribonucleic acid is considered to be the most important target molecule, as it is necessary for maintenance of reproductive integrity of the cell. However, whatever the critical target, it is assumed to be directly affected by the ionizing radiation that causes alteration of the molecular structure. The most powerful direct effect is produced by high linear energy transfer (LET) radiation therapy. To produce intermediate radiation products, the photon may interact with cellular water to produce oxygen free radicals. Although the free radicals are relatively short-lived, they do interact with biologically important molecular molecules to produce molecular damage. Free radicals, however, can also revert to molecular oxygen. Thus, the likelihood of interaction as opposed to reversion can be modified by reaction with molecular oxygen, prolonging the life of the reactive species.

All radiation effects are random, whether they are direct or indirect. The random event is important in understanding the general nature of cell killing. While assuming that DNA is the critical target for radiation effect, one must recognize that a cell damaged by radiation may divide once or more before all the progeny are incapable of subsequent division. Thus, a radiated cell may not appear damaged until it prepares for cell division. At the time of cell division a number of events may occur. The cell may die while undergoing division; it may produce unusual cellular forms owing to aberrant attempts at division; it may be unable to divide but physiologically survive; it may divide, producing one or more generations of daughter cells before these offspring become reproductively sterile; or it may suffer no damage. Because radiation damage is random, if radiation produces one lethal lesion per cell, on the average, some cells will have one lesion, some will have more than one lesion, and some will have no lethal damage. The proportion of cells that have no lethal events is e^{-1}, or a survival fraction of 0.37. The dose required to reduce the survival fraction to this 37 per cent on an

exponential curve is known as the D_0, and it is related to the slope of the exponential survival curve. The smaller the dose required to reduce the survival fraction to 37 per cent, the more sensitive are the cells to radiation. The survival curves of mammalian cells have a "shoulder" at low doses but an exponential relationship at higher doses. The shoulder demonstrates a reduced efficiency of cell killing at low radiation doses (Fig. 28–10).

There is no difference between the survival curve characteristics of normal tissue and malignant tissue. The survival characteristics of most tumor tissue resemble those of the normal tissue of origin. Following cellular radiation, the damage may be modified and not lead to cell death. Alteration or modification of cell damage is referred to as cellular repair. Repair may be categorized as potentially lethal damage repair and sublethal damage repair. Potentially lethal damage ultimately will lead to cell death. However, when the radiation conditions are modified to permit repair, those cells that would normally have died do not. Postradiation conditions that suppress cell division are most favorable to repair of potentially lethal damage, since they permit time for repair to occur. The repair of potentially lethal damage may be the factor that provides the degree of variability in cellular

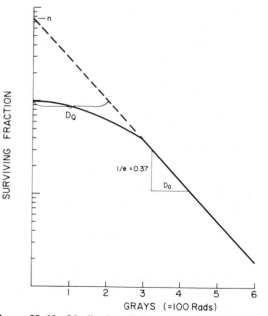

Figure 28–10. Idealized radiation survival curve. (From Hellman, S.: *In* DeVita, V. T., Hellan, S., and Rosenberg, S. A. (Eds.): Principles and Practice of Oncology. Philadelphia, J. B. Lippincott Co., 1982, p. 112. Used by permission.)

susceptibility to radiation. The shoulder on the radiation survival curve occurs as the cell, when subjected to low-energy radiation, is able to repair some of the radiation damage (sublethal damage repair). Dividing the dose of radiation into two fractions separated in time permits reappearance of the shoulder when radiation survival curves are constructed (Weichselbaum et al., 1977). Thus, two doses of radiation separated in time are less effective than the same total dose given at one time.

Molecular oxygen is the most important modifier of the biologic effect of ionizing radiation (Mottram, 1936; Read, 1952; Gray et al., 1953). Greater doses of radiation are required under hypoxic conditions as compared with situations in which the cells are well oxygenated (Belli et al., 1967) (Fig. 28–11). The oxygen enhancement ratio (OER) is a ratio of the dose required for equivalent cell killing in the absence of oxygen as compared with the presence of oxygen. The OER of different cells varies from about 2.5 to 3.5. This indicates that, for a given cell survival level, three times as much radiation is required under hypoxic conditions as under conditions of good cell oxygenation. Very low oxygen tension must be reached before hypoxia has a protective effect. The exact mechanism of the oxygen effect is not known. However, current thinking indicates that oxygen affects the interaction of the initial chemical products of radiation with the biologic materials of the target. Oxygen favors free radical formation, whereas sulfhydryl compounds shorten the half-life of free radicals, returning them to an innocuous state. Every tumor has areas in which cells are well oxygenated and areas in which cells are poorly oxygenated. If all tumors do contain hypoxic regions that may ultimately produce tumor regrowth, for cure to be effected by radiation these hypoxic cells must return to a level of oxygenation wherein they are sensitive to radiation therapy. Laboratory studies have shown that immediately following single-dose radiation, the surviving tumor cells are largely those that were originally hypoxic.

Radiation therapists have long known that fractionation, or division of the radiation into multiple small dosages, allows for more effective tumor control without excessive complications. The relationship between the acute effects of radiation therapy and the delayed impact appears to be dependent upon the scheme of fractionation chosen by the radiotherapist, the source and energy of radiation, and the volume of tissue treated. Acute effects appear to be primarily dependent upon time, whereas the late effects appear to be primarily influenced by the total dose and the size of the individual treatment fractions. It is important that the dose rate be kept moderate. Homogeneity of dosage is also important, a problem that is encountered with interstitial radiation. In the absence of adequate implant geometry, the tumor is exposed to unnecessary hot spots and to areas that receive less than adequate irradiation.

The acute radiation effects seem to be primarily on those tissues that are rapidly renewed, such as skin, oropharyngeal mucosa, small intestine, rectum, bladder mucosa, and vaginal mucosa. The cells of these tissues are rapidly proliferating, and, when they are subjected to fractionated radiation, the processes of repair, repopulation, and recruitment all are involved. The effect upon those cells that are rapidly dividing is dependent on the balance between the cell birth rate and the cell death rate and is influenced by the time allowed for repopulation of cells that are killed. The effect is therefore very dependent upon protraction, or the time over which the radiation is given. The late effects are the dose-limiting effects that restrict radiation therapy. These include fibrosis, necrosis, fistula formation, ulceration that fails to heal, and specific organ damage, such as spinal cord transection and so forth. They do not appear to depend upon the rapid proliferation of cells for repopulation. The late effects

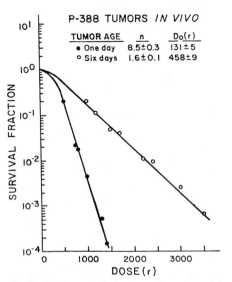

Figure 28–11. In vivo survival curves for oxic and hypoxic tumor cells. (From Hellman, S.: In DeVita, V. T., Hellman, S., and Rosenberg, S. A. (Eds.): Principles and Practice of Oncology. Philadelphia, J. B. Lippincott Co., 1982, p. 113. Used by permission.)

are not dependent upon protraction but are dependent upon the total-dose radiation and the size of the radiation fraction. Since the parameters of fractionation and protraction are varied, the acute radiation effect may be dissociated from the late radiation effect.

The therapeutic index is the relationship between the desired and the undesired effects of any treatment (Goodman and Gilman, 1970). Altering time-dose relationships by fractionation, protraction, or split-course technique; using interstitial treatment; and manipulating the target volumes are techniques of the radiotherapist to maximize the therapeutic index. Most radiotherapists deliver the radiation in fractions of between 180 and 250 rads per day. Experience has shown that this will produce tumor control without excessive acute or delayed effects. The fraction size that is tolerated in terms of the acute effects appears to be directly dependent upon the volume irradiated, the amount and type of the dose, the surrounding normal tissue, and the age of the patient. Patients are frequently given small breaks during the treatment interval to allow for repopulation and recruitment of cells. This may also allow time for tumor regression by reoxygenation of previously anoxic tissue. The split-course technique is an attempt to formalize and extend these treatment breaks (Scanlon, 1980; Parson et al., 1980b). Often, several weeks without treatment are inserted into the middle of a program to diminish the acute effects. There is some evidence that split-course techniques used without any increase in the total dose of radiation may be associated with lessened tumor control (Parson et al., 1980a).

Tumor volume is important in radiation therapy. The larger the volume that must be irradiated, the smaller the dose that is tolerated. Alternatively, the larger the volume of tumor, the greater the dose required for tumor control. This may be the single factor that explains the ability of radiation therapy to control very small tumor volumes but to be frequently ineffective in controlling large tumor volumes. The radiotherapist, in planning field size and radiation course, distinguishes between gross tumor involvement and subclinical extension into apparently normal surrounding tissues. The large number of cells present in the clinically evident tumor requires very high doses of radiotherapy, as noted previously. However, it is proposed that subclinical extension may be controlled with lower doses of radiation, as these cells are frequently well oxygenated and most rapidly dividing.

In order to achieve this goal, radiation therapists have developed a variety of techniques to establish tumor control. The *shrinking-field technique* provides the largest potential tumor bed with a moderate dose of radiation and then reduces the target volume to the tumor and increases the dose. A modification of the shrinking-field technique is the *boost technique*, in which the maximized tolerated dose is given to a specific tumor volume and then localized radiation therapy is used to raise the dose within the tumor bed. The surrounding normal tissues, which limit the dose of radiation given, may be so closely adjacent to the tumor that any target volume that includes the tumor must also, of necessity, include the surrounding normal tissues. This may contribute to complications and be a dose-limiting factor in the delivery of tumoricidal radiation therapy. It should be noted that radiation rarely fails at the periphery of the tumor, where cells are small in number and well vascularized. However, it frequently fails in the center of the tumor, where there is a large volume of tumor cells existing in a minimal oxygen environment. Surgery is often limited by the necessity to preserve adjacent normal tissues. Thus, surgery may fail at the periphery while it controls the tumor in the hypoxic center of the large-volume mass. Giving radiation prior to surgery would maximize the impact of these two treatments, with preoperative radiation sterilizing cells at the margin of the resection and surgery removing the bulk of the tumor volume. This concept, although attractive theoretically, has yet to be established in practice.

Principles of Chemotherapy

Chemotherapy is used for the treatment of systemic disease and should be used to cure disease rather than to merely suppress the symptomatology. The total burden of cancer cells in the body appears to influence the outcome of treatment. When chemotherapy is utilized in repetitive dosing, the net tumor cell kill per treatment is the sum of the surviving cells plus the regrowth of the tumor cell population during the interval between treatments. It has been demonstrated that anticancer drugs kill cancer cells by first-order kinetics. A given dose of agent will kill a constant fraction of a population of cells regardless of the size of that cell population (Skipper et al., 1964). If 100,000 cells are reduced to 1 cell after a treatment, then, when 1 billion cells are present at the initiation of treatment, by law of first-order reaction, treatment will leave 1000 residual cells, assuming that the larger population has an equal number of sensitive and resistant cell lines. Thus, it would appear that the chance of killing the last surviving cancer cell is greater when the population size is small. It must be remembered that the growth fraction increases with decreasing tumor size (Simpson-Herren et al., 1974; Mendelsohn, 1960). Furthermore, the chance of drug-resistant cell lines being present in any tumor mass is related to the inherent mutation rate of that tumor cell population (Luria and Delbruck, 1943). Therefore, the appearance of drug-resistant cells varies directly with tumor mass, and the chance of having multiple drug-resistant lines and an enhanced percentage of drug-resistant cells increases with the mass of tumor burden (Goldie and Coldman, 1979).

These are important observations when applied to the human tumor system, and they provide the rationale for combination chemotherapy in preference to single-agent therapy against tumor cell populations that have a constant growth fraction. The inclusion of a small number of resistant tumor cells in a large tumor mass may not influence the initial response to chemotherapy, but this occurrence does explain why patients who have complete remissions are not always cured. The killing effect of cancer chemotherapeutic agents has a selectivity for cancer cells over normal host cells. While the cancer cells do not divide at a rate faster than that of their normal tissue counterpart, the population of cancer cells usually has a higher growth fraction (Mendelsohn, 1960). Most anticancer agents share two properties: They effect cell kill by altering DNA synthesis, and they do not kill cells that are resting unless such cells will divide following drug exposure.

The major reason for treatment failure appears to be drug resistance. Resistance to drugs occurs in cell populations because some cells are resistant initially to the agent or agents chosen, or because resistant cell lines appear under the pressure of exposure to the drugs that are being used (Brockman, 1975; Freireich et al., 1966; DeVita et al., 1975; Hutchison, 1963). This is different from treatment failure in radiotherapy, as primary resistance to radiotherapy is rarely seen. It should be recognized that a single surviving cancer cell will lead to the death of the host. Consequently, the appearance of a cell from a sanctuary or the presence or selection of a resistant mutant line seems to be the major cause of chemotherapy failure (Skipper, 1978; Furth and Kahn, 1937; Goldin et al., 1956). It is believed that the probability of resistant cells increases as tumor size increases (Goldie and Coldman, 1979). The likelihood of at least one resistant cell occurring in a population may change from low to high over a very short interval of tumor growth. The greater the mutation rate, the earlier cell resistance is likely to occur (Law, 1952; Luria and Delbruck, 1943; Skipper et al., 1972). This becomes clearer when it is recognized that to reach a mass of 1 billion cells (the lower limits of tumor recognition), a single cancer cell must go through between 27 and 30 doublings (DeVita et al., 1975). The lethal tumor body burden for humans is thought to be 10^{12} cells (Brockman, 1975). Only ten additional doublings will increase the cell burden from 10^9 to 10^{12}. The assumption has been made that when metastases are visible, some cells may have spontaneously mutated to drug resistance by the time the patient presents for treatment. Thus, there is a theoretical advantage in initiating treatment when the cell population is small, the growth fraction is high, and the likelihood of de novo cell lines' resistance to treatment is minimal. Clinicians, therefore, have begun to consider the use of postoperative adjunctive chemotherapy (Schabel, 1976, 1977).

CELL CYCLE KINETICS AND ANTINEOPLASTIC AGENTS

The cell cycle can be divided into four stages. As the cells divide they pass through a G-1 phase, an S or DNA synthetic phase, a G-2 phase, and a mitotic phase. The G-1 phase is a "gap" arresting phase between cell division and the DNA synthetic phase, and G-2 is a gap between the S phase and mitosis. The G-1 phase appears to be most important for control of cell growth. It is in G-1 that external conditions determine whether cycling cells will continue in the proliferative cycle or whether they will be switched into a G-0, or resting, phase. The external conditions have less effect on the other portions of the cell cycle. Cells usually transit the cycle and then enter into G-0 (quiescence) only during periods of suboptimal conditions. That point in the G-1 phase at which it is determined whether the cell will continue in the cyclic proliferation or whether it will enter the G-0 cycle has been termed the restriction point (Pardee, 1974). There is a considerable body of evidence to suggest that events in G-1 are particularly sensitive to environmental conditions and that the ability of individual cells to progress past this restriction point differs. Transit of G-1 can be delayed for extended periods under adverse conditions without the cells ever entering S or G-0 (Pledger et al., 1978). The restriction point, or event, is sensitive to external influences that will determine whether or not a cell will cycle and thus how fast a population of cells will grow. Neoplastic cells are less dependent on these external influences than are nonmalignant cells. Little is known about the biochemistry of the G-1 portion of the cell cycle. Synthesis of proteins and RNA is necessary for transit of the G-1 phase, making the events of G-1 sensitive to agents that interfere with the necessary enzymatic events (Murakami and Masui, 1980).

One of the primary problems facing the urologic oncologist is the treatment of disease once metastatic deposits have established growth. Although the ideal would be to destroy malignant cells at any point during the multistep sequence from primary tumor to formation of established metastatic lesions, frequently the patients have established metastases at the time of clinical diagnosis. Thus, the approach should be aimed at the control of the metastatic deposit. The occurrence of interlesional cellular heterogeneity and the increasing heterogeneity within any single metastatic deposit with time suggests that the cells within the metastatic lesion can be quite diverse in their responses to treatment. Thus, it is important for any assay of new agents to include identification of therapies that circumvent the problem of tumor cell diversity.

One of the current methods for evaluating the impact of chemotherapeutic agents on specific tumors is the clonogenic soft agar assay. This involves dispersing tumor cells from surgical biopsy specimens and placing them in soft agar to evaluate the effect of various chemotherapeutic agents on the cells from individual metastatic lesions (Buick, 1980). These assays are based on the ability of dispersed, clonogenic cells to propagate in vitro. These assays, however, have failed to fulfill the goals set by their proponents. Few cells proliferate in vitro; usually, less than 1 per cent of the seeded cells undergo replication. Thus, the tumor cells that grow represent only a minor subpopulation within the tumor. If the metastatic cell subpopulations vary significantly in their clonogenic potential, the stem cell assay will be unable to evaluate any therapeutic response of the tumor cell subpopulations that cannot grow in vitro but that may be life-threatening in the intact tumor-bearing host. It may be that the in vitro soft agar assay is valuable not as a predictive test, not to identify agents that are effective in controlling tumor growth in the intact tumor-bearing host, but to predict agents that are not effective in inhibiting tumor cell growth (Poste, 1982).

Once metastasis is established, the timing of therapy and its effect on the tumor cell subpopulation may be critical to determine whether the tumor can be controlled by the chosen therapy. If the therapy has controlled the majority, but not all, of the tumor cell subpopulations in a polyclonal tumor, the surviving subpopulations may become phenotypically unstable secondary to absence of the regulatory interactions that exist among the subpopulations. The regulatory interactions that exist in an untreated tumor mass may establish an equilibrium state that can be deregulated or circumvented by effective removal of certain "stabilizing" cell subpopulations. Therapy may disturb this equilibrium, restricting subpopulation adversity, which in turn produces new tumor cell variants from the surviving subpopulations. Regrowth of the new tumor cell variants would continue until a new regulatory level of cellular diversity was achieved. Retreatment would be effective only if it were capable of eliminating surviving subpopulations before they had time to produce new variants. Therapeutic systems must take these questions into account. The initial problem is whether therapy will increase the phenotypic instability of the tumor cell subpopulation by restricting cell subpopulation diversity within the heterogeneous tumor and its metastatic deposits. The second question is whether the therapeutic diversification of the residual surviving cells can be inhibited by a series of different therapeutic regimens applied in rapid succession.

PRINCIPLES OF COMBINATION CHEMOTHERAPY

Use of combination chemotherapy has been promoted, as these combinations (1) may provide maximum cell kill in a range of toxicity that is tolerated by the host, (2) may provide a broader range of coverage to control de novo cell lines in the multicellular tumor population, and (3) may prevent or reduce the development of new resistant cell lines. Four principles apply in the selection of combination chemotherapy programs (DeVita, 1981):

1. Drugs that are known to be partially effective when used alone must be those that are selected for combination. Drugs that produce some fraction of a complete remission are preferable to those that may produce only a partial response.

2. If several drugs of a single class are

available, selection should be based on toxicity that does not overlap the toxicity of other drugs included in the combination. Such selection may lead to a wider range of side effects and greater discomfort for the patient; however, it minimizes the risk to any single organ system and reduces the potential for death from drug toxicity.

3. Each drug chosen should be used at optimum dosing schedule.

4. Those drug combinations that are selected should be given at consistent intervals. The interval between cycles should be the narrowest possible, in order to allow the recovery of sensitive normal target tissue but reduce the chance of repopulation by tumor cells.

Combination chemotherapy is given cyclically, with the recognition that the bone marrow has a storage compartment capable of supplying mature cells to the peripheral blood for 8 to 10 days after the stem cell pull has ceased to function. Events seen in the peripheral blood are 6 to 7 days behind events that occur in the bone marrow. In patients who have received no previous treatment, thrombocytopenia and leukopenia are usually seen on the ninth and tenth days after the initial dosing, with the lowest counts being identified on the eighteenth to nineteenth day, and recovery occurring between the twenty-first and twenty-eighth days. Previous treatment with either radiotherapy or other chemotherapy may shorten the time to leukopenia and thrombocytopenia and also prolong the recovery period.

The limiting factor in most postoperative adjuvant treatments is that patients who would not recur will be exposed to potentially lethal cytotoxic drugs only to extend treatment benefit to those who would recur.

Principles of Treatment Selection: Local and Regional Versus Systemic

The urologic clinician, when treating a patient with genitourinary malignancy, must initially determine the extent of disease. Once this has been established, treatment can be selected.

All the therapies available for the management of malignant disease produce their effect by different mechanisms and, as such, may be complementary when used simultaneously or in sequence. Surgery produces control of malignant disease by complete eradication of the primary tumor. It should be considered a local treatment only. Radiation therapy induces a fractional kill per unit dose; however, the fraction is not a constant but is dependent upon tumor oxygenation and repair of radiation damage. The ability of radiation therapy to control a malignant site is limited by the mass of tumor and its relationship to normal vital structures. Chemotherapy is systemic and produces tumor control by killing a percentage of the exposed cells at any given dose irrespective of the absolute number of tumor cells. Hormonal deprivation induces a fractional cell kill dependent only on the number of hormone-dependent cells within the tumor burden.

One can examine these various modalities and consider that rational combinations of therapy might effect maximal disease control. However, the ability of these modalities to interact depends upon the effectiveness of each one independently. In other words, although it has been postulated that surgical debulking may increase the growth fraction of residual disease and make it more sensitive to subsequent chemotherapy, current clinical observations would argue instead for cytoreductive chemotherapy initially, to be followed by surgical removal of residual disease.

CRITERIA FOR USE OF ADJUVANT THERAPY

The combined use of two treatment modalities, either simultaneously or sequentially, requires that the two therapies be synergistic (i.e., that they, when used in combination, enhance the effect over that achieved when each is used separately) or that they be independently effective. When two treatments are to be used in combination, the urologic clinician must select those that have different modalities of disease control and thus are complementary and not competing. Few studies exist to identify the relative impact of single-modality therapy versus combination therapy, and one must compare single-arm trials in order to determine the relative benefit. Nonetheless, there are some data to strongly support the combination of regional therapy to control microscopic regional extension and radical surgery to control the large-volume, organ-confined disease. This argument is most compelling when one examines current views of the management of transitional carcinoma of the bladder. Two schools of thought exist—the school that argues that preoperative radiation therapy is of no survival benefit, and the one that claims that preoperative radiation therapy does provide a significant survival advantage. The argument rests not on the ability of either surgery or radiation to control disseminated disease, but on the ability of these two treatments in combination to provide enhanced local control.

There is a single institutional study from the M. D. Anderson Hospital in which patients with Stage 0 or Stage A carcinoma of the bladder received radical surgery either preceded or not preceded by external-beam radiation therapy (Bracken et al., 1981). One hundred and nine patients were evaluated. Fifty-six patients received 5000 rads prior to cystectomy. Preoperative radiation eradicated all tumor in 36 per cent, and no patient who was P_0 after radiation ever had recurrent disease. However, 11 per cent of the 53 nonirradiated patients were also P_0 at the time of cystectomy. When local recurrence rates are examined, a strong argument can be made for the ability of radiation therapy to control either micrometastatic disease or tumor dissemination, as occurred through manipulation at the time of radical cystectomy. Local pelvic recurrence was noted in only 3.5 per cent of the patients who received 5000 rads preoperatively, as compared with 9.5 per cent of those who were not irradiated. Thus, the argument can be made that external-beam radiation therapy may reduce local recurrence rates.

PRINCIPLES OF EVALUATING TREATMENT RESPONSE

The clinician, when examining the impact of therapy, must ascertain that the anatomic extent of disease in each patient was accurately assessed prior to treatment. While survival is the end point in determining any treatment, there may be competing risks of death in the individual undergoing malignant disease control, or there may be subsequent treatments that are applicable in theory, each of which may affect the disease course. In such cases, it may be appropriate to use as a criterion the first evidence of disease beyond the anatomic limits that was present at the initiation of treatment to determine the impact of that treatment. Survival and time to first evidence of treatment failure have different end points. In the consideration of these two end points in patients with metastatic prostate carcinoma or with node-positive prostate carcinoma, it is evident that there are distinct differences in the apparent disease control.

The magnitude of this problem is most clearly demonstrated in determining the effectiveness of initial treatment in a disease such as prostatic adenocarcinoma, in which subsequent radiotherapy, androgen deprivation, and chemotherapy may each alter the disease course independently. Further, the clinical investigator may use disease-free survival rather than crude survival in data analysis. When comparing treatments proposed by different investigators, the clinician must ensure that apparent differences in treatment are not produced in part by different methods of data analysis. The ultimate test of a proposed treatment protocol rests in a well-designed clinical trial, in which equivalently staged patients are randomly assigned to one of two or more therapeutic strategies. Such a trial removes the bias that can unknowingly be introduced in a single-arm, single-institution clinical experiment.

An awareness that inaccurate staging, biologic variability, and variation in response criteria each contributes to differences in reported treatment efficacy will aid the clinician as he attempts to identify optimum treatment for the urologic malignancies.

References

Theories of Carcinogenesis

Baltimore, D.: Tumor viruses. 1974 Cold Spring Harbor Symp. Quant. Biol., *39*:1187, 1975.

Berenblum, I.: Theoretical and practical aspects of the two-stage mechanism of carcinogenesis. *In* Griffin, A. C., and Shaw, C. R. (Eds.): Carcinogens: Identification and Mechanisms of Action. New York, Raven Press, 1979, pp. 25–36.

Binns, A., and Meins, F., Jr.: Habituation of tobacco pith cells for factors promoting cell division is inheritable and potentially reversible. Proc. Natl. Acad. Sci. USA, *70*:2620, 1973.

Butler, T. P., and Gullino, P. M.: Quantitation of cell shedding into efferent blood of mammary adenocarcinoma. Cancer Res., *35*:512, 1975.

Chew, E. C., Josephson, R. K., and Wallace, A. C.: Morphologic aspects of the arrest of circulating cancer cells. *In* Weiss, L. (Ed.): Fundamental Aspects of Metastasis. Amsterdam, North-Holland Publishing Co., 1976, pp. 121–150.

Day, E. D., Planinisek, J. A., and Pressman, D.: Localization in vivo of radioiodinated anti-rat fibrin antibodies and radioiodinated rat fibrinogen in the Murphy rat lymphosarcoma and in other transplantable rat tumors. J. Natl. Cancer Inst., *22*:413, 1959.

Dingemans, K. P.: Invasion of liver tissue by blood-borne mammary carcinoma cells. J. Natl. Cancer Inst., *53*:1813, 1974.

Everson, T. C., and Cole, W. H.: Spontaneous Regression of Cancer. Philadelphia, W. B. Saunders Co., 1966.

Farber, E. E.: Carcinogenesis—cellular evolution as a unifying thread: Presidential address. Cancer Res., *33*:2537, 1973.

Folkman, J.: Tumor angiogenesis. Adv. Cancer Res., *19*:331, 1974.

Folkman, J.: Tumor angiogenesis. *In* Becker, F. F. (Ed.): Biology of Tumors: Cellular Biology and Growth. Vol. 3. New York, Plenum Press, 1975, pp. 355–388.

Folkman, J., and Cotran, R.: Relation of endothelial proliferation to tumor growth. Int. Rev. Exp. Pathol., *16*:207, 1976.

Foulds, L.: Neoplastic Development. New York, Academic Press. Vol. I, 1959; Vol. II, 1975.

Gershon, R. K., Carter, R. L., and Lane, N. J.: Studies on homotransplantable lymphomas in hamster: IV. Observations on macrophages in the expression of tumor immunity. Am. J. Pathol., *51*:1111, 1967.

Harnden, D. G.: Cytogenetics of human neoplasia. *In* Mulvihill, J. J., Miller, R. W., and Fraumeni, J. F., Jr. (Eds.): Progress in Cancer Research and Therapy. Vol. 3. Genetics of Human Cancer. New York, Raven Press, 1977, pp. 87–204.

Hart, I. R., and Fidler, I. J.: Cancer invasion and metastasis. Q. Rev. Biol., *55*:121, 1980.

Hart, I. R., and Fidler, I. J.: The implications of tumor heterogeneity for studies on the biology and therapy of cancer metastasis. Biochim. Biophys. Acta, *651*:37, 1981.

Hatanaka, M.: Transport of sugars in tumor cell membranes. Biochim. Biophys. Acta, *355*:77, 1974.

Hecht, F., and McCaw, B. K.: Chromosome instability syndrome. *In* Mulvihill, J. J., Miller, R. W., and Fraumeni, J. F., Jr. (Eds.): Progress in Cancer Research and Therapy. Vol. 3. Genetics of Human Cancer. New York, Raven Press, 1977, pp. 105–123.

Knudson, A. G.: Mutation and cancer. Adv. Cancer Res., *17*:317, 1973.

Knudson, A. G.: Genetic influences in human tumors. *In* Becker, F. F. (Ed.): Cancer: A Comprehensive Treatise. Vol. 1. New York, Plenum Press, 1975, pp. 59–74.

Knudson, A. G., and Strong, L. C.: Mutation and cancer: A model for Wilms' tumor of the kidney. J. Natl. Cancer Inst., *48*:313, 1972.

Kramer, R. H., and Nicholson, G. L.: Invasion of vascular endothelial cell monolayers and underlying matrix by metastatic human cancer cells. *In* Schweiger, H. G. (Ed.): International Cell Biology. New York, Springer-Verlag, 1981, pp. 794–799.

Magee, P. N.: The relationship between mutagenesis, carcinogenesis, and teratogenesis. *In* Scott, D., Bridges, B. A., and Sobels, F. (Eds.): Progress in Genetic Toxicology. Vol. 2. Amsterdam, Elsevier, 1977, pp. 15–27.

McKinnell, R. G., Deggins, B. A., and Labat, D. D.: Transplantation of pluripotent nuclei from triploid frog tumors. Science, *165*:394, 1969.

Miller, E. C., and Miller, J. A.: The mutagenicity of chemical carcinogens: correlations, problems and interpretations. *In* Hollaender, A. (Ed.): Chemical Mutagens: Principles and Methods for Detection. Vol. 1. New York, Plenum Press, 1971, pp. 83–119.

Miller, J. A.: Concluding remarks on chemicals and chemical carcinogenesis. *In* Griffin, A. C., and Shaw, C. R. (Eds.): Carcinogens: Identification and Mechanisms of Action. New York, Raven Press, 1979, pp. 455–469.

Miller, J. A., and Miller, E. C.: Ultimate chemical carcinogens as reactive mutagenic electrophiles. *In* Hiatt, H. H., Watson, J. D., and Winsten, J. A. (Eds.): Origins of Human Cancer. New York, Cold Spring Harbor Laboratory, 1977, pp. 605–627.

Mootse, G., Agostino, D., and Cliffton, E. E.: Alterations in fibrinogen, plasminogen and inhibitors of plasmin with the growth of V2 carcinoma in rabbits. J. Natl. Cancer Inst., *35*:567, 1965.

Mulvihill, J. J.: Congenital and genetic diseases. *In* Fraumeni, J. F., Jr. (Ed.): Persons at High Risk of Cancer. New York, Academic Press, 1975, pp. 3–35.

Nakamura, K., Kawaguchi, T., Asahina, S., et al.: Electron microscopic studies on extravasation of tumor cells and early foci of hematogenous metastases. Gann, *20*:57, 1977.

Nicolson, G. L.: Cancer metastasis: Organ colonization and the cell surface properties of malignant cells. Biochim. Biophys. Acta. In press.

Nowell, P. C.: The clonal evolution of tumor cell populations. Science, *194*:23, 1976.

Pardee, A. B.: Cell division and a hypothesis of cancer. J. Natl. Cancer Inst., *14*:7, 1964.

Pierce, G. B., and Cox, W. F.: Neoplasms as caricatures of tissue renewal. *In* Saunders, G. F. (Ed.): Cell Differentiation and Neoplasia. New York, Raven Press, 1978, pp. 57–66.

Pitot, H. C., and Heidelberger, C.: Metabolic regulatory circuits and carcinogenesis. Cancer Res., *23*:1694, 1963.

Poste, G.: Experimental systems for analysis of the malignant phenotype. Cancer Metastasis Rev., *1*:141, 1982.

Poste, G., Doll, J., Brown, A. B., et al.: A comparison of the metastatic properties of B16 melanoma clones isolated from cultured cell lines, subcutaneous tumors and individual lung metastases. Cancer Res., *42*:2770, 1982.

Reich, E., Rifkin, D., and Shaw, E. (Eds.): Proteases and Biological Control. New York, Cold Spring Harbor Laboratory, 1975.

Rinkus, S. J., and Legator, M. S.: Chemical characterization of 465 known or suspected carcinogens and their correlation with mutagenic activity in the Salmonella typhimurium system. Cancer Res., *39*:3289, 1979.

Stevens, L. C.: The development of transplantable teratocarcinomas from intratesticular grafts of pre- and post-implantation mouse embryos. Dev. Biol., *21*:364, 1970.

Sugarbaker, E. V.: Patterns of metastasis in human malignancies. Cancer Biol. Rev., *2*:235, 1981.

Temin, H. M.: On the origin of RNA tumor viruses. Harvey Lect., *69*:173, 1975.

Todaro, G. J.: RNA tumor virus genes (virogenes) and transforming genes (oncogenes): genetic transmission, infectious spread, and modes of expression. *In* Hiatt, H. H., Watson, J. D., and Winsten, J. A. (Eds.): Origins of Human Cancer. New York, Cold Spring Harbor Laboratory, 1977, pp. 1169–1196.

Tooze, J. (Ed.): The Molecular Biology of Tumor Viruses. New York, Cold Spring Harbor Laboratory, 1973.

Warren, B. A.: Environment of the blood-borne tumor embolus adherent to vessel wall. J. Med., *4*:150, 1973.

Weinstein, I. B.: Current concepts of mechanisms of chemical carcinogenesis. Bull. N. Y. Acad. Med., *54*:366, 1978.

Weinstein, I. B., Yamaguchi, N., and Gebert, R.: Use of epithelial cell cultures for studies on the mechanism of transformation by chemical carcinogens. In Vitro, *11*:130, 1975.

Weisburger, J. H.: Chemical carcinogenesis. *In* Holland, J. S., and Frei, E. (Eds.): Cancer Medicine. Philadelphia, Lea & Febiger, 1973, pp. 45–90.

Winkelhake, J. L., and Nicolson, G. L.: Determination of adhesive properties of variant metastatic melanoma cells to BALB/3T3 cells and their virus-transformed derivatives by a monolayer attachment assay. J. Natl. Cancer Inst., *56*:285, 1976.

Wood, S., Jr.: Pathogenesis of metastasis formation observed in vivo in the rabbit ear chamber. Arch. Pathol., *66*:550, 1958.

Principles for Determining the Extent of Disease

Anderstrom, C., Johansson, S., and Nilsson, S.: Significance of lamina propria invasion on the prognosis of patients with bladder tumors. J. Urol., *124*:23, 1980.

Bracken, R. B., Johnson, D. E., and Samuels, M. L.: Alpha feto-protein determinations in germ cell tumors of the testis. Urology, 6:382, 1975.

Bracken, R. B., McDonald, M. W., and Johnson, D. E.: Cystectomy for superficial bladder cancer. Urology, 18:459, 1981.

Braunstein, G. D., Vaitukaitis, J. L., Carbone, P. P., and Ross, G. T.: Ectopic production of human chorionic gonadotropin by neoplasms. Ann. Intern. Med., 78:39, 1973.

Brenckman, W. D., Lastinger, L. B., and Sedor, F.: Unpredictable fluctuations in serum acid phosphatase activity in prostatic cancer. JAMA, 245:2501, 1981.

Gleason, D. F., and Mellinger, G. T.: Prediction of prognosis for prostatic adenocarcinoma by combined histological grading and clinical staging. J. Urol., 111:58, 1974.

Grossman, B., Batata, M., Hilaris, B., and Whitmore, W. F., Jr.: 125-I implantation for carcinoma of the prostate: Further followup of the first 100 cases. Urology. In press.

Heney, N. M., Ahmed, S., Flanagan, M. J., Frable, W., Corder, M. P., Hafermann, M. D., and Hawkins, I. R.: Superficial bladder cancer: Progression and recurrence. J. Urol., 130:1083, 1983.

Kramer, S. A., Cline, W. A., Farnham, R., Carson, C. C., Cox, E. B., Hinshaw, W., and Paulson, D. F.: Prognosis of patients with stage D1 prostatic adenocarcinoma. J. Urol., 125:817, 1981.

Lange, P. H., McIntire, K. R., Waldmann, T. A., et al.: Serum alpha-fetoprotein and human chorionic gonadotropin in the diagnosis and management of nonseminomatous germ-cell testicular cancer. N. Engl. J. Med., 295:1237, 1976.

Lange, P. H., McIntire, K. R., Waldmann, T. A., et al.: Alpha-fetoprotein and human chorionic gonadotropin in the management of testicular tumors. J. Urol. In press.

Maier, J. G., and Sulak, M. H.: Radiation therapy in malignant testis tumors. I: Seminoma; II: Carcinoma. Cancer, 32:1212, 1974.

McIntire, K. R., Waldmann, T. A., Moertel, C. G., et al.: Serum alpha-fetoprotein in patients with neoplasms of the gastrointestinal tract. Cancer Res., 35:991, 1975.

Mizejewski, G. J., Young, S. R., and Allen, R. P.: Alpha-fetoprotein: Effect of heterologous antiserum on hepatoma cells in vitro. J. Natl. Cancer Inst., 54:1361, 1975.

Moore, M. R., Vogel, C. L., Walton, K. N., et al.: The use of human chorionic gonadotropin and alpha-fetoprotein in evaluation of testicular tumors. Am. Soc. Clin. Oncol. (Abstract No. C-12), 1976.

Paulson, D. F.: The role of endocrine therapy in the management of prostate cancer. In Skinner, D. G., and deKernion, J. B. (Eds.): Genitourinary Cancer. Philadelphia, W. B. Saunders Co., 1978.

Paulson, D. F.: Assessment of the anatomic extent and biologic hazard of prostatic adenocarcinoma. Urology, 15:537, 1980a.

Paulson, D. F.: The prognostic role of lymphadenectomy in adenocarcinoma of the prostate. Urol. Clin. North Am., 7:615, 1980b.

Paulson, D. F., Cline, W. A., and Hinshaw, W.: Extended field radiation therapy vs. delayed hormonal therapy in node positive prostatic adenocarcinoma. J. Urol., 127:935, 1982.

Selli, C., Hinshaw, W., Woodard, B., and Paulson, D. F.: Stratification of risk factors in renal cell carcinoma. Cancer, 52:899, 1983.

Shepheard, B. G. F.: Alpha-fetoprotein and teratomas of the testis. Proc. R. Soc. Med., 67:307, 1974.

Sogani, P. C., Herr, H. W., Bains, M. S., and Whitmore, W. F., Jr.: Renal cell carcinoma extending into inferior vena cava. J. Urol., 130:660, 1983.

Swanson, D. A., Orovan, W. L., Johnson, D. E., and Giacco, G.: Osseous metastases secondary to renal cell carcinoma. Urology, 18:556, 1981.

Vaitukaitis, J. L., and Ross, G. T.: Recent advances in the evaluation of gonadotropic hormones. In Cruger, W. P., Coggin, C. H., Hancock, E. W., et al. (Eds.): Ann. Rev. Med., 24:295, 1973.

Vaitukaitis, J. L., Braunstein, G. D., and Ross, G. T.: A radioimmunoassay which specifically measures human chorionic gonadotropin in the presence of human luteinizing hormone. Am. J. Obstet. Gynecol., 113:751, 1972.

Treatment of Malignant Disease

Adams, G. E., and Dewez, D. L.: Hydrated electrons and radiobiological sensitization. Biochem. Biophys. Res. Commun. 12:473, 1963.

Adams, G. E., Ahmed, L., Fielden, E. M., et al.: The development of some metronidazoles as hypoxic cell sensitizers. Cancer Clin. Trials, 3:37, 1980.

Belli, J. A., Dicus, G. J., and Bonte, F. J.: Radiation response of mammalian tumor cells. 1. Repair of sublethal damage in vivo. J. Natl. Cancer Inst., 38:673, 1967.

Donaldson, S. C., Glick, J. M., and Wilbur, J. R.: Adriamycin activating a recall phenomenon after radiation therapy. Ann. Intern. Med., 81:407, 1974.

Goodman, L. S., and Gilman, A.: The Pharmacological Basis of Therapeutics. New York, The Macmillan Co., 1970, p. 21.

Gray, L. H.: Radiation biology and cancer. In Cellular Radiation Biology. M.D. Anderson Hospital and Tumor Institute, 18th Symposium on Fundamental Cancer Research. Baltimore, Williams & Wilkins Co., 1965, pp. 7–25.

Gray, L. H., Coger, A. D., Ebert, M., et al.: The concentration of oxygen dissolved in tissues at the time of irradiation as a factor in radiotherapy. Br. J. Radiol., 26:638, 1953.

Mottram, J. C.: Factors of importance in radiosensitivity of tumors. Br. J. Radiol., 9:606, 1936.

Parson, J. T., Bova, F. J., and Million, R. R.: A reevaluation of the University of Florida split-course technique for squamous carcinoma of the head and neck. Int. J. Radiat. Oncol. Biol. Phys., 6:1645, 1980a.

Parson, J. T., Thar, T. L., Bova, F. J., et al.: An evaluation of split-course irradiation for pelvic malignancies. Int. J. Radiat. Oncol. Biol. Phys., 6:175, 1980b.

Pinkel, D.: Actinomycin D in childhood cancer: a preliminary report. Pediatrics, 23:342, 1959.

Read, J.: The effect of ionizing radiation on the broad beam root: the dependence of the x-ray sensitivity on dissolved oxygen. Br. J. Radiol., 25:89, 1952.

Scanlon, P.: Split-dose radiotherapy: The original premise. Int. J. Radiat. Oncol. Biol. Phys., 6:527, 1980.

Upton, A. C., Randolph, M. L., and Conklin, J. W.: Late effects of fast neutrons and gamma rays in mice as influenced by the dose rate of irradiation: Induction of neoplasia. Radiat. Res., 41:467, 1970.

Weichselbaum, R., Little, J. B., and Nove, J.: Response of human osteosarcoma in vitro to irradiation: evidence for unusual cellular repair activity. Int. J. Radiat. Biol., 31:295, 1977.

Principles of Chemotherapy

Brockman, R. W.: Circumvention of resistance. Pharmacologic basis of cancer chemotherapy. 27th Annual Symposium on Fundamental Research, University of Texas, M. D. Anderson Hospital and Tumor Institute. Baltimore, Williams & Wilkins Co., 1975, pp. 691–711.

Buick, R. M.: In vitro clonogenicity of primary human tumor cells: Quantitation and relationship to tumor stem cells. In Salmon, S. E. (Ed.): Cloning of Human Tumor Stem Cells. New York, Alan R. Liss, 1980, pp. 15–22.

DeVita, V. T., Jr., Young, R. C., and Canellos, G. P.: Combination versus single-agent chemotherapy: review of the basis of selection of drug treatment of cancer. Cancer, 35:98, 1975.

Freireich, E. J., Gehan, E. A., Rall, D. P., et al.: Quantitative comparison of toxicity of anticancer agents in mouse, rat, dog, monkey and man. Cancer Chemother. Rep., 50:219, 1966.

Furth, J., and Kahn, M. C.: The transmission of leukemia of mice with a single cell. Am. J. Cancer, 31:276, 1937.

Goldie, J. H., and Coldman, A. J.: A mathematic model for relating the drug sensitivity of tumors to the spontaneous mutation rate. Cancer Treat. Rep., 63:1727, 1979.

Goldin, A., Venditti, J. M., Humphries, S. R., et al.: Influences of the concentration of leukemic inoculum on the effectiveness of treatment. Science, 123:840, 1956.

Hutchison, D. J.: Cross-resistance and collateral sensitivity studies in cancer chemotherapy. In Haddow, A., and Weinhouse, S. (Eds.): Advances in Cancer Research. Vol. 7. New York, Academic Press, 1963, pp. 235–350.

Law, L. W.: Origin of the resistance of leukemic cells to folic acid antagonists. Nature, 169:628, 1952.

Luria, S. E., and Delbruck, M.: Mutations of bacteria from virus sensitivity to virus resistance. Genetics, 28:491, 1943.

Mendelsohn, M. L.: The growth fraction: A new concept applied to tumors. Science, 132:1496, 1960.

Murakami, H., and Masui, H.: Hormonal control of human colon carcinoma cell growth in serum-free medium. Proc. Natl. Acad. Sci., 77:3464, 1980.

Pardee, A. B.: A restriction point for control of normal animal cell proliferation. Proc. Natl. Acad. Sci., 71:1286, 1974.

Pledger, W. J., Stiles, C. D., Antoniades, H. N., et al.: An ordered sequence of events is required before BALB/c-3T3 cells become committed to DNA synthesis. Proc. Natl. Acad. Sci., 75:2839, 1978.

Poste, G.: Experimental systems for analysis of the malignant phenotype. Cancer Metastasis Rev., 1:141, 1982.

Sato, G. H., and Ross, R.: Hormones and Cell Culture: A and B. New York, Cold Spring Harbor Laboratory, 1979.

Schabel, F. M.: Concepts from systemic treatment of micrometastases developed in murine systems. Am. J. Roentgenol. Radium Ther. Nucl. Med., 127:500, 1976.

Schabel, F. M.: Rationale for adjuvant chemotherapy. Cancer, 39:2875, 1977.

Simpson-Herren, L., Sanford, A. H., and Holmquist, J. P.: Cell population kinetics of transplanted Lewis lung carcinoma. Cell Tissue Kinet., 7:349, 1974.

Skipper, H. E.: Reasons for success and failure in treatment of murine leukemias with the drugs now employed in treating human leukemias. Cancer Chemotherapy. Vol. 1. Ann Arbor, Mich., University Microfilms Int., 1978, pp. 1–166.

Skipper, H. E., Hutchison, D. J., Schabel, F. M., Jr., et al.: A quick reference chart on cross-resistance between anticancer agents. Cancer Treat. Rep., 56:493, 1972.

Skipper, H. E., Schabel, F. M., Jr., and Wilcox, W. S.: Experimental evaluation of potential anticancer agents. XII. On the criteria and kinetics associated with "curability" of experimental leukemia. Cancer Chemother. Rep., 35:1, 1964.

Yen, A., and Pardee, A. B.: Exponential 3T3 cells escape in mid-G1 from their high serum requirement. Exp. Cell Res., 116:103, 1978.

Principles of Combination Chemotherapy

Bracken, R. B., McDonald, M. W., and Johnson, D. E.: Cystectomy for superficial bladder cancer. Urology, 18:459, 1981.

DeVita, V. T.: The consequences of the chemotherapy of Hodgkin's disease: The 10th Annual David A. Karnofsky Lecture. Cancer, 47:1, 1981.

Pilch, Y. H.: Tumor immunology. In Pilch, Y. H. (Ed.): Surgical Oncology. New York, McGraw-Hill Book Co., 1983, pp. 142–163.

CHAPTER 29

Renal Tumors

JEAN B. deKERNION, M.D.

INTRODUCTION

Tumors, by definition, represent "new growths" that may be either benign or malignant, solid or cystic, primary or secondary, and intrinsic or extrinsic but that always involve the organ under consideration. In consideration of the kidney, primary attention is focused upon the parenchymal neoplastic disorders intrinsic to the kidney—predominantly malignancies, which are of greatest importance, with reference as well to benign tumors of the kidney, malignancies metastatic to the kidney, and uncommon renal neoplastic disorders. Wilms' tumor, the common renal malignancy of childhood, is dealt with elsewhere in this volume, as are neuroblastoma, the multiplicity of renal cystic disorders, and primary retroperitoneal tumors.

HISTORICAL CONSIDERATIONS

The evolution of knowledge about renal tumors is in actuality the history of surgical daring in a microcosm. Autopsy information relative to renal disorders was scant, and it was only the introduction of nephrectomy and other subsequent surgical interventions for renal diseases that provided the clinical information and histopathologic insight that form the basis of our current concepts of renal tumors. Thus, the historical data available to us date back little more than 100 years.

Harris (1882) reported on 100 surgical extirpations of the kidney, a sufficient number to permit some sort of analysis of clinical, surgical, and pathologic features of renal disorders that require surgery. The first documented nephrectomy was apparently accomplished by Wolcott

in 1861, who operated with the mistaken assumption that the tumor mass was a hepatoma. In 1867, Spiegelberg removed a kidney incidentally in the course of excising an echinococcus cyst. The first planned nephrectomy—for persistent ureteral fistula—was performed by Gustav Simon in 1869, and his patient survived with cure of the fistula. It was only one year later (1870) that the first planned nephrectomy was successfully accomplished in the United States, by John Gilmore of Mobile, Alabama—on this occasion as treatment for atrophic pyelonephritis and persistent urinary infection (Glenn, 1980).

With surgical intervention, tissue became available to pathologists for histologic interpretation. Unfortunately, such interpretation was not always accurate, and there were often serious professional differences of opinion. According to Carson (1928), the first accurate gross description of kidney tumors dates to 1826, with Konig's observations. In 1855, Robin had examined solid tumors apparently arising in the kidney and concluded that renal carcinoma arose from renal tubular epithelium. This interpretation was confirmed by Waldeyer in 1867. Unfortunately, theoretical and practical considerations of renal tumors were confused by Grawitz (1883), who contended that such apparent renal tumors arose from adrenal rests within the kidney. He introduced the terminology "struma lipomatodes aberrata renis" as descriptive nomenclature for the tumors of clear cells that he believed were derived from the adrenal gland. He based his conclusions not only on the fatty content, analogous to that seen in the adrenals, but also on the location of the tumors beneath the renal capsule, the approximation to the adrenals, the lack of similarity of the cells to uriniferous tubules, and the demonstration of amyloid not unlike that seen with adrenal degeneration.

This histogenetic concept was adopted by subsequent investigators, and pathologists of the era readily embraced the idea that renal tumors truly arose from the adrenals. In 1894, Lubarch endorsed the idea of there being a suprarenal origin of renal tumors, and the term "hypernephroid tumors," indicating origin above the kidneys, was advocated by Birch-Hirschfeld (Birch-Hirschfeld and Doederlein, 1894). It was this semantic and conceptual mistake that led to the introduction of the term "hypernephroma," which predominates in the literature describing parenchymal tumors of primary renal origin.

Weichselbaum and Greenish (1883) described renal adenomas containing both papillary and alveolar cellular types. Some clarification of the histopathology of renal tumors is derived from the work of Albarran and Imbert (1903), and the four-volume contribution of Wolff (1883), written between 1883 and 1928, adds further historical significance to our understanding of renal tumors today (Glenn, 1980).

CLASSIFICATION

An appropriate, simple, and all-inclusive classification of renal tumors has eluded surgical pathologists and urologic surgeons alike over the past century. Even with the elimination of hydronephrosis and various inflammatory tumefactions of the kidney, such as xanthogranulomatous pyelonephritis, from the category, the spectrum of renal tumors remains extremely broad. Various classifications have been adopted in an effort to acknowledge and include the various new growths of diverse causes that can afflict the human kidney.

Certainly, the most comprehensive classification of renal tumors is that offered by Deming and Harvard (1970) in a previous edition of this text. These authorities establish 11 categories of renal tumors, with multiple subdivisions embracing virtually every known new growth that may involve the kidney—common, uncommon, or rare—and including the various renal cystic disorders as well as the pararenal retroperitoneal tumors that may involve the kidney secondarily. This classification is reproduced here (Table 29–1) because it provides the most succinct presentation of renal tumors, yet retains accuracy and inclusiveness.

Another approach has been taken by other authors: Only new solid parenchymal growths arising primarily in the kidney have been considered. Lakey (1975), for example, subdivides renal neoplasms into benign and malignant tumors, classifying these neoplasms as shown in Table 29–2. When one considers that the vast majority of benign renal tumors represent the various cystic disorders, with few solid lesions, one can focus attention on the category of renal malignancies. Within the past decade, arguments have been made for the classification of malignant renal neoplasms into four categories: *nephroblastoma* and other embryonic renal malignancies; *nephrocarcinoma,* the generic term for adult renal parenchymal malignancies; *urothelial malignancies* of the renal pelvis; and *other malignancies* of the renal substance, capsule, or perirenal structures. Such a simplistic subcategorization of renal malignancies offers considerable appeal.

An effort must be made, however, to provide a classification that is both complete and uncomplicated, embracing all the lesions that predispose to renal mass or new growth. Such a simplified classification was proposed by Glenn (1980) (Table 29–3). *Benign tumors* include those of the renal capsule (such as fibroma), renal parenchymatous adenomas, vascular tumors, the various cystic lesions and dysplasias, heteroplastic and mesenchymal tumors, and even the various hydronephroses. *Tumors of the renal pelvis,* not a primary consideration here, include the benign papillomas as well as transitional, squamous, and adenocarcinomatous malignancies. *Pararenal tumors* are those that involve the kidney by extension and invasion, and they may be either benign or malignant. *Embryonic tumors* comprise predominantly nephroblastoma (Wilms' tumor) and the embryonic or mesotheliomatous carcinomas and sarcomas of childhood. *Nephrocarcinoma* is the generic category that includes adult renal parenchymatous malignancies, primarily the classic "hypernephroma" and papillary adenocarcinoma. The category of *other malignancies* embraces the relatively rare mesenchymal malignancies, such as the various sarcomas, hemangiopericytomas, infiltrative malignancies such as myeloma, and secondary or metastatic malignancies manifesting within the renal substance. To Glenn's original classification has been added the *oncocytoma.* Though most of these tumors behave as benign neoplasms, it seems inappropriate to classify oncocytoma as such, in view of the uncertainty in diagnosis and the occasional documentation of metastases: hence, its classification as a separate neoplasm.

TABLE 29–1. Classification of Renal Tumors (Deming and Harvard)

1. Tumors of the Renal Capsule
   Fibroma
   Leiomyoma
   Lipoma
   Mixed
2. Tumors of the Mature Renal Parenchyma
   Adenoma
   Adenocarcinoma
     (hypernephroma)
     (Renal cell cancer)
     (Alveolar carcinoma)
3. Tumors of the Immature Renal Parenchyma
   Nephroblastoma (Wilms')
   Embryonic carcinoma
   Sarcoma
4. Epithelial Tumors of the Renal Pelvis
   Transitional cell papilloma
   Transitional cell carcinoma
   Squamous cell carcinoma
   Adenocarcinoma
5. Cysts
   Solitary
   Unilateral multiple
   Calyceal
   Pyogenic
   Calcified
   Tubular ectasia
   Tuberous sclerosis
   Cystadenoma
   Papillary cystadenoma
   Dermoid
   Pararenal and perirenal cysts
     Hydrocele renalis
     Lymphatic
     Wolffian
   Malignant
6. Vascular Tumors
   Hemangioma
   Hamartoma
   Lymphangioma

7. Neurogenic Tumors
   Neuroblastoma
   Sympathicoblastoma
   Schwannoma
8. Heteroplastic Tissue Tumors
   Adipose
   Smooth muscle
   Adrenal rests
   Endometriosis
   Cartilage
   Bone
9. Mesenchymal Derivatives
   Connective Tissue
     Fibroma
     Fibrosarcoma
     Osteogenic sarcoma
   Adipose Tissue
     Lipoma
     Liposarcoma
   Muscle Tissue
     Leiomyoma
     Leiomyosarcoma
     Rhabdomyosarcoma
10. Pararenal and Perirenal Solids Tumors
    Lipoma
    Sarcomas
      Liposarcoma
      Fibrosarcoma
      Lymphangiosarcoma
    Cancer
    Teratoma
    Lymphoblastoma
    Neuroblastoma
    Hodgkin's disease
11. Secondary Tumors
    Cancer
    Sarcoma
    Blastoma
    Granuloma
    Thymoma
    Testicular
    Renal

TABLE 29–2. LAKEY'S CLASSIFICATION OF
RENAL TUMORS

Benign Tumors
  Adenoma
  Fibroma
  Lipoma
  Leiomyoma
  Angioma
  Rhabdomyoma
  Neurofibroma
  Dermoid
  Endometriosis
  Angiomyolipoma (hamartoma)

Malignant Tumors
  Nephroblastoma (Wilms' tumor)
  Adenocarcinoma, renal cell carcinoma
  Sarcomas
    Fibrosarcoma
    Liposarcoma
    Leiomyosarcoma
    Osteogenic sarcoma
  Lymphoblastoma
    Lymphomas, myeloma
  Secondary malignant tumors

TABLE 29–3. SIMPLIFIED CLASSIFICATION
OF RENAL TUMORS

1. Benign Tumors
   Renal capsule
   Renal parenchyma
   Vascular tumors
   Cystic lesions, dysplasia, hydronephrosis
   Heteroplastic, mesenchymal tumors

2. Tumors of Renal Pelvis
   Benign papilloma
   Transitional and squamous cell carcinomas, adenocarcinomas

3. Pararenal Tumors
   Benign
   Malignant

4. Embryonic Tumors
   Nephroblastoma (Wilms' tumor)
   Embryonic, mesotheliomatous tumors
   Sarcomas

5. Nephrocarcinoma
   Renal cell carcinoma, adenocarcinoma,
     "hypernephroma"
   Papillary cystadenocarcinoma

6. Other Malignancies
   Primary: mesenchymal, hemangiopericytoma, myeloma
   Secondary: metastatic lesions

7. Oncocytoma

BENIGN RENAL TUMORS

Benign renal tumors may arise from any of the multiple cell types within and around the kidney. Renal cysts are perhaps the most common benign renal mass lesion (Fig. 29–1). Approximately 70 per cent of asymptomatic renal mass lesions are simple cysts and are of no clinical significance (Lang, 1973). The major import of most benign lesions lies in either their growth to a large size creating clinical symptoms, or their differential diagnosis from malignant renal tumors (see below) (Fig. 29–2). Cysts may be single or multiple and unilateral or bilateral. As discussed later, modern uroradiographic techniques can distinguish renal carcinoma from simple cysts with great accuracy. Occasionally, especially in the case of complex cysts, the true cystic nature of the lesion may be determined only at surgery. It is beyond the scope of this discussion to cite each case report associated with the myriad rare benign tumors; we will concentrate on those that are found more commonly and those that are associated with symptoms or bear similarities to malignant tumors.

CORTICAL ADENOMAS

Renal cortical adenomas (Fig. 29–3) are commonly encountered at autopsy and are benign tumors both clinically and histologically. Bell (1950) found a direct correlation between size and malignant potential, noting that tumors less than approximately 3 cm in size had little propensity for metastatis. However, in his series of 62 tumors less than 3 cm in diameter, three had metastasized. Murphy and Mostofi (1970) concluded that renal adenomas are benign tumors, distinguishable from true adenocarcinomas. An alternative view was presented by Bennington and Beckwith (1975), who argued that all tubular cell adenomas are malignant, simply representing an early stage of renal carcinoma growth.

The etiology of renal cortical adenomas is unclear. Owing to the frequency with which they are encountered in autopsy specimens as well as their frequency in males, an endocrine relationship has been suggested. No definite etiologic factor has been recognized, however, and no absolute association with the presence of frank renal cell carcinoma has been established.

The renal adenoma is characterized by uniform acidophilic or clear cells, with monotonous nuclear and cellular characteristics. Symptoms are unusual and are encountered only when the

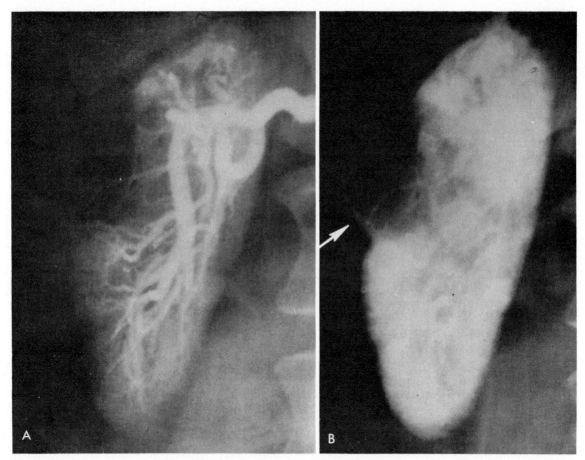

Figure 29–1. Simple renal cyst. *A*, Selective arteriogram demonstrating parenchymal defect and avascularity. *B*, Nephrographic phase of arteriogram confirming hypovascularity and demonstrating "beak" sign of renal cyst (arrow).

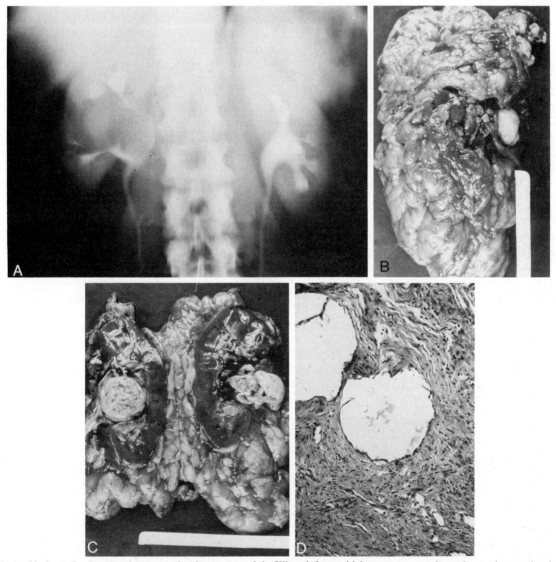

Figure 29–2. *A,* Pyelogram demonstrating large parapelvic filling defect, which was compound on ultrasonic examination. *B,* A smooth glistening wall of cyst protruding through renal pelvis. *C,* Sagittal section demonstrating laminated, compound cyst. *D,* Microscopic section showing pure cystic nature of the mass.

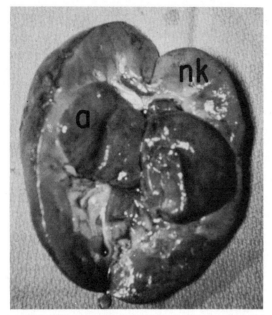

Figure 29–3. Benign adenoma *(a)* located in central portion of bivalved normal kidney *(nk)*.

tumor erodes the collecting system or adjacent vessels. Most renal adenomas are discovered incidentally. The computerized tomography and arteriography characteristics are often indistinguishable from those of small renal adenocarcinomas, except for the general absence of arteriovenous fistulae, venous pooling, and calcification.

The clinician is often faced with a dilemma when the small, 3-cm renal parenchymal tumor is diagnosed. Although segmental resection or wedge resection may be appropriate, the true tendency for multiplicity is uncertain, and the final characterization of the mass as an adenoma usually awaits careful tissue sectioning. For this reason, most diagnosed renal parenchymal tumors are treated as true renal cell carcinomas.

RENAL HAMARTOMAS (ANGIOMYOLIPOMA)

Renal hamartomas (Fig. 29–4) are benign tumors that may occur as an isolated phenomenon or as part of the syndrome associated with tuberous sclerosis. Approximately 80 per cent of patients with the diagnosis of hamartoma have some or all of the other stigmata of tuberous sclerosis. This is a disease that is both hereditary and familial and is characterized by mental retardation, epilepsy, and adenoma sebaceum. In these patients, hamartomas may also be found in the brain, eye, heart, lung, and bone (McCullough et al., 1971). Patients with tuberous sclerosis require careful screening for the presence of renal tumors.

Renal hamartomas are frequently bilateral. They are often yellow and gray and have a propensity for profuse hemorrhage, large size, and multiplicity (Fig. 29–5). Microscopically, the tumor is named for the three primary components—unusual abnormal blood vessels, clusters of adipocytes, and sheets of smooth muscle. Pleomorphism is common, and mitotic figures, although rarely seen, can be prominent (Fig. 29–6) (Colvin and Dickersin, 1978). While no case of widespread metastases has been reported, metastasis to regional lymph nodes has been documented (Bloom et al., 1982).

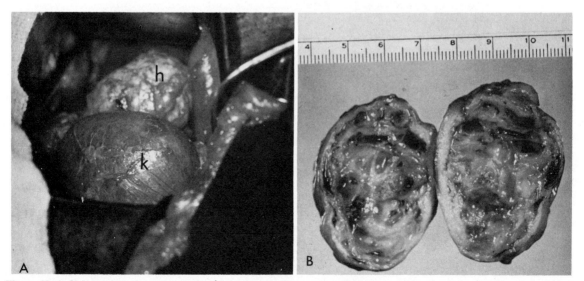

Figure 29–4. Hamartoma of renal capsule. *A,* At surgery, hamartoma *(h)* is seen arising from the capsule of the kidney *(k)*. *B,* Gross appearance of excised hamartoma suggests multiple cellular elements of tumor.

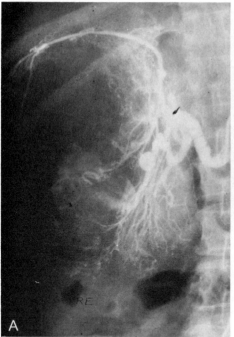

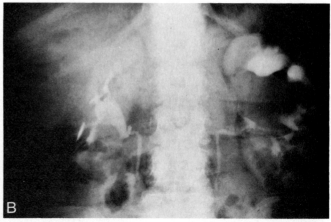

Figure 29–5. *A,* A 60-year-old woman with no evidence of tuberous sclerosis presented with hemorrhage into a large right flank tumor. Exploration and biopsy revealed hamartoma. *B,* One year after percutaneous angioinfarction of right renal hamartoma, also demonstrating central hamartoma in left kidney, unchanged in one year.

Because of the multiplicity of these tumors and their propensity for bilaterality, conservative surgery is often imperative. The angiographic pattern of the tumor is not sufficiently typical to reliably separate it from renal carcinoma. However, the high fat content allows for a distinctive pattern on the computerized tomography scan, with areas having the density corresponding to areas of fatty tissue (DaPonte et al., 1983). This typical CT picture has led some authors to suggest that surgical exploration and biopsy are no longer necessary if all CT criteria are met (Lingeman et al., 1982). While computerized tomography has aided in the differential diagnosis of this tumor, errors in diagnosis have been made, and reliance upon CT alone should be recommended with caution (Shapira et al., 1983).

The treatment of the isolated tumor is complete surgical excision. However, in the patient with bilateral tumors or a nonresectable tumor, percutaneous angioinfarction may control growth of the tumor and hemorrhage (Lieberman et al., 1983). The urgency for excision of the tumor must be tempered by its benign course and by its frequent propensity for very slow growth.

FIBROMAS

Fibrous tissue is found in the renal parenchyma, the perinephric tissues, and the renal capsule, and fibromas may arise from any of these structures. Glover and Buck (1982) reviewed the eight reported cases of medullary fibroma and noted that most have occurred in women. These are rare tumors that are uniformly benign and occasionally are difficult to separate from fibrosarcomas of the retroperitoneum. They are often on the periphery of the kidney and may have to grow to a large size before becoming clinically obvious. Symptoms are rare and are usually associated with either distortion of the collecting system or growth outside the confines of the renal fossa, though hematuria is common in patients with medullary fibromas.

The tumors are large, are adherent to the kidney, and often resemble uterine fibroids. They are microscopically benign, with sheets of fibroblasts or a loose myxomatous stroma. Angiographically, they are generally hypovascular but have no specific radiographic characteristics to distinguish them from hypovascular malignant tumors. A radical nephrectomy is usually performed because of the uncertainty of the diagnosis, but awareness of their benign nature warrants partial nephrectomy in selected cases.

LIPOMAS

Renal lipomas are among the rarest of renal tumors. Their origin is unclear, but they probably originate from fat cells within the renal

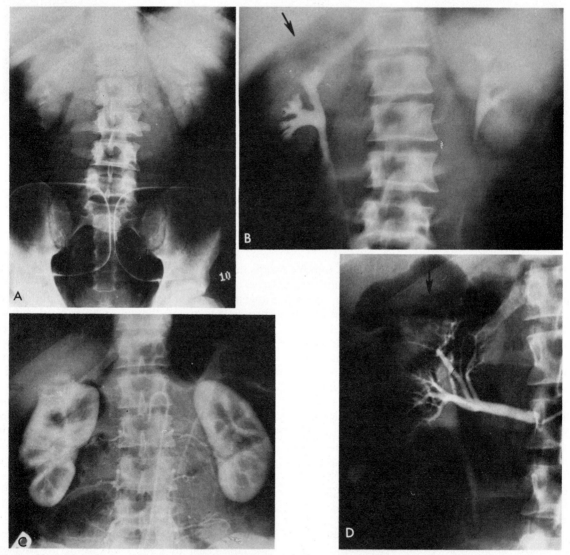

Figure 29–6. Hamartoma of kidney suggesting malignancy. *A,* Intravenous pyelogram is not diagnostic in patient with microscopic hematuria and hypertension. *B,* Tomogram discloses defect in renal outline and parenchyma at right upper pole (arrow). *C,* Nephrographic phase of arteriogram confirms presence of tumor with neovascularity. *D,* Neovascularization (arrow) is confirmed on selective renal arteriography.

Illustration continued on opposite page

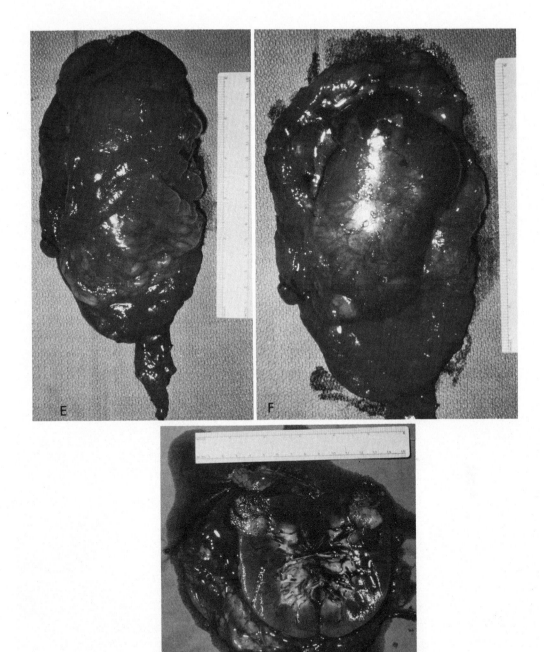

Figure 29–6 *Continued E,* Gross specimen from right radical nephrectomy embraces Gerota's fascia, perinephric fat, and kidney. *F,* After Gerota's fascia and the perinephric fat have been opened, tumor is visible at the upper pole of the right kidney. *G,* On sectioning of the kidney, tumor is seen to be intrinsic to the renal substance, with suggestion of invasion.

Illustration continued on following page

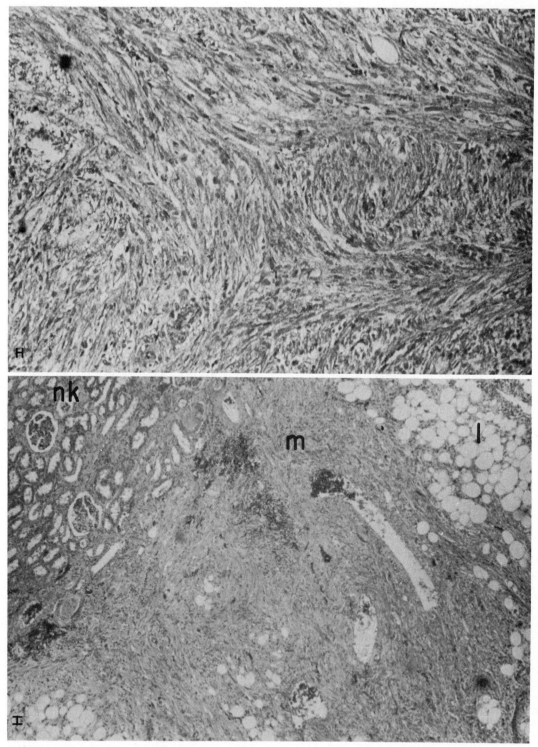

Figure 29–6 *Continued H,* Histologic appearance of fibromyomatous elements of tumor. *I,* Normal kidney *(nk)* is seen with adjacent myomatous *(m)* and lipomatous *(l)* elements of intrinsic tumor, diagnosed as angiofibromyolipoma (hamartoma).

capsule or parenchyma (Robertson and Hand, 1941). Dineen et al. (1983) recently reported a case of lipoma and reviewed the literature, documenting 18 cases of proven intrarenal lipoma. The tumor typically occurs in middle-aged females, grows to a large size, and has pain as its presenting symptom, with hematuria occurring in some patients. A malignant potential has been suggested but has not been proved. The gross characteristics are those of any lipoma. The tumors are confined within the renal capsule, in contrast to the perirenal lipomas, which are extracapsular. The tumors have the greasy feeling of all lipomas, pale lobules being interposed with streaks consisting of blood vessels. Microscopically the cells are uniform fat cells with peripherally placed nuclei surrounded by thin plasma membranes. The treatment is surgical excision, usually requiring total nephrectomy.

Commonly, these lipomas have other cellular elements (Robertson and Hand, 1941) and can be classified as variants of angiomyolipoma. These should not be classified as pure lipomas, but they have the same clinical significance and the same benign course.

Perinephric lipomas are difficult or impossible to separate from intrarenal lipomas and may arise from perinephric fat or in adjacent areas of the retroperitoneum (Pfeiffer and Gandin, 1946). These tumors are often huge, and excision without nephrectomy is seldom possible. CT scan should show the typical fat density, allowing preoperative consideration of conservative excision.

OTHER BENIGN TUMORS

Since the kidney is a complex organ consisting of many cell types within and surrounding the renal capsule, virtually every classification of benign tumor has been reported. Myomas, lymphangiomas, and hemangiomas have been found.

One of the rarest but most fascinating tumors is the functional renin-secreting juxtaglomerular tumor. It was first described by Robertson et al. (1967), and approximately ten cases have been described in the literature. The tumors arise from the juxtaglomerular cells (Orjauvik et al., 1975) in young patients, who present typically with hypertension, elevated serum renin levels, and hyperaldosteronism. Presence of the tumor is suspected in individuals with an extremely high differential renal vein/renin ratio with no other obvious cause for hypertension. The tumors are typically very small, seldom more than 2 or 3 cm in diameter, and often are not detectable radiographically. Occasionally, the segments of the kidney harboring the tumor can be identified by selective renal vein sampling (Bonnin et al., 1977). Grossly, the tumors are gray-yellow with hemorrhagic areas and microscopically are typical hemangiopericytomas. Electron microscopic studies reveal the characteristics of the juxtaglomerular cells, and tumor extracts may be shown to contain high concentrations of renin (Colvin and Dickersin, 1978).

This tumor is always benign and should be distinguished from the generally larger, nonfunctional, and sometimes malignant typical renal hemangiopericytoma.

MALIGNANT RENAL TUMORS

Renal Cell Carcinoma

INCIDENCE

Renal cell carcinoma is a relatively rare tumor, accounting for approximately 3 per cent of adult malignancies. In a recent report from the National Cancer Institute, approximately 18,000 new cases of renal carcinoma were predicted to occur in 1984 (Silverberg, 1984). Little evidence suggests that the tumor is increasing in incidence, though it may be detected in earlier stages than previously. The tumor is more common among urban dwellers and is more common in males, with a male-to-female ratio of approximately 2:1. Familial renal carcinoma has been reported, affecting as many as five family members. Patients with von Hippel–Lindau disease have a higher incidence of carcinoma (Lauritsen, 1975), and patients with polycystic kidney disease appear to have a predisposition for development of the tumor, although this has not been firmly established. Renal carcinoma is a tumor of adults, occurring primarily in the fifth to the seventh decades of life, but it may occasionally occur in the younger age groups.

ETIOLOGY

The tumor seems to arise from the proximal convoluted tubule, the same cell of origin as that for renal adenomas (Tannenbaum, 1971). Although a number of etiologic agents have been identified in animal models (Bennington and Beckwith, 1975), no specific agent has been definitely incriminated as causative of human renal carcinoma. Epidemiologic studies have incriminated tobacco, though the specific carcinogen has not been described (Weir and Dunn, 1970; Kantor, 1977). A high incidence of renal carcinoma has been noted in men who smoke pipes or cigars (Kantor, 1977). The typical renal cell carcinoma can be produced in the adult Syrian hamster by chronic treatment with diethylstilbestrol (Kirkman and Bacon, 1949), but the hormone has not been shown to cause renal carcinoma in humans.

No definitive relationship between occupational and industrial carcinogens and renal carcinoma has been documented. Male cigarette smokers exposed to industrial contaminants of cadmium have been reported to have a slightly increased risk of developing the tumor (Kolonel, 1976). No other relationship has been reported, although research in this area has been limited. The radiographic agent Thoratrast was reported to be associated with a high incidence of renal carcinoma in one study (Wenz, 1967). At the present time, there is a paucity of studies regarding the cause of renal carcinoma, and few hypotheses seem to warrant extensive investigation.

PATHOLOGY

Renal cell carcinomas are typically round, varying in size from tumors several centimeters in diameter to tumors that almost fill the abdomen (Figs. 29–7 and 29–8). They generally do not have a true histologic capsule but almost always have a pseudocapsule composed of compressed parenchyma and fibrous tissue. The amount of hemorrhage and necrosis varies greatly, but few tumors are uniform in gross appearance. Areas of yellowish or brownish soft tumor are usually interposed between sclerotic or fibrotic areas and patches of hemorrhage and necrosis. Multiple cysts are found not infrequently, probably resulting from segmental necrosis and resorption. The collecting system is generally displaced and often is invaded. Gerota's fascia seems to provide a barrier against local spread but may be compressed and invaded. Calcification may occur and can be stippled or may occur in a plaque-like arrangement. Renal carcinoma is typically unilateral, but bilaterality, either synchronous or asynchronous, occurs in approximately 2 per cent of cases (Moertel et al., 1961). Von Hippel–Lindau disease is characteristically associated with the presence of multiple and bilateral renal carcinomas (Greene and Rosenthal, 1951). As noted further on, the tumor frequently extends into

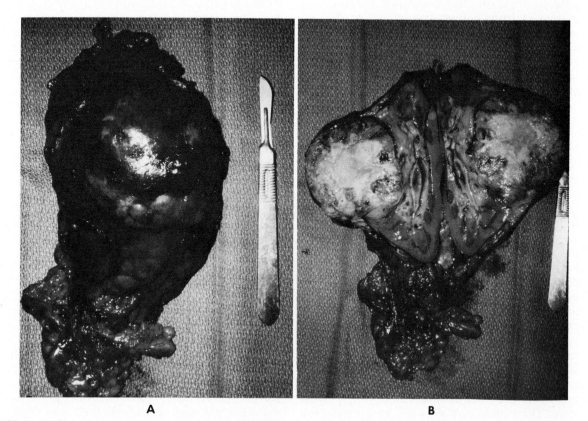

| A | B |

Figure 29–7. *A,* Radical nephrectomy specimen with Gerota's fascia intact. *B,* Specimen opened to reveal massive tumor.

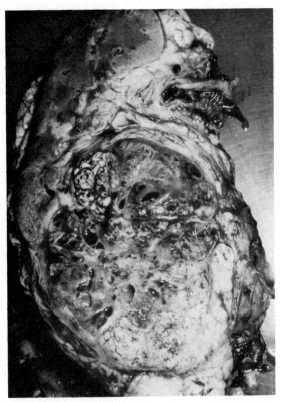

Figure 29–8. Typical renal cell carcinoma with thick pseudocapsule.

the renal vein as a thrombus, which may be propagated for varying distances into the inferior vena cava. The more malignant and larger tumors can invade locally, with extension into the surrounding muscles and direct invasion into adjacent organs.

Microscopic Features. In recent years, electron microscopic studies have identified the proximal tubular cell as the origin of renal cell carcinoma. The proximal tubular cell has multiple surface microvilli, giving the brush border characteristic, and contains a more complex cytoplasm than the more distal tubular cells. The ultrastructural characteristics of the proximal cell are found in varying degrees in most renal carcinomas. However, brush borders are usually not fully developed and are present on only some cells. The origin of the tumor from proximal tubular cells has been supported by a number of investigators (Tannenbaum, 1971; Fisher and Horvat, 1972; Sun et al., 1977). The detailed ultrastructure of the various cell types composing the classic renal carcinoma has been carefully detailed by Colvin and Dickersin (1978).

The characteristic light microscopic feature of renal carcinoma is the clear cell (Fig. 29–9).

These are rounded or polygonal cells with abundant cytoplasm, which stain very poorly and contain a cholesterol-like substance as well as neutral lipids and phospholipids. Few tumors contain only clear cells, however; a granular cell component is usually present in varying degrees and may actually compose the major portion of the tumor (Fig. 29–10). These cells have eosinophilic cytoplasm and abundant mitochondria. Some tumors contain primarily spindle cells, which may resemble pleomorphic mesenchymal cells (Fig. 29–11); they may make difficult the differentiation from fibrosarcoma. The three common cell types—clear cells, granular cells, and spindle cells—may occur alone or in varying combinations in the same tumor. The reason for the multiplicity of cell types is unknown. Other than that discussed earlier, Wallace and Nairn (1972) have demonstrated brush border antigens on renal tumors, characteristic of proximal tubular cells, and the absence of the distal tubular Tamm-Horsfall antigen. Renal carcinomas may exhibit a variety of microscopic growth patterns. Tumors may grow in solid sheets or trabecular patterns or may form alveoli. Less commonly, tumors demonstrate papillary growth or tubular patterns.

A number of authors have related various types of grading systems to prognosis, perhaps the first being Hand and Broders (1932). Within a given stage, however, the microscopic grading seems to have less significance than in some tumors. Nonetheless, tumors with nuclei resembling normal cells demonstrate a low malignant potential in contrast to the bizarre heterogeneous nuclei typical of spindle cell tumors, which are associated with a worse prognosis. A great disparity in survival has not been demonstrated between patients whose tumors contain clear cells and those with granular cells. However, tumors composed mainly of spindle cells seem to have a worse prognosis (Colvin and Dickersin, 1978).

CLINICAL PRESENTATION

Nature has provided a well-protected environment for the human kidney, and its only expression to the outside environment is through its primary product, the urine. Pain cannot be expected to occur unless the tumor invades surrounding areas or obstructs the outflow of urine owing to hemorrhage and subsequent formation of blood clots. It is therefore not surprising that the presenting signs and symptoms are often those related to local invasion or distant metastases. The classic triad of pain, hematuria, and a flank mass is certainly a

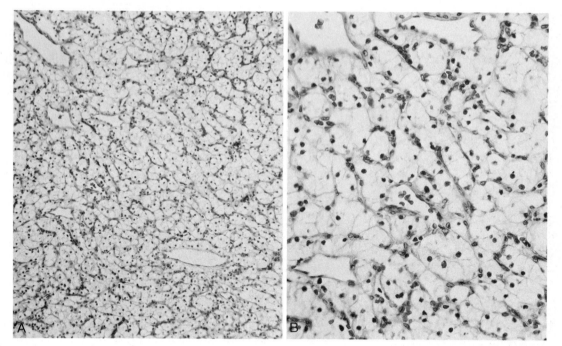

Figure 29–9. *A*, Typical pattern of clear cell carcinoma with small nuclei and clear cytoplasm (× 125). *B*, Higher power magnification showing pure clear cell pattern (× 313).

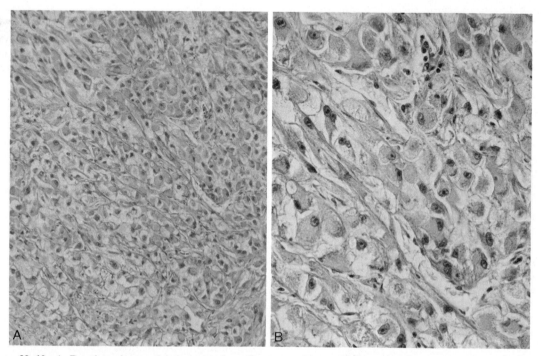

Figure 29–10. *A*, Renal carcinoma showing granular cell pattern with small nuclei and granular cytoplasm (× 125). *B*, Higher power magnification emphasizing typical granular cell pattern (× 313).

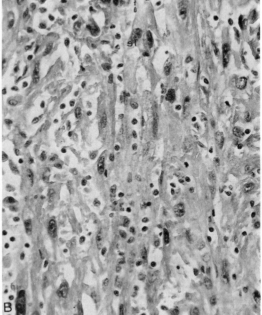

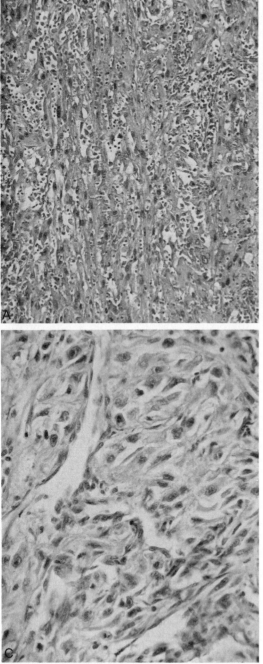

Figure 29–11. *A*, Low-power magnification of sarcomatous pattern of renal carcinoma showing spindle cell variety (× 125). *B*, Higher power magnification of same lesion demonstrating similarity to sarcomatoid cells (× 313). *C*, Similar pattern in another renal carcinoma (× 313).

TABLE 29–4. INCIDENCE OF SYMPTOMS IN 180
PATIENTS WITH RENAL CELL CARCINOMA

Symptom	Per Cent
Classic triad	10
Pain	41
Hematuria	38
Mass	24
Weight loss	36
Fever	18
Hypertension	22
Hypercalcemia	6

reliable clinical symptom complex but is found in few patients and generally indicates far advanced disease. One or two of these symptoms or signs are commonly associated with renal carcinoma (Table 29–4). The most frequent findings are pain or hematuria secondary to the primary tumor, but symptoms due to metastatic disease probably occur more frequently. Weight loss, fever, night sweats, and the sudden development of a varicocele in the male are not uncommon findings. Hypertension is known to occur, but it is unclear whether this is due to segmental renal artery occlusion or to elaboration of renin or renin-like substances.

Few tumors are associated with such diverse paraneoplastic syndromes. Hematopoietic disturbances, endocrinopathies, and biochemical aberrations have all been associated with renal malignancy. These myriad syndromes and their relative incidences are listed in Table 29–5 (Chisholm, 1974). Erythrocytosis has long been recognized as a sign of renal carcinoma and occurs in approximately 3 per cent of patients with elevated red blood cell count. This has been presumed to be secondary to an erythropoietin-like substance (Thorling, 1972). The leukocyte and platelet counts are usually normal.

TABLE 29–5. INCIDENCE OF SYSTEMIC SYNDROMES IN
PATIENTS WITH RENAL CELL CARCINOMA

Effect	Ratio	Per Cent
Raised erythrocyte sedimentation rate	362/651	55.6
Hypertension	89/237	37.5
Anemia	473/1300	36.3
Cachexia, weight loss	338/979	34.5
Pyrexia	164/954	17.2
Abnormal liver function	65/450	14.4
Raised alkaline phosphatase	64/434	10.1
Hypercalcemia	44/886	4.9
Polycythemia	43/1212	3.5
Neuromyopathy	13/400	3.2
Amyloidosis	12/573	2.0

From Chisholm, G. D.: Ann. N.Y. Acad. Sci., *230*:403, 1974.

Hypercalcemia is often the most troublesome secondary manifestation of renal carcinoma (Plimton and Gelhorn, 1956). Although the exact incidence is unclear, it sometimes accounts for the primary presenting symptoms of weight loss, fatigue, and generalized weakness. Parathyroid-like hormone production by primary renal tumors has been reported (Goldberg et al., 1964), though the hypercalcemia is seldom controlled by removal of the primary tumor, indicating production of the substance by metastatic sites. Hypercalcemia is also often secondary to extensive skeletal metastases with generalized osteolysis.

The most common paraneoplastic syndrome associated with renal carcinoma is hepatic dysfunction, which has been reported in approximately 20 per cent of patients with renal carcinoma in the absence of hepatic metastases (Utz et al., 1970). The etiology of the syndrome is unclear, but it is characterized by hepatosplenomegaly, prolonged prothrombin time, elevated alkaline phosphatase values, and, sometimes, elevated serum haptoglobin levels. Following removal of the primary lesion, liver function may return to normal, but serologic aberrations may recur with the clinical appearance of tumor recurrence. The presence of this hepatopathy appears to be a dire prognostic sign, and few such patients survive 5 years (Boxer et al., 1978).

In an excellent review of the problem of paraneoplastic syndrome, Sufrin et al. (1977) documented elevated peripheral renin blood levels in patients with high-stage and high-grade lesions. Following nephrectomy, the plasma renin levels sometimes return to normal, and the authors suggest that this may be a useful measure of occult disease. Elevation of the erythrocyte sedimentation rate resulting from renal carcinoma has also been reported by several authors, and such elevation has been correlated with a poor prognosis (Böttiger, 1970; Kaufman and Mims, 1966). However, the lack of specificity of this test has precluded its wide use in diagnosis and follow-up of renal cancer patients.

RADIOGRAPHIC DIAGNOSIS

The rapid evolution of uroradiography has provided the urologist with a number of diagnostic tests designed primarily to determine whether a renal mass lesion exists and to separate solid renal mass lesions from the more common benign renal cysts. Controversy exists regarding the reliability of each method and its place in the decision-making process as well as the extent to which each can provide the most cost-effective preoperative information.

The traditional intravenous pyelography with infusion nephrotomography remains the primary diagnostic step in most institutions. Combined with ultrasound and percutaneous cyst puncture, the diagnostic accuracy in differentiating a cyst versus a solid lesion approaches 100 per cent (Lang, 1977). Very few purely cystic lesions will prove to harbor renal carcinoma. This small group of cystic tumors can be identified in almost every case by cyst aspiration and injection of contrast material (Fig. 29–12). Clear fluid that has no malignant cells and a low fat and protein content, and low lactic acid

dehydrogenase aspirated from a cyst with smooth walls, are almost absolute evidence of the absence of malignancy (Figs. 29–13 and 29–14) (Lang, 1977). The only consistent difference between a cyst containing a tumor and a hemorrhagic benign cyst is the presence of malignant cells. Since detection of low-grade tumors may be difficult in aspirated old blood, the presence of blood in a cyst must raise the index of suspicion sufficiently to prompt further diagnostic tests.

The radionuclide scan is often underutilized in the study of small renal mass lesions (Fig. 29–15). Its major role is reserved for the patient with a homogeneous small parenchymal mass

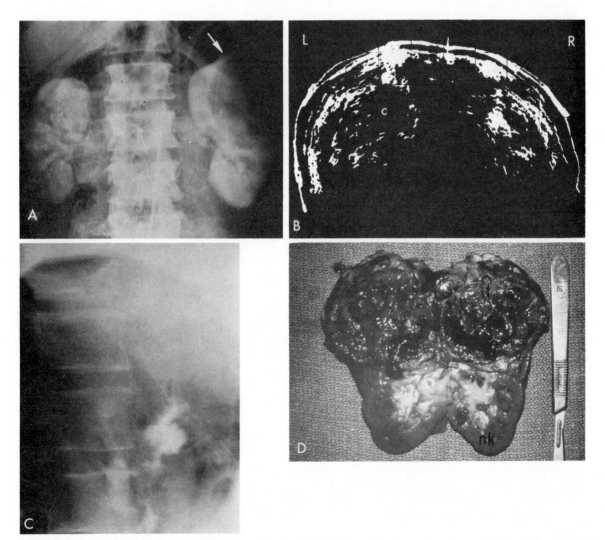

Figure 29–12. Nephrocarcinoma presenting as renal cyst. *A,* Nephrographic phase of aortogram discloses hypovascular tumor with "beak" sign (arrow). *B,* Ultrasound study suggesting cyst *(c)* of upper pole of left kidney. *C,* Needle puncture with injection of contrast medium indicates the solid nature of the lesion and suggests malignancy. *D,* Massive tumor of the upper pole proved to be papillary adenocarcinoma, with normal kidney *(nk)* below.

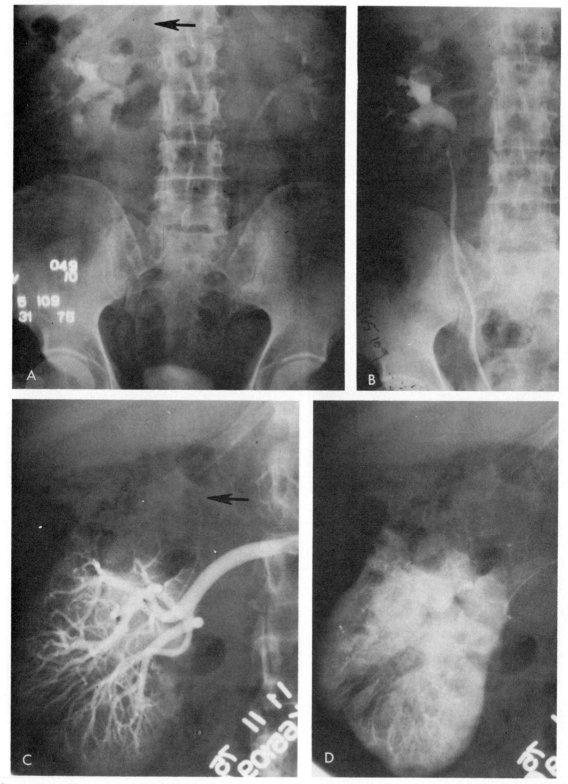

Figure 29–13. Renal cyst. *A*, Intravenous pyelogram suggests mass (arrow) at upper pole of right kidney. *B*, Retrograde pyelogram confirms presence of mass distorting upper calyx. *C*, Selective arteriogram confirms the avascular nature of the mass (arrow). *D*, Nephrographic phase of arteriogram is confirmatory.

Illustration continued on opposite page

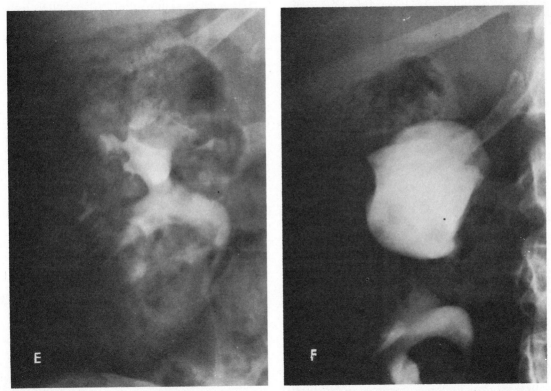

Figure 29–13 *Continued E*, Under fluoroscopic control, the collecting system is opacified on intravenous pyelography. *F*, Needle puncture of cyst is accomplished with aspiration of contents and injection of contrast material, demonstrating the relatively smooth outline of the uncomplicated benign renal cyst.

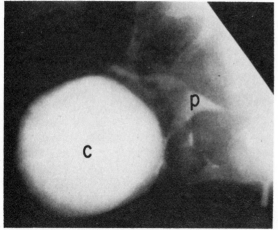

Figure 29–14. Simple renal cyst *(c)* after needle puncture, aspiration, and instillation of contrast with simultaneous intravenous pyelogram to opacify renal collecting system *(p)*.

that does not have the characteristics of a cyst or a tumor but may suggest the presence of a renal parenchymal rest. Uniform distribution of the radioisotope in the area of the suspected renal mass is a reliable indicator of the absence of tumor.

Selective renal arteriography has remained for decades the final diagnostic step in the evaluation of renal mass lesions. In most centers, it has been employed in the patient whose initial diagnostic study, perhaps supplemented by echography, suggested the presence of solid components in a renal mass. The number of tests interposed between the initial step and the arteriogram vary but often exceed the requirements for a cost-effective diagnosis. The morbidity of percutaneous selective renal angiography by the Seldinger technique is minimal in skilled hands. However, femoral artery false aneurysms, distal arterial emboli, hemorrhage, and impairment of renal function secondary to the contrast media have been reported. Loss of renal function is a special danger in patients who already have intrinsic renal disease, patients with a solitary kidney harboring a large tumor, and patients with diabetes mellitus. The classic angiographic picture of renal cell carcinoma is shown in Figures 29–16 and 29–17. Neovascularity, arteriovenous fistulae, pooling of contrast media, and accentuation of capsular vessels are the hallmarks of renal cell carcinoma. However, all spectra of the angiographic picture

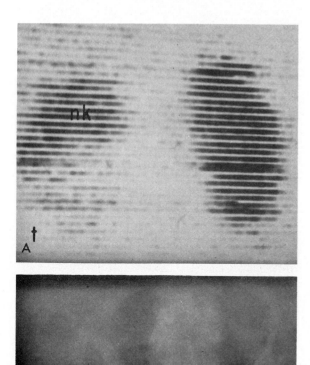

Figure 29–15. Radioisotope renal scan. *A,* Normal renal uptake on left and at upper pole of right kidney *(nk),* with poor uptake or "cold" area at right lower pole, indicating tumor *(t). B,* Concurrent intravenous pyelogram is inconclusive.

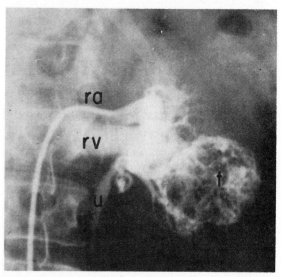

Figure 29–16. Selective renal arteriogram *(ra)* demonstrating neovascularization of renal tumor *(t),* early filling of renal vein *(rv),* and opacification of renal pelvis and ureter *(u)*.

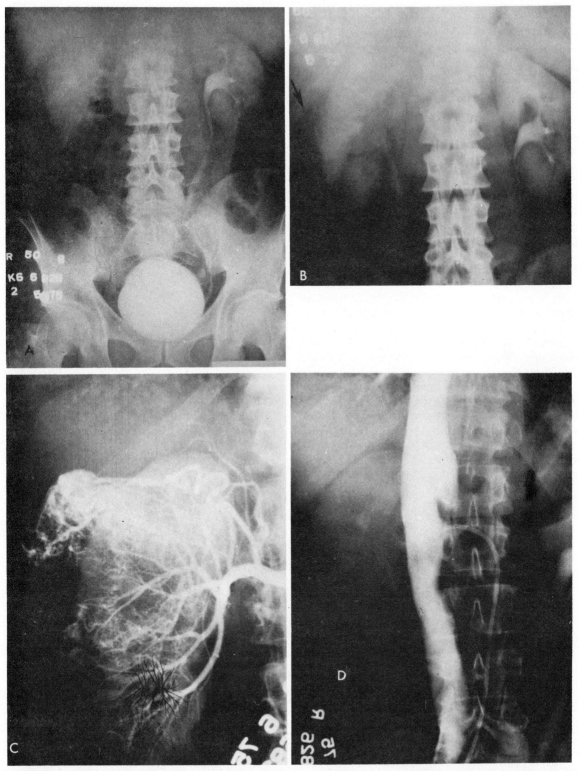

Figure 29–17. Typical nephrocarcinoma. *A,* Routine intravenous pyelogram discloses poor function of right kidney. *B,* Tomography aids in identifying parenchymal defect (arrow) at the lateral aspect of the right kidney. *C,* Selective arteriogram establishes the diagnosis of tumor. *D,* ˘   ˘ogram discloses no evidence of tumor involvement.

exist, and hypovascular tumors often pose a difficult diagnostic problem. The infusion of epinephrine to constrict normal vessels without constricting the tumor vessels often obviates this difficulty. Properly performed, the selected renal arteriogram remains an accurate method for the diagnosis of renal carcinoma (Fig. 29–18).

The development of computerized axial tomography, which offers a number of specific advantages over other methods, has demanded a complete re-evaluation of the traditional approaches to diagnosis (Fig. 29–19). Although infusion of contrast material and ingestion of contrast are important components, the procedure is less invasive than angiography or cyst puncture (Figs. 29–20 and 29–21). Second, the density of the mass lesions can now be accurately measured, usually obviating the need for ultrasonography or cyst puncture. Third, the test is an outpatient procedure, in contrast to angiography, which requires hospitalization. Finally, more thorough staging information is obtained from computerized tomography than from any of the other diagnostic methods (Figs. 29–22 to 29–24).

Numerous authors have compared computerized tomography to angiography for evaluation of renal mass lesions and have concluded that tomography is superior both in accuracy and in cost-effectiveness (Mauro et al., 1982; Karp et al., 1981; Kothari et al., 1981). Jaschke et al. (1982) correlated preoperative staging of 125 renal carcinomas with the angiographic and pathologic findings. The CT scan correctly di-

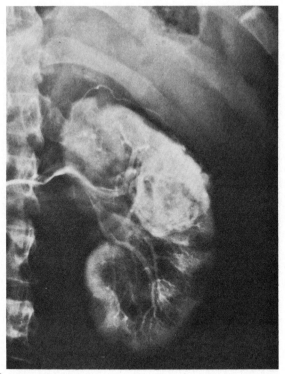

Figure 29–18. Typical arterial phase of selective renal angiogram demonstrating renal carcinoma in solitary kidney as well as multiple small cysts. Typical pattern of puddling of contrast is noted.

agnosed renal vein involvement in 91 per cent, vena caval extension in 97 per cent, perirenal extension in 79 per cent, lymph node metastases in 87 per cent, and extension to adjacent organs in 96 per cent of patients. Richie et al. (1983)

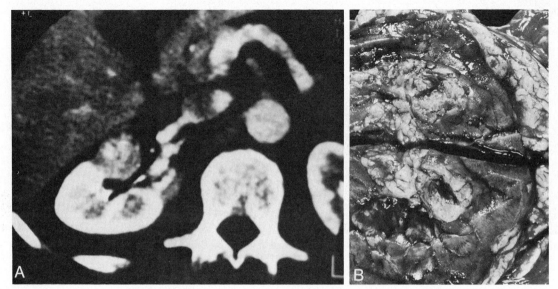

Figure 29–19. *A,* CAT scan demonstrating incidentally diagnosed small tumor in right kidney. *B,* Surgical specimen showing small typical renal cell carcinoma.

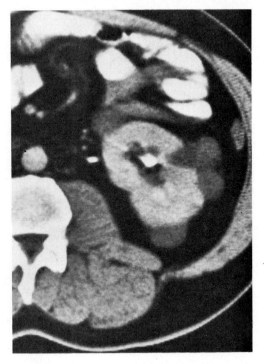

Figure 29–20. CAT scan demonstrating multiple benign renal cysts with density indicating clear fluid.

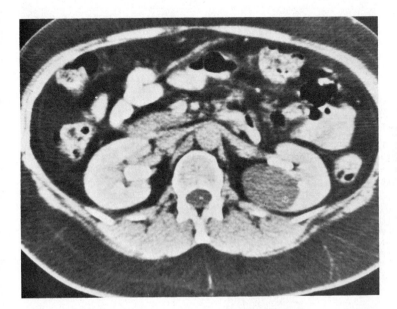

Figure 29–21. CAT scan demonstrating normal left kidney and large posterior left renal cyst with smooth wall and density consistent with clear fluid.

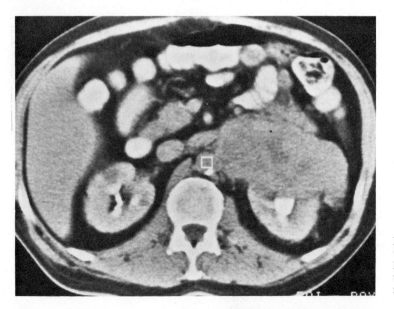

Figure 29–22. CAT scan demonstrating two small cysts in the right kidney and a large solid mass in the left kidney extending over the aorta and filling the left renal vein.

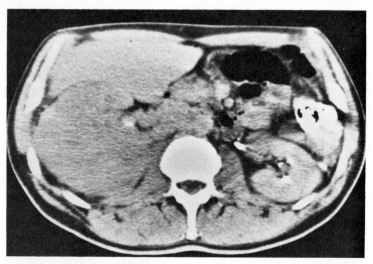

Figure 29–23. Huge right renal cell carcinoma with involvement of pericaval and interaorta-caval lymph nodes, proven at surgery.

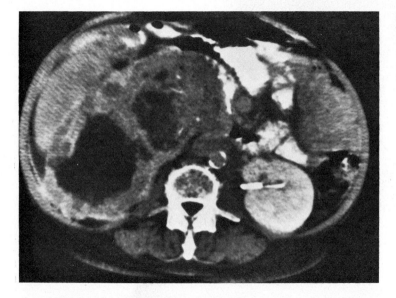

Figure 29–24. Large right renal mass, mixed solid and cystic on ultrasound. CAT scan demonstrates a renal cell carcinoma with extensive central necrosis and involvement of adjacent lymph nodes.

studied not only the staging accuracy but also the diagnostic reliability of CT scan in 45 patients compared with that of the angiogram. The tests were similar in diagnostic accuracy (95 per cent versus 85 per cent) and detection of renal vein extension, but CT scan was more accurate in detection of regional lymph node metastases. The sensitivity of the CT scan was further supported by Raval and Lamki (1983). The CT scan detected occult renal carcinoma in five patients whose tumors were not found by other diagnostic tests.

In the excellent article by Lang (1984), the relative accuracy of enhanced CT scan compared with other diagnostic studies was determined in a prospective fashion. In addition to accurately separating cystic from solid lesions, properly performed, enhanced computerized tomography can detect tumor extension through the capsule or into surrounding structures. Extension to the renal vein and vena cava can be determined with great accuracy, obviating the need for the traditional venacavography. Extension to the regional lymph nodes is a poor prognostic sign, and few patients are cured surgically. Computerized tomography can detect extensive regional lymph node involvement in many patients. From the data presented by Lang, it appears that, as a single diagnostic study, computerized tomography is the most cost-effective method of evaluating a suspected renal mass lesion. Utilizing the rapid-enhancement method suggested by Lang, further staging information seems plausible. However, certain pitfalls of computerized tomography have also become apparent. While extension through the capsule is often accurately diagnosed, a number of false positive findings will occur. The test will not detect limited lymph node involvement, and a small but disconcerting number of patients will seem to have involved lymph nodes that prove to be normal at surgery. One must be careful not to deny patients the potential for surgical cure on the basis of these false positive readings. Nonetheless, the new-generation CT scanners have provided us with a single test for diagnosis and staging of renal tumors that is minimally invasive and cost-effective.

The place of angiography, therefore, has become somewhat uncertain. Computerized tomography gives no information regarding the renal vasculature. Therefore, angiography remains the primary diagnostic test in the patient with a suspected tumor in the solitary kidney, when parenchymal-sparing surgical procedures are anticipated. Second, although differentiation of primary versus metastatic lesions is dif-

ficult even with angiography, the typical hypovascular angiographic appearance of a lesion metastatic to the kidney at least raises the suspicion of the clinician and may alter treatment plans. Computerized tomography has no way to distinguish lesions according to their vascularity. Third, a small number of patients will have an equivocal density reading on the CT scan and will require angiography for clarification of the nature of the renal lesion. Finally, the presence of a small lesion in the contralateral kidney is easily identified on a properly performed angiogram. Whether computerized tomography can recognize these small lesions with equal accuracy is uncertain.

STAGING

The staging system most commonly employed in the United States is Robson's modification of the system of Flocks and Kadesky (Fig. 29–25) (Robson et al., 1968). The limitations of the system become obvious when it is noted that survival of patients with Stage II tumor is equal to that of patients with Stage III tumor in some series, indicating an inappropriate assignment of prognostic factors. The placement of renin vein, vena caval, and lymph node involvement into the Stage III group accounts for this apparent contradiction, owing to the inclusion of all levels of renal vein extension. The TNM system proposed by American Joint Committee for Cancer Staging and End Result Reporting separates venous involvement from lymph node invasion and quantitates each. As such, this seems to be an improvement over the currently employed system (Table 29–6). In this system, tumors extending into the capsule are grouped with those extending into the renal vein in the T_3 category but are separated by subclasses (T_{3a}, T_{3b}, T_{3c}). The quantitation of the extent of lymph node involvement is another important refinement. The TNM system, however, is complicated, and the optimal way to combine subgroups into meaningful staging groups is still controversial.

Clinical staging of renal carcinoma has been alluded to in the discussion on diagnosis. Regional staging with computerized tomography is valuable but sometimes misleading, and the true local and regional extent of the tumor is most accurately determined by the pathologist. Evaluation for the presence of distant metastases is important in light of the recognized incurability of patients with metastatic disease. Renal carcinoma blood-borne metastases may be manifested in any organ system, but the most common sites are the lung, liver, subcutaneous

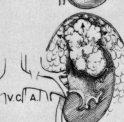

STAGING OF RENAL CELL
CARCINOMA

STAGE I

TUMOR WITHIN CAPSULE

STAGE II

TUMOR INVASION OF
PERINEPHRIC FAT (CON-
FINED TO GEROTA'S
FASCIA)

STAGE III

TUMOR INVOLVEMENT OF
REGIONAL LYMPH NODES
AND/OR RENAL VEIN
AND CAVA

STAGE IV

ADJACENT ORGANS OR
DISTANT METASTASES

Figure 29–25. Staging of nephrocarcinoma as proposed by Holland, in accord with schemes of Robson, Murphy, and Flocks and Kadesky. (From Holland, J. M.: Cancer, *32*:1030, 1973. Reproduced with permission of author and publishers.)

TABLE 29–6. STAGE CLASSIFICATION OF
RENAL CELL CARCINOMA

Tumor Stage	Robson*	TNM†
No primary	—	T_0
Small primary, minimal distortion	A	T_1
Large tumor, renal distortion	A	T_2
Involving perinephric tissues	B	T_{3a}
Involving renal vein	C	T_{3b}
Involving renal vein and infradiaphragmatic vena cava	C	T_{3c}
Invading adjacent structures	D	T_4
Involving superior vena cava	C	—
No nodes involved	A,B	N_0
Single, ipsilateral node involved	C	N_1
Involvement of multiple regional nodes	C	N_2
Fixed regional nodes	C	N_3
Involved juxtaregional nodes	C	—
Distant metastases	D	M_1

*Robson, C. J., Churchill, B. M., and Anderson, W.:
Trans. Am. Assoc. Genitourin. Surg., *60*:122, 1968.

†Beahrs, O. H., and Myers, M. H. (Eds.): American
Joint Committee on Cancer: Manual for Staging of Cancer.
2nd ed. Philadelphia, J. B. Lippincott Co., 1983, p. 178.

tissue, and central nervous system. The extent
of the preoperative evaluation in the asymptomatic patient must emphasize cost-effectiveness.
In a study at this institution, no patient with
normal liver function tests and a nonpalpable
liver was found to have metastases on the radionuclide liver-spleen scan (Lindner et al., 1983).
Similarly, no patient without symptoms of skeletal involvement and with normal alkaline phosphatase and serum calcium values had detectable skeletal metastases on radionuclide bone
scan. An appropriate preoperative evaluation,
therefore, seems to comprise a routine chest x-
ray, liver function tests, serum calcium measurement, and history and physical examination.

PROGNOSTIC FACTORS

The factors that have been associated with
a poor prognosis in renal cell carcinoma are
renal vein involvement, extension to regional
lymph nodes, extension through Gerota's fascia,
involvement of contiguous organs, and distant
metastases (deKernion and Berry, 1980). Although renal vein extension has long been
thought to be associated with a poor prognosis
(Myers et al., 1968), some studies have failed
to show this correlation (Skinner et al., 1972;
Selli et al., 1983). This may be due to the
emphasis in recent years on complete excision
of the renal veins and on preoperative identification of renal vein extension. In a recent study,
Hoehn and Hermanek (1983) quantitated renal

vein extension according to whether the main
renal vein was involved or whether only microscopic extension was present. The authors found
a significant increase in local recurrence and
metastases in patients with extension into the
main renal vein, but no prognostic importance
could be attributed to microscopic vein involvement. In future development of staging systems,
this important distinction must be considered.

Involvement of the regional lymph nodes
draining the renal parenchyma is a dire prognostic sign, associated with a 5-year survival rate
of from 0 to 30 per cent (deKernion, 1980a).
The extent of lymphatic dissemination is no
doubt important, and those who survive seem
to be patients with very limited early lymphatic
involvement. The implications with respect to
the extent of the surgical procedure are discussed later. Invasion through Gerota's fascia
and into the perinephric fat was perhaps a
greater detriment to survival prior to the widespread adoption of radical nephrectomy with
complete excision of Gerota's fascia. Even after
the excision of Gerota's fascia, extension of
tumor into the perinephric fat decreases the 5-
year survival rate to approximately 45 per cent
(Skinner et al., 1972; Siminovitch et al., 1983).
Tumor extension to contiguous organs is rarely
associated with 5-year survival even after radical
surgical excision. The significance of local tumor
persistence or recurrence is reflected in our
study of patients with metastatic renal carcinoma (deKernion et al., 1978). Those who had
incomplete tumor excision owing to extension
into Gerota's fascia had a much poorer prognosis than even those who developed distant
metastases without local tumor recurrence. The
size of the renal tumor is only indirectly correlated with survival (Böttiger, 1970). Size is perhaps important only in discerning renal adenomas from true renal carcinomas, a subject
discussed previously.

SURGICAL TREATMENT OF LOCALIZED
RENAL CARCINOMA

Surgery remains the only effective method
of treatment of primary renal carcinoma, and
the objective of the procedure must be to excise
all tumor with an adequate surgical margin.
Simple nephrectomy was practiced for decades
but has been supplanted by radical nephrectomy, which is presumed, (although not absolutely proved), to increase the surgical cure rate
(Robson, 1963; Patel and Lavengood, 1978).
Though the definition varies, radical nephrectomy generally implies the excision of Gerota's
fascia and its contents, including the kidney and

the adrenal gland. This accomplishes several objectives: First, the adrenal gland, which is not infrequently involved, is excised; second, lymphatic metastases, which may diffuse through the perirenal fat, are removed; and third, a more adequate margin away from the tumor is achieved, especially when the tumor invades the perirenal fat. More adequate renal vein division is also accomplished. Since these appear to be important factors in determining survival, especially invasion of the perinephric fat, cure can be expected to be seriously compromised if microscopic or gross tumor is left in Gerota's fascia. Although the true increase in survival realized by radical nephrectomy versus simple nephrectomy is often debated, the radical nephrectomy has become the standard method of surgical therapy.

Regional lymphadenectomy is often added to radical nephrectomy, and increased survival has been attributed to removal of involved lymph nodes (Robson, 1963; Peters, 1980). As noted earlier, regional node extension is an important prognostic factor seldom associated with long-term cure. It is generally impossible to assess the impact of lymph node involvement on survival, since other factors usually exist. Survival in patients who have unresectable lymph nodes approaches zero, but some authors have reported survival when limited lymph node involvement is successfully resected. Skinner and colleagues (1972) found a 17 per cent 10-year survival in those with lymph node involvement. The greatest survival—30 per cent of patients alive at 10 years following extensive lymphadenectomy—was reported by Robson (1963). However, Hultén and coworkers (1969) found no survivors when involved regional lymph nodes were excised.

Interpretation of the literature is difficult, since the number and location of involved lymph nodes are often not stated as fully as other important factors, such as the type of primary operation performed. However, it is possible that the improved survival that has occurred since the advent of radical nephrectomy with lymphadenectomy stems from the complete excision of the primary tumor rather than from excision of the regional nodes. Several characteristics of renal carcinoma argue against a therapeutic role for lymphadenectomy. First, the tumor metastasizes through the blood stream and the lymphatic system with equal frequency, and most patients with positive lymph nodes eventually have blood-borne metastases. Second, the lymphatic drainage of renal carcinoma is variable and may occur anywhere in the retroperitoneum. Third, many patients without

metastases to regional lymph nodes develop disseminated metastases (deKernion, 1980a). However, as pointed out by Marshall and Powell (1982) and confirmed by our own experience, most tumors initially metastasize to lymph nodes in the renal hilum or in the paracaval or para-aortic area immediately adjacent to the hilum. Although an occasional patient will have a distant retroperitoneal lymph node as the first site of metastasis, one can encompass the most probable first and second drainage areas by performing a limited lymph node dissection—paracaval and interaortacaval for right-sided tumors, and para-aortic and interaortacaval for left-sided tumors. Although the practical therapeutic value of this approach is still uncertain owing to the factors mentioned, it can be accomplished simply and provides valuable staging information.

The surgical technique of radical nephrectomy has been described by a number of authors (Stewart, 1975; deKernion, 1980b). The surgical approach is guided more by individual preference than by necessity. The transperitoneal approach through a subcostal incision allows early ligation of the renal artery and vein prior to tumor manipulation. This is an essential technical consideration in the management of renal carcinoma (i.e., early ligation of the artery and vein), and, to be acceptable, any approach must incorporate it. Other transabdominal incisions have also been employed with a similar intent of early ligation of the vessels.

The thoracoabdominal incision described by Chute et al. (1949) is commonly practiced and is especially suitable for large tumors in the upper pole of the kidney. This may include extraperitoneal or intraperitoneal incision as a disadvantage and perhaps an increased postoperative morbidity and increased time. The dorsolumbar osteoplastic flap described by Nagamatsu (1950) also provides excellent exposure. In many cases, a flank incision through the eleventh intercostal space or a supracostal incision allows excellent exposure without entering the pleural cavity and can be performed extraperitoneally. We have employed this approach for many small tumors and tumors in the lower pole and have found it to be associated with minimal postoperative morbidity, provided the costovertebral ligaments of the eleventh rib are divided adequately, allowing the rib to be deflected downward (deKernion, 1980b). The urologic surgeon should be skilled in a number of approaches, tailoring the incision to the body habitus of the patient and the size and position of the renal tumor.

Since the advent of sophisticated angiographic methods, preoperative occlusion of the renal artery has been advocated as an adjunct to the surgical procedure. Hemorrhage is reduced, especially in patients with very large tumors supplied by many parasitized vessels. The renal vein can be ligated prior to dissection of the renal artery, and a host immune stimulation has been attributed to renal infarction (Hirsh et al., 1979). However, a salutary effect on survival has not been demonstrated, and the procedure can be associated with complications that may compromise the ability of the patient to tolerate surgery, including pain, ileus, sepsis, and dislocation of the infarcting coil. Early ligation of the renal artery and vein can be safely performed without preoperative infarction, and little evidence suggests that the latter is an appropriate preoperative measure. However, it may be a reasonable adjunct in patients with large vascular tumors.

The long-term outcome following surgical therapy for renal carcinoma depends upon many factors, including tumor stage, grade, and histologic type and the surgical procedure. Data, therefore, are difficult to compare, and the use of various staging systems compounds the difficulty. Some general statements, however, can be made with respect to the efficacy of radical nephrectomy.

After radical nephrectomy for Stage I renal carcinoma, 5-year survival ranges from 60 to 82 per cent, compared with the 5-year survival for Stage II of approximately 47 to 80 per cent (Robson et al., 1968; Skinner et al., 1972; Böttiger, 1970; McNichols et al., 1981). In the series reported by Robson (1963), in which all patients underwent radical nephrectomy and extensive lymphadenectomy after careful preoperative selection, the survival of patients with Stage II tumors (extension through the capsule) was identical to that for those with Stage I disease, presumably owing to a more thorough excision of the tumor and a decreased local tumor recurrence. Individuals with Stage III tumors have an expected survival of between 35 and 51 per cent, depending upon the number of patients included in the category because of renal vein involvement without lymph node extension or extracapsular extension. As mentioned earlier, patients with extension to the contiguous organs have a very poor outlook, and those with distant metastases have virtually no chance of surviving 5 years (see further on).

Radiation therapy has been used as a preoperative or postoperative surgical adjunct. Several early reports showed an increased survival with the use of preoperative radiotherapy (Cox et al., 1970; Richie, 1966). A randomized study

conducted by Werf-Messing (1973) compared the results of 3000 rads of preoperative therapy with those of no therapy. Five-year survival was not improved, although the onset of local recurrence was postponed. Thus far, no study has demonstrated effectiveness of preoperative radiotherapy for renal carcinoma.

The purpose of postoperative radiotherapy is to sterilize any existing microscopic or gross tumor. A number of studies have used varying doses of radiotherapy to the renal fossa following nephrectomy but have not shown a significantly improved survival (Peeling et al., 1969). Indeed, survival after postoperative radiotherapy was diminished in the study by Finney (1973). For similar reasons, radiotherapy for regional lymph node extension was not proved to be of significant value. Although occasionally a large tumor may be reduced in size by preoperative therapy, no evidence currently exists to support the routine use of radiotherapy in renal carcinoma other than palliative treatment of skeletal metastases.

TUMOR IN THE SOLITARY KIDNEY AND BILATERAL RENAL TUMORS

Renal cell carcinoma may occur in the patient who has a solitary kidney, the other kidney either congenitally absent or having been removed for benign disease (Fig. 29–26). Bilateral neoplasms may also occur, either synchronously or asynchronously (Fig. 29–27). A clearer understanding of the renal vasculature and more sophisticated surgical approaches now usually make it possible to excise the tumor, leaving the patient with sufficient parenchyma to maintain life without dialysis. The standard partial nephrectomy in vivo, combined with regional hypothermia, is the most common approach. Autotransplantation following ex vivo excision is now commonplace in many large centers. However, the enthusiasm for this approach has diminished considerably, and most tumors are now excised from the solitary kidney without the need for the "workbench" approach.

Excision of tumor in the solitary kidney is associated with excellent short-term results (Marberger et al., 1981; Zincke and Swanson, 1982). Initial studies suggested that survival was significantly better in patients with tumor in the solitary kidney versus those with synchronous or asynchronous tumor in the opposite kidney (approximately 70 per cent versus 50 per cent (Wickham, 1975). A recent report by Topley et al. (1983), however, suggested that 5-year survival was poor only in those with asynchronous bilateral tumors (38 per cent) compared with unilateral tumors in a solitary kidney (71 per

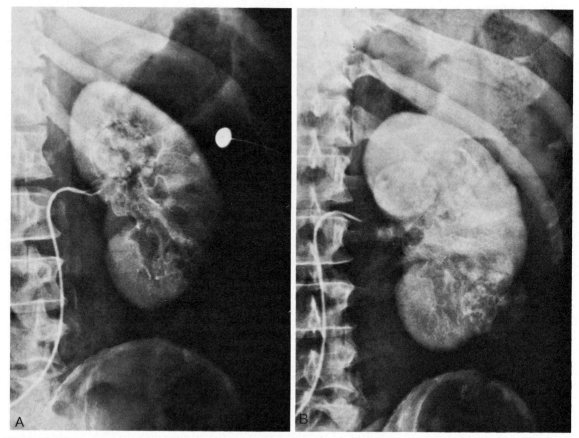

Figure 29–26. *A,* Selective left renal angiogram demonstrating three renal cell carcinomas. *B,* Oblique view uncovers another tumor in the upper pole on the posterior aspect of the kidney.

cent) and bilateral synchronous tumors (71 per cent). This conclusion was supported by the cumulative experience from this institution (Smith et al., 1984). Twenty patients with tumor in the solitary kidney and 18 patients with bilateral renal carcinoma were treated by partial nephrectomy in vivo (21) or ex vivo incision and autotransplantation. Radical nephrectomy with dialysis was the treatment in three patients. A number of conclusions were possible from this

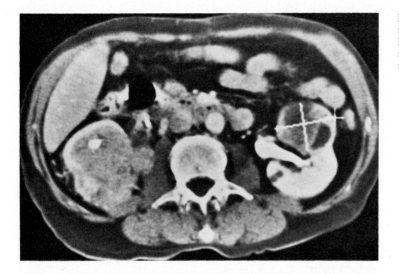

Figure 29–27. Bilateral renal cell carcinoma in a 61-year-old man with microhematuria. Patient underwent partial left nephrectomy and, subsequently, right radical nephrectomy.

study. First, complete removal of the tumor, whether in the solitary kidney or of bilateral renal tumors, was associated with a 72 per cent tumor-free survival at 3 years. Second, the survival was independent of whether the patient had tumor in the opposite kidney. Third, overall crude survival for patients with bilateral renal tumors that were completely excised was 57 per cent. Fourth, survival was dependent upon the stage of the local tumor. Eighty per cent of patients with Stage I tumors have survived 3 years, versus 50 per cent of patients with Stage II tumors. Fifth, ex vivo surgery is seldom necessary, and most patients can be adequately managed in vivo with regional hypotheramia. Finally, though bilateral nephrectomy with dialysis is seldom necessary, it should be an option offered to selected patients in the modern era of hemodialysis and transplantation.

While the short-term results have been uniformly good, the success of aggressive surgery in long-term cure has been questioned. The report by Topley et al. (1983) indicated a crude 5-year survival of 70 per cent following removal of tumor in the solitary kidney or of bilateral renal tumors. Even assuming a more modest long-term cure rate, the evidence currently supports the aggressive surgical management of tumor in the solitary kidney with preservation of renal parenchyma sufficient to sustain a good quality of life.

INFERIOR VENA CAVAL EXTENSION

Propensity for renal carcinoma to invade the renal veins and extend into the main renal vein as a tumor thrombus is well recognized. Continued growth of the thrombus into the vena cava occurs in a small number of cases, usually without direct invasion of the vessel (Fig. 29–28). The importance of delineating the extent of venous involvement is therefore obvious, and either inferior venacavogram or computerized axial tomography is essential in preoperative evaluation of renal tumors. Vena caval extension was considered to be a dire prognostic sign in the past, associated with little prospect for surgical cure. However, since the recognition of the importance of caval extension and aggressive surgical treatment, it is realized that most patients can still be cured surgically (Shefft et al., 1978).

The anatomic and surgical considerations in the patient with vena caval extension have been reviewed by Clayman and associates (1980). In this excellent review, 1-year survival of patients following surgical removal of vena caval extension was 75 per cent. This study and others attested to the wisdom of surgical removal of the vena caval thrombus even when the tumor extended into the right atrium, and the surgical approaches to accomplish vena caval thrombus excision have been thoroughly described (Cummings, 1982; Marshall et al., 1984). A limited infracaval extension, once recognized, is easily managed (deKernion and Smith, 1984). However, supradiaphragmatic and right atrial extension require an extended operation, often with cardiopulmonary bypass. While this has been accomplished and is technically feasible, little is known about the long-term survival of these patients.

The experience at our institution was reviewed to crystallize the extent of intervention appropriate in patients with massive vena caval thrombus (Cherrie et al., 1982). The prognosis was proved to be dependent upon the known factors, including local extension of tumor and regional lymph node involvement. The combined experience at this institution and the published literature indicate that 35 per cent of patients with lymph node involvement survived 2 years after nephrectomy and excision of vena caval thrombus, compared with 81 per cent of patients without lymph node extension. Similarly, no patient with distant metastases survived 3 years after nephrectomy with vena caval thrombus removal. Surgical results also seemed to be dependent upon the superior extent of the tumor thrombus, and patients with infradiaphragmatic extension seemed to have a prognosis similar to those with low-stage tumors, though numbers of patients in our study were too small to properly analyze this factor.

It therefore appears that removal of vena caval thrombus in the patient without regional or distant metastatic disease is the indicated surgical endeavor and is associated with an excellent prospect for cure. Extended operations for tumor in the supradiaphragmatic cava or right atrium seem to result in few long-term cures but may be palliative in some patients. However, they seem warranted only in the absence of any other local or distant dissemination.

Occasionally, the tumor may invade the wall of the vena cava. Resection of the vena cava is feasible, with preservation of a sleeve to accommodate venous drainage. This is most practical in patients with right-sided renal tumors, since the left renal vein can drain through the spermatic vein. The anatomic considerations and surgical approaches have been described (Clayman et al., 1980; McCullough and Gittes, 1975), but the procedure is rarely indicated.

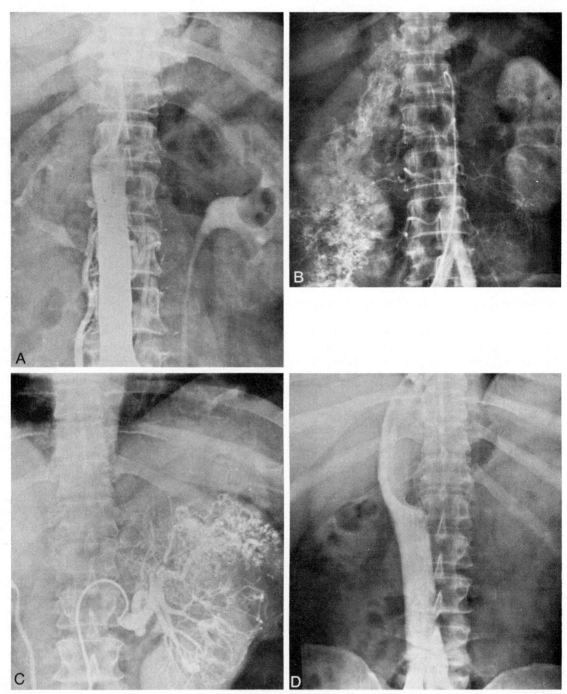

Figure 29–28. *A*, Arterial pattern in a large thrombus extending from a right renal tumor through the renal vein and into the inferior vena cava. *B*, Filling defect created by the thrombus. *C*, Angiogram in another patient demonstrating a large left renal carcinoma with arterial pattern of tumor extension into the left renal vein. *D*, Filling defect created by extension into the vena cava. Both patients were successfully treated surgically.

LOCALLY INVASIVE RENAL CARCINOMA

The propensity for renal carcinoma to grow to large size locally and to disseminate prior to diagnosis results in many patients presenting with large primary tumors that invade adjacent structures. Such patients usually present with pain, generally from invasion of the posterior abdominal wall, nerve roots, or paraspinous muscles. Liver extension is uncommon, and intrahepatic metastases occur more often than does local extension. The capsules of large tumors may indent and compress adjacent liver parenchyma but seldom actually grow by direct extension into the liver. Duodenal and pancreatic invasion is an extremely poor prognostic sign, and this author is not aware of any such patients being surgically cured. The propensity for the tumors to parasitize vessels accounts for the frequent extension into the large bowel, mesentery, and colon.

Since surgical therapy is the only effective management for this tumor, extended operations are sometimes indicated. Complete excision of the tumor, including excision of the involved bowel, spleen, or abdominal wall muscles, is essential. En bloc partial hepatectomy is rarely curative but may occasionally be worthwhile, since no other therapeutic options exist. Partial excision of the large primary tumor, or "debulking," is seldom, if ever, indicated. Only 12 per cent of patients who underwent incomplete excision of locally extensive tumor were alive at 12 months in a report from this institution (deKernion et al., 1978). Most reports suggest that less than 5 per cent of patients with extension into adjacent viscera survive 5 years after surgery. However, it is unclear in these reports which patients underwent complete excision, and the extent of involvement is often not stated. It is appropriate, therefore, to individualize when choosing patients for such extended radical nephrectomy. Preoperative staging by computerized tomography may spare the patient an unnecessary operation that is incapable of removing all or even most of the invasive tumor.

The role of radiation therapy in locally extensive carcinoma has been debated. Standard preoperative adjunctive radiotherapy has been shown in several early series to improve survival (Cox et al., 1970; Richie, 1966). However, a subsequent study by Werf-Messing (1973) compared therapy of 3000 rads preoperatively with no preoperative therapy. Survival was not influenced at 5 years, though the radiotherapy seemed to delay the time to local renal fossa recurrence. Large tumors may sometimes be decreased in size by radiotherapy, and nonresectable left-sided renal tumors may occasionally become resectable after such therapy, but delivery of effective radiotherapy to right renal tumors is difficult owing to the proximity of the liver.

As noted previously, routine postoperative radiotherapy, although an attractive concept for sterilizing minimal residual tumor, has not been shown to influence overall survival. It still seems appropriate, however, to utilize postoperative radiotherapy in selected patients after excision of locally invasive tumors. When tumor is known to have been left behind in the renal fossa or adjacent structures, postoperative radiotherapy may occasionally retard regrowth of tumor mass. The involved area should be carefully marked with metal clips to direct the radiotherapy. The frequency with which this postoperative therapy will be effective is uncertain, and the specter of distant dissemination dampens enthusiasm for all such locoregional therapies.

Many tumors are very extensive and involve the retroperitoneum extensively as well as adjacent viscera. As noted earlier, debulking seems to have little beneficial effect. Chemotherapeutic or hormonal agents have not been successful (see further on). Innovative approaches are sometimes useful in controlling symptoms in these patients.

Since the development of the sophisticated angiographic techniques and the availability of radioactive seeds, it is possible to direct high-dose radiotherapy through the arterial supply directly into the tumor. Multiple tumor vessels can be entered selectively, and radioactive seeds can be placed deep in the tumor. Currently, ^{125}I seeds may be the most effective method, because of the low-energy emission that allows selective high-dose irradiation to the tumor while sparing adjacent normal tissues. The procedure can be repeated as often as necessary to achieve complete tumor implantation, and doses of 10,000 rads can be delivered safely. This approach, occasionally with the addition of external radiotherapy and intra-arterial chemotherapy, was utilized in 22 patients with locally extensive renal carcinoma. Survival of these patients was 59 per cent at 2 years and 33 per cent of the patients at risk for 5 years. Distant metastases were unaffected. However, survival was improved and significant local palliation was achieved. Tumor size was decreased in all patients, and control of hemorrhage, control of pain, and weight gain were achieved in 80 per cent of cases. Toxicity was mild.

This appears to be a reasonable approach to the patient with a large, symptomatic non-resectable primary renal carcinoma, especially in the absence of distant metastases (Lang and deKernion, 1981). Renal artery infarction with inert materials will also occasionally provide a significant palliation. The major problem is the postinfarction syndrome (see earlier) and the risk of hemorrhage of the necrotic tumor. Serial infarction of the tumor with selection of segmental branches minimizes the postinfarction syndrome and the risk of rupture. We have employed this approach in several patients, with marked reduction in size of the tumor and at least temporary palliation.

TREATMENT OF METASTATIC RENAL CARCINOMA

Palliative or Adjunctive Nephrectomy. Approximately 30 per cent of patients have metastases at the time the diagnosis of renal carcinoma is first made, and early reports suggested that removal of the primary lesion induces regression of the metastases. This approach has been widely embraced by urologists and performed both for the purpose of control of symptoms and for the purpose of regression of metastatic sites.

The term "palliative nephrectomy" is best reserved for the operation performed for the control of severe symptoms. This procedure seems to be most effective in patients with severe hemorrhage, severe pain, paraneoplastic syndromes, and compression of adjacent viscera. The frequency with which each of these specific symptoms is controlled, however, is unclear, and modern methods, including angioinfarction, seldom make this the only palliative alternative. Patients with metastases at the time of presentation have an average survival of approximately 4 months, and only 10 per cent can be expected to survive 1 year (deKernion et al., 1979). The surgical mortality from the operation must also be superimposed on the potential benefits. Nonetheless, palliative nephrectomy is occasionally warranted for control of severe symptoms, especially for profuse hemorrhage.

The term "adjunctive nephrectomy" has been adopted to describe removal of the primary tumor in the patient with metastases, for the purpose of either prolonging survival or causing regression of metastatic lesions. Although a common practice for many years, the procedure has recently come under more careful scrutiny.

At the present time, no uniformity of opinion exists regarding its efficacy. The known spontaneous regression of renal tumors has been cited as support for the practice of adjunctive nephrectomy. Regression occurs in renal tumors only rarely, in perhaps 0.4 per cent of patients, or 1 in 250 (Montie et al., 1977). Some reports are even more pessimistic, such as that from the Mayo Clinic, in which no patient underwent regression in the 533 patients reviewed (Myers et al., 1968). Following adjunctive nephrectomy, regression can be expected to occur in less than 1 per cent of patients (Montie et al., 1977). Such regressions are often short-lived, and the mortality rate ranges from 2 to 15 per cent, mainly dependent upon patient selection. On the basis of this information, it seems difficult to support routine practice of adjunctive nephrectomy.

Improvement of patient survival by removal of a large primary tumor has been also cited in support of adjunctive nephrectomy. No study has thus far been reported in which patients are properly stratified and then randomized to undergo adjunctive nephrectomy versus no nephrectomy. However, in a study from this institution, survival of patients undergoing nephrectomy was identical to the survival for the general population of patients with renal carcinoma, suggesting that the nephrectomy had minimal impact on the outcome (deKernion et al., 1978).

Adjunctive nephrectomy is therefore no longer practiced in many centers on a routine basis, though some authors still support its application in selected patients (Fried, 1977). Indeed, the procedure may have application in certain clinical settings. Five-year survival seems to be improved in patients who have excision of solitary renal metastases (Middleton, 1967; O'Dea et al., 1978). It may be appropriate, therefore, to recommend nephrectomy with excision of solitary metastasis in this select group of patients, though micrometastases are likely to be present at other sites. Similarly, as part of an experimental study, adjunctive nephrectomy may be appropriate. Finally, the heterogeneity of renal cell carcinoma and its variable natural history defy therapeutic generalizations. Patients with limited pulmonary metastases, a resectable primary lesion, and a normal performance status seem to have a survival greater than others with metastatic disease. In a review of patients at this institution, those in this category had a 5-year survival of approximately 30 per cent following adjunctive nephrectomy and various postoperative treatment programs. The impact of the postoperative treatment programs is unclear, but the data indicated that some effect was independent of these systemic therapies. The impact of the adjunctive nephrectomy can also be questioned, since a similar group of patients who did not undergo nephrectomy have not been followed. However, in young healthy patients who meet these specific criteria, adjunctive nephrectomy may be appropriate, especially if it is part of a planned treatment program. It has become obvious that the entire question of the role of adjunctive nephrectomy must constantly be reassessed in careful clinical studies.

Angioinfarction-Nephrectomy. The concept of percutaneous angiographic infarction of renal carcinoma followed by nephrectomy was based primarily upon the theory of stimulation of host immune response, aided by the ease with which angiographic infarction can be performed. The most extensive experience has been that of Swanson et al. (1983). One hundred patients with renal carcinoma were treated by infarction-nephrectomy. Twenty-eight per cent of the patients had partial or complete regression of distant metastases. Of the evaluable patients, 7 had a complete response, 8 had partial regression, and 13 had stabilization of tumors for at least 1 year. Eighty-eight patients received progesterone therapy following nephrectomy. The median survival did not seem to be greater than in those treated by adjunctive nephrectomy alone. Patient selection was important, since only those most likely to respond were included. Patients who responded were almost invariably those who had pulmonary metastases, and these are the patients who most commonly respond to any form of therapy and also most commonly undergo spontaneous regression of metastases. These are the same patients who were cited previously as a favored

group that can be expected to do well for a prolonged period of time. A randomized study under way, however, has thus far shown no advantage in patients who underwent prenephrectomy infarction (Crawford et al., 1982).

The complications of infarction are significant. Nephrectomy is usually performed 3 to 5 days after infarction. During that time, the postinfarction syndrome is encountered in most patients, including severe abdominal pain, nausea, diarrhea, fever, and paralytic ileus. Hypertension and severe sepsis may also occur. Unintentional embolization of peripheral vessels has been observed occasionally. It therefore seems that wide advocacy of this aggressive and perhaps hazardous approach must await further results of randomized trials.

Chemotherapy. The traditional modern management of advanced solid tumors has been with cytotoxic agents. In spite of the remarkable advances realized in other tumors, renal cell carcinoma has remained refractory to these agents. A number of drugs have been used as single agents (Table 29–7) (deKernion and Lindner, 1982). These drugs have been used in various dosage schedules, and responses have been measured by disparate criteria. The lack of therapeutic efficacy, however, is apparent. A major complicating factor in interpretation of these and other trials is the unusual natural history of renal cell carcinoma, which may remain stable for varying intervals. Partial regression and stabilization of previously growing lesions are not uncommon, irrespective of the therapeutic intervention, and natural-history factors are often impossible to separate from results of therapy.

Vinblastine appears to be the most commonly employed single agent. Hrushesky and Murphy (1977) reported a 25 per cent objective

TABLE 29–7. SINGLE-AGENT CHEMOTHERAPY OF METASTATIC RENAL CELL CARCINOMA

Drug	No. Patients	Response	
		COMPLETE	PARTIAL
4'(9-acridinylamine) methanesulfon-m-aniside	37	0	1
Baker's antifol	17	1	0
Methotrexate	20	0	2
Ifosfamide	15	0	1
Cyclophosphamide (high-dose)	12	0	0
Methyl-GAG	76	1	6
Chloroethyl-cyclohexy-nitrosourea	23	0	4
5-Fluorouracil	12	0	0
Hydroxyurea	24	0	1
Vinblastine	15	0	2
Actinomycin D	65	0	1
Triazimate	59	1	2
Cis-platinum	32	0	0

response, superior to any other single agent or combination of agents. We have noted partial regression in only 1 of 16 patients treated with vinblastine.

The data in Table 29–8 indicate that no more than approximately 15 per cent of patients will demonstrate a response to single-agent chemotherapy, with virtually no prospect of complete regression or cure. The therapeutic significance of this low level of activity must be questioned in view of the natural history of the tumor. It nonetheless appears appropriate to offer some patients with disseminated metastases a trial of single-agent chemotherapy, with vinblastine sulfate or CCNU being the most suitable choices.

Since single agents have generally not been proved to be effective, and since combination therapy depends upon the combined efficacy of the agents, responses to combination chemotherapy have been expectedly low (Table 29–8) (deKernion and Lindner, 1982). Several studies suggest a somewhat better response with combinations, especially when vinblastine is one of the agents. However, toxicity is compounded and the response is usually of short duration. It does not, therefore, appear to be appropriate to routinely recommend combination cytotoxic agents. However, carefully constructed prospective clinical trials are still important and provide the best hope for identifying effective treatment regimens.

In vitro testing of chemotherapeutic agents has been suggested as a means of identifying effective agents for specific patients. Day and associates (1981) utilized explanted renal carcinoma tumors implanted into athymic mice. The tumors in the mice demonstrated an identical chemosensitivity pattern to that observed in vitro. The human tumor stem cell or clonogenic assay described by Salmon and associates (1978) has been studied to test its application in renal carcinoma. The most extensive experience was

reported by Lieber (1984), who successfully cultured human renal tumors in soft agar. Response to single agents was rarely noted, and thus far no correlation has been demonstrated between the assay and the actual clinical response. The author concluded that the assay is not yet an accurate clinical aid, but remains an important research tool.

Hormonal Therapy. The basis for hormone treatment of advanced renal carcinoma was the demonstration of its efficacy against an estrogen-induced clear cell tumor in the adult Syrian hamster (Kirkman and Bacon, 1949). A review of the clinical literature by Bloom (1973) showed an objective response of approximately 15 per cent in patients with metastatic renal carcinoma. However, this represented a summary of Phase II trials of varying patient selection and criteria of response. In a review of 110 patients at our institution, no patients had a response to progestational agents (deKernion et al., 1978). Though no reports have substantiated the role of progesterones, the paucity of side effects and the lack of effective cytotoxic treatment have prompted propagation of its use as the agent of choice. Side effects include nausea, vomiting, breast tenderness, and uterine bleeding, but these are seldom sufficient to cause cessation of therapy.

The variability of response has been attributed to varying dosage schedules. Although no good study has compared the types of progesterones or the dosage schedules, an orally administered divided dose of 160 mg per day of Provera is well tolerated and is the frequent choice. Medroxyprogesterone acetate is administered twice weekly and is well tolerated.

A number of other hormonal agents have been employed, but progesterones appear to be the only agents with therapeutic efficacy (Table 29–9) (deKernion and Lindner, 1982). As a method of selecting patients for hormone therapy, progesterone receptors on renal tumors

TABLE 29–8. RESULTS OF MULTIPLE-AGENT CHEMOTHERAPY OF METASTATIC RENAL CELL CARCINOMA

Drugs	No. Patients	Response	
		COMPLETE	PARTIAL
Vinblastine, chloroethyl-cyclohexy-nitrosourea	93	3	9
Vinblastine, methyl-chloroethyl-cyclorohexy-nitrosourea	15	0	1
Vinblastine, methotrexate, bleomycin	14	0	5
Vinblastine, methotrexate, bleomycin, tamoxifen	14	0	5
Vinblastine, cyclophosphamide, 5-fluorouracil	10	0	0
Vinblastine, cyclophosphamide, hydroxyurea, medroxyprogesterone acetate, prednisone	45	1	6
Cyclophosphamide, 5-fluorouracil, vincristine, methotrexate	18	0	0
Vinblastine, cyclophosphamide, doxorubicin, bleomycin, bacillus Calmette Guérin	14	0	3

TABLE 29–9. HORMONAL THERAPY OF METASTATIC RENAL CELL CARCINOMA

Agent	No. Patients	Response	
		COMPLETE	PARTIAL
Medroxyprogesterone acetate	116	7	4
Testosterone	48	0	0
Tamoxifen	106	0	2
Nafoxidine	39	2	2
Estramustine phosphate	16	0	0

have been measured. In a study by Concolino and associates (1978), several patients with progesterone receptors did respond while those without receptors did not. Others are now studying the significance of surface receptors. However, in the current climate of skepticism regarding the antitumor effect of progesterone, enthusiasm for receptor research has waned.

In summary, progesterones continue to be a method of management in the absence of more effective agents. However, it is important to note that no proper study has proved the efficacy of these agents in management of advanced renal carcinoma.

Immunotherapy. The theory supporting immunotherapy is that host immune functions play a role in tumor control, and that these immune functions can be further stimulated. Immunotherapy has been reported to have a role in management of some tumors, especially in control of minimal residual disease (Mathé, 1978), but has not proved effective in causing regression of advanced metastatic cancer. However, the unusual natural history of renal carcinoma, including spontaneous regression, delayed growth of metastatic lesions, and varying tumor doubling times, suggests that host immune factors may be important. Though many studies of immune functions have been conducted in patients with renal cancer, no firm evidence has been found to implicate host immunity as the regulating factor in tumor growth. This is partly due to our ignorance of the intricacies of the host immune response during malignant transformation and tumor growth. However, the hypothesis still remains testable, and a number of modalities have been used.

The most commonly used approach has been the use of *active nonspecific immunotherapy,* and the agent has been bacillus Calmette Guérin (BCG). Minton and associates (1976) reported partial regression in four of nine patients with pulmonary metastases treated with intradermal BCG. Morales and Coworkers (1982) observed response in five of eight patients treated, but neither series has been expanded into a formal Phase II trial. Other studies similarly suggested that BCG had a low level of clinical activity (Brosman, 1977), but no rigidly conducted trial has thus far supported the efficacy of this agent.

Numerous methods of *active specific immunotherapy* have been employed. Tykkä (1981) treated 31 patients after nephrectomy with a soluble fraction of autologous tumor polymerized with ethylchlorformiate. The agent was given intradermally along with purified protein derivative tuberculin or *Candida* antigen as an adjuvant. Complete regression of pulmonary metastases occurred in 6 of 16 patients with pulmonary metastases, and survival seemed to be increased over that of a control group. The patient population was somewhat heterogeneous, and selection of controls presented a problem of interpretation. Prager and associates (1981) developed a similar approach mixing autologous irradiated cells polymerized with dichlorodiphenyl trichloroethane injected percutaneously. Survival of 27 treated patients was improved significantly over that of the control group.

Based upon animal studies, a clinical trial was conducted by Schapira and associates (1979) using irradiated autologous cells with *C. parvum* as an adjuvant injected intradermally. Subsequently, McCune and associates (1981) treated 14 patients and reported partial regression in 5 with metastatic renal carcinoma. A randomized Phase III trial was conducted based upon these data. Following adjunctive nephrectomy, patients were randomized to receive either Megace or the immunotherapy that was injected intradermally weekly for 8 weeks. Partial or complete responses were noted in 10 per cent of the immunotherapy group versus 4 per cent of those receiving the progesterone. Patients who responded were those with either pulmonary or subcutaneous metastases who had a good performance status and an intact immune response measured by a positive response to DNCB skin test (McCune et al., in press). Importantly, this randomized allocation to progesterone therapy failed to demonstrate any significant clinical effect in patients receiving the hormone.

Several methods of *adoptive immunotherapy* have been employed in patients with advanced renal cancer. Transfer factor was utilized by Bukowski and associates (1979), combined with other modalities, in patients with measurable metastatic renal carcinoma. One patient of nine treated with transfer factor alone had a complete response, and two of eight patients treated with transfer factor plus BCG had partial regression. One complete regression and four partial regressions were noted in 14 patients treated with a combination of transfer factor, progesterone, and chloro-ethyl-cyclohexo-nitrosourea.

Xenogeneic ribonucleic acid extracted from immunized animals has been shown to be effective in a number of animal models. A Phase II trial was conducted in patients with renal carcinoma who were treated with RNA extracted from the lymphoid organs of sheep that had been immunized with human renal cell carcinoma. No patient had a complete regression and seven had only partial responses, most of which would be classified as only minimal response by current criteria (Ramming and deKernion, 1977). Although patients with pulmonary metastases only initially did better than the matched control group, by 4 years all patients had died of metastatic disease (deKernion and Ramming, 1980). Richie and associates (1981) obviated the problem of degradation of the RNA by human tissue ribonucleases. The patients' leukocytes were incubated in vitro with the xenogeneic RNA and subsequently reinfused. Several patients demonstrated a response, but the efficacy of RNA administered by any route is still questionable.

The *interferons* are glycoproteins produced by human cells in response to viral infections or other inducers. The antiviral and antineoplastic activity seems to be mediated by direct tumor cytotoxicity or by indirect cytotoxicity through natural killer cell stimulation, or by both (Stehm et al., 1982). The interferons have shown some efficacy against a number of human malignancies, including multiple myeloma, breast cancer, and lymphoma (Gutterman et al., 1979; Merigan et al., 1978), and several studies have recently been conducted in patients with renal cell carcinoma. At this institution, an extended Phase II trial of alpha interferon was performed in patients with measurable metastatic renal carcinoma. Of 34 evaluable patients, a complete response was noted in 1, partial responses in 4, and minimal responses in 6. In addition, eight patients had prolonged (more than 6 months) stabilization of previously growing metastases

(deKernion et al., 1983). A study by Quesada and associates (1982) in 13 renal carcinoma patients treated with human leukocyte interferon reported a partial response in 1 patient, minimal response in 3, and stabilization in 2 others. In a Phase I trial at our institution using fibroblast interferon, one patient with renal carcinoma achieved a marked partial regression that was maintained for almost 2 years (Sarna et al., 1982).

In an attempt to improve on the observed response rate, a Phase II trial combining weekly vinblastine (0.1 mg per kg) with alpha interferon (3 million units IM daily 5 days a week) has been recently completed (Figlin et al., in press). Of 23 evaluable patients, 1 had a partial response, 4 had minimal responses, and three had stabilization of growth. The overall efficacy, therefore, was similar to that achieved by interferon alone, and vinblastine, with its added toxicity, seemed to be unassociated with clinical gain.

The interferons therefore have unquestionable activity against renal carcinoma. However, most patients who respond are those with limited metastases, and especially limited pulmonary metastases. The low level of clinical response requires further trials with newer and less expensive interferons, perhaps combined with other agents.

Sarcomas of the Kidney

Sarcomas constitute only about 2 to 3 per cent of malignant tumors of the kidney but increase in incidence with advancing age (Farrow et al., 1968; Saitoh et al., 1982). The most common presenting signs and symptoms are essentially those of a large renal carcinoma, i.e., pain, a flank mass, and hematuria (Fig. 29–29).

The differentiation from renal adenocarcinoma is usually difficult or impossible. Sarcomas present as solid masses, and the angiographic pattern is generally one of a hypovascular solid tumor without arteriovenous fistulae. Leiomyosarcomas are the most common variety, composing about 60 per cent of the total incidence of sarcomas. Sixty-six cases were identified by Niceta and coworkers (1974) and were most common in women in the fourth to sixth decades of life.

Treatment for leiomyosarcoma, as with any sarcoma, is radical nephrectomy. This is especially important since these tumors can seldom be definitely differentiated from renal adenocarcinoma. The prognosis is generally poor

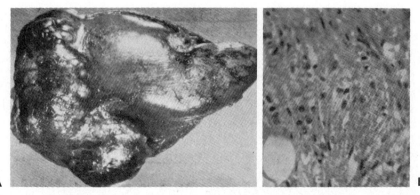

Figure 29–29. Sarcoma of renal capsule. *A,* Massive tumor arising from renal capsule. *B,* Histologic diagnosis of fibrosarcoma.

when patients are treated with surgery alone. Adjuvant chemotherapy may be beneficial. Beccia et al. (1979) treated a patient with adjuvant chemotherapy, and the individual survived 4 years without evidence of recurrence. Two patients were treated by Helmbrecht et al. (1974) with adjuvant radiation and chemotherapy in addition to surgery. In view of the experience with other sarcomas, doxorubicin is perhaps the most logical agent for adjuvant therapy and definitive treatment.

Osteogenic sarcomas are extremely rare tumors of the kidney. The genesis of such tumors is problematic, and osteogenic differentiation may occur in various sarcomatoid renal cell tumors (Moon et al., 1983). These tumors contain calcium and are rock-hard or may have a sunburst calcification. The presence of extensive calcification in a rather hypovascular tumor should suggest the presence of this rare lesion. The tumor may metastasize to bone and pose a problem as to whether the tumor in the kidney is a metastasis or truly a primary lesion. Biggers and Stewart (1979) reviewed the literature and recorded seven cases, detailing the clinical and pathologic features of the tumor. The poor prognosis was emphasized, and although radical nephrectomy is the treatment of choice, few patients are cured.

Virtually every other variety of sarcoma has been described in the kidney. Liposarcomas represent about 19 per cent of renal sarcomas and are often confused with angiomyolipomas or with very large benign primary lipomas. These tumors occur generally in the fifth and sixth decades of life and are usually of large size (Economou et al., 1984). Carcinosarcoma of the kidney has been described in several cases and is composed of classic renal cell carcinoma components in addition to fibrosarcomatous elements (Rao et al., 1977). Fibrosarcoma has been

described and is easily mistaken for leiomyoma or leiomyosarcoma (Kansara and Powell, 1980). Fibroxanthosarcoma (Chen, 1979) and angiosarcoma (Allred et al., 1981) have also been described. Rhabdomyosarcoma is one of the rarest renal neoplasms and was associated with hypertension in a case reported by Selvaggi et al. (1979). One patient with rhabdomyosarcoma has been treated in recent years at our institution and succumbed to metastatic disease 14 months after radical nephrectomy.

One of the most thorough studies of the incidence and metastatic pattern of sarcomas was made by Saitoh et al. (1982). In 2651 cases of renal tumors, they reported an incidence of sarcomas of 1 per cent. Nine were leiomyosarcoma, five were rhabdomyosarcoma, and five were fibrosarcoma. The most common sites of metastases were the liver, lymph nodes, and lung.

Surgery is the only potentially curative method of treating these rare tumors. The survival following surgery alone, however, is extremely poor. The success that has been realized by intra-arterial doxorubicin therapy combined with radiation provides at least a testable hypothesis for the adjuvant treatment of these tumors. The patient illustrated in Figure 29–30 had a poorly differentiated sarcoma of the kidney that completely regressed following doxorubicin and external radiotherapy, and the residual fibrous mass was subsequently excised. The patient is free of disease 2 years after surgery. Although adjuvant intravenous doxorubicin following nephrectomy has not been proved to be of value, the current experience suggests that this may be a reasonable approach.

Malignant fibrous histiocytoma is the most common soft tissue sarcoma in adults. Seven such tumors arising in the kidney have been reported. The tumors usually grow to large size

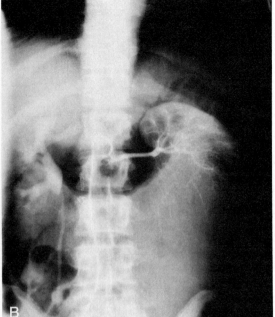

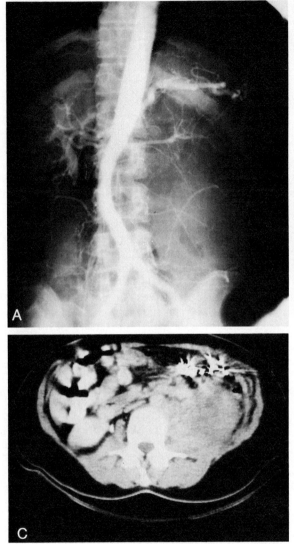

Figure 29–30. *A,* Aortic flush phase demonstrating huge left flank mass in a 36-year-old woman with flank pain. Note aortic displacement. *B,* Selective left renal arteriogram showing typical hypovascular pattern associated with sarcomas. *C,* CAT scan demonstrating the large tumor fixed to the posterior abdominal wall and paraspinous muscles, proven to be a poorly differentiated sarcoma by biopsy.

and may be clinically and angiographically indistinguishable from renal cell carcinoma. The histology is similar to histiocytomas arising in other areas. Therapy is radical nephrectomy, but local recurrence is frequent. Radiotherapy may be effective (Osamura et al., 1978; Raghavaiah et al., 1980).

Hemangiopericytoma

The renin-secreting tumors of the kidney, discussed previously, are usually small benign tumors that produce severe hypertension. These are often histologically hemangiopericytomas. However, renal and perirenal hemangiopericy-

toma may exist, may grow to large size, and may develop a malignant potential. Local or distant metastases have been reported in approximately 15 per cent of patients (Glenn, 1980). Ordonez et al. (1982) described a hemangiopericytoma extending into the vena cava as a thrombus. DiEsidio et al. (1980) reported a retroperitoneal hemangiopericytoma that metastasized to the liver, kidney, and abdominal cavity. A major concern with these tumors is their profuse vascularity. Smullens et al. (1979) described catheter embolization of hemangiopericytoma of the retroperitoneum in two patients, which greatly facilitated their safe removal. When these tumors are confined to the kidney, the most appropriate treatment is radical nephrectomy.

Lymphoblastoma

Malignancies of the lymphoma type, including reticulum cell sarcoma, lymphosarcoma, and leukemia, are uncommon and generally occur in the kidney as only one manifestation of the systemic disease. Knoepp (1956) identified a primary lymphosarcoma of the kidney treated, apparently successfully, with radical nephrectomy. Silber and Chang (1973) also reported a primary lymphoma of the kidney. Leukemia generally involves the kidney in an infiltrative pattern, producing hematuria, enlarged kidneys, and progressive renal failure.

The treatment of these processes is generally the indicated systemic treatment for that particular disease. Nephrectomy is seldom, if ever, indicated except in the case of a solitary lesion or in the patient with severe symptoms, such as uncontrollable hemorrhage.

Since the treatment of these lesions is not the primary purview of the urologist, his major concern rests in the diagnosis of renal involvement by these systemic diseases and in their separation from other renal mass lesions. Hartman et al. (1982) related pathologic findings with radiologic findings in 21 patients with renal lymphoma. The radiographic picture depended upon the pattern of involvement and the size, number, and distribution of the lesions. They concluded that the lymphoma initially grows between the nephrons and subsequently expands and produces the typical lymphomatous masses.

Computed tomography appears to be the method of choice in diagnosing renal lymphoma (Heiken et al., 1983). The initial nodular lesions, which later become confluent, are best detected with contrast medium administration. Four patterns of involvement were documented by computed tomography by Heiken and associates: (1) multiple intraparenchymal nodules, (2) direct contiguous lymph node masses, (3) solitary renal lesions, and (4) diffuse infiltration (Heiken et al., 1983). Jafri et al. (1982) described similar findings in 16 patients with non-Hodgkin's lymphomas of the kidney. CT was accurate in determining the size and location of the tumor and was useful in evaluating the response to systemic therapy. Various patterns of involvement, including solitary nodules, multiple nodules, focal infiltration, diffuse infiltration, contiguous extension, and renal enlargement, were noted. Retroperitoneal adenopathy was identified by CT scan in all the patients. Others have suggested that the findings of renal infiltration and multiple intraparenchymal nodules associated with retroperitoneal adenopathy

should raise the possibility of renal lymphoma. At the present time, computed tomography appears to be the most reliable way to diagnose renal involvement by lymphoma and to monitor the progress of therapy.

Metastatic Tumors

The kidney is a frequent site of metastatic deposits from a variety of solid tumors and hematologic malignancies. The high blood flow, profuse vascularity, and fertile soil of the renal parenchyma provide a hospitable environment for deposition and growth of malignant cells.

Metastases to the kidney are seldom clinically identified and are most often discovered at autopsy. They are, in that sense, often clinically inconsequential, since the nature of the metastatic disease militates against the removal of an isolated renal metastasis. In a review of 5000 autopsies, Klinger (1951) found 21 cases of metastases from lung carcinoma (Fig. 29–31).

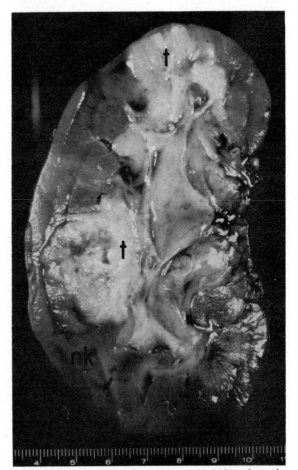

Figure 29–31. Metastatic carcinoma of the kidney from the lung, demonstrating the diffuse invasive character of metastatic tumor *(t)* in normal renal substance *(nk)*.

Olsson (1971) reported that 20 per cent of patients dying of lung cancer had renal metastases, 40 per cent of which were bilateral. These tumors are often small and multiple, and it has been estimated that as many as 19,000 persons annually may have lung cancer with secondary renal metastases. While these tumors seldom present with clinical symptoms, massive hemorrhage has been reported (Walther et al., 1979). Virtually every other solid neoplasm may metastasize to the kidney, including ovarian, bowel, and breast malignancies. Lymphoma and lymphoblastoma are among the most common metastatic lesions of the kidney. These usually present as multiple nodules, but occasionally single nodules and diffuse infiltration have been reported (Kyaw and Koehler, 1969). Metastatic or secondary lesions within the kidney generally produce few symptoms. Flank pain and hematuria may occur, but pyelographic identification is difficult to distinguish from primary renal neoplasms. Arteriographically, these tumors are usually round and hypovascular, without the discrete neovascularity and other angiographic characteristics associated with primary renal cell carcinoma (Fig. 29–32).

Whether renal carcinoma frequently metastasizes to the opposite kidney is controversial. The same malignant propensity that caused a tumor in one kidney could be reasonably expected to give rise to another primary lesion in the opposite kidney. The short-term results (cited previously) following excision of tumor in the contralateral kidney (synchronously or asynchronously) seem to be better than survival following excision of a solitary metastasis. However, no serologic or histologic method has been devised to accurately determine whether such tumors are metastatic or de novo lesions.

Renal Oncocytoma

Renal oncocytoma has recently become a recognized clinical and pathologic entity. The tumor is characterized by a histologic pattern of large eosinophilic cells with a granular cytoplasm and typical polygonal form. Mitoses are rare and the cells have a benign ultrastructure, characterized by a profusion of mitochondria. Grossly, the tumors have a typical appearance, usually tan or light brown in color, well-circumscribed, round, encapsulated, and containing a central dense fibrous band with fibrous trabeculae extending out in a stellate pattern. Necrosis and hypervascular areas are absent (Fig. 29–33). Electron microscopy demonstrates the abundance of mitochondria with endoplasmic reticulum or Golgi apparatus, distinguishing this cell type from the low-grade renal carcinoma cell (Landier et al., 1979). The typical cell appearance suggests an origin from the proximal tubular cells (Merino and Livolsi, 1982). The exact incidence of oncocytoma as compared with other renal tumors is unknown, owing to the recent identification of the distinct pathologic nature of the tumor. It occurs more commonly in males than in females and has generally the same age incidence as that of renal cell carcinoma. Tumors vary in size and may be quite large. Clinical presentation is generally associated with flank pain, and although hematuria is not a characteristic, a number of patients have this as their presenting symptom. The incidence in 253 renal tumors was 5.3 per cent as reported by Merino and Livolsi (1982) and approximately 3 per cent in the report of Lieber et al. (1981).

The tumors are typically unifocal, though several case reports of multifocal oncocytoma have been reported. Warfel and Eble (1982) reported a case in which more than 200 small renal oncocytomas were found in a bilateral distribution. Persky et al. (1982) and Moura and Nasciment (1982) also reported cases of bilateral oncocytoma.

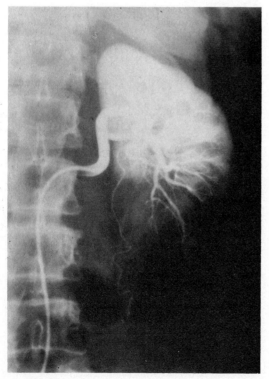

Figure 29–32. Arteriogram demonstrating hypovascular mass in left kidney. This proved to be a solitary metastasis of lymphoblastoma.

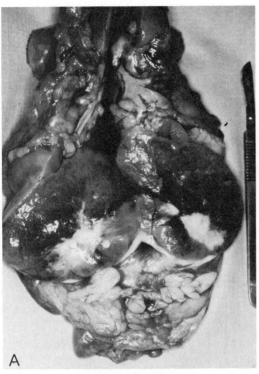
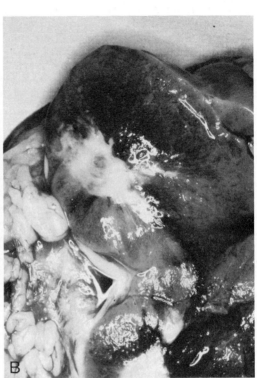
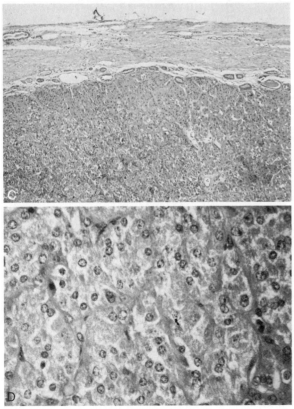

Figure 29–33. *A* and *B,* Gross appearance of a typical oncocytoma. The tumor was well circumscribed, light tan, and smooth, with no hemorrhage or necrosis. *C,* Microscopic pattern of the same tumor showing typical benign-appearing oncocytes (× 125). *D,* Higher power magnification demonstrating monotonous oncocytes with round nuclei, granular cytoplasm, and absence of mitotic figures (× 313).

The typical radiographic appearance is one of the clinical hallmarks of this neoplasm and has been largely responsible for its identification as a specific clinical entity. The pyelographic appearance is one of a circumscribed solid mass of varying size and location in the kidney. The arterial phase of the angiogram reveals a typical "spoke-wheel" or stellate pattern seldom associated with venous pooling or arteriovenous fistulae (Bonavita et al., 1981). However, the typical angiographic picture is not always identified, and the angiogram may be indistinguishable from that of a hypovascular renal cell carcinoma. No typical computerized tomography picture has been identified.

Numerous reports have demonstrated the benign nature of true renal oncocytoma (Merino and Livolsi, 1982; Bonavita et al., 1981; Lingeman et al., 1983; van der Walt et al., 1983). The largest experience was reported by Lieber et al. (1981) from the Mayo Clinic. Ninety cases satisfying the histologic criteria of renal oncocytoma were studied. None of the 62 patients with Grade I tumors developed metastases, but four patients with Grade II tumors died of metastatic disease. Barnes and Beckman (1983) indicated the importance of distinguishing oncocytomas from tumors that were histologically intermediate between oncocytoma and renal carcinoma. They identified a small group of tumors that resembled oncocytomas but also contained some characteristics of renal carcinoma. Some renal carcinomas had areas that microscopically resembled oncocytomas, and this finding was confirmed in the report by Lieber et al. (1981).

The management of renal oncocytomas therefore must be colored by these two characteristics: the unreliability of angiographic pattern, and the presence of malignant elements and oncocytoma cells in the same tumor. Clearly, a reliable preoperative diagnosis of renal oncocytoma merits an attempt at more conservative surgery, i.e., partial nephrectomy. However, as pointed out by Lieber et al. (1981), needle aspiration biopsy and even frozen-section diagnosis are insufficient for a secure diagnosis of oncocytoma. Radical nephrectomy is still the safest method of therapy unless contraindicated by other factors (e.g., solitary kidney, small size, poor renal function).

References

Albarran, J., and Imbert, L.: Les Tumeurs du Rein. Paris, Masson et Cie, 1903.

Allred, C. D., Cathey, W. J., and McDivitt, R. W.: Primary renal angiosarcoma: a case report. Hum. Pathol., 12:665, 1981.

Barnes, C. A., and Beckman, E. N.: Renal oncocytoma and its cocongeners. Am. J. Clin. Pathol., 79:312, 1983.

Beccia, D. J., Elkurt, R. J., and Rane, R. J.: Adjuvant chemotherapy in renal leiomyosarcoma.. Urology, 13:652, 1979.

Bell, E. T.: Renal Disease. 2nd ed. Philadelphia, Lea & Febiger, 1950, p. 435.

Bennington, J. L., and Beckwith, J. B.: Tumors of the kidney, renal pelvis and ureter. Atlas of Tumor Pathology. Washington, D. C., Armed Forces Institute of Pathology, 1975, Fasc. 12.

Biggers, R., and Stewart, J.: Primary renal osteosarcoma. Urology, 13:674, 1979.

Birch-Hirschfeld, F. V., and Doederlein, A.: Zentralbl. Krankh. Horn. Sex. Org., Vol. 3, 1894.

Bloom, D. A., Scardino, P. T., Ehrlich, R. M., and Waisman, J.: Significance of lymph nodal involvement in renal angiomyelolipoma. J. Urol., 128:1292, 1982.

Bloom, H. J.: Hormone induced and spontaneous regression of metastatic renal cancer. Cancer, 32:1006, 1973.

Bonavita, J. A., Pollack, H. M., and Banner, M. P.: Renal oncocytoma: further observations and literature review. Urol. Radiol., 2:229, 1981.

Bonnin, J. M., Cain, M. D., Jose, J. S., Mukherjee, T. M., Perrett, L. V., Scroop, G. C., and Seymour, A. E.: Hypertension due to a renin-secreting tumor localized by segmental renal vein sampling. Aust. N. Z. J. Med., 7:630, 1977.

Böttiger, L. E.: Prognosis in renal carcinoma. Cancer, 26:780, 1970.

Boxer, R. J., Waisman, J., Lieber, M. M., Mampaso, F. M., and Skinner, D. G.: Non-metastatic hepatic dysfunction associated with renal carcinoma. J. Urol., 119:468, 1978.

Brosman, S.: Non-specific immunotherapy in GU cancer. In Proceedings of Chicago Symposium. Chicago, Franklin Institute Press, 1977, p. 97.

Bukowski, R. M., Groppe, D., Reimer, R., Weick, J., and Hewlett, J. S.: Immunotherapy (IT) of metastatic renal cell carcinoma. Abstract C-457. Proc. Am. Assoc. Cancer Res. Am. Soc. Clin. Oncol., 20:402, 1979.

Carson, W. J.: Tumors of the kidney: Histologic study. Trans. Sect. Urol. A. M. A., 1928.

Chen, K. T.: Fibroxanthosarcoma of the kidney. Urology, 13:439, 1979.

Cherrie, R. J., Goldman, D. G., Lindner, A., and deKernion, J. B.: Prognostic implications of vena caval extension of renal cell carcinoma. J. Urol., 128:910, 1982.

Chisholm, G. D.: Nephrogenic ridge tumors and their syndromes. Ann. N. Y. Acad. Sci., 230:403, 1974.

Chute, R., Soutter, L., and Kerr, W.: The value of thoracoabdominal incision in the removal of kidney tumors. N. Engl. J. Med., 241:951, 1949.

Clayman, R. V., Gonzalez, R., and Fraley, E. E.: Renal cell carcinoma invading the inferior vena cava: clinical review and anatomical approach. J. Urol., 123:157, 1980.

Colvin, R. B., and Dickersin, G. R.: Pathology of renal tumors. In Skinner, D. G., and deKernion, J. B. (Eds.): Genitourinary Cancer. Philadelphia, W. B. Saunders Co., 1978.

Concolino, G., Marocchi, A., Conti, C., Tenaglia, R., DiSilverio, F., and Bracci, U.: Human renal cell carcinoma as a hormone dependent tumor. Cancer Res., 38:4340, 1978.

Cox, C. E., Lacy, S. S., Montgomery, W. G., and Boyce, W. H.: Renal adenocarcinoma: a 28 year review with emphasis on rationale and feasibility of preoperative radiotherapy. J. Urol., *104*:51, 1970.

Crawford, E. D., Gottesman, J. E., Grossman, B., and Scardino, P. T.: Renal infarction-nephrectomy for metastatic renal cancer: A Southwest Oncology Group Study. Presented at Annual Meeting of Southcentral Section of American Urological Association, New Orleans, 1982.

Cummings, K. B.: Surgical management of renal cell carcinoma with extension into the vena cava. *In* Crawford, E. E., and Borden, T. A. (Eds.): Genitourinary Cancer Surgery. Philadelphia, Lea & Febiger, 1982, pp. 70–85.

DaPonte, D., Zungri, E., Algaba, F., and Sole-Balcells, F.: Angiomyolipome rénal isolé—etude de 10 cas. J. Urol. Nephrol., *89*:267, 1983.

Day, J. W., Shrivastav, S., Lin, G., Bonar, R. A., and Paulson, D. F.: In vitro chemotherapeutic testing of urologic tumors. J. Urol., *125*:490, 1981.

deKernion, J. B.: Lymphadenectomy for renal cell carcinoma: therapeutic implications. Urol. Clin. North Am., *7*:697, 1980*a*.

deKernion, J. B.: Radical nephrectomy. *In* Ehrlich, R. E. (Ed.): Modern Techniques in Surgery. New York, Futura, pp. 1–14, 1980*b*.

deKernion, J. B., and Berry, D.: The diagnosis and treatment of renal cell carcinoma. Cancer, *45*:1947, 1980.

deKernion, J. B., and Lindner, A.: Treatment of advanced renal cell carcinoma. In Kuss, R., Murphy, G., Khoury, S., and Karr, J. (Eds.): Proceedings of the First International Symposium on Kidney Tumors. New York, Alan R. Liss, 1982, p. 614.

deKernion, J. B., and Ramming, K. P.: The therapy of renal adenocarcinoma with immune RNA. Invest. Urol., *17*:378, 1980.

deKernion, J. B., and Smith, R. B.: The kidney and adrenal glands. In Paulson, D. F. (Ed.): Genitourinary Surgery. Vol. 1 New York, Churchill Livingstone, 1984, pp. 1–153.

deKernion, J., Lindner, A., Figlin, R., Sarna, G., and Smith, R. B.: The treatment of metastatic renal cell carcinoma with a human leukocyte interferon. Proceedings of 19th Congress of Societé Internationale d'Urologie. J. Urol., *130*:1063, 1983.

deKernion, J. B., Ramming, K. P., and Smith, R. B.: Natural history of metastatic renal cell carcinoma: a computer analysis. J. Urol., *120*:148, 1978.

Deming, C. L., and Harvard, B. M.: Tumors of the kidney. *In* Campbell, M. F., and Harrison, J. H. (Eds.): Urology. Vol. 2. 3rd ed. Philadelphia, W. B. Saunders Co., 1970, p. 884.

DiEsidio, M., Gadaleta, A., Monina, M., and Cappeletti, V.: Retroperitoneal hemangiopericytoma. Presentation of a case with recurrence and multiple metastases. Radiol. Med. (Torino), *66*:331, 1980.

Dineen, M. K., Venable, D. D., and Misra, R. P.: Pure intrarenal lipoma—report of a case and review of the literature. Presented at the Annual Meeting, Southeastern Section of the American Urologic Association, Florida, 1983.

Economou, J. S., Lindner, A., Smith, R. B., Ehrlich, R. M., and deKernion, J. B.: Management of genitourinary sarcomas in adults. J. Urol. In press.

Farrow, G. M., Harrison, E. G., Utz, D. C., and Remine, W. H.: Sarcomas and sarcomatoid and mixed malignant tumors of the kidney in adults. Cancer, *22*:545, 1968.

Figlin, R. A., deKernion, J. B., Maldazys, J., and Sarna, G. P.: Human leukocyte interferon (IFN/vinblastine (VBL) therapy for metastatic renal cell carcinoma (RCCa). Proc. Am. Soc. Clin. Oncol. In press.

Finney, R.: The value of radiotherapy in the treatment of hypernephroma—a clinical trial. Br. J. Urol., *45*:258, 1973.

Fisher, E. R., and Horvat, B.: Comparative ultrastructural study of so-called renal adenoma and carcinoma. J. Urol., *108*:382, 1972.

Freed, S. Z.: Nephrectomy for renal cell carcinoma with metastases. Urology, *9*:613, 1977.

Glenn, J. F.: Renal tumors. *In* Harrison, J. H., Gittes, R. F., Perlmutter, A. D., et al. (Eds.): Campbell's Urology. 4th ed. Philadelphia, W. B. Saunders Company, 1980.

Glover, S. D., and Buck, A. C.: Renal medullary fibroma: a case report. J. Urol., *127*:758, 1982.

Goldberg, M. F., Tashjian, A. H., Order, S. C., and Dammin, G. J.: Renal adenocarcinoma containing a parathyroid hormone–like substance and associated with marked hypercalcemia. Am. J. Med., *36*:805, 1964.

Grawitz, P.: Die sogenannten Lipome der Niere. Virchows Arch. [Pathol. Anat.] *93*:39, 1883.

Greene, L. F., and Rosenthal, M. H.: Multiple hypernephromas of the kidney in association with Lindau's disease. N. Engl. J. Med., *244*:633, 1951.

Gutterman, J., Yap, Y., Buzdar, A., Alexanian, R., Hersh, E., Cabanillas, F., and Greenberg, S.: Leukocyte interferon (IF) induced tumor regression in patients (PTS) with breast cancer and B cell neoplasms. Abstract 674. Proc. Am. Assoc. Cancer Res. Am. Soc. Clin. Oncol., *20*:167, 1979.

Hand, J. R., and Broders, A. C.: Carcinoma of the kidney: the degree of malignancy in relation to factors bearing on prognosis. J. Urol., *28*:199, 1932.

Harris, R. P.: An analytical examination of 100 cases of extirpations of the kidney. Am. J. Med. Sci., *84*:109, 1882.

Hartman, D. S., Davis, C. J., Goldman, S. M., Friedman, A. C., and Fritzsche, P.: Renal lymphoma: radiologic-pathologic correlation of 21 cases. Radiology, *144*:759, 1982.

Heiken, J. P., Gold, R. P., Schnur, M. J., King, M. J., Bashist, B., and Glazer, H. S.: Computed tomography of renal lymphoma with ultrasound correlation. J. Comput. Assist. Tomogr., *7*:245, 1983.

Helmbrecht, L. J., and Cosgrove, M. D.: Triple therapy for leiomyosarcoma of the kidney. J. Urol., *112*:581, 1974.

Hersh, E. M., Wallace, S., Johnson, D. E., and Bracken, R. B.: Immunological studies in human urological cancer. *In* Johnson, D. E., and Samuels, M. L. (Eds.): Cancer of the Genitourinary Tract. New York, Raven Press, 1979.

Hoehn, W., and Hermanek, P.: Invasion of veins in renal cell carcinoma—frequency, correlation and prognosis. Eur. Urol., *9*:276, 1983.

Hrushesky, W. J., and Murphy, G. P.: Current status of the therapy of advanced renal carcinoma. J. Surg. Oncol., *9*:277, 1977.

Hultén, L., Rosencrantz, T., Seeman, L., Wahlquist, L., and Ahrén, C.: Occurrence and localization of lymph node metastases in renal cell carcinoma. Scand. J. Urol. Nephrol., *3*:129, 1969.

Jafri, S. Z., Bree, R. L., Amendola, M. A., Glazer, G. N., Schwab, R. E., Francis, I. R., and Borlaza, G.: CT of renal and perirenal non-Hodgkin lymphoma. Am. J. Radiol., *138*:1101, 1982.

Jaschke, W., van Kaick, G., Peter, S., and Palmtas, H.: Accuracy of computed tomography in staging of kidney tumors. Acta Radiol. [Diagn.] (Stockh.), *23*:593, 1982.

Kansara, V., and Powell, I.: Fibrosarcoma of the kidney. Urology, *16*:419, 1980.

Kantor, A. F.: Current concepts in the epidemiology and

etiology of primary renal cell carcinoma. J. Urol., *117*:415, 1977.

Karp, W., Ekelund, L., Olafsson, G., and Olsson, A.: Computed tomography, angiography and ultrasound in staging of renal carcinoma. Acta Radiol. [Diagn.] (Stockh.), *22*:625, 1981.

Kaufman, J. J., and Mims, M. M.: Tumors of the kidney. *In* Ravitch, M. M., Ellison, E. H., Julian, O. C., Thal, A. P., and Wangensteen, O. H. (Eds.): Current Problems in Surgery. Chicago, Yearbook Medical Publishers, 1966, pp. 1–44.

Kirkman, H., and Bacon, R. L.: Renal adenomas and carcinomas in diethylstilbestrol treated male golden hamsters. Anat. Rec., *103*:475, 1949.

Klinger, M. E.: Secondary tumors of the genitourinary tract. J. Urol., *65*:144, 1951.

Knoepp, L. F.: Lymphosarcoma of the kidney. Surgery, *39*:510, 1956.

Kolonel, L. N.: Association of cadmium with renal cancer. Cancer, *37*:1782, 1976.

Kothari, K., Segal, A. J., Spitzer, R. M., and Peartree, R. J.: Preoperative radiographic evaluation of hypernephroma. J. Comput. Assist. Tomogr., *5*:702, 1981.

Kyaw, M., and Koehler, P. R.: Renal and perirenal lymphoma: arteriographic findings. Radiology, *93*:1055, 1969.

Lakey, W. H.: Tumors of the kidney. *In* Karafin, L., and Kendall, A. R. (Eds.): Urology. Vol. 2. New York, Harper & Row, 1975.

Landier, J. F., Desligneres, S., Boccon-Gibod, L., and Steg, A.: Renal oncocytomas. Sem. Hop. Paris, *55*:1275, 1979.

Lang, E.: Comparison of dynamic and conventional computed tomography, angiography and ultrasonography in the staging of renal cell carcinoma. Radiology. In press.

Lang, E., and deKernion, J. B.: Transcatheter embolization of advanced renal cell carcinoma with radioactive seeds. J. Urol., *126*:581, 1981.

Lang, E. K.: Asymptomatic space occupying lesions of the kidney: a programmed sequential approach and its impact on quality and cost of health care. South. Med. J., *70*:277, 1977.

Lang, E. K.: Roentgenographic assessment of asymptomatic renal lesions. Radiology, *109*:257, 1973.

Lauritsen, J. G.: Lindau's disease: a study of one family through six generations. Acta Chir. Scand., *139*:482, 1975.

Lieber, M. M.: Soft agar colony formation assay for in vitro chemotherapy sensitivity testing of human renal cell carcinoma: Mayo Clinic experience. J. Urol., *131*:391, 1984.

Lieber, M. M., Tomera, K. M., and Farrow, G. M.: Renal oncocytomas. J. Urol., *125*:481, 1981.

Lieberman, S. F., Keller, F. S., Pearse, H. D., Fuchs, E. F., Rosch, J., and Barry, J. M.: Percutaneous vasoocclusion for non-malignant renal lesions. J. Urol., *129*:805, 1983.

Lindner, A., Goldman, D. G., and deKernion, J. B.: Cost effective analysis of prenephrectomy radioisotope scans in renal cell carcinoma. Urology, *22*:127, 1983.

Lingeman, J. E., Donohue, J. P., Madrua, J. A., and Selke, F.: Angiomyolipoma: emerging concepts in management. Urology, *20*:566, 1982.

Lingeman, J. E., Eble, J. N., and Donohue, J. P.: Renal oncocytomas: clinical and pathologic features. Presented at American Urologic Association Meeting, Las Vegas, 1983.

Marberger, M., Pugh, R. C. B., Auvert, J., Bertermann, H., Costantini, A., Gammelgaard, P. A., Petterson, S., and Wickham, J. E. A.: Conservative surgery of renal carcinoma: the EIRSS experience. Br. J. Urol., *53*:528, 1981.

Marshall, F., and Powell, K. C.: Lymphadenectomy for renal cell carcinoma: anatomical and therapeutic considerations. J. Urol., *128*:677, 1982.

Marshall, F. F., Reitz, B. A., and Diamond, D. A.: New technique for management of renal cell carcinoma involving right atrium: hypothermia and cardiac arrest. J. Urol., *131*:103, 1984.

Mathé, G.: Systemic immunotherapy in shifting from the Middle Ages to the Renaissance. I. The multiplication of randomized trials showing significant effect of active immunotherapy on residual minimal disease. Cancer Immunol. Immunother., *5*:149, 1978.

Mauro, M. A., Wadsworth, D. E., Stanley, R. J., and McClennan, B. L.: Renal cell carcinoma: angiography in the CT era. Am. J. Radiol., *139*:1135, 1982.

McCullough, D. L., and Gittes, R. F.: Ligation of the renal vein in the solitary kidney: effects on renal function. J. Urol., *113*:295, 1975.

McCullough, D. L., Scott, R., Jr., and Seybold, H. M.: Renal angiomyelolipoma (hamartoma): review of the literature and report of 7 cases. J. Urol., *105*:32, 1971.

McCune, C. S., deKernion, J. B., Huben, R. P., and Pontes, E.: Specific immunotherapy vs. Megace for metastatic renal cell carcinoma. A prospective randomized trial. J. Urol. In press.

McCune, C. S., Schapira, D. V., and Henshaw, E. C.: Specific immunotherapy of advanced renal carcinoma: evidence for the polyclonality of metastases. Cancer, *47*:1984, 1981.

McNichols, D. W., Segura, J. W., and deWeerd, J. H.: Renal cell carcinoma: long term survival and late recurrence. J. Urol., *126*:17, 1981.

Merigan, T. C., Sikora, K., Breeden, J. H., Levy, R., and Rosenberg, S. A.: Preliminary observations on the effect of human leukocyte interferon in non-Hodgkin's lymphoma. N. Engl. J. Med., *299*:1449, 1978.

Merino, M. J., and Livolsi, V. A.: Oncocytomas of the kidney. Cancer, *50*:1852, 1982.

Middleton, R. G.: Surgery for metastatic renal cell carcinoma. J. Urol., *97*:973, 1967.

Minton, J. P., Pennline, K., Nawrocki, J. F., Kibbey, W. E., and Dodd, M. C.: Immunotherapy of human kidney cancer. Abstract C-258. Proc. Am. Assoc. Cancer Res. Am. Soc. Clin. Oncol., *17*:301, 1976.

Moertel, C. G., Dockerty, M. B., and Baggenstoss, A. H.: Multiple primary multiple malignant neoplasms. III. Tumors of multicentric origin. Cancer, *14*:238, 1961.

Montie, J. E., Stewart, B. H., Straffon, R. A., et al.: The role of adjunctive nephrectomy in patients with metastatic renal cell carcinoma. J. Urol., *117*:272, 1977.

Moon, T. D., Dexter, D. F., and Morales, A.: Synchronous independent primary osteosarcoma and adenocarcinoma of the kidney. Urology, *21*:608, 1983.

Morales, A., Wilson, J. L., Pater, J. L., and Loeb, M.: Cytoreductive surgery and systemic bacillus Calmette-Guerin therapy in metastatic renal cancer: a phase II trial. J. Urol., *127*:230, 1982.

Moura, A. C., and Nasciment, A. G.: Renal oncocytoma: report of a case with unusual presentation. J. Urol., *127*:311, 1982.

Murphy, G. P., and Mostofi, F. K.: Histologic assessment and clinical prognosis of renal adenoma. J. Urol., *103*:31, 1970.

Myers, G. H., Fehrenbaker, L. G., and Kellais, P. P.: Prognostic significance of renal vein invasion by hypernephroma. J. Urol., *100*:420, 1968.

Nagamatsu, G.: Dorso-lumbar approach to kidney and adrenal with osteoplastic flap. J. Urol., *63*:569, 1950.

Niceta, T., Lavengood, R. W., Jr., Fernandes, M., and Tozzo, P. J.: Leiomyosarcoma of the kidney: review of the literature. Urology, *3*:270, 1974.

O'Dea, M. J., Zincke, H., Utz, D. C., and Bernatz, P. E.: The treatment of renal cell carcinoma with solitary metastases. J. Urol., *120*:540, 1978.

Olsson, C. A.: Pulmonary cancer metastatic to the kidney: a common renal neoplasm. J. Urol., *105*:492, 1971.

Ordonez, N. G., Bracken, R. B., and Stroehlein, K. B.: Hemangiopericytoma of the kidney. Urology, *20*:191, 1982.

Orjauvik, O. S., Aas, M., Fauchald, P., Hovig, T., Oystese, B., Brodwall, E. K., and Flatmark, A.: Renin-secreting renal tumor with severe hypertension. Acta Med. Scand., *197*:329, 1975.

Osamura, R. Y., Watanabe, K., Yoneyama, K., and Hayashi, T.: Malignant fibrous histiocytoma of the renal capsule: light and electron microscopic study of a rare tumor. Virchows Arch. [Pathol. Anat.], *380*:377, 1978.

Patel, N. P., and Lavengood, R. W.: Renal cell carcinoma: natural history and results of treatment. J. Urol., *119*:722, 1978.

Peeling, W. B., Martell, B., and Shepheard, B. G.: Postoperative irradiation in the treatment of renal cell carcinoma. Br. J. Urol., *41*:23, 1969.

Persky, L., Fu, Y. S., and Chidi, J.: Unusual presentation of renal oncocytoma. Presented at American Urologic Association, Kansas City, 1982.

Peters, P.: The role of lymphadenectomy in the management of renal cell carcinoma. Urol. Clin. North Am., *7*:705, 1980.

Pfeiffer, G. E., and Gandin, M. M.: Massive perirenal lipoma with report of a case. J. Urol., *56*:12, 1946.

Plimton, C. H., and Gelhorn, A.: Hypercalcemia in malignant disease without evidence of bone destruction. Am. J. Med., *21*:750, 1956.

Prager, M. D., Baechtel, F. S., Peters, P. C., Brown, G. L., and Greene, C. L.: Specific immunotherapy of human metastatic renal cell carcinoma. Abstract 647. Proc. Am. Assoc. Cancer Res. Am. Soc. Clin. Oncol., *22*:163, 1981.

Quesada, J. R., Gutterman, J. U., Swanson, D., and Trinidade, A.: Antitumor effects of partially pure human leukocyte interferon in renal cell carcinoma. Abstract 562. Proc. Am. Assoc. Cancer Res., Am. Soc. Clin. Oncol., *23*:143, 1982.

Raghavaiah, N. V., Mayer, R. F., Hagitt, R., and Soloway, M. S.: Malignant fibrous histiocytoma of the kidney. J. Urol., *123*:951, 1980.

Ramming, K. P., and deKernion, J. B.: Immune RNA therapy for renal cell carcinoma: survival and immunologic monitoring. Ann. Surg., *186*:459, 1977.

Rao, M. S., Lotuaco, L. G., and McGregor, D. H.: Carcinosarcoma of the adult kidney. Postgrad. Med. J., *53*:408, 1977.

Raval, B., and Lamki, N.: Computed tomography in detection of occult hypernephroma. CT, *7*:199, 1983.

Richie, E. W.: The place of radiotherapy in the management of parenchymal carcinoma. J. Urol., *95*:313, 1966.

Richie, J. P., Garnick, M. B., Seltzer, S., and Bettman, M. A.: Computerized tomography scan for diagnosis and staging of renal cell carcinoma. J. Urol., *129*:1114, 1983.

Richie, J. P., Wang, B. S., Steele, G. D., Jr., Wilson, R. E., and Mannick, J. A.: In vivo and in vitro effects of xenogeneic immune ribonucleic acid in patients with advanced renal cell carcinoma: a phase I study. J. Urol., *126*:24, 1981.

Robertson, P. W., Klidjiian A., Harding, L. K., Walters, G., Lee, M. R., and Robb-Smith, A. H.: Hypertension due to a renin-secreting renal tumor. Am. J. Med., *43*:963, 1967.

Robertson, T. D., and Hand, J. R.: Primary intrarenal lipoma of surgical significance. J. Urol., *46*:458, 1941.

Robson, C. J.: Radical nephrectomy for renal cell carcinoma. J. Urol., *89*:37, 1963.

Robson, C. J., Churchill, B. M., and Anderson, W.: The results of radical nephrectomy for renal cell carcinoma. Trans. Am. Assoc. Genitourin. Surg., *60*:122, 1968.

Saitoh, H., Shimbo, T., Wakabayashi, T., Takeda, M., and Ogishima, K.: Metastases of renal sarcoma. Tokai J. Exp. Clin. Med., *7*:365, 1982.

Salmon, S. E., Hamburger, A. W., Soehnlen, B., Durie, B. G. M., Alberts, D. S., and Moon, T. E.: Quantitation of differential of sensitivity of human tumor stem cells to anti-cancer drugs. N. Engl. J. Med., *298*:1321, 1978.

Sarna, G., Figlin, R., Bryson, Y., Mauritzon, N., and Cline, M.: A phase I trial of human lymphoblastoid interferon (HuLyINF) administered intermittently. Abstract C-155. Proc. Am. Soc. Clin. Oncol., *1*:39, 1982.

Schapira, D. V., McCune, C. S., and Henshaw, E. C.: Treatment of advanced renal cell carcinoma with specific immunotherapy consisting of autologous tumor cells and *C. parvum*. Abstract C-234. Proc. Am. Assoc. Cancer Res. Am. Soc. Clin. Oncol., *20*:348, 1979.

Schapira, R. A., Skinner, D. G., Stanley, P., and Edelbrock, H.: Renal tumors associated with tuberous sclerosis: the case for aggressive surgical management. Presented at 78th Annual Meeting of the American Urologic Association, Las Vegas, April 1983.

Selli, C., Hinshaw, W. M., Woodard, B. H., and Paulson, D. F.: Stratification of risk factors in renal cell carcinoma. Cancer, *52*:899, 1983.

Selvaggi, F. P., Fabiano, G., and Cantcroce, S.: Hypertensive renal rhabdomyosarcoma. Eur. Urol., *5*:371, 1979.

Shefft, P., Novick, A. C., Straffon, R. A., and Stewart, B. H.: Surgery for renal cell carcinoma extending into the inferior vena cava. J. Urol., *120*:28, 1978.

Silber, S. J., and Chang, C. Y.: Primary lymphoma of the kidney. J. Urol., *110*:282, 1973.

Silverberg, E.: Cancer statistics, 1984. Cancer, *34*:7, 1984.

Siminovitch, J. M., Montie, J. E., and Straffon, R. A.: Prognostic indicators in renal adenocarcinoma. J. Urol., *130*:20, 1983.

Skinner, D. G., Pfister, R. F., and Colvin, R.: Extension of renal cell carcinoma into the vena cava: the rationale for aggressive surgical management. J. Urol., *107*:711, 1972.

Smith, R. B., deKernion, J. B., Ehrlich, R. M., Skinner, D. G., and Kaufman, J. J.: Bilateral renal cell carcinoma and renal cell carcinoma in the solitary kidney. J. Urol., *132*:450, 1984.

Smullens, S. N., Scotti, D., Osterholm, J., and Weiss, A.: Preoperative embolization of retroperitoneal angiopericytomas as an aid in their removal. Proc. Am. Assoc. Cancer Res., *20*:394, 1979.

Stehm, E. R., Kronenberg, L. H., Rosenblatt, H. M., Bryson, Y., and Merigan, T. C.: Interferon: immunobiology and clinical significance. Ann. Intern. Med., *96*:80, 1982.

Stewart, B. H.: Radical nephrectomy. *In* Stewart, B. H. (Ed.): Operative Urology: The Kidney, Adrenal Gland and Retroperitoneum. Baltimore, The Williams & Wilkins Co., 1975.

Sufrin, G., Mirand, E. A., Moore, R. H., et al.: Hormones in renal cancer. J. Urol., *117*:433, 1977.

Sun, C. N., Bissada, N. K., White, H. J., and Redman, J. F.: Spectrum of ultrastructural patterns of renal cell carcinoma. Urology, *9*:195, 1977.

Swanson, D., Johnson, D. E., von Eschenbach, A. C., Chuang, V. P., and Wallace, S.: Angioinfarction plus nephrectomy for metastatic renal cell carcinoma—an update. J. Urol., *130*:449, 1983.

Tannenbaum, M.: Ultrastructural pathology of human renal cell tumors. Pathol. Annu., *6*:249, 1971.

Thorling, E. B.: Paraneoplastic erythrocytosis and inappropriate erythropoietin production. Scand. J. Haematol. (Suppl.), *17*:1, 1972.

Topley, M., Novick, A. C., and Montie, J. E.: Long term results following partial nephrectomy for localized renal adenocarcinoma. Presented at American Urologic Association Annual Meeting, Las Vegas, 1983.

Tykkä, H.: Active specific immunotherapy with supportive measures in the treatment of advanced palliatively nephrectomised renal adenocarcinoma. A controlled clinical study. Scand. J. Urol. Nephrol. (Suppl.), *63*:1, 1981.

Utz, D. C., Warren, M. M., and Gregg, J. A.: Reversible hepatic dysfunction associated with hypernephroma. Mayo Clin. Proc., *45*:161, 1970.

van der Walt, J. D., Reid, H. A., Rigdon, R. A., and Shaw, J. H.: Renal oncocytoma. A review of the literature and report of an unusual multicentric case. Virchows Arch. [Pathol. Anat.], *398*:291, 1983.

van der Wurf-Messing, B.: Carcinoma of the kidney. Cancer, *32*:1056, 1973.

Wallace, A. C., and Nairn, R. C.: Renal tubular antigens in kidney tumors. Cancer, *29*:977, 1972.

Walther, P. J., Marks, L. S., Stern, D., and Smith, R. B.: Renal metastasis of adenocarcinoma of the lung: massive hematuria managed by therapeutic embolization. J. Urol., *122*:398, 1979.

Warfel, K. A., and Eble, J. N.: Renal oncocytomatosis. J. Urol., *127*:1179, 1982.

Weichselbaum, A., and Greenish, R. W.: Pasadenome der Neire. Med. Jahrb. Vien. Vol. 213, 1883.

Weir, J. M., and Dunn, J. E., Jr.: Smoking and mortality: a prospective study. Cancer, *25*:105, 1970.

Wenz, W.: Tumors of the kidney following retrograde pyelography with colloidal thorium dioxide. Ann. N. Y. Acad. Sci., *145*:806, 1967.

Wickham, J. E. A.: Conservative renal surgery for adenocarcinoma. The place of bench surgery. Br. J. Urol., *47*:25, 1975.

Wolff, J.: Die Lehre von der Krebskronsheit. Von den altesten Zeiten bis zur Gagenwart. *In* Adenome der Neire. Med. Jahrb. Vien, Vol. 213, 1883.

Zincke, H., and Swanson, S. K.: Bilateral renal cell carcinoma: influence of synchronous and asynchronous occurrence on patient survival. J. Urol., *128*:913, 1982.

CHAPTER 30

Transitional Cell Cancer: Upper Tracts and Bladder

MICHAEL J. DROLLER, M.D.

INTRODUCTION

In recent years, many advances have been made in our understanding of the biology of transitional cell cancer. In several instances, this has led directly to changes in an approach to therapy. In many respects, however, transitional cell cancers of both the upper tract and the bladder remain poorly defined entities.

For example, although urothelial cancers may assume any one of several different forms (in situ, superficial, or infiltrative), our knowledge of what determines or reflects ultimate tumor behavior remains limited: We do not yet know why different forms of transitional cell cancer occur or whether their development follows the same or separate but interrelated pathways; we cannot predict whether a tumor will remain regionally confined or whether cancer cells will metastasize; moreover, we are ignorant as to the timing of these events in the overall course of a patient's disease.

Many of the problems associated with selecting the most effective treatment for the various forms of urothelial cancer reflect this situation. Not only are the answers to such questions likely to be critical in determining the most effective treatments for each of these cancers, but also it is probably only within this context that the efficacy of such treatments can be assessed.

The purpose of this chapter is to review current concepts of the epidemiology, natural history, staging, methods of diagnosis, and approaches to treatment of the various forms of transitional cell cancer as they involve various structures in the urinary tract. Attention will focus upon those factors that may determine distinct behavioral patterns of the various forms of transitional cell cancer at each organ site. The results of various treatments will be assessed in this context. This will constitute the basis for a discussion of those treatments that are at present viewed as controversial. Taken together, these may permit the determination of those areas that may prove fruitful for future investigation.

TRANSITIONAL CELL CANCER OF THE BLADDER

Epidemiology

INCIDENCE AND MORTALITY PATTERNS

New diagnoses of bladder cancer will comprise 37,000 cases in the United States in 1983 to 1984 (American Cancer Society, 1983). Of these, 27,000 will involve males and 10,000 will involve females. Generally, age-adjusted incidence rates for males have varied between 2 and 8 per 100,000, and incidence rates for females have ranged between 1 and 2.5 per 100,000 (Fig. 30–1) (Matanoski and Elliott, 1981). The overall incidence in populations over 40 years of age has been found to be approximately 20 per 100,000. Bladder cancer has also been found to occur nearly twice as frequently in white males as in black males and with a 44 per cent greater incidence in white females than in black females (Davies, 1977).

Age-incidence curves demonstrate an increase at a constant rate throughout adult life for both whites and blacks of both sexes, but the incidence for women born after 1920 is higher than that for women born prior to this

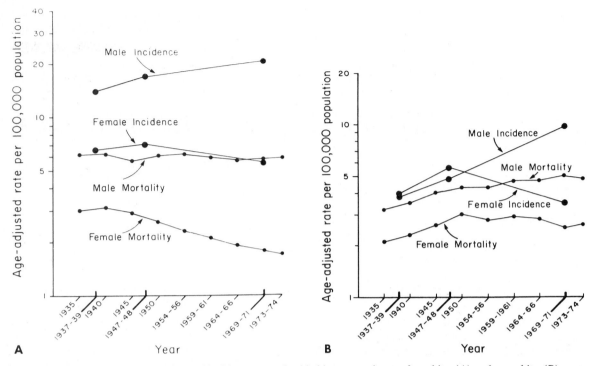

Figure 30–1. Age-adjusted mortality and incidence rates for bladder cancer by sex for white *(A)* and nonwhite *(B)* races (incidence adapted from First–Third National Cancer Surveys; mortality representing U.S. rates 1935–1974).

   Data from these surveys show stable mortality but rising incidence of bladder cancer in white males; increase in both rates (with incidence increasing at a faster rate) in nonwhite males; decrease in incidence in females of all races; and a stable (nonwhite) or declining (white) mortality in females. The increased incidence in males without similar increases in mortality may represent the type of bladder cancer that develops in response to environmental carcinogens (superficial papillary proliferative lesions that are not generally life-threatening). Corresponding decreased incidences in females may represent decreased exposure to some environmental carcinogens despite the hypothetical effects of increased smoking. (From Matanoski, G. M., and Elliott, E. A.: Epidemiol. Rev., *3*:203, 1981. Based on Devesa, S. S., and Silverman, D. T.: J. Natl. Cancer Inst., *60*:545, 1978. Used by permission.)

date (Fig. 30–2) (Hoover and Cole, 1971; Devesa and Silverman, 1978). This may reflect the influence that specific risk factors (smoking, industrial exposure, artificial sweeteners) have had for individual subpopulations in accordance with changing patterns of exposure during different periods of time. In addition, correlations between mortality rates and geographic distribution in the United States have demonstrated that residence in urban areas and location in the northeastern United States, where chemical industries are found in high concentration, are serious risk factors for development of bladder cancer (Blot and Fraumeni, 1978; Hoover and Fraumeni, 1975).

   The epidemiologic significance of mortality rates has been more difficult to assess (Fig. 30–3). Despite previous reports that males had a higher mortality rate than females, recent studies have described essentially identical 3- and 5-year survivals for both sexes (63 per cent and 60 per cent for males, 57 per cent and 56 per

cent for females, respectively) (Burbank and Fraumeni, 1970). Similarly, despite differences in incidence rates between blacks and whites, mortality rates have been more nearly identical (Wynder and Goldsmith, 1977).

   At first glance, these differences can be interpreted as reflecting either differences in treatment, shorter time to diagnosis, or differences in disease expression (i.e., initially localized in 75 per cent of whites versus 50 per cent of blacks) (Wynder and Goldsmith, 1977). However, it is equally plausible that the proportion of life-threatening forms of the disease has remained relatively constant despite an overall increased incidence of all bladder cancer cases (incorporating both superficial and infiltrative forms of disease). This would imply that environmental risk factors induced an increase only in the less aggressive, superficial (proliferative) forms of disease, while the more aggressive (infiltrative) forms of cancer were more strongly affected by host factors and by their own intrin-

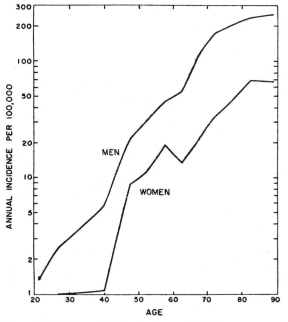

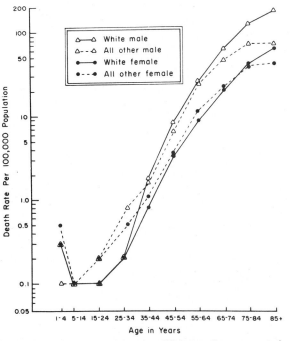

Figure 30–2. Annual incidence curves of bladder cancer per 100,000 population by age and sex (International list No. 181).

These curves clearly show an increased incidence of bladder cancer at a constant rate throughout adult life. Bladder cancer is more common in men than in women in each nation studied, with a ratio well over 2:1 in the United States. (From Cole, P., et al.: N. Engl. J. Med., *284*:129, 1971. Used by permission.)

Figure 30–3. Age-specific mortality rates for cancers of urinary organs by race and sex.

These curves demonstrate an increased death rate from bladder cancer with age from 25 years through all remaining age groups. The peak under age 5 years represents an increased death rate from kidney neoplasma. Death rates at older ages represent primarily cancers of the bladder. Mortality rates are higher for males than for females in all age groups. Deaths in nonwhite groups generally exceed those in white groups at younger ages (till ages 35 to 44 years). The relative roles of environmental and host factors in producing the types of cancers that lead to death as indicated in these figures are unknown. (From National Center for Health Statistics. Vital Statistics of the United States, 1975, Vol. II, Part A. Hyattsville, Md., 1979. Used by permission.)

sic characteristics regardless of the presence or absence of environmental factors. This would explain how the latter, as possibly more independent of the effects of external factors, might be more likely to remain constant. Epidemiologic testing of this hypothesis seems strongly indicated.

RISK FACTORS

Environmental Agents. Several factors have been implicated etiologically in the development of bladder cancer. Study of their mechanism of action has led to the concept that neoplastic transformation is a multistep phenomenon that reflects an interaction between processes known as initiation and promotion (Fig. 30–4). According to Farber (1981), "The various steps are characterized by cell populations that represent stages in the cellular evolution from normal, through initiated, pre-neoplastic cells, to highly malignant neoplasia."

"Initiation" is a process in which biochemical lesions are introduced into nuclear deoxyribonucleic acid (DNA) and other cellular macromolecules (Brooker 1980; Cohen, 1979). This process is thought to be rapid and to

require at least one cell cycle to produce an irreversible state. In most instances, metabolic conversion to chemically active derivatives, known as ultimate carcinogens, is required for initiation (Miller, 1978). The reactive derivative appears to be a positively charged molecule or "electrophilic reactant" that can interact with electron-dense sites on cellular DNA (Farber, 1981). Resultant lesions are then responsible for mispairing of nucleotide bases and subsequent mutations that lead to carcinogenesis (Lawley, 1976). Some have therefore suggested that a substance has to be activated within close proximity to the target cell in order to alter that cell's DNA (King, 1982). Initiation may thus require enzymatic activation of stable carcinogens by uroepithelial cells, while other enzymes capable of metabolizing these reactive derivatives to prevent carcinogenesis may balance

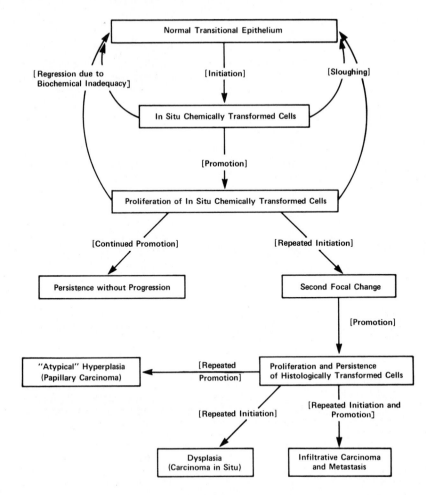

Figure 30–4. Mechanisms of carcinogenesis in bladder cancer.

Theoretical concepts of carcinogenesis in transitional cell cancer include a process known as "initiation," by which initial neoplastic transformation occurs, and one known as "promotion," by which cell replication is stimulated and neoplastic changes induced by initiation are fixed in place. Multiple steps of initiation and promotion may be needed to generate histologically recognizable transitional cell cancers. Regression or maturation may conceivably occur in the early phases of transformation in transitional cell cancer, possibly because the abnormal cells are sloughed into the urine and normal cells then take their place. In later phases, however, after repetitive initiation and promotion have taken place, regression and maturation may be less likely to occur. Interruption at different stages in the multiple steps involved in these processes may fix in place a certain phase of neoplastic transformation. Biochemical details of these processes are at present largely unknown. (Adapted from Droller, M. J.: Monogr. Urol., *3*:131, 1982. Used by permission.)

these effects. Processes that decrease the cell's capacity for DNA repair or that accelerate cell replication may enhance carcinogenesis by stabilizing any carcinogenic damage. This could explain the cumulative effects of carcinogens in the genesis of bladder cancer.

In contrast, the process of "promotion" is one in which selective stimulation of initiated cells leads to their proliferation and fixes in place any DNA changes brought about by initiation (Fig. 30–4) (Hiatt et al., 1977). Promotion, thought to be reversible until a tumor has actually developed, appears to require long periods of continued exposure to the promoting agent and may be cumulative for both a single and for several promoting agents (Cohen, 1979; Hicks, 1980).

Substances that promote tumor development are generally thought to cause only cell proliferation, or hyperplasia. Such cells lack those characteristics that permit uncontrolled growth and dissemination. Only when initiation

has taken place can promotion therefore presumably lead to the phenotypic expression of cancer. On the other hand, initiation by itself is also insufficient. According to Farber (1981), initiated cells have to be selectively stimulated to undergo focal hyperplasia: "The essence of promotion is the selective stimulation of initiated cells to grow relative to the surrounding cells, i.e., the creation of a differential growth environment, leading to focal proliferation (amplification or expansion) of the initiated cell population." Each sequence of focal change followed by selective proliferation brings the overall process closer to the overt development of cancer (Farber, 1981). Although the first sequence appears to be environmentally dependent, and initial focal proliferations may regress or mature to normal tissue, later sequences become self-generating and particular focal changes then persist and expand into the development of a preneoplastic state (Farber and Cameron, 1980). Repetitive exposures of the transitional epithelium to initiating and promoting agents may then be necessary for the development of clinically recognizable cancer (Hicks and Chowaniec, 1977; Hicks, 1980). In essence, the development of cancer appears to be a multistage process (Fig. 30–4).

These concepts are directly applicable to an analysis of factors that have been implicated in the genesis of bladder cancer. Thus, most, if not all, of these factors have a long latency period and their effects are cumulative. In addition, tumor incidence appears to be proportional to the dose of a given carcinogen, a relationship that may be modified if the reaction between the ultimate carcinogen and DNA is lethal to the cell rather than mutagenic (Hicks, 1981). This balance proscribes a greater carcinogenic hazard from the cumulative effects of low doses of environmental carcinogens than from a single high-dose exposure. Less clear is the question of whether the patient has an innate predisposition for, or resistance against, the development of cancer, and whether environmental factors play an initiator or promoter role either in the type of cancer that develops or in whether a cancer will be generated at all.

Animal models of carcinogen-induced bladder cancer have for the most part demonstrated the development of superficial papillary disease. Even when tumors have become invasive in these models, metastases have been rare (Cohen, 1979; Hicks and Chowaniec, 1977; Jacobs, et al., 1977). Corresponding clinical observations have suggested that carcinogens may be associated largely with the development of superficial disease. Progression to invasion in these instances has often been observed only in a smaller number of patients in whom host factors may conceivably have played a more prominent role (Matanoski and Elliott, 1981; Devesa and Silverman, 1978). That many patients with no known carcinogenic exposure develop the more aggressive types of bladder cancer without any prior history of superficial disease (Kaye and Lange, 1982; Prout, 1982) implies the possible primary importance of unknown host factors in the genesis of these more aggressive forms of disease.

INDUSTRIAL CARCINOGENS. In 1895, Rehn reported that workers involved in the manufacture of the fuchsin dye aniline were at risk for the development of bladder cancer (Rehn, 1895). Subsequently, the intermediates 2-naphthylamine and benzidine, rather than the aniline dye itself, were shown to be responsible for these instances of bladder cancer (Case et al., 1954).

Demonstrations of the role of carcinogens in experimental tumor development were unsuccessful until Hueper induced bladder cancer in dogs with beta-naphthylamine (Hueper et al., 1938). Other investigators then demonstrated that direct contact between carcinogens and transitional epithelium was necessary for bladder tumors to develop (McDonald and Lund, 1954; Scott and Boyd, 1953).

Similar associations with a variety of aromatic amines (beta-naphthylamine, 4-aminobiphenyl, 4-nitrobiphenyl, 2-naphthylamine, and benzidine) were subsequently reported (Case et al., 1954; Morrison and Cole, 1976). Variation in risk ratios for these chemicals was suggested to be based upon exposure time, ingestion dosages, urothelial metabolic capabilities (activation or deactivation), and possible intrinsic host susceptibility or resistance to neoplastic transformation (Farber, 1981; Hicks, 1981).

Epidemiologists have estimated that occupational exposures in high-risk industries accounted for 18 to 34 per cent of the overall bladder cancer experience in male populations (Cole et al., 1972; Cole, 1973). The subtlety of some of these associations was suggested by observations that carcinogen exposure might occur only during specific phases of manufacture (Case and Hosker, 1954), while tumors would be seen only after long latency periods (Armenian and Lilienfeld, 1974; Hoover and Cole, 1973; Wynder et al., 1963). Indeed, the highest risk was found to occur 40 to 50 years after exposure to industrial carcinogens (Cole et al., 1972), and longer exposure to carcinogen only shortened the latency period without substantially increasing risk (Case et al., 1954).

Tumor development in this context has not been limited to industrial carcinogen exposure. Recent studies have reported that azo dyes found in sewage could be broken down into aromatic amines by a variety of bacteria, including *E. coli* (Oyasu and Hopp, 1974). According to these reports, nitrosamines could be formed from nitrites and secondary amines under the acidic conditions in the stomach or by bacterial synthesis from dietary sources (e.g., nitrates and nitrites used as chemical food preservatives) within the urinary tract proper (Wolf, 1973; Oyasu and Hopp, 1974; Chapman et al., 1981). In fact, N-nitrosation and the formation of nitrosamines could take place at any site where nitrates, secondary amines, and nitrate-reducing bacteria occurred together (Hicks et al., 1977). Therefore, carcinogen exposure could not only derive from purely exogenous sources but could also reflect the production of endogenous aromatic amines, their metabolism by intestinal bacterial flora, or their activation by the urothelium itself (Radomski and Brill, 1970; Hicks et al., 1977).

Despite the tendency to view each of these associations as cause-effect phenomena, Hicks (1981) has suggested that bladder tumors that arise in this context do so as the result of "multiple sequential exposures to low doses of one or more carcinogens or by initiation of the neoplastic process by a low dose of a carcinogen followed by promotion with a co-factor that itself may not necessarily be a carcinogen." Taken together with the cumulative effect of large numbers of environmental carcinogens and the prolonged latency periods that have characterized intervals between exposure and cancer expression, these associations have supported the involvement of a multistep process in carcinogenesis.

CIGARETTE SMOKING. The association between cigarette smoking and bladder cancer was first noted in the mid-1950's when Lilienfeld reported a fourfold excess risk for development of bladder cancer among male smokers when compared with nonsmokers (Lilienfeld et al., 1956). Subsequent investigations reported that mortality rates were comparably increased (Best, 1966). More recent studies have suggested that 30 to 40 per cent of bladder cancer cases could be directly associated with cigarette smoking (Cole et al., 1971) and that this might even overshadow the influence of occupational carcinogens (Hoover and Cole, 1971).

The amount of smoking, the length of time from the onset of smoking, and the degree of inhalation have each been correlated with an increased risk and mortality from bladder cancer (Wynder and Goldsmith, 1977; Hoover and Cole, 1971; Wynder et al., 1963). Men who smoked one-half to two packs per day doubled their risk for developing bladder cancer, while those who smoked more than two packs per day tripled their risk, regardless of whether filter or nonfilter brands were used. Correspondingly, a decreased risk was found in men who had smoked for less than 20 to 30 years (Howe et al., 1980), although cessation had to have occurred 7 to 15 years before the risk was found to have been reduced (Wynder and Goldsmith, 1977). The use of other forms of tobacco in which no inhalation took place was not associated with an increased incidence of disease.

Women who smoke have also been found to have a significant excess risk for developing bladder cancer (Wynder and Goldsmith, 1977; Howe et al., 1980; Hoover and Cole, 1971).

However, only more recent cohorts of women have shown the predicted increased incidence of bladder cancer relative to the incidence in comparable cohorts of men (Campbell, 1973). Failure to demonstrate this risk in earlier studies was probably related to the later time at which women started smoking as well as to possible differences in their earlier patterns of inhalation (Lilienfeld et al., 1956; Cole et al., 1971). Given the probable latency that may exist between the onset of cigarette smoking, its overall quantity and duration, and the development of bladder cancer (Armstrong and Doll, 1975) and the assumption that the 1925 female birth cohort was the first to smoke cigarettes in a manner comparable to that of men (Haenszel et al., 1956), some have predicted that major increases in bladder cancer among women will not be seen before 1993.

Two pathways of carcinogenesis have been suggested to account for the association between bladder cancer and cigarette smoking. In one, high concentrations of tryptophan metabolites (see below) were found in the urine of cigarette smokers (Wolf, 1973; Kerr et al., 1965). Several studies, however, failed to confirm this association (Brown et al., 1970). Others hypothesized the presence of bladder carcinogens in cigarette smoke (Hecht et al., 1976; Wynder et al., 1963). For example, 2-naphthylamine and nitrosamines have been shown to be bladder carcinogens that are absorbed in the lungs and excreted in the urine (Hoffman et al., 1969; Hecht et al., 1976). Although present in cigarette smoke in only minute amounts, the cumulative effect of such carcinogens, especially in the presence of other potential environmental carcinogens, might create a situation in which neoplastic transformation would be likely to occur.

ARTIFICIAL SWEETENERS. Controversy concerning the putative carcinogenic nature of sodium cyclamate and sodium saccharine has centered on conflicting evidence from both animal and human studies. Both substances have been found to have carcinogenic activity as either initiators (cyclamates) or promoters (saccharine and cyclamates) in the etiology of bladder tumors in rodents (Price et al., 1970; Hicks and Chowaniec, 1977). Critics of these studies suggested that the doses of each substance used (500 to 700 times those used by humans) were clinically irrelevant and that carcinogenic effects were shown only after exposure in utero or in the neonatal period (Price et al., 1970; Isselbacher and Cole, 1977). On the other hand, proponents of these studies, rationalizing that dosages had to be increased in animal studies in order to shorten the latency period of carcinogenicity and make tumor development evident during an animal's short life expectancy, suggested that carcinogenicity is an intrinsic property of a chemical and that dosage is irrelevant if a carcinogenic effect at any dose can be demonstrated (Sontag, 1980).

Cyclamates were not used widely in the United States until 1963 and were withdrawn in 1969 because of incriminating data regarding their carcinogenicity. Because the population of cyclamate users has not yet experienced a sufficiently long latency, it may be too early to evaluate any effects on bladder cancer development from this period of use (Matanoski and Elliott, 1981).

In contrast, saccharine has been used for many years by diabetics, but no excess clinical risk of bladder cancer development has yet been documented (Armstrong and Doll, 1975; Kessler, 1970). Moreover, no significant differences have been seen between bladder cancer patients and controls in amount, duration, or frequency of use of non-nutritive sweetener (Kessler and Clark, 1978; Connolly et al., 1978; Wynder and Stellman, 1980; Morrison and Buring, 1980). Some have suggested that selected subgroups (nonsmoking females, male heavy smokers) may indeed have an excess risk, even if this does not characterize the general population (Hoover and Strasser, 1980). This remains to be confirmed.

The widespread acceptance of these substances by nondiabetic populations is a relatively recent phenomenon. Since the latency period for development of bladder cancer may be long, it is currently impossible to determine any overall enhanced carcinogenic risk for the general public.

COFFEE DRINKING. An association between bladder cancer and coffee consumption has been based upon inconclusive findings (Cole, 1971; Simon et al., 1975). Either the true risk is too low to detect epidemiologically or the high frequency of coffee drinking in the general population has made the actual risk difficult to discern (Marrett et al., 1983). That coffee intake is also often associated both with smoking and with artificial sweeteners may further confuse pertinent observations. Those correlates that have been reported have been weak, and dose-response relationships have not been well documented (Morrison, 1978; Fraumeni et al., 1971).

SCHISTOSOMIASIS. Geographic differences in the incidence of squamous cell cancer relative to transitional cell cancer probably reflect differences in the incidence of schistosomiasis in these areas (Brand, 1979; Oyasu and Hopp, 1974). In Egypt, for example, where 70 per cent of bladder cancers are of the squamous cell type, the prevalence of schistosomiasis is as high as 45 per cent (Hinder and Schmaman, 1969). In this regard, higher levels of ova have been found in the bladder wall of patients having squamous cell cancer compared with patients having transitional cell cancer (Hinder and Schmaman, 1969). In each case, bladder cancers have been associated with infestations that were severe and long-standing (Gelfand et al., 1967).

The chronic irritation and resultant epithelial proliferation associated with the deposition of schistosome eggs in the bladder wall ultimately could be misdirected into abnormal hyperplasia and metaplasia. A spontaneous chromosomal error in regenerative cells could then become the initiating carcinogenic focus (Brand, 1979). The concomitant chronic foreign body reaction and fibrosis have been postulated to block lymphatics and thereby permit carcinogenic chemicals or metabolites to accumulate (Brand, 1979).

Several observations, however, have suggested that schistosomal infestation alone may be insufficient cause for carcinogenesis. For example, although ova have been found along the entire length of bilharzial ureters, evidence of neoplasia has been rare (Wallace, 1981). Explanations have invoked either a more prolonged tumor latency in the ureter or the possibility that bilharzial ova act only as promoters and require initiators to generate the multistep process of tumor development. Nitrites, which are used as fertilizers in areas in which schistosomiasis is endemic, have been suggested as one possible source of nitrosamines in the bladder (Wallace, 1981).

Bacterial infections leading to the production of nitrosamines as proximate carcinogens have also been suggested to play a role in the genesis of these cancers (Chevlen et al., 1979; El-Menzabani et al., 1979; Magee and Barnes, 1967). Bacteria have been found to be a rich source of nitrate reductase, which may reduce nitrates to nitrites that react in turn with amines in the urine to form carcinogenic nitrosamines (Hawksworth and Hill, 1971; El-Menzabani et al., 1979). In addition, *E. coli* and *Pseudomonas,* commonly present in the bladder of bilharzial patients, have been found to have a high level of beta-glucoronidase (Barber et al., 1951, Beall and Grant, 1952). Hydrolysis of conjugated inactive carcinogens to active carcinogens by this enzyme and their exposure to an already damaged urothelium might contribute further to the genesis of bilharzial bladder cancer (El-Aaser et al., 1979, Norden and Gelfand, 1972).

CHRONIC IRRITATION AND INFECTION. On the basis of observations in schistosomiasis, a strong association has also been postulated to exist between chronic irritation or infection and the development of both transitional cell and squamous cell cancer in nonschistosomal bladders. The predominant association in these instances has been between the existence of a neurogenic bladder, the need for chronic indwelling catheters, the concomitant presence of chronic infection, and the resultant genesis of squamous cell carcinoma (Kaufman et al., 1977; Broecker et al., 1981). For example, Kaufman observed squamous cancer on random biopsy in 6 of 62 spinal cord injury patients, 5 of whom were among 25 who had had indwelling urethral catheters for more than 10 years. Squamous metaplasia was more common in those catheterized for more than 10 years (80 per cent) compared with those catheterized for shorter periods (40 per cent) and those not catheterized at all (20 per cent). Similar findings were made in the urethra of these patients (67 per cent, 36 per cent, and 44 per cent, respectively).

The predisposition of such patients to bacterial infection, stones, chronic foreign body reactions, and obstruction has been associated with an estimated 16 to 20 times higher risk for development of squamous cell cancer (El-Masri et al., 1981; Melzak, 1966). In addition, patients with defunctionalized bladders who develop pyocystis have been suggested to be at risk for tumor development if their condition is of long duration (Garvin et al., 1977). In one study of 36 patients at risk for development of squamous carcinoma under such circumstances, squamous metaplasia was seen in 90 per cent of those with chronic infected bladder and in 64 per cent of those with a postdiversion bladder. The need for continued urine flow to these bladders and the role of prolonged exposure to extrinsic urinary carcinogens in these instances remains to be clarified (Moloney et al., 1981).

PHENACETIN AND ANALGESIC ABUSE. Phenacetin as an analgesic and antipyretic has been in common use since its introduction in 1887 (Flower et al., 1980). It was not until 1965, however, that Hultergren described five patients with transitional cell cancer of the renal pelvis, all of whom had ingested 5 to 15 kg of phenacetin during a 10-year period (Hultergren et al., 1965). Bengtsson then reported nine patients with transitional cell tumors of the renal pelvis

and two with transitional cell tumors of the bladder, all of whom had ingested large quantities of phenacetin (Bengtsson et al., 1968). Subsequent reports indicated that most of these patients were female (reversing the male preponderance that was usually seen in transitional cell cancer) and that nearly half of them had consumed more than 5 kg of compound analgesic (Gankeer and deRuiter, 1979; Angervall et al., 1969; Juusela, 1973; Rathert et al., 1975; Wahlqvist, 1980). Similar findings in Australia and New Zealand confirmed the association between phenacetin and the development of both upper tract and bladder transitional cell cancer (Taylor, 1972; Mahoney et al., 1977).

The overall risk of developing bladder cancer in this setting was estimated to be 2.6:1 (McCredie et al., 1983), with the risk increasing to 4:1 if as much as 2 kg of phenacetin had been ingested (Fokkens, 1979). Latency was estimated to range between 15 and 20 years for upper tract tumors, with a longer induction period for patients who developed bladder cancer (Tosi and Movin, 1977; Johansson and Wahlqvist, 1977).

The precise mechanism by which analgesic compounds induce transitional cell carcinoma is unclear. Phenacetin is an aniline derivative, and its carcinogenicity may be related to its ortho-hydroxyamine metabolites (Buck et al., 1966; Prescott, 1970; Rathert et al., 1975). Others have suggested that drugs compounded with the phenacetin, such as caffeine, may play a role in tumor development. Whether the nephrotoxic effect of phenacetin is what creates a predilection for tumor development in the kidney is unclear (Taylor, 1972). Similarly unclear is whether cigarette smoking may enhance this risk (Mahoney et al., 1977). Some have suggested that smoking's effect on the kidney might induce an alteration in the metabolism of phenacetin, which might then in turn lead to carcinogenesis (Kuntzman et al., 1977).

Acetaminophen (Tylenol) is metabolized to paracetamol, the same substance that is a product of phenacetin metabolism (Prescott, 1970). At present, however, an association between Tylenol ingestion and transitional cell cancer has not been demonstrated. Whether the time interval is still too short to demonstrate an association in this setting remains to be determined.

CYCLOPHOSPHAMIDE. An increased incidence of bladder cancer has been reported to follow use of cyclophosphamide after a relatively short latency (Pearson and Soloway, 1978; Seltzer et al., 1978). Patients with systemic lupus erythematosus and rheumatoid arthritis treated with cyclophosphamide have been found to have a 3 per cent incidence of bladder cancer and a nine times higher risk for developing bladder cancer than comparable groups not taking this drug (Plotz et al., 1979; Fairchild et al., 1979). In a recent review of 16 cases of cyclophosphamide-associated bladder cancers, intervals of 6 to 13 years were seen between initiation of treatment and diagnosis of tumor; 11 patients had had antecedent hemorrhagic cystitis, and 13 cases of invasive tumors were documented (Durkee and Benson, 1980).

Others, however, have suggested that an association between cyclophosphamide ingestion and bladder tumor development has not been proved (Pearson and Soloway, 1978). First, many of these patients have been exposed to a variety of carcinogenic treatments (radiotherapy, other chemotherapeutic agents). In addition, administration of cyclophosphamide to experimental animals in the presence of other carcinogens did not enhance the development of bladder tumors (Hicks et al., 1975). Nonetheless, cyclophosphamide creates a setting that is hypothetically conducive to bladder carcinogenesis. Its administration leads to epithelial necrosis within 24 hours, followed by rapid regeneration and hyperplasia (Koss, 1967; Goldman and Warner, 1970). This may set the stage for exposure to the alkylating action of cyclophosphamide metabolites, with ensuing repetitive initiation and promotion ultimately leading to tumor development. Proof of this mechanism requires further study.

ONCOGENIC VIRUSES. A potential association between viral infection and bladder cancer was initially based on reports that viruses could be isolated from transitional cell tumors and could be shown to produce cytopathic changes in tissue culture cells (Fraley et al., 1974a). Such cells appeared to contain virus-like particles that resembled those in the original tumor (Fraley et al., 1974b), and sera from patients with transitional cell tumors appeared to prevent the cytopathic changes induced by these viruses in tissue culture (Elliott et al., 1973; Fraley et al., 1974a).

Other studies questioned the significance of these observations. The potentially oncogenic oncornaviruses were found to be common contaminants of tissue culture, and polyomaviruses were found to cause only asymptomatic infections in humans and were not found to be associated with tumor development (Gardner et al., 1971; Gardner, 1973).

Interest in the role of viruses in bladder cancer has recently been resurrected by descriptions of so-called oncogenes. The original oncogene hypothesis suggested that cancer arose from viral genes inserted into germ cells and that activation by mutagenic events during aging and exposure to carcinogens would induce tumor development (Huebner and Todaro, 1969). This concept supported earlier suggestions that the viral genes associated with transitional cell cancer might be transmitted vertically in man and activated by environmental physical or chemical factors (Fraley et al., 1974a).

Recently described oncogenes in bladder tumor cell lines and the resultant production of increased levels of abnormal proteins have been suggested to be responsible for the phenotypic expression of neoplastic transformation (Cooper, 1982). Although attempts to identify similar oncogenes in fresh bladder tumor tissue have thus far generally been unsuccessful (Feinberg et al., 1983), the repeated demonstration of these oncogenes in bladder cancer cell lines continues to support their suggested importance in malignant transformation of transitional epithelium. Particularly intriguing have been reports that oncogenes are not alien to the host cell but are believed to have arisen from the cell's own genome (Eva et al., 1982; Pulciani et al., 1982) and that such so-called proto-oncogenes may be an intrinsic part of every vertebrate cell (Aaronson, 1984).

Oncogenes activated as the result of carcinogen stimulation may serve as growth factors and growth factor receptors and may regulate cell growth through their enzyme capabilities. A single oncogene, however, may only induce cell proliferation (Bishop and Varmus, 1982). Several may be required to produce an oncogene cascade and induce transformation, with the ultimate expression of clinical cancer (Hunter, 1984). Hence, the apparent association between oncogenes and the multistep process of initiation and promotion, proliferation and fixation of altered DNA base-pairing, in the genesis of bladder cancer by bladder carcinogens. It remains to be seen whether the oncogene cascade is pertinent in only a select group of patients who may then have the propensity for the development of bladder cancer after exposure to environmental carcinogens, whether the presence of oncogenes is alone sufficient for tumor development, or whether these structures constitute a limited or integral part of the overall process of neoplastic transformation.

PELVIC IRRADIATION. Women who have received pelvic irradiation for functional uterine bleeding or cervical cancer have been found to be two to four times more likely to develop bladder cancer (Palmer and Sprate, 1956). In a recent retrospective study of patients treated for cervical carcinoma and followed for as long as 25 years, there was a 57 times greater risk than that for the general female population for developing bladder cancer (Duncan et al., 1977). Comparable, though less striking, findings have been made in women successfully treated for uterine or cervical cancer by intracavitary radium (McIntyre and Pointon, 1971). Whether these trends will persist, however, remains to be seen (Iokhens and Hop, 1979).

Host Factors

GENETIC PREDISPOSITION. A genetic predisposition for the development of bladder cancer has not been proved (Lynch and Walzak, 1980; Sharma et al., 1976). McCullough described families in which transitional cell bladder carcinoma developed in 6 of 34 relatives who survived beyond the age of 30 years (McCullough et al., 1975). Purtilo described 11 cases of transitional cell carcinoma in five unrelated families in which afflicted patients were younger than in nonfamilial cases (Purtilo et al., 1979). Although familial clustering of transitional cell carcinoma appeared to be consistent with an autosomal dominant trait (Sharma et al., 1976), many suggested that familial clustering could just as well have reflected the commonality of environmental factors (Morganti et al., 1956).

Increased frequencies of particular HLA antigens (A9,B5, and CW4) among patients with bladder cancer as compared with controls may indicate a propensity among certain patient populations to develop bladder cancer in response to environmental stimuli (Arce et al., 1978; Editorial, 1979). On the other hand, certain subgroups of patients may be predestined to develop bladder cancer regardless of extrinsic factors. The multistage concept of bladder cancer development and the possible role of oncogenes in bladder cancer may both be relevant in this regard. If oncogenes originate from normal cells ("proto-oncogenes") and are highly conserved, they probably play critical roles in normal cell processes. Errors in DNA base-pairing induced by initiators, and proliferation and fixation of these errors by promoters, may produce a pool of cancer cells with a particular point mutation—chromosomal translocation (Bishop and Varmus, 1982; Reddy et al., 1982). Activation of an oncogene cascade may produce a situation of unregulated neoplastic transformation and cell proliferation (Levinson et al., 1978; Taparowsky et al., 1982; Aaronson, 1984).

What determines an individual patient's theoretical predisposition to point mutations and putative oncogene activation, and what determines the type of cancer likely to develop by such mechanisms, are entirely unknown. In this regard, it would be useful to obtain information concerning the type of bladder cancer (superficial or invasive) that has been observed in such instances, whether a given allele predisposes to a particular form of the disease, or whether exposure to environmental factors alters the type of cancer that is seen.

TRYPTOPHAN METABOLITES. An unusual rate of excretion of aromatic tryptophan metabolites was described in patients with bladder cancer nearly 40 years ago (Ekman and Strombeck, 1947). Subsequent studies showed that at least 50 per cent of bladder cancer patients without known carcinogen exposure excreted abnormal levels of kynurenine, acetyl kynurenine, kynurenic acid, and 3-hydroxykynurenine in the urine (Brown et al., 1960) and that such patients, when given a loading dose of L-tryptophan, excreted increased amounts of the metabolites as compared with controls (Wolf, 1973). Of particular interest were findings that patients with occupational bladder cancer did not demonstrate abnormal tryptophan metabolism and that patients studied after removal of their tumor persisted in their abnormal tryptophan metabolite excretion (Oyasu and Hopp, 1974).

The mechanism by which an abnormality of tryptophan metabolism is associated with bladder cancer is unknown. Although tryptophan metabolites are aromatic, attempts to induce bladder tumors in mice by administering tryptophan metabolites either orally or parenterally have failed (Bryan and Springberg, 1966; Bryan, 1969, 1971). Since more than 99 per cent of the administered dose was excreted unmetabolized in the urine, it was suggested that tryptophan metabolites might require a local abnormality in the bladder to function as promoters of carcinogenesis. In other studies, however, animals fed tryptophan together with 2-acetylaminofluorine (another promoting carcinogen) developed bladder cancers, and animals maintained on a pyridoxine-deficient diet and administered the carcinogen did the same (Melicow et al., 1964); however, animals given only the carcinogen did not (Dunning et al., 1950; Morrison, 1978). Taken together, tryptophan metabolites may be incomplete carcinogens that require the coordinating influence of one or more factors to cause bladder cancer (Bryan, 1977).

Clinical observations have further complicated this picture. For example, only 17 per cent of bladder cancer patients in Boston had abnormal tryptophan metabolism, whereas 47 per cent of bladder cancer patients in Wisconsin had abnormal metabolism (Wolf, 1973). In addition, tryptophan metabolites were found to be excreted in increased amounts in patients with other types of cancer as well as in patients with a variety of non-neoplastic diseases (Brown et al., 1960; Wolf, 1973; Ambarelli and Rubino, 1962; Rose, 1967).

Because pyridoxine (vitamin B_6) appeared to correct the abnormal excretion of tryptophan metabolites by bladder cancer patients (Brown et al., 1960; Romas et al., 1976), some suggested that pyridoxine deficiency might play a role in the carcinogenic effects of tryptophan metabolites. The immune response has also been suggested to have an influence in this regard. Thus, bladder cancer patients who could not respond positively to skin test antigens were found to have abnormal tryptophan metabolism as well, whereas those who could respond tended to have normal tryptophan metabolism (Romas et al., 1976). Administration of pyridoxine to those bladder cancer patients who were anergic reversed their immunologic skin response defect and corrected tryptophan metabolite excretion. Whether this ultimately affected tumor progression, however, is unclear. Recent studies of possible benefits from pyridoxine administration in preventing superficial bladder cancer recurrence did not demonstrate a prophylactic effect and suggest that further assessment of this phenomenon is indicated (Byar et al., 1977).

GALACTOSYL TRANSFERASE. The enzymatic capability of the transitional epithelium either to activate or to inhibit the carcinogenic character of various substances may also be important in the epidemiology of bladder cancer. For example, cell surface galactosyl transferase has been associated with cell differentiation, cell recognition, and cell adhesion (Shur and Roth, 1975). In addition, this enzyme has been observed to increase in tissue culture cells after they have been virally transformed (Morgan and Bossman, 1974). A nearly tenfold increase in the specific activity of this enzyme has been demonstrated in exfoliated neoplastic cells from the urine of rats with carcinogen-induced bladder tumors, and biopsy samples of human transitional cell tumors have been found to have greater galactosyl transferase activity than non-neoplastic vesical mucosa (Plotkin et al., 1977, 1979). The unresolved question is whether enzyme induction occurs as a result of neoplastic transformation or whether varying enzymatic activities reflect the propensity of an epithelium to respond to potential environmental carcinogens and become transformed.

In sum, a variety of host and environmental factors may interact in predisposing an individual to the development of bladder cancer. Although initiating factors in bladder cancer may require the briefest of exposures of an appropriately prepared target for their impact, promoting factors may require prolonged exposures and may act cumulatively to achieve their carcinogenic effect.

What role environmental versus host factors have in the development of a particular form of bladder cancer is unclear. Conceivably, environmental factors may predispose to the development only of superficial proliferative disease, in which the majority of patients are not at mortal risk. In contrast, host factors may predispose to the rapid development of infiltrative tumors, in which the majority of patients are diagnosed later in the course of their disease and may therefore be more likely to succumb. Varying interactions between these distinct forms of disease may occur when environmental carcinogens induce the phenotypic expression of disease to which the host has been genetically predisposed. The role of oncogenes in these interactions may be critical. How environmental stimuli interact with putative oncogenes in the genesis of a neoplastic process, however, remains to be clarified. In addition, these mechanisms must be interpreted in the context of the multistep processes of repetitive initiation and promotion thought to be responsible for bladder carcinogenesis. While much remains to be learned of these putative interactions, it seems reasonable to limit exposure to those factors in which a clear risk for tumor development has been demonstrated.

Biology and Natural Behavioral Patterns

THEORETICAL CONSIDERATIONS

Bladder cancer is not a single disease. Rather, it probably represents a spectrum of distinct processes in which developmental pathways may or may not be interrelated (Fig. 30–5) (Droller, 1981, 1982). Originally, the apparent linear histologic spectrum of in situ, superficial, and infiltrative bladder cancer prompted the concept that all bladder cancer progresses through a sequence of events in which initially

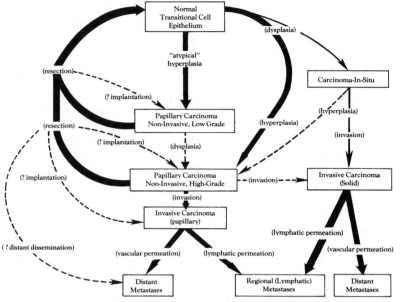

Figure 30–5. Hypothetical pathways in the natural history of bladder cancer.

The variable courses of superficial and invasive transitional cell cancers of the bladder are schematized. The theoretically likely occurrence of each pathway is symbolically represented by the size of the directional arrows.

Epithelial hyperplasia in the absence of dysplasia may lead to the development of superficial low-grade papillary tumors. Multiplicity or recurrence of these tumors implies either pre-existing generalized neoplastic field changes or implantation of tumor cells at the time of resection or from prior shedding. The primary occurrence of dysplasia may lead to the development of higher-grade intraepithelial lesions—carcinoma in situ. Subsequent hyperplasia may lead to proliferation of these cells, which may then directly infiltrate through the basement membrane into the lamina propria and extend in the form of a solid cluster of cells into the muscularis and perivesical fat. The occurrence of hyperplasia followed by progressive dysplasia may lead to the generation of papillary tumors that are of higher grade and that may penetrate the lamina propria, thereby giving rise to mixed papillary/solid infiltrative carcinomas.

The natural history of disease is probably established by early events in neoplastic transformation, in which tumor cells assume the biochemical characteristics that ultimately determine both their histologic appearance and their clinical course. The critical stages are probably those that involve early lamina propria penetration and vascular and lymphatic infiltration. The timing of these events, especially those that give rise to distant metastatic disease, is entirely unknown. (From Droller, M. J.: Curr. Probl. Surg., *18*:209, 1981. Used by permission.)

superficial tumors become invasive, infiltrate the lamina propria, extend to superficial muscle and then to deep muscle, finally penetrate the perivesical fat, and ultimately metastasize to distant sites (Friedell et al., 1977; Prout, 1979; Skinner, 1977). Observations in animal models of carcinogen-induced bladder cancer appeared to support this concept (Friedell, 1976; Friedell et al., 1977; Jacobs et al., 1977). Thus, histologic proliferation and hyperplasia were followed by infiltration in an apparently orderly sequence. Further support was provided by observations in these models that bladder tumor development was a multistage process involving initiation and promotion, and that transformation of a normal cell to a malignant cell involved an inexorable progression once the appropriate mutational events had occurred. In these examples, the continuum led from preneoplasia to hyperplasia (reversible), to atypical hyperplasia (possibly irreversible), to carcinoma in situ and eventual infiltration (both irreversible) (Cohen, 1979; Hicks, 1981; Cohen et al., 1984).

Clinical observations, however, have suggested a variability of developmental pathways rather than a single, inexorable sequence of events. For example, although over 70 per cent of bladder cancer cases occur in superficial form (Greene et al., 1973; Varkarakis et al., 1974), only a small proportion of these patients have been observed to progress to invasive disease (Cutler et al., 1982). Moreover, the majority of patients with muscle-invasive cancer, most of whom have reached this advanced stage upon initial clinical presentation (Kaye and Lange, 1982; Prout, 1982b), do not have a previous history of clinically diagnosed superficial disease.

Some have suggested that the more malignant growths developed their unique capacity for invasion at the very beginning, whereas the less aggressive growths never developed this capability; the former would therefore be more likely to progress fairly early in their development, while the latter would in most instances remain superficial and regionally confined without ever progressing (Jewett, 1977; Prout, 1977; Marshall, 1956; Cooper, 1975; Droller, 1981).

What determines these distinctions is unknown. That promotional factors weigh more heavily in determining a course of proliferation and hyperplasia is one possibility. Another is that the cascade of oncogenes necessary for complete neoplastic transformation has not been generated, such that only cell proliferation can occur, and that dysplasia will occur only if additional oncogene activation for dysplasia takes place. The more critical and basic event that results in neoplastic transformation has also not been defined. Clayson described cancer as "a group of cells which had permanently lost [their] ability to respond to some or all of the mechanisms which in the normal organism control the number and position of the cell type from which the tumor arose" (Clayson, 1975). However, "neoplastic transformation [has] to do much more than just increase mitotic rate; the cell [has] to acquire properties which enable it to penetrate the basement membrane and exist in the subepithelial environment" (Clayson, 1975). This capability may be the fulcrum upon which the clinical course of bladder cancer may turn, and it may define which pathway a particular bladder cancer will follow.

FORMS OF BLADDER CANCER AND THEIR BEHAVIOR

Epithelial Atypia or Dysplasia. A major objective in the study of the biology of bladder cancer has been to define the concept of "preneoplastic" changes in an otherwise morphologically normal epithelium and to understand the significance of such lesions in the presumed continuum between normal transitional epithelium and bladder cancer (Friedell, 1976). Exploration of this concept has invoked two primary questions. First, can such lesions be recognized visually by any technology? Second, does the presence of a particular lesion designated as "preneoplastic" imply the inevitable progression to cancer, the probability that cells somewhere in the bladder will give rise to cancer, or the equally plausible possibility that the lesion may regress if the inciting condition is eliminated? (Cohen et al., 1984.)

In dealing with the first question, some have suggested that a "preneoplastic" lesion is composed of "a proliferation of cells with characteristic but non-neoplastic histological and cytological features that are associated in space or time with the development of . . . carcinoma of the same histologic type. [Although] the constituent cells are atypical, . . . individually and collectively they do not look like malignant cells" (Cohen et al., 1984; Friedell, 1976). The terms "urothelial atypia" and "dysplasia" have been used to describe these lesions, and they have been categorized according to their morphologic severity as being mild, moderate, or severe (Murphy and Soloway, 1982). Lesions of the lowest grade have not been readily distinguished from reactive, regenerating, and reparative urothelium. Those of highest grade have been difficult to distinguish from unequivocal carcinoma in situ.

Scanning and transmission electron microscopy have been used to identify these lesions. In normal urothelium, surface cells have been characterized as having mainly microridges and an occasional microvillus (Tannenbaum et al., 1978). Such cells have appeared to be capable of phagocytizing bacteria, and telolysosomes have commonly been observed. This has been contrasted to well-differentiated tumors, in which surface cells contain numerous pleomorphic microvilli rather than microridges, and in which telolysosomes have been seen only rarely. Urothelial biopsy specimens characterized as "preneoplastic" but apparently normal by light microscopy have been found to have numerous microvilli, and the question as to whether such lesions are then irreversible has been posed.

In addressing this question, Friedell (1981) has advanced the concept of a histologic diagnostic threshold for bladder cancer as an index influenced by both qualitative and quantitative abnormalities. According to this concept, when proliferative lesions are seen to be "atypical" with only minimal hyperplasia, such lesions would have to show marked qualitative cellular and nuclear abnormalities before a diagnosis of cancer would be made (Cohen et al., 1984). If only a slight or moderate qualitative abnormality of basal or intermediate cells is present, a diagnosis of dysplasia would be made if there were no appreciable increase in the number of these cells. The diagnostic threshold for malignancy would not be reached in these instances if epithelium was only hyperplastic and without nuclear or cellular abnormalities. Therefore, lesions such as von Brunn's nests, cystitis cystica, and cystitis glandularis have been referred to collectively as proliferative cystitis and not as "preneoplastic" lesions (Friedell, 1981). Such lesions have not been associated with inevitable tumor development and, although frequently found in patients with bladder cancer, have also been seen in normal bladder, appearing to increase in frequency with age (Wiener et al., 1979).

The use of scanning or transmission electron microscopy to determine whether morphologic indices demonstrated by such lesions indicate irreversibility and possibly also inevitable progression to neoplasia remains the subject of much study and controversy. Some have suggested that a variety of precursor lesions may exist, some of which may be reversible, others of which may develop into cancers without metastatic potential, while still others of which may become neoplastic and pose major risk to patients who express these types of cells. Thus, Weinstein et al. (1979) have suggested that those lesions described as "atypical" may be the precursors of lower-grade transitional cell cancers, whereas other areas may give rise to high-grade carcinoma in situ (see further on).

Most information regarding the biologic significance of epithelial atypia, vis-à-vis correlations with tumor developmental patterns, has been based upon studies in animal models. One example of this is the apparent biologic significance of the development of pleomorphic microvilli in chemical carcinogenesis in such models (Jacobs et al., 1976; Cohen et al., 1976). Short microvilli of uniform size and shape have been observed on the luminal surface of normal urothelium (Hicks, 1975; Weinstein et al., 1976), and pleomorphic microvilli have been described on human bladder cancer cells (Fulker et al., 1971), with the degree of pleomorphism increasing with increasing tumor grade (Jacobs et al., 1976; Hicks and Chowaniec, 1978). As the transitional epithelium in the carcinogenesis models evolved through simple hyperplasia to nodular and papillary hyperplasia, and from noninvasive carcinoma ultimately to invasive carcinoma, the critical visual indication of malignancy was the appearance of such pleomorphic microvilli on the luminal surface of cells in the hyperplastic lesions (Jacobs et al., 1976; Cohen et al., 1976). This was associated, in turn, with the irreversibility of such lesions and their progression to cancer. Pleomorphic microvilli were then found to be present on all carcinomas induced by a variety of carcinogens in several species (Shirai et al., 1977; Hicks and Chowaniec, 1978). They could also be seen in cells obtained from the urine of animals with early "preneoplastic" changes, long before clearly malignant cells were seen (Jacobs et al., 1976).

Comparable attempts to correlate "premalignant" morphologic changes with ultimate cancer development in clinical situations have been hampered by the lack of access to the earliest phases of tumor development and restriction to study of static samples rather than an evolving continuum. Pleomorphic microvilli have been present on exfoliated transitional cancer cells but have not been seen in cells from normal patients or in those with non-neoplastic proliferative conditions (bacterial cystitis, cyclophosphamide hemorrhagic cystitis) (Cohen et al., 1984). The presence of atypical cells at the margin of superficial tumors has been associated with ultimate progression to cancer in 10 to 15 percent of cases, compared with less than 5 percent progression when normal epithelium was present at the margin of comparable tumors (Althausen et al., 1976). Findings of atypical cells in random biopsies of sites distant from a presenting tumor, even when these areas were endoscopically normal, have been associated with a greater likelihood of recurrence and in many instances of recurrence with progression (Smith et al., 1983; Wolf and Hojgaard, 1983). However, others have not observed a consistent predictive pattern for ultimate cancer development in the setting of atypia on random biopsy (Cutler et al., 1982). What therefore still is lacking is an identification of that feature which is consistently and reliably detectable and which indicates the point at which progression is inevitable and irreversible if untreated.

Carcinoma In Situ (Flat). Insight into the natural history of bladder cancer was provided in 1952 by Melicow, who suggested that carcinoma in situ was a distinct cancer entity that represented bladder cancer's earliest stage (Fig. 30–6) (Melicow, 1952). Because carcinoma in situ generally appeared to culminate in the development of metastases in these instances, others suggested that this entity, though noninvasive, represented a highly aggressive neoplastic diathesis (Melamed et al., 1964, Utz et al., 1970).

For example, Melamed described 25 patients with flat carcinoma in situ, 24 of whom had had prior tumors (Melamed et al., 1964). Of 12 treated with resection and radiation but not cystectomy, 9 (75 per cent) progressed to invasive cancer. Similarly, Utz observed that of 62 patients with flat carcinoma in situ seen after their primary bladder cancer had been treated by resection and fulguration, 82 per cent developed recurrence and 73 per cent developed infiltrative cancers (Utz et al., 1973). Twenty-four (40 per cent) of these patients were dead of their disease within 5 years.

Similar observations on the seemingly aggressive nature of this entity were also made when flat carcinoma in situ was present in the absence of previous or concomitant gross tumor. Anderson reported 15 patients with carcinoma in situ, 12 of whom (80 per cent) developed invasive bladder cancer within 3 years (Anderson, 1973). Similarly, Daly observed 18 patients with positive urinary cytology with no evidence of overt tumor at cystoscopy, 11 of whom (61 per cent) developed invasive cancer within 19

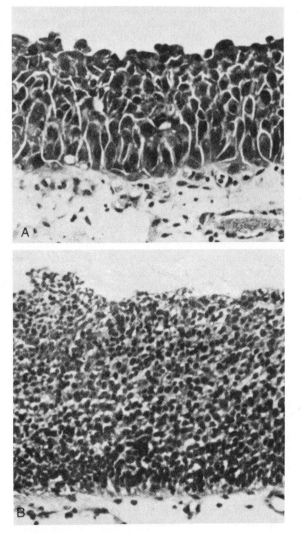

Figure 30–6. Carcinoma in situ.

A and *B*, Considered to be the earliest stage in tumor development, carcinoma in situ represents intraepithelial neoplastic transformation in which changes in cellular morphology occur without extension of cells into the lumen of the bladder or penetration through the basement membrane into the lamina propria. The neoplastic change may give rise either to small or to large cells with atypical nuclei. Epithelial thickness is markedly increased in all cases.

Cohesiveness between adjacent cells and adherence to the basal membrane may be decreased, predisposing cells to slough into the lumen of the bladder. Since the basal membrane may therefore be denuded by the sloughing of its epithelial layer, the diagnosis of carcinoma in situ is occasionally easier to make on a cytologic preparation than with a histologic biopsy. (From Koss, L.G.: Tumors of the urinary bladder. *In* Firminger, H. I. (Ed.): Atlas of Tumor Pathology. Washington, D.C., Armed Forces Institute of Pathology, Fascicle II, 1975. Used by permission.)

months of diagnosis (Daly, 1976). Equally ominous were findings by Riddle in 12 patients with extensive and symptomatic flat carcinoma in situ, 9 of whom had unsuspected lamina propria infiltration at cystectomy (Riddle, 1975).

Of 11 patients treated by radiation alone, only 1 remained alive at 18 months. Similarly, Whitmore observed that diffuse carcinoma in situ with vesical irritability was associated with the later development of infiltrating cancer in 50 to 80 per cent of instances (Whitmore, 1979).

On the other hand, several reports indicated that the presence of carcinoma in situ by itself might not imply as ominous a prognosis as was initially suggested. For example, Koss and Melamed found 13 cases of carcinoma in situ among 503 men who were being followed after exposure to xenylamine, a potent bladder carcinogen (Koss et al., 1969). A latency period of negative cytology ranging from several months to 8 years was followed by a variable period of positive urinary cytology without histologic confirmation of in situ cancer (Melamed et al., 1960; Koss et al., 1969). Within the subsequent 11 to 77 months, only 7 of the 13 men who had developed positive urinary cytologies developed invasive cancer. Although thirty-five others in this group had developed invasive bladder cancer in the absence of documented carcinoma in situ (Koss et al., 1974), only half the patients who initially had developed carcinoma in situ ultimately progressed to invasive disease, and this only after a relatively prolonged time and in a highly selected group.

Similar observations were made by Farrow, who reported 27 patients with persistently positive urinary cytology and in whom the average duration of symptoms before the first positive cytologic examination had been 32 months (Farrow et al., 1977). Only 3 patients in this group (11 per cent) developed invasive carcinoma, while 24 other patients with carcinoma in situ who were under observation for an average of 33 months did not progress to invasive disease. When a second group of patients with carcinoma in situ was assessed, disease in 40 per cent (25 of 62) was found not to progress during 5 years of follow-up (Utz et al., 1970). Riddle noted that such patients tended to have lesser symptomatology and to maintain a relatively benign course (Riddle, 1975).

These disparate observations may reflect the occurrence of different types of flat carcinoma in situ, the one being relatively innocuous and the other more pervasive and aggressive (Cooper et al., 1973). The process of intraepithelial neoplastic transformation may entail the development of two types of tumor cells: those that have limited capacity for "atypical" hyperplasia but no capacity at all for further progression (so-called terminal differentiation) (Weinstein et al., 1980) and those that have the enzymatic capacity for penetration into the bladder wall (Riddle, 1975; Droller and Walsh, 1984). Weinstein et al. (1980, 1984) have suggested that cancers arising in bladders of patients harboring relatively poorly differentiated carcinomas in situ elsewhere in the bladder are not uncommonly of low or moderate grade. The developmental pathway that has led to such "atypical hyperplasia" has therefore been suggested as being distinct from that which has produced the carcinoma in situ. They have further suggested that the progression of carcinoma in situ itself into a solid invasive tumor is not an inevitable event, even though such lesions may be endowed with the capacity to evolve into malignant cancers (Weinstein et al., 1984). Indeed, two forms of carcinoma in situ have been proposed to exist. One represents the progenitor lesion of solid cancer with infiltrative capabilities. The other, so-called carcinoma paradoxicum, represents those areas of carcinoma in situ that lack the capacity to evolve further into invasive cancers. Findings that 20 per cent of 21 bladders removed for diffuse carcinoma in situ were found to contain microscopic zones of invasion into the lamina propria are particularly relevant in this regard (Farrow et al., 1976). A more recent analysis of 70 cystectomy specimens in which the bladder was removed for clinically evident flat carcinoma in situ alone disclosed that 24 (34 per cent) had T_1 lesions, and that three patients had died of metastatic disease within 4 years (Farrow and Utz, 1982). More recent studies have confirmed these observations (Kakizoe et al., 1984). In addition, these studies have noted a lower incidence of dysplasia or carcinoma in situ in the setting of multiple superficial papillary transitional cell cancers, especially when these have also tended to be of lower grade. Moreover, growth of carcinoma in situ was actually found to be bidirectional, both extending into the bladder lumen and invading the lamina propria. Such findings support suggestions that multiple pathways may characterize bladder cancer development (Droller, 1981) and that initial intraepithelial neoplastic transformation probably produces different types of carcinoma in situ with varying biologic and malignant potential.

Taken together, the different forms of carcinoma in situ include those that lack the capability to infiltrate and therefore probably pose little immediate threat for progression (Weinstein, 1979) and those that are dysplastic and extensive, may have the capability to infiltrate the submucosal connective tissue and underlying muscle (Riddle, 1975; Weinstein, 1982), and carry with them the risk of progression to a life-threatening situation.

Superficial Transitional Cell Cancers. The majority of patients with transitional cell cancer present with superficial papillary disease (Greene et al., 1973; Varkarakis et al., 1974). In assessing the clinical implications of "superficial" disease there are two major questions that must be considered. The first concerns the likelihood of tumor recurrence. The second and more important concerns the likelihood of tumor progression.

The term "superficial" has traditionally been applied both to those tumors that have remained confined to the mucosa (Fig. 30–7) and to those that have extended into the lamina propria (Fig. 30–8). Penetration of the basement membrane, however, may represent an enzymatic capability not shared by all cells composing each of these tumor types. This distinction, moreover, may indicate potential differences in ultimate biologic behavior and risk for progression.

The structural integrity of normal urothelium is maintained by intercellular junctions (Pauli et al., 1977), cytoskeletal architecture (Weinstein and Pauli, 1981), and stromal-epithelial interactions (Pauli and Weinstein, 1982). Invasion of cancer cells implies disintegration of these factors. Tumor cell surface enzymes and secreted proteases can digest collagens, elastins, glycoproteins, and proteoglycans of the connective tissue stroma (Strauli, 1980; Liotta et al., 1979; Pauli and Weinstein, 1982). The basement membrane at sites of invasion is either fragmented or absent, and new capillary proliferation may be induced near the tumor-stromal interface (Chodak et al., 1980, 1981; Tatematsu et al., 1978; Weinstein et al., 1984).

Determination of these capabilities may ultimately reside in the carcinogenic activation of particular oncogenes in an oncogenic cascade. Activation of a single oncogene may lead to multifocal cell proliferation without accompanying capabilities for infiltration. Activation of a second oncogene may result in the generation of more dysplastic cells with invasive capabilities, amplification of uncontrolled growth, and ultimate tumor progression (Bishop and Varmus, 1982; Hamlyn and Sikora, 1983). Taken together, the term "superficial" bladder cancer may actually refer to two separate forms of disease in which risk of recurrence and risk of progression may be quite distinct.

Clinically, the risk for recurrence and that for progression have been associated with several factors. These have included tumor grade, initial tumor multicentricity, and presence of various epithelial changes at sites either adjacent to or distant from the primary tumor. However,

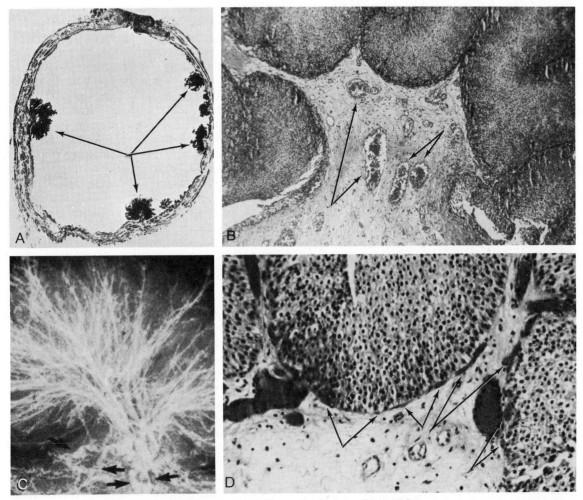

Figure 30–7. Superficial transitional cell cancer: mucosally confined tumors (Stage T$_A$).

A, Low-grade papillary transitional cell cancer appears to be the most common manifestation of neoplastic transformation, consisting of the multicellular, proliferative epithelium being thrown into papillary excrescences that extend into the bladder lumen (arrows). In addition to the multiple superficial papillary tumors that may be seen, numerous diffuse areas of papillary hyperplasia may appear. *B and C,* Each tumor contains a central vascular core with connective tissue stroma (arrows). *D,* At higher magnification, the epithelial basement membrane appears to be intact and is rarely, if ever, penetrated by neoplastic cells. The vasculature that penetrates the central core of these tumors extends microtributaries that lie immediately subjacent to the epithelial basal layer (arrows). (*A* from Koss, L. G.: Tumors of the urinary bladder. *In* Firminger, H. I. (Ed.): Atlas of Tumor Pathology. Washington, D.C., Armed Forces Institute of Pathology, Fascicle 11, 1975; used by permission of Dr. R. O. K. Schade, Newcastle-upon-Tyne, England, and Dr. L. G. Koss. *B* from Sarma, K. P.: Br. J. Urol., *53:*228, 1981. Used by permission.)

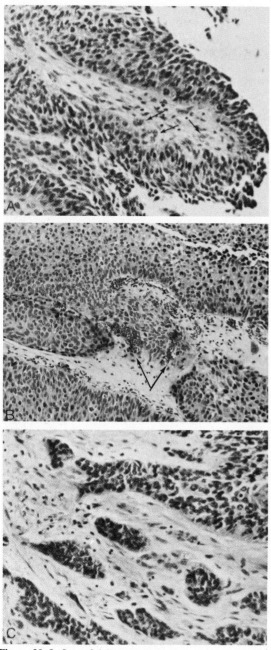

Figure 30–8. Superficial transitional cell carcinoma: lamina propria invasion (Stage T_1).

A, Neoplastic transformation may lead to the generation of cells with the capability to penetrate through the epithelial basement membrane into the lamina propria (arrows). B, Since the microvasculature is immediately subjacent to the basement membrane, cells that infiltrate the lamina propria may readily come into direct contact with blood vessels (arrows). The ability of cells to infiltrate the lymphatics and vasculature (C), therefore, is not a matter of the depth to which the cells must penetrate the lamina propria but rather a matter of the enzymatic capabilities of these cells upon reaching vessels that lie in their immediate vicinity. (A and C from Koss, L.G.: Tumors of the urinary bladder. In Firminger, H. I. (Ed.): Atlas of Tumor Pathology. Washington, D.C., Armed Forces Institute of Pathology, 1975, Fascicle 11. Used by permission.)

the major distinction that determines the likelihood of simple recurrence or recurrence with progression appears to be whether penetration of the lamina propria has already occurred (Anderstrom et al., 1980; Heney et al., 1983). Since this distinction is usually apparent at the time of initial clinical presentation, the potential natural history of superficial disease in the individual patient may in many instances represent a fait accompli.

A recent longitudinal study by the National Bladder Cancer Collaborative Group A (NBCCGA) of patients with newly diagnosed superficial bladder tumors observed that 65 per cent of 120 patients with histologically documented superficial tumors confined to the mucosa were disease-free at 12 months, while 52 per cent and 46 per cent were disease-free at 24 and 36 months, respectively (Cutler et al., 1982). Similar observations were made in patients with lamina propria invasion. However, only 4 patients (3 per cent) with mucosally confined tumors subsequently developed recurrence with muscle invasion. In contrast, of 78 patients whose initial "superficial" tumor had invaded the lamina propria, progression to muscle invasion occurred in 19 patients (24 per cent), and nearly two thirds of these became manifest within 1 year of initial diagnosis (Cutler et al., 1982; Heney et al., 1982).

Initial multiplicity of superficial disease has generally been associated only with the likelihood of simple recurrence in each type of tumor. In patients with mucosally confined tumors, the presence initially of a single tumor was associated with a 67 per cent likelihood of recurrence, contrasting with a 90 per cent likelihood of recurrence in patients who initially had multiple tumors (Cutler et al., 1982). In addition, the interval between initial appearance of tumor and first recurrence was shorter for patients with multiple tumors than for those with a single lesion. Although recurrence in the setting of initial multiplicity of disease may possibly have reflected incomplete resection of tumors because of their multiplicity, it was more probably indicative of the multicentric presence of endoscopically undetectable disease that became clinically apparent only after additional proliferation had been allowed to take place. Comparable observations were made for tumors that were not mucosally confined (Barnes et al., 1967; Varkarakis et al., 1974; Cutler et al., 1982; Greene et al., 1973).

Diffuseness of epithelial involvement, though related to multiplicity, has appeared to relate more directly to recurrence with progression and, in turn, to tumor that was less likely to be mucosally confined. In describing diffuseness of mucosal involvement with neoplastic change, the NBCCGA reported that while only 31 of 186 newly diagnosed patients (17 per cent) had either moderate or severe dysplasia at sites away from the presenting tumor, 23 per cent of these patients never achieved initial disease-free status (Cutler et al., 1982). In contrast, 98 per cent of patients with no nontumor abnormality, more often the case in mucosally confined disease, readily achieved disease-free status. In this regard, Althausen observed that of the 30 per cent of patients with initially superficial transitional cell tumors who developed muscle infiltration 5 years after diagnosis, the majority appeared to have had some mucosal abnormality in the epithelium adjacent to the primary lesion (Althausen et al., 1976). Of 78 patients whose tumor biopsy samples permitted an analysis of the adjacent epithelium, 12 (15 per cent) had carcinoma in situ, and 10 (83 per cent) of these developed muscle invasion within 5 years. In contrast, 41 patients (53 per cent) had normal epithelium at the margin of the initial presenting tumor, and only 3.8 per cent of these patients progressed to muscle invasion. Intermediate within these groups were 25 patients (32 per cent) who had atypical epithelium at the tumor margin, and only 11.5 per cent went on to develop invasive cancer. These observations were congruent with earlier studies in which "proliferative lesions" (flat carcinoma in situ or epithelial atypia) occurred in only 26 per cent of patients with papillary tumors (or those confined to the mucosa) but occurred in 60 per cent of patients with infiltrating tumors (Eisenberg et al., 1960). The ominous prognostic significance of carcinoma in situ, and possibly also of severe epithelial dysplasia, in selected mucosal biopsies from normal-appearing urothelium has also been well documented in several other investigations (Koss et al., 1977; Murphy et al., 1979; Smith et al., 1983; Wolf and Hojgaard, 1983).

The grade of tumor on initial presentation also has appeared to be related to diffuseness of epithelial involvement and has seemed to be an important predictor of recurrence with a higher probability of progression in both forms of disease (Fig. 30–9). Whereas 75 per cent of patients with histologic Grade 1 tumors (usually mucosally confined) are likely to be disease-free at 12 months, only 55 per cent of patients with Grade 3 tumors initially (more often superficially infiltrative lesions) have been found to be disease-free at that time (Cutler et al., 1982; Anderson, 1973; Varkarakis et al., 1974; Narayana et al., 1983). This may be associated with the extent of epithelial involvement as well as recurrence. Thus, in one study 5 of 33 patients with Grade 1 carcinoma (15 per cent), 17 of 29 patients with Grade 2 carcinoma (59 per cent), and 10 of 13 patients with Grade 3 carcinoma (77 per cent) showed significant urothelial abnormalities at sites distant from the presenting tumor (Heney et al., 1978). More recent reports have shown that 2 per cent of 92 Grade 1 patients, 11 per cent of 79 Grade 2 patients, and 45 per cent of 31 Grade 3 patients with mucosally confined lesions showed progression of disease, usually within 2 years of diagnosis (Heney et al., 1983). This coincided with 38 per cent of 94 Grade 1 patients, 55 per cent of 69 Grade 2 patients, and 66 per cent of 20 Grade 3 patients who showed moderate or severe dysplasia in selected mucosal biopsies. In T_1 tumors, 0 of 7, 6 of 29 (21 per cent), and 13 of 27 (48 per cent) of Grades 1, 2, and 3 lesions, respectively, showed similar progression (Heney et al., 1983). As important have been findings that a change in grade from 1 or 2 to 3 may herald the progression of disease in patients with lamina propria invasion (England et al., 1981). Of 192 patients with T_1 disease in one series, the majority of the 30 per cent whose lesions ultimately progressed were found either to have advanced-grade tumors or to develop a higher grade tumor during the course of their initially superficial disease.

Findings on urinary cytopathology have mirrored each of these observations. A greater proportion of patients with Grade 3 primary superficial tumors, usually more characteristic of those that had invaded the lamina propria, were found to have positive cytologies (Cutler et al., 1982). Only 50 per cent of Grade 1 tumor–bearing patients with positive cytologies were disease-free at 12 months compared with 68 per cent of similar patients whose cytologies were negative. Similarly, only 38 per cent of Grade 2 tumor–bearing patients with positive cytologies were disease-free in comparison with 64 per cent of Grade 2 patients whose cytologies were negative; two thirds of patients with Grade 3 disease had positive cytologies, and only 50 per cent of these were disease-free. The most probable interpretation of these findings was that a positive cytology in the presence of low-grade papillary tumors reflected the presence of epithelial cancer that was not necessarily visible endoscopically, and that the higher the grade of clinically apparent disease, the more likely it was to represent the presence, possibly subclinically, of more diffuse urothelial involvement. This would be particularly likely in the setting of Grade 1 papillary disease in which carcinoma

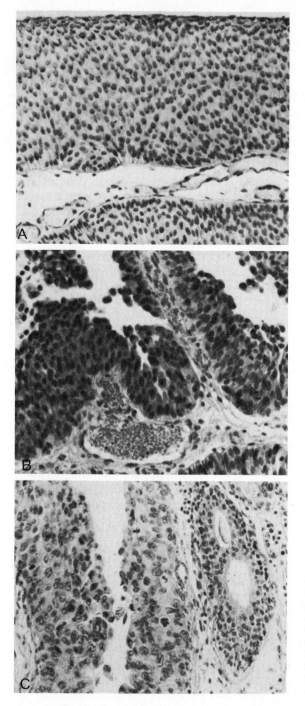

Figure 30–9. Grading of transitional cell carcinoma.

Grade 1 tumor cells are characterized by a relatively small homogeneous nuclear size and a minimal degree of variation in nuclear shape *(A)*. There is still some evidence of maturation from the basal cell layers to the most superficial layer, even though there is an increase in the number of cells composing the entire epithelial cell layer. Grade 2 tumor cells demonstrate greater variability in both nuclear size and shape *(B)*. Exfoliation of abnormal cells from the epithelial surface can occasionally be seen. Grade 3 tumor cells show a striking variability in nuclear size, shape, and cytoplasmic area *(C)*. No evidence of maturation proceeding from the basal layer to the superficial layer of cells is apparent. Numerous mitoses are evident throughout these cell layers. (From Friedell, G. H., et al.: Urol. Clin. North Am., *3*:53, 1976. Used by permission.)

or carcinoma in situ elsewhere in the urothelium was the source of cancer cells rather than the endoscopically obvious lower-grade papillary tumor.

The mechanism of tumor recurrence in all of these cases has generally been assumed to reflect instability of the urothelium and broad-field urothelial changes. However, some have suggested that recurrence in some instances may represent tumor cell implantation (Boyd and Burnand, 1974; Weldon and Soloway, 1975) rather than de novo development from unrecognized but already transformed sites (Prout, 1982b). Experimentally, instillation of carcinogen-induced tumor cells into chemically or cautery traumatized bladders led consistently to superficial tumor development and indicated the validity of this possibility (Weldon and Soloway, 1975). Clinically, a higher incidence of recurrent superficial tumors at the bladder dome suggested the possibility that tumor cells shed during resection and held at the dome by surface tension might be responsible for the tumor recurrence that was observed (Boyd and Burnand, 1974, Heney et al., 1982). That random biopsies documented normal mucosa at other sites in the bladder in the majority of patients with mucosa-confined superficial bladder tumors at the time of initial presentation (Heney et al., 1978; Cutler et al., 1982) suggested either that other potential foci of neoplastic change were not histologically detectable at initial tumor presentation or that implantation is an important mechanism of recurrence in many of these instances. The possible importance of this mechanism in other than recurrence of simple superficial disease remains to be determined.

Taken together, the higher the grade and the more diffuse the involvement of the mucosa, the greater is the likelihood of disease recurrence with possible progression in all types of superficial disease (Narayana et al., 1983). The critical distinction in behavioral patterns between mucosally confined disease, when recurrence is usually seen, and infiltrative "superficial" disease, when recurrence with progression is more likely to occur (Anderstrom et al., 1980), may reside in the greater enzymatic capabilities of the latter types of tumor and a consequent more aggressive potential.

Muscle-Infiltrative Cancers. The survival rate in patients with advanced muscle-invasive cancer, unamenable to other than palliative treatment, was reported by Marshall and Whitmore to be less than 3 per cent at 1 year from the time of diagnosis, and 92 per cent of these patients failed to survive 6 months (Marshall and Whitmore, 1956). In addition, only 35 per cent of these patients survived 1 year after the onset of symptoms, 5.4 per cent survived 3 years, and 2.7 per cent survived 5 years (Marshall, 1956). Even when treatment seemed possible, at least 50 per cent of such patients died within 18 months of diagnosis and only 20 to 40 per cent survived as long as 5 years (Marshall and McCarron, 1977; Whitmore, 1980).

Treatment failures have as often been due to distant metastatic disease as to local recurrence (Whitmore, 1980; Prout et al., 1979). Correspondingly, when tumors were regionally invasive, tumor deaths correlated directly with the frequency of vascular and lymphatic invasion within the bladder muscle wall (Bell et al., 1971;

McDonald and Thompson, 1948; Soto et al., 1977).

The major questions in muscle-invasive bladder cancer have therefore focused upon whether a tumor may already have metastasized at the time it is initially diagnosed and what factors determine this occurrence. Several observations are important in this regard. The first is that only 10 to 30 per cent of initially superficial tumors have actually been found to progress to muscle invasion (Fulker et al., 1971; Cutler et al., 1981; Varkarakis et al., 1974). The second is that the majority of patients with muscle-invasive disease are found to have this stage of tumor at their initial presentation (Kaye and Lange, 1982; Hopkins et al., 1983). The third is that at least 50 per cent of these patients fail with distant metastatic disease within 2 years of radical therapy (Prout et al., 1979).

Explanations for these observations have focused on two hypotheses. One postulates that these tumors develop sequentially but rapidly from superficial disease and penetrate the bladder wall prior to the development of clinically recognizable symptoms. Another suggests that the majority of these tumors follow a separate developmental pathway that consists largely of rapid infiltration of the bladder muscularis; accordingly, protrusion into the bladder lumen (the "superficial" component of the disease) occurs only later in the life of the tumor, and it is only then that the tumor expresses itself clinically.

The first of these explanations, implicating a relentless sequential progression of disease, was suggested by Melicow, who demonstrated carcinoma in situ in bladders that contained muscle-invasive tumors (Melicow, 1952). The concept was reinforced by Farrow and coworkers, who reported that 20 per cent of cases of carcinoma in situ had microfoci of lamina propria infiltration (Farrow et al., 1976). Various studies of chemical carcinogenesis in animal models of bladder cancer also supported the concept of a continuum of tumor progression (Jacobs et al., 1977; Cohen et al., 1984).

On the other hand, the rapid systemic progression of these tumors, the implication that metastasis may have occurred early in the course of tumor progression, and the fact that the majority of superficial tumors do not progress all suggest the existence of a separate developmental pathway for muscle-invasive tumors that may be entirely different from that postulated for tumors confined to the mucosa. This mechanism may possibly be more akin to that for "superficial" tumors that have infiltrated the lamina propria. The 20 per cent incidence of lymphatic involvement by tumors that had penetrated only the lamina propria (9 of 47), with 66 per cent of these patients (6 of 9) dying within 5 years of cystectomy, supports this possibility (Jewett et al., 1964). In effect, once a tumor has expressed its local aggressiveness by infiltration into or through the bladder wall, it may also have expressed its capacity to metastasize. Although the temporal aspects of this process in bladder cancer are unknown, the relatively short symptomatic history of patients with muscle-infiltrative disease and the early appearance of distant disease suggest that progression and metastasis may take place early in the overall developmental history.

In examining these possibilities, it is also important to consider the type of muscle-invasive disease represented by patients who have responded well to standard therapeutic regimens. In such instances, muscle infiltration may not be the *sine qua non* that predicts the likelihood of treatment failure. Indeed, histologic correlates possibly reflective of behavioral distinctions between different muscle-infiltrative tumor diatheses have been described. These include tumor architecture, patterns of cellular infiltration into and through the bladder wall, and apparent involvement of bladder wall vasculature and lymphatics.

The significance of tumor architecture in the context of tumor behavior was first addressed by Aschner, who distinguished between tumors that were papillary and those that were not (Aschner, 1928). Although he suggested that tumor infiltration rather than tumor architecture determined treatment success, subsequent reports demonstrated that papillary tumors infiltrated muscle layers only superficially whereas tumors with a more solid pattern generally appeared to infiltrate more deeply (Figs. 30–10 and 30–11; see Table 30–8) (Pryor, 1973; Prout, 1982b). Correspondingly, papillary tumors with infiltration were associated with a 35 per cent 5-year survival, whereas solid tumors with infiltration had an 18 per cent 5-year survival (McDonald and Thompson, 1948). In addition, papillary tumors appeared more commonly to invade the bladder wall in a "broad-front" pattern, which was characterized by seemingly cohesive masses of tumor cells sharply demarcated from the muscle and stroma (Soto et al., 1977). In contrast, solid or nodular tumors appeared more often to penetrate the bladder wall in a tentacular pattern in which cords or clusters of tumor cells extended in finger-like projections between muscle fascicles (Soto et

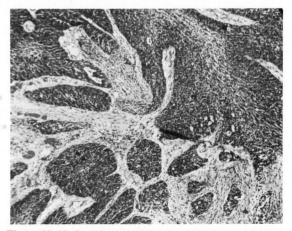

Figure 30–10. Invasive transitional cell carcinoma: "broad-front" infiltrative pattern.

Muscle-invasive transitional cell cancers can have either a papillary architecture or a solid, nodular architecture. Papillary tumors tend to invade the muscle more superficially and to penetrate the bladder wall in a "broad-front" or cohesive mass of cells. These tumors appear less likely to penetrate the vasculature or lymphatics of the bladder wall and have been described as more radiosensitive than their more solid counterparts. (From Droller, M. J., and Walsh, P. C.: Urology, 22:2, 1983. Used by permission.)

al., 1977). The greater depth of penetration by less cohesive clusters of cells appeared to imply that solid tumors might be more likely to metastasize. Observations that solid tumors were accompanied by vascular infiltration two to three times as often as their papillary infiltrative

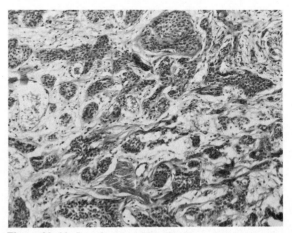

Figure 30–11. Invasive transitional cell carcinomas: tentacular infiltrative pattern.

Tumors with a solid or nodular architecture appear to arise from dysplastic masses of cells that extend with finger-like, tentacular processes deep into the muscularis, and often through the muscularis to the perivesical fat. These tumors have been observed to infiltrate the bladder wall vasculature or lymphatics twice as often as their papillary counterparts. (From Droller, M. J., and Walsh, P. C.: Urology, 22:2, 1983. Used by permission.)

counterparts supported this impression (Soto et al., 1977; Bell et al., 1971; Prout, 1982b). Corresponding survivals of 11 per cent in those with vascular involvement and 38 per cent in those with no vascular involvement demonstrated the ominous implications that solid, more deeply infiltrative tumors appeared to have (McDonald and Thompson, 1948; Sjolin et al., 1976; Bell et al., 1971). Recent clinical observations that 75 per cent of all patients with solid tumors were found to have lymphatic invasion while only 25 per cent of patients with papillary invasive tumors had similar invasion further supported these suggestions (Fig. 30–12; see Table 30–8) (Prout, 1982a; Slack and Prout, 1980; Heney et al., 1984).

Taken together, the association of papillary architecture with more superficial penetration by cohesive clusters of cells and less frequent involvement of blood vessels may indicate a pathway of tumor development characterized predominantly by atypical hyperplasia and cellular proliferation with less aggressive behavior (Droller, 1981). When metastases occur in these cases, they may represent late events in the overall course of tumor progression. In contrast, the association of a more solid architecture with deeper penetration of less cohesive cell clusters and more frequent blood vessel and lymphatic involvement may indicate a pathway of development in which distant dissemination is more likely to occur, possibly early in tumor development. Further characterization of these dis-

tinctions may ultimately permit a more precise definition of the variety of tumor diatheses that are seen.

SUMMARY SCHEME OF BLADDER CANCER BIOLOGY

Variability in the clinical course of different forms of bladder cancer suggests that differences in intrinsic characteristics may find phenotypic expression through distinct, though possibly interrelated, developmental pathways (see Fig. 30–5). If cellular proliferation predominates, it may give rise to superficial papillary lesions that are not particularly aggressive, even if already infiltrative when diagnosed. If cellular dysplasia takes place, its phenotypic expression may involve proliferation into more solid infiltrative lesions that are likely to be more aggressive.

Differences between such tumors, whether superficial or invasive, may reflect changes both in cell surface characteristics and in enzymatic capabilities. Thus, development of aggressive infiltrative disease may involve modification of intercellular communications (McNutt et al., 1971; Sheridan, 1970), which may lead to alteration of cell-to-cell cohesion so that cells may enter into anchorage-independent growth (Weinstein et al., 1976; Edelman, 1976). The associated production of extracellular proteases from such cells may then permit degradation of the basal lamina and underlying connective tissue elements so that invasion of the bladder wall can take place (Fidler, 1978; Kuettner and Pauli, 1978; Pauli and Weinstein, 1982; Weinstein et al., 1984). The ultimate cause of these differences may reside in the specific oncogene or set of oncogenes that are activated. Thus, a single activation may result in only a proliferative process; additional activations may be required for the development of a proliferative, dysplastic, more aggressive neoplastic process (Bishop and Varmus, 1982; Hamlyn and Sikora, 1983).

The same considerations may be applicable in estimating the likelihood of metastases. Experimental studies have suggested that undifferentiated tumors are more likely to shed cells directly into lymphatics and blood vessels (Kleinerman and Liotta, 1977; Suzuki et al., 1978) and that rapid cell division, a characteristic of more anaplastic tumors, may favor cellular detachment (Weiss, 1977). Observations that cells at the periphery of a tumor may exhibit tissue invasiveness (Carr et al., 1976) coincide clinically with findings of malignant cells in effluent venous blood in several tumor systems (Golinger et al., 1977). This may be especially perti-

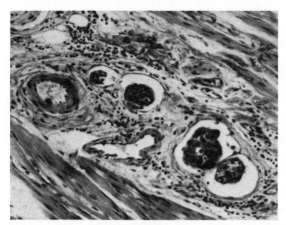

Figure 30–12. Lymphatic infiltration by muscle-invasive tumors.

The precise time or stage at which vascular and lymphatic invasion takes place is unknown. If this event is purely a reflection of intrinsic tumor behavior, it may occur early in the development of neoplasia. Most often, it accompanies high-grade tumors that have penetrated deeply into the muscularis or into the perivesical fat. (From Jewett, H. J., et al.: J. Urol., 92:668, 1964. Used by permission.)

nent in bladder cancer in those instances of early infiltration in which dysplastic tumor cells may be seen within vascular or lymphatic channels and may then also be seen to have metastasized through the bladder wall (Jewett and Cason, 1948).

These considerations have led to the generation of a schema for the development of the different forms of bladder cancer (Droller, 1980). Epithelial hyperplasia in the absence of dysplasia may lead to superficial low-grade papillary tumors. Recurrence of tumors may signify the presence of similar proliferative cellular foci that express themselves at different times after the initial tumor has been resected (Prout, 1982b). Recurrence may also represent implantation of tumor cells onto other areas of the bladder mucosa either at the time of resection or from prior intravesical shedding of tumor cells (Soloway, 1983).

The occurrence of hyperplasia and dysplasia together may signal the development of higher-grade papillary lesions that, though still predominantly proliferative, may have a greater tendency to extend into the lamina propria in the form of "papillary invasion." The same enzymatic machinery necessary for such penetration may also permit these tumors to infiltrate lymphatic or vascular structures.

The occurrence of dysplasia alone, in the absence of hyperplasia, may lead to histologically recognizable flat carcinoma in situ. This may remain as in situ disease, slough to be replaced by normal or other abnormal cells, or invade the lamina propria (Weinstein et al., 1980; Farrow et al., 1976). Hyperplasia in such instances may lead to nodular protrusion of neoplastic cells into the bladder lumen and concomitant extension of tumor cells into lamina propria and muscle. Conceivably, these cells may also penetrate lymphatics or vascular structures without ever growing to any major extent into the bladder lumen until late in their course. Therefore, such tumors may not necessarily present clinically until they are far advanced. If hyperplasia occurs early in these instances, tumors may express both papillary and solid features, may protrude into the bladder lumen as well as into the bladder wall early in their development, and may therefore become clinically manifest before muscle infiltration and lymphatic or vascular permeation has taken place.

Although clinical course in the majority of these forms of disease is likely to be determined by the earliest events in neoplastic transformation, genetic drift in a heterogeneous population of cells may in some instances account for a change from the expected pattern of development. The occasional change in tumor grade of superficial lesions may reflect such an occurrence. The course of patients with their first superficial tumor who may ultimately have progressive cancer is more prolonged than it is in patients who have had multiple recurrent tumors (Cutler et al., 1982). This is strongly suggestive of the greater likelihood of sequential activation of multiple oncogenes because of the increased cell proliferation that occurs; it may be what actually permits clinical expression of more aggressive, less differentiated tumors when earlier tumors were low grade. That such progression does not appear to characterize tumor diatheses in a majority of cases suggests that the earliest events in the development of a particular tumor determine its biologic potential in most instances, that genetic drift and its influence on tumor behavior may be a factor to consider only in a substantially smaller number of instances, and that tumor cell homogeneity rather than heterogeneity, vis-à-vis oncogene activation, may actually be more the norm in most patients. Thus, all cells in a given tumor will generally express the same oncogene complement and therefore share the same potential intrinsic behavior through multiple recurrences.

The critical stages are probably those that involve early infiltration by dysplastic cells, since this is also likely to be an expression of the potential for vascular and lymphatic infiltration. Penetration into the muscle layers may simply reflect a further expression of this potential.

Use of this schema may assist in an understanding of the patterns of tumor behavior that are commonly seen, help to identify additional factors that indicate which developmental pathway a particular tumor may follow, and assist in attempts to intervene in an appropriate and timely fashion in treating various forms of the disease.

Staging of Bladder Cancer

EVOLUTION OF PRESENT STAGING SYSTEMS

Distinctions in the behavioral patterns of bladder tumors and observations of the results of various forms of therapy have led to the evolution of staging systems in bladder cancer (Fig. 30–13; Table 30–1). Such systems are helpful in establishing prognosis for a given lesion, assigning particular therapy for that le-

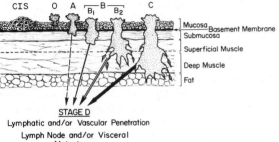

STAGE D
Lymphatic and/or Vascular Penetration
Lymph Node and/or Visceral Metastases

Figure 30–13. Schematic staging system for bladder cancer. This diagram depicts different stages of bladder cancer. Superficial lesions $(0, A, B_1)$ are drawn as papillary growths with a "broad-front" invasive pattern, while more deeply invasive lesions (B_2, C) are drawn as solid growths that infiltrate in a more tentacular fashion. Staging in this diagram also indicates a lesser (O,A,B_1) or a greater (B_2, C) likelihood of lymphatic or vascular penetration and resultant regional or distant metastatic disease by the size of arrows leading to Stage D. (CIS = carcinoma in situ; Stage 0 = papillary configuration with no extension into the lamina propria; Stage A = papillary configuration with extension into the lamina propria; Stage B_1 = extension into the superficial muscle layer with a broad-front invasion of cohesive masses of cells; Stage B_2 = extension into the deep muscle with tentacular infiltration; Stage C = extension through the muscle into the perivesical fat; Stage D = metastatic disease that is either regional (D_1) or distant (D_2). (From Droller, M. J.: Curr. Probl. Surg., *18*:209, 1981. Used by permission.)

sion, and assessing the results of therapy from the response of similar tumors in other patients.

Distinctions between different patterns of tumor behavior were initially based on tumor grade. Albarran (1892) suggested that prognosis could be based upon distinct macroscopic and microscopic appearances that distinguished differentiated from undifferentiated epithelial bladder tumors. Subsequently, Broders (1922) noted that malignant tumors of the bladder epithelium varied in behavior and prognosis according to the proportion of undifferentiated cells that they contained.

Geraghty (1922) was the first to describe a direct relationship between the depth of invasion and the occurrence of metastases. However, this type of system was not adopted till 1946, when Jewett and Strong first demonstrated the clinical usefulness of a staging schema based on the extent of tumor penetration through the bladder wall. In this system (based initially upon autopsy findings), bladder tumors could be separated into three groups. Stage A comprised tumors with only submucosal invasion, and 100 per cent of these were described as potentially curable. Stage B consisted of tumors with muscle invasion, and 86.6 per cent of these were

TABLE 30–1. STAGING SYSTEMS OF BLADDER CANCER

Jewett 1946	Jewett 1952	Marshall 1952	Bladder Cancer Staging (Clinical-Pathologic)	American Joint Committee UICC—1974 CLINICAL	American Joint Committee UICC—1974 PATHOLOGIC
			No tumor definitive specimen	T_0	P_0
		0	Carcinoma in situ	TIS	PIS
A	A		Papillary tumor—no invasion	T_A	P_A
		A	Papillary tumor—lamina propria invasion	T_1	P_1
B	B_1	B_1	Superficial } muscle invasion	T_2	P_2
	B_2	B_2	Deep	T_{3A}	P_3
C	C	C	Invasion of perivesical fat	T_{3B}	P_3
		D_1	Invasion of contiguous viscera	T_4	P_4
			Involvement of pelvic nodes		N_{1-3}
		D_2	Involvement of juxtaregional nodes		N_4
			Distant metastases		M_1

Staging systems for bladder cancer have been based upon observations of the clinical course of different tumors in association with their depth of penetration through the bladder wall at presentation. Initial observations distinguished between superficial invasion (Stage A), muscle invasion (Stage B), and invasion into perivesical fat (Stage C), suggesting that superficial tumors did not carry the same ominous prognosis that deeply invasive tumors did. Subsequently, a clinical distinction was found between superficial muscle invasion (Stage B_1), which had a more benign prognosis, and deep muscle invasion (Stage B_2), which had a more ominous prognosis. A distinction was also noted between superficial tumors that had invaded the lamina propria (Stage A) and those that had remained confined to the mucosa (Stage 0).

The TNM system was then introduced to include stages for carcinoma in situ (TIS) and to distinguish between papillary tumors without lamina propria invasion (T_A) and those that had invaded the lamina propria (T_1). Stages in which deep muscle invasion or invasion into perivesical fat $(T_{3A}$ and T_{3B}, respectively) had occurred were combined, and the distinction between superficial muscle invasion (T_2) and deep muscle invasion (T_{3A}) was maintained.

Some have recently suggested that all muscle-invasive disease $(T_2$ and $T_{3A})$ is the same and is to be distinguished from tumor that has penetrated into perivesical fat (T_{3B}). Because previous studies have shown that superficial muscle invasion may in many instances be comparable to lamina propria invasion rather than to deep muscle invasion and may not necessarily have an ominous prognosis, the clinical significance of this distinction remains to be confirmed.

From Droller, M. J.: Curr. Probl. Surg., *18*:209, 1981. Used by permission.

"potentially curable." Stage C comprised tumors with perivesical extension, and only 26 per cent of these were considered "curable."

Subsequent analysis of segmental cystectomy or total cystectomy specimens prompted the suggestion that tumors that had invaded muscle only superficially (Stage B_1) behaved like tumors that had invaded only the lamina propria (Stage A), whereas those that were deeply invasive of the muscle (Stage B_2) behaved like those that had extended perivesically (Stage C) (Jewett and Cason, 1948; Jewett and Lewis, 1948).

Marshall extended this classification by distinguishing a stage for superficial disease in which no submucosal infiltration had occurred (Stage 0), and a stage in which lymph node involvement was already present (Stage D) (Marshall, 1952). He also confirmed Jewett's observation of the clinically important distinction between superficial (Stage B_1) and deep (Stage B_2) muscle invasion.

The American Joint Committee and the Union Internationale Contre Cancer (UICC) restructured this classification so that tumors invading deep muscle and those extending through the deep muscle into perivesical fat were grouped as one stage (T_3), distinct from those that had invaded muscle only superficially (T_2) (Mostofi et al., 1973; Sobin, 1978; Wallace et al., 1975). Recently, however, Johnson suggested a clinical distinction between tumors that were deeply invasive of muscle and those that had penetrated the perivesical fat (Johnson, 1985). This implied that maintaining separate T_{3A} and T_{3B} stages for such tumors might be clinically useful. He also indicated that the difficulty in distinguishing clinically between superficial and deep muscle invasion made such attempts a meaningless exercise, an impression that confirmed suggestions by the WHO–UICC Staging Committees (Chisholm et al., 1980). However, other reports have proposed that superficial muscle invasion may reflect a tumor diathesis distinct from that associated with deep infiltration, and this has been supported by numerous clinical experiences (see further on). The distinction between different forms of muscle-invasive disease has therefore been retained in most centers and continues to be a clinically useful one.

The UICC has also suggested that tumors that infiltrated and those that did not infiltrate the lamina propria should be grouped as a single stage (T_1). However, Jewett observed that 20 per cent of tumors that had penetrated the lamina propria showed lymphatic permeation; two thirds of these were also found to have metastasized through the bladder wall via these lymphatics. He contended that this was a unique stage of disease that should be regarded as different from that of tumors confined to the mucosa (Jewett and Eversole, 1960; Jewett et al., 1964). Similarly, Pryor (1973) suggested several stages of superficial disease: P_A, in which true papillary in situ tumor was present (88 per cent 3-year survival); P_{1A}, in which there was breakthrough of the basement membrane by papillary disease and infiltration of the stromal core of the tumor (77 per cent 3-year survival); and P_{1B}, in which infiltration of the true lamina propria had occurred (64 per cent 3-year survival). The NBCCGA has recently reported upon the greater tendency of lamina propria–invasive tumors to progress in comparison with the minimal tendency of tumors confined to the mucosa to do the same (Cutler et al., 1982). This further supports the need to separate superficial tumors confined to the mucosa with no infiltration (Stage T_A) from those that have invaded the lamina propria (Stage T_1) (Prout, 1982b).

ADDITIONAL FACTORS INFLUENCING THE STAGING OF BLADDER CANCERS

Staging Errors. The usefulness of staging systems has been limited by the lack of accuracy in assessing the clinical extent of disease (Table 30–2) (Schmidt and Weinstein, 1976; Kenny et al., 1970; Marshall, 1952; Prout, 1975). When tumors have been clinically staged as superficial (0, A, or B_1), operative pathologic staging has demonstrated an understaging error of approximately 25 per cent and an accuracy of only 50 to 80 per cent. When tumors have been clinically staged as more deeply invasive (B_2 and C), accuracy on subsequent pathologic assessment has ranged between 15 and 33 per cent, and 20 to 30 per cent of cases have actually proved to be Stage D. Moreover, lesions clinically staged as more advanced have been overstaged in 20 per cent of cases.

In this context, the most relevant questions clinically involve not so much the confirmation of arbitrary anatomic distinctions between tumors that a staging system imposes, but rather the reliability of predicting which tumors are most likely to progress and which patients are likely to benefit from regional therapy. These questions pertain largely to those stages of disease that lie in the middle of the bladder cancer spectrum (Stages B_1, B_2, and C), in which the cumulative clinical staging error has ranged be-

TABLE 30–2. CLINICAL STAGING ERRORS IN BLADDER CANCER

Investigator	Clinical Stage	Patients (No.)	Operative Stage		
			O, A, B$_1$	B$_2$, C	D
Marshall (1952)	O, A, B$_1$	29	19 (66%)*	7 (24%)†	3 (10%)‡
Prout (1975)		40	19 (48%)	13 (33%)	8 (20%)
Whitmore (1977)		66	52 (79%)	10 (15%)	4 (6%)
Kenny (1970)		34	21 (62%)	10 (29%)	3 (9%)
Marshall (1952)	B$_2$, C	67	9 (13%)§	25 (37%)*	33 (49%)‡
Prout (1975)		66	13 (20%)	31 (47%)	22 (33%)
Whitmore (1977)		65	0 (0)	41 (63%)	24 (37%)
Kenny (1970)		21	2 (10%)	16 (76%)	3 (14%)

*Number in parentheses represents percentage of accurately staged tumors.
†Number in parentheses represents percentage of understaged tumors.
‡Number in parentheses represents percentage of unrecognized Stage D tumors.
§Number in parentheses represents percentage of overstaged tumors.
Clinically staged superficial lesions (Stages O, A, or B$_1$) have been accurately staged in only 50 per cent to 80 per cent of instances. Pathologic demonstration of actual Stages B$_2$ and C in clinically staged superficial lesions has ranged between 15 per cent and 33 per cent, whereas unrecognized metastases (Stage D) have been found in 6 per cent to 20 per cent of these cases. In contrast, lesions clinically staged as more advanced (Stages B$_2$ and C) have been overstaged in up to only 20 per cent of patients, while unrecognized metastases in such lesions have ranged between 14 per cent and 49 per cent.
From Droller, M. J.: Curr. Probl. Surg., *18*:209, 1981. Used by permission.

tween 20 and 40 per cent (Prout, 1982a; Marshall and Whitmore, 1956).

Distinctions in Muscle-Invasive Disease. Initial staging systems separated muscle-invasive tumors into those that had penetrated superficially and those that had invaded deeply. Some have suggested, however, that this distinction may be meaningless (Johnson, 1985; Richie et al., 1975; Skinner, 1977). This impression has been based on observations that clinical distinctions between these stages may be impossible (Chisholm et al., 1980) as well as the assumption that any degree of muscle infiltration may have a deleterious influence on survival.

This view may be too simplistic, however. Other features of muscle-invasive tumors have been shown to distinguish apparently aggressive cancers from those that may be less aggressive (see earlier). Tumors with a papillary histologic appearance have been found to penetrate the muscularis more superficially than tumors with a solid or nodular appearance (Soto et al., 1977; Prout, 1982a). This difference has been correlated with a lesser or greater likelihood of blood vessel and lymphatic infiltration in these respective tumor types (only half as often in more superficially invasive as in more deeply invasive tumors) (Bell et al., 1971; Slack and Prout, 1980). Corresponding differences in survival of patients with these tumor types have also been seen. For example, patients with tumors of a papillary configuration in one report had a 91 per cent 3-year and a 48 per cent 5-year survival rate, whereas patients whose tumors had a solid histologic pattern were found to have only a 30 per cent 3-year and a 12 per cent 5-year survival rate (Pryor, 1973).

These findings have also been associated with the type of response to a variety of therapeutic modalities. Papillary, more superficially infiltrative disease has been found more likely to be downstaged, and often totally eliminated, by radiation therapy; nodular, more deeply infiltrative disease has not (Slack et al., 1977; Prout, 1975). Tumors with superficial muscle invasion have also often been found to be amenable to a variety of forms of regional therapy (transurethral resection, segmental cystectomy), whereas those with deep muscle invasion have generally failed the same treatments (Brice et al., 1956; Cordonnier, 1974; Wajsman et al., 1975; Whitmore et al., 1977; Utz et al., 1973; Resnick and O'Connor, 1973; Milner, 1954).

Muscle infiltration by itself, therefore, does not appear to be the only determinant of therapeutic efficacy. In this regard, Prout (1975) has stated

. . . if muscle invasion were the sole factor that determined curability, any local attack on the tumor would be curative providing it removed or destroyed the tumor. This is clearly not the case. Bladder carcinoma that spreads into muscle kills the host because cells have the capability of invading lymphatics and blood vessels [and then successfully metastasizing]. But not all muscle invasive tumors contain cells with this capability. Recognition of those factors associated with the likelihood of vascular or lymphatic infiltration [and capability of successful distant spread] will permit more accurate staging of disease and more precise [determination] of appropriate therapy.

Tumor Multicentricity and Grade. The rapidity of tumor recurrence in conjunction with diffuseness of epithelial involvement has been termed polychronotopism (Whitmore, 1979; Prout, 1979). Both spatial and temporal components of a tumor diathesis have been shown to be important in predicting the probability that a particular superficial tumor diathesis will progress (see earlier) (Cutler et al., 1982).

Cellular differentiation is also of importance. Low-grade lesions appear less likely to recur rapidly or to become invasive than high-grade lesions (Cutler et al., 1982). Thus, only 19 per cent of Grade 1 superficial lesions progressed to invasion in one series of patients, whereas 69 per cent of Grade 3 tumors developed infiltrating cancer, half of them within 6 months (Limas et al., 1979). That there are far fewer high-grade, truly superficial tumors than low-grade tumors may reflect this phenomenon and confers additional importance on this criterion in the assessment of superficial disease. Indeed, the relative rarity of high-grade superficial lesions implies that when high-grade lesions are seen, they represent the few instances in which potentially invasive disease is clinically apparent at an earlier stage of tumor development. These suggestions are supported by findings that patients with well-differentiated tumors had a 3-year survival of 67 per cent in one series, whereas only 50 per cent of patients with poorly differentiated tumors survived 1 year and only 20 to 30 per cent survived 3 years (Sjolin et al., 1976).

Variability in the course of different forms of carcinoma in situ also supports this concept. Diffuse disease has been associated with a 20 per cent incidence of microscopic infiltration (Farrow et al., 1976). Relentless clinical progression in the setting of diffuse disease has also been described (Droller and Walsh, 1983). The same has seemed less likely to occur with lower-grade or unifocal in situ disease and simple epithelial atypia (Heney et al., 1978; Friedell et al., 1982). Taken together, the extent of disease, even when superficial, may have to be considered in assessing possibilities of ultimate clinical course.

Surface Blood Group Antigens. Surface blood group antigens, which are oligosaccharides attached to lipoproteins at the outer surface of the cell membrane, are normally expressed on the membranes of human epithelial and endothelial cells in many organs and are present on normal transitional epithelial cells of the urinary bladder (Kovarik et al., 1968; Limas and Lange, 1980). DeCenzo et al. (1975) were the first to observe that deletion of blood group antigens from the surface of bladder tumor cells signaled an ominous clinical course, whereas retention of these antigens appeared to predict a favorable prognosis (DeCenzo et al., 1975; Prout and Weinstein, 1982).

Subsequent studies indicated that morphologically similar superficial bladder tumors could be separated with respect to their invasive potential on the basis of the presence or absence of naturally occurring surface blood group antigens (Fig. 30–14) (Limas et al., 1979). Thus, progression to invasion was infrequent in bladders with tumors that had retained surface blood group antigens but was common when deletion of antigens had occurred (Neuman et al., 1980). In a review of several studies, the presence of blood group antigens in low-grade lesions was correlated with the likelihood of progression in less than 3 per cent of cases (Catalona, 1981). This coincided with findings that low-grade tumors confined to the mucosa had less than a 3 per cent likelihood of becoming invasive (Cutler et al., 1982). Absence of surface blood group antigens was associated with the likelihood of progression in 65 per cent of patients (Catalona, 1981). Exclusion of low-grade tumors from this analysis further increased the predictive value for progression of such diatheses to 88 per cent. In addition, 100 per cent of 62 random biopsies in patients with antigen-positive tumors were also positive, whereas only 27 per cent of 41 random biopsies in patients with antigen-negative tumors were positive (Stein, 1981). Thus, the test appeared to reflect a process that had involved broad areas of the urothelium.

The red cell adherence test has seemed most useful in identifying patients with an optimistic prognosis. It has been less successful in identifying patients who theoretically should undergo cystectomy at a time when tumor is still superficial but likely to penetrate the bladder wall and metastasize. Enthusiasm for the clinical usefulness of such testing has been tempered by findings that "loss" of reactivity for blood group antigens is not an "all or none" phenomenon; that the level of reactivity may be influenced by subtle differences in methodology or by particular conditions, such as squamous metaplasia or previous radiation therapy; and that the threshold for positive or negative test results by either red cell adherence or immunoperoxidase methods is based on semiquantitative evaluations, is subjective, and is likely to vary for different observers (Lange and Limas,

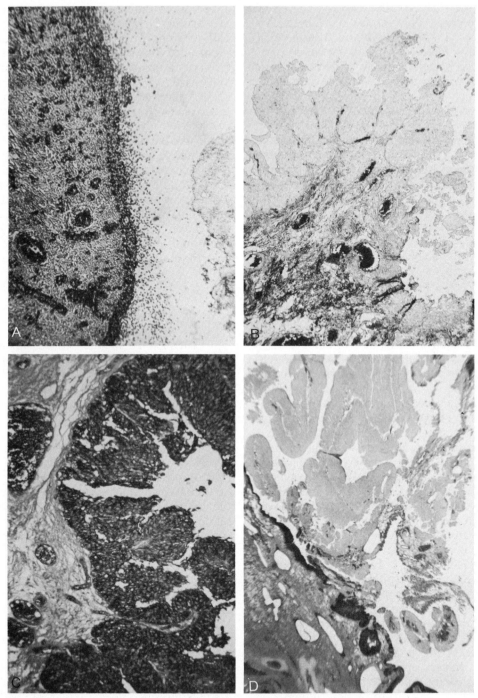

Figure 30–14. Surface blood group antigens as markers for transitional cell cancers.

The presence or absence of surface blood group antigens has been used as an indication of the probable recurrence or progression of superficial transitional cell cancers. Assays that have been used include the red cell adherence assay (*A* and *B*) and the immunoperoxidase assay (*C* and *D*). Staining by adherent red cells or by enzyme activity indicates retention of antigens and likelihood of benign tumor behavior. Lack of staining indicates antigen deletion and more likely recurrence and progression. Further refinements of these techniques are necessary before they can achieve general applicability in the determination of suitable therapy for patients with superficial transitional cell cancers. (*A*, Normal uroepithelium and adherent red cells; *B*, red cell adherence–negative superficial papillary tumor with normally labeled control areas on vascular endothelium; *C*, peroxidase labeling of superficial papillary tumor; *D*, peroxidase-negative tumor and peroxidase-positive normal epithelium.) (*A* and *B* from Emmott, R. C., et al.: J. Urol., *125*:26, 1981; *C* and *D* from Wiley, E. L., et al.: J. Urol., *128*:276, 1982. Used by permission.)

1980; Emmott et al., 1981; Wiley et al., 1982; Weinstein et al., 1979; Limas and Lange, 1980; Flanigan et al., 1983; Wolk and Bishop, 1983). Attention to these concerns is warranted if such testing is to become capable of detecting which superficial tumors potentially place their host at risk.

THE THOMSEN-FRIEDENREICH ANTIGEN (T-ANTIGEN). This surface antigen is represented in masked form on normal urothelium (Coon et al., 1982). T-antigen and surface blood group antigens behave as independent variables in human bladder (Weinstein et al., 1984). In one study, patients who had blood group antigen deletion with normal T-antigen expression had few recurrences and a 16 per cent incidence of subsequent invasion (Weinstein et al., 1984). Those with abnormal T-antigen expression (either T-antigen positive or cryptic T-antigen negative) had a nearly 65 per cent incidence of recurrence with invasion (Summers et al., 1983). Whether or not this antigen will have sufficient specificity and sensitivity to provide adequate positive predictive value, and whether it will be as subject to the whims of methodology as ABH blood group antigen detection has been, will determine its usefulness in predicting tumor course and designing suitable therapy.

Tumor Karyotype and Marker Chromosomes. An apparent progressive increase in modal chromosome number with tumor dedifferentiation has been observed in a number of studies (Falor and Ward, 1973; Shigematsu, 1965). In such studies, only 20 per cent of cells in invasive tumors have been found to have a modal chromosome number. This is in contrast to noninvasive cancers, in which more than 50 per cent of the cells have had a simple modal number (Falor, 1971). However, correlations between anaplasia, chromosome number and appearance, and development of more progressive tumors have been based upon analysis of different types of tumors in different patients rather than upon analysis of progressive tumors in the same patient. Therefore, whether chromosomal changes in superficial tumors will actually be shown to indicate potential infiltration and metastases remains to be determined.

The presence of marker chromosomes rather than chromosomal number may be more important in determining ultimate tumor course. In a 10-year analysis of the chromosomes in noninvasive papillary carcinomas, tumors without markers did well, whereas those with markers behaved aggressively (Summers et al., 1981). Moreover, the triad of tetraploidy, chromosomal markers, and submucosal invasiveness

appeared to indicate a prognosis poor enough to warrant early cystectomy (Falor and Ward, 1978; Sandberg, 1984). That superficial tumors often were shown to have a single marker chromosome in many cells of the same tumor (Falor and Ward, 1977) and there was maintenance of karyotypic profile of each tumor through many recurrences (Falor and Ward, 1976) suggested that the karyotypic profile and biologic activity of the disease in many instances are consistently maintained and may determine the clinical course (Farsund et al., 1983).

Ultimately, many if not all of these considerations may be factored into a clinically useful, more highly developed staging system for bladder cancer. This will be predicated upon the additional understanding of the biology of disease these factors are found to provide.

Methods of Diagnosis

Diagnosis in bladder cancer involves not only establishment of the presence of disease but also identification of factors that characterize its behavior and predict its course.

SYMPTOMS

Hematuria, either gross or microscopic, is the most common presenting symptom in bladder cancer, occurring in 85 per cent of patients (Varkarakis et al., 1974). Neither the number of lesions nor their size or stage is related to the amount of hematuria seen at initial presentation. Only rarely accompanied by other symptoms, such hematuria is usually referred to as "painless."

On the other hand, urgency, frequency, and strangury, as indicative of vesical irritability, may also reflect the presence of cancer, usually of a diffuse flat carcinoma in situ (Utz et al., 1970; Melamed et al., 1964; Utz and Zincke, 1974). Microscopic hematuria is commonly seen in this setting.

The mean duration of symptoms before diagnosis of tumor has generally ranged between 3 and 8 months (Varkarakis et al., 1974; Marshall, 1956). In the case of diffuse carcinoma in situ, vesical irritability has usually been present for a matter of months, but positive cytologies may have been present for years without associated symptoms in the setting of focal disease.

DIAGNOSTIC PROCEDURES

Cystoscopy and Transurethral Resection. Cystoscopy and transurethral resection are the mainstays in the diagnosis of transitional cell cancer. The purpose of cystoscopy is to identify the presence of tumor and characterize its gross appearance as papillary, sessile, or nodular (Fig. 30–15). Multiplicity and size of lesions can also provide important prognostic information. In the case of carcinoma in situ, slightly raised velvety erythematous areas may be seen. These areas may be diffuse and blend gradually with hyperemic atypical mucosa, or they may be sharply demarcated from normal mucosa. Bladder irritability or spasticity during cystoscopy may indicate the presence of diffuse carcinoma in situ; such spasticity is less common when gross lesions are present in the absence of in situ disease.

Transurethral resection (Fig. 30–16) permits pathologic confirmation of diagnosis. Both superficial and deep biopsy samples must be separately assessed to determine the depth to which a tumor may have penetrated the bladder wall. In addition, tumor architecture, cellular grade, pattern of infiltration, and possible involvement of lymphatics and vasculature can be assessed and then used to determine the appropriate course of therapy and possible prognosis. If a lesion is clearly superficial endoscopically, resection should be done with a light hand. In

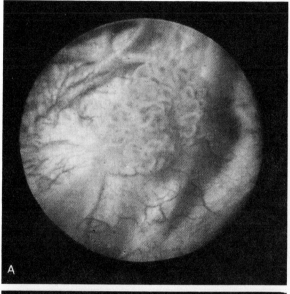

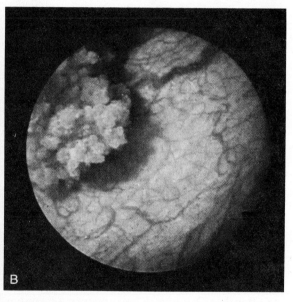

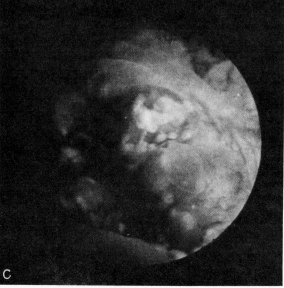

Figure 30–15. Endoscopic appearance of transitional cell cancers.

Superficial papillary tumors are represented by frond-like papillary outgrowths of hypertrophied transitional epithelium, with each papillary excrescence composed of several layers of epithelial cells surrounding a vascular connective tissue core (*A* and *B*). The base of these lesions is frequently characterized by prominent blood vessels but an otherwise normal-appearing bladder mucosa. Occasional hypervascularization and mucosal erythema in the vicinity of a papillary tumor may indicate the presence of carcinoma in situ *(B)*. Discrete foci of raised, velvety, erythematous lesions may also indicate the presence of in situ disease.

Nodular or solid tumors, endoscopically described as sessile, appear as cauliflower-like masses that blend into the surrounding mucosa and give the impression of having more tumor subjacent to an otherwise normal or erythematous epithelium *(C)*. Areas of necrosis may occasionally be seen. (From Bauer, K. M.: Cystoscopic Diagnosis. Philadelphia, Lea & Febiger, 1969. Used by permission.)

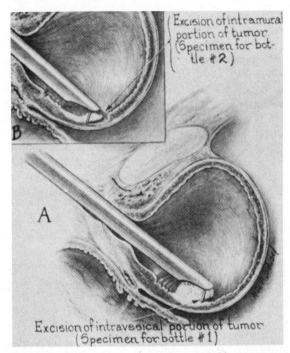

Excision of intramural portion of tumor (Specimen for bottle #2)

B

A

Excision of intravesical portion of tumor (Specimen for bottle #1)

Figure 30–16. Transurethral resection of bladder tumors. Fractional excision of a bladder tumor requires resection of both the superficial portions of the tumor and its deeper components. Because of the need to assess the extent of tumor penetration, care should be taken to include muscle in the deep biopsy specimen without introducing cautery artifact. On the other hand, when a lesion is clearly superficial the subjacent bladder wall usually is thin, and care should therefore be taken not to perforate the bladder wall. (From Jewett, H. J.: J. Urol., *82*:92, 1959. Used by permission.)

these instances, the bladder wall is unlikely to be thickened, and perforation may be more likely to occur.

Random Biopsy. The influence of spatial multicentricity on prognosis (Pomerance, 1972) has prompted the increasing use of urinary cytology and multiple random biopsy to evaluate the entire urothelium at the time of initial or recurrent tumor presentation. Biopsy samples are obtained with a cold-cup biopsy forceps at the margin of any visible lesion and of endoscopically normal or suspicious areas of the bladder and prostatic urethra (NBCCGA, 1977). Findings of epithelial atypia or carcinoma in situ at such sites may indicate a more ominous prognosis (Althausen et al., 1976; Heney et al., 1978; Cooper et al., 1977).

Urinary Cytology. Urinary cytology can assist in defining the spatial extent of urothelial cancer (Fig. 30–17). Though introduced in 1945 (Papanicolaou and Marshall, 1945), it was not until the clinical importance of carcinoma in situ was appreciated some years later that the clinical usefulness of cytologic evaluation was recognized.

The reliability of urinary cytology may depend upon both the extent of a tumor diathesis and the degree of cellular anaplasia. Low-grade tumors are often found to have a negative urinary cytology because of the tendency toward a normal cellular appearance. In one report, only 3 per cent of low-grade papillary tumors showed cancer cells in the cytologic smear, whereas more than 50 per cent of Grade 2 and the majority of Grades 3 and 4 tumors had a positive reading (Esposti and Zajicek, 1972). Moreover, the distinction between low-grade tumors and traumatic or inflammatory conditions may lead to false positive readings in as many as 15 per cent of samples (Geisse and Tweeddale, 1978; Allegra et al., 1972).

If high-grade tumor cells are present in the cytologic specimen from a patient in whom the only cystoscopically visible lesion is a superficial low-grade carcinoma, a lesion of higher grade in addition to the endoscopically visible lesion may be present either in the bladder or elsewhere in the urinary tract (Friedell et al., 1982). In those instances in which visible tumor remains elusive despite persistently positive cytology, the prostate gland, prostatic urethra, upper urinary tracts, or portions of the bladder that might be inaccessible to direct visualization (anterior dome, bladder diverticulum) may be the source of the neoplastic cells.

The yield of positive cytologic specimens is enhanced when bladder washings rather than voided specimens are obtained (Friedell et al.,

Figure 30–17. Urinary cytology in bladder cancer. Cytologic samples from bladders with varying types and grades of bladder cancer are depicted in this composite. Critical characteristics relate to the irregular appearance of the cell nucleus, clumped and marginated chromatin pattern, and prominent nucleolar structure. Inflammatory conditions may interfere with interpretation of low-grade tumors and occasionally with diagnosis of squamous cell cancers. *A,* Normal transitional epithelium, voided. *B,* Normal transitional epithelium, barbotaged. *C,* Grade 1 transitional cell tumor. *D,* Grade 2 transitional cell tumor. *E,* Grade 3 transitional cell tumor. *F,* Carcinoma in situ. *G,* Squamous cell cancer. *H,* Adenocarcinoma of rectum infiltrating bladder. (From Tweeddale, D., and Dee, A. L.: *In* Harrison, J. H., et al. (Eds.): Campbell's Urology. 4th ed. Philadelphia, W. B. Saunders Co., 1979. Used by permission.)

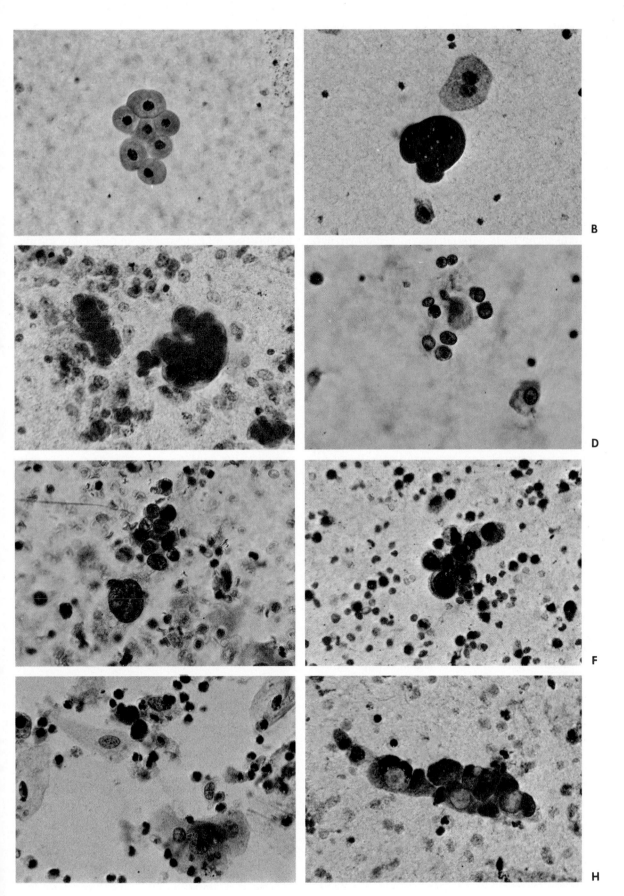

B

D

F

H

1982). Reasons for this include better preservation of cells, better cellular yield, better representation of the bladder epithelium, and less contaminating background debris. In addition, low-grade papillary tumors may be more likely to shed papillary fronds that are more readily interpretable as cancer.

Urinary cytology has not been particularly useful as a screening procedure for bladder cancer in the general population. Farrow and coworkers (1977) observed positive cytologic findings in only 106 of 35,000 cytologic specimens in patients without previous bladder neoplasm who were being seen for a variety of presumably non-neoplastic urologic problems. Although these specimens were obtained in the absence of cytoscopic evidence of neoplasm, carcinoma in situ was ultimately diagnosed in two thirds. Overall, cytologic examination has been found to be far more productive when a selected, potentially at-risk population has been identified.

Recent reports have focused on the use of computerized systems to assist in the diagnosis of malignant cells in voided or aspirated urines. Special fluorescent labeling techniques have been used in such instances to discriminate between normal and cancerous cells in an automated and standardized system (Collste et al., 1979; Koss et al., 1975; Tribukait et al., 1979). Highly differentiated tumors in these reports have usually appeared to be euploid, whereas decreased differentiation has been characterized by an aneuploid appearance. Chromosome studies and quantitative determination of DNA content of individual cell nuclei have confirmed these readings.

Average cell size for normal cells has been found to be practically twice that of tumor cells, while nuclear area has been comparable in benign and malignant cells. Therefore, the ratio of nuclear area to total cell area is important in distinguishing malignant from benign cells. The presence of denser chromatin granules and coarse nuclear granularity in cancer cells has appeared to be of greater importance than other descriptors in the visual identification of the cancer cells. This methodology may prove to be highly useful in both screening and diagnosis because of its rapidity, objectivity, and reproducibility.

Recent studies in prostate cancer have developed the concept of "relative nuclear roundness," which might be used as an index in distinguishing between cancers of lesser or greater malignant potential (Diamond et al., 1982). Assessment of how closely a cancer's nuclei in histologic cross section approximated a perfect circle was correlated with the ultimate clinical course in patients with Stage B_1 and A_2 prostate cancer. With this approach, more accurate retrospective separation between those tumors that demonstrated metastatic potential and those that did not was possible than had been the case in an analysis of these same histologic sections by other grading systems (Epstein et al., 1984). Although heterogeneity of cells in a given cancer and artifacts in obtaining and processing tissue were noted as possible limitations in the general applicability of this method, further development may permit its application to the prospective assessment of various forms of transitional cell cancer. Moreover, application of fluorescent labeling techniques and flow cytometry to the concept of nuclear roundness may ultimately permit automated determination of the prognosis of a given lesion.

Bimanual Palpation. In 1922, Geraghty stated that no patient with a palpable bladder tumor had been cured of disease. This concept became the basis for the Jewett staging system (Jewett, 1977), the strength of which rested on the ability to distinguish clinically by bimanual examination and resection between superficial disease and disease that had penetrated through the muscularis to the perivesical tissue (Fig. 30–18).

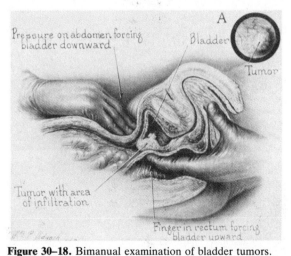

Figure 30–18. Bimanual examination of bladder tumors.

The depth of penetration of bladder tumors, as determined by bimanual examination under anesthesia, originally was an important adjunct in assessing tumor stage. Although fraught with inaccuracy, bimanual palpation remains useful in determining whether a bladder mass is fixed to the pelvic wall, whether it is palpable prior to and following transurethral resection, or whether it is not palpable and hence suggestive of a lower stage of disease. (From Jewett, H. J.: In The Cyclopedia of Medicine, Surgery, Specialties. Philadelphia, F. A. Davis Co., 1950. Used by permission.)

However, Marshall (1952) observed that preoperative estimate of tumor extent was accurate in only 81 per cent of patients. Subsequent studies indicated that bimanual examination could not accurately gauge the level of infiltration. Understaging of superficial tumors $(0, A, \text{ and } B_1)$ ranged as high as 33 per cent (Marshall, 1952; Schmidt and Weinstein, 1976; Whitmore, 1977), and overstaging of more extensive tumors (B_2 or C) occurred in 15 per cent (see Table 30–2). Bimanual examination is therefore now used mostly in determining whether or not a mass is palpable and whether it is fixed in the pelvis. The absence of palpable induration implies that a tumor may be superficial. A palpable mass with histologic evidence of tumor in muscle almost always indicates deep penetration (Skinner, 1977).

Bimanual examination must be performed with the patient totally relaxed by general or spinal anesthesia. Under the best of circumstances, bimanual examination will not reveal lymph node involvement. It also cannot distinguish between benign and malignant fixation of the bladder in patients with previous radiation fibrosis or pelvic inflammatory disease. When bimanual examination fails to detect fixation, however, and a previously palpable mass is no longer palpable after transurethral resection, it is possible that the tumor is truly superficial and, even if invasive of muscle, may be amenable to surgical cure.

Radiographic Assessment of Bladder Cancer

EXCRETORY UROGRAPHY. Intravenous pyelography may be used to determine the presence of lesions in the upper tracts and whether or not ureteral obstruction has occurred (Friedland et al., 1983). The latter may signify an infiltrative bladder cancer near the ureteral orifice or at the base of the bladder (Fig. 30–19).

The appearance of rigid deformity of the bladder wall during the cystogram phase of the excretory urogram may indicate deep infiltration by a bladder tumor with fixation of that portion of the bladder wall. Although 75 per cent of bladder tumors greater than 1 cm in diameter may be seen on the cystogram phase of the intravenous pyelogram, the absence of a radiolucent bladder mass does not reliably exclude the presence of a bladder tumor.

FRACTIONAL CYSTOGRAPHY. Exposures are made as fractionated amounts of x-ray contrast are withdrawn from a bladder that has been filled with 200 ml of contrast medium. The normal bladder wall usually collapses concentrically. A rigid or fixed bladder wall does not

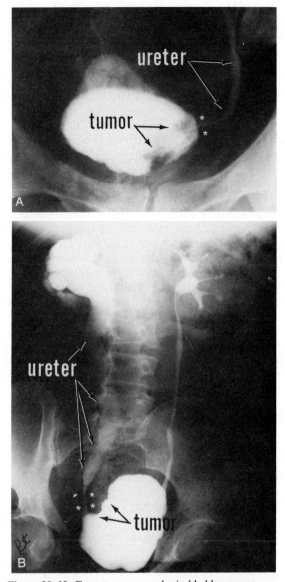

Figure 30–19. Excretory urography in bladder cancer.

The intravenous pyelogram can sometimes demonstrate the presence of a neoplasm in the bladder during its cystogram phase. *A,* When the neoplasm occurs at or near a ureteral orifice (arrows), the absence of ureteral obstruction (asterisks) may imply that the lesion is not invasive. *B,* In contrast, when ureteral obstruction is seen (asterisks), the likelihood of deep invasion of the bladder wall by the tumor (arrows) is increased. The urogram permits the delineation of abnormalities of the upper tracts as well. (From Droller, M. J.: Curr. Probl. Surg., *18*:209, 1981. Used by permission.)

collapse. The absence of successive concentric images has been said to characterize the bladder wall at the site of tumor infiltration. However, false positive images have been found to occur in the setting of previous bladder surgery or when a benign cause for extravesical fixation of the bladder wall exists (Connolly et al., 1967). Double or triple contrast materials have been used in variations of fractional cystography to visualize the bladder and to demonstrate tumors in bladder diverticula.

PELVIC ARTERIOGRAPHY. Pelvic arteriography may demonstrate a vascular stain in some invasive lesions. The tumor itself, though often relatively avascular, may be outlined by a soft tissue shadow with deformity of the vessels feeding the tumor (Gittes, 1979). Corkscrew vessels and venous lakes may be associated with poorly differentiated invasive lesions.

Although pelvic arteriography may be useful in defining perivesical infiltration, false positive findings have occurred in the presence of inflammatory bladder disease or prior pelvic surgery. False negative results have occurred when small invasive tumors were relatively avascular or when tumors invaded the prostate. This procedure is therefore not commonly employed.

PEDAL LYMPHANGIOGRAPHY. Pedal lymphangiography has been used to detect metastases in pelvic lymph nodes. Important features of such studies have included (1) evidence of lymphatic obstruction through a lack of lymph node filling 24 hours after injection of contrast; (2) peripheral defects in lymph nodes; and (3) enlargement of lymph nodes with a foamy appearance, suggesting reactive hyperplasia, fatty infiltration, or lymphoproliferative disorders (Winterberger and Murphy, 1974). Using such criteria, as many as 25 per cent false positive and 15 per cent false negative readings have been reported. Others have reported a concordance of 80 per cent between lymphography and subsequent operative node histology (Turner et al., 1976).

The first lymph node metastases from bladder tumors appear in the obturator nodes (Smith and Whitmore, 1981). Although the visualization of these nodes by pedal lymphangiography has been controversial, several reports have suggested that these nodes could indeed be readily identified (Merrin et al., 1977; Heney et al., 1978; Zoretic et al., 1983; Kaplan, 1983). Pedal lymphangiography has therefore recently been used in conjunction with percutaneous needle aspiration of suspicious lymph nodes to diagnose metastatic disease prior to surgical exploration (Zoretic et al., 1983; Boccon-Gibod et al., 1984). In these reports, aspiration material adequate for evaluation was obtained in 80 per cent of cases with positive lymphangiograms, and 40 per cent of these were positive for cancer. The usefulness of this method is clearly limited by the sensitivity and specificity of lymphangiography. Microscopic disease, inflammatory changes, and total replacement of lymphoid tissue by metastatic deposits will influence the accuracy of diagnosis. As an adjunct in preoperative staging, however, needle aspiration appears to have a potentially important role.

COMPUTERIZED TOMOGRAPHY (CT) SCANNING. Computerized tomography with enhancement by intravenous x-ray contrast and transurethral introduction of air has proved useful in determining whether a primary bladder tumor has led to bladder wall thickening, whether there has been perivesical tumor extension, whether pelvic lymph nodes are enlarged, and whether tumor is present at sites not readily accessible by other means (Fig. 30–20). This technique has been used most effectively when no prior resection, open surgery, or radiation has taken place. Major limitations have centered on the inability to identify superficial microscopic muscle invasion (Hodson et al., 1979). Further technical development to permit clinical appreciation of this critical stage of disease is of major importance.

Purely superficial tumors do not appear on CT scanning to lead to bladder wall thickening, and often the vascular stalk can be clearly distinguished. In addition, there is no visible limitation to the distensibility of the bladder in the area of the tumor. Muscle-invasive cancer is usually associated with thickening and deformity of the vesical wall and often a loss of the smooth serosal contour. Early Stage C (T_{3B}) lesions have been identified by a loss of definition of the margin of perivesical fat as compared with uninvolved portions of the bladder (Seidelmann et al., 1977; Husband and Hodson, 1981).

Detection of pelvic lymph node enlargement by CT scanning has been used in conjunction with thin-needle aspiration to determine the presence of nodal metastases. Enlargement alone is not diagnostic of the presence of cancer, and absence of enlargement does not exclude the presence of micrometastases (Seidelmann et al., 1977).

CT scanning has been particularly useful in those instances in which anatomic assessment of a particular bladder lesion has not been possible by other means. Thus, evaluation of the intramural ureter or of a diverticulum that may harbor a transitional cell tumor has been made possible by CT scanning when other methods were ineffective (Fig. 30–21).

SONOGRAPHY. The continued development of ultrasound with either transurethral or trans-

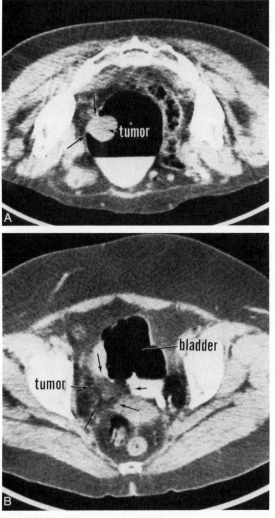

route (Resnick et al., 1984; Matouschek, 1984; Jaeger et al., 1984). Because these techniques have not been fully refined, it is too soon to tell whether the limitations that have characterized CT scanning will also characterize the use of sonography in these settings.

MAGNETIC RESONANCE IMAGING. In the not too distant future, magnetic resonance imaging (MRI) will supplant many of our present techniques in accurately assessing the extent of cancer in a noninvasive manner. Based upon differences in magnetic resonance signals produced by protons following their excitation by varying radio-frequency pulses, the relative position, density, and biochemical environment of

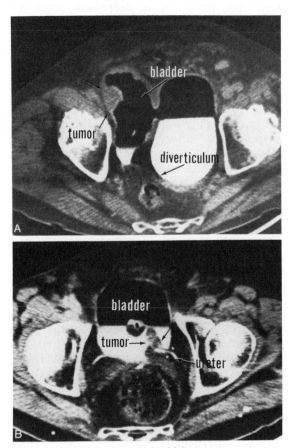

Figure 30–20. CT scanning in bladder cancer.

CT scanning, aided by double contrast amplification (introduction of air via urethral catheter and intravenous injection of contrast), can be used to examine the contour of the bladder and intraluminal lesions of the bladder wall when the bladder is in its distended and relaxed state. *A,* Absence of bladder wall thickening implies the presence of superficial disease, although microscopic penetration into the lamina propria and between muscle fascicles cannot be excluded. *B,* Bladder wall thickening under and at the margins of a lesion implies extension of tumor through the wall of the bladder with possible involvement of perivesicular structures (arrows). Attempts should be made to perform CT scanning prior to any instrumentation of the bladder wall so that inflammatory thickening of the bladder wall does not interfere with interpretation of stages. (From Droller, M. J.: Curr. Probl. Surg., *18*:209, 1981. Used by permission.)

rectal access may provide additional means of diagnosing bladder cancer and assessing the extent of disease (Nakamura and Nijuma, 1980; Holm et al., 1976; Schuller et al., 1982). The most sensitive approach with this modality at present appears to involve the transurethral

Figure 30–21. CT scanning in bladder cancer.

CT scanning is particularly useful in the diagnosis of bladder cancer when anatomic localization of a tumor is not possible by other methods. *A,* When a diverticulum is present that cannot be evaluated by endoscopic means, CT scanning may assist in the delineation of lesions both in the bladder and in its diverticulum and may indicate whether a particular lesion is invasive of the diverticular or bladder wall (arrows). *B,* A bladder tumor at or near a ureteral orifice (arrows) may be shown by CT scanning to be superficial and not to obstruct the ureteral orifice (asterisks). (From Droller, M. J.: Curr. Probl. Surg., *18*:209, 1981. Used by permission.)

the protons can be computed (Williams and Hricak, 1984). This can produce images, often with sufficient anatomic discrimination, to permit distinctions between neoplastic and normal tissue. Although preliminary application of this technique in tumor involvement of the bladder wall has not been consistently accurate (Resnick et al., 1984), bladder tumors appear to have a signal intensity higher than bladder muscle, which conceivably can determine their depth of penetration into the bladder wall (Williams and Hricak, 1984). Inaccuracies comparable to those that have been seen with CT scanning and transrectal or abdominal ultrasonography indicate the need for further evaluation and refinement of this modality. Whether such development will result in a decreased need for extensive resection and a consequent effect on the course of disease because of fewer surgical manipulations remains to be seen.

Urinary Tumor Markers

MONOCLONAL ANTIBODIES. The development of hybridoma techniques has generated much interest in the potential for developing monoclonal antibodies against tumor-specific antigens in a variety of cancers (Kohler and Milstein, 1975). Numerous investigators began to implement this technology in bladder cancer, with a threefold purpose. The first was to identify tumor-specific antigens in bladder cancer, possibly distinguishing between antigens characteristic of a low-grade, low-stage disease from those of high-grade, high-stage disease. The second was to use antibodies formed against these antigens as a means to diagnose the presence of metastases by tagging such antibodies with radioisotopes. The third, of greatest potential importance, was to exploit such antibodies in the treatment of disseminated disease using radiolabeled ligands.

Exploitation of these technologies in such directions would clearly be dependent upon the actual existence of tumor-specific antigens, their relative homogeneity within an individual patient, and the possible homogeneity, at least at some level, between different tumors in different patients (Droller, 1984).

Preliminary studies have suggested that monoclonal antibodies might indeed be produced against membrane components of bladder tumor cells (Fradet et al., 1984). These antibodies have been used in preliminary studies to distinguish between low-grade and high-grade bladder cancers. Others have produced monoclonal antibodies that have been used to identify putative tumor-specific antigens in transitional cell cancer cell lines and in clinical specimens.

The validity of these assertions and their more general applicability remain to be confirmed.

CARCINOEMBRYONIC ANTIGEN (CEA). CEA is a glycoprotein that has been found to be elevated in urine in association with urothelial cancer (Hall et al., 1972). Urine levels in these studies have been found to be independent of tumor size, differentiation, or depth of infiltration.

Plasma levels, however, have not correlated with urinary levels. Moreover, urinary tract infections, transurethral resection, and the presence of an ileal conduit were each associated with elevated CEA levels (Lattimer, 1976). It therefore appears that neither urinary nor plasma CEA levels are particularly useful as indices of the presence or extent of bladder cancer.

RHEUMATOID FACTOR. Rheumatoid factor (RF) is a gamma globulin antibody-like substance of high molecular weight produced in response to antigen-antibody complexes. Elevated titers of RF have been reported in advanced stages of bladder cancer (Gupta et al., 1979) and have been correlated with the blocking of lymphocyte-mediated cytotoxicity, clinical staging, and tumor recurrence (Pyrhonen et al., 1976). In one study, the presence of RF was associated with tumor recurrence in 77 per cent of cases; its absence was associated with recurrence in only 14 per cent of cases. Elevated titers were not observed in benign urinary diseases.

MISCELLANEOUS SUBSTANCES. A number of substances, including β-glucuronidase (Boyland et al., 1955), plasminogen activators (Hisazumi et al., 1973), fibrinogen degradation products (Wajsman et al., 1975), and tumor-specific proteins (Gozzo et al., 1977), have been examined in the urine of patients with bladder cancer. To date, specificity of these substances for bladder cancer and their clinical usefulness in the evaluation of disease remain to be established.

Host Immune Response.

Little is known of the influence of bladder cancer on the host immune response. Identification of the presence of tumor-associated antigens has involved either direct attempts to prepare specific antisera or monoclonal antibodies (Gozzo et al., 1977) or examination of lymphocyte activity as an indirect index of the presence of tumor through presumed stimulation of an immune response (Bean et al., 1974; Bubenick et al., 1970; Hakala et al., 1974; O'Toole et al., 1974). Although initial results suggested that tumor stage could be correlated with lymphocyte cytotoxicity, that successful treatment with radiation resulted in abrogation of lymphocyte cytotoxic response, and that return of lymphocyte cytotoxicity implied tumor recurrence, findings in individual patients were highly variable and results have generally been inconclusive.

Depression of the cellular immune response in patients with advanced bladder cancer has also been suggested to be a useful index in characterization of the neoplastic diathesis. Decreased responses or increased suppressor cell activity were observed in mixed lymphocyte culture in association with a patient's tumor status (Nishio et al., 1979; Cummings et al., 1978). Technical variability and lack of specificity have limited the clinical applicability of these tests.

Others have examined skin test antigen response and delayed hypersensitivity as a correlate of immune response capabilities. Generally, depressed or absent responses to a variety of skin test or recall antigens have been seen in association with advanced cancer (Catalona and Chretien, 1973; Olssen et al., 1974). Such tests, however, have been too insensitive and nonspecific to use as an index for an individual patient's clinical course.

Studies of regional lymph nodes in patients with bladder cancer have correlated histologic appearance and in vitro functional activity of lymphocytes with stage of disease. Thus, 19 of 22 patients whose nodes appeared to be "stimulated" survived 5 years, whereas only 5 of 25 patients whose nodes appeared as either "unstimulated" or depleted of lymphocytes survived (Herr et al., 1976). In these studies, patient lymph node lymphocytes did not function in either a stimulatory or a responder capacity in mixed lymphocyte culture. These depressed responses were more pronounced in patients whose tumors had progressed outside the bladder.

At present, the role of the immune response in tumor development and progression remains unclear. Whether depression of this response represents a cause or an effect of advanced disease is entirely unknown. In addition, no test currently available is sufficiently specific to permit assessment of disease status in the individual patient (Droller, 1984; 1985a).

Treatment Modalities

TREATMENT OF SUPERFICIAL BLADDER CANCER

Surgery. Transurethral resection is the mainstay of "curative" treatment for superficial bladder cancer. However, "cure" of a solitary superficial cancer is predicated on the remainder of the urothelium being normal both by random biopsy and by urinary cytology. Initial treatment of superficial transitional cell cancer therefore depends upon a full evaluation of the urothelium at the time of initial tumor resection. If multiple foci of transitional cell cancer are found in the bladder, more broadly based therapeutic approaches are indicated (see further on).

Survival of patients with solitary low-grade, low-stage tumors approaches normal life expectancy (Nichols and Marshall, 1956). In these instances, transurethral resection is entirely satisfactory treatment for control of the tumor (Barnes et al., 1967). If there is recurrence in these instances, progression is unlikely to occur (Greene et al., 1973; Varkarakis et al., 1974; Cutler et al., 1982). Such recurrent tumors are then again amenable to simple transurethral resection for control of disease.

The presence of epithelial atypia or carcinoma in situ at the margin of a superficial tumor implies the potential for rapid development of muscle-invasive disease (Anderson, 1973; Althausen et al., 1976; Heney et al., 1978; Pomerance, 1972). In addition, if multiple biopsies disclose carcinoma in situ at other foci in the bladder, the more diffuse spatial extent of the tumor diathesis may imply more rapid recurrence, possibly with rapid progression (Cutler et al., 1982; Schade and Swinney, 1968). Such findings may signal the need for a more radical therapeutic approach than simple transurethral resection (see further on).

The pathologist assumes an important role in determining not only the grade of the lesion but also whether invasion of the lamina propria has already occurred. Lamina propria invasion has been found to indicate a potentially more ominous tumor behavior, 25 to 30 per cent of such lesions ultimately progressing. This is in comparison with lesions confined to the mucosa, in which only 2 to 4 per cent progress (Anderson, 1973; Anderstrom et al., 1980; Pryor, 1973; Cutler et al., 1982). In addition, high-grade lesions have been shown to have a poorer prognosis than low-grade lesions when a superficial tumor has penetrated the lamina propria (Pryor, 1973; Cutler et al., 1982). Such findings imply the need for close surveillance and possibly more aggressive intervention, especially if a lower-grade, mucosally confined tumor was initially present.

The capacity of tumors to be extensive both spatially and temporally indicates the need for systematic endoscopic evaluation of the bladder at regular intervals and assessment, when indicated, of the entire urothelium (upper tracts as well as prostatic urethra). Standard protocols call for endoscopic evaluation every 3 months. Urinary cytology is an additional effective means of screening for possible tumor recurrence in these instances.

At interval assessment, either no tumor will have recurred or recurrent tumor will have remained superficial and of low grade. As most recurrences develop within 2 years of initial presentation (Varkarakis et al., 1974), it is not unreasonable to prolong the interval between repeat evaluations in those patients in whom initial tumor evaluation indicated the presence of low-risk disease and in whom no visible or cytologic recurrence has been demonstrated during the first 2 years of follow-up.

Intravesical Chemotherapy. Rapid tumor recurrence, development of a higher grade of lesion, invasion of the lamina propria, or occurrence of a positive cytology in the setting of low-grade disease may signal the development of a possibly more aggressive tumor diathesis. The potential for progression in these instances has prompted some to suggest cystectomy when these changes occur (see further on). Others have favored a trial of intensive intravesical chemotherapy for control of disease in these situations (Table 30–3). An appreciation of the natural history of bladder cancer is critical in attempting to decide between these options.

The chance of a tumor recurring and then invading muscle ranges from 2 to 4 per cent for a tumor initially confined to the mucosa (Stage T_A) to approximately 30 per cent for a tumor that has penetrated into the lamina propria (T_1)

(Cutler et al., 1982). Patients who present initially with multiple tumors appear more likely to experience recurrence than those who present with a solitary lesion. However, recurrences are likely to remain superficial. Patients with abnormal mucosal biopsies have been found to have more than twice the likelihood of a subsequent tumor (40 per cent) than those whose biopsies were normal (15 per cent) (Soloway et al., 1978; Murphy et al., 1979). However, these tumors too were likely to be superficial.

The influence of histologic grade on recurrence has been suggested by findings that 75 per cent of patients with initial Grade 1 tumors will be disease-free at 1 year compared with only 55 per cent of patients with initial Grade 3 lesions (Cutler et al., 1982). However, if the initial tumor is T_1, a Grade 3 lesion will have a 45 per cent likelihood of progressing to muscle invasion, whereas a Grade 1 lesion will have less than a 15 per cent likelihood of progression (Anderstrom et al., 1980).

The major rationale for the routine use of intravesical chemotherapy is to treat residual foci of disease after transurethral resection of the primary lesion and to prevent the possible development of recurrences from tumor cells that may have been seeded onto a traumatized epithelium during resection (Soloway, 1980, 1983). Other instances in which intravesical chemotherapy has been used successfully have included (1) the presence of multifocal tumors that are not controllable by endoscopic resection alone, (2) medical contraindications to repeated anesthesia, (3) multifocal carcinoma in situ localized to the bladder, and (4) tumors not amenable to endoscopic resection. A variety of

TABLE 30–3. Intravesical Chemotherapy for Superficial (T_A–T_1) Bladder Cancer

Agent	Dosage	Regimen	Results
Thiotepa	30–60 mg (1 mg/ml H$_2$O)	weekly × 4–6, then monthly	30% complete response* 20–30% partial response
Mitomycin C	40 mg (1 mg/ml H$_2$O)	weekly × 8, then monthly	45% complete response† 33% partial response
Adriamycin (doxorubicin)	40–50 mg (1–2 mg/ml saline)	weekly × 4, then monthly	55–65% complete response‡
Epodyl	1 per cent solution, 60 ml	weekly × 6, then monthly	30% complete response§
BCG	120 mg/50 ml saline‖	weekly × 5–6, then monthly	60–80% complete response¶

*50% likelihood of successful prophylaxis.
†67% complete response in previously untreated patients, 25% complete response in previous thiotepa failures.
‡Possible early recurrence on cessation of therapy.
§Demonstrated early and only in patients without lamina propria invasion.
‖With or without 5 mg intradermally.
¶Possible recurrence in ureter or prostatic urethra; long-term course not yet known.
Intravesical Chemotherapeutic Agents: The variety of agents that have been used intravesically, their dosages, and the percentage of complete and partial responses as gleaned from several reports are shown. Responses appear, in general, to be comparable among the various agents examined.

chemotherapeutic agents have been applied successfully both in treatment of existing disease and in prophylaxis against recurrence.

THIOTEPA (TRIETHYLENETHIOPHOSPHORAMIDE). Thiotepa, an alkylating agent, was initially described in the early 1960's for intravesical treatment primarily of tumors that were so multiple as to be unresectable or that had recurred so rapidly as to make repetitive anesthesia unfeasible (Jones and Swinney, 1961; Veenema et al., 1962). In these as well as in subsequent reports, superficial bladder tumors were partially or completely destroyed in approximately 30 to 50 per cent of patients (Nocks et al., 1979; Veenema et al., 1969, 1974; Koontz et al., 1981). Most recently, the NBCCGA reported that patients receiving thiotepa had a significantly better chance of being tumor-free at 1 year (66 per cent) than did a randomized control group (40 per cent) (Koontz et al., 1981; Heney et al., 1983) (Fig. 30–22).

An initial response to thiotepa appeared to indicate that a patient's neoplastic diathesis might respond to a prophylactic course of this agent as well (Koontz et al., 1981; Nocks et al., 1979). Patients with a successful initial response to weekly thiotepa had an overall recurrence rate of only 44 per cent (8/18) when treated prophylactically with monthly thiotepa. This compared with a 79 per cent recurrence rate (19/24) when treatment consisted of transurethral resection alone. The delay to recurrence was 15 months in patients who responded to thiotepa versus 4 months in those who were initially untreated. The frequency of new tumors was also decreased in these groups (0.33 and 1.78 yearly recurrence, respectively).

Suggestions that tumor cell implantation

Figure 30–22. Duration of disease-free status for patients receiving thiotepa.

Evaluation of intravesical thiotepa in the management of superficial transitional cell carcinoma of the bladder by the NBCCGA is depicted. Patients rendered free of disease by resection were randomized either to receive thiotepa prophylaxis for a 2-year period or to undergo no further treatment. At 24 months, 53 per cent of the prophylactic group had remained free of tumor, compared with 27 per cent of the control group *(A)*. Ultimately, 29 patients in the prophylactic group and 34 control patients experienced recurrence, but time to first recurrence was significantly longer in the prophylaxis group *(A)*. Exclusion of patients who had been treated successfully with thiotepa prior to randomization disclosed that 43 per cent of the prophylactic group and 18 per cent of the control group had not experienced recurrence at 24 months *(B)*. Similar examination of post-therapy patients disclosed that 67 per cent of the prophylactic group and 44 per cent of the control group were free of disease at 24 months, differences that were not statistically significant *(C)*.

It is important to note in this study that all curves ultimately became congruent. Of additional note is that disease-free curves for treatment-prophylaxis *(B)* and treatment-responsive, nonprophylaxis (control) patients *(C)* were identical, implying an influence of intrinsic tumor behavior on treatment results. In addition, prophylactic thiotepa did not appear to inhibit progression or development of invasive carcinoma. Moreover, progression to invasion occurred frequently among patients with flat carcinoma in situ, and thiotepa did not affect this at all. Treatment in all groups lasted for only 2 years. Whether prolonged treatment would have altered these results is unknown. (From Prout, G. R., et al.: J. Urol., *130*:677, 1983. Used by permission.)

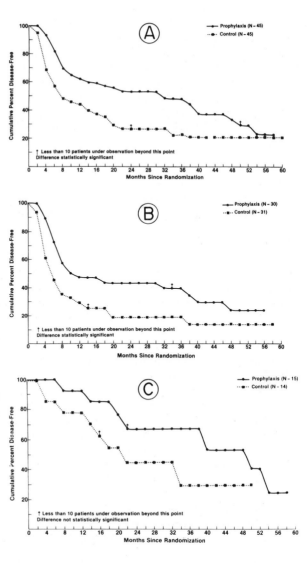

might account for tumor recurrence (Weldon and Soloway, 1975; Boyd and Burnand, 1974) prompted the prophylactic use of thiotepa immediately following transurethral resection of the primary tumor in several studies (Burnand et al., 1976; Gavrell et al., 1978). Patients treated with 30 mg of thiotepa (in 60 ml of water) twice daily for 3 days postoperatively experienced a decreased recurrence rate from 9.5 months before treatment to 33 months after (Gavrell et al., 1978). If the patient was maintained on thiotepa indefinitely, the recurrence-free interval increased to 41 months. In a similar study of 19 patients who were treated immediately postoperatively with 90 mg of thiotepa (in 100 ml of water for 30 minutes), 11 (58 per cent) experienced recurrence. This compared with a recurrence of 97 per cent in 31 of 32 untreated patients. Only 1 of 19 (5 per cent) had recurrence in the bladder vault, whereas 27 of 32 (84 per cent) untreated patients had such recurrence (Burnand et al., 1976). No treated patients developed recurrence limited to the vault, compared with seven control patients who did. Continued use of thiotepa in patients whose tumor recurred did not diminish the frequency of recurrence, implying chemical insensitivity in this subgroup of tumors.

Thiotepa has also been used to treat carcinoma in situ. In one study, 42 per cent (5/12) of patients developed negative urine cytology after two courses of treatment (Koontz et al., 1981), while in another study 40 per cent (16/40) of patients with carcinoma in situ treated with transurethral fulguration and thiotepa had a complete initial response (Prout, 1982c).

The successes described in these reports obscured the fact that when such treatment failed to control flat carcinoma in situ, it might lead to catastrophic results in a majority of patients. Thus, 21 of 40 patients in one series, and 7 of 8 patients in another, developed muscle invasion, metastatic disease, or extension to the prostate within an average of 27 to 32 months despite intensive thiotepa treatment (Prout, 1982c; Droller and Walsh, 1984).

The ultimate progressive course of disease may reflect the intrinsic nature of the tumor diathesis rather than failure of thiotepa therapy. Thus, the incidence of tumor progression was greater in patients who had multiple recurrences than in those who had only an occasional tumor (England et al., 1981). In addition, patients who initially had T_1 tumors, tumor multicentricity, or high-grade disease appeared more likely to undergo progression (England et al., 1981; Zincke et al., 1983). In such instances, progres-

sion could be inexorable, so that despite the appearance of disease control during early phases of therapy, such control might be illusory (Prout et al., 1983). Factors that indicate a possibly more aggressive tumor diathesis (high-grade, lamina propria invasion, diffuse carcinoma in situ) have often been found to predict these failures. Aside from these instances, the use of thiotepa may be highly effective against recurrent and multiple superficial disease both therapeutically and prophylactically.

Most current treatment protocols call for a 6- to 8-week course of thiotepa (30 mg in 30 ml of water) if superficial tumor recurrence takes place within 6 months. A similar protocol is recommended for patients with high-grade lesions, lamina propria invasion, or carcinoma in situ (especially if extensive or symptomatic). In these latter instances, however, patients might be considered candidates for early cystectomy because of the potential aggressiveness of their diathesis (Droller and Walsh, 1984).

Patients are generally advised to restrict fluid intake for 12 hours prior to thiotepa instillation in order to prevent dilution of the agent by diuresis. After 8 weekly treatments, monthly instillations are given for 2 years, followed by bimonthly treatments for 1 year. If no recurrence develops, treatments may be discontinued. Cytologic and cystoscopic monitoring is imperative throughout this course. Persistent positive cytology despite intensive treatment may indicate the presence of tumor at sites inaccessible to intravesical chemotherapy or tumor progression despite negative endoscopic appearance (Droller and Walsh, 1984; Prout et al., 1983; Green et al., 1984).

Major toxicities of thiotepa have included leukopenia, thrombocytopenia, anemia, and occasional cystitis and fever (Hisazumi et al., 1975; Nieh et al., 1978). Most of these appear to be related to systemic absorption and may therefore be associated either with inflammatory mucosal disease or with recurrent tumor (Lunglmayr and Czech, 1971; Mitchell, 1971). This may necessitate temporary interruption or complete cessation of therapy.

MITOMYCIN C. The use of mitomycin C has achieved an approximate 50 per cent complete response rate and a 30 per cent partial response rate in the treatment of superficial bladder tumors (Bracken et al., 1980; Soloway et al., 1981). This compound, obtained from *Streptomyces caespitosus*, must be activated in vivo by NADPH-dependent reduction of its quinone group before it can cross-link with DNA and inhibit DNA synthesis (Prout, 1984). Low-grade tumors have appeared to be more responsive (10/18 complete and 6/18 partial) than have high-grade tumors (1/11 complete and 3/11 partial) (Mishina et al., 1975). In addition, of patients who failed thiotepa treatment (the majority with high-grade cancers and nearly 40 per cent with multifocal carcinoma in situ) an overall response rate of 75 per cent has been observed with mitomycin C (45 per cent complete and 30 per cent partial) (Soloway and Ford, 1983; Huland et al., 1984). However, failures, with ensuing progression, have appeared to be more common in these instances (Droller, 1983; Droller and Walsh, 1984), suggesting the need to be somewhat circumspect over the long term.

Side effects have included vesical irritability and occasional contraction of bladder capacity. Systemic effects have been minimal, presumably because the molecule is too large to be absorbed. Present protocols use 40 mg mitomycin C in 50 to 60 ml water intravesically in regimens identical to those used with thiotepa.

ADRIAMYCIN (DOXORUBICIN). Adriamycin, an antibiotic prepared either by aerobic fermentation of *Streptomyces peucetius* var. *caesius* or by chemical synthesis from daunomycin, has yielded a response rate similar to that seen with thiotepa and mitomycin C (Edsmyr, 1981). Early reports on the use of 40 mg Adriamycin per 20 ml saline biweekly disclosed a 65 to 70 per cent response rate (Soloway, 1983). In other studies, the number of recurrent tumors was decreased from 72 per cent to 39 per cent (Abrams et al., 1981), and a 74 per cent remission was obtained in 19 patients who had previously failed other treatments (Edsmyr et al., 1980).

Treatment initiated 1 week after surgery and then given at 3-week intervals for a total of eight treatments (60 mg Adriamycin in 50 ml water) led to a decrease in recurrence from 75 per cent prior to onset of therapy to 18 per cent following Adriamycin prophylaxis (Edsmyr, 1981). In another study, in which 11 of 27 patients were thiotepa failures and 16 had T_1 disease, 55 per cent of patients maintained a complete response to Adriamycin with negative cytology (Garnick, 1983). Jakse observed that 85 per cent of superficial tumors that were blood group antigen–negative responded to Adriamycin and demonstrated no evidence of tumor progression (Jakse et al., 1983). At least two thirds of these might have been expected to progress during the interval of follow-up (Limas et al., 1979; Neuman et al., 1980). In addition, control of carcinoma in situ was seen in two thirds of cases over the short term (Jakse et al.,

1981). However, longer follow-up is necessary to confirm the persistence of these results and the efficacy of treatment (Jakse et al., 1984; Garnick et al., 1984).

In many instances, Adriamycin treatment has produced remission only during therapy, and tumor recurrence has been observed upon cessation of treatment. Because of minimal absorption through the bladder wall, systemic toxicity has been negligible (Jacobi and Thuroft, 1981).

BACILLUS CALMETTE-GUÉRIN (BCG). BCG (a preparation of killed or attenuated tubercle bacillus) was introduced as a means of treating superficial bladder cancers by recruitment of immune response mechanisms (Pang and Morales, 1982; Morales et al., 1976). However, its effect may be mediated instead by induction of an inflamatory reaction in the epithelial layer (Connolly, 1983).

Initial reports of the effects of intravesical BCG treatments and concomitant intradermal BCG injection described a substantial decrease in recurrence of superficial tumors (Eidinger and Morales, 1976; Morales et al., 1976). In a subsequent prospectively randomized study, intravesical BCG (120 mg in 50 ml of normal saline weekly for 5 weeks, with concomitant intradermal inoculations of 5 mg) decreased recurrence rates from 11 in 24 (46 per cent) in controls to 5 in 23 (22 per cent) in treated patients and prolonged disease-free intervals (Lamm et al., 1981). When BCG was used in prophylaxis, tumor frequency was found to be decreased from 2.97 tumors per patient month in controls to 0.75 tumor per patient month in the BCG-treated group (Lamm et al., 1981). In comparing thiotepa with BCG, the latter (in a regimen of six weekly intravesical treatments with Tice strain BCG without concomitant intradermal inoculation, then every other week for 3 months, then monthly for 2 years) completely inhibited tumor recurrence in all patients (Brosman, 1982). In contrast, 9 of 19 (40 per cent) patients treated with thiotepa had a recurrence within 24 months. Of 12 patients who had been thiotepa failures, 10 had complete tumor disappearance after BCG therapy.

Carcinoma in situ has also appeared to respond to BCG. Morales (1980) reported elimination of in situ disease in 5 of 7 patients who remained tumor-free for 12 to 33 months. Brosman (1982) reported that 5 of 7 patients had complete resolution of cellular atypia after weekly instillations of BCG for 18 weeks. Herr reported that 11 of 17 (65 per cent) patients with flat carcinoma in situ associated with papillary tumors developed negative cytology and improvement in irritative symptoms for an 18-month period after BCG treatment. This contrasted with similar improvement in only 2 of 24 (8 per cent) patients with comparable disease who were treated with transurethral resection (TUR) alone (Herr et al., 1983). Recent observations on 24 patients with only flat carcinoma in situ and no papillary disease demonstrated that 19 (79 per cent) were free of disease for more than 1 year following treatment with TUR and intravesical BCG alone (Herr, 1983). Over 33 per cent of patients who had responded in these studies had failed prior intravesical therapy, usually with thiotepa.

Standard dosages (depending upon the strain of bacillus used) range between 10^9 and 10^{11} organisms instilled in 40 ml saline. Recent studies have suggested that the number of viable organisms instilled may determine therapeutic efficacy (Kelly et al., 1984). Given identical numbers of organisms, the efficacy of Tice and Pasteur strains appears comparable (Lamm et al., 1981; Morales et al., 1976; Herr et al., 1983). Additional studies have suggested that BCG may be administered orally and still achieve its therapeutic effect (Netto and Lemos, 1983, 1984). How this works is entirely unknown, and reports on this effect are preliminary. Confirmation of these observations is strongly indicated so that suitable application in superficial or even invasive bladder cancer can be expedited.

Toxicities of BCG instillation have included dysuria, hematuria, urinary frequency, fever, and malaise (Brosman, 1982; Morales, 1984). Isoniazid has been administered for persistent fevers, but systemic tuberculosis has thus far not been observed.

BLEOMYCIN. Bleomycin has been used only sparingly in the intravesical treatment of superficial bladder cancer. In one study, complete responses were observed only in patients with small superficial tumors (Bracken et al., 1977). In patients with more extensive disease initially considered unresectable, bleomycin in some instances rendered the tumors amenable to transurethral resection. However, none of these patients achieved a complete response, and the overall partial response rate was only 36 per cent. Intense cystitis and the occurrence of cystitis cystica have limited this drug's clinical usefulness.

EPODYL (TRIETHYLENE GLYCODIGLYCEROL ETHER). Initial results with 1 per cent Epodyl in treating superficial bladder cancers compared favorably with those of thiotepa. Complete or partial benefit was recorded in 66 per cent of patients in one study (Nielsen and Thybo, 1979); in another, 19 of 63 (30 per cent) patients had a complete response, while 20 of 63 (32 per cent) were failures from the start (Riddle, 1981). Only patients who did not have lamina propria invasion responded to treatment and patients who responded were found to do so early (Riddle, 1981; Fitzgerald et al., 1979).

Late recurrence was found predominantly in patients whose tumors showed only a partial response during early treatment (Nielsen and Thybo, 1979). Of 20 patients who responded initially and then relapsed, 7 of 8 deaths were due to bladder cancer. Of 24 patients who completely failed Epodyl treatment, 13 of 17 deaths were due to bladder cancer, while 19 patients required radical therapy (Riddle, 1981).

Occasional severe chemical cystitis has limited the general use of this agent. Although its systemic absorption is presumed to be minimal because of its molecular size, and potential systemic side effects have therefore not been observed, inability to test for serum Epodyl levels has prevented its authorization for use in the United States.

SYSTEMIC CHEMOTHERAPY FOR SUPERFICIAL DISEASE. Administration of chemotherapeutic agents systemically to achieve topical therapeutic concentrations in the urinary tract has had mixed results. Oral administration of methotrexate (50 mg weekly) was found to reduce the recurrence rate of tumors significantly from 2.6 to 1.2 in 11 of 16 patients (Hall et al., 1981). Approximately 40 per cent of the methotrexate was excreted within 24 hours. In a similar study, cyclophosphamide (1 gm per m^2 every 3 weeks) produced a complete response in 12 of 15 patients who received the drug for 3 to 12 months (England et al., 1981a). Whether such patients are at risk for later development of transitional cancer through exposure to cyclophosphamide metabolites remains to be seen.

SYSTEMIC PROPHYLAXIS OF SUPERFICIAL TUMOR

Pyridoxine. Pyridoxine (vitamin B_6) has been suggested as a means of preventing recurrent superficial transitional cell cancer because of its apparent ability to restore urinary tryptophan metabolite levels to normal (Brown et al., 1960). After an initial recurrence rate similar to that for placebo, pyridoxine-treated patients appeared to have decreased recurrence rates (Byar et al., 1977). Whether this resulted from adjustment of tryptophan metabolism, and whether this effect represents potential long-term efficacy, require further evaluation. In these studies, the recurrence percentage was 60.4 for placebo patients and 46.9 for pyridoxine patients, results that suggested a trend but were not statistically significant. Although it was suggested that the interval to development of a second tumor (rather than initial tumor recurrence) was altered by pyridoxine (Soloway, 1984), recent studies have suggested that pyridoxine at the levels examined may not influence recurrent tumor development.

Retinoic Acid. Retinoids (vitamin A and its analogs) have been described as potent substances in the control of cellular differentiation and proliferation (Bollag, 1979; Sporn and Roberts, 1983). They have also been found to suppress experimental carcinogenesis in vivo, development of phenotypically malignant cells in vitro, and proliferation of fully transformed and invasive neoplastic cells in vivo (Sporn, 1983).

The most extensively studied of these agents, 13-*cis*-retinoic acid, has been found to inhibit the extent of tumor development in an experimental model of carcinogen-induced bladder cancer, but it has had less effect on tumor incidence (Sporn et al., 1977). Other studies in a model of invasive bladder cancer demonstrated a decreased incidence of both total bladder neoplasms in all animals and the severity of tumor involvement of each bladder (Becci et al., 1981).

The ultimate application of retinoids clinically may involve prevention of disease through suppression of malignant transformation or extension of latency. As such, retinoids have been suggested to function in an "antipromotion" capacity, and they may therefore be most effective against superficial cancers, especially in those most likely to be more extensive and to progress. Their limitation, however, may be their toxicity (Sporn, 1983). An early clinical study of retinoic acid (80 to 100 mg/day) in eight patients with diffuse papillomatosis showed response in only one case, but angular stomatitis and alopecia limited therapy (Zingg and Sulmoni, 1972). Because of the theoretical usefulness of this agent, further developmental efforts seem highly indicated.

Laser Therapy. Adaptation of laser technology to bladder cancer therapy is in its infancy. The laser transmits a wavelength of light at a particular energy, which, when absorbed as heat, may coagulate blood vessels, kill tumor cells, and lead to sloughing of necrotic tumor tissue (Staehler and Hofstedter, 1979; Hofstedter, 1981). Its theoretical advantage may rest in its capability to eradicate recurrent or multiple superficial tumors without the need for anes-

thesia and with minimal blood loss or trauma to surrounding and underlying normal tissue. Major disadvantages have been the inaccessibility of some tumors to treatment because of their location out of direct line of the laser beam, and the lack of tissue for pathologic assessment.

Recent studies have proposed the use of hematoporphyrin derivative (HPD), a strong photosensitizing agent, in conjunction with lasers to treat bladder cancers (Benson et al., 1982; Tsuchiya et al., 1983; Kelly and Snell, 1976). This has been based upon observations of laser-catalyzed tumor destruction by this compound (Dougherty et al., 1975, 1978; Hayata et al., 1982) and findings that HPD is accumulated and retained in greater amounts by malignant than by normal cells (Gomer and Dougherty, 1979; Kessel, 1981).

HPD accumulation and photodestruction have recently been applied in the treatment of bladder tumors, and some have suggested that preferential HPD localization might also occur in premalignant cells that were not endoscopically visible (Kelly and Snell, 1976; Hisazumi et al., 1983; Benson et al., 1982). The diagnostic and therapeutic potential implicit in tumor-selective HPD retention, both for the bladder and for the upper tracts, is under continued investigation. Problems that remain to be solved include expansion of the narrow photoradiation field, which limits extensive therapy in the bladder; the length of time required for photoradiation treatment; and epidermal sensitization to light, which necessitates lengthy protection from sunlight (Benson et al., 1983).

Irradiation. Generally, external irradiation has not been effective in the treatment of superficial disease, largely because of the likelihood of recurrence (Caldwell, 1976). On the other hand, interstitial radiation has recently been used with apparent success in several studies. In one report, radioactive gold grains or tantalum wire were used to treat 180 patients with superficial disease (Williams et al., 1981). Only 10 per cent of T_1 patients and 16 per cent of T_2 patients experienced recurrence. Use of radium implants for solitary T_1 lesions led to an 18 per cent recurrence rate compared with a 75 per cent recurrence rate in similar patients treated by resection alone (Van der Werf–Messing, 1981). The relapse was at the site of prior tumor in 46 per cent of the resection-only patients and in 11 per cent of the radium-treated group. It was 8 per cent at other sites in the former group and 6 per cent in the latter. In addition, relapse was more often multiple in the resection-only group (18 per cent versus 1 per cent). Initial therapeutic failure in these studies led to full-course radiation and/or cystectomy in 20 per cent of radium-treated patients and 65 per cent of resection-only patients. During a 10-year follow-up, 90 per cent of the radium-treated patients and only 50 per cent of the resection-only patients remained free of distant metastases (Van der Werf–Messing, 1984). Clinical T_1 lesions in these studies corresponded to pathologic T_1 tumors in 86 per cent of cases; the remaining 14 per cent were pathologic T_2 tumors.

The fact that these results are so drastically different from those obtained with other treatments or reported from other centers, however, makes them difficult to interpret. Although tumor selection may have played a role, results such as these warrant further evaluation, preferably in the context of a prospective randomized investigation.

In other work, placement of a radium capsule in a urethral catheter balloon has been used to treat patients who had failed endoscopic resection (Hewitt et al., 1981). Of 55 patients, 10 ultimately required cystectomy, while progression occurred in only 2 patients. Carcinoma in situ was present in 15 of these patients.

Although tumor recurrence may impose some restrictions on the treatment of superficial cancers by such irradiation, the apparent efficacy of this modality in selected instances would appear to justify its further clinical study.

TREATMENT OF MUSCLE-INVASIVE TRANSITIONAL CELL CANCER

Only 15 to 30 per cent of patients with muscle-invasive bladder cancers have been documented to progress from initially superficial disease (Varkarakis et al., 1974). What proportion of these individuals actually harbored invasive disease that was unrecognized at the time of diagnosis is unknown (Droller, 1983a). However, the majority of patients with muscle-invasive bladder cancer are diagnosed with this stage of disease at their initial presentation (Kaye and Lange, 1982), and a history of symptoms in such patients is relatively short when reviewed retrospectively (Marshall, 1956).

The rapidity of tumor progression may account for the minimal symptomatology at the earliest stages of tumor development in these instances. In addition, although aggressive regional therapy is usually instituted soon after the diagnosis is made, at least 50 per cent of patients die of distant metastases within 1½ to 2 years of treatment (Marshall and McCarron, 1977; Whitmore, 1980). That these metastases are usually not recognized at the time of initial presentation may indicate that dissemination takes place early in tumor development but that there has not been sufficient time for it to declare itself. Alternative explanations suggest either that metastases are spread as the result of the type of regional therapy applied or that metastases already present subclinically at initial diagnosis of the primary disease are stimulated by treatment-induced compromise of host defenses. The entire question concerning the nature of host-tumor interactions and their effect upon the clinical expression of metastatic disease is still unanswered. It is clearly one that must be considered if we are to understand when certain patients may ultimately not benefit from aggressive regional treatments.

Previous reports suggested that survival of patients with high-stage tumors, if not amenable to radical treatment, was less than 3 per cent within 1 year of diagnosis (Marshall, 1956). Even with treatment, substantial increments in survival in many of these patients were often not obtained (Marshall and McCarron, 1977; Whitmore, 1983). Moreover, as presumed improvements in treatment that might have been expected to increase survivals were introduced, potential therapeutic benefits were not realized (Marshall and McCarron, 1977).

The problem in this form of disease has been to distinguish between cancers that, though infiltrative, were still confined to the bladder and those that were not. An understanding of the different patterns of tumor development and identification of those factors that might characterize the particular pathway a bladder cancer has followed (see earlier) might permit application of appropriate treatments to the bladder cancer that is present. If this could be done, benefits of a particular treatment would "not be concealed through inappropriate application to patients who either are doomed to failure because they already have a systemic disease or who do not truly require a particular [radical] form of treatment" (Caldwell, 1976).

Segmental Cystectomy. Segmental cystectomy has achieved its greatest success in the treatment of highly localized superficial bladder cancer (Stages A and B_1) (Table 30–4) (Cummings et al., 1978b; Whitmore, 1983; Utz et al., 1973). Five-year survivals for superficial stages (including superficial muscle invasion, Stage B_1) have ranged between 50 and 70 per cent. In contrast, survivals for deeply invasive cancers (Stages B_2–C) have generally varied between 10 and 35 per cent (Novick and Stewart, 1976; Evans and Texter, 1975; Brannan et al., 1978).

TABLE 30–4. FIVE-YEAR SURVIVAL FOR BLADDER CANCER PATIENTS TREATED BY SEGMENTAL CYSTECTOMY

Authors	Number	Five-Year Survival (%)				Operative Mortality (%)
		TIS/T$_1$ (O/A)	T2 (B$_1$)	T$_{3A}$ (B$_2$)	T$_{3B}$ (C)	
Marshall et al. (1956)	115	63 (40/64)		22 (11/50)		6.5
Riches (1960)	88	58 (7/12)	36 (16/44)		0 (0/6)	7
Magri (1962)	104	80 (8/10)	38 (10/26)		26 (5/19)	10
Jewett et al. (1964)	133	70 (16/23)	30	8 (4/48)		—
Masina (1965)	72	82	50	38		8.5
Cox et al. (1969)	59	61	27	17		—
Resnick and O'Conor (1973)	102	71 (20/28)	77 (10/13)	18 (3/16)	12.5 (2/24)	2
Ulz et al. (1973)	187	68 (17/25)	47 (18/38)	40 (14/35)	29 (11/38)	1.5
Evans and Texter (1975)	47	69	43	0		0
Novick and Stewart (1976)	50	67	53	20		0
Cummings et al. (1978b)	98	79 (31/38)	80 (17/21)	45 (10/22)	6 (1/17)	—
Brannan et al. (1978)	45	79	80	45		—

Survivals in Patients Treated with Segmental Cystectomy: Segmental cystectomy has had the greatest success when applied to superficial, unifocal bladder cancers, extending from low-stage lesions (Stage A) through superficial muscle infiltration (Stage B$_1$). No effect on tumor recurrence would be expected. Survivals may in many instances reflect intrinsic tumor behavior in these highly selected cases rather than solely the results of therapy.

Adapted from Whitmore, W. F., Jr.: Semin. Urol., *1*:34, 1983; and from Utz, D. C., and DeWeerd, J. H.: Genitourinary Cancer.

The greatest success even in superficial disease has been with low-grade lesions, in which there was recurrence in only 30 per cent of cases, as compared with high-grade lesions, in which recurrence was seen in 80 to 100 per cent of cases (Schoborg et al., 1979). Corresponding 5-year survivals in these groups were 86 per cent and 40 per cent, respectively, suggesting the more aggressive intrinsic nature of high-grade lesions, even when apparently still superficial.

Indications for segmental cystectomy have generally included the histologically well-documented presence of a solitary neoplasm at least 3 cm distant from the bladder neck, inaccessibility of the lesion to transurethral resection, or location of tumor in a vesical diverticulum (Brannan et al., 1978). Contraindications have included recurrent or multiple tumors, the presence of flat carcinoma in situ, involvement of the bladder neck in women or invasion of the prostatic urethra in men, extravesical extension of disease, prior irradiation, and inadequate vesical volume (Jardin and Vallancien, 1984).

Continued arguments in favor of segmental cystectomy for infiltrative cancer have been based upon the assumption that the poor results of total cystectomy were just as likely to have been obtained with partial cystectomy, and the good results with cystectomy were in many instances as likely to have been seen with partial cystectomy. In both cases the intrinsic nature of the disease may have been a major factor in determining outcome. In this context, the likelihood of vesical recurrence would probably be the most important consideration in determining whether segmental cystectomy was insufficient treatment. What is clearly needed is a means of defining the true extent of disease, the probability of its regional confinement, and its potential for having already disseminated or possibly recurring as the manifestation of a broader neoplastic field change. The selection of patients for this modality is therefore critical in obtaining a satisfactory clinical outcome (Pontes and Lopez, 1984; Jardin and Vallancien, 1984).

If segmental cystectomy is undertaken, tumor spill must be avoided and cystotomy should be done as far away from the tumor as possible. Preoperative biopsies to assess margins free of disease may complement frozen-section assessment of margins at surgery. A ureter in proximity to the tumor should be reimplanted rather than allowed to compromise the extent of cancer surgery. Precise mucosal apposition at closure may be important, so that any abnormal mucosa is not inadvertently buried in the bladder wall. Theoretically, suprapubic catheter drainage may permit extravesical seeding of tumor. Therefore, postoperative urethral drainage may be preferable. The roles of preoperative radiation and regional lymphadenectomy as supportive therapy when segmental cystectomy is performed have not been evaluated.

Continued follow-up of these patients with cystoscopy and urinary cytology is mandatory. The frequency of these examinations should be the same as for superficial cancers treated transurethrally. The development of dysplasia mandates more frequent assessment. In addition, pelvic CT scan, magnetic resonance imaging (if available), and mucosal biopsy are indicated if recurrence is suspected.

Cystectomy. Surgical treatments of muscle-invasive bladder cancer initially involved either segmental or total cystectomy, the latter being feasible only after satisfactory urinary diversion could be accomplished with acceptable morbidity and mortality (Leadbetter and Cooper, 1950). Despite these attempts, however, most realized the dismal outlook that deep muscle invasion implied (Table 30–5) (Jewett and Cason, 1948; Jewett and Lewis, 1948). In early series, total cystectomy for tumors with deep muscle invasion was found to produce a 20 per cent 2-year and a 10 to 15 per cent 5-year survival (Marshall and Whitmore, 1956; Brice et al., 1956). Therapeutic "success" in some instances was alleged to be due to a 3 to 5 per cent "freak" survival in patients who were left untreated (Marshall and McCarron, 1977), and some surgical failures were thought to be due to difficulties with urinary diversion. Within this framework, 5-year survivals in surgical patients treated after 1952 seemed better than survivals in patients treated before 1952. This was suggested to reflect better patient selection and improvements in perioperative care (Marshall and McCarron, 1977; Radwin, 1980; Prout, 1975). Similar findings were reported in a more recent review: Forty-eight per cent of patients with clinical T_3 disease treated with cystectomy alone in an earlier series died of bladder cancer, compared with 46 per cent of those treated with 2000 rads preoperatively in a subsequent series

(Smith et al., 1982). Hospital mortality in these groups was 14 per cent and 2 per cent, respectively, indicating improvement in delivery of treatment rather than improvement in control of disease (Montie et al., 1984).

In each of these studies, therapeutic failures with tumor recurrence were thought to reflect the presence of peripheral tumor processes beyond surgical margins, local implantation of tumor cells at the time of surgery, and vascular or lymphatic dissemination of viable tumor cells as a result of surgical manipulation (Whitmore, 1980; Powers and Palmer, 1968).

Radiation Therapy. The development of high-energy, external-beam irradiation provided a modality to treat transitional cell cancer that theoretically could counter the events that had led to surgical failure. A major additional attraction was that it allowed maintenance of voiding and sexual function.

Initial enthusiasm for this modality prompted its use as the sole treatment for bladder cancer (Table 30–6). So-called definitive radiation therapy utilized 6000 to 7000 rads from a cobalt source administered in 7 to 8 weeks either by rotation or by multiple fields. This produced 5-year survivals ranging between 14 and 37 per cent for patients who were clinically staged as having B_2 or C cancers (Goffinet et al., 1975; Caldwell, 1976; Miller and Johnson, 1973). However, only 20 to 25 per cent of tumors in these studies appeared to be totally radiosensitive. The remaining patients had tumor persistence and then either were required to undergo radical surgery or, more usually,

TABLE 30–5. SURVIVAL IN BLADDER CANCER PATIENTS FOLLOWING SIMPLE OR RADICAL CYSTECTOMY*

Investigators	STAGE B_1		STAGE B_2		STAGE C	
	3-Year	5-Year	3-Year	5-Year	3-Year	5-Year
Cystectomy						
Brice et al. (1956)		25/68 (37%)	8/63 (13%)	7/63 (11%)		8/88 (9%)
Jewett et al. (1964)		2/4 (50%)		2/12 (16%)		5/43 (12%)
Cox et al. (1969)	8/13 (62%)	5/11 (45%)	2/5 (40%)	2/5 (40%)	3/12 (25%)	2/11 (18%)
Poole-Wilson and Barrard (1971)	13/44 (30%)	8/32 (25%)	(combined with Stage B_1)		2/10 (20%)	1/8 (12%)
Long et al. (1972)			6/11 (55%)	6/11 (55%)	2/20 (10%)	2/20 (10%)
Pomerance (1972)	11/20 (55%)	3/23 (13%)	9/21 (38%)	6/21 (29%)	5/41 (12%)	1/41 (2%)
Cordonnier (1974)		10/19 (52%)		4/14 (28%)		5/28 (18%)
Wajsman et al. (1976)	20/28 (72%)	14/28 (50%)	24/64 (38%)	21/64 (32%)		
Radical cystectomy						
Long et al. (1972)		3/4 (75%)		1/4 (25%)		5/10 (50%)
Whitmore (1977)		18/30 (60%)		8/31 (26%)		2/19 (11%)
Pearse et al. (1978)		9/14 (64%)		6/12 (50%)		3/15 (20%)
Montie et al. (1984)						
(clinically staged)		21/24 (87%)		11/18 (61%)		11/18 (61%)
(pathologically staged)		5/8 (62%)		14/19 (73%)		8/14 (57%)

*Expressed as number and percentage of patients.

TABLE 30–6. SURVIVAL IN BLADDER CANCER PATIENTS AFTER EXTERNAL-BEAM RADIATION THERAPY

| Investigator | Survival, Clinical Stage B₂–C* | | Regional Failure* |
	3-YEAR	5-YEAR	
Friedman (1959)	5/32 (15%)	4/21 (19%)	37/55 (67%)
Crigler et al. (1966)	24/59 (41%)	13/46 (28%)	136/201 (68%)
Frank (1970)		8/26 (31%)	
Edsmyr et al. (1967)	18/40 (48%)	1/9 (11%)	34/101 (34%)
Miller (1977)		14/71 (21%)‡	29/75 (39%)
		12/66 (18%)§	
Morrison (1975)		35/128 (28%)	44/85 (41%)
Goffinet (1975)	55/123 (45%)‡	(35%)‡	176/358 (50%)
	33/95 (35%)§	(25%)§	
Cummings et al. (1976)		5/14 (36%)	17/25 (68%)
Birkhead et al. (1976)	8/29 (28%)	5/28 (18%)	
Rider and Evans (1976)	41/162 (25%)	29/162 (18%)	44/66 (33%)
Wallace and Bloom (1976)	24/85 (28%)	18/85 (21%)	
Hope-Stone et al. (1981)	110/220 (50%)	83/220 (38%)†	38/95 (40%)

*Number of patients and percentage.
†An additional ten patients had salvage cystectomy.
‡Stage B₂ patients only.
§Stage C patients only.

succumbed to their disease. Moreover, a substantial proportion of those patients whose tumors appeared initially to be radiosensitive subsequently developed tumor recurrence. These persons also then required radical salvage surgery.

Because of these failures, supporters of so-called definitive radiation suggested that this modality be reserved for those whose tumors demonstrate a response to a trial dose of radiation (Hope-Stone, 1984). The rationale and criticisms of this approach are discussed further on (Droller, 1985b).

Integrated Radiation and Cystectomy. The failure of radiation alone to cure disease in the majority of these cases—but its theoretical advantage in controlling regional disease when cystectomy alone might have failed—prompted suggestions that limited radiation might be combined with cystectomy so as to optimize the benefits of each. Thus, surgery would remove the primary lesion that clinically was presumed to be regionally "confined," while radiation would theoretically kill tumor cells disseminated either locally or systemically at the time of surgery, eradicate microscopic pelvic disease already present, and destroy transected peripheral tumor extensions or tumor cells left behind at the time of surgery (Hoye and Smith, 1961; Inch et al., 1970; Potter, 1975). A number of investigations in animal cancer models provided convincing experimental evidence that supported these ideas (Powers and Palmer, 1968).

Initial implementation of preoperative radiation utilized a protocol in which patients received 4000 rads in 4 to 6 weeks followed by

radical cystectomy (Table 30–7) (Whitmore et al., 1977a; Whitmore, 1980; Smith et al., 1982). When patients with clinical Stage B₂ and C tumors treated with this protocol were compared with those in a historical group of clinically comparable patients who had undergone cystectomy alone, apparent marked improvements in 5-year survival (34 per cent versus 16 per cent) and decreases in pelvic recurrence (24 per cent versus 37 per cent) were seen. Noteworthy in both groups were the comparable incidences of distant metastases to bone, lungs, or liver.

Subsequent protocols that incorporated 2000 rads in 5 days followed immediately by cystectomy produced results that were comparable to those seen with 4000 rads (Whitmore et al., 1977b; Whitmore, 1980). Interestingly, radiation portal size did not influence 5-year survivals (58 per cent with 2000 rads, small field from 1966 to 1971 versus 43 per cent with 2000 rads, large field from 1971 on) even though an apparent (but not significant) gradual decrease in pelvic recurrence rate (20 per cent with small field versus 17 per cent with large field) was noted (Smith et al., 1982). Failures in each instance were still due largely to distant metastatic disease.

Interest in definitive radiation persisted, both because of patient reluctance to accept loss of voiding and sexual function and because of improvements in delivery of radiation that appeared to minimize earlier complications (contracted bladders, vesical hemorrhage, bowel irritability, and stenosis) (Caldwell, 1976; Miller and Johnson, 1973). This prompted several pro-

TABLE 30–7. SURVIVAL OF BLADDER CANCER PATIENTS FOLLOWING
PREOPERATIVE RADIATION AND CYSTECTOMY*

Investigator and Institution	Radiation Dosage	Survival† Stages B$_2$–C	Regional Failures	Operative Mortality
Miller and Johnson (1973) M.D. Anderson Hospital	5000 rad/5 wk	37/92 (35%) (old) 19/35 (53%) (new)	15/92 (16%)	3/92 (3%)
van der Werf-Messing (1973) Rotterdam	4000 rad/4 wk	21/52 (40%)	7/54 (13%)	7/54 (13%)
DeWeerd and Colby (1973) Mayo Clinic	4800 rad/5 wk	51/94 (54%) 3-yr 23/45 (51%)		6/152 (2%)
Wallace and Bloom (1976) Royal Marsden Hospital	4000 rad/4 wk	32/77 (41%) 3-yr 25/77 (33%)		6/77 (8%)
Reid et al. (1976) Royal Victoria Hospital	2000 rad/4 days	56/92 (60%) 3-yr 38/92 (41%)		18/135 (13%)
Prout (1976) National Cooperative Study	4500 rad/4½ wk	20/60 B$_2$ (33%) 2/22 C (10%)	3/32 (10%)	
Whitmore (1977) Sloan-Kettering	2000 rad/5 days 4000 rad/4 wk	18/43 (41%) 17/50 (34%)	12/86 (14%) 19/119 (16%)	8/86 (9%) 13/119 (11%)

*Presented as number and percentage of patients.
†Unless indicated, represents 5-year survival rate.

spective randomized trials, in which the results of "definitive" full-course radiation were compared with results of preoperative radiation and cystectomy (Miller, 1977; Wallace and Bloom, 1976). Wallace and Bloom observed 28 per cent and 21 per cent 3-year and 5-year survivals for 85 patients receiving full-course radiation. This compared with 41 per cent and 33 per cent 3-year and 5-year survivals in 77 patients given preoperative irradiation followed by cystectomy. A rapid decrease in the number of patients who were free of disease was seen in each group during the first year after treatment, but many patients who had received radiation alone and were considered "survivors" ultimately required salvage cystectomy. Thus, of 85 patients treated with full-course radiation, 18 came to salvage cystectomy and 60 per cent of these survived. If these patients were removed from analysis, 5-year survival of the radiation therapy only group was 24 per cent compared with 44 per cent for the group undergoing planned combined therapy. Miller and Johnson (1973) reported a similar 51 per cent actuarial 5-year survival for patients receiving preoperative irradiation and cystectomy compared with only a 14 per cent actuarial survival for patients treated with "definitive" irradiation. In addition, many of the latter group subsequently required salvage cystectomy for cure of disease. That combined radiation and cystectomy offered the greatest opportunity for cure of disease was subsequently confirmed in other studies (DeWeerd and Colby, 1973; Reid et al., 1976; Sagerman et al., 1980; Skinner, 1980; Hall and Heath, 1981; Mohiuddin and Kramer, 1981).

Van der Werf–Messing (1973, 1979) suggested that tumor downstaging, presumably as a result of radiation, signified a positive influence on prognosis. In T$_3$ patients, stage reduction after 4000 rads was associated with 5-year survivals of 80 per cent compared with less than 30 per cent if no downstaging was seen. In T$_1$ and T$_2$ patients, however, similar apparent benefits in association with stage reduction were not obtained. The Urologic Cancer Research Group reported that 51 per cent of patients with clinical Stage B$_2$ or C disease survived 5 years if no tumor (P$_0$) was found in the surgical specimen after radiation. This compared with an actuarial survival of 26 per cent in patients who were found to have persistent tumor (in which case radiation did not appear to affect survival) (Fig. 30–23) (Prout, 1975; Prout et al., 1970, 1973; Slack et al., 1977). The Institute of Urology reported 3-year survival rates of 62 per cent for patients with an apparent complete response to radiation (P$_0$) compared with 14 per cent for patients who showed no apparent response (P$_2$, P$_3$) (Fig. 30–24) (Bloom, 1981; Bloom et al., 1982). Similarly, others described an apparently radiosensitive subgroup of tumors that appeared to have a corresponding improved prognosis (Blandy et al., 1980; Hope-Stone et al., 1981; Miller, 1977; Reid et al., 1976; Boileau et al., 1980).

The implications of these findings were supported by observations that patients who were forced to undergo salvage cystectomy after definitive irradiation for recurrent clinical Stage T$_2$ or T$_3$ disease seemed to have an unexpectedly favorable prognosis if their initial tumor ap-

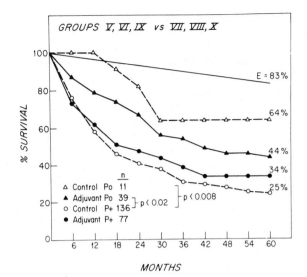

Figure 30–23. Tumor downstaging and survival in muscle-invasive bladder cancer.

Results from the Urologic Cooperative Group demonstrated that patients whose cystectomy specimens showed no tumor pathologically following radiation (adjuvant P_0) had a significantly enhanced survival (44 per cent) when compared with patients with persistent tumor in the cystectomy specimen, regardless of whether or not the latter group had received preoperative irradiation (Control or Adjuvant P+, 25 per cent and 34 per cent, respectively). Although survival in nonirradiated patients who were found to have no tumor in the cystectomy specimen was greater than in all other groups (control P_0, 64 per cent), numbers were too few to calculate statistical significance. (From Prout, G. R., Jr.: Urol. Clin. North Am., *3*:149, 1976. Used by permission.)

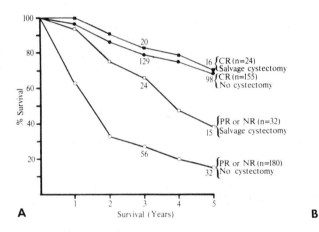

A

B

Figure 30–24. Tumor downstaging with definitive radiotherapy and estimates of survival.

Apparent responsiveness to radiation therapy (4000 R or 6000 R) has been associated with enhanced survival in patients who have had either downstaged tumor or no tumor remaining in the bladder (P_0–P_2). Even if tumor recurred in these instances, such patients appeared to have benefited if they were then able to undergo salvage cystectomy. That these patients were clinically staged and that invasion of muscle was not always a histologic criterion for inclusion in these treatment groups may be important in interpreting such results. The difference in survival between partial or complete tumor regression and no response with preoperative irradiation, and a similar favorable response in comparison with no response with full-course radiotherapy, was significant in each group (p <0.01). *A*, Survival results with or without salvage cystectomy for complete (CR) or partial (PR) responders among all patients treated with radiation, as reported by Blandy et al. *B*, Survival results in the same study for clinically staged T_3 patients. *C*, Results with either 4000 R and immediate cystectomy or salvage cystectomy after 6000 R of presumed definitive radiation according to pathologic stage, as reported by Bloom et al. (*A* and *B* from Blandy, J. P., et al.: Br. J. Urol., *52*:506, 1980. *C* from Bloom, H. J. G., et al.: Br. J. Urol., *54*:136, 1982. Used by permission.)

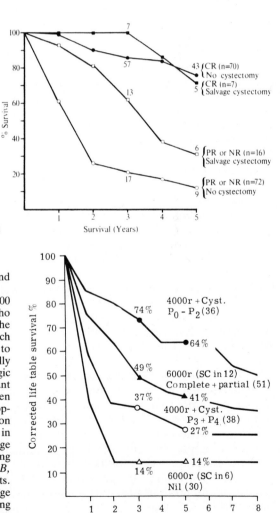

C

peared to have been radiosensitive and downstaged (Fig. 30–24) (Bloom et al., 1982; Blandy et al., 1980; Hope-Stone et al., 1981).

Planned Definitive Radiation/Salvage Cystectomy. The implications of tumor downstaging prompted suggestions that radiation might be used to identify patients with radiosensitive tumors who might have a prognostic advantage (Bloom, 1981; Veenema et al., 1981). Others carried this concept further by suggesting that radiation could be used to select those patients likely to be cured *solely* by radiation therapy, and that surgery might then be applied in a salvage format, if necessary, for tumor recurrence (Veenema et al., 1981; Shipley, 1984).

Reports that newer techniques of external irradiation had produced crude survivals (27 per cent [36/132] for T_2; 38 per cent [83/220] for T_3; 9 per cent [24/262] for T_4) that were comparable to those obtained with planned preoperative radiation and cystectomy (Blandy et al., 1980; Hope-Stone et al., 1981; Bloom et al., 1982) provided impetus for this approach. In addition, survivals appeared to be enhanced when an initial complete response to radiation was seen (Hope-Stone et al., 1981; Bloom et al., 1982; Goodman et al., 1981). Thus, 70 per cent of patients with complete response (observed in 48 per cent of 132 T_2 patients, in 42 per cent of 220 T_3 patients, and in 6 per cent of 262 T_4 patients) survived 5 years compared with only 18 per cent of patients with partial or no response.

This optimistic presentation of data obscured the fact that over 50 per cent of each of these groups were not downstaged. Five-year survivals for these individuals were only 9 per cent and 10.5 per cent for T_2 and T_3 patients, respectively, and even less if such patients were unable to undergo cystectomy. Moreover, only 30 per cent of all T_2 and T_3 patients survived on the basis of full-course radiation, the majority surviving only if total response had been seen (Blandy et al., 1980).

Despite these concerns, some persisted in suggesting that if bladder and sexual function could be preserved an attempt at definitive radiation to obtain a cure, even if in only a small proportion of patients, was a reasonable treatment approach. The effects of preliminary radiation therapy (3000 to 4000 rads) could be assessed by a change in gross tumor size, decrease in ureteral obstruction (if present), or downstaging of tumor on microscopic evaluation, and these could then serve as indications to proceed to a full course (6500 to 7000 rads) of radiation. When this approach was used, 57

per cent (17/30) of clinical Stage T_3 patients who received split-course, full-dose radiation survived 5 years (crude survival) (Veenema et al., 1981). An additional five of seven patients with T_3 disease who received 3000 to 4000 rads and conservative surgery for incomplete response survived 5 years (crude survival) for an apparent combined 60 per cent (22/37) 5-year crude survival. Of these patients, 55 per cent (21/37) with initial microscopically documented T_3 tumors who experienced radiation-associated tumor downstaging ultimately came to cystectomy; 64 per cent (28/44) required cystectomy for control of their disease; and 55 per cent were therapeutic failures. These findings were not unlike those in other reports, in which five-year survivals with full-course radiation for complete responders, partial responders, and nonresponders were 62 per cent, 27 per cent, and 14 per cent, respectively (Bloom, 1981).

In those patients who failed radiation, salvage cystectomy purportedly still enhanced survival (40 per cent versus 12 per cent for patients who did not undergo cystectomy) (Blandy et al., 1980). In addition, stage-for-stage survivals in patients who underwent cystectomy in the salvage setting were the same as those in patients who underwent planned cystectomy after preoperative irradiation (Crawford and Skinner, 1980; Whitmore, 1980). Patients who failed radiation with superficial disease had a 60 to 65 per cent survival, while those who failed with invasive disease had a 15 to 25 per cent survival after cystectomy (Smith and Whitmore, 1981a).

Morbidity and mortality with salvage cystectomy were suggested to approximate that seen in patients undergoing planned preoperative irradiation and cystectomy (Smith and Whitmore, 1981a; Swanson et al., 1981; Crawford and Skinner, 1980). Indeed, while mortality approximated 3 or 4 per cent, the only increase in morbidity in such studies involved the incidence of wound infection. Others, however, reported a 10 to 20 per cent mortality when such patients underwent salvage cystectomy (Blandy et al., 1980; Goodman et al., 1981). Moreover, many patients either were medically unable to undergo radical surgery or had tumors that were found to be technically unresectable. In these instances, survivals were only one-third those in patients who underwent satisfactory salvage cystectomy. Therefore, enthusiasm for the efficacy of definitive radiation in controlling various forms of bladder cancer was dampened by the likelihood of tumor recurrence and the risks imposed by radiation when cystectomy became necessary in the salvage setting.

Interstitial Radiation. Several reports have

suggested that radium implants in T_2 tumors produced survivals at least as good as other treatments (Van der Werf–Messing, 1978). Important prognostic factors included cellular differentiation and tumor architecture. A high degree of differentiation and a papillary configuration implied improved prognosis. Patients in these studies were selected on the basis of extent of tumor and overall clinical condition. Less than 20 per cent of tumors treated were found pathologically to be Stage T_3.

In a more recent review of this work, it appeared that actuarial survival was most influenced by the degree of differentiation, the frequency of abnormalities on intravenous pyelography, and the need for repeated transurethral resection of recurrent cancer (Van der Werf–Messing, 1984). Although satisfactory treatment might conceivably have been accomplished by transurethral resection alone, a corresponding analysis of the same treatment for T_1 tumors appeared to discount this possibility (Van der Werf–Messing et al., 1984). Thus, there were multiple recurrences in 40 per cent of the resection-only group compared with only 2 per cent in the radium-treated patients. Cystectomy or full-course radiation had to be provided to 60 per cent of the resection-only patients and to only 18 per cent of those patients who received radium. In addition, salvage treatment became impossible because of the development of metastases in 50 per cent of the resection-only group compared with only 10 per cent of the radium-treated patients.

Estimated survival in the radium group approximated 90 per cent (of 95 evaluable patients: 196 patients were treated initially) compared with only 20 per cent (involving 13 patients of an initial 143 patients) in the resection-only group for T_1 disease (Van der Werf–Messing et al., 1984). In this regard, it was interesting that the first recurrence in a higher category than T_1 appeared in 22 per cent of the resection-only patients compared with only 1.5 per cent in the radium group. Conclusions as to the efficacy of radium implantation for superficial muscle-infiltrative disease await prospectively randomized study with appropriate stratification of tumor type.

Controversies and Unresolved Questions

RADIATION THERAPY. A number of questions have arisen concerning interpretation of the results with radiation and the primacy of this modality in treating bladder cancer. Foremost has been whether radiation actually provides any therapeutic benefit above what has been achieved with surgery alone (Radwin, 1980; Droller, 1983c). When successes in small selected patient population subgroups are excluded (see later), the majority of patients with muscle-invasive bladder cancers treated with radiation and surgery have continued to fail. That uniform therapies have led to variable results implies heterogeneity in the natural behavior of the muscle-invasive bladder cancers being treated. In addition, other factors have emerged to challenge the more traditional interpretations of successes that have been attributed to the use of radiation therapy.

Methodologic Flaws. Interpretations of the efficacy of radiation have been based largely upon estimates of improved survival and decreased incidence of pelvic recurrence. However, these estimates have been based upon comparisons between nonconcurrent series of patients, and no randomized prospective studies have been done comparing surgery alone with radiation plus surgery. Presumed improvements as a result of radiation, however, may actually reflect better surgery and perioperative treatment (McCarron and Marshall, 1979; Marshall and McCarron, 1977; Prout, 1975). This possibility has been strongly supported by several recent retrospective reviews of the results of contemporary cystectomy, which are as impressive, even in older patients, as earlier results with radiation and cystectomy together (Skinner et al., 1984; Skinner and Lieskovsky, 1984; Montie et al., 1984).

In addition, patient selection has probably played an important role in results that have been obtained. If, at the time of surgery, extensive disease led to exclusion of a patient from fulfilling the combined protocol, a bias in favor of survivals in the combined-therapy group would have been introduced. Similarly, those not faring well enough during radiation to continue with combined-treatment protocols would, by their exclusion, also have biased results in favor of combined therapy. Those who remained in the combined-treatment protocols would have introduced a correspondingly favorable bias for this regimen by constituting a better group of treatment candidates. The influence of such factors was implied in results reported by the Urologic Cancer Research Group (Prout, 1975). Only 50 per cent of patients randomized to receive radiation and cystectomy completed the protocol, whereas 60 per cent of those randomized to cystectomy alone completed treatment. Survivals of clinically staged T_2–T_3 patients in these groups were not significantly different (37 per cent and 31 per cent, respectively). Similar difficulties were encountered in the Institute of Urology Study, in which 21 per cent of patients were unable to undergo cystectomy and were eliminated in an analysis of results (Wallace and Bloom, 1976).

Staging errors may also have played a role in the results that were described. For example, in several reports, histologic confirmation of muscle invasion was not a necessary criterion for entry to protocol (Miller and Johnson, 1973; Van der Werf–Messing, 1979). If the designation "invasion" included lamina propria infiltration, prognosis would have been more favorable regardless of therapy, and results would have been skewed in favor of that particular treatment. In addition, patients in some reports were for the most part only clinically staged, often just by bimanual palpation (Blandy et al., 1980; Hope-Stone et al., 1981). If results were reported for overstaged tumors, when in fact the lesions were of lower stage, an additional bias in favor of combined therapy would have been introduced.

Tumor Downstaging and Survival. The benefits of radiation-induced tumor downstaging have also been questioned (Droller, 1983c). For example, such benefits have appeared to be confined in some studies to patients with clinical Stage T_3 disease (Van der Werf–Messing, 1973, 1979). Possibly, T_2 patients were advantaged to begin with, so that a potential beneficial influence of radiation was obscured. However, it is unclear why T_3 patients who were downstaged did so much better than those who were not downstaged, especially since failures in each instance were usually due to distant metastatic disease.

Perhaps T_3 patients who appeared to be downstaged actually represented a heterogeneous assortment of tumor stages. Since staging in these reports often did not require histologic confirmation of muscle invasion, clinical overstaging could have produced artificially improved results (Wallace and Bloom, 1976; Miller, 1977; Van der Werf–Messing, 1979). Even when retrospective reviews demonstrated muscle invasion in 80 per cent of patients who had been clinically staged as having T_3 disease, depth of infiltration could not be documented and there was no indication as to which of these patients were benefited by their treatment. Thus, Van der Werf–Messing (1979) observed that the prognosis of patients with stage reduction was similar both when there was carcinoma in the muscle of the biopsy specimen and when there was no demonstrable involvement. However, it is difficult to conceive that this could be interpreted as demonstrating only the efficacy of radiation. Rather, it would seem to support the possibility that some of these tumors were

actually of superficial stage to begin with. Otherwise, if radiation plays no role in decreasing the incidence of metastases (Whitmore, 1980), it would be difficult to explain how the same number of patients with presumed T_3 disease prior to radiation did not ultimately develop metastases. Indeed, separate findings that lymph node involvement was associated with 40 per cent of deaths in patients with T_3 disease and with only 7 per cent of deaths in patients with more superficial invasive tumors stress the importance of this possibility in the interpretation of results (Van der Werf–Messing, 1979). Corresponding differences have been described for the development of distant metastases (19 per cent in T_3 versus 7 per cent in superficial invasive disease).

Findings of no tumor (P_0) in the surgical specimen after radiation appeared to confer even more special survival advantage. However, only 25 of 42 (62 per cent) such patients reported by Van der Werf–Messing (1979) had cancer in the muscle on initial biopsy, implying that some of these patients might have been "curable" by transurethral resection alone. The Urologic Oncology Group reported that 30 to 35 per cent of clinical Stage B_2–C patients with muscle involvement in the initial biopsy specimen had no tumor in the bladder after 4000 rads. Only 8 to 10 per cent of patients who had been treated with transurethral resection alone were found to have no remaining tumor at cystectomy (Prout, 1975; Prout et al., 1973; Slack et al., 1977). This implies that radiation had "cured" 25 per cent of patients with muscle-invasive tumors. Actuarial survival of patients with no tumor in their surgical specimen following radiation (51 per cent) was significantly better than survival of those patients with tumor remaining (26 per cent) (Prout et al., 1973).

The critical question, however, is whether these patient groups were truly comparable. Patients whose tumors appeared to be sensitive to radiation were not compared with those whose tumors were similarly downstaged to P_0 by resection alone. Yet, the latter group appeared to have an even greater survival advantage than the irradiated P_0 group (Prout, 1975).

Further evidence that tumor heterogeneity might be important in the overall interpretation of these results was provided by observations that papillary transitional cell tumors might be more "radiosensitive" than solid tumors (Prout, 1975; Slack et al., 1977). The NBCCGA observed that 42 per cent of patients with papillary tumors were graded P_0 after radiation compared with only 30 per cent for patients with solid tumors (Cummings, 1979; Slack and Prout, 1982). However, preoperative irradiation eradicated tumor from 40 per cent of B_1 patients and 32 per cent of B_2 and C patients (Slack and Prout, 1980); in nonirradiated individuals, P_0 patients were primarily those staged clinically as B_1 (Table 30–8). This suggested that such tumors were more likely to be superficial. Other studies indicated that papillary tumors, even when within muscle, were more superficially than deeply invasive, a feature that may well have influenced results that supposedly reflected the effects of therapy (Pryor, 1973; Soto et al., 1977). In addition, papillary tumors were found to invade the bladder wall lymphatics and vasculature only half as often as solid tumors (Table 30–8) (Soto et al., 1977; Prout, 1982b). This coincided with findings that the majority of instances of vascular invasion involved bladders in which tumor had not been eradicated.

Each of these factors could account for the apparently lower incidence of distant failure in tumors that appeared to be more "radiosensitive." Indeed, 39 of 45 solid tumors and only 6 of 45 papillary tumors showed lymphatic permeation in one series (Table 30–8). In another series, of 159 patients receiving 5000 rads preoperatively, 56 (35 per cent) had no tumor in their cystectomy specimen (Boileau et al., 1980). Of these, 41 per cent (12/29) were Stage B_1, 34 per cent (13/38) were Stage B_2, and 24 per cent (11/45) were Stage C disease. Although tumor appearance evidently did not account for significant differences in survival in this report,

no residual tumor characterized 46 per cent of papillary lesions and 37 per cent of solid lesions. In addition, patients with lymphatic involvement only in their preoperative specimen had an 80 per cent 5-year survival compared with a 20 to 40 per cent survival in those who had lymphatic involvement in their postoperative specimen as well.

Finally, in studies of the efficacy of radiotherapy, survival curves of patients relative to those of nonirradiated patients were depressed for patients with solid tumors and elevated for patients with papillary tumors. Even when radiation eradicated solid tumors, survivals were similar to those for irradiated patients with residual papillary tumors and less than those for irradiated patients with no residual papillary tumors. This implied that the papillary nature of the tumor and its intrinsic behavior, rather than the response to irradiation, may have determined the likelihood of survival.

The apparent therapeutic impact of tumor downstaging may reflect the intrinsic nature of a tumor and its particular invasive characteristics rather than solely an effect of therapy. Prout (1982a) has noted that the absence of tumor in the surgical specimen as the presumed result of radiation may actually fail to protect the patient from death from bladder cancer, even though more of these patients seem to have been advantaged by a P_0 finding. Along similar lines, Bloom has concluded that the variability of treatment response in patients with clinical T_3 disease may be "indicative of a generally favor-

TABLE 30–8. STAGING DISTINCTIONS BETWEEN SOLID AND PAPILLARY BLADDER CANCER

Condition	Stage	Solid Tumor		Papillary Tumor	
		NUMBER	%	NUMBER	%
Pathologic stages	No tumor	8	9	2	6
(Cystectomy specimen)	O–A	6	7	3	8
In nonirradiated patients	B_1	10	11	10	28
	B_2	27	30	7	19
	C	22	24	7	19
	D_1	17	19	7	19
Clinical stages	B_1	19	28	27	53
(TUR specimen)	B_2	28	42	20	39
Prior to irradiation	C	17	25	4	8
In irradiated patients	D_1	3	4	0	0
Lymphatic invasion					
Nonirradiated	Present	39	43	6	17
	Absent	52	57	30	83
Irradiated	Present	38	54	14	33
	Absent	33	46	29	67

Stages and Lymphatic Involvement by Papillary and Solid Transitional Cell Cancers: Distinct shifts of the majority of papillary tumors toward more superficial stages and of solid tumors toward more deeply infiltrative stages are apparent. In addition, lymphatic involvement is more commonly seen in solid tumors and has been shown in earlier studies to correspond to depth of infiltration.
Adapted from Slack, N. N., and Pront, G. R., Jr.: AUA Monogr., *1*:213, 1982.

able biologic responsive tumor," largely signifying "variation in natural history of deeply invasive bladder cancer" rather than effectiveness of a therapeutic regimen (Bloom et al., 1982).

Pelvic Recurrence. The effect of radiation on pelvic recurrence of tumor has been suggested by a reported decrease in such recurrence in T_3 patients from 28 per cent (38/136) in those who had undergone cystectomy alone to 16 per cent (19/119) and 14 per cent (12/86) in patients who had received either 4000 or 2000 rads of preoperative irradiation, respectively (Whitmore et al., 1977a; Whitmore, 1980; Batata et al., 1980, 1981). In addition, the greatest decrease in pelvic recurrence appeared to be in patients who had experienced tumor downstaging.

However, these differences were apparent only after a 5-year observation period and were substantially less at intervals of 1 and 2 years (Whitmore, 1980). This was also true when pelvic and extrapelvic recurrences were examined together. Therefore, since extrapelvic recurrence alone in high-stage disease was not affected by preoperative irradiation—10 in 70 (14 per cent) with cystectomy alone versus 14 in 61 (23 per cent) with 4000 rads and 11 in 57 (19 per cent) with 2000 rads—the apparent lower incidence of pelvic recurrence over the 5-year period in patients undergoing radiation might just as easily have reflected, at least in part, compromised survival in those patients who rapidly developed distant metastatic disease and were therefore eliminated from long-term follow-up.

In this regard, Smith has shown that when first recurrence is outside the pelvis after cystectomy, clinical or subclinical pelvic disease has only rarely appeared to have had time to develop (Smith et al., 1982). Moreover, enlargement of pelvic irradiation fields did not appear to decrease deaths with clinical lymph node metastases, and high-grade tumors were associated with a higher incidence of death in the presence of clinically tumor-positive lymph nodes regardless of whether radiation had led to tumor downstaging (Van der Werf–Messing, 1979). This suggests that interpretations of putative radiosensitivity of tumors based upon findings of a 6 per cent (2/36) incidence of positive nodes in the presence of a good response of the primary tumor to irradiation as opposed to a 34 per cent (13/38) incidence of positive nodes in radioresistant cases may have been spurious (Bloom, 1981). Instead, the indolent nature in some forms of the disease may have been as significant as the putative role of radiation in decreasing the incidence of pelvic recurrence. Prout and Coworkers (1979) indicated that 39 of 50 (78 per cent) patients who developed metastases did so within 1 year of surgery, that 37 of these were outside the soft tissues of the pelvis, and that, within this time, radical pelvic surgery had been successful in controlling local pelvic disease with or without adjuvant radiotherapy.

Findings that lymph node involvement was unchanged in patients with T_3 disease whether or not radiation therapy had been administered—14 in 64 (22 per cent) for cystectomy alone versus 7 in 50 (14 per cent) for 4000 rads and 9 in 52 (17 per cent) for 2000 rads—added to the dilemma (Slack and Prout, 1982). That so-called radiation-sensitive papillary tumors had been observed to be more superficially invasive and less likely to have penetrated the bladder wall and lymphatics (Soto et al., 1977) may also have made them less likely to involve pelvic structures and would explain the discrepancy.

In a recent review of this subject, Whitmore and Batata (1984) have suggested that preoperative radiation was of value only in T_3N_0 lesions that were radio-responsive (downstaged) and in which local recurrence alone was likely to be the cause of treatment failure. This would have applied to only 20 per cent of their T_3 patients, even if an optimum response was assumed. The persistent impression was that although radiation may have some benefit, this might be restricted to only a small group of patients, the selection of whom would be critical in maximizing anticipated success from such treatment. Beneficial effects may be either undetermined or unpredictable by available clinical criteria.

Not all series have demonstrated particularly high incidences of pelvic recurrence. A pelvic recurrence rate of only 7 per cent was noted by Prout in patients undergoing cystectomy alone between 1967 and 1975 (Prout et al., 1979). A similar finding of 9 per cent incidence of pelvic recurrence was noted for comparable patients at the Cleveland Clinic (Montie et al., 1984).

Definitive Radiation. Findings that 70 to 75 per cent of those patients achieving a complete response to radical radiotherapy survived 5 years, and that 40 to 45 per cent of those with only a partial response and therefore requiring salvage cystectomy for recurrent tumor also survived 5 years (Hope-Stone, 1984), have been used to support protocols in which infiltrative bladder cancer could be treated by radiation alone and cystectomy performed only in those patients who failed to respond or who relapsed after initial response. Proponents of this approach have argued further that if 30 to 40 per cent of all patients survive 5 years following radiotherapy alone (Blandy et al., 1980; Smith, 1984), and if 40 per cent of all patients who undergo cystectomy (with or without adjunctive radiation) die of metastases within 1 to 2 years of diagnosis (Prout et al., 1979), cystectomy will be therapeutic in only 20 to 30 per cent of such patients, being unnecessary in the former group and inadequate in the latter.

A further analysis of such statements, however, suggests a different interpretation. For example, in those studies that compared "definitive" radiation with preoperative irradiation and cystectomy in a prospective, randomized fashion, 5-year survivals not only were substantially less in the former group but also required salvage cystectomy in a large number of patients (Bloom et al., 1982; Miller, 1977). Therefore, apparent 5-year survival with definitive radiation therapy as reported in other studies (Hope-Stone, 1984; Blandy et al., 1980) might not necessarily have been tantamount to cure. Rather, those patients with aggressive disease probably died of metastatic cancer within 1 to 2 years of treatment (Prout et al., 1979), while those with less aggressive disease survived, regardless of whether regional disease was present. The implied bias in such observations was further supported by the impression that less aggressive tumors would be those more likely to be resectable in the event of persistence or recurrence. This would be compatible with survivals of only 10 to 15 per cent in patients treated only with "definitive" radiation whose tumors became unresectable. This compares with survivals far greater in those who were then able to undergo salvage cystectomy (Bloom et al., 1982; Hope-Stone et al., 1981; Miller, 1977). Both of these factors would favor patients with less aggressive cancers, possibly skewing interpretations in favor of treatment efficacy of radiation when tumor heterogeneity may have been largely responsible for reported results.

Tumor downstaging would also enter into this analysis. The Institute of Urology reported 3-year survival rates of 62 per cent for patients with a complete response to radiation compared with 14 per cent for those who showed no response (Bloom et al., 1982). Comparable observations were made for those patients requiring salvage cystectomy for tumor recurrence (Blandy et al., 1980; Hope-Stone, 1984). However, in those patients downstaged by resection

alone, survival ranged between 60 and 70 per cent (Slack et al., 1977), again suggesting that tumor type may have biased results in favor of whatever manner of therapy was applied. In further support were other findings that the form of primary tumor (T_1 or $T_{2/3}$ disease) appeared to determine the ultimate clinical course after radiation therapy, even though all recurrent tumors were muscle-invasive ($T_{2/3}$) prior to cystectomy (Droller and Walsh, 1983). With the ultimate dependence of many of such patients on salvage cystectomy, it is not unreasonable to suspect that the natural history of disease in the individual may have been the major determinative factor in the course of the disease. The need for comparable concurrent groups of control patients to evaluate the influence of natural history of disease on such results is therefore indicated not only by this possibility but also by observations that survival rates in responders and nonresponders to radiation who actually then undergo cystectomy may ultimately be comparable (Slack et al., 1977; Bloom et al., 1982).

Leaving aside such theoretical considerations, is there something actually wrong with an approach in which radiation is given, tumor response is evaluated, and cystectomy is reserved for those who need it? Some have suggested that "there is nothing to be lost and everything to be gained by carrying out a watching policy. . . . Many patients will thus be spared the perils and discomfort of radical surgery and their overall life-span will not be jeopardized" (Hope-Stone, 1984). Unfortunately, the realities that have been observed do not fully support this position. In most reports, radiation alone has been insufficient treatment for the majority of patients, over 50 per cent still requiring cystectomy. In addition, full-course radiation may weaken the tolerance for major surgery and in many instances eliminate patients from consideration for this modality. Then, if cystectomy cannot be done, survival will be extremely poor, averaging only 10 to 15 per cent (Bloom et al., 1982; Hope-Stone, 1984).

The factor of age must also be considered. In the Institute of Urology series, 5-year survivals of cystectomy patients were 40 per cent in those younger than 60 years and only 22 per cent in those older than 65 years (Bloom et al., 1982). In those patients undergoing salvage cystectomy in the London Hospital series, 5-year survivals were 70 per cent for those under 55 years of age and only 23 per cent for those over 65 years (Hope-Stone, 1984). In these instances, full-course radiation may sufficiently delay cystectomy so that when cystectomy is eventually needed, a possibility in a large number of patients, the patient's age may compromise suitability for surgery and expectations for a successful result.

In addition, operative morbidity and mortality of salvage cystectomy are not inconsiderable. Although cystectomy is a feasible undertaking in the elderly (Skinner et al., 1984), several reports have described a 10 to 15 per cent mortality of cystectomy in the salvage setting (Blandy et al., 1980). Since radiation may also create the impression that a bladder is not resectable, it may further compromise a patient's legitimate chance for a surgical cure. Finally, a delay in regional excision may permit tumor progression and metastasis to take place if this has not already occurred at initial presentation. This situation may be especially likely if only a partial response to radiation is seen and a longer time allowed to elapse before recurrence or persistence is recognized.

Taken together, definitive radiation may sound like a more attractive solution to the problem of invasive bladder cancer than it actually is. Few patients respond without recurrence for a substantial length of time. For those who do, side effects may still weaken them substantially and may compromise their quality of life. For those who respond only temporarily or not at all, cystectomy may carry a higher morbidity and mortality and may not be available to the patient who has become medically less sound either because of radiation itself or because of advancing age. The influence of the natural history of bladder cancer must also be considered in any interpretation of these situations. This is why appropriate control patients are needed to justify conclusions that may otherwise be inaccurate or incomplete.

In sum, the role of radiation in the treatment of invasive bladder cancer remains unclear. What is needed is a means to characterize the nature of invasive tumors to determine whether they are regionally confined and therefore amenable to control and cure by cystectomy (either with or without radiation). This information may also be useful in determining whether certain tumors are susceptible to irradiation, in which case they may not require additional treatment.

Treatment for muscle-invasive disease is in a state of flux. Most would suggest that all muscle-invasive tumors require cystectomy, with or without preoperative irradiation. They would also agree that technical surgical advances have

reached their maximum capability in effectively controlling regional disease. The role of radiation therapy as an adjunct to cystectomy, however, needs to be clarified. Its additive effect to regional therapeutic success is unclear, but it appears to have no role in the prevention of distant disease. The possibility that radiation may ultimately limit the maximal use of systemic therapy has even prompted some to abandon radiation rather than compromise a patient's options. Further characterization of tumors that invade the bladder wall may provide solutions to these problems by defining which tumor patients may be likely to benefit from radiation and which should bypass this modality.

PELVIC LYMPHADENECTOMY. The incidence of regional lymph node metastases is less than 10 per cent in P_2 disease, approximately 20 per cent in P_3 disease, and greater than 40 per cent in P_4 disease (Whitmore, 1983). Corresponding incidences of distant metastases have been 20 to 30 per cent in P_2 disease, 40 to 50 per cent in P_3 disease, and greater than 60 per cent in P_4 disease (Whitmore, 1983). Although lymph node metastases have generally implied a limited prospect of cure with surgery (Smith and Whitmore, 1981b; Bloom et al., 1982), some have observed that vascular dissemination may occur independent of lymphatic spread and that lymphatic involvement may not necessarily signify concomitant vascular spread (Whitmore, 1983).

While pelvic lymphadenectomy at the time of cystectomy has generally been viewed as a diagnostic procedure, several anecdotal reports have suggested that lymph node dissection may in some cases also be therapeutic. Thus, 10 to 20 per cent of patients achieved greater than 5-year survival in the presence of minimal microscopic nodal disease when lymphadenectomy was performed (Whitmore and Marshall, 1962; Dretler et al., 1972; Laplante and Brice, 1973). Recently, a dramatic 35 per cent projected 5-year survival following a "meticulous" lymph node dissection was reported for patients with limited microscopic disease in regional nodes (Skinner, 1982).

These results contrast with the experience reported by Whitmore, in which the overall impact of pelvic lymph node dissection on cure rates in T_3 disease was reflected by 5-year survivals of only 7 per cent of patients when lymph nodes were involved by tumor (Smith and Whitmore, 1981b; Whitmore, 1983). Over 80 per cent of these patients died of bladder cancer— 38 per cent died of distant disease alone, 25 per cent died with only pelvic recurrence, and the remainder died with both. Interestingly, these results were within range of the "freak" survivals that had been described by Marshall in patients with untreated deeply invasive disease, 5 to 10 per cent of whom survived for 5 or more years (Marshall and McCarron, 1977). The negative influence of lymphatic involvement on expected survival was also demonstrated by the NBCCGA (Slack and Prout, 1982). Although only 17 per cent of papillary tumors had involvement of bladder wall lymphatics compared with 43 per cent of solid tumors, expected survivals were poor in each group despite radiation therapy and pelvic lymphadenectomy.

In sum, lymphadenectomy may provide therapeutic benefit to a small proportion of patients who have only microscopic nodal involvement by tumor. Lymphadenectomy may theoretically provide palliation in some patients by decreasing pelvic recurrence (Smith et al., 1982; Smith and Whitmore, 1981b), though this has not been seen in all instances (Montie et al., 1984). Moreover, tumor recurrence at distant sites is probably not influenced by lymphadenectomy. Although lymphadenectomy in the majority of patients may assist only in determining prognosis, its ease of performance and the theoretical therapeutic benefit it may yield in a selected subgroup of patients make it an appropriate procedure to perform at the time of cystectomy.

Role of Prostatic Involvement and Urethrectomy. Primary transitional cell cancer of the prostate has been seen rarely, representing at most 1 to 4 per cent of all prostate tumors (Ray et al., 1977; Black et al., 1974). Stromal invasion has usually been present in these instances, and prognosis has been poor.

Involvement of the prostate by transitional cell carcinoma has been found to occur in 10 to 15 per cent of cases of bladder cancer (Schellhammer et al., 1977; Chibber et al., 1981). Over half of these have been associated with invasive bladder cancer, while 40 per cent have been seen in the setting of diffuse flat carcinoma in situ (Seemayer et al., 1975).

Tumor patterns have included ductal involvement alone or combined ductal and acinar (glandular) involvement (Johnson et al., 1972; Schellhammer et al., 1977). Each of these patterns has occurred with or without stromal infiltration, but when infiltration has been seen, both ductal and acinar involvement has also usually been present (Chibber et al., 1981). Stromal involvement in the absence of overlying epithelial cancer has generally signified retroperitoneal penetration by infiltrative cancer

originating in the bladder. In one study, stromal infiltration was found most frequently in association with high-stage and locally metastatic tumors (17/22) (Schellhammer et al., 1977). In contrast, two thirds of cases with limited in situ patterns were seen only in association with low-stage tumors.

Survival in those patients with only ductal-nonstromal involvement (55 per cent) has been twice that for all other groups (Seemayer et al., 1975; Chibber et al., 1981). The likelihood of survival has appeared to be greater when only in situ disease was present; it has been poor when stromal involvement was seen. In those few instances in which prostatic stromal invasion has been present in the setting of low-stage bladder cancer, survivals have been less than might have been anticipated from treatment of the bladder tumor alone. In the setting of otherwise localized high-stage bladder tumors, the 10 to 20 per cent 5-year survival when prostate has been involved is comparable to that reported for patients with limited nodal metastases (Chibber et al., 1981; Kirk et al., 1979).

Patients with prostatic involvement by tumor have been found to have a 30 per cent incidence of urethral involvement as well (Schellhammer et al., 1977). The same has been observed for those with diffuse flat carcinoma in situ of the bladder (Faysal, 1980). Otherwise, only 5 to 10 per cent of urethras have been found to have carcinoma, even if bladders had multiple tumors or tumors had encroached on the bladder neck. For example, a series of 110 cystectomies with simultaneous elective urethrectomies (in which neither prostate involvement nor diffuse carcinoma in situ was present) demonstrated only a 5 per cent incidence of urethral carcinoma in situ and an 8 per cent incidence of uroepithelial atypia (Schellhammer and Whitmore, 1976). This suggested that the risk of leaving residual cancer if urethrectomy was not performed in these patients was small. Even when immediate urethrectomy was performed, 60 per cent (3/5) of patients with urethral carcinoma in situ and 55 per cent (5/9) of patients with epithelial atypia died of their primary bladder cancer (Schellhammer and Whitmore, 1976). Urethrectomy therefore did not appear to enhance survival.

On the other hand, delayed urethrectomy in those patients who subsequently manifest urethral carcinoma may not be a curative procedure. In one series of 27 delayed urethrectomies for cancer, in which 12 specimens had infiltrative disease and 11 specimens had carcinoma in situ, 100 per cent of the former and 73 per cent of the latter died of cancer within 5 years of urethrectomy (Schellhammer and Whitmore, 1976). Moreover, 7 of 27 (27 per cent) patients who had urethrectomy for known urethral cancer later had tumors in the glandular urethral remnant (Schellhammer et al., 1976). The lethal implications of carcinoma when it develops in a retained urethra have prompted some to advocate that total urethrectomy be performed routinely in conjunction with cystectomy (Schellhammer et al., 1976). Arguments in favor of this approach have been based on the minimal surgical risk, absence of functional and anatomic sacrifice, and risks of later tumor recurrence in the retained urethra (Ahlering et al., 1984).

However, others have suggested that urethrectomy is indicated only in the setting of diffuse carcinoma in situ or prostatic involvement by the bladder cancer. Otherwise, the incidence of urethral cancer is too low to justify routine urethral excision. If this option is chosen, compulsive monitoring of the urethra by cytologic assessment of urethral washings is mandatory. This may permit detection of recurrence when it is presumably still superficial and may enable possibly curative delayed urethrectomy (Beahrs et al., 1984; Zabbo and Montie, 1984).

TRANSITIONAL CELL CANCER IN BLADDER DIVERTICULA. A higher incidence of transitional cell cancers (2.9 to 6.7 per cent) has been reported to occur within bladder diverticula than in the normal bladder (Kelalis and McLean, 1967; Knappenberger et al., 1960). This may reflect either enhanced activation of urinary carcinogens through prolonged exposure to uroepithelial enzymes in the diverticulum or prolonged contact of the diverticular epithelium to carcinogens contained within the stagnant diverticular urine (Gittes, 1979). It may also involve retention of detritus and debris, which may produce chronic irritation within the diverticulum. Although detailed experimental and clinical proof for these possibilities is lacking, Gerridzen (1982) reported on 48 diverticula, 5 of which had tumors and 12 of which showed chronic inflammation.

Tumors in a diverticulum have been thought to have a worse prognosis than comparable tumors within the normal bladder. Absence of the normal bladder muscle layers has been suggested to permit extension of an infiltrative tumor more easily into the perivesical tissues. Whether the normal muscle layers truly represent a barrier against such infiltration, however, is unknown. It is probably more likely that those characteristics that determine tumor cell penetration of the basement membrane and invasion to begin with also determine prognosis. The thinner wall of the diverticulum may only permit earlier expression of a potentially aggressive diathesis. However, it is unlikely that this determines whether that diathesis will be more or less malignant.

Earlier reports that 84 per cent of patients with tumors in diverticula survived less than 1 year after the onset of symptoms (Kelalis and McLean, 1967) might therefore be reinterpreted in view of subsequent observations of an 80 per cent 2-year survival for patients with noninvasive tumors within a diverticulum and a 30 per cent 2-year survival for patients with invasive tumors in these structures (Montagne and Boltuch, 1976). Such results are virtually the same as those for comparable stages of tumor in the bladder proper.

Careful examination of any diverticulum is mandatory. In the event that a narrow diverticular neck does not permit endoscopic evaluation, CT scanning may provide adequate visualization. Although cytology from the diverticulum may be difficult to obtain in these instances, lavage of diverticular urine may furnish a suitable specimen.

When a diverticular tumor has been diagnosed endoscopically, confirmatory cold-cup biopsies should be taken, and multiple biopsies of the surrounding bladder mucosa should be performed to exclude tumor involvement at other sites. Extensive transurethral resection of the diverticular lesion should be discouraged for fear of perforating the diverticular wall.

Tumor excision requires open diverticulectomy with removal of a generous rim of peridiverticular bladder tissue. Care should be taken not to spill any of the diverticular contents at surgery. Ipsilateral lymph node dissection in continuity with the specimen may be indicated when the tumor is of high grade or is sessile. In these instances, preoperative irradiation may also be considered. Cystectomy usually is unnecessary unless other areas of the bladder are involved by infiltrative tumor.

METASTATIC DISEASE

Distant metastases, occurring largely in bone, lung, and liver, are the major cause of treatment failure in patients with muscle-invasive bladder cancer (Prout et al., 1979). At least 50 per cent of patients with muscle-invasive cancer have clinically demonstrable metastases within 1½ to 2 years after cystectomy. That such metastases were not clinically detectable at

TABLE 30–9. SINGLE-AGENT CHEMOTHERAPY FOR METASTATIC BLADDER CANCER

Agent	N*	CR*	PR (>50%)*	Per Cent	Range†	95% Confidence Limits
cis-platinum	60 (320)	2	23	42 (30)	17–55	29–55
Cytoxan	56 (98)	5	10	27 (31)	6–58	16–40
Methotrexate	123 (236)	5	30	28 (29)	0–40	21–38
Adriamycin	246 (223)	6	41	19 (18)	0–71	14–24
Mitomycin C	52 (42)	2	10	23 (13)	0–21	13–37
5-FU	131 (75)	4	18	17 (35)	0–70	11–25
VM-26	65 (108)	3	8	17 (16)	9–21	9–28
Bleomycin	70 (79)	3	5	11 (5)	10–15	5–21
VP-16	9 (29)	0	1	11 (0)		0–48
Vinblastine	9 (38)	0	1	11 (16)		0–48
Vincristine	11	0	3	27		6–61
Hexamethylmelamine	21	1	8	43		22–66

*N = number of patients; CR and PR = complete and partial response, respectively.
†When two or more series of more than five patients each.
Systemic Chemotherapy of Metastatic Bladder Cancer: A variety of chemotherapeutic agents have been used either singly, or in combination, in treating both regional and distant metastatic bladder cancer. Selected ranges of results with these agents are presented. Generally, positive responses have been of only short duration.
Adapted from Yagoda, A.: Semin. Urol., *1*:60, 1983; and from Stump, D. C., and Corder, M. P.: AUA Monogr., *1*:305, 1982.

the time of initial therapy suggests either that distant metastases antedated cystectomy or that surgical manipulation led to distant dissemination. If distant dissemination occurs early in tumor development, tumor manipulation at surgery as a mechanism for further dissemination may be irrelevant. Repeated transurethral resection of tumors has not been associated with an increased incidence of metastatic disease, even in studies of anaplastic, muscle-invasive tumors (Prout et al., 1979). Thus, the varying intrinsic character of tumors may account in most instances for occurrence of distant metastatic disease, an event that may have taken place early in tumor development.

Several cytotoxic agents have been found to be effective either in controlling progressive tumor growth or in inducing partial regression of disease. These have included cis-diamminedichloroplatinum II (cis-platinum), 5-fluorouracil, cyclophosphamide (Cytoxan), methotrexate, doxorubicin (Adriamycin), and vinblastine sulfate (Yagoda, 1983; Stump and Corder, 1982) (Tables 30–9 and 30–10).

In the testing of these agents, response rate has traditionally been defined as > 50 per cent reduction in the totaled products of all tumor measurements (at least 2 diameters) lasting for at least 1 month (Yagoda, 1983). Tumor response with single-agent therapy has ranged between 15 and 40 per cent, and with combination regimens it has ranged between 25 and 50 per cent (Yagoda, 1983; Stump and Corder, 1982). Though at first glance impressive, these percentages are somewhat misleading. For the most part, any response seen with these agents

TABLE 30–10. COMBINATION-AGENT CHEMOTHERAPY FOR METASTATIC BLADDER CANCER

Agent	N*	CR*	PR (>50%)*	Per Cent	Range†	95% Confidence Limits
CDDP + Cytoxan	26 (102)	0	15	58 (26)		37–77
CDDP + Cytoxan + Adriamycin	19 (202)	2	11	68 (46)	44–90	43–87
CDDP + Adriamycin + 5-FU	16 (44)	0	10	63 (44)		35–85
Cytoxan + Adriamycin	33	2	7	27	17–50	13–46
Adriamycin + 5-FU	84	7	27	40	35–50	30–52
Cytoxan + Adriamycin + 5-FU	3	0	2	67		9–99
Adriamycin + VM-26	29	0	5	17		6–36

*N = number of patients; CR and PR = complete and partial response, respectively.
†When two or more series of more than five patients each.
Adapted from Yagoda, A.: Semin. Urol., *1*:60, 1983; and from Stump, D. C., and Corder, M. P.: AUA Monogr., *1*:305, 1982.

has applied to only a small group of patients, has usually been partial, and has been short-lived.

Attempts to improve on these results have incorporated the use of soft-agar clonogenic assays to identify single or combination agents to which a particular patient's tumor cells might be more sensitive (Salmon and Von Hoff, 1981; Stanisic et al., 1983). Clinical implementation of information derived from such observations, however, has not yet led to noticeably improved tumor response or patient survival. Moreover, technical difficulties with these assays and their interpretation have prevented their generalized clinical applicability (Lieber, 1984).

The continued use of cytotoxic agents and reports of partial responses both systemically and regionally when the bladder has not been removed warrant some familiarity with the suggested mechanism of action of these agents as well as with their potential toxicities. Since muscle-invasive bladder cancer is often a systemic problem when it is initially diagnosed, judicious use of existing agents in new combinations and identification of new agents are of major import if we are to be successful in decreasing the incidence of failures due to distant disease.

Chemotherapeutic agents have been placed into specific categories based upon their mechanism of action (Corder et al., 1984). Alkylating agents (cyclophosphamide, cis-platinum, thiotepa) act by substituting an alkyl group for hydrogen in organic molecules. This produces defects in intrastrand and interstrand DNA cross-linking with resultant breaks in DNA during replication. These agents act upon resting and actively dividing cells and are therefore cell cycle phase–nonspecific. Antimetabolites (5-fluorouracil, hexamethylmelamine, methotrexate) act through their structural similarity to natural biosynthetic molecules, either competing with these substances to alter enzyme function or becoming incorporated into molecules and preventing their function in normal cell activity (Corder et al., 1984). These substances are cell cycle phase–specific agents. Cytotoxic antibiotics (doxorubicin, mitomycin) all are derived from soil-borne *Streptomyces,* act by inhibition of DNA synthesis, and are cell cycle phase–nonspecific. Plant-derived antimitotics (podophyllotoxins, vinca alkaloids) either affect DNA, RNA, and protein synthesis or are cell cycle phase–specific for mitosis.

Cis-Platinum. Cis-platinum is an alkylating agent that inhibits DNA replication, probably by intrastrand cross linkage. Serum half-life has been found to be approximately 60 to 70 hours, 25 per cent of the drug being excreted in the urine every 24 hours. The usual intravenous dosage has ranged between 1 and 1.6 mg per kg every 3 weeks (Yagoda, 1983).

The maximum response of bladder cancer to cis-platinum has occurred within 2 to 3 doses, and remissions have lasted 5 to 7 months (Yagoda et al., 1976). A 40 per cent overall response rate has been seen (Stump and Corder, 1982), and the average survival for responders has been 7 months longer than for nonresponders (Herr, 1980).

Nausea and vomiting have usually occurred within 2 to 4 hours after administration of the drug and have persisted for 6 to 12 hours. Their severity has occasionally been decreased by heavy sedation prior to and during drug infusion. Anorexia has also been common. Dose-related nephrotoxicity (renal tubular necrosis occurring primarily in the proximal tubule) and ototoxicity have been seen after repeated doses. Each of these can be either prevented or minimized with adequate hydration and mannitol diuresis (Yagoda et al., 1976). Less common toxicities have included hypomagnesemia, peripheral neuropathy, mild myelosuppression, and Raynaud's phenomenon.

Methotrexate. Methotrexate is a folate antagonist that binds to dihydrofolate reductase and prevents the production of adequate intracellular levels of tetrahydrofolic acid. DNA and RNA production is similarly inhibited. It has been used in doses ranging between 50 and 200 mg every 2 weeks (Stump and Corder, 1982).

Most remissions have occurred within 2 to 3 weeks and have persisted for a median duration of 6 months (Natale et al., 1981). Overall response rates have been 28 per cent with 5 complete and 30 partial responses in 123 patients (Stump and Corder, 1982). Approximately 50 per cent of the drug is excreted, mostly unchanged, in the urine in the first 4 to 6 hours.

Major toxicities have included myelosuppression, anemia, stomatitis, glossitis, gastrointestinal ulcerations, alopecia, and hepatotoxicity (Hall et al., 1974; Turner et al., 1977). Salicylates and some antibiotics have been observed to enhance toxicity both by blocking renal tubular secretion and by displacing protein-bound methotrexate; oral anticoagulants have been found to be potentiated by the action of methotrexate. Citrovorum can be administered to minimize and even block the toxic side effects of this compound.

Doxorubicin. Doxorubicin (Adriamycin) is an antineoplastic antibiotic that intercalates between nucleotide pairs in the DNA helix. In addition, superoxide formation may lead to a direct toxic effect on the cell membrane. Average dose has been 45 to 75 mg per m^2 every 3 weeks. The plasma half-life is 24 hours, and over 40 per cent is excreted in the biliary tract in 7 days (corresponding urinary excretion is only 10 per cent).

Objective evidence of response has been seen in 15 to 35 per cent of patients, and 50 per cent have described improved performance status and weight gain (Cross et al., 1976; Yagoda et al., 1977). Overall, 6 complete and 41 partial responses have been seen in 246 patients, for a total response rate of 19 per cent (Stump and Corder, 1982). Major side effects have included nausea, vomiting, anorexia, alopecia, myelosuppression, and cardiomyopathy. Most of these have been dose-related, with decreased dosages limiting side effects.

Vinblastine. Vinblastine sulfate is a vinca alkaloid that inhibits mitosis by arresting the cell cycle in metaphase. It also affects DNA-dependent and RNA-dependent polymerases. Therapeutic effects in bladder cancer have been comparable to those seen with doxorubicin (Yagoda, 1983). The primary excretory route is via the biliary tract with a cumulative urinary excretion of only 10 to 20 per cent. Side effects have included bone marrow suppression, peripheral neuropathy and paresthesias, occasional jaw pain, and urinary retention.

Mitomycin C. Mitomycin C is an antibiotic agent in which DNA replication is inhibited by blockage of intrastrand cross linkage after its conversion in vivo to an alkylating agent. Response rates have varied between 13 and 37 per cent, with an overall response rate of 23 per cent in 52 patients (Stump and Corder, 1982; Holland et al., 1973). Decrease in tumor size has been reported to follow direct intra-arterial infusion (Burn, 1966; Sullivan, 1962). Major toxicity has included delayed myelosuppression, and this usually has occurred 28 to 35 days after administration of drug.

Cyclophosphamide (Cytoxan). Cyclophosphamide is an alkylating agent that has been reported to have an overall response rate of 27 per cent (Yagoda, 1977; Stump and Corder, 1982). It has been used in combination with cis-platinum to achieve a partial additive effect, but response rates have usually been short-lived. Long-term responses of 6 to 12 months without maintenance therapy have been described but have been largely anecdotal. Cyclophosphamide must be metabolized before it becomes cytotoxically active. Dose modification may be necessary in renal failure, since metabolites are excreted renally (Corder et al., 1984). The usual dose is 1.0 to 1.2 mg/m^2 intravenously every 3 weeks. Myelosuppression and occasional upper tract hemorrhage have been reported and have been dose-related. Bladder toxicity (fibrosis, telangiectasis, hemorrhagic cystitis) has not been dose-related.

5-Fluorouracil. 5-Fluorouracil is an antimetabolic DNA base analog that has been used in several studies at doses as high as 500 mg every 10 days (Stump and Corder, 1982). There have been only 22 objective responses in 131 patients with bladder cancer, for a response rate of 17 per cent. Major toxicities have included myelosuppression and gastrointestinal inflammation. This agent is metabolized intracellularly to 5-fluorodeoxyuridylate and by the liver to inactive metabolites, 80 per cent of which are excreted by the kidney.

Combinations of Agents. Most agents individually have had limited reproducible or predictable activity against metastatic bladder cancer. When agents have been used in combination, some increases in response rates have been reported, but minimal impact on survival has been observed (see Table 30–10).

Additional approaches in the use of various agents have included adjuvant chemotherapy and regional chemotherapy, neither of which has achieved well-documented therapeutic responses (Corder et al., 1984). Because of the systemic nature of many forms of bladder cancer at the time of initial clinical diagnosis, identification of effective agents in attempts to achieve long-term disease-free survival remains an urgent priority.

Other Forms of Bladder Cancer

ADENOCARCINOMA

Adenocarcinoma of the bladder represents less than 1 per cent of muscle-invasive tumors (Jacobo et al., 1977; Mostofi, 1968) (Fig. 30–25). Its origins are either at the bladder base near the trigone or, when its origin is the urachus, at the dome.

The source of adenocarcinoma at the base of the bladder is unclear. Histologic rests of intestinal or cloacal mucosa in the wall of the bladder have been suggested to undergo malignant degeneration, but this theory has been based upon analyses of bladder exstrophy patients, in whom a high incidence of adenocarcinoma has been observed (O'Kane and Megaw, 1968). Another source may be areas of cystitis

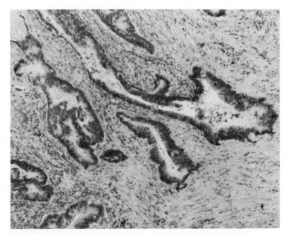

Figure 30–25. Adenocarcinoma of the bladder.
These cancers either may involve the trigone and posterior wall of the bladder in patients who have a history of infection, cystitis glandularis, or cystitis cystica or may arise as a result of neoplastic transformation of the urachus with penetration of adenocarcinoma into the dome of the bladder. Mucin often can be demonstrated in cells of these tumors, which histologically assume a typical glandular pattern. (From Friedel, G. H., et al.: Urol. Clin. North Am., *3*:53, 1976. Used by permission.)

glandularis, in which irritative stimuli may lead to neoplastic degeneration. Alternatively, the urothelium may undergo metaplasia to produce glandular epithelium, a possibility based upon the cloacal origin of the transitional epithelium (Mostofi, 1954; Foot, 1944).

Nonurachal adenocarcinoma that invades muscle has usually been treated by radical cystectomy (Thomas et al., 1971). Adjunctive preoperative irradiation has not been found to be valuable in this tumor, and radiation alone has proved ineffective (Jacobo et al., 1977).

The urachus as the source of adenocarcinoma at the bladder dome is more readily understood. It is this form that has been associated with the appearance of mucus in the urine. Although diagnosis is based upon endoscopy and biopsy in each case, CT scan may be particularly helpful in urachal tumors, since the major part of the tumor mass may be outside the bladder in the area of the urachal remnant.

The primary approach in treatment of urachal adenocarcinoma is regional excision. Wide resection of midline tissues, extending to the umbilicus and including a broad rim of normal bladder at the dome, is indicated. Adjunctive preoperative irradiation may be unnecessary, but its role in these cases is impossible to assess.

The prognosis of the disease in patients in whom tumor is more advanced and beyond the extent of surgical excision is uniformly poor,

and neither radiation nor chemotherapy has been found to be effective.

SQUAMOUS CELL CARCINOMA

Squamous cell carcinoma of the bladder represents only 5 to 8 per cent of bladder tumors (Newman et al., 1968; Mostofi, 1968), and these are to be distinguished from those transitional cell tumors that display "squamous" or "epidermoid" cellular characteristics (Fig. 30–26). The latter lesions usually reflect higher stage cancers and an ominous prognosis, whereas pure squamous cell cancers in the absence of transitional cell tumors may actually be well differentiated and less far advanced.

Squamous cell carcinoma has been associated etiologically with chronic inflammation. The presence of chronic infection, especially in the setting of calculi or an indwelling catheter, is thought to favor the transformation of transitional cell epithelium into squamous epithelium by a process known as squamous metaplasia. However, squamous metaplasia alone does not necessarily portend the development of squamous cell carcinoma. Proliferation of areas of squamous metaplasia may lead to the development of leukoplakia, a condition that has been suggested to represent a premalignant state at nongenitourinary sites (Connery, 1953). However, leukoplakia and squamous metaplasia are normal findings in as many as 30 per cent of women (Widran et al., 1974).

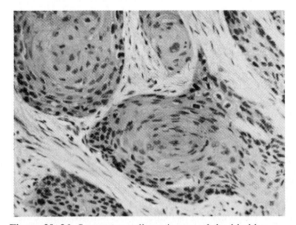

Figure 30–26. Squamous cell carcinoma of the bladder.
These tumors may arise from squamous metaplasia of transitional epithelium with subsequent neoplastic transformation of these cells. They may occur in either low or high grade and are therefore distinguishable from transitional cell cancers of high grade that are sometimes found to contain squamous elements. Characteristic features include typical squamoid elements with keratin pearls. (From Friedel, G. H., et al.: Urol. Clin. North Am., *3*:53, 1976. Used by permission.)

The role of infection in the etiology of squamous cell carcinoma has not yet been clarified. Certain bacteria may convert nitrates to nitrites and nitrosamines—potent carcinogens of the urothelium (Brand, 1979). Foreign body irritation (indwelling catheter, calculi) may induce proliferation that, in conjunction with carcinogens, may favor neoplastic transformation. Whether retinoids or some other factor determine the development of squamous cell versus transitional cell cancer in this setting is unknown.

The natural history of squamous cell carcinoma may involve early infiltration, and prognosis in these instances is poor. Jewett observed that even superficial squamous cell carcinoma of the bladder may frequently be associated with permeation of the perivesical lymphatics (Jewett et al., 1964).

Results with cystectomy have often been poor. Although this may represent the rapidity of tumor progression once neoplastic transformation has taken place, it more probably reflects the possibility that accurate endoscopic diagnosis was obscured by concomitant long-term infection and irritation, so that tumor growth, though possibly indolent, was recognized only later in its course. Cytologic examination may be difficult, if not impossible, in this setting because the character of injury to the urothelium by infection or trauma may mimic the cytologic picture of squamous neoplasia (Tweeddale and Dee, 1979).

Periodic bimanual examination and CT scan of the bladder in patients at risk for development of squamous cancer may assist in determining whether increased thickening of the bladder wall, possibly due to cancer, is taking place. However, such findings may signal that the tumor has already infiltrated the bladder muscle. A high index of suspicion is probably the most effective means of obtaining an accurate, timely diagnosis. Routine random biopsy in patients known to be at risk may be justified in order to confirm the presence of disease at earlier stages.

Some reviews of surgical experience with squamous cell carcinoma have presented surprisingly good results (Richie et al., 1976). Radical cystectomy was curative in half these cases and was even found to be effective in 20 per cent of patients with Stage D disease. These results implied a slow evolution of metastatic disease in the setting of regionally extensive cancer. Other studies reported a 16 per cent 5-year survival with radiation and cystectomy, and failure to control local disease in 92 per cent of

cancer deaths (Jones et al., 1980). However, even in these instances, only 8 per cent of patients developed distant metastases.

Squamous cell cancer associated with schistosomiasis has shown a similar response to therapy, with 80 per cent of recurrences appearing regionally after cystectomy (Chevlen et al., 1979). Five-year survivals of 35 per cent when lymph nodes were free of cancer contrasted with survivals of 18 per cent when tumor was found in unilateral obturator or iliac nodes, and 0 per cent when other nodes were involved.

The role of radiation therapy in this form of cancer is unclear. Use of 4000 rads in a hyperfractionation regimen preoperatively in schistosomal squamous cell cancer doubled disease-free survival from 25 per cent to 50 per cent in the initial 2-year postoperative interval when compared with surgery alone (Chevlen et al., 1979). Less information is available on the use of radiation in other forms of squamous cell cancer. Therefore, although it has been used as an adjunct to surgery, its need has not been well documented.

BLADDER SARCOMA

Sarcoma of the bladder in adults is extremely rare, accounting for less than 1 per cent of adult bladder tumors. Leiomyosarcoma, a malignancy arising in the smooth muscle cells in the bladder wall, is the predominant histologic cell type. There is no known association with other bladder pathology or systemic disease, and the etiology of this entity is entirely unknown.

The rarity of the condition makes it impossible to establish treatment guidelines. Radical surgery has been used effectively in some cases (Gittes, 1979). Interestingly, 5-year survivals as high as 50 per cent have been observed following partial cystectomy (Khoury and Gilloz, 1984). In contrast, carcinoleiomyosarcomas have an extremely poor prognosis, with metastasis usually present at the time of initial diagnosis. The use of surgery in conjunction with chemotherapy, which has radically altered the management of sarcomas in children, may ultimately negate the need for overly radical surgery and permit local excisional surgery to be equally effective.

Palliative Management of Bladder Cancer

Intractable hemorrhage may occur in patients with bladder cancer and may be especially troublesome when previous full-course radiation has been administered. When tumor is the source of bleeding in these cases, resection and extensive fulguration may successfully stop the hemorrhage. However, when bleeding persists despite thorough fulguration, other measures are needed.

When a diffuse hemorrhagic cystitis is seen and hematologic coagulation and platelet factors are determined to be normal, evacuation of clots and continuous bladder irrigation to prevent further bladder distention caused by clot retention may be sufficient to cause cessation of bleeding.

When bleeding persists, instillation of 1 to 2 per cent silver nitrate by continuous flow may sclerose bladder microvasculature and prevent further hemorrhage. This treatment is well tolerated without anesthetic and creates little risk. On the other hand, when hemorrhage and clot formation do not cease, instillation of formalin may be necessary (Brown, 1969; Firlit, 1973; Kumar et al., 1975). Anesthesia is needed in these instances because of the pain and bladder spasm that may result from formalin.

Formalin in the bladder causes precipitation of cellular proteins of the bladder mucosa and fixes and occludes telangiectatic and capillary vessels (McGuire et al., 1974). A 100 per cent formalin solution is actually the equivalent of a 37 per cent solution of the gas formaldehyde. The 10 per cent formalin (3.7 per cent formaldehyde) solution that was originally used to treat hemorrhagic cystitis was attended by numerous complications, such as acute tubular necrosis, papillary necrosis, and hydronephrosis (Godec and Gleich, 1983). When concentrations of less than 4 per cent formalin have been used, complications have been minimal and control of hemorrhage has usually been achieved (Fair, 1974; Shah and Albért, 1973).

When formalin is used, a preliminary cystogram is necessary to rule out reflux. A combination of reverse Trendelenburg position and intraureteral occlusive Fogarty catheters can be used if reflux is present (Droller, 1980). Contact times of 10 to 15 minutes with the bladder filled under gravity at pressures not greater than 15 cm are usually sufficient to control hemorrhage. A catheter for continuous bladder irrigation is left indwelling in such patients. It is important that patients be closely monitored so that inadvertent bladder distention does not occur. Bleeding should cease within 48 hours after instillation.

Patients may occasionally benefit from intravenous infusion of vasopressin (0.4 U/ml/min) (Pyritz et al., 1978). Although potential side effects of hypertension, bradycardia, coronary or peripheral arterial insufficiency, and free-water retention must be considered in the elderly patient, use of vasopressin may sufficiently reduce the degree of hemorrhage until other therapeutic measures have time to take effect.

Embolization of hypogastric arteries has been suggested as a means of controlling severe hemorrhage. Such treatment has often been ineffective, and reported results have been inconsistent. Urinary diversion without cystectomy may permit bladder decompression and prevent the presumed astringent effects of urine on the source of hemorrhage. The reported efficacy of this procedure must be tempered by the risk these patients may have for major surgery.

Control of hemorrhage has also been reported by use of the Helmstein balloon (Glashan, 1975). In order to generate sufficient intravesical pressure with this technique, systolic blood pressure must be exceeded, and this may require epidural anesthesia because of the duration for which sustained pressure is needed. Occasionally, repeated treatments are necessary, making this form of therapy cumbersome.

TRANSITIONAL CELL CANCER OF THE RENAL PELVIS AND URETER

Epidemiology

INCIDENCE AND MORTALITY

Transitional cell cancer of the renal pelvis accounts for only 7 per cent of all kidney tumors (Campbell, 1963; Lucke and Schlumberger, 1957) and 5 per cent of all urothelial tumors (Nocks et al., 1982). The incidence of primary ureteral tumors is even more rare, accounting for only 1 to 25 per cent of all cancers of the upper urinary tract (Bennington and Beckwith, 1975; Foord and Ferrier, 1939). Overall figures of the anatomic distribution of uroepithelial tumors have been quoted as: bladder, 90 per cent; urethra, 6 to 8 per cent, and renal pelvis/ureter, 2 to 4 percent (Batata and Grabstald, 1976). When rates are standardized per 100,000 by age intervals, a steady increase in renal pelvic and ureteral tumors occurs with age in both males and females (Fraley, 1978), with males predominating for both renal pelvic (2 to 3:1) and ureteral (2 to 4:1) tumors (Abeshouse, 1956; Hawtrey, 1971).

The occurrence of upper tract transitional

cell cancer implies a 30 to 50 per cent likelihood for subsequent development of transitional cell cancer of the bladder (Kakizoe et al., 1980). When both renal pelvic and ureteral cancers are present simultaneously, the probability of bladder cancer increases to 75 per cent (Kakizoe et al., 1980). In each instance, the predominant location of bladder cancer is on the same side as the upper tract lesion. This suggests either that implantation of tumor cells shed from the proximal tumor is responsible for the bladder cancer recurrence or that bladder epithelial cells on that side of the trigone share characteristics with the ipsilateral upper tract urothelium, which makes them equally susceptible to neoplastic transformation. An additional possibility is that the carcinogenic stimuli first appear in the bladder at highest concentration on the side of the upper tract lesion but are then diluted by urine from the contralateral side.

The development of upper tract uroepithelial cancer implies a 2–4 per cent chance for the development of transitional cell cancer in the contralateral collecting system (Babaian and Johnson, 1980). Similarly, the appearance of transitional cell cancer of the bladder suggests only a 2 to 3 per cent likelihood for subsequent development of upper tract tumor (Babaian and Johnson, 1980; Schellhammer and Whitmore, 1976). Since a majority of patients with advanced bladder cancer may not survive long enough to manifest upper tract tumors and since the incidence of ureteral carcinoma in situ at cystectomy is approximately 10 per cent (Whitmore, 1983), the actual risk of upper tract tumor development might be greater if more patients with bladder cancer survived.

Mortality from renal pelvic or ureteral cancers reflects the stage at which they are diagnosed (see further on). Approximately half of patients in each group present with superficial disease and half with more advanced disease. Appropriate treatment in the former group permits essentially normal life expectancy. Most patients composing the latter group fail to survive longer than 2 to 3 years after diagnosis (Cummings, 1980).

ETIOLOGY

Chemical Carcinogens. The relatively low incidence of tumors of the upper tract may reflect the rapid transit of potential chemical carcinogens through the upper tracts in comparison with their stasis in the bladder. In addition, upper tract epithelial enzymes may activate conjugated forms of these carcinogens so that, although they are inactive during upper tract transit, their activated form is at high enough concentration to promote tumor development by the time they reach the bladder. On the other hand, some substances (phenacetin, bracken fern) have been strongly associated with the development of upper tract tumors to the relative exclusion of bladder tumors. In these instances, enzymes in the upper tracts may detoxify active carcinogens as they pass to the bladder, so that their carcinogenic activity is virtually limited to the upper tracts.

Several reports have documented an association between exposure to industrial carcinogens and the occurrence of uroepithelial tumors of the ureter and pelvis (Gittes, 1979). The mechanism of tumor induction in these situations is probably identical to that for bladder tumors.

Balkan Nephropathy. Balkan nephropathy is a slowly progressive inflammation of the renal interstitium that may ultimately lead to renal failure (Petkovic et al., 1972). It affects inhabitants of the Balkan countries (Yugoslavia, Rumania, Bulgaria, and Greece) and has been associated with the development of tumors of the renal pelvis and ureters (Petkovic et al., 1971).

Patients with Balkan nephropathy develop upper tract tumors that are generally slow-growing, superficial, largely proliferative lesions that are not particularly aggressive. Bladder involvement is rare, with incidence ratios of upper tract tumors to bladder tumors being as great as 40:1 (Petkovic et al., 1971). What initiates or promotes the development of these tumors is unknown. However, the pathway by which these tumors develop is probably one of cellular proliferation. Because of their multiplicity and bilaterality, these tumors are best managed by conservative regional therapies that are designed to maximize retention of renal function (Petkovic, 1972).

Analgesic Nephropathy. An association between ingestion of analgesic compounds and development of renal pelvic cancers was first reported in Sweden (Hultergren et al., 1965; Hoybye and Nielsen, 1971) and subsequently confirmed in Australia (Adam et al., 1970; Mahoney et al., 1977). To date, similar associations have not been described in many other geographic areas. Although the mechanism of tumor induction in this setting is unknown, studies on the metabolism of phenacetin, the agent most commonly present in those analgesic compounds that have been implicated, have documented the homology of orthoaminophenols (the major phenacetin metabolites) with aromatic amines (Rathert et al., 1975). Recent years have witnessed an increased use of acetaminophen (Tylenol), which is an analog of phenacetin metabolites. Whether this will be associated with the development of upper tract transitional cell cancer after a sufficient latency period has elapsed, and what quantities may be necessary to demonstrate this potential association, remain to be determined.

At least half of patients with these cancers have been found to have consumed more than 5 kg of compound analgesics (Mahoney et al., 1977). However, a similar number have smoked more than 15 cigarettes per day for at least 20 years, suggesting perhaps a mixed etiology. The incidence of carcinoma of the renal pelvis has been calculated to be nine times greater in kidneys damaged by analgesics than in those with nonanalgesic inflammatory disease (Taylor, 1972; Mahoney et al., 1977). In addition, phenacetin-associated renal pelvic cancers have been estimated to occur approximately 11 years earlier than those upper tract cancers not associated with analgesic abuse (Bengtsson et al., 1978). When patients with analgesic nephropathy have ceased phenacetin ingestion, progression of renal damage has stopped, but risk of tumor development has remained (Johansson and Wahlqvist, 1979).

Ratios of renal parenchymal compared with renal pelvic carcinoma (4 to 8:1) and those of bladder compared with renal pelvic urothelial tumors ($> 10:1$) have been reversed in analgesic abusers (Schmauz and Cole, 1974; Bengtsson et al., 1968; Rathert et al., 1975). Moreover, the fact that the preponderance of these tumors occurs in females reverses the normal male:female distribution usually seen in upper tract cancer but reflects the gender proportion of analgesic abusers. The age at onset of the disease in females is lower than that in non–drug-related renal pelvic tumors. The same is not true for the disease when seen in males (Taylor, 1972).

Approximately 30 to 50 per cent of these tumors when initially diagnosed are squamous cell, but they appear to originate in transitional epithelium (Gittes, 1979). The chronic inflammation associated with the nephropathy or the ischemia associated with the papillary necrosis often seen in this condition may be responsible for these squamous changes.

Bladder cancers have not been seen as frequently as upper tract disease in this context (Goakeer and DeRuiter, 1979; Mahoney et al., 1977). Possibly, the active carcinogens responsible for development of such tumors are detoxified by the upper tract epithelium by the time they reach the bladder. Alternatively, an important cocarcinogenic condition present in the renal pelvis may not be present in the bladder (Vaught and King, 1979).

Inflammation and Infection. Chronic irritation of the renal pelvis has been associated with the development of squamous cell carcinoma. These tumors account for 7 per cent of renal pelvic cancers. Although long-standing infection may contribute to the development of cancer in these instances (Gittes, 1979; Booth et al., 1980), particular organisms with the capacity to metabolize substances in the urine into carcinogens may be required. More than half these patients have a history of renal calculi, but less than 1 per cent of patients with calculi are later found to have renal pelvis squamous cell carcinoma (Clayman et al., 1983).

While the presence of calculus may conceivably increase chronic irritation and thereby promote neoplastic development, there is no evidence that patients with staghorn calculi are more prone to the development of upper tract tumors. The precise mechanism of development of tumors in this setting remains unclear.

Cigarette Smoking. Recent studies have described a substantial risk for upper tract transitional cell cancer development in association with cigarette smoking, with the greatest risk appearing among the heaviest smokers (McLaughlin, in press; Booth et al., 1980; Morrison and Cole, 1982). The mechanism of tumor induction is probably the same as that suggested for bladder cancer associated with cigarette smoking.

Natural History of Disease

The concepts that were useful in understanding the natural histories of different forms of bladder cancer may be equally applicable in characterizing various forms of transitional cell cancer of the upper urinary tract. The underlying concept is that different patterns of tumor development may determine the unique clinical course that a particular tumor of the upper tract will follow. Thus, one can envision processes of initiation and promotion resulting in neoplastic transformations in the upper tract, which may lead to proliferation of the urothelium without dysplasia, dysplasia without proliferation, or a combination of the two.

If the proliferative pathway is followed, low-grade lesions may develop that do not pose a major risk to the patient (Droller, 1981). Only

25 per cent of patients with solitary papilloma have been described as developing a more aggressive cancer (Bennington and Beckwith, 1975; Grabstald et al., 1971; Nocks et al., 1982). Even in the setting of multiple papillomas, which may be taken to reflect multicentricity of a proliferative developmental pathway, only half such patients have progressed to infiltrative cancers (Cummings, 1980).

The benign nature of the proliferative pathway is suggested further by correlations between tumor architecture and tumor stage. The majority of papillary renal pelvic tumors were found in one series to be of low stage (30/43—70 per cent), whereas only a few were of high stage (5/43—12 per cent) (Grabstald et al., 1971). Similarly, the majority of papillary ureteral tumors were of low stage (27/42—64 per cent) (Heney et al., 1981). In both instances, survivals approached normal life expectancy.

On the other hand, if neoplastic transformation leads predominantly to dysplasia, resultant tumor cells may have the capability to invade the basement membrane and penetrate the renal pelvic or ureteral wall (Droller, 1981). Proliferative progression of such cells may then lead to infiltrative cancers with a more ominous prognosis. The majority of upper tract uroepithelial tumors that were solid or nonpapillary were found in one series to be high-grade lesions (12/14—86 per cent), while the majority of papillary or proliferative tumors were found to be of lower or less dysplastic grade (33/42—78 per cent) (Heney et al., 1981). Correspondingly, the majority of solid renal pelvic tumors (22/25—88 per cent) and ureteral tumors (9/14—64 per cent) were also of high stage (Grabstald et al., 1971; Nocks et al., 1982; Heney et al., 1981).

The dysplastic pathway has also been associated with more diffuse involvement of the urothelium by cancer. Thus, 20 of 33 (60 per cent) Grade 3 renal pelvic tumors and 12 of 20 (60 per cent) Stage D tumors had carcinoma in situ at the margin of the primary lesion (Grabstald et al., 1971; Nocks et al., 1982). In contrast, the majority of low-stage tumors (21/31—68 per cent), which were also of low grade and largely proliferative, had only mild or moderate atypia. Similar observations for ureteral cancers demonstrated that 14 of 19 (74 per cent) Grade 3 lesions had carcinoma in situ adjacent to the primary tumor, whereas only 20 per cent of patients with Grade 2 lesions had any abnormality present (Heney et al., 1981). Conversely, 15 of 16 (94 per cent) patients with normal epithelium at the tumor margin had low-stage, low-grade lesions, whereas 11 of 18 (61 per cent) patients with carcinoma in situ of the adjacent urothelium had high-stage, high-grade lesions (Heney et al., 1981). Varying degrees of urothelial atypia and even frank carcinoma were observed at sites distant from the primary tumor as the stage and grade of the primary tumor increased (McCarron et al., 1982; Mahadevia et al., 1983; Kakizoe et al., 1980, 1981).

The aggressive nature of predominantly dysplastic lesions has been suggested by observations of a more limited 5-year survival of Grade 3 tumors (20 per cent) compared with Grade 2 tumors (90 per cent) and Grade 1 tumors (100 per cent) of the renal pelvis (Grabstald et al., 1971; Booth et al., 1980; Nocks et al., 1982). Corresponding 5-year survivals for Grades 3, 2, and 1 tumors in the ureter of 30 per cent, 80 per cent, and 100 per cent, respectively, confirm this suggestion (Heney et al., 1981; Booth et al., 1980).

Taken together, upper tract uroepithelial tumors, like bladder tumors, may develop along several pathways. Were there but a single pathway by which initial neoplastic transformation led to superficial proliferative disease while foci of dysplastic cells within such lesions produced infiltrative cancer and metastasis, one might expect a higher incidence of advanced tumors in the renal pelvis, because of the later presentation of clinically manifest symptoms from tumors in this location and a higher proportion of superficial tumors in the ureter because of the likelihood of earlier expression of obstructive symptomatology from even more benign tumors in this location. However, virtually equal numbers of superficial and infiltrative cancers have been observed in both the renal pelvis and the ureter at initial tumor diagnosis. Therefore, the likelihood of multiple, possibly interacting pathways of tumor development under various conditions needs to be considered in an approach to the staging and treatment of upper tract tumors.

Pathologic Grading and Staging

Staging systems of uroepithelial tumors of the renal pelvis and ureter have been based upon considerations of the natural history of disease and the efficacy of various therapies. Though comparable in many respects to staging systems described for bladder cancer, unique structural aspects of the renal pelvis and ureter have led to several differences in the classification schema as they pertain to the upper tracts (Fig. 30–27).

The most widely used staging system is predicated upon whether tumor has invaded the thin, smooth muscle wall of the renal pelvis or ureter and whether it has extended into the surrounding tissues (Batata and Grabstald, 1976; Grabstald et al., 1971). Group 1 renal pelvic tumors, accounting for 14 per cent of renal pelvic tumors (Wagle et al., 1974), are histologically benign papillomas. In the absence of tumors elsewhere in the urinary tract, none of these patients has been found to develop regional recurrence or distant metastases follow-

ing nephrectomy and partial ureterectomy. Group 2 renal pelvic tumors, constituting 27 per cent of renal pelvic tumors, consist of carcinomas without demonstrable subepithelial invasion, those with focal microscopic invasion, or papillomas with carcinoma in situ either within a papilloma or elsewhere in the renal pelvic mucosa. In these instances, carcinoma in situ has generally been localized and has not appeared to have the same degree of dysplasia that has characterized the more diffuse form of disease seen in the bladder. None of the patients in this group has been found to develop regional or distant recurrence following partial nephro-

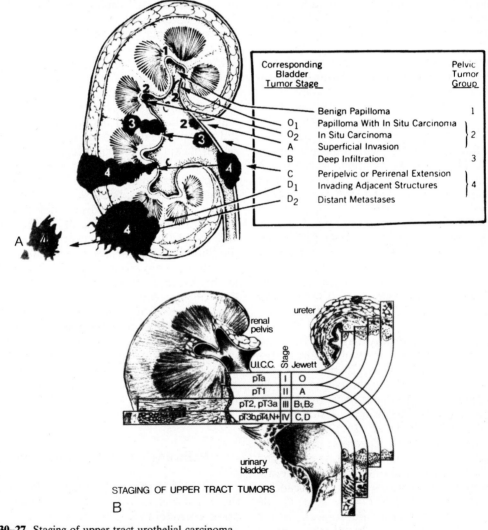

Figure 30–27. Staging of upper tract urothelial carcinoma.

A, Initial staging systems separated benign papilloma (Group 1) from those tumors that either were in situ or had superficial invasion (Group 2; Stages 0–A). Deep infiltration was categorized as Group 3 (Stage B). Perirenal or peripelvic extension and invasion of adjacent structures were categorized as Group 4 (stages C–D$_1$). *B*, Recent adjustments of this system have correlated these stages with those in bladder cancer (B). (*A* from Grabstald, H., et al.: J.A.M.A., *218*:845, 1971; *B* from Cummings, K. B.: Urol. Clin. North Am., 7:569, 1980. Used by permission.)

ureterectomy if there were no associated bladder or ureteral tumors. Group 3 renal pelvic tumors, constituting 28 per cent of renal pelvic tumors, consist of carcinomas that, though still confined to the kidney, have infiltrated the pelvic wall or renal parenchyma or both. Despite this greater extension, 75 per cent 5-year survivals have been described for patients with these tumors. This suggests that infiltration in the upper tract may not have as much potential for distant dissemination as appears to be the case for bladder cancer (Zincke and Neves, 1984), or that sufficient numbers of cases were not available to permit identification of tumor subgroups with more aggressive biologic potential. In contrast, Group 4 renal pelvic tumors, accounting for 31 per cent of tumors at this site, are the most virulent tumors. These extend beyond the renal pelvis or parenchyma and invade peripelvic and perirenal fat, lymph nodes, hilar vessels, and adjacent or distant tissues. Five-year survivals in this group have been less than 5 to 10 per cent.

Subgroups of all of these categories have incorporated neoplastic multicentricity (Grabstald et al., 1971). Group A within each category includes no tumors other than the presenting lesion. Group B has other tumors present. In each of the four categories, the presence of other tumors implies a more pervasive diathesis and a more ominous course, probably because multicentricity has more commonly been seen in higher stage and higher grade tumors, in which prognosis was likely to be poor to begin with.

In a recent report, Cummings and coworkers (1975) updated attempts to incorporate cellular grade with tumor stage and arrived at comparable conclusions (Fig. 30–27). Stage 1 tumors were noninvasive, Stage 2 tumors had superficial submucosal invasion, Stage 3 tumors invaded the renal pelvic muscle or renal substance, and Stage 4 tumors extended through the adventitia of the pelvis or through the kidney capsule. Corresponding survivals for low-stage (1 and 2) or high-stage (3) lesions were 80 per cent and 30 per cent, respectively (Cummings et al., 1975). No Stage 4 patient survived. Within each of these stages, Grade 1 cells had normal cellular morphology, Grade 2 cells had minimal pleomorphism, Grade 3 cells had significant pleomorphism with mitoses and giant cells, and Grade 4 cells showed extreme pleomorphism (Cummings et al., 1975). Corresponding survivals by grade were 80 per cent and 20 per cent for low-grade (1 and 2) and high-grade (3) tumors, respectively. Generally, higher grades corresponded to higher stages;

thus, no patients with Grade 3 tumors were found to exhibit Stage 1 or 2 disease (Cummings, 1980). Similar findings as to grade and stage were reported by Booth and associates (1980), who also indicated that tumor multiplicity might predispose to a more ominous prognosis.

Similar considerations for staging have been applied to transitional cell carcinoma of the ureter (Fig. 30–27) (Batata et al., 1975; Batata and Grabstald, 1976). Tumors confined to the mucosa or submucosa (Stage A), accounting for 50 to 60 per cent of primary ureteral tumors (Batata et al., 1975), have been associated with a 90 per cent 5-year survival. Those with muscle invasion (Stage B) or penetration through the entire ureteral wall (Stage C), constituting 10 per cent and 20 per cent of ureteral tumors, respectively, have been found to determine 40 to 50 per cent and 10 to 20 per cent 5-year survivals, respectively. All patients with involvement of periureteral soft tissues (Stage D), accounting for 15 per cent of ureteral tumors, died of their disease. Similar results have been reported in more recent reviews (McCarron et al., 1983).

Tumor grade has been found to correlate with these stages for ureteral cancer. Thus, 74 per cent of Stages A and B tumors were Grade 1 or 2 histologically, whereas 64 per cent of Stage C tumors were Grade 3 or 4 (Bloom et al., 1970; Batata et al., 1975; Hawtrey, 1971). Corresponding 5-year survivals ranged between 50 and 80 per cent for Grades 1 and 2 tumors and between 0 and 16 per cent for Grades 3 and 4 tumors across all stages (Bloom et al., 1970; Batata et al., 1975).

Correspondingly, the likelihood of regional lymph node involvement and distant metastases in ureteral cancer seems to be directly related to tumor stage. No Stage A patient has been found to develop metastatic disease, whereas most patients with lesions in regional lymphatics had tumors that had invaded deeply into or through muscle (Batata et al., 1975). Patients with Stage B or C disease demonstrated distant metastases in 40 per cent and 75 per cent of instances, respectively.

Methods of Diagnosis

SYMPTOMS

Hematuria is the initial presenting symptom in the majority of individuals with upper tract transitional cell cancer (Grabstald et al., 1971). It is also the most common symptom, occurring in 60 to 75 per cent of patients (Bloom et al., 1970; Babaian and Johnson, 1980).

Flank pain, thought to be secondary to local invasion and resultant ureteral obstruction, has been characterized as a dull ache that is often nonradiating. Paradoxically, this symptom has occurred more often with renal pelvic (36 per cent) than with ureteral tumors (17 per cent) (McCarron et al., 1983). In the event of active bleeding with clot formation, colic rather than a dull ache may accompany the acute obstruction (Gittes, 1979).

A small proportion of patients (7 per cent) may present with constitutional symptoms, such as weight loss and anorexia. Invariably, this has been associated with advanced disease (Mc-Carron et al., 1983). Approximately 10 to 15 per cent of patients may be asymptomatic, and the lesion may then be discovered on radiographic evaluation of presumably unrelated problems (Babaian and Johnson, 1980).

Physical examination may confirm costovertebral angle tenderness. An abdominal mass has been palpable in 5 to 15 per cent of patients (Strong and Pearse, 1976). For the most part, however, there are no physical findings that are pathognomonic.

DIAGNOSTIC PROCEDURES

Excretory Urography. Excretory urography is abnormal in the majority of cases of upper tract tumors (Figs. 30–28 to 30–31). Such studies demonstrate either an intraluminal filling defect or nonfunction secondary to obstruction by clot or tumor mass (Richie, 1978). Although total nonvisualization is likely to indicate invasive ureteral cancer, this finding in itself has not been found to predict the extent of a tumor and its invasiveness with consistent accuracy (McCarron et al., 1983). Thus, although in several series nonvisualization was the most common radiographic finding encountered with ureteral cancers (37 per cent), invasive disease was indicated in only 60 to 80 per cent of instances (McCarron et al., 1983; Bloom et al., 1970; Scott and McDonald, 1970). Nonvisualization was also associated with 20 per cent of neoplasms of the renal pelvis, of which only one third were found to be of high stage (McCarron et al., 1983).

Hydronephrosis with or without hydroureter has been seen in 35 per cent of such patients, and ureteral filling defects without obstruction have been observed in 20 per cent (Richie, 1978). In the setting of a normal urogram, 85 per cent of patients with upper tract neoplasm have had a low-stage tumor, while only 10 to 15 per cent have had a high-stage tumor (Bloom et al., 1970).

In the absence of total obstruction, the "wine goblet" or meniscus shape has been found to be important in distinguishing a ureteral tumor from a nonopaque calculus (Figs. 30–30 and 30–31) (Bergman et al., 1961). In these instances, the ureter is flattened or collapsed distal to the stone, the same not being the case when a tumor is present.

Retrograde Pyelography. Retrograde pyelography has been useful in confirming the presence of filling defects in the renal pelvis or ureter in 75 per cent of cases (Strong and Pearce, 1976). In the presence of obstruction or in the face of inadequate excretion of contrast and nonvisualized "phantom" calyces, this is especially important for obtaining an outline of the entire upper urinary tract (Figs. 30–28 to 30–31) (Brennan and Pollack, 1979). In addition, it may complement excretory urography in ascertaining the presence of multiple tumors and in better delineating the filling defects seen in 50 per cent of patients with renal pelvic neoplasms and 12 per cent with ureteral neoplasms (Fig. 30–32) (McCarron et al., 1983).

At the time of retrograde study, selective aspirated or barbotaged urine samples can be obtained for cytologic analysis (see further on). A suspicious lesion can also be brushed to obtain a more definitive specimen for pathologic analysis (Blute et al., 1981).

Sonography. Sonography has been useful in distinguishing nonopaque calculi from soft tissue defects in the renal pelvis (McCarron et al., 1983). It will not distinguish between other soft tissue masses, such as sloughed papillae, blood clots, or matrix "calculi." Examination of the ureter by sonography is more difficult than examination of the renal pelvis and is less reliable.

CT Scanning. Computerized tomography has been used to outline filling defects of upper tract tumors, especially of the calyces and renal pelvis (Figs. 30–28 and 30–29). Moreover, CT scanning has provided a means to distinguish between transitional cell cancer of the renal pelvis and renal cell cancer (Gatewood et al., 1982). The criteria for transitional cell cancer upon which these distinctions have been based include the following: (1) appearance of a solid mass in the renal pelvis and/or in a ballooned calyx, with displacement and compression of the renal sinus fat; (2) minimal enhancement after intravenous injection of iodinated contrast material; (3) trapping of contrast material in curvilinear calyceal spaces or in compressed collecting ducts around the periphery of the tumor; (4) delayed enhancement of the renal paren-

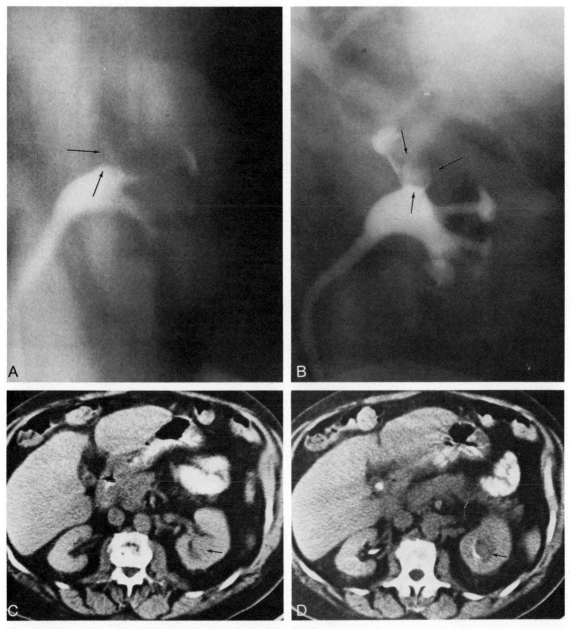

Figure 30–28. Radiographic assessment of calyceal transitional cell cancer.

   A, Intravenous pyelography in this patient disclosed incomplete filling of the upper pole calyx of the left kidney (arrows). *B,* Retrograde pyelography disclosed a filling defect in this calyx, with the remainder of the collecting system being apparently normal (arrows). *C,* CT scans confirmed the presence of a mass in the upper portion of the renal collecting system displacing renal sinus fat (arrow). *D,* The mass was well defined after opacification of the surrounding renal parenchyma and showed minimal visual enhancement (arrow). A thin semilunar sliver of contrast material surrounded the medial margin of the mass. (From Gatewood, O. B., et al.: J. Urol., *127*:876, 1982. Used by permission.)

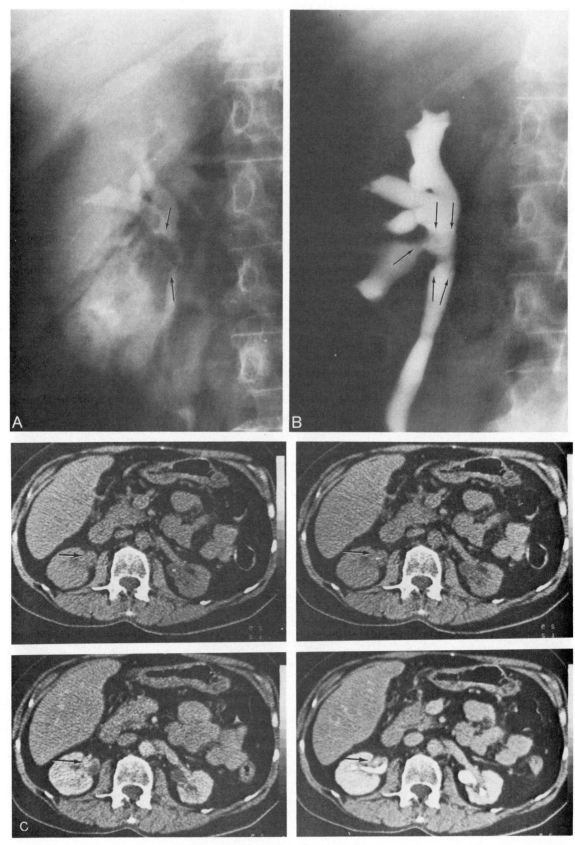

Figure 30–29. *See legend on opposite page.*

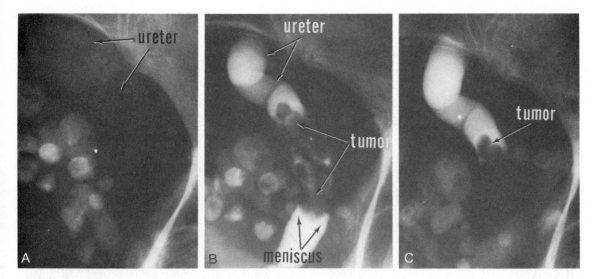

Figure 30–30. Ureteral transitional cell cancer.

A, Radiographic evaluation of this female patient, who had complained of left-sided, nonradiating back pain, disclosed markedly delayed and diminished function of the left kidney with a dilated left collecting system (arrows; spherical opacities are diverticuli seen on earlier barium enema). *B,* Retrograde pyelography confirmed the dilatation of the collecting system and demonstrated a characteristic meniscus filling defect in the lower ureter inferior to the ureteral mass (arrows). *C,* Drainage films confirmed the obstruction secondary to the intrinsic ureteral mass. At surgery, the ureter was found to contain a superficially infiltrative papillary transitional cell cancer. No other areas of neoplasia or epithelial atypia were seen, and the patient has not experienced tumor recurrence.

chyma surrounding larger lesions due to retention of contrast in obstructed tubules; and (5) preservation of reniform contour of the kidney.

Renal Angiography. Renal angiography may demonstrate encasement of intrarenal arteries, hypertrophy of the artery to the renal pelvis, and the presence of a tumor vascular blush for cancers larger than 3 cm in diameter (Fig. 30–33) (Cummings et al., 1975). Others have suggested this technique to distinguish a filling defect in the renal pelvis due to an indentation by an elbow of the main arterial tree, an arterial aneurysm, or a congenital vascular malformation (Gittes, 1979).

Antegrade Pyelography. Antegrade pyelography should be reserved for those instances in which intravenous pyelography or retrograde studies have been unsuccessful in establishing a diagnosis (Firstater, 1965). It should be undertaken only with the understanding that tumor spill may occur through the puncture site (Tomera et al., 1982). Generally, this procedure has not been found to be necessary for diagnosis.

Ureteroscopy and Nephroscopy. Transurethral ureteroscopy has been described as a useful adjunct in the diagnosis of ureteral and renal pelvic lesions (Bush et al., 1979). The rapid advances in development of flexible ureteroscopes and nephroscopes will undoubtedly make these procedures more common in the diagnosis of upper tract tumors (Bagley et al., 1983). So too, percutaneous nephroscopy may soon be adapted to the diagnosis and possibly even the treatment of upper tract tumors.

The potential risk of tumor spill with the

Figure 30–29. Radiographic assessment of upper ureteral infiltrative uroepithelial cancer.

Intravenous pyelogram showed incomplete filling of lower pole calyces in the right kidney of a patient with a prolonged history of recurrent infections. *A,* The ureteral pelvic junction and upper ureteral contour were ragged and "moth-eaten" (arrows). Retrograde pyelogram disclosed a normal lower pole calyx with a narrow infundibulum that appeared to be encased. *B,* The moth-eaten appearance of the upper ureter and ureteral pelvic junction was confirmed (arrows). *C,* Unenhanced views on computed tomography showed a mass in the renal pelvis (1 and 2, arrows). Following contrast injection, slight enhancement of the renal pelvic mass could be detected, but with increasing enhancement of the parenchyma and opacification of the collecting system and pelvis the mass could be distinguished more clearly (3 and 4, arrows). (From Gatewood, O. B.: Contemp. Issues CAT Scan., in press. Used by permission.)

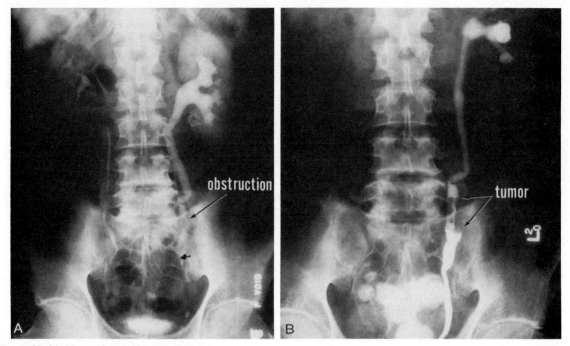

Figure 30–31. Ureteral transitional cell cancer.

A, Upon presentation with gross, painless hematuria, this male patient was found to have a partially obstructed left kidney, with obstruction at the level of the common iliac artery. *B*, Retrograde pyelography disclosed a filling defect, which at surgery was found to represent deeply invasive transitional cell cancer. No other areas of uroepithelial atypia were seen. The patient died of metastatic cancer 2 years after surgery.

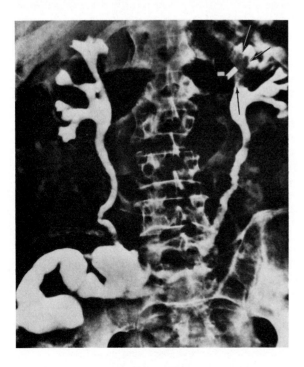

Figure 30–32. Upper tract tumor recurrence with previous bladder cancer.

This patient had had muscle-invasive transitional cell cancer of the bladder and had undergone cystectomy and ileal loop urinary diversion. Microscopic hematuria prompted the present loopogram, which disclosed multiple small filling defects in the ureter and a prominent filling defect in the upper pole calyx of the left kidney (arrows). Pathologic assessment confirmed the presence of a large transitional cell cancer in the upper pole calyx and ureteritis cystica in the ureter. (From Friedland, G. W., et al.: Uroradiology: An Integrated Approach. New York, Churchill Livingstone, 1983. Used by permission.)

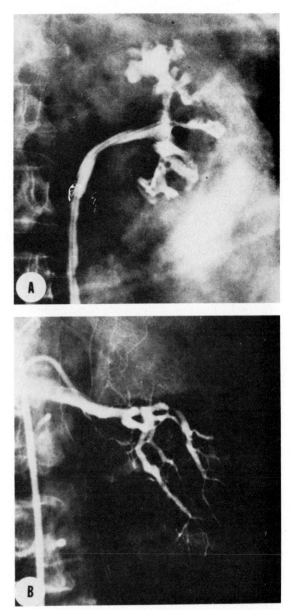

Figure 30–33. Arteriography in upper tract transitional cell cancer.

A, Intravenous pyelography in this patient with microscopic hematuria had demonstrated irregular contours of calyces and infundibula, a finding that was confirmed on retrograde pyelography. In this study, narrow infundibula were seen in many calyces, suggesting fixation and encasement. *B,* Renal arteriography demonstrated this encasement as well as occlusion of many arteries. Pathology studies disclosed extensive infiltrating cancer that had involved all of the infundibula. The small round filling defects seen retrograde are air bubbles. (From Friedland, G. W., et al.: Uroradiology: An Integrated Approach. New York, Churchill Livingstone, 1983. Used by permission.)

use of percutaneous diagnostic modalities may be more than a hypothetical consideration (Tomera et al., 1982). In 11 patients examined by intraoperative nephroscopy, 2 developed local recurrence of noninvasive low-grade tumors within 6 months to 3 years. However, in another series of 33 patients in whom the collecting system was opened for the purpose of diagnosis and treatment, there was no evidence of tumor implantation in the wound during short-term follow-up (McCarron et al., 1983). The fact that methods of renal pelvic examination were sufficiently different in these reports could explain the varying results. It is clear, however, that the

potential import of tumor spill can best be documented in low-grade neoplasms, since regional recurrence in high-grade invasive tumor may reflect the natural history of the disease. Until further information is available, methods that involve opening an otherwise intact collecting system must be used with caution.

Magnetic Resonance Imaging. As was the case in bladder cancer, many see a very important role developing for magnetic resonance imaging in detecting a variety of conditions involving the kidney (Williams and Hricak, 1984). This would be directly applicable to transitional cell cancer of the renal pelvis vis-à-vis its distinction from renal cell carcinoma and the possibility of exploiting the use of contrast media in rendering accurate diagnoses. The multiplanar capabilities of magnetic resonance imaging would also make it useful in the diagnosis of ureteral lesions. The relative stability of the retroperitoneum would prevent possible movement artifacts from interfering with accurate diagnosis. Further evaluation of this modality, however, is necessary to confirm these impressions.

Upper Tract Cytology. The presence of a radiolucent filling defect on x-ray studies may require cytologic studies to document the presence of cancer. Appropriate upper tract urine samples can be obtained either from voided urines or from washings obtained at the time of retrograde pyelographic examination. Brush biopsies can be used when cytologic findings are negative or show only well-differentiated cells when a high-grade malignancy is suspected.

In a review of 100 histologically documented renal pelvic tumors, a high correlation between tumor stage, grade, and cytologic sediment smears was obtained (Blute et al., 1981; McCarron et al., 1983). As might be expected, false negative studies occurred in 80 per cent of low-grade, low-stage lesions. Conversely, 60 per cent of high-grade lesions exhibited positive or strongly suspicious readings. In a more recent study of 30 upper tract carcinomas, a similarly high percentage of apparently normal urine sediments was seen in the presence of well-differentiated tumors, while a high percentage of positive tests was obtained in cases of high-grade carcinoma (McCarron et al., 1983). Cytologic samples obtained by barbotage have been said to provide a more reliable sampling of the upper tract when neoplasia is present (Leistenschneider and Nagel, 1980; Zincke et al., 1976). In these instances, accuracy of cytologic diagnosis increased from 35 to 60 per cent with voided urine, to 60 to 70 per cent with urine collected passively by catheter, to 80 to 90 per cent with lavaged samples. Diagnostic considerations in the interpretation of urinary cytologies from the upper tract are otherwise similar to those described for bladder cancer.

Surface Blood Group Antigens. Recent retrospective analyses have demonstrated a strong correlation between the presence of surface blood group antigens and the absence of invasive disease in carcinomas of the renal pelvis and ureter (Gruber et al., 1982; Hall et al., 1982). The same concept has been used in applying the surface blood group antigen test in cytologic specimens, but with mixed results

(Gruber et al., 1982). If a suitable sample can be obtained only at the time of surgery, the clinical usefulness of this method may be limited. However, percutaneous and cytologic methods may ultimately provide preoperative samples. This will enable these techniques to be used in further defining the intrinsic nature and potential behavior of an upper tract neoplasm so that an appropriate therapeutic decision can be made. The test may also be applicable to brush biopsy specimens in which the grade of tumor is unclear but the presence or absence of blood group antigens may determine whether conservative surgery is indicated.

Treatment

SURGERY

Simple nephrectomy was originally the procedure of choice for tumors of the renal pelvis. In these instances, recurrence in the ipsilateral ureteral stump was as high as 84 per cent (Colston, 1935; Kimball and Ferris, 1934; Kirwin, 1941). This demonstrated the necessity of removing the entire ureter and a periureteral segment of the bladder at the time of nephrectomy for such lesions (Deming and Harvard, 1970).

Subsequent reports indicated that survival of patients with urothelial tumors of the renal pelvis and ureter was determined predominantly by anatomic stage and histologic grade of the cancer rather than the specific surgical approach that was used (Batata and Grabstald, 1976; Batata et al., 1975; Mills and Vaughn, 1983; McCarron et al., 1983; Grabstald et al., 1971). Thus, results of complete nephroureterectomy with bladder cuff excision and results of partial ureterectomy were equally good for low-stage, low-grade tumors and equally dismal for less differentiated, more invasive cancers. The unresolved question concerned the likelihood of tumor recurrence in the ipsilateral system, depending upon the type of surgery performed and the type of tumor that was present.

Extent of Surgery for Renal Pelvic Tumors. The similarity of results in treating low-stage, low-grade renal pelvic tumors by either partial nephrectomy or total nephroureterectomy (McCarron et al., 1983) has prompted an emphasis on the former so that renal function might be preserved if anatomically consistent with adequate extirpative cancer surgery. The necessity to attempt preservation of renal function in the context of a solitary kidney, renal insufficiency, or bilateral low-stage cancer has been a further indication for segmental excision

(Montie, 1979). The choice of this approach makes it obligatory to establish that a tumor is truly unifocal and of low stage and low grade. In these instances, urinary cytology is likely to be negative, so that retrograde brush biopsy histology in conjunction with radiographic monitoring of the lesion may be of primary importance in a decision in favor of segmental excision.

In contrast, high-grade tumors, which are also likely to be of high stage and to have positive cytology (Nocks et al., 1982), have generally been found to have multiple areas involved by neoplastic changes. It may therefore be impossible to determine suitable margins of excision if partial nephrectomy is contemplated. This was highlighted in one recent series in which 5 of 9 (56 per cent) and 5 of 8 (62 per cent) patients treated by segmental or local resection and partial nephrectomy, respectively, developed local recurrence (Zincke and Neves, 1984).

In another series, 90 per cent of patients with high-grade, high-stage, but regionally confined lesions in the renal pelvis treated with less than total excision of the upper tract ultimately died of cancer, whereas only 30 per cent of those treated with total excision died of their disease (McCarron et al., 1983). In this regard, Koss has described dysplastic changes to occur in the epithelium of the collecting ducts in some patients with high-stage renal pelvic or calyceal tumors (Mahadevia et al., 1983). Recognition of the true extent of disease in such patients at the time of surgery may thus be impossible. Concerns that a 5-year follow-up may be insufficient to determine the success of partial excision are also relevant in this regard (Clayman et al., 1983). Thus, if the time between surgery and recurrence is 2 to 3 years and the survival time for more aggressive recurrent disease is also 2 to 3 years, patients would still be expected to survive 5 years, even if recurrence took place.

Similar considerations will affect the decision whether to remove the entire ureter when high-stage renal pelvic tumors are present. Recurrence of tumor in the ureteral stump has been found in 30 to 60 per cent of such cases when only partial nephroureterectomy was performed (Kakizoe et al., 1980; Richie, 1978; Williams and Mitchell, 1973a; Strong and Pearse, 1976). Because such recurrence is usually silent, and early detection therefore rare, the majority of patients die of their recurrent tumor. It thus appears that total nephroureterectomy is indicated in high-stage, high-grade renal pelvic cancers.

Total ureteral excision implies removal of a cuff of bladder at the ureteral orifice as well. In one report, only 5 of 17 (29 per cent) patients who had adequate excision of a cuff of bladder developed bladder tumors, whereas 12 of 20 (60 per cent) patients who had inadequate cuff excision developed bladder carcinoma (Williams and Mitchell, 1973b). In 12 patients, these tumors were in the region of the ureteral orifice, and 13 of these lesions were of the same histologic grade as the original pelvic tumor.

Some have suggested that radical nephroureterectomy may be more effective therapy for high-stage disease than simple total nephroureterectomy (Johansson et al., 1976; Johansson and Wahlqvist, 1979; Cummings, 1980). Of all patients who underwent simple nephroureterectomy and who succumbed to their disease, local tumor recurrence was seen in 43 per cent. In addition, the 5-year survival rate for patients with Stages C and D disease who underwent radical nephrectomy was 74 per cent compared with 37 per cent in patients treated with simple nephrectomy.

Systematic regional lymph node dissection has not been found to enhance the effectiveness of surgery if tumors are of high grade or high stage, since in these instances the overall results are so poor to begin with (Grabstald et al., 1971). In one report, all patients with high-stage renal pelvic carcinoma who had positive regional nodes died of metastatic cancer within 1 year despite total removal of all adjoining renal pelvic and para-aortic nodes (McCarron et al., 1983). Correspondingly, lymph node involvement is uncommon in low-stage disease and lymphadenectomy is therefore unlikely to remove additional tumor. Lymph node dissection at the time of nephrectomy may offer prognostic information but little, if any, therapeutic benefit.

In summary, the procedure of choice for most renal pelvic transitional cell cancers and all high-stage cancers is total nephroureterectomy with excision of the ipsilateral periureteral cuff of bladder mucosa. The rarity of synchronous bilateral neoplasia, the low incidence of asynchronous development of contralateral upper tract tumors, and the increased risk of tumor recurrence in the ipsilateral ureter distal to the original tumor are the rationale for this approach. Contemplation of anything less than total excision must take into account potential risk for tumor recurrence anywhere in the upper tract unit. In other than unifocal, low-grade, low-stage renal pelvic tumors, the probable extensive involvement of both contiguous and noncontiguous sites and even of collecting tubule epithelium would appear to make segmental excision an entirely unnecessary option and to create a potentially serious risk.

Recent developments in obtaining safe transurethral and percutaneous access to the upper tract have provided hypothetical regional treatment options heretofore impossible in a practical sense. Conceivably, low-stage lesions might be amenable to fulguration or resection, obviating the need for open surgery, even if conservative. Such patients would then be placed into surveillance programs, much as has been the case with bladder cancer. The critical caveat in these situations is whether sufficient information can be obtained about the neoplastic diathesis to permit accurate evaluation of the urothelium and its potential for tumor recurrence, infiltration, or progression. Recurrence rates of 50 to 60 per cent even for low-grade lesions in conservatively treated renal units (Zincke and Neves, 1984) must be taken into account in adopting this approach. On the other hand, the greater maintenance of anatomic integrity and a closed system may decrease the recurrence rates that were previously seen with pyelotomy and pyeloscopy (Tomera et al., 1982). Therefore, as long as potential risks are understood, the natural history of disease considered, and the likelihood of tumor development at other urothelial sites weighed, study of this approach may be indicated in view of the benefits it might introduce.

Extent of Surgery for Ureteral Cancer. Similar considerations are important in treating urothelial cancers in the ureter. In general, the more proximal the location of the primary tumor, the more likely is distal recurrence to ensue (Babaian and Johnson, 1980; Kakizoe et al., 1980). In proximal ureteral cancers, distal recurrence may be seen in as many as 50 per cent of patients in whom only partial ureterectomy had been performed (Mazeman, 1976; Wallace et al., 1981). On the other hand, as one proceeds distally in the ureter, the risk of malignant disease developing proximally is lessened (Babaian and Johnson, 1980).

When tumors involve the upper ureter, therefore, considerations are the same as those that applied to renal pelvic cancers. Segmental excision may be appropriate for low-stage lesions if the character of such lesions can be documented without question. For high-stage lesions, the greater likelihood of multifocal disease and distal ureteral recurrence implies the need for total nephroureterectomy. Anything less may compromise expectations for tumor-free survival.

In the distal ureter, several studies have described successful management of low-grade, noninvasive tumors by partial ureterectomy and ureteral reimplantation (Brown and Roumani, 1974; Kretkowski and Derrick, 1973; Mazeman, 1976; Babaian and Johnson, 1980). The same may hold for invasive disease at this site, since the chance of developing malignant disease above the level of ureteral resection would appear to be remote (Babaian and Johnson, 1980; Bloom et al., 1970). Thus, no differences were seen in 5-year survivals of patients with ureteral cancer whether they had undergone complete nephroureterectomy (47 per cent 5-year survival) or partial ureterectomy (55 per cent 5-year survival) (Batata et al., 1975).

If a primary neoplasm is identified in the ureter and disease in the renal pelvis or more proximal ureter can be excluded, segmental excision may be feasible. This certainly appears to be the case in low-stage disease and may also be so in high-stage disease. Because of possible tumor recurrence below the line of resection, constant vigilance for new tumors is mandatory (Babaian and Johnson, 1980; Bloom et al., 1970; Williams and Mitchell, 1973). Arguments for performing segmental excision must also be weighed against findings that 50 per cent of patients may have multiple lesions, with at least half of these being unsuspected. Nonetheless, segmental excision with conservation of renal tissue seems to be an appropriate course in many instances of distal ureteral cancer, especially since the intrinsic behavior of a particular tumor may determine recurrence and overall survival regardless of the therapeutic procedure (Bloom et al., 1970).

Transureteral fulguration and even resection of superficial low-grade ureteral tumors may also be possible. The impact of this capability on the management of possible tumor recurrence, tumor progression, and patient survival, however, is unknown at present. Therefore, periodic follow-up with urinary cytology, intravenous pyelography, and, when indicated, ureteronephroscopy is necessary when this course of treatment is chosen.

Bladder Evaluation and Management in the Setting of Upper Tract Urothelial Cancers. Because of the risk of tumor recurrence in the bladder, patients with a history of upper tract cancer require continued endoscopic surveillance following their primary procedure. The incidence of concurrent or subsequent bladder tumors in one series was 28 per cent in association with renal pelvic cancers, 55 per cent in association with ureteral cancers, and 75 per cent in association with multiple renal pelvic and ureteral cancers (Kakizoe et al., 1981). In other series, 20 to 50 per cent of patients with tumors of the renal pelvis or ureter were found to have had associated bladder tumors before, during, or after the primary tumor had been treated (Grabstald et al., 1971; Williams and Mitchell, 1973a,b; Grace et al., 1968; Wagle et al., 1974; Batata and Grabstald, 1976; Say and Hori, 1974). Bladder tumors have been found to appear within 5 to 12 months in 60 per cent of patients and within 13 to 18 months in 20 per cent, yielding an 80 per cent total recurrence in just 1½ years (Williams and Mitchell, 1973a,b; Grabstald et al., 1971). Cystoscopic evaluation of the bladder should therefore be done at 3-month intervals for a period of 2 years, just as is done in follow-up of primary bladder cancer. This should be sufficient in the majority of instances to detect whether tumor recurrence in the bladder has taken, or is likely to take, place.

Although the risk for developing contralateral disease is small and the likelihood of developing upper tract tumors when bladder tumors occurred initially is also small, pyelographic assessment of the upper tract(s) on an annual basis seems appropriate. Urinary cytology may also be useful in following these patients, especially if the previous neoplasm was of higher grade.

Management of the Ureteral Remnant. The continued assessment of patients with upper tract tumors who have not had excision of the ureteral stump is particularly difficult, since progression of a recurrent tumor in the ureteral stump may proceed unnoticed. At the very least, retrograde injection of contrast agent into the ureteral stump should be done at endoscopic follow-up every 6 months. At these times, lavage samples for urinary cytology should also be obtained,

Gittes (1979) has suggested that the ureteral stump be removed at the time that any other surgery in the area of the bladder is contemplated. This view may be tenable in the setting of prior low-grade disease. The alternative is to remove the stump regardless of whether any other surgery is contemplated. This view is based on the possibility that by the time tumor recurrence is clinically apparent, it may have progressed beyond the stage at which satisfactory cancer surgery is still possible. The likelihood of this occurrence may be sufficient indication in the face of previous high-grade, high-stage disease to warrant removal of the ureteral stump electively.

The availability of the ureteroscopic capabilities has provided a new alternative in the follow-up of these patients. Whether this method will be a more sensitive diagnostic modality than direct aspiration cytology remains to be determined.

INTRAPELVIC/URETERAL CHEMOTHERAPY

Recent advances in endoscopic instrumentation and an increased use of topical chemotherapeutic agents for the control of superficial disease in the bladder have prompted attempts to treat superficial tumors of the upper tract by chemotherapeutic agents instilled directly into the ureter or renal pelvis in a retrograde fashion.

Initial application of this modality has been in highly selected clinical situations, such as recurrent disease in a solitary kidney, occurrence of synchronous bilateral superficial disease, or surgical/anesthetic risk for a particular patient. In each of these instances, it is critical to ascertain that the tumor in question is truly superficial. Ultimate efficacy and potential risks of the use of these agents in such a therapeutic approach will require thorough assessment.

An additional potential access to the upper tracts is through the use of percutaneous techniques with instillation of chemotherapeutic agents in an antegrade fashion. This approach may also provide the opportunity of treating superficial recurrent transitional cell cancers of the ureter and renal pelvis with resection or fulguration. Such methods assume the capability of characterizing the nature of a tumor diathesis, since these techniques will violate an otherwise intact collecting system and may induce regional or distant dissemination of an otherwise relatively benign cancer (Tomera et al., 1982).

Other Cancers of the Upper Tract

SQUAMOUS CELL CARCINOMA

Squamous cell carcinoma of the upper urinary tract constitutes less than 15 per cent of tumors of the renal pelvis and a smaller percentage of ureteral tumors (Deming and Harvard, 1970). This form of cancer has been suggested to arise in areas of chronic irritation. Thus, the majority of squamous cell cancers have been associated with chronic infection, and generally these cancers have been reported in the setting of pre-existing calculus or leukoplakia as well (Higgins, 1953). Although the presence of calculous disease in the absence of other potentially carcinogenic factors (exposure to carcinogens, infection of the upper tracts) does not necessarily imply an increased risk for squamous cell carcinoma, these tumors have been associated with the presence of a calculus in over 50 per cent of cases (Deming and Harvard, 1970).

Of further interest have been findings of squamous cell carcinoma in the lower ureter in association with schistosomiasis (Dimmette et al., 1956). In these cases, a direct association of such tumors with chronic inflammation and irritation in schistosome-induced refluxing ureters has been postulated. No cases of upper urinary tract squamous cell carcinomas have been seen in this setting. Although etiologic mechanisms have been suggested to be similar to those associated with squamous cell carcinoma of the bladder in each of these instances, experimental proof of their existence remains to be obtained.

The diagnosis of squamous cell carcinoma is usually made when the tumor is already far advanced. This may reflect both the lack of specificity of symptoms associated with tumor development and their lack of distinction from symptoms of calculi, infection, and chronic irritation. The diagnosis should be suspected when a deformity appears in the parenchyma of a kidney containing a long-standing calculus (Gittes, 1979). As opposed to a renal parenchymal tumor, squamous cell carcinoma of the renal pelvis usually spreads in a scirrhous or tentacular fashion without capsule formation and invades rapidly without deforming the renal outline (Bennington and Beckwith, 1975). The value of cytologic examination is limited in these instances because of the frequency of suspicious cells in the setting of chronic inflammation. Xanthogranulomatous pyelonephritis can also obscure the diagnosis of squamous cell carcinoma.

Ultrasonography and CT scanning may permit greater definition of these conditions. Needle aspirates of suspicious areas may also be used to determine whether neoplasia is present.

Radical surgery has rarely been effective therapy because of the advanced stage of disease by the time diagnosis is made. Somewhat greater success has been observed with squamous carcinoma of the ureter. In these instances, diagnosis may have been made at an earlier stage of disease because of earlier occurrence of obstructive symptoms. However, reports are too few to permit meaningful assessment.

MESENCHYMAL TUMORS

Occasionally, vermiform masses may be seen within the ureter. These are histologically distinct from papillary uroepithelial tumors, since they consist of polypoid masses of mesenchymal tissue that are covered with a thin layer of benign urothelium (Bennington and Beckwith, 1975). Although they may initially be indistinguishable from their pedunculated uroepithelial counterparts, radiographically they may be characterized by an elongated and narrow polypoid tumor (either with a single branch or with several thin branches) extending from a common stalk (Gittes, 1979). Cytologic examinations and brush biopsies are negative for tumor in these instances. Treatment consists only of local excision of the polyp at its base. Recurrence is rare, and no neoplastic potential has been documented.

When malignant mesenchymal tumors have been diagnosed, they usually have already metastasized. The prognosis of these patients is uniformly poor (Gittes, 1979). Such lesions include leiomyosarcoma, hemangiosarcoma, and lymphosarcoma.

TUMORS METASTATIC TO THE COLLECTING SYSTEM

Metastases to the upper urinary tract have arisen from such varied sources as stomach, prostate, breast, lung, and cervix. In addition, involvement by a variety of lymphomas has been described. These metastatic tumors appear as discrete masses that usually are localized within the upper tract wall. They may thus be differentiated from metastases to the retroperitoneum, which usually are clinically and radiographically indistinguishable from retroperitoneal fibrosis. The most common symptoms are hematuria and obstruction. All levels of the ureter or renal pelvis or both have been involved by such metastases with equal frequency (Gittes, 1979).

Occasionally, metastatic renal cell carcinoma occurs in the ureteral stump after radical nephrectomy (Sinner, 1959). These lesions usually present clinically with gross hematuria, and diagnosis may be made by cystoscopy and pelvic CT scanning. Urinary cytology may be diagnostic for the presence of exfoliated renal cancer cells. Treatment in these situations is usually a futile exercise.

INTRINSIC NON-NEOPLASTIC URETERAL MASSES

Endometriosis. Endometriosis may be an important cause of ureteral obstruction in females, and it is usually associated with extensive disease elsewhere in the pelvis. Although endometrial implants in the wall of the bladder may account for menstrual hematuria, this may also occur in association with erosion of functional endometrial tissue through the wall of the ureter. Endometriosis is usually seen as an extrinsic compression of the ureter. At surgery, a "chocolate cyst" appears to have been formed, usually in the area of the pelvic ureter (Gittes, 1979). Treatment ranges from medical hormonal manipulation to surgery, depending upon the severity of disease and the results of medical therapy.

Ureteritis Cystica. Ureteritis cystica is an uncommon process in which small cysts or blebs are scattered along the uroepithelial lining of the ureter (Fig. 30–32). They may be confused with multiple ureteral tumors. However, urinary cytology and brushings will be negative. These lesions rarely produce hematuria or obstruction. Although the etiology of these cysts is unknown, they are thought to represent degeneration of the cell nests of von Brunn, resulting in epithelium-lined cysts in the submucosa that are similar to those found in the renal pelvis and the bladder as the result of chronic infection (Carroll, 1963). Treatment should be directed toward control of infection. Surgical therapy is not indicated.

References

Bladder Urothelial Carcinoma

Aaronson, S. A.: Transforming genes of retroviruses and human cancer cells. *In* Fortner, J. G., and Rhoads, J. E. (Eds.): Accomplishments in Cancer Research, 1983. Philadelphia, J. B. Lippincott, 1984, p. 139.

Abrams, P. H., Choa, R. G., Gaches, C. G. C., et al.: A controlled trial of single dose intravesical adriamycin in superficial bladder tumors. Br. J. Urol., 53:585, 1981.

Ahlering, T. E., Lieskovsky, G., and Skinner, D. G.: Indications for urothrectomy in men undergoing single stage radical cystectomy for bladder cancer. J. Urol., 131:657, 1984.

Albarran, J.: Les Tumeurs de la Vessie. Paris, G. Steinheil, 1892, p. 41.

Allegra, S. R., Broderick, P. A., and Corvese, N. L.: Cytologic and histogenetic observations in well-differentiated transitional cell carcinoma of the bladder. J. Urol., 107:777, 1972.

Althausen, A. F., Prout, G. R., Jr., and Daly, J. J.: Noninvasive papillary carcinoma of the bladder associated with carcinoma in situ. J. Urol., 116:575, 1976.

Ambarelli, V., and Rubino, A.: Some aspects of tryptophan-nicotinic acid chain in Hodgkin's disease. Relative roles of tryptophan loading and vitamin A. Supplementation on urinary excretion of metabolites. Haematol. Latiner, 5:49, 1962.

American Cancer Society: Cancer Statistics. CA, 33:2, 1983.

Anderson, C. K.: Current topics on the pathology of bladder cancer. Proc. R. Soc. Med., 66:283, 1973.

Anderstrom, C., Johansson, S., and Nilsson, S.: The significance of lamina propria invasion on the prognosis of patients with bladder tumors. J. Urol., 124:23, 1980.

Angervall, L., Bengtsson, U., Zetterlund, C. G., et al.: Renal pelvic carcinoma in a Swedish district with abuse of a phenacetin-containing drug. Br. J. Urol., 41:401, 1969.

Arce, S., Lopez, R., Almaguer, M., et al.: HL-A antigens and transitional cell carcinoma of the bladder. Mater. Med. Pol., 10:98, 1978.

Armenian, H. K., and Lilienfeld, A. M.: The distribution of incubation periods of neoplastic diseases. Am. J. Epidemiol., 99:92, 1974.

Armstrong, B., and Doll, R.: Bladder cancer mortality in diabetics in relation to saccharin consumption and smoking habits. Br. J. Prev. Soc. Med., 29:73, 1975.

Aschner, P. W.: The pathology of vesical neoplasms. Its evaluation in diagnosis prognosis. JAMA, 91:1697, 1928.

Bagley, D. H., Huffman, J. L., and Lyon, E. S.: Combined rigid and flexible ureteropyeloscopy. J. Urol., 130:243, 1983.

Barber, M., Brooksbank, B. W. L., and Kuper, S. W. A.: Staphylococcal phosphatase, glucuronidase, and sulphatase. J. Pathol. Bacteriol., 63:57, 1951.

Barnes, R. W., Bergman, R. T., Hadley, H. L., et al.: Control of bladder tumors by endoscopic surgery. J. Urol., 97:864, 1967.

Batata, M. A., Chu, F. C., Hilaris, B, S., Whitmore, W. F., Kim, Y. S., and Lee, M. Z.: Bladder cancer in men and women treated by radiation therapy and/or radical cystectomy. Urology, 18:15, 1981.

Batata, M. A., Whitmore, W. F., Jr., Chu, F. C., Hilaris, B. S., Unal, A., and Chung, S.: Patterns of recurrence in bladder cancer treated by irradiation and/or cystectomy. Int. J. Radiat. Oncol. Biol. Phys., 6:155, 1980.

Beahrs, J. R., Fleming, T. R., and Zincke, H.: Risk of local urethral recurrence after radical cystectomy for bladder cancer. J. Urol., 131:264, 1984.

Beall, D., and Grant, G. A.: Preparation of β-glucuronidase from E. coli. Rev. Can. Biol. Exp., 11:51, 1952.

Bean, M. A., Pees, H., Fogh, J., et al.: Cytotoxicity of lymphocytes from patients with cancer of the urinary bladder: detection by a ^{3}H-proline microcytotoxicity test. Int. J. Cancer, 14:186, 1974.

Becci, P. J., et al.: N-butyl-N-(4-hydroxybutyl) nitrosamine-induced urinary bladder cancer in C57BL/6 × DBA/2F¹ mice as a useful model for study of chemoprevention of cancer with retinoids. Cancer Res., 41:927, 1981.

Bell, J. T., Burney, S. W., and Friedell, G. H.: Blood vessel invasion in human bladder cancer. J. Urol., 105:675, 1971.

Bengtsson, U., Angervall, L., Ekman, H., et al.: Transitional cell tumors of the renal pelvis in analgesic abusers. Scand. J. Urol. Nephrol., 2:145, 1968.

Bengtsson, U., Johansson, S., and Angervall, L.: Malignancies of the urinary tract and their relation to analgesic abuse. Kidney Int., 13:107, 1978.

Benson, R. C., Jr., Farrow, G. M., Kinsey, J. H., et al.: Detection and localization of in situ carcinoma of the bladder with hematoporphyrin derivative. Mayo Clin. Proc., 57:548, 1982.

Benson, R. C., Jr., Kinsey, J. H., Cortese, D. A., et al.: Treatment of transitional cell carcinoma of bladder with hematoporphyrin derivative phototherapy. J. Urol., 130:109, 1983.

Best, E. W. R.: A Canadian Study of Smoking and Health. Ottawa, Dept. of Natl. Health and Welfare, 1966, p. 137.

Birkhead, B. M., Conley, J. G., and Scott, R. M.: Intensive radiotherapy of locally advanced bladder cancer. Cancer, 37:2746, 1976.

Bishop, J. M., and Varmus, H.: Functions and origins of retroviral transforming genes. *In* Weiss, R., Teich, N., Varmus, H., and Coffin, J. (Eds.): RNA Tumor Viruses. Cold Springs Harbor Laboratory Monograph Series, 1982.

Black, M. M., Leis, H. P., Jr., and Shone, B.: Cellular hypersensitivity to breast cancer. Cancer, 33:952, 1974.

Blandy, J. P., England, H. R., Evans, S. J., Hope-Stone, H. F., Mair, G. M., Mantell, B. S., Oliver, R. T., Paris, A. M., and Resdon, R. A.: T3 bladder cancer—the case for salvage cystectomy. Br. J. Urol., 52:506, 1980.

Bloom, H. J. G.: Preoperative intermediate-dose radiotherapy and cystectomy for deeply invasive carcinoma of the bladder: rationale and results. In Bladder Cancer: Principles of Combination Therapy. Oliver, R. T. D., Hendry, W. F., and Bloom, H. J. G., London, Butterworth, 1981, p. 151.

Bloom, H. J. G., Hendry, W. F., Wallace, D. M., and Skeet, R. G.: Treatment of T3 bladder cancer: controlled trial of pre-operative radiotherapy and radical cystectomy versus radical radiotherapy. Second report and review (for the Clinical Trials Group, Institute of Urology). Br. J. Urol., 54:136, 1982.

Blot, W. J., and Fraumeni, J. F., Jr.: Geographic patterns of bladder cancer in the United States. J. Natl. Cancer Inst., 61:1017, 1978.

Boccon-Gibod, L., Katz, M., Cochard, B., et al.: Lymphography and percutaneous fine needle node aspiration biopsy in the staging of bladder carcinoma. J. Urol., 132:24, 1984.

Boileau, M. A., Johnson, D. E., Chan, R, C., and Gonzalez, M. O.: Bladder carcinoma: Results with preoperative radiation therapy and radical cystectomy. Urology, 16:569, 1980.

Bollag, W.: Retinoids and cancer. Cancer Chemother. Pharmacol., 3:207, 1979.

Booth, C. M., and Kellett, M. J.: Intravenous urography in the follow-up of carcinoma of the bladder. Br. J. Urol., 53:246, 1981.

Boyd, P. J. R., and Burnand, K. G.: Site of bladder-tumor recurrence. Lancet, 2:1290, 1974.

Boyland, G., Wallace, D. M., and Williams, D. C.: Activity of sulfatase and β-glucuronidase in urine, serum, and bladder tissue. Br. J. Cancer, 9:62, 1955.

Bracken, R. B., Johnson, D. E., Rodriguez, L., et al.: Treatment of multiple superficial tumors of bladder with intravesical bleomycin. Urology, 9:161, 1977.

Bracken, R. B., Johnson, D. E., von Eschenback, A. C., et al.: Roile of intravesical mitomycin C in management of superficial bladder tumors. Urology, 16:11, 1980.

Brand, K. G.: Schistosomiasis-cancer: Etiological considerations: A review. Acta Trop. (Basel), 36:203, 1979.

Brannan, W., Ochsner, M. G., Fuselier, H. A., Jr., and Landry, G. R.: Partial cystectomy in the treatment of transitional cell carcinoma of the bladder. J. Urol., 119:213 1978.

Brice, M., Marshall, V. F., Green, J. L, et al.: Simple total cystectomy for carcinoma of the urinary bladder: one hundred fifty-six consecutive cases—five years later. Cancer, 9:576, 1956.

Broders, A. C.: Epithelioma of the genitourinary organs. Ann. Surg., 75:574, 1922.

Broecker, B. H., Klein, F. A., and Hackler, R. H.: Cancer of the bladder in spinal cord injury patients. J. Urol., 125:196, 1981.

Brookes, P.: Chemical carcinogenesis. Br. Med. Bull., 36:1, 1980.

Brosman, S. A.: Experience with BCG in patients with superficial bladder carcinoma. J. Urol., 128:27, 1982.

Brown, R. B.: A method of management of inoperable carcinoma of the bladder. Med. J. Aust., 1:23, 1969.

Brown, R. R., Price, J. M., Satter, E. J., et al.: The metabolism of tryptophan in patients with bladder cancer. Acta Union Intern. Contre Cancrum, 16:299, 1960.

Brown, R. R., Price, J. M., Burney, S. W., et al.: Lack of effect of smoking on the excretion of tryptophan metabolites by man. Cancer Res., 30:611, 1970.

Brown, R. R., Price, J. M., Satter, E. J., et al.: The metabolism of tryptophan in patients with bladder cancer. Acta Union Intern. Contre Cancrum, 16:299, 1960.

Bryan, G. T.: Pellet implantation studies of carcinogen compounds. J. Natl. Cancer Inst., 43:255, 1969.

Bryan, G. T.: The role of urinary trytophan metabolites in the etiology of bladder cancer. Am. J. Clin. Nutr., 24:841, 1971.

Bryan, G. T.: The pathogenesis of experimental bladder cancer. Cancer Res., 37:2813, 1977.

Bryan, G. T., and Springberg, P. D.: Role of the vehicle in the genesis of bladder carcinomas in mice by the pellet implantation technique. Cancer Res., 26:105, 1966.

Bubenick, J., Perlmann, P., and Helmstein, K.: Cellular and humoral immune responses to human urinary bladder carcinomas. Int. J. Cancer, 5:310, 1970.

Buck, H., Hauser, P. K., and Rudiger, W.: Uber die Ausseheidung eines noch nicht beschriebenen Penacetin metaboliten bein Menschen und beiden ratte. Arch. Pathol. Pharmacol., 253,25, 1966.

Buick, R. N., Stanisic, T. H., Fry, S. E., et al.: Development of an agar-methyl-cellulose clonogenic assay for cells in transitional cell carcinoma of the human bladder. Cancer Res., 39:5051, 1979.

Burbank, F., and Fraumeni, J. F., Jr.: Synthetic sweetener consumption and bladder cancer trends in the United States. Nature, 227:296, 1970.

Burn, J.: Intra-arterial infusion in malignant disease of the pelvis. In Second Symposium on Methotrexate in the Treatment of Cancer, Worrall, M., and Espiner, H. J. (Eds.): Bristol, Wright, 1966, p. 58.

Burnand, K. G., Boyd, P. J. R., Mayo, M. E., et al.: Single dose intravesical Thiotepa as an adjuvant to cystodiathermy in the treatment of transitional cell bladder carcinoma. Br. J. Urol., 48:55, 1976.

Byar, D., and Blackard, C.: Comparisons of placebo pyridoxine, and topical thiotepa in preventing recurrence of stage I bladder cancer. Urology, 10:556, 1977.

Caldwell, W. L.: Radiotherapy: definitive integrated and palliative therapy. Urol. Clin. North Am., 3:129, 1976.

Campbell, H. J.: Cancer of the bladder experiences of a health maintenance organization. Urology, 2:637, 1973.

Carr, I., McGinty, F., and Norris, P.: The fine structure of neoplastic invasion: invasion of liver, skeletal muscle and lymphatic vessels by the Rd/3 tumour. J. Pathol., 118:91, 1976.

Case, R. A. M., and Hosker, M. E.: Tumour of the urinary bladder as an occupational disease in the rubber industry in England and Wales. Br. J. Prev. Soc. Med., 8:39, 1954.

Case, R. A. M., Hosker, M. E., McDonald, D. B., et al.: Tumours of the urinary bladder in workmen engaged in the manufacture and use of certain dyestuff intermediates in the British chemical industry. Part I. The role of aniline, benzidine, alpha-naphthylamine and beta-naphthylamine. Br. J. Ind. Med., 11:75, 1954.

Catalona, W. J.: Practical utility of specific red cell adherence test in bladder cancer. Urology, 18:113, 1981.

Catalona, W. J., and Chretien, P. B.: Correlation among host immunocompetence and tumor stage, tumor grade and vascular permeation in transitional carcinoma. J. Urol., 110:526, 1973.

Chapman, J. W., Connolly, J. G., and Rosenbaum, L.: Occupational bladder cancer: A case-controlled study.

In Connolly, J. G. (Ed.): Carcinoma of the Bladder. New York, Raven Press, 1981, p. 45.

Chevlen, E. M., Airward, H. K., Ziegler, J. L., et al.: Cancer of the bilharzial bladder. Int. J. Radiat. Oncol. Biol. Phys., *5*:921, 1979.

Chibber, P. J., McIntyre, M. A., Hindmarsh, J. R., et al.: Transitional cell carcinoma involving the prostate. Br. J. Urol., *53*:605, 1981.

Chisholm, G. D., Hindmarsh, J. R., Howatson, A. G., et al.: TNM (1978) in bladder cancer: Use and abuse. Br. J. Urol., *52*:500, 1980.

Chodak, G. W., Haudenschild, C., Gittes, R. S., et al.: Angiogenic activity as a marker of neoplastic and pre-neoplastic lesions of the human bladder. Ann. Surg., *192*:762, 1980.

Chodak, G. W., Scheiner, C. J., and Zetter, B. R.: Urine from patient with transitional cell carcinoma stimulates migration of capillary endothelial cells. N. Engl. J. Med., *305*:869, 1981.

Clayson, D. B.: Experimental studies in urothelial cancer. *In* Cooper, E. H., and Williams, R. E. (Eds.): The Biology and Clinical Management of Bladder Cancer. London, Blackwell Scientific Publications, 1975.

Cohen, S. M.: Urinary bladder carcinogenesis: Initiation-promotion. Semin. Oncol., *6*:157, 1979.

Cohen, S. M., Greenfield, R. E., Jacobs, J. B., and Friedell, G. H.: Precancerous and noninvasive lesions of the urinary bladder. *In* Carter, R. L. (Ed.): Precancerous States. New York, Oxford Press, 1984, p. 278.

Cohen, S. M., Jacobs, J. B., Arai, M., et al.: Early lesions in experimental bladder cancer: Experimental design and light microscopic findings. Cancer Res., *36*:2508, 1976.

Cole, P.: Coffee-drinking and cancer of the lower urinary tract. Lancet, *1*:1335, 1971.

Cole, P.: A population-based study of bladder cancer. *In* Doll, R., and Vodopija, I. (Eds.): Host Environment Interactions in the Etiology of Cancer in Man. Lyon, IARC, 1973, p. 83.

Cole, P., Hoover, R., and Friedell, G. H.: Occupation and cancer of the lower urinary tract. Cancer, *29*:1250, 1972.

Cole, P., Monson, R. R., Haning, H., et al.: Smoking and cancer of the lower urinary tract. N. Engl J. Med., *284*:129, 1971.

Collste, L. G., Darzynkiewicz, L., Traganos, F., et al.: Cell-cycle distribution of urothelial tumour cells as measured by flow cytometry. Br. J. Cancer, *40*:872, 1979.

Connery, D. B.: Leukoplakia of the urinary bladder and its association with carcinoma. J. Urol., *69*:121, 1953.

Connolly, J. G.: Letter to Editor. J. Urol., *130*:368, 1983.

Connolly, J. G., Challis, T. W., Wallace, D. M., et al.: An evaluation of the fractionated cystogram in the assessment of infiltrating tumors of the bladder. J. Urol., *98*:356, 1967.

Connolly, J. G., Rider, W. D., Rosenbaum, L., et al.: Relation between the use of artificial sweeteners and bladder cancer. Can. Med. Assoc. J., *119*:408, 1978.

Coon, J., Weinstein, R. S., and Summers, J.: Blood group precursor T antigen expression in human urinary bladder carcinoma. Am. J. Clin. Pathol., *77*:692, 1982.

Cooper, E. H.: Biology of human bladder cancer. *In* Cooper, E. H., and Williams, R. E. (Eds.): The Biology and Clinical Management of Bladder Cancer. London, Blackwell, Scientific Publications, 1975, p. 65.

Cooper, G. M.: Cellular transforming genes. Science, *217*:801, 1982.

Cooper, J. A., and Hunter, T.: Regulation of cell growth and transformation by tyrosine-specific kinases: The search for important cellular substrate proteins. Curr. Top. in Microbioi. Immunol. *107*:125, 1983.

Cooper, P. H., Wajsman, J., Johnston, W. H., and Skinner, D. G.: Severe atypia of transitional epithelium and carcinoma of the urinary bladder. Cancer, *31*:1055, 1973.

Cooper, T. P., Wheelis, R. F., Correa, R. J., et al.: Random mucosal biopsies in the evaluation of patients with carcinoma of the bladder. J. Urol., *117*:46, 1977.

Corder, M. P., McFadden, D. B., and Stump, D. C.: Chemotherapy of advanced transitional cell carcinoma of the bladder. *In* Smith, P. H., and Prout, G. R. (Eds.): Bladder Cancer. London, Butterworth, 1984, p. 240.

Cordonnier, J. J.: Simple cystectomy in the management of bladder carcinoma. Arch. Surg., *108*:19, 1974.

Cox, C. E., Cass, A. S., and Boyce, W. H.: Bladder cancer: a 26 year review. J. Urol., *101*:550, 1969.

Crawford, E. D., and Skinner, D. G.: Salvage cystectomy after irradiation failure. J. Urol., *123*:32, 1980.

Crigler, C. M., Miller, L. S., Guinn, G. A., et al.: Radiotherapy for carcinoma of the bladder. J. Urol., *96*:55, 1966.

Cross, R. J., Glashan, R. W., Humphrey, C. S., et al.: Treatment of advanced bladder cancer with adriamycin and 5-fluorouracil. Br. J. Urol., *48*:609, 1976.

Cummings, K.: Current concepts in the management of patients' invasive bladder carcinoma. Semin. Oncol., *6*:220, 1979.

Cummings, K. B., Kodera, Y., and Bean, M. A.: In vitro immune parameters in relation to clinical course in transitional cell carcinoma. Natl. Cancer Inst. Monogr., *49*:119, 1978a.

Cummings, K. B., Mason, J. T., Correa, R. J., Jr., and Gibbons, R. P.: Segmental resection in the management of bladder carcinoma. J. Urol., *119*:56, 1978b.

Cummings, K. B., Taylor, W. J., Correa, R. J., et al.: Observations on definitive cobalt radiation for cure in bladder carcinoma: 15-year follow-up. J. Urol., *115*:152, 1976.

Cutler, S. J., Heney, N. M., and Friedell, G. H.: Longitudinal study of patients with bladder cancer: factors associated with disease recurrence and progression. *In* Bonney, W., and Prout, G. (Eds.): AUA Monographs. Vol. I: Bladder Cancer. Baltimore, The William & Wilkins Co., 1982, p. 35.

Daly, J. J.: Carcinoma in situ of the urothelium. Urol. Clin. North Am., *3*:87, 1976.

Davies, J. M.: Two aspects of the epidemiology of bladder cancer in England and Wales. Proc. R. Soc. Med., *70*:411, 1977.

DeCenzo, J. M., Howard, P., and Irish, C. E.: Antigenic deletion and prognosis of patients with stage A transitional cell bladder carcinoma. J. Urol., *114*:874, 1975.

Devesa, S. S., and Silverman, D. T.: Cancer incidence and mortality trends in the United States: 1935–74. J. Natl. Can. Inst., *60*:545, 1978.

DeWeerd, J. H., and Colby, M. Y., Jr.: Bladder carcinoma treated by irradiation and surgery: Interval report. J. Urol., *109*:409, 1973.

Diamond, D. A., Berry, S. J., Jewett, H. J., et al.: A new method to assess metastatic potential of human prostate cancer: Relative nuclear roundness. J. Urol., *128*:729, 1982.

Dougherty, T. J., Grindey, G. B., Fiel, R., et al.: Photo-radiation therapy. II. Cure of animal tumors with hematoporphyrin and light. J. Natl. Cancer Inst., *55*:115, 1975.

Dougherty, T. J., Kaufman, J. E., Goldfarb, A., et al.: Photoradiation therapy for the treatment of malignant tumors. Cancer Res., *38*:2628, 1978.

Dretler, S. R., Ragsdale, B. D., and Leadbetter, W. F: The value of pelvic lymphadenectomy in the surgical treatment of bladder cancer. Trans. Am. Assoc. Genitourin. Surg., *64*:79, 1972.

Droller, M. J.: Hemorrhagic cystitis. *In* Kaufman, J. (Ed.): Current Therapy. Philadelphia, W. B. Saunders Co., 1980, p. 207.

Droller, M. J.: Bladder cancer. Curr. Probl. Surg., *18*:205, 1981.

Droller, M. J.: Bladder cancer. Monogr. Urol., *3*:131, 1982.

Droller, M. J.: Radiation therapy in bladder cancer. *In* Murphy, G. P. (Ed.): Proceedings of the First International Meeting on Bladder Cancer. 1983a.

Droller, M. J.: Intravesical chemotherapy in the management of carcinoma in situ of the urinary bladder. World J. Urol., *1*:103, 1983b.

Droller, M. J.: The controversial role of radiation therapy as adjunctive treatment of bladder cancer. J. Urol., *129*:897, 1983c.

Droller, M. J.: Immunotherapy in genitourinary neoplasia. Urol. Clin. North Am., *11*:643, 1984.

Droller, M. J.: Immunotherapy in genitourinary neoplasia: current status. J. Urol., *133*:1, 1985a.

Droller, M. J.: The case against definitive radiation therapy in the treatment of infiltrative bladder cancer. World J. Urol., in press, 1985b.

Droller, M. J., and Walsh, P. C.: Therapeutic efficacy of salvage cystectomy. Do results reflect natural history of bladder cancer? Urology, *22*:118, 1983.

Droller, M. J., and Walsh, P. C.: Is topical chemotherapy safe and effective in the management of flat carcinoma-in-situ of the bladder? Presented at Annual AUA Meeting, New Orleans, 1984.

Duncan, R. E., Bennett, D. W., Evans, A. T., et al.: Radiation-induced bladder tumors, J. Urol., *118*:43, 1977.

Dunning, W. F., Curtis, M. R., and Maun, M. E.: The effect of added dietary tryptophan on the occurrence of 2-acetylaminofluorene induced liver and bladder cancer in rats. Cancer Res., *10*:454, 1950.

Durkee, C., Benson, R., Jr.: Bladder cancer following administration of cyclophosphamide. Urology, *16*:145, 1980.

Edelman, G. M.: Surface modulation in cell recognition and cell growth. Science, *192*:218, 1976.

Editorial: Genetic association with bladder cancer. Br. Med. J., *2*:514, 1979.

Edsmyr, F.: Intravesical therapy with doxorubicin in patients with superficial bladder tumors. *In* Oliver, R. T. D., Hendry, W. F., and Bloom, H. J. G. (Eds.): Bladder Cancer: Principles of Combination Therapy. London, Butterworth, 1981, p. 107.

Edsmyr, F., Berlin, T., Duchek, M., et al.: Intravesical therapy with adriamycin in patients with superficial bladder tumors. Eur. Urol., *6*:132,-1980.

Edsmyr, F., Jacobsson, F., Dahl, O., et al.: Cobalt 60 teletherapy of carcinoma of the bladder. Acta Radiol., *6*:81, 1967.

Eidinger, D., and Morales, A.: Treatment of superficial bladder cancer in man. Ann. N. Y. Acad. Sci., *277*:239, 1976.

Eisenberg, R. B., Roth, R. B., and Weinberg, M. H.: Bladder tumors and associated proliferative mucosal lesions. J. Urol., *84*:544, 1960.

Ekman, B., and Strombeck, J. P.: Demonstration of tumorigenic decomposition products of 2,3-azotoluene. Acta Physiol. Scand., *14*:43, 1947.

El-Aaser, A. A., El-Menzabani, M. M., Higgy, N. A., et al.: A study on the aetiological factors of bilharzial bladder cancer in Egypt. 3. Urinary β-glucuronidase. Eur. J. Cancer Clin. Oncol., *15*:573, 1979.

Elliott, A. Y., Fraley, E. E., Cleveland, P., et al.: Isolation of RNA virus from papillary tumors of the human renal pelvis. Science, *179*:393, 1973.

El-Masri, W. S., and Fellows, G.: Bladder cancer after spinal cord injury. Paraplegia, *19*:265, 1981.

El-Menzabani, M. M., El-Aaser, A. A., and Zakhary, N. I.: A study on the aetiological factors of bilharzial bladder cancer in Egypt: 1. Nitrosamines and their precursors in urine. Eur. J. Cancer Clin. Oncol., *15*:287, 1979.

Emmott, R. C., Droller, M. J., and Javadpour, N.: Studies of ABO (H) surface antigen specificity: carcinoma in situ and nonmalignant lesions of the bladder. J. Urol., *125*:26, 1981.

England, H. R., Molland, E. A., Oliver, R. T. D., et al.: Systemic cyclophosphamide in flat carcinoma in situ of the bladder. *In* Oliver, R. T. D., Hendry, W. F., and Bloom, H. J. G. (Eds.): Bladder Cancer: Principles of Combination Therapy. London, Butterworth, 1981a.

England, H. R., Paris, A. M. I., and Blandy, J. P.: The correlation of T_1 bladder tumor history with prognosis and follow-up requirements. Br. J. Urol., *53*:593, 1981b.

England, H. R., Paris, A. M. I., and Blandy, J. P.: Intravesical thiotepa as adjuvant to cystodiathermy in multiple recurrent Superficial bladder tumors. *In* Oliver, R. T. D., Hendry, W. F., and Bloom, H. J. G. (Eds.): Bladder Cancer: Principles of Combination Therapy. London, Butterworth, 1981c.

Epstein, J. I., Berry, S. J., and Eggleston, J. C.: Nuclear roundness factor: A predictor of progression in untreated stage A_2 prostate cancer. Cancer, *54*:1666, 1984.

Esposti, P. L., and Zajicek, J.: Grading of transitional cell neoplasms of the urinary bladder from smears of bladder washings: A critical review of 326 tumors. Acta Cytol., *16*:529, 1972.

Eva, A., Robbins, K. C., Andersen, P. R., et al.: Cellular genes analogous to retroviral *onc* genes are transcribed in human tumour cells. Nature, *295*:116, 1982.

Evans, R. A., and Texter, J. H., Jr.: Partial cystectomy in the treatment of bladder cancer. J. Urol., *114*:391, 1975.

Fair, W. R.: Formalin in the treatment of massive bladder hemorrhage: techniques, results, and complications. Urology, *3*:573, 1974.

Fairchild, W. V., Spence, C. R., Solomon, H. D., et al.: The incidence of bladder cancer after cyclophosphamide therapy. J. Urol., *122*:163, 1979.

Falor, W. H.: Chromosomes in non-invasive papillary carcinoma of the bladder. JAMA, *216*:791, 1971.

Falor, W. H., and Ward, R. M.: DNA banding patterns in carcinoma of the bladder. JAMA, *226*:1322, 1973.

Falor, W. H., and Ward, R. M.: Fifty-three month persistence of ring chromosome in noninvasive bladder carcinoma. Acta Cytol., *20*:272, 1976.

Falor, W. H., and Ward, R. M.: Prognosis in well-differentiated noninvasive carcinoma of the bladder based on chromosomal analysis. Surg. Gynecol. Obstet., *144*:515, 1977.

Falor, W. H., and Ward, R. M.: Prognosis in early carcinoma of the bladder based on chromosomal analysis. J. Urol., *119*:44, 1978.

Farber, E.: Chemical carcinogenesis and urinary bladder. *In* Connolly, J. G. (Ed.): Carcinoma of the Bladder. New York, Raven Press, 1981, p. 67.

Farber, E., and Cameron, R.: Sequential analysis of cancer development. Adv. Cancer Res. *31*:125, 1980.

Farrow, G. M., and Utz, D. C.: Observations on microinvasive transitional cell carcinoma of the urinary bladder. Clin. Oncol., *1*:609, 1982.

Farrow, G. M. Utz, D. C., and Rife, C. C.: Morphological and clinical observations of patients with early bladder cancer treated with total cystectomy. Cancer Res., *36*:2495, 1976.

Farrow, G. M., Utz, D. C., Rife, C. C., et al.: Clinical observations on 69 cases of in situ carcinoma of the urinary bladder. Cancer Res., *37*:2794, 1977.

Farsund, T., Laerum, O. D., and Hostmark, J.: Ploidy disturbance of normal-appearing bladder mucosa in patients with urothelial cancer: Relationship to morphology. J. Urol., *130*:1076, 1983.

Faysal, M. H.: Urethrectomy in men with transitional cell carcinoma of the bladder. Urology, *16*:23, 1980.

Feinberg, A. P., Vogelstein, B., Droller, M. J., et al.: Mutation affecting the 12th amino acid of the c-Ha-ras oncogene product occurs infrequently in human cancer. Science, *220*:1175, 1983.

Fidler, I. J.: Tumor heterogeneity and biology of cancer invasion and metastasis. Cancer Res., *38*:2651, 1978.

Firlit, C. F.: Intractable hemorrhagic cystitis secondary to extensive carcinomatosis: management with formalin solution. J. Urol., *110*:57, 1973.

Fitzgerald, J. M., Khan, O., Oliver, R. T. D., and Riddle, P. R.: Longterm followup in patients with superficial bladder tumors treated with intravesical epodyl. Br. J. Urol., *51*:545, 1979.

Flanigan, R. C., King, C. T., Clark, T. D., et al.: Immunohistochemical demonstration of blood group antigens in neoplastic and normal human urothelium: A comparison with standard red cell adherence. J. Urol., *130*:499, 1983.

Flower, R. J., Mercada, S., and Vane, J. R.: Analgesic-antipyretics and anti-inflammatory agents: drugs employed in the treatment of gout. *In* Goodman, A., and Gilman, A. G. (Eds.): The Pharmacological Basis of Therapeutics. New York, Macmillan, 1980.

Fokkens, W.: Phenacetin abuse related to bladder cancer. Environ. Res., *20*:192, 1979.

Foot, N. C.: Glandular metaplasia of the epithelium of the urinary tract. South. Med. J., *37*:137, 1944.

Fradet, Y., Cordon-Cardo, C., Whitmore, W. F., Jr., et al.: Bladder tumor heterogeneity defined by tissue typing with monoclonal antibodies. Proc. Am. Urol. Assoc. 79th Annual Mtg., 1984.

Fraley, E. E., Elliott, A. Y., Castro, A. E., et al.: Ribonucleic acid virus associated with human urothelial tumors: Significance for diagnosis and treatment. J. Urol., *111*:378, 1974a.

Fraley, E. E., Elliott, A. Y., Cleveland, P., and Stern, N.: RNA virus associated with human transitional cell cancers of the urinary tract. Minn. Med., *57*:871, 1974b.

Frank, H. G.: Policy and results of treatment by radiotherapy of carcinoma of the bladder in Leeds. Clin. Radiol., *21*:425, 1970.

Fraumeni, J. F., Jr., Scotto, J., and Dunham, L. J.: Coffee-drinking and bladder cancer. Lancet, *2*:1204, 1971.

Friedell, G. H.: Carcinoma, carcinoma in situ, and "early lesions" of the uterine cervix and the urinary bladder: Introduction and definitions. Cancer Res., *36*:2482, 1976.

Friedell, G. H.: Precancerous lesions of the urinary bladder. Acta Endoscop., *11*:53, 1981.

Friedell, G. H., Hawkins, I. R., Ahmed, S. W., and Schmidt, J. D.: The role of urinary tract cytology in the detection and clinical management of bladder cancer. *In* Bonney, W. W., and Prout, G. R. (Eds.): Bladder Cancer. AUA Monographs. Baltimore, The William & Wilkins Co., 1982, p. 49.

Friedell, G. H., Jacobs, J. B., Nagy, G. K., et al.: The pathogenesis of bladder cancer. Am. J. Pathol., *89*:431, 1977.

Friedland, G. W., Filly, R., Goris, M. L., et al.: Uroradiology: An Integrated Approach. London, Churchill Livingstone, 1983.

Friedman, M.: Supervoltage (2MVp) rotation irradiation of cancer of the bladder. Radiology, *73*:191, 1959.

Fulker, M. J., Cooper, E. H., and Tanaka, T.: Proliferation and ultrastructure of papillary transitional cell carcinoma of the human bladder. Cancer, *27*:71, 1971.

Gankeer, H. A., and deRuiter, H. J.: Carcinoma of the renal pelvis following the abuse of phenacetin-containing analgesic drugs. Br. J. Urol., *51*:188, 1979.

Gardner, S. D.: Prevalence in England of antibody to human polyomavirus (BK). Br. Med. J., *1*:77, 1973.

Gardner, S. D., Field, A. M., Colemen, D. V., et al.: New human papovavirus (BK) isolated from urine after renal transplantation. Lancet, *1*:1253, 1971.

Garnick, M. B.: Intravesical chemotherapy for superficial bladder carcinoma. *In* Garnick, M. B., and Richie, J. P. (Eds.): Urologic Cancer: A Multidisciplinary Perspective. New York, Plenum Press, 1983, p. 101.

Garnick, M. B., Schade, D., Israel, M., et al.: Intravesical doxorubicin for prophylaxis in management of recurrent superficial bladder carcinoma. J. Urol., *131*:43, 1984.

Garvin, D. D., Weber, C. H., Jr., and Polsky, M. S.: Carcinoma in the defunctionalized bladder: Report of a case and review of the literature. J. Urol., *117*:669, 1977.

Gavrell, G. J., Lewis, R. W., Meehan, W. L., and Leblanc, G. A.: Intravesical thiotepa in the immediate postoperative period in patients with recurrent transitional cell carcinoma of the bladder. J. Urol., *120*:410, 1978.

Geisse, L. J., and Tweeddale, D. N.: Pre-clinical cytological diagnosis of bladder cancer. J. Urol., *120*:51, 1978.

Gelfand, M., Weinberg, R. W., and Castle, W. M.: Relationship between carcinoma of the bladder and infestation with *Schistosoma haematobium*. Lancet, *1*:1249, 1967.

Geraghty, J. T.: Treatment of malignant disease of the prostate and bladder. J. Urol., *7*:33, 1922.

Gerridzen, R. G., and Futter, N. G.: Ten year review of vesical diverticula. Urology, *20*:33, 1982.

Gittes, R. F.: Tumors of the bladder. *In* Harrison, J. H., Gittes, R. F., Perlmutter, A., Stamey, T. A., and Walsh, P. C. (Eds.): Campbell's Urology. Philadelphia, W. B. Saunders Co., 1979, p. 1033.

Glashan, R. W.: A critical review of the management of bladder neoplasia using a modified form of Helmstein's pressure therapy. Br. J. Urol., *47*:57, 1975.

Godec, C. J., and Gleich, P.: Intractable hematuria and formalin. J. Urol., *130*:688, 1983.

Goffinet, D. R., Schneider, M. J., Glatstein, E. J., et al.: Bladder cancer: results of radiation therapy in 384 patients. Radiology, *117*:149, 1975.

Goldman, R. L., and Warner, N. E.: Hemorrhagic cystitis and cytomegalic inclusions in the bladder associated with cyclophosphamide therapy. Cancer, *25*:7, 1970.

Golinger, R. C., Gregorio, R. M., and Fisher, E. R.: Tumor cells in venous blood draining mammary carcinomas. Arch. Surg., *112*:707, 1977.

Gomer, C. J., and Dougherty, T. J.: Determination of [^{3}H]- and [^{14}C] hematoporphyrin derivative distribution in malignant and normal tissue. Cancer Res., *39*:146, 1979.

Goodman, G. B., Hislop, T. G., Elwood, J. M., et al.: Conservation of bladder function in patients with invasive bladder cancer treated by definitive irradiation and selective cystectomy. Int. J. Radiat. Oncol. Biol. Phys., *7*:569, 1981.

Gowing, N. F. C.: Urethral carcinoma associated with cancer of the bladder. Br. J. Urol., *32*:428, 1960.

Gozzo, J. J., Gottschalk, K., O'Brien, P., et al.: Use of heterogenous and monospecific antisera for the diagnosis of bladder cancer. J. Urol., *118*:748, 1977.

Green, D. F., Robinson, M. R. G., Glashan, R., et al.: does intravesical chemotherapy prevent invasive bladder cancer? J. Urol., *131*:33, 1984.

Greene, L. F., Hanash, K. A., and Farrow, G. M.: Benign papilloma or papillary carcinoma of the bladder? J. Urol., *110*:205, 1973.

Gupta, N. P., Malavija, A. N., and Singh, S. M.: Rheumatoid factor: correlation with recurrence in transitional cell carcinoma of the bladder. J. Urol., *121*:417, 1979.

Haenszel, W., Shimkin, M. B., and Thiller, H. P.: Tobacco smoking patterns in the United States. Public Health Monograph 45. Washington, D. C., 1956.

Hakala, T. R., Lange, P. H., Castro, A. E., et al.: Antibody induction of lymphocyte-mediated cytotoxicity against human transitional cell carcinomas of the urinary tract. N. Engl. J. Med., *291*:637, 1974.

Hall, R. R., and Heath, A. B.: Radiotherapy and cystectomy for T₃ bladder carcinoma. Br. J. Urol., *53*:598, 1981.

Hall, R. R., Bloom, H. J. G., Freeman, J. E., et al.: Methotrexate treatment for advanced bladder cancer. Br. J. Urol., *46*:431, 1974.

Hall, R. R., Herring, D. W., Gibb, I., et al.: Prophylactic oral methotrexate therapy for multiple superficial bladder carcinoma. Br. J. Urol., *53*:582, 1981.

Hall, R. R., Laurence, D. J., Darcy, D., et al.: Carcinoembryonic antigen in the urine of patients with urothelial carcinoma. Br. Med. J., *3*:609, 1972.

Hamlyn, P., and Sikora, K.: Oncogenes. Lancet, *2*:236, 1983.

Hawksworth, G. M., and Hill, J. J.: Bacteria and the N-nitrosation of secondary amines. Br. J. Cancer, *25*:520, 1971.

Hayata, Y., Kato, H., Konaka, C., et al.: Hematoporphyrin derivative and laser photoradiation in the treatment of lung cancer. Chest, *81*:269, 1982.

Hecht, S. S., Tso, T. C., and Hoffman, D.: Selective reduction of tumorigenicity of tobacco smoke IV. Approaches to the reduction of N-nitrosamines and aromatic amines. Proc. Third World Conf. on Smoking and Health. Washington, D. C., DHEW Pub. # (NIH) 76-1221, 1976, p. 535.

Heney, N. M., Ahmed, S., Flanagan, M. J., et al.: Superficial bladder cancer: Prognosis and recurrence. J. Urol., *130*:1083, 1983.

Heney, N. M., Daly, J., Prout, G. R., et al.: Biopsy of apparently normal urothelium in patients with bladder cancer. J. Urol., *120*:559, 1978.

Heney, N. M., Nocks, B. N., Daly, J. J., et al.: T_a and T₁ bladder cancer: Location, recurrence, and progression. Br. J. Urol., *54*:152, 1982.

Heney, N. M., Proppe, K., Prout, G. R., Jr., et al.: Invasive bladder cancer: Tumor configuration, lymphatic invasion, and survival. J. Urol., *130*:895, 1983.

Herr, H.: Cisdiamminedichloride platinum II in the treatment of advanced bladder cancer. J. Urol., *123*:853, 1980.

Herr, H. W.: Carcinoma in situ of the bladder. Semin. Urol., *1*:15, 1983.

Herr, H. W., Bean, M. A., and Whitmore, W. F., Jr.: Prognostic significance of regional lymph node histology in cancer of the bladder. J. Urol., *115*:264, 1976.

Herr, H. W., Pinsky, C. M., Whitmore, W. F., Jr., et al.: Effect of intravesical BCG on carcinoma in situ of the bladder. Cancer, *51*:1323, 1983.

Hewitt, C. B., Babiszewski, J. F., and Antunez, A. R.: Update on intracavitary radiation in the treatment of bladder tumors. J. Urol., *126*:323, 1981.

Hiatt, H. A., Watson, J. D., and Winsten, J. A. (Eds.): Origins of Human Cancer. Vol. 4. Cold Spring Harbor Conferences on Cell Proliferation, 1977.

Hicks, R. M.: The mammalian urinary bladder: An accommodating organ. Biol. Rev., *50*:215, 1975.

Hicks, R. M.: Multistage carcinogenesis in the urinary bladder. Br. Med. Bull., *36*:39, 1980.

Hicks, R. M.: Carcinogenesis in the urinary bladder: A multi-stage process. *In* Connolly, J. G. (Ed.): Carcinoma of the Bladder. New York, Raven Press, 1981, p. 75.

Hicks, R. M., and Chowaniec, J.: The importance of synergy between weak carcinogens in the induction of bladder cancer in experimental animals and humans. Cancer Res., *37*:2943, 1977.

Hicks, R. M., and Chowaniec, J.: Experimental induction, histology and ultrastructure of hyperplasia and neoplasia of the urinary bladder epithelium. Int. Rev. Exp. Pathol., *18*:199, 1978.

Hicks, R. M., Wakefield, J., Saint, S. T. J., and Chowaniec, J.: Evaluation of a new model to detect bladder carcinogens or co-carcinogens: Results obtained with saccharin, cyclamate, and cyclophosphamide. Chem. Biol. Interact., *11*:225, 1975.

Hicks, R. M., Walters, C. L., Elsebai, I., et al.: Demonstration of nitrosamines in human urine: preliminary observations on a possible etiology for bladder cancer in association with chronic urinary tract infections. Proc. R. Soc. Med., *70*:413, 1977.

Hinder, R. A., and Schmaman, A.: Bilharziasis and squamous carcinoma of the bladder. S. Afr. Med. J., *43*:617, 1969.

Hisazumi, H., Naito, K., and Misaki, T.: Fibrinolytic activity in normal and cancerous tissues of the bladder. Invest. Urol., *11*:28, 1973.

Hisazumi, H., Uchibayaski, T., Naito, K., et al.: The prophylactic use of Thiotepa and urokinase in transitional cell carcinoma of the bladder: a preliminary report. J. Urol., *114*:394, 1975.

Hisazumi, H., Misaki, T., and Miyoshi, N.: Photoradiation therapy of bladder tumors. J. Urol., *130*:685, 1983.

Hodson, N. J., Husband, J. E., and MacDonald, J. S.: The role of computed tomography in the staging of bladder cancer. Clin. Radiol., *30*:389, 1979.

Hoffman, D., Masuda, Y., and Wynder, E. L.: α-naphthylamine and β-naphthylamine in cigarette smoke. Nature, *221*:254, 1969.

Hofstedter, A.: Endoscopica Zerstorung von Blasentunoren mi laser. Urologe, *20*:317, 1981.

Holland, J. F., Scharlau, C., Gailani, S., et al.: Vincristine treatment of advanced cancer: a cooperative study of 392 cases. Cancer Res., *33*:1258, 1973.

Holm, H. H., Kristensen, J. K., Rasmussen, S. N., et al.: Abdominal Ultrasound. Baltimore, University Park Press, 1976.

Hoover, R., and Cole, P.: Temporal aspects of occupational bladder carcinogenesis. N. Engl. J. Med., *288*:1040, 1973.

Hoover, R., and Cole, P.: Population trends in cigarette smoking and bladder cancer. Am. J. Epidemiol., *94*:409, 1971.

Hoover, R., and Fraumeni, J. F., Jr.: Cancer mortality in U.S. counties with chemical industries. Environ. Res., *9*:196, 1975.

Hoover, R. N., and Strasser, P. H.: Artificial sweeteners and human bladder cancer: preliminary results. Lancet, *1*:837, 1980.

Hope-Stone, H. F.: Radiotherapy in the management of invasive bladder cancer. In Smith, P. H., and Prout, G. R. (Eds.): Bladder Cancer. London, Butterworth, 1984, p. 203.

Hope-Stone, H. F., Blandy, J. P., Oliver, R. T. D., and England, H.: Radical radiotherapy and salvage cystectomy in the treatment of invasive carcinoma of the bladder. In Oliver, R. T. D., Hendry, W. F., and Bloom, H. J. G. (Eds.): Bladder Cancer: Principles of Combination Therapy. London, Butterworth, 1981, p. 127.

Hopkins, S. C., Ford, K. S., and Soloway, M. S.: Invasive bladder cancer: Support for screening. J. Urol., 130:61, 1983.

Howe, G. R., Burch, J. D., Miller, A. B., et al.: Tobacco use, occupation, coffee, various nutrients, and bladder cancer. Natl. Cancer Inst., 64:701, 1980.

Hoye, R. C., and Smith, R. R.: The effectiveness of small amounts of preoperative irradiation in preventing the growth of tumor cells disseminated at surgery. Cancer, 14:284, 1961.

Huebner, R. J., and Todaro, G. J.: Oncogenes of RNA tumor viruses as determinants of cancer. Proc. Natl. Acad. Sci., 64:1087, 1969.

Hueper, W., et al.: Experimental production of bladder tumors in dogs by administration of beta-naphthylamine. J. Indust. Hyg. Toxicol., 20:46, 1938.

Huland, H., Otto, U., Droese, M., et al.: Long term mitomycin C instillation after transurethral resection of superficial bladder carcinoma: Influence on recurrence, progression, and survival. J. Urol., 132:27, 1984.

Hultergren, N., Lagengren, C., and Ljungqvist, A.: Carcinoma of the renal pelvis in papillary necrosis. Acta Clin. Scand., 130:314, 1965.

Hunter, T.: The proteins of oneogenes. Sci. Am., Aug. 1984, p. 70.

Husband, J. E., and Hodson, N. J.: Computerized axial tomography for staging and assessing response of bladder cancer to treatment. In Oliver, R. T. D., Hendry, W. F., Bloom, H. J. G. (Eds.): Bladder Cancer: Principles of Combination Therapy. London, Butterworth, 1981, p. 27.

Inch, W. R., McCredie, J. A., and Sutherland, R. M.: Effect of x-radiation to tumor bed on local recurrence. Front. Radiat. Ther. Oncol., 5:30, 1970.

Iokhens, W., and Hop, W. C.: Radiation-induced bladder tumors. J. Urol., 121:690, 1979.

Isselbacher, K. J., and Cole, P.: Saccharin—the bitter sweet. N. Engl. J. Med., 296:1348, 1977.

Jacobi, G. H., and Thuroft, J. W.: Prophylactic intravesical doxorubicin instillation after TUR of superficial transitional cell tumors: 3 years experience. In Oliver, R. T. D., Hendry, W. F., and Bloom, H. J. G. (Eds.): Bladder Cancer: Principles of Combination Therapy. London, Butterworth, 1981, p. 85.

Jacobo, E., Loening, S., Schmidt, J. D., et al.: Primary adenocarcinoma of the bladder: a retrospective study of 20 patients. J. Urol., 117:54, 1977.

Jacobs, J. B., Arai, M., Cohen, S. M., et al.: Early lesions in experimental bladder cancer: Scanning electron microscopy of cell surface markers. Cancer Res., 36:2512, 1976.

Jacobs, J. B., Arai, M., Cohen, S. M., et al.: A long-term study of reversible and progressive urinary bladder cancer lesions in rats fed N-[4-(5-nitro-2-furyl)-2-thiazolyl] formamide. Cancer Res., 37:2817, 1977.

Jaeger, N., Radeke, H. W., and Weissbach, L.: Transurethral sonography—a non–invasive method to determine the infiltration of bladder tumors. In Kuss, R., et al. (Eds.): Bladder Cancer. New York, Alan R. Liss, 1984, p. 237.

Jakse, G., Hofstadter, F., and Marberger, H.: Intracavitary doxorubicin hydrochloride therapy for carcinoma in situ of the bladder. J. Urol., 125:185, 1981.

Jakse, G., Hofstadter, F., Engelman, U., and Jacobi, G. H.: ABH-antigenicity of transitional cell carcinoma of the urinary bladder in patients subjected to topical chemoprophylaxis. World J. Urol., 1:82, 1983.

Jakse, G., Hofstadter, F., and Marburger, H.: Topical doxorubicin hydrochloride therapy for carcinoma in situ of bladder: Follow-up. J. Urol., 131:41, 1984.

Jardin, A., and Vallancien, G.: Partial cystectomy for bladder tumors. In Kuss, R., et al. (Eds.): Bladder Cancer. New York, Alan R. Liss, 1984, p. 387.

Jewett, H. J.: Cancer in the bladder: Diagnosis and staging. Cancer, 32:1072, 1973.

Jewett, H. J.: The historical development of the staging of bladder tumors: personal reminiscences. Urol. Surv., 27:37, 1977.

Jewett, H. J., and Cason, J. F.: Infiltrating carcinoma of the bladder: curability by segmental resection. South. Med. J., 41:158, 1948.

Jewett, H. J., and Eversole, S. L., Jr.: Carcinoma of the bladder: characteristic modes of local invasion. J. Urol., 83:383, 1960.

Jewett, H. J., and Lewis, E.: Infiltrating carcinoma of bladder: curability by total cystectomy. J. Urol., 60:107, 1948.

Jewett, H. J., and Strong, G. H.: Infiltrating carcinoma of the bladder: relation of depth of penetration of the bladder wall to incidence of local extension and metastases. J. Urol., 55:366, 1946.

Jewett, H. J., King, L. R., and Shelley, W. M.: A study of 365 cases of infiltrating bladder cancer: relation of certain pathological characteristics to prognosis after extirpation. J. Urol., 92:668, 1964.

Johansson, S., and Wahlqvist, L.: Tumours of urinary bladder and ureter associated with abuse of phenacetin-containing analgesics. Acta Pathol. Microbiol. Scand. (A), 85:768, 1977.

Johansson, S., and Wahlqvist, L.: A prognostic study of urothelial renal pelvic tumors. Cancer, 43:2525, 1979.

Johnson, D. E., Hogan, J. M., and Ayala, A. C.: Transitional cell carcinoma of the prostate: A clinical and monphological study. Cancer, 29:287, 1972.

Johnson, D. E.: Personal communication, 1985.

Jones, H. C., and Swinney, J.: Thiotepa in the treatment of tumours of the bladder. Lancet, 2:615, 1961.

Jones, M. A., Bloom, H. J. G., Williams, G., Trott, P. A., and Wallace, D. M.: The management of squamous cell carcinoma of the bladder. Br. J. Urol., 52:511, 1980.

Juusela, H.: Carcinoma of the renal pelvis and its relationship to analgesic abuse. Ann. Chir. Gynaecol. Fenn., 62:386, 1973.

Kakizoe, T., Matsumoto, K., Nishio, Y., et al.: Analysis of 90 step-sectioned cystectomized specimens of bladder cancer. J. Urol., 131:467, 1984.

Kaplan, W. D.: Ileopelvic lymphoscintigraphy. Semin, Nucl. Med., 13:42, 1983.

Kaufman, J. M., Fam, B., Jacobs, S. C., et al.: Bladder cancer and squamous metaplasia in spinal cord injury patients. J. Urol., 118:967, 1977.

Kaye, K. W., and Lange, P. H.: Mode of presentation of invasive bladder cancer: reassessment of the problem. J. Urol., 128:31, 1982.

Kelalis, P. P., and McLean, P.: The treatment of diverticulum of the bladder. J. Urol., 98:349, 1967.

Kelley, D. R., Ratliff, T. L., Shapiro, A., et al.: Intravesical BCG for superficial bladder cancer. Proc. Am. Urol. Assoc. Mtg., New Orleans, May 1984, abst. 539.

Kelly, J. F., and Snell, M. E.: Hematoporphyrin derivative:

A possible aid in the diagnosis and therapy of carcinoma of the bladder. J. Urol., *115*:150, 1976.

Kenny, G. M., Hardner, G. J., and Murphy, G. P.: Clinical staging of bladder tumors. J. Urol., *104*:720, 1970.

Kerr, W. K., Barkin, M., Levers, P. E., et al.: The effect of cigarette smoking on bladder carcinogens in man. Can. Med. Assn. J., *93*:1, 1965.

Kessel, D.: Transport and binding of hematoporphyrin derivative and related porphyrins by murine leukemia L1210 cells. Cancer Res., *41*:1318, 1981.

Kessler, I. I.: Cancer mortality among diabetics. J. Natl. Cancer Inst., *44*:673, 1970.

Kessler, I. I., and Clark, J. P.: Saccharin, cyclamate, and human bladder cancer. JAMA, *240*:349, 1978.

Khoury, S., and Gilloz, A.: Non–transitional cell carcinoma of the bladder in adults. *In* Kuss, R., et al. (Eds.): Bladder Cancer. New York, Alan R. Liss, 1984, p. 275.

King, C. M.: The origins of urinary bladder cancer. *In* Bonney, W. W., and Prout, G. R., Jr., (Eds.): AUA Monographs. Vol. I: Bladder Cancer. Baltimore, The Williams & Wilkins Co., 1982, p. 13.

Kirk, D., Hinton, C. E., and Shaldon, C.: Transitional cell carcinoma of the prostate. Br. J. Urol., *51*:575, 1979.

Kleinerman, J., and Liotta, L.: Release of tumor cells. *In* Day, S. (Ed.): Progress in Cancer Research and Therapy. Vol. 5. New York, Raven Press, 1977, p. 135.

Knappenberger, S. T., Uson, A. C., and Melicow, M. M.: Primary neoplasms occurring in vesical diverticular: a report of 18 cases. J. Urol., *83*:153, 1960.

Kohler, G., and Milstein, C.: Continuous cultures of fused cells secreting antibody of predefined specificity. Nature (Lon.), *256*:495, 1975.

Koontz, W. W., Jr., Prout, G. R., Jr., and Minnis, J. E.: The use of intravesical thiotepa in the management of noninvasive carcinoma of the bladder. J. Urol., *125*:307, 1981.

Koss, L. G.: A light and electron microscopic study of the effects of a single dose of cyclophosphamide on various organs in the rat. Lab. Invest., *16*:44, 1967.

Koss, L. G., Bartels, P. H., Bibbo, M., et al.: Computer discrimination between benign and malignant urothelial cells. Acta Cytol., *19*:378, 1975.

Koss, L. G., Melamed, M. R., and Kelly, R. E.: Further cytologic and histologic studies of bladder lesions in workers exposed to para-aminodephenyl: progress report. J. Natl. Cancer Inst., *43*:233, 1969.

Koss, L. G., Nakanishi, I., and Freed, S. Z.: Non–papillary carcinoma in situ and atypical hyperplasia in cancerous bladders. Further studies of surgically removed bladders by mapping. Urology, *9*:442, 1977.

Koss, L. G., Tiamson, E. M., and Robbins, M. A.: Mapping cancerous and precancerous bladder changes. A study of the urothelium in ten surgically removed bladders. JAMA, *227*:281, 1974.

Kovarik, S., Davidsohn, I., and Stejksal, R.: ABO antigens in cancer: detection with mixed cell agglutination reaction. Arch. Pathol., *86*:12, 1968.

Kuettner, K. E., and Pauli, B. U.: Resistance of cartilage to normal and neoplastic invasion. *In* Horton, J. E., Tarpley, T. M., Jr., and Davis, W. E. (Eds.): Mechanisms of Localized Bone Loss. Arlington, Va., Information Retrieval, 1978, p. 251.

Kumar, S., Rosen, P., and Grabstald, H.: Intravesical formalin for the control of intractable bladder hemorrhage secondary to cystitis or cancer. J. Urol., *114*:540, 1975.

Kuntzman, R., Partuck, E. J., Kaplan, S. A., et al.: Phenacetin metabolism: Effect of hydrocarbons and cigarette smoking. Clin. Pharmacol. Ther., *22*:757, 1977.

Lamm, D. L., Thor, D. E., Winters, W. D., et al.: BCG immunotherapy of bladder cancer: inhibition of tumor recurrence and associated immune response. Cancer, *48*:82, 1981.

Lange, P. H., and Limas, C.: Tissue blood-group antigen testing in transitional cell carcinoma of the bladder (Letter). J. Urol., *124*:304, 1980.

Laplante, M., and Brice, M., II: The upper limits of hopeful application of radical cystectomy for vesical carcinoma: does nodal metastasis always indicate incurability? J. Urol., *109*:261, 1973.

Lattimer, J. K.: Carcinoembryonic antigen and bladder carcinoma. J. Urol., *115*:46, 1976.

Lawley, P. D.: Carcinogenesis by alkylating agents. *In* Searle, C. E. (Ed.): Chemical Carcinogens. Washington, D.C., American Chemical Society, 1976, p. 366.

Leadbetter, W. F., and Cooper, J. F.: Regional gland dissection for carcinoma of the bladder: A technique for one-stage cystectomy, gland dissection, and bilateral uretero-enterostomy. J. Urol., *63*:242, 1950.

Levinson, A. D., Opperman, H., Levintow, L., et al.: Evidence that the transforming gene of avian sarcoma virus encodes a protein kinase associated with a phosphoprotein. Cell, *15*:561, 1978.

Lieber, M. M.: In vitro culture and chemotherapy sensitivity testing of human transitional cell carcinoma. Urol. Clin. North Am., *11*:725, 1984.

Lilienfeld, A. M., Levin, M. L., and Moore, G. E.: The association of smoking with cancer of the urinary bladder in humans. Arch. Intern. Med., *98*:129, 1956.

Limas, C., and Lange, P. H.: Altered reactivity for A, B, and H antigens in transitional cell carcinoma of the urinary bladder. A study of mechanisms involved. Cancer, *46*:1366, 1980.

Limas, C., Coon, J., IV, Lange, P. H., and Weinstein, R. S.: ABH antigens in human urinary bladder carcinomas: detection and clinical applications. *In* Bonney, W. W., and Prout, G. R., Jr. (Eds): AUA Monographs. Vol. I: Bladder Cancer. Baltimore, The William & Wilkins Co., 1980, p. 69.

Limas, C., Lange, P. H., Fraley, E. E., et al.: A, B, H antigens in transitional cell tumors of the urinary bladder: correlation with the clinical course. Cancer, *44*:2099, 1979.

Liotta, L. A., Abe, S., Robey, P. D., et al.: Preferential digestion of basement membrane collagen by enzyme derived from a metastatic murine tumor. Proc. Nat. Acad. Sci., *76*:2268, 1979.

Long, R. T. L., Grummon, R. A., Spratt, J. S., et al.: Carcinoma of the urinary bladder (comparison with radical, simple, and partial cystectomy and intravesical formalin). Cancer, *29*:98, 1972.

Lunglmayr, G., and Czech, K.: Absorption studies on intraluminal Thiotepa for topical cytostatic treatment of low-stage bladder tumors. J. Urol., *106*:72, 1971.

Lynch, H. T., and Walzak, M. P.: Genetics in urogenital cancer. Urol. Clin. North Am., *7*:815, 1980.

Magee, P. N., and Barnes, J.: Carcinogenic nitroso compounds. Adv. Cancer Res., *10*:163, 1967.

Magri, J.: Partial cystectomy: a review of 104 cases. Br. J. Urol., *34*:74, 1962.

Mahoney, J. F., Storey, B. G., Ibarez, R. C., and Stewart, J. H.: Analgesic abuse, renal parenchymal disease, and carcinoma of the kidney or ureter. Aust. N. Z. J. Med., *7*:463, 1977.

Marrett, L. D., Walter, S. D., and Miegs, J. W.: Coffee drinking and bladder cancer in Connecticut. Am. J. Epidemiol., *117*:113, 1983.

Marshall, V. F.: The relation of the preoperative estimate to the pathologic demonstration of the extent of vesical neoplasms. J. Urol., *68*:714, 1952.

Marshall, V. F.: Symposium on bladder tumors: current clinical problems regarding bladder tumors. Cancer, 9:543, 1956.

Marshall, V. F., and McCarron, J. P., Jr.: The curability of vesical cancer: greater now or then? Cancer, 37:2753, 1977.

Marshall, V. F., and Whitmore, W. F., Jr.: The surgical treatment of cancer of the urinary bladder. Cancer, 9:609, 1956.

Masina, F.: Segmental resection for tumors of the urinary bladder: ten years follow-up. Br. J. Surg., 52:279, 1965.

Matanoski, G. M., and Elliott, E. A.: Bladder cancer epidemiology. Epidemiol. Rev., 3:203, 1981.

Matouschek, E.: Experimental studies on intravesical ultrasonography. In Kuss, R., et al. (Eds.): Bladder Cancer. New York, Alan R. Liss, 1984, p. 227.

McCarron, J. P., Jr., and Marshall, V. F.: The survival of patients with bladder tumors treated by surgery: Comparative results of an old and a recent series. J. Urol., 122:322, 1979.

McCredia, M., Stewart, J. H., Ford, J. M., et al.: Phenacetin-containing analgesics and cancer of the bladder or renal pelvis in women. Br. J. Urol., 55:220, 1983.

McCullough, D. L., Lamm, D. L., McLaughlin, A. P., et al.: Familial transitional cell carcinoma of bladder. J. Urol., 113:629, 1975.

McDonald, D. F., and Lund, R. R.: The role of urine in vesical carcinoma. I. Experimental confirmation of the urogenous theory of pathogenesis. J. Urol., 71:560, 1954.

McDonald, J. R., and Thompson, G. J.: Carcinoma of the urinary bladder: a pathological study with special reference to invasiveness and vascular invasion. J. Urol., 60:435, 1948.

McGuire, E. J., Weiss, R. M., Schiff, M., Jr., and Lytton, B.: Hemorrhagic radiation cystitis: treatment. Urology, 3:204, 1974.

McIntyre, D., and Pointon, R. C.: Vesical neoplasms occurring after radiation treatment of the uterine cervix. J.R. Coll. Surg., (Edinb.), 16:141, 1971.

McNutt, N. S., Hershberg, R. A., and Weinstein, R. S.: Further observations on the occurrence of nexuses in benign and malignant human cervical epithelium. J. Cell. Biol., 51:805, 1971.

Melamed, M. R., Koss, L. G., Ricci, A., et al.: Cytohistological observations on developing carcinoma of the urinary bladder in man. Cancer, 13:67, 1960.

Melamed, M. R., Voutsa, N. G., and Grabstald, H.: Natural history and clinical behavior of in situ carcinoma of the human urinary bladder. Cancer, 17:1533, 1964.

Melicow, M. M.: Histological study of vesical urothelium intervening between gross neoplasm in total cystectomy. J. Urol., 68:261, 1952.

Melicow, M. M., Uson, A. C., and Price, T. D.: Bladder tumor induction in rats fed 2-acetamidofluorene (2-AAF) and a pyridoxine-deficient diet. J. Urol., 91:520, 1964.

Melzak, J.: The incidence of bladder cancer in paraplegia: Paraplegia, 4:85, 1966.

Merrill, R. W., Brown, H. E., and Rose, J. F.: Bladder carcinoma treated by partial cystectomy: A review of 54 cases. J. Urol., 122:471, 1979.

Merrin, C.: Current studies at Roswell Park Memorial Institute. In Cooperative Studies Discussion Group—Bladder Cancer. Bethesda, Md., National Cancer Institute, 1976, p. 4.

Merrin, C., Wajsman, Z., Baumgartner, G., et al.: The clinical value of lymphangiography: are the nodes surrounding the obturator nerve visualized? J. Urol., 117:762, 1977.

Miller, E. C.: Some current perspectives on chemical carcinogenesis in humans and experimental animals. Cancer Res., 38:1479, 1978.

Miller, L. S.: Bladder cancer superiority of preoperative irradiation and cystectomy in clinical stages B2 and C. Cancer (Suppl. 2), 39:973, 1977.

Miller, L. S., and Johnson, D. E.: Megavoltage irradiation for bladder cancer: Alone, postoperative, or preoperative? Proceedings of 7th National Cancer Conference, 1973, p. 771.

Milner, W. A.: The role of conservative surgery in the treatment of bladder tumors. Br. J. Urol., 26:275, 1954.

Mishina, T., Oda, K., Munata, S., et al.: Mitomycin C bladder instillation therapy for bladder tumors. J. Urol., 114:217, 1975.

Mitchell, R. J.: Intravesical thiotepa in the treatment of transitional cell bladder carcinoma. Br. J. Urol., 43:185, 1971.

Mohiuddin, M., and Kramer, S.: Preoperative radiotherapy for bladder cancer: A perspective. Urology, 17:515, 1981.

Moloney, P. J., Fenster, H. N., and McLoughlin, M. C.: Carcinoma in the defunctionalized urinary tract. J. Urol., 126:260, 1981.

Montagne, D. K., and Boltuch, R. L.: Primary neoplasms in vesical diverticula: Report of 10 cases. J. Urol., 116:41, 1976.

Montie, J. R., Straffon, R. A., and Stewart, B. H.: Radical cystectomy without radiation therapy for carcinoma of the bladder. J. Urol., 131:477, 1984.

Morales, A.: Treatment of carcinoma in situ of the bladder with BCG. A phase II trial. Cancer Immunol. Immunother., 9:69, 1980.

Morales, A.: Long-term results and complications of intracavitary bacillus Calmette Guerin therapy for bladder cancer. J. Urol., 132:457, 1984.

Morales, A., Eidinger, D., and Bruce, A. W.: Intracavitary bacillus Calmette-Guerin in the treatment of superficial bladder tumors. J. Urol., 115:180, 1976.

Morgan, H. R., and Bossman, H. B.: Alterations of surface properties of chick embryo fibroblasts infected with four Rous sarcoma viruses producing distinctive cell transformations. Proc. Soc. Exp. Biol. Med., 146:1146, 1974.

Morganti, G., Gianferrai, L., Cresseri, A., Arrigoni, G., and Lovati, G.: Recherches clinico-statistiques et genetiques sur les neoplasies de la vessie. Acta Genet., 6:306, 1956.

Morrison, A. S.: Geographic and time trends of coffee imports and bladder cancer. Eur. J. Cancer, 14:51, 1978.

Morrison, A. S., and Buring, J. E.: Artificial sweeteners and cancer of the lower urinary tract. N. Engl. J. Med., 302:537, 1980.

Morrison, A. S., and Cole, P.: Epidemiology of bladder cancer. Urol. Clin. North Am., 3:13, 1976.

Morrison, R.: The results of treatment of cancer of the bladder. A clinical contribution to radiobiology. Clin. Radiol., 26:67, 1975.

Morrison, R.: Cancer of the urinary bladder—Epidemiology and aetiology. Urol. Res., 6:183, 1978.

Mostofi, F. K.: Potentialities of bladder epithelium. J. Urol., 71:705, 1954.

Mostofi, F. K.: Pathology and spread of carcinoma of bladder. JAMA, 206:1764, 1968.

Mostofi, F. K., Sobin, L. H., and Torloni, H.: Histologic Typing of Urinary Bladder Tumours. Geneva, WHO, 1973.

Murphy, W. M., Nagy, G. R., Rao, M. K., et al.: "Normal" urothelium in patients with bladder cancer. Cancer, 44:1050, 1979.

Murphy, W. M., and Soloway, M. J.: Developing carcinoma (dysplasia) of the urinary bladder. Pathol. Annu., 17:197, 1982.

Nakamura, S., and Nijuma, T.: Staging of bladder cancer by ultrasonography: A new technique by transurethral intravesical scanning. J. Urol., 124:341, 1980.

Narayana, A. S., Loening, S. A., Slymen, D. J., et al.: Bladder cancer: Factors affecting survival. J. Urol., 130:56, 1983.

Natale, R. B., Yagoda, A., Watson, R. E., et al.: Methotrexate: An active drug in bladder cancer. Cancer, 47:1246, 1981.

National Bladder Cancer Collaborative Group A (NBCCGA): Surveillance, initial assessment, and subsequent progress of patients with superficial bladder cancer in a prospective longitudinal study. Cancer Res., 37:2907, 1977.

Netto, N. R., Jr., and Lemos, G. C.: Comparison of treatment methods for prophylaxis of recurrent superficial bladder tumors. J. Urol., 129:33, 1983.

Netto, N. R., Jr., and Lemos, G. C.: Bacillus Calmette Guerin immunotherapy of infiltrating bladder cancer. J. Urol., 132:675, 1984.

Neuman, A. J., Jr., Carleton, C. E., Jr., and Johnson, S.: Cell surface A, B, or O (H) blood group antigens as an indicator of malignant potential in stage A bladder carcinoma. J. Urol., 124:27, 1980.

Newman, D. M., Brown, J. R., Jay, A. C., et al.: Squamous cell carcinoma of the bladder. J. Urol., 100:470, 1968.

Nichols, J. A., and Marshall, V. F.: The treatment of bladder carcinoma by local excision and fulguration. Cancer, 9:17, 1956.

Nieh, P. T., Daly, J. J., Heaney, J. A., et al.: The effect of intravesical thiotepa on normal and tumor urothelium. J. Urol., 119:59, 1978.

Nielsen, H. V., and Thybo, E.: Epodyl treatment of bladder tumors. Scand. J. Urol. Nephrol., 13:59, 1979.

Nishio, B., Horii, A., Morikawa, Y., et al.: Studies of the nonspecific cellular immune response in patients with urinary bladder carcinoma. Invest. Urol., 16:336, 1979.

Nocks, B. N., Nieh, P. T., and Prout, G. R., Jr.: A longitudinal study of patients with superficial bladder carcinoma successfully treated with weekly intravesical thiotepa. J. Urol., 122:27, 1979.

Norden, D. A., and Gelfand, M.: Bilharzia and bladder cancer, an investigation of urinary β-glucuronidase associated with S. haematobium infection. Trans. R. Soc. Trop. Med. Hyg., 66:864, 1972.

Novick, A. C., and Stewart, B. H.: Partial cystectomy in the treatment of primary and secondary carcinoma of the bladder. J. Urol., 116:570, 1976.

O'Kane, H. O., and Megaw, J. M.: Carcinoma in the exstrophic bladder. Br. J. Surg., 55:631, 1968.

Olssen, C. A., Chute, R., and Rao, C. N.: Immunologic reduction of bladder cancer recurrence rate. J. Urol., 111:173, 1974.

O'Toole, C., Perlmann, P., Unsgaard, B., et al.: Cellular immunity to human urinary bladder carcinoma. I. Correlation to clinical stage and radiotherapy. Int. J. Cancer, 10:77, 1972.

Oyasu, Y., and Hopp, M. L.: The etiology of cancer of the bladder. Surg. Gynecol. Obstet., 138:97, 1974.

Palmer, J. P., and Sprate, D. W.: Pelvic carcinoma following irradiation for benign gynecological diseases. Am. J. Obstet. Gynecol., 72:497, 1956.

Pang, A. S. D., and Morales, A.: Immunoprophylaxis of a murine bladder cancer with high dose BCG immunizations. J. Urol., 127:1006, 1982.

Papanicolaou, G. N., and Marshall, V. F.: Urine sediment

smears as a diagnostic procedure in cancers of the urinary tract. Science, 101:519, 1945.

Pauli, B. U., and Weinstein, R. S.: Correlations between cell surface protease activities and abnormalities of occludens junctions in rat bladder carcinoma in vitro. Cancer Res., 42:2289, 1982.

Pauli, B. U., Weinstein, R. S., Alroy, J., et al.: Ultrastructure of cell junctions in SANST-induced urothelial tumors in urinary bladder of Fischer rats. Lab. Invest., 37:609, 1977.

Pearse, H. D., Reed, R. R., and Hodges, C. V.: Radical cystectomy for bladder cancer. J. Urol., 119:216, 1978.

Pearson, R. M., and Soloway, M. S.: Does cyclophosphamide induce bladder cancer? Urology, 11:437, 1978.

Plotkin, G. M., Brigham, S. C., and Wolf, G.: Uridine-5'-diphosphate galactose: Glycoprotein galactosyl transferase activity in exfoliated bladder epithelial cells in rats fed N-[4-(5-nitro-2-furyl)-2-thiazolyl] formamide. Cancer Biochem. Biophys., 2:59, 1977.

Plotkin, G. M., Wides, R. J., Gilbert, S. L., et al.: Galactosyl transferase activity in human transitional cell carcinoma lines and in benign and neoplastic human bladder epithelium. Cancer Res., 39:3856, 1979.

Plotz, P. H., Klippel, J. H., Decker, J. L., et al.: Bladder complications in patients receiving cyclophosphamide for systemic lupus erythematosus or rheumatoid arthritis. Ann. Intern. Med., 91:221, 1979.

Pomerance, A.: Pathology and prognosis following total cystectomy for carcinoma of bladder. Br. J. Urol., 44:451, 1972.

Pontes, J. E., and Lopez, R.: Tumor recurrence following partial cystectomy. In Kuss, R., et al. (Eds.): Bladder Cancer. New York, Alan R. Liss, 1984, p. 387.

Poole-Wilson, D. S., and Barrard, R. J.: Total cystectomy for bladder tumors. Br. J. Urol., 43:16, 1971.

Potter, J. F.: Preoperative irradiation and surgery. Cancer, 35:84, 1975.

Powers, W. E., and Palmer, L. A.: Biologic basis of preoperative radiation treatment. Am. J. Roentgenol., 102:176, 1968.

Prescott, L. F.: The absorption, metabolism, excretion, and CNS effects of phenacetin. In Kincaid-Smith, P., and Fairley, K. F. (Eds.): Renal Infection and Renal Scarring. Melbourne, Mercedes, 1970, p. 359.

Price, J. M., Biava, C. G., Oser, B. L., et al.: Bladder tumors in rats fed cyclohexylamine or high doses of a mixture of cyclamate and saccharin. Science, 167:1131, 1970.

Prout, G. R., Jr.: The surgical management of bladder carcinoma. Urol. Clin. North Am., 3:149, 1975.

Prout, G. R., Jr.: Bladder carcinoma and a TNM system of classification. J. Urol., 117:583, 1977.

Prout, G. R., Jr.: Classification and staging of bladder carcinoma. Semin. Oncol., 6:189, 1979.

Prout, G. R., Jr.: Classification and staging of bladder carcinoma. In Bonney, W. W., and Prout, G. R. (Eds.): AUA Monographs. Vol I: Bladder Cancer. Baltimore, The Williams & Wilkins Co., 1982a.

Prout, G. R., Jr.: Heterogeneity of superficial bladder cancer. In Bonney, W. W., and Prout, G. R. (Eds.): AUA Monographs. Vol. I: Bladder Cancer. Baltimore. The Williams & Wilkins Co., 1982b.

Prout, G. R., Jr.: The results of conservative treatment in patients with carcinoma in situ of the bladder. Proc. ASCO. (Abst. 424), 183, 1982c.

Prout, G. R., Jr.: Superficial bladder cancer. In Smith, P. H., and Prout, G. R. (Eds.): Bladder Cancer. London, Butterworth, 1984, p. 151.

Prout, G. R., Jr., and Weinstein, R. S.: Cell membranes

and blood group antigens: an overview. *In* Bonney, W. W., and Prout, G. R., (Eds.): AUA Monographs. Vol. I: Bladder Cancer. Baltimore, The Williams & Wilkins Co., 1982, p. 63.

Prout, G. R., Jr., Griffin, P. P., and Shipley, W. U.: Bladder carcinoma as a systemic disease. Cancer, *43*:2532, 1979.

Prout, G. R., Jr., Koontz, W. W., Jr., Coombs, L. J., et al.: Long-term fate of 90 patients with superficial bladder cancer randomly assigned to receive or not to receive thiotepa. J. Urol., *130*:677, 1983.

Prout, G. R., Jr., Slack, N. H., and Bross, I. D. J.: Irradiation and 5-fluorouracil as adjuvants in the management of invasive bladder carcinoma. A cooperative group report after 4 years. J. Urol., *104*:116, 1970.

Prout, G. R., Jr., Slack, N. H., and Bross, I. D. J.: Preoperative irradiation and cystectomy for bladder carcinoma: IV. Results in a selected population. Proceedings of 7th National Cancer Conference, 1973, p. 783.

Pryor, J. P.: Factors influencing the survival of patients with transitional cell tumours of the urinary bladder. Br. J. Urol., *45*:586, 1973.

Pulciani, S., Santos, E., Lauver, A. V., et al.: Oncogenes in solid human tumours. Nature, *300*:539, 1982.

Purtilo, D. T., McCarthy, B., Young, J. P. S., and Friedell, G. H.: Familial urinary bladder cancer. Semin. Oncol., *6*:254, 1979.

Pyrhonen, S., Timonen, T., Heikkinen, A., et al.: Rheumatoid factor as an indicator of serum blocking activity and tumor recurrences in bladder tumors. Eur. J. Cancer, *12*:87, 1976.

Pyritz, R., Droller, M. J., and Saral, R.: Use of vasopressin in the control of hemorrhage in the control of cyclophosphamide-induced cystitis. J. Urol., *120*:253, 1978.

Radomski, J. L., and Brill, E.: Bladder cancer induction by aromatic amines: role of N-hydroxymetabolites. Science, *167*:992, 1970.

Radwin, H. M.: Radiotherapy and bladder cancer: a critical review. J. Urol., *124*:43, 1980.

Rathert, P., Melchor, H., and Lutzeyer, W.: Phenacetin: a carcinogen for the urinary tract? J. Urol., *113*:653, 1975.

Ray, B., Canto, A., and Whitmore, W. F., Jr.: Experience with primary carcinoma of the male urethra. J. Urol. *117*:591, 1977.

Reddy, E. P., Reynolds, R. K., Santos, E., et al.: A point mutation is responsible for the acquisition of transforming properties by the T_{24} human bladder carcinoma oncogene. Nature, *300*:143, 1982.

Rehn, L.: Ueber blasentumoren bei fuchsinarbeitern. Arch. Kind Chir., *50*:588, 1895.

Reid, E. C., Oliver, J. A., and Fishman, I. J.: Preoperative irradiation and cystectomy in 135 cases of bladder cancer. Urology, *8*:247, 1976.

Resnik, M. I., Kursh, E. D., and Bryan, P. D.: Nuclear magnetic resonance imaging in bladder cancer. *In* Kuss, R., et al. (Eds.): Bladder Cancer. New York, Alan R. Liss, 1984, p. 255.

Resnik, M. I., and O'Conor, V. J., Jr.: Segmental resection for carcinoma of the bladder: review of 102 patients. J. Urol., *109*:1007, 1973.

Riches, E.: Choice of treatment in carcinoma of the bladder. J. Urol., *84*:472, 1960.

Richie, J. P., Skinner, D. G., and Kaufman, J. J.: Radical cystectomy for carcinoma of the bladder: 16 years' experience. J. Urol., *113*:186, 1975.

Richie, J. P., Waisman, J., Skinner, D. G., et al.: Squamous

carcinoma of the bladder: treatment by radical cystectomy. J. Urol., *115*:670, 1976.

Riddle, P. R.: Flat carcinoma in situ of the bladder. Br. J. Urol., *47*:829, 1975.

Riddle, P. R.: The use of intravesical ethoglucid in the management of superficial bladder tumors. *In* Oliver, R. T. D., Hendry, W. F., and Bloom, H. J. G. (Eds.): Bladder Cancer: Principles of Combination Therapy. London, Butterworth, 1981, p. 63.

Rider, W. D., and Evans, D. H.: Radiotherapy in the treatment of recurrent bladder cancer. Br. J. Urol., *48*:595, 1976.

Romas, N. A., Ionascu, L., Ionescu, G., et al.: Anergy and tryptophan metabolism in bladder cancer. J. Urol., *115*:387, 1976.

Rose, D. P.: The influence of sex, age, and breast cancer on tryptophan metabolism. Clin. Chim. Acta, *18*:221, 1967.

Sagerman, R. H., Yu, W. S., Ryoo, M. C., King, G. A., Chung, C. T., and Ismmanuel, I. G.: Integrated preoperative irradiation and radical cystectomy. Int. J. Radiat. Oncol. Biol. Phys., *6*:607, 1980.

Salmon, S. E., and Von Hoff, D. D.: In vitro evaluation of anticancer drugs with the human tumor stem cell assay. Semin. Oncol., *8*:377, 1981.

Sandberg, A. A.: Karyotypic findings in bladder carcinoma. *In* Smith, P. H., and Prout, G. R. (Eds.): Bladder Cancer. London, Butterworth, 1984, p. 46.

Schade, R. O. K., and Swinney, J.: Pre-cancerous changes in bladder epithelium. Lancet, *2*:943, 1968.

Schellhammer, P. F.: Urethral meatal carcinoma following cystourethrectomy for bladder carcinoma. J. Urol., *115*:61, 1976.

Schellhammer, P. F., and Whitmore, W. F., Jr.: Transitional cell carcinoma of the urethra in men having cystectomy for bladder cancer. J. Urol., *115*:56, 1976.

Schellhammer, P. F., Bean, M. A., and Whitmore, W. F., Jr.: Prostatic involvement by transitional cell carcinoma: pathogenesis, patterns, and prognosis. J. Urol., *118*:399, 1977.

Schmauz, R., and Cole, P.: Epidemiology of cancer of the renal pelvis and ureter. J. Natl. Cancer Inst., *52*:1431, 1974.

Schmidt, J. D., and Weinstein, S. H.: Pitfalls in clinical staging of bladder tumors. Urol. Clin. North Am., *3*:107, 1976.

Schoborg, T. W., Sapolsky, J. L., and Lewis, C. W., Jr.: Carcinoma of the bladder treated by segmental resection. J. Urol., *122*:473, 1979.

Schuller, J., Walther, V., Schmidt, E., et al.: Intravesical ultrasound tomography in staging bladder cancer. J. Urol., *128*:264, 1982.

Scott, W. W., and Boyd, H. L.: Carcinogenic effects of beta-naphthylamine on normal and substituted isolated sigmoid loop bladder of dogs. J. Urol., *70*:914, 1953.

Seemayer, T. A., Knaack, J., Thelmo, W. L., et al.: Further observations on carcinoma in situ of the urinary bladder: Silent but extensive intraprostatic involvement. Cancer, *36*:514, 1975.

Seidelmann, F. E., Cohen, W. N., and Bryan, P. J.: Computed tomographic staging of bladder neoplasms. Radiol. Clin. North Am., *15*:419, 1977.

Seltzer, S. E., Benazzi, R. B., and Kearney, G. P.: Cyclophosphamide and carcinoma of bladder. Urology, *11*:352, 1978.

Shah, B. C., and Albert, D. J.: Intravesical instillation of formalin for the management of intractable hematuria. J. Urol., *110*:519, 1973.

Sharma, S. K., Bapva, B. C., and Singh, S. M.: Familial profile of transitional cell carcinoma. Br. J. Urol., *48*:442, 1976.

Sheridan, J. D.: Low resistance junctions between cancer cells in various solid tumors. J. Cell. Biol., *45*:91, 1970.

Shigematsu, S.: Significance of the chromosome in vesicle cancer. Proc. 13th Cong. Soc. Intl. d'Urologie. Edinburgh, Livingstone, 1965, p. 111.

Shipley, W. U.: Full dose irradiation for invasive bladder cancer: prognostic factors and technique. Urology *23*:95, 1984.

Shirai, T., Murasaki, G., Tatematsu, M., et al.: Early surface changes of the urinary bladder epithelium of different animal species induced by N-butyl-(4-hydroxybutyl) nitrosamine. Gann, *68*:203, 1977.

Shur, B. D., and Roth, S.: Cell surface glycosyltransferases. Biochem. Biophys. Acta, *415*:473, 1975.

Simon, D., Yen, S., and Cole, P.: Coffee drinking and cancer of the lower urinary system. J. Natl. Cancer Inst., *54*:587, 1975.

Sjolin, K. E., Nyholm, K., and Trautner, K.: Studies of transitional cell tumours of the bladder: Prognosis and causes of death. Acta Pathol. Microbiol. Scand. (A), *84*:361, 1976.

Skinner, D. G.: Current state of classification and staging of bladder cancer. Cancer Res., *37*:2838, 1977.

Skinner, D. G.: Current perspectives in the management of high-grade invasive bladder cancer. Cancer, *45*:1866, 1980.

Skinner, D. G.: Management of invasive bladder cancer: a meticulous pelvic node dissection can make a difference. J. Urol., *128*:34, 1982.

Skinner, D. G., and Lieskovsky, G.: Contemporary cystectomy with pelvic node dissection compared to preoperative radiation therapy plus cystectomy in management of invasive bladder cancer. J. Urol., *131*:1069, 1984.

Skinner, E., Lieskovsky, G., and Skinner, D. G.: Radical cystectomy in the elderly patient. J. Urol., *131*:1065, 1984.

Slack, N. H., and Prout, G. R., Jr.: Heterogeneity of invasive bladder carcinoma and different responses to treatment. J. Urol., *123*:644, 1980.

Slack, N. H., and Prout, G. R., Jr.: Heterogeneity of invasive bladder carcinoma and different responses to treatment. *In* Bonney, W. W., and Prout, G. R. Jr. (Eds.): AUA Monographs. Vol. I: Bladder Cancer. Baltimore, The Williams & Wilkins Co., 1982, p. 213.

Slack, N. H., Bross, I. D., and Prout, G. R., Jr.: Five-year followup results of a collaborative study of therapies for carcinoma of the bladder. J. Surg. Oncol., *9*:393, 1977.

Smith, G., Elton, R. A., Beynon, L. L., et al.: Prognostic significance of biopsy results of normal-looking mucosa in cases of superficial bladder cancer. Br. J. Urol., *55*:665, 1983.

Smith, J. A., Jr., and Whitmore, W. F., Jr.: Salvage cystectomy for bladder cancer after failure of definitive irradiation. J. Urol., *125*:643, 1981a.

Smith, J. A., and Whitmore, W. F., Jr.: Regional lymph node metastasis from bladder cancer. J. Urol., *126*:591, 1981b.

Smith, J. A., Jr., Batata, M., Grabstald, H., Sogani, P. C., Herr, H. W., and Whitmore, W. F., Jr.: Preoperative irradiation and cystectomy for bladder cancer. Cancer, *49*:869, 1982.

Smith, P. H.: Invasive bladder cancer: A lethal enigma. *In* Smith, P. H., and Prout, G. R., Jr. (Eds.): Bladder Cancer. London, Butterworth, 1984, p. 223.

Sobin, L. H.: The WHO histological classification of urinary bladder tumors. Urol. Res., *6*:193, 1978.

Soloway, M. S.: Rationale for intensive chemotherapy for superficial bladder cancer. J. Urol., *123*:461, 1980.

Soloway, M. S.: Surgery and intravesical chemotherapy in the management of superficial bladder cancer. Semin. Urol., *1*:23, 1983.

Soloway, M. S.: Systemic therapy for superficial bladder cancer. Urology, *23*:88, 1984.

Soloway, M. S., and Ford, K. S.: Subsequent tumor analysis of 36 patients who have received intravesicle mitomycin C for superficial bladder cancer. J. Urol., *130*:74, 1983.

Soloway, M. S., Murphy, W. M., DeFuria, D., et al.: The effect of mitomycin C on superficial bladder cancer. J. Urol., *125*:646, 1981.

Soloway, M. S., Murphy, W. M., Rao, M. K., et al.: Serial multiple-site biopsies in patients with bladder cancer. J. Urol., *120*:57, 1978.

Sontag, J. M.: Experimental identification of genitourinary carcinogens. Urol. Clin. North Am., 7:803, 1980.

Soto, E. A., Friedell, G. H., and Tiltman, A. J.: Bladder cancer as seen in giant histologic sections. Cancer, *39*:447, 1977.

Sporn, M. B.: Retinoids and suppression of carcinogenesis. Hosp. Pract., *18*:83, 1983.

Sporn, M. B., Roberts, A. B.: The role of retinoids in differentiation and carcinogenesis. Cancer Res., *43*:3034, 1983.

Sporn, M. B., et al.: 13-cis-retinoic acid: Inhibition of bladder carcinogenesis in the rat. Science, *195*:487, 1977.

Staehler, G., and Hofstedter, A.: Transurethral laser irradiation of urinary bladder tumors. Eur. Urol., *5*:64, 1979.

Stanisic, T. H., Owens, R., and Graham, A. R.: Use of clonal assay in determination of urothelial drug sensitivity in carcinoma in situ of bladder: clinical correlations in 5 patients. J. Urol., *129*:949, 1983.

Stein, B.: Specific red cell adherence: Immunologic evaluation of random mucosal biopsies in carcinoma of the bladder. J. Urol., *126*:37, 1981.

Strauli, P.: A concept of tumor invasion. *In* Straley, P., Barrett, A. J., and Baici, A. (Eds.): Proteinases and Tumor Invasion. New York, Raven Press, 1980, p. 1.

Stump, D. C., and Corder, M. P.: Chemotherapeutic approaches to transitional cell carcinoma of the bladder. III. Invasive and metastatic disease. *In* Bonney, W. W., and Prout, G. R., Jr. (Eds.): AUA Monographs. Vol. I: Bladder Cancer. Baltimore, The Williams & Wilkins Co., 1982, p. 305.

Sullivan, R. D.: Intra-arterial methotrexate therapy: the dose, duration, and route of administration studies of methotrexate in clinical cancer chemotherapy. *In* Porter, R., and Wiltshaw, E. (Eds.): First Symposium on Methotrexate in the Treatment of Cancer. Bristol, Wright, 1962, p. 50.

Summers, J. L., Coon, J. S., and Ward, R. M., et al.: Prognosis in carcinoma of the urinary bladder based on tissue ABH and T antigen status and karyotype of the initial tumor. Cancer Res., *43*:934, 1983.

Summers, J. L., Falor, W. H., and Ward, R.: A 10-year analysis of chromosomes in non-invasive papillary carcinoma of the bladder. J. Urol., *125*:177, 1981.

Suzuki, N., Withers, H. R., and Williams, M.: DNA content, cell size, and malignancy (Abstract 741). Proc. Am. Assn. Cancer Res., *19*:186, 1978.

Swanson, D. A., von Eschenback, A. C., and Johnson, D. E.: Salvage cystectomy for bladder carcinoma. Cancer, *47*:2275, 1981.

Tannenbaum, M., Tannenbaum, S., and Carter, H. W.: SEM, BEI and TEM ultrastructural characteristics of normal, pre-neoplastic, and neoplastic human transitional epithelia. *In* Scanning Electron Microscopy, Vol. 2, SEM Inc., A.M.F. O'Hare, Illinois, 1978, p. 949.

Taparowsky, W., Suard, Y., Fasano, O., et al.: Activation of the T_{24} bladder carcinoma transforming gene is linked to a single amino acid change. Nature, *300*:762, 1982.

Tatematsu, M., Cohen, S. M., Fukushima, S., et al.: Neovascularization in benign and malignant urinary bladder epithelial proliferative lesions of the rat observed in situ by scanning electron microscopy and autoradiography. Cancer Res., *38*:1792, 1978.

Taylor, J. S.: Carcinoma of the urinary tract and analgesic abuse. Med. J. Aust., *1*:407, 1972.

Thomas, D. G., Ward, A. M., and Williams, J. L.: A study of 52 cases of adenocarcinoma of the bladder. Br. J. Urol., *43*:4, 1971.

Tosi, S. E., and Movin, L. J.: Bladder tumor associated with phenacetin abuse. Urology, *9*:59, 1977.

Tribukait, B., Gustafson, H., and Esposti, P.: Ploidy and proliferation in human bladder tumors as measured by flow-cytofluorometric DNA-analysis and its relations to histopathology and cytology. Cancer, *43*:1742, 1979.

Tsuchiya, A., Obara, N., Miwa, M., et al.: Hematoporphyrin derivative and laser photoradiation in the diagnosis and treatment of bladder cancer. J. Urol., *130*:79, 1983.

Turner, A. G., Hendry, W. F., MacDonald, J. S., and Wallace, D. M.: The value of lymphography in the management of bladder cancer. Br. J. Urol., *48*:579, 1976.

Turner, A. G., Hendry, W. F., and William, G. B.: The treatment of advanced bladder cancer with methotrexate. Br. J. Urol., *49*:673, 1977.

Tweeddale, D., and Dee, A. L.: Cytopathology of the urinary tract. *In* Harrison, J. H., Gittes, R. F., Perlmutter, A., Stamey, T. A., and Walsh, P. C. (Eds.): Campbell's Urology. Philadelphia, W. B. Saunders Co., 1979, p. 1071.

Utz, D. C., and Zincke, H.: The masquerade of bladder cancer in situ as interstitial cystitis. J. Urol., *111*:160, 1974.

Utz, D. C., Hanash, K. A., and Farrow, G. M.: The plight of the patient with carcinoma in situ of the bladder. J. Urol., *103*:160, 1970.

Utz, D. C., Schmitz, S. E., Fugelso, P. D., and Farrow, G. M.: A clinicopathologic evaluation of partial cystectomy for carcinoma of the urinary bladder. Cancer, *32*:1075, 1973.

Van der Werf–Messing, B.: Carcinoma of the bladder treated by preoperative irradiation followed by cystectomy. Cancer, *32*:1084, 1973.

Van der Werf–Messing, B.: Carcinoma of the bladder $T_3N \times MO$ treated by preoperative irradiation followed by cystectomy: Third report of the Rotterdam Radio-Therapy Institute Cancer, *36*:718, 1978.

Van der Werf–Messing, B.: Preoperative irradiation followed by cystectomy to treat carcinoma of the urinary bladder category T_3NX_1O-4MO. Int. J. Radiat. Oncol. Biol. Phys., *5*:3975, 1979.

Van der Werf–Messing, B.: Carcinoma of the urinary bladder (Category $T_1N \times Mo$) treated either by radium implant or by transurethral resection only. Int. J. Radiat. Oncol. Biol. Phys., *7*:299, 1981.

Van der Werf–Messing, B.: Interstitial radium therapy of superficial bladder cancer (category T_1MXMO and T_2MXMO). *In* Smith, P. H., and Prout, G. R. (Eds.): Bladder Cancer. London, Butterworth, 1984, p. 191.

Van der Werf–Messing, B., Menon, P. S., and Hop, W. C. J.: Interstitial radiotherapy of carcinoma of the bladder at the Rotterdam Radiotherapy Institute. *In* Kuss, R., et al. (Eds.): Bladder Cancer. New York, Alan R. Liss, 1984, p. 71.

Varkarakis, M. J., Gaeta, J., Moore, R. H., et al.: Superficial bladder tumor: aspects of clinical progression. Urology, *4*:414, 1974.

Veenema, R.J., Dean, A. L., Jr., Roberts, M., et al.: Bladder carcinoma treated by direct instillation of thiotepa. J. Urol., *88*:60, 1962.

Veenema, R. J., Dean, A. L., Jr., Usom, A. C., et al.: Thiotepa bladder instillation: therapy and prophylaxis for superficial bladder tumors. J. Urol., *101*:711, 1969.

Veenema, R. J., Harisiadis, L., Chang, C., Puchner, P., Romas, N., Wechsler, M., and Guttman, R.: Bladder carcinoma: preliminary external radiotherapy used as a means for selecting complete treatment. *In* Connolly, J. G. (Ed.): Carcinoma of the Bladder. New York, Raven Press, 1981, p. 183.

Veenema, R. J., Romas, N. A., and Fingerhut, B.: Chemotherapy for bladder cancer. Urology, *3*:135, 1974.

Wahlqvist, L.: Chemical carcinogenesis—a review and personal observations with special reference to the role of tobacco and phenacetin in the production of urothelial tumours. *In* Pavone-Macaluso, M., et al. (Eds.): Bladder Tumors and Other Topics in Urological Oncology. New York, Plenum Press, 1980, p. 47.

Wajsman, Z., Merrin, C. S., Chu, T. M., et al.: Evaluation of biological markers in bladder cancer. J. Urol., *114*:879, 1975a.

Wajsman, Z., Merrin, C., Moore, R., et al.: Current results from treatment of bladder tumors with total cystectomy at Roswell Park Memorial Institute. J. Urol., *113*:806, 1975b.

Wallace, D. M.: Fundamental concepts in urothelial neoplasia. *In* Connolly, J. G. (Ed.): Carcinoma of the Bladder. New York, Raven Press, 1981, p. 7.

Wallace, D. M., and Bloom, H. J. G.: The management of deeply infiltrating (T_3) bladder carcinoma: controlled trial of radical radiotherapy versus preoperative radiotherapy and radical cystectomy (first report). Br. J. Urol., *48*:587, 1976.

Wallace, D. M., Chisholm, G. D., and Hendry, W. F.: T. N. M. classification for urological tumours (U.I.C.C.)—1974. Br. J. Urol., *47*:1, 1975.

Weinstein, R. S.: Origin and dissemination of human urinary bladder carcinoma. Semin. Oncol., *6*:149, 1979.

Weinstein, R. S.: Intravesical dissemination and invasion of urinary bladder carcinoma. *In* Bonney, W. W., and Prout, G. R., Jr. (Eds.): AUA Monographs. Vol. I: Bladder Cancer. Baltimore, The Williams & Wilkins Co., 1982, p. 27.

Weinstein, R. S., Alroy, J., Farrow, G. M., et al.: Blood group isoantigen deletion in carcinoma in situ of the urinary bladder. Cancer, *43*:661, 1979.

Weinstein, R. S., Coon, J. S., and Pauli, B. U.: Characterization of urinary bladder cancer cells. *In* Smith, P. H., and Prout, G. R. (Eds.): Bladder Cancer. London, Butterworth, 1984, p. 12.

Weinstein, R. S., Merk, F. B., and Alroy, J.: Structure and function of intercellular junctions in cancer. Adv. Can. Res., *23*:23, 1976.

Weinstein, R., Miller, A. W., III, and Pauli, B. V.: Carcinoma in situ: comments on the pathology of a paradox. Urol. Clin. North Am., *18*:523, 1980.

Weinstein, R. S., and Pauli, B. U.: Cell relationships in epithelia. *In* Koss, L. G., and Coleman, D. V. (Eds.): Advances in Clinical Cytology. London, Butterworth, 1981, p. 160.

Weiss, L.: Cell detachment and metastasis. *In* Stansly, P.

G., and Sato, H. (Eds.): Cancer Metastasis, Approaches to the Mechanism, Prevention and Treatment. Tokyo, Tokyo University Press, 1977, p. 25.

Weldon, T. E., and Soloway, M. S.: Susceptibility of urothelium to neoplastic cellular implantation. Urology, 5:824, 1975.

Whitmore, W. F., Jr.: Assessment and management of deeply invasive and metastatic lesions. Cancer Res., 37:2756, 1977.

Whitmore, W. F., Jr.: Management of bladder cancer. Curr. Probl. Cancer, 4:1, 1979.

Whitmore, W. F.: Integrated irradiation and cystectomy for bladder cancer. Br. J. Urol., 52:1, 1980.

Whitmore, W. F., Jr.: Management of invasive bladder neoplasms. Semin. Urol., 1:34, 1983.

Whitmore, W. F., Jr., and Batata, M. A.: Status of integrated irradiation and cystectomy for bladder cancer. Urol. Clin. North Am., 11:681, 1984.

Whitmore, W. F., Jr., and Marshall, V. F.: Radical total cystectomy for cancer of the bladder: 230 consecutive cases five years later. J. Urol., 87:853, 1962.

Whitmore, W. F., Jr., Batata, M. A, Ghoneim, M. A, Grabstald, H., and Unal, A.: Radical cystectomy with or without prior irradiation in the treatment of bladder cancer. J. Urol., 118:184, 1977a.

Whitmore, W. F., Jr., Batata, M. A., Hilaris, B. S., Reddy, G. N., Unal, A., Ghoneim, M. A., Grabstald, H., and Chu, F.: A comparative study of 2 preoperative radiation regimens with cystectomy for bladder cancer. Cancer, 40:1077, 1977b.

Widran, J., Sanchez, R., and Gruhn, J.: Squamous metaplasia of the bladder: a study of 450 patients. J. Urol., 112:479, 1974.

Wiener, D. P., Koss, L. G., Lablay, B., et al.: The prevalence and significance of Brunn's nests, cystitis cystica, and squamous metaplasia in normal bladders. J. Urol., 122:317, 1979.

Wiley, E. L., Mendelsohn, G., Droller, M. J., and Eggleston, J.: CEA and blood group substances in bladder cancer. J. Urol., 128 (2):276, 1982.

Williams, G. B., Trott, P. A., and Bloom, J. H. G.: Carcinoma of the bladder treated by interstitial irradiation. Br. J. Urol., 53:221, 1981.

Williams, R. D., and Hricak, H.: Magnetic resonance imaging in urology. J. Urol., 132:641, 1984.

Williams, R. E.: Treatment in transitional cell carcinoma. In Cooper, E. H., et al. (Eds.): The Biology and Clinical Management of Bladder Cancer. London, Blackwell Scientific Publications, 1975.

Winterberger, A. R., and Murphy, G. P.: Correlation of B-scan ultrasonic laminography in bladder tumors. Vasc. Surg., 8:169, 1974.

Wolf, H.: Studies on the role of tryptophan metabolites in the genesis of bladder cancer. Acta Chir. Scand. (Suppl.), 433:154, 1973.

Wolf, H., and Hojgaard, K.: Urothelial dysplasia concomitant with bladder tumours as a determinant factor for future new occurrences. Lancet, 2:134, 1983.

Wolk, F. N., and Bishop, M. C.: The specific red cell adherence test in transitional cell carcinoma of the bladder before and after radiotherapy in patients with blood group A. J. Urol., 130:71, 1983.

Wynder, E. L., and Goldsmith, R.: The epidemiology of bladder cancer—a second look. Cancer, 40:1246, 1977.

Wynder, E. L., and Stellman, S. D.: Artificial sweetener use and bladder cancer: a case-control study. Science, 207:1214, 1980.

Wynder, E. L., Onkerdonk, J., and Mantel, N.: An epidemiological investigation of cancer of the bladder. Cancer, 16:1388, 1963.

Yagoda, A.: Future implications of phase 2 chemotherapy trials in ninety-five patients with measurable advanced bladder cancer. Cancer Res., 37:2775, 1977.

Yagoda, A.: Chemotherapy of metastatic bladder cancer. Cancer, 45:1879, 1980.

Yagoda, A.: Chemotherapy for advanced urothelial cancer. Semin. Urol., 1:60, 1983.

Yagoda, A., Watson, R. C., Gonzales-Vitale, J. C., et al.: Cis-dichlorodiammineplatinum (II) in advanced bladder cancer. Cancer Treat. Rep., 60:917, 1976.

Yagoda, A., Watson, R. E., Grabstald, H., et al.: Adriamycin (NSC-12327) and cyclophosphamide (NSC-26271) in advanced bladder cancer. Cancer Treat. Rep., 61:97, 1977.

Zabbo, A., and Montie, J. E.: Management of the urethra in men undergoing radical cystectomy for bladder cancer. J. Urol., 131:267, 1984.

Zincke, H., Garbeff, P. J., and Beahrs, J. R.: Upper urinary tract transitional cell cancer after radical cystectomy for bladder cancer. J. Urol., 131:50, 1984.

Zincke, H., Utz, D. C., Taylor, W. F., et al.: Influence of thiotepa and doxorubicin instillation at time of transurethral surgical treatment of bladder cancer in tumor recurrence: a prospective, randomized, double-blind controlled trial. J. Urol., 129:505, 1983.

Zingg, H., and Sulmoni, A.: Chemotherapy in superficial neoplasms of the bladder. S. Afr. Med. J., 46:916, 1972.

Zoretic, S. N., Wajsman, Z., Beckley, S. A., et al.: Filling of the obturator nodes in pedal lymphangiography: Fact or fiction. J. Urol., 129:533, 1983.

Upper Tract Urothelial Carcinoma

Abeshouse, B. S.: Primary benign and malignant tumors of the ureter; review of the literature and report of one benign and 12 malignant tumors. Am. J. Surg., 91:237, 1956.

Adam, W. R., Dawborn, J. K., Price, G. C., et al.: Anaplastic transitional cell carcinoma of the renal pelvis in association with analgesic abuse. Med. J. Aust., 1:1108, 1970.

Babaian, R. J., and Johnson, D. E.: Primary carcinoma of the ureter. J. Urol., 123:357, 1980.

Bagley, D. H., Huffman, J. L., and Lyon, E. S.: Combined rigid and flexible ureteropyeloscopy. J. Urol., 130:243, 1983.

Batata, M., and Grabstald, H.: Upper urinary tract urothelial tumors. Urol. Clin. North Am., 3:79, 1976.

Batata, M. A., Whitmore, W. F., Hilaris, B. J., et al.: Primary carcinoma of the ureter: a prognostic study. Cancer, 35:1626, 1975.

Bengtsson, U., Angervall, L., Ekman, H., et al.: Transitional cell tumors of the renal pelvis in analgesic abusers. Scand. J. Urol. Nephrol., 2:145, 1968.

Bengtsson, U., Johansson, S., and Angervall, L.: Malignancies of the urinary tract and their relation to analgesic abuse. Kidney Int., 13:107, 1978.

Bennington, J. L., and Beckwith, J. B.: Tumors of the kidney, renal pelvis, and ureter. In Atlas of Tumor Pathology. Washington, D.C., Armed Forces Institute of Pathology, Fascicle 12, 1975.

Bergman, H., Fridenberg, R. M., and Sayegh, V.: New roentgenologic signs of carcinoma of the ureter. Am. J. Roentgenol., 86:707, 1961.

Bloom, N. A., Vidone, R. A., and Lytton, B.: Primary carcinoma of the ureter—a report of 102 new cases. J. Urol., 103:590, 1970.

Blute, R., Gittes, R., and Gittes, R. F.: Renal brush biopsy: survey of indications, technique, and results. J. Urol., 126:146, 1981.

Booth, C. M., Cameron, K. M., and Pugh, R. C. B.: Urothelial carcinoma of the kidney and ureter. Br. J. Urol., 52:430, 1980.

Brennan, R. E., and Pollack, H.: Nonvisualized ("phantom") renal calyx: causes and radiological approach to diagnosis. Urol. Radiol., 1:17, 1979.

Brown, H. E., and Roumani, G. K.: Conservative surgical management of transitional cell carcinoma of the upper urinary tract. J. Urol., 112:184, 1974.

Bush, I. M., Zamora, S., John T., et al.: Transurethral endoscopic surgery of the ureter and renal pelvis. Presented at AUA Annual Meeting, New York, 1979.

Campbell, M. F. (Ed.): Urology. 2nd ed. Philadelphia, W. B. Saunders Co., 1963, p. 942.

Carroll, G.: Nontuberculous infections of the urinary tract. In Campbell, M. F. (Ed.): Urology. 2nd ed. Philadelphia, W. B. Saunders Co., 1963, p. 399.

Clayman, R. V., Lange, P. H., and Fraley, E. E.: Cancer of the upper urinary tract. In Javadpour, N. (Ed.): Principles and Management of Urologic Cancer. Baltimore, The Williams & Wilkins Co., 1983.

Colston, J. A. C.: Complete nephroureterectomy: a new method employing the principle of electrocoagulation of the intramural portion of the ureter. J. Urol., 33:110, 1935.

Cummings, K. B.: Nephroureterectomy: rationale in the management of transitional cell carcinoma of the upper urinary tract. Urol. Clin. North Am., 7:569, 1980.

Cummings, K. B., Correa, R. J., Gibbons, R. P., et al.: Renal pelvic tumors. J. Urol., 113:158, 1975.

Deming, E. L., and Harvard, B. M.: Tumors of the kidney. In Campbell, M. F. and Harrison, J. H. (Eds.), Urology. 3rd ed., Philadelphia, W. B. Saunders Co., 1970, p. 930.

Dimmette, R. M., Sproat, J. F., and Sayegh, E. S.: The classification of carcinoma of the urinary bladder associated with schistosomiasis and metaplasia. J. Urol., 75:680, 1956.

Dodson, H. I.: Urological Surgery. St. Louis, C. V. Mosby Co., 1956, p. 308.

Droller, M. J.: Bladder cancer. Curr. Probl. Surg., 18:209, 1981.

El-Menzabani, M. M., El-Aaser, A. A., and Zakbary, N. I.: A study on the aetiological factors of bilharzial bladder cancer in Egypt. A. Nitrosamines and their precursors. Eur. J. Cancer, 15:287, 1979.

Firstater, M.: Tumors of the ureter. J. Urol. Nephrol., 71:893, 1965.

Foord, A. G., and Ferrier, P. A.: Primary carcinoma of the ureter, with report of seven cases. JAMA, 112:596, 1939.

Fraley, E. C.: Cancer of the renal pelvis. In Skinner, E. G., and deKernion, J. B. (Eds.): Genitourinary Cancer. Philadelphia, W. B. Saunders Co., 1978, p. 134.

Gatewood, O. M. B., Goldman, S. M., Marshall, F. F., and Siegelman, S. S.: Computerized tomography in the diagnosis of transitional cell carcinoma of the kidney. J. Urol., 127:876, 1982.

Gittes, R. F.: Tumors of the ureter and renal pelvis. In Harrison, J. H., Gittes, R. F., Perlmutter, A., Stamey, T. A., and Walsh, P. C. (Eds.): Campbell's Urology. 4th ed. Philadelphia, W. B. Saunders Co., 1979, p. 1010.

Goakeer, H. A., and DeRuiter, H. J.: Carcinoma of the renal pelvis following the abuse of phenacetin-containing analgesic drugs. Br. J. Urol., 51:188, 1979.

Grabstald, H., Whitmore, W. F., Jr., and Melamed, M.: Renal pelvic tumors. JAMA, 218:845, 1971.

Grace, D. A., Taylor, W. N., Taylor, J. N., and Winter, C. C.: Carcinoma of the renal pelvis—a 15 year review. J. Urol., 98:566, 1968.

Gruber, M. B., Becker, S. N., Warren, N. M., et al.: Specific red cell adherence test applied to tumors of ureter and renal pelvis. Urology, 19:361, 1982.

Hall, L., Faddoul, A., Saberi, A., et al.: The use of the red cell surface antigen to predict the malignant potential of transitional cell carcinoma of the ureter and renal pelvis. J. Urol., 127:23, 1982.

Hawtrey, C. E.: Fifty-two cases of primary ureteral carcinoma: a clinical-pathologic study. J. Urol., 105:188, 1971.

Heney, N. M., Nocks, B., Daly, J., et al.: Prognostic factors in carcinoma of the ureter. J. Urol., 125:632, 1981.

Higgins, C. C.:Tumors of the renal pelvis: a review of 47 cases. Ann. Surg., 137:95, 1953.

Hoybye, G., and Nielsen, O. E.: Renal pelvis carcinoma in phenacetin abusers. Scand. J. Urol. Nephrol., 5:190, 1971.

Hultengren, N., Lagergren, C., and Ljungqvist, A.: Carcinoma of the renal pelvis in renal papillary necrosis. Acta Chir. Scand., 130:314, 1965.

Johansson, S., and Wahlqvist, L.: a prognostic study of urothelial renal pelvis tumors. Cancer, 43:2525, 1979.

Johansson, S., Angervall, L., Bengtsson, U., et al.: A clinicopathologic study of epithelial tumors of the renal pelvis. Cancer, 37:1376, 1976.

Kakizoe, T., Fujita, J., Murase, T., et al.: Transitional cell carcinoma of the bladder in patients with renal pelvic and ureteral cancer. J. Urol., 124:17, 1980.

Kakizoe, T., Fujita, J., Tatsuro, M., et al.: Transitional cell carcinoma of the bladder in patients with renal pelvic and ureteral cancer. J. Urol., 125:25, 1981.

Kimball, F. N., and Ferris, H. W.: Papillomatous tumor of the renal pelvis associated with similar tumors of the ureter and bladder. J. Urol., 31:257, 1934.

Kinder, C. H., and Wallace, D. M.: Recurrent carcinoma of the ureteric stump. Br. J. Surg., 50:202, 1962.

Kirwin, T. J.: Papillary carcinoma of the renal pelvis. Surg. Gynecol. Obstet., 73:759, 1941.

Kretkowski, R. C., and Derrick, F. C., Jr.: Primary ureteral tumors. Reconsideration of management. Urology, 1:36, 1973.

Leistenschneider, W., and Nagel, R.: Lavage cytology of the renal pelvis and ureter with special reference to tumors. J. Urol., 124:597, 1980.

Lucke, B., and Schlumberger, H. G.: Tumors of the kidney, renal pelvis, and ureter. In Atlas of Tumor Pathology. Washington, D.C., Armed Forces Institute of Pathology, Section 8, 1957.

Mahadevia, P. S., Karwa, G. L., and Koss, L. G.: Mapping of urothelium in carcinomas of the renal pelvis and ureter: a report of nine cases. Cancer, 51:890, 1983.

Mahoney, J. F., Storey, B. G., Ibanez, R. C., et al.: Analgesic abuse, renal parenchymal disease and carcinoma of the kidney or ureter. Aust. N. Z. J. Med., 7:463, 1977.

Mazeman, E.: Tumours of the upper urinary tract calyces, renal pelvis, and ureter. Eur. Urol., 2:120, 1976.

McCarron, J. P., Jr., Chasko, S. B., and Gray, G. F., Jr., Systematic mapping of nephroureterectomy specimens removed for urothelial cancer. Pathological findings and clinical correlations. J. Urol., 128:243, 1982.

McCarron, J. P., Mullis, C., and Vaughn, E. D., Jr.: Tumors of the renal pelvis and ureter: current concepts and management. Semin. Urol., 1:75, 1983.

McLaughlin, J.: Etiology of cancer of the renal pelvis. In press.

Mills, C., and Vaughn, E. D.: Carcinoma of the ureter:

Natural history, management, and 5-year survival. J. Urol., *129*:275, 1983.

Montie, J. E.: Preservative surgery for carcinoma of the upper urinary tract. Bale, T. B. (Ed.): AUA Update Series. Vol. 1, p. 5, 1981.

Morrison, A. S., and Cole, P.: Urinary tract. *In* Schottenfeld, D., and Fraumeni, J. F., Jr. (Eds.): Cancer Epidemiology and Prevention. Philadelphia, W. B. Saunders Co., 1982, p. 925.

Nocks, B., Heney, N. M., Daly, J., et al.: Transitional cell carcinoma of renal pelvis. Urology, *19*:479, 1982.

Petkovic, S. D.: A plea for conservative operation for ureteral tumors. J. Urol., *107*:220, 1972.

Petkovic, S., Mutavdzic, M., Petronic, V., et al.: Tumors of the renal pelvis and ureter: clinical and etiologic studies. J. Urol., *44*:1, 1972.

Petkovic, S., Mutavdzic, M., Petronic, V. L., and Markovic, V.: Tumors of the renal pelvis and ureter: clinical and etiologic studies. J. Urol. Nephrol. (Paris), *77*:429, 1971.

Rathert, P., Melchior, H., and Lutzeyer, W.: Phenacetin: a carcinogen for the urinary tract? J. Urol., *113*:653, 1975.

Richie, J. P.: Management of ureteral tumors. *In* Skinner, D. G., and deKernion, J. P. (Eds.): Genitourinary Cancer. Philadelphia, W. B. Saunders Co., 1978, p. 150.

Say, C. C., and Hori, J. M.: Transitional cell carcinoma of the renal pelvis. J. Urol., *112*:438, 1974.

Scott, W. W., and McDonald, D. F.: Tumors of the ureter. *In* Campbell, M. F., and Harrison, J. H. (Eds.): Urology. 3rd ed. Philadelphia, W. B. Saunders Co., 1970, p. 978.

Sinner, W.: Die Karzinominnpfmetastase am Uretesstumpf nach Nephrectomie eines solides Nierenkarzinoms. J. Urol., *52*:673, 1959.

Strong, D. W., and Pearse, H. D.: Recurrent urothelial tumors following surgery for transitional cell carcinoma of the upper urinary tract. Cancer, *38*:2173, 1976.

Taylor, J. S.: Carcinoma of the urinary tract and analgesic abuse. Med. J. Aust., *1*:407, 1972.

Tomera, K. M., Leary, F. J., and Zincke, H.: Pyeloscopy in urothelial tumors. J. Urol., *127*:1088, 1982.

Vaught, J. B., and King, C. M.: Phenacetin studies, Science, *206*:637, 1979.

Wagle, D. G., Moore, R. H., and Murphy, G. P.: Primary carcinoma of the renal pelvis. Cancer, *33*:1642, 1974.

Wallace, M. A., Wallace, D. M., Whitfield, H. N., et al.: The late results of conservative surgery for upper tract urothelial carcinomas. Br. J. Urol., *53*:537, 1981.

Whitmore, W. F., Jr.: Management of invasive bladder neoplasms. Semin. Urol., *1*:34, 1983.

Williams, C. B., and Mitchell, J. P.: Carcinoma of the renal pelvis: a review of 43 cases. Br. J. Urol., *45*:370, 1973a.

Williams, C. B., and Mitchell, J. P.: Carcinoma of the ureter—a review of 54 cases. Br. J. Urol., *45*:377, 1973b.

Zincke, H., Aquilo, J., Farrow, G., et al.: Significance of urinary cytology in the early detection of transitional cell cancer of the upper urinary tract. J. Urol., *116*:781, 1976.

Zincke, H., and Neves, R. J.: Feasibility of conservative surgery for transitional cell cancer of the upper urinary tract. Urol. Clin. North Am., *11*:717, 1984.

CHAPTER 31

Benign and Malignant Tumors of the Male and Female Urethra

STANLEY C. HOPKINS, M.D.C.M., F.R.C.S.(C)
HARRY GRABSTALD, M.D.

Tumors of the Female Urethra

BENIGN URETHRAL LESIONS

Urethral Caruncle

The urethral caruncle is the most common benign tumor in the female urethra. These papillary excrescences have been mentioned in female subjects since the 16th century. Sharpe (1750) excised the first caruncle with total relief of symptoms.

These lesions are most frequently found in the postmenopausal period. They characteristically present as a reddened, tender, polypoid excrescence protruding from the inferior portion of the urethral meatus. Symptoms may be nonspecific. Dysuria, frequency, dyspareunia, hematuria, and a pressure sensation in the perineum are not infrequent clinical presentations (Grabstald, 1973). In some cases there may be no presenting symptoms (Novak and Woodruff, 1979).

On histologic examination, these excrescences are composed of a highly vascularized fibroplastic connective tissue stalk heavily infiltrated with leukocytes. Overlying is an epithelium that is either transitional or squamous cell in type. Three arbitrary forms of urethral caruncles are described as papillomatous, angiomatous, and granulomatous.

The papillomatous lesion is covered by varying amounts of transitional and stratified squamous epithelium. Occasionally, epithelium-lined crypts may appear as deep-seated nests of epithelial cells in cross section. These areas may be confused with carcinoma (Mostofi, 1979).

The angiomatous caruncle is more vascular, but overall is similar to the papillomatous type. The granulomatous caruncle lacks epithelial hyperplasia and is almost entirely composed of granulation tissue.

Symptomatic lesions are successfully managed by complete excision and light fulguration of the base. Caruncles that are not suspicious or symptomatic can be left untreated (Grabstald, 1973).

Cysts

Congenital periurethral cysts are rare. They may arise from vestigial remnants of the müllerian or mesonephric duct systems, or from the primitive urogenital sinus. An embryologic origin for these cysts can usually be identified by the histologic appearance of the lining epithelium unless there is gross distortion by infection (Das, 1981).

Acquired inclusion cysts of the urethral

1441

epithelium are common and usually small. These cysts frequently arise as a result of inflammatory occlusion of the urethral glands resulting from childbirth, chronic irritation, or surgical trauma. The cysts are often totally asymptomatic and discovered only upon routine pelvic examination. Occasionally, the patient may complain of perineal pain, dysuria, an obstructed stream, dyspareunia, a vaginal discharge, or a palpable mass (Das, 1981).

In the adult, spontaneous rupture is rare and may be complicated by abscess formation. Marsupialization of symptomatic uninfected cysts can provide satisfactory treatment. Total excision of the cyst wall is usually necessary (Das, 1981).

Fibrous Polyps

Fibrous polyps can arise in the folds of the female urethra. These polyps may be difficult to differentiate from a granulomatous caruncle (see earlier) (Novak and Woodruff, 1979). Local excision and light fulguration of the base is the treatment of choice.

Condylomata Acuminata

Condylomata acuminata have been known since ancient times. These papillary lesions characteristically occur on the moist mucocutaneous regions of the external genitalia. It is currently accepted that a member of the papova group of viruses is the underlying causative agent. In either sex, condylomata are most frequent in young adults 20 to 40 years of age, although lesions in children as young as 3 years have been seen (Powell, 1978).

Sexual contact appears to be the primary mode of spread, reflecting its predominance in the age population at risk for sexual promiscuity. Coitus at an earlier age and multiple sexual partners have contributed to the increasing incidence of this venereally transmitted disease (Powell, 1978).

In gross appearance, the condyloma is a gray, pale yellow or pinkish excrescence that may exist as a solitary lesion or form multiple disfiguring and enlarging masses. The cauliflower-like appearance is due to multiple branching epithelial processes. They are characterized histologically by relatively abundant epithelium covering a scanty amount of poorly vascularized tissue. Leukocyte infiltration of the stalk is heavy.

In females, condylomata are seldom found outside the genitoanal areas. These warts may be extensive, and spread into the anus and rectum is frequent. Growth into the female genital system, including the fourchette and lower vagina inside the hymenal ring, is also common. Involvement of the upper vagina and cervix is less frequent. Occasionally, these warts may involve the urethra and bladder (although rarely) as well (Petterson et al., 1976). Massive pelvic disease has resulted in ureteral and bowel obstruction and lower extremity edema.

In contrast to the common wart, condylomata acuminata may harbor a potential for malignant transformation. In the vulva, up to 16 per cent of squamous cell cancers may have preceding or coexisting condylomata acuminata. In addition, there have been the occasional reports of condylomata associated with the Buschke-Lowenstein tumor, a condyloma-like neoplasm arising in the vulva that may be distinguished from condylomata acuminata by its deep penetration of adjacent tissue (Powell, 1978).

Symptoms of urethral or bladder involvement may include a painful visible lesion at the meatus, urethral discharge, hematuria, pyuria, or persistent bladder and urethral irritation.

Transurethral resection and fulguration of the base is adequate for most lesions arising in the urethra or bladder (Petterson et al., 1976). Topical chemotherapeutic agents have gained in popularity over the past decade, and in the female, thiotepa and 5-fluorouracil have been employed with good result (Weimar et al., 1978; Powell, 1978). Recently, carbon dioxide laser therapy has been introduced as a method of treatment (Fuselier et al., 1980; Rosemberg et al., 1981).

Rarely, extensive intraurethral and intravesical condylomata may follow a malignant recurring course necessitating cystectomy (Kleiman and Lancaster, 1962; Lewis et al., 1962). Topical agents and autogenous vaccine (Ablin and Curtis, 1975) therapy should be kept in mind before radical excision is performed (Petterson et al., 1976).

CARCINOMA OF THE FEMALE URETHRA

Incidence

Carcinoma arising from the female urethra represents one of the few epithelial cancers that occur more frequently in women than in men. This group of pleomorphic neoplasms is uncommon; slightly more than 1200 cases are in the literature. Probably many more are unreported (McCrea, 1952; Ruch et al., 1952; Fagan and Hertig, 1955; Grabstald et al., 1966; Blath and Boehm, 1973; Bracken et al., 1976; Allen and Nelson, 1978; Elkon et al., 1980; Turner and Hendry, 1980; Hopkins et al., 1983).

The peak incidence occurs in the fifth and sixth decades. Tumors may arise at any age and have been found in children as young as 4 years and in women in the ninth decade (Roberts and Melicow, 1977; Ray and Guinan, 1979).

These neoplasms appear to be more common in Caucasians. Ray and Guinan (1979) reported 85 per cent occur in white, 12 per cent in black, and 4 per cent in Latin American–origin women. Others have suggested that the racial predilection is less distinct and that the reported white to non-white proponderance is more likely a reflection of the population referral base to individual reporting institutions (Hopkins et al., 1983).

Anatomy and Histology

The female urethra is less complex than its male counterpart. The various epithelial surfaces found along its length, however, reflect the multiple histologic characteristics of the neoplasms seen (Grabstald, 1973). The distal two thirds of the urethra is lined by stratified squamous epithelium that continues externally onto the vulva. The proximal third is lined by transitional epithelium, which merges internally with the bladder. Beneath the mucosa are submucosal connective tissue, elastic fibers, spongy venous sinuses, and the periurethral Skene's glands. These glands are usually concentrated in the perimeatal region but may extend along the entire urethral length. The glands and their ducts are lined by pseudostratified and stratified columnar epithelium. Deep to the submucosa lies the urethral smooth muscle that is continuous with the inner longitudinal muscle of the detrusor.

The lymphatics of the distal urethra along with those of the vulva drain into the superficial and deep inguinal lymph nodes. Those of the more proximal urethra drain into the pelvic chains, including the external iliac, internal iliac, and obturator lymph nodes (Hand, 1970).

Etiology

The causes for urethral carcinoma remain unknown. Urethral caruncles and fibrous pol-yps, which are known manifestations of chronic urethral irritation, can occur in association with urethral carcinoma (2–11 per cent) (Marshall et al., 1960; Allen and Nelson, 1978). It has been inferred that chronic urethral irritation from micturition, coitus, pregnancy, or recurrent infection may predispose some females to develop urethral carcinoma, although no direct causal relationship has been documented (Fagen and Hertig, 1955; Monaco et al., 1958; Marshall et al., 1960; Severino et al., 1977).

Histopathology

The vast majority of primary urethral carcinomas in the female are squamous cell (68 per cent), adenocarcinoma (18 per cent), transitional cell carcinoma (8 per cent), and melanoma (4 per cent) (Zeigerman and Gordon, 1970). Neoplasms associated with, or occurring within, a diverticulum have a different histologic distribution (see later). Unusual tumors arising from the urethra include mucoid carcinoma, cloacogenic carcinoma, and myoblastoma (Menville and Counsellor, 1935; Roberts and Melicow, 1977).

In assigning location of origin to these tumors, various similar terminologies have been applied. Grabstald et al. (1966) classified tumors limited to the distal third of the urethra as distal. When other than the anterior third was involved, the tumors were classified as posterior or entire. In that series, there was essentially an equal number of carcinomas arising either anteriorly or along the entire urethra (Fig. 31–1). Roberts and Melicow (1977) categorized site of origin into (three) zones according to predominance of occurrence. Again, approximately one half of tumors arose from the distal urethra or vulvourethral junction.

FEMALE URETHRA

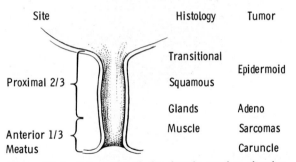

Figure 31–1. Schematic of the female urethra showing normal epithelial distribution and prevalent tumor types.

Diagnosis

HISTORY

The symptoms and signs of female urethral carcinoma are usually vague or nondiagnostic, and the time interval between onset of symptoms to diagnosis by the clinician is frequently long. This delay may range from days to greater than 5 years, with the average time to diagnosis being 5 to 6 months (Staubitz et al., 1955; Monaco et al., 1958; Grabstald et al., 1966). Urethral bleeding or spotting is the most common presenting symptom. Gross hematuria is rare (Bracken et al., 1976). Other symptoms may mimic benign disease. Urinary frequency (25 per cent), dysuria (30 per cent), urinary obstruction (39 per cent), and perineal pain (10 per cent) are relatively common. Urinary incontinence (4 per cent), vaginal discharge (5 per cent), and dyspareunia are less frequent (Johnson, 1982). Occasionally, a neoplasm has been discovered as an incidental finding during evaluation of a diverticulum or a caruncle, or for some other urologic problem.

PHYSICAL EXAMINATION

Examination of the female urethra should be included in the routine urologic physical examination. Tumors arising from the distal or mid-urethra can present as a papillary excrescence protruding from the meatus. Because they may be grossly similar, an early neoplasm can be mistaken for a urethral caruncle, although this is rare (Marshall et al., 1960). A collar-like ring of induration or a persistent ulceration or

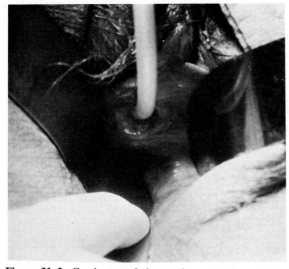

Figure 31–2. Carcinoma of the urethra extending to the anterior vaginal wall inferiorly. The induration extends superiorly to the pubic ramus.

erosion of the urethra is always suspect for carcinoma.

In the more advanced disease stage, a urethral neoplasm eroding into the vaginal vault may be difficult to distinguish from a primary vaginal carcinoma on the basis of physical examination alone (Fig. 31–2). Examination of the groin and lower limbs is necessary to evaluate regional lymph node status and for evidence of lymphatic or venous stasis, and edema.

LABORATORY STUDIES

Urinalysis may show the presence of red blood cells or leukocytes, and culture may yield greater than 10^5 colonies of one or more organisms. Urine cytologic examination may be positive, but usually is of academic interest owing to the advanced state of the majority of these neoplasms. Anemia and hypoalbuminemia can occur secondary to the effects of chronic infection. Urinary obstruction may also cause azotemia (Grabstald, 1973).

RADIOLOGY

Retrograde urethrography (RUG) may demonstrate a luminal filling defect, obstruction, urethral diverticulum, or urethrovaginal fistula, but is frequently nondiagnostic. Intravenous pyelogram (IVP) may be normal or show lateral deviation of the ureters in the presence of gross retroperitoneal lymphadenopathy. Lymphangiogram may detect gross pelvic lymph node metastases. Computerized axial tomography (CT) has recently shown promise for assessing pelvic node status. The inability of lymphangiography and CT scans to detect micrometastases and the potential for false positives (secondary to inflammation) and false negatives are well-known inherent weaknesses of these noninvasive techniques.

Anteroposterior and lateral chest films, whole lung tomography, and CT scan of the chest are usually negative, since distant metastases are infrequent, occurring in less than 10 per cent of the patients at presentation (Grabstald et al., 1966).

BIOPSY

Biopsy should be obtained from all suspicious urethral lesions. Tumors arising at the meatus or perimeatal region should be completely excised. Proximal urethral tumors can be biopsied transurethrally. Transvaginal biopsy may be necessary, but one would recommend this only to confirm or deny vaginal involvement (or origin) or when there is an obvious vaginal tumor.

The bladder, especially the neck area, must

be carefully evaluated in proper urethral tumor staging. Primary bladder cancer with urethral extension or vice versa must be documented.

CLINICAL STAGING

Grabstald (1966) has proposed a clinical staging system:

Stage 0 —In situ (limited to mucosa)
Stage A—Submucosal (not beyond submucosa)
Stage B—Muscular (infiltrating periurethral muscle)
Stage C—Periurethral
    1. Infiltrating muscular wall of vagina
    2. Infiltrating muscular wall of vagina with invasion of vaginal mucosa
    3. Infiltrating other adjacent structures such as bladder, labia, and clitoris
Stage D—Metastasis
    1. Inguinal lymph nodes
    2. Pelvic lymph nodes below bifurcation of aorta
    3. Lymph nodes above bifurcation of aorta
    4. Distant

This is based on the following:

1. Inspection, including careful examination of the urethra, labia, vagina, groin, and lower extremities;
2. Palpation, including bimanual examinations with the patient under anesthesia to evaluate the extent of induration and fixation and to attempt to determine pelvic and inguinal lymph node status;
3. Cystourethroscopy, including biopsy of the primary tumor and adjacent normal-appearing areas;
4. Additional biopsy of vagina, labia, and inguinal nodes as suggested by inspection, palpation, and cystourethroscopy.

This system has become accepted because of its simplicity and its practical application toward therapy.

DIFFERENTIAL DIAGNOSIS

The differential diagnosis of urethral carcinoma in the female includes urethral erosion, ulceration, periurethral abscess, traumatic urethral fistula, tuberculosis, condylomata acuminata, urethral prolapse, fibrous polyp, and urethral caruncle (Zeigerman and Gordon, 1970).

Treatment

The relative infrequency of these neoplasms has resulted in a lack of uniformity in treatment.

Many methods have been proposed. These have included transurethral resection or local excision, partial to total urethrectomy, external-beam radiation therapy, intracavitary radiation or brachytherapy, simple cystourethrectomy to anterior exenteration with or without inguinal lymph node dissection, and vulvectomy.

In general, tumor stage and location are more important in determining survival than is histopathologic character (Sullivan and Grabstald, 1978), although some authors have suggested that histologic type may also influence prognosis (Zeigerman and Gordon, 1970). As a rule, an anterior carcinoma has a generally better prognosis than the posterior or entire urethral tumor (Grabstald et al., 1966), although for either, size of the primary, resultant depth of invasion and, obviously, node status have significant prognostic importance (Bracken et al., 1976).

SURGERY: ANTERIOR URETHRAL CARCINOMA

Tumors arising from the distal third of the urethra and limited to the mucosa (Stage 0) or involving the submucosa (Stage A) have been successfully managed by a good transurethral resection (Sullivan and Grabstald, 1978). Neoplasms infiltrating the urethral muscularis (Stage B) or the small lesion infiltrating the periurethral tissue (Stage C) may be managed by partial urethrectomy if an adequate margin of normal tissue can be obtained. It has been suggested that partial or subtotal urethrectomy for these more infiltrating lesions may result in stress or total incontinence. This fear has not been justified (Grabstald, 1982).

The 5-year survival for patients with distal one-third tumors appropriately treated with good surgical therapy should be 90 per cent or better.

SURGERY: POSTERIOR OR ENTIRE URETHRAL CARCINOMA

Neoplasms arising from the posterior or involving the entire urethra have a more dismal prognosis. These tumors are almost always of higher stage, and greater than 50 per cent of patients have (pelvic) nodal involvement (Johnson, 1982). Examination of the abdominal contents and pelvic lymph nodes is mandatory prior to surgical removal, for gross involvement of iliac or obturator nodes precludes exenteration. For patients harboring a more localized tumor, the treatment of choice has been anterior exenteration and urinary diversion, although results have been poor. Accumulated 5-year survival ranges between 10 and 17 per cent, and local tumor recurrence is extremely high (66 to

100 per cent), accounting for much of the morbidity and mortality. Death may frequently result from sepsis, hemorrhage, or inanition in the absence of tumor dissemination (Grabstald et al., 1966; Zeigerman and Gordon, 1970; Desai et al., 1973; Chu, 1973).

Recently, an integrated approach using external-beam radiation (2000–5000 rads) followed by anterior exenteration and urinary diversion has been recommended (Bracken et al., 1976; Sullivan and Grabstald, 1978; Johnson, 1982). Other authors have proposed a triad approach using interstitial brachytherapy to the tumor (3000–4000 rads) with field external-beam radiation therapy (2000–3000 rads) prior to or following surgery (Hopkins et al., 1983). For patients whose tumor encroaches upon or involves the inferior pubic rami or the symphysis pubis, en bloc resection including the pubic rami plus pelvic musculature may be required (Klein et al., 1983). The morbidity of this procedure is such that it requires careful case selection.

TREATMENT OF INGUINAL LYMPH NODES

Inguinal lymphadenopathy in the female harboring a distal urethral neoplasm may range between 10 and 56 per cent (Riches and Cullen, 1951; Grabstald et al., 1966; Desai et al., 1973). Grabstald and others noted inguinal lymph node involvement in 60 to 88 per cent of patients with clinically palpable groin nodes (Grabstald, 1973; Desai et al., 1973) and recommended that bilateral groin dissection should be restricted to the patient with clinically abnormal inguinal nodes at presentation, or if delayed adenopathy follows surgery. Excisional biopsy of suspicious nodes is mandatory. Prophylactic lymphadenectomy has not been proved to be better than therapeutic node dissection in carefully followed patients, and has generally been discouraged (Levine, 1980; Johnson, 1982).

RADIATION THERAPY

Orthovoltage external-beam and radium intracavitary radiation were used to treat urethral neoplasms early in this century (Grabstald et al., 1966). Results were discouraging. Local failure approached 100 per cent and severe complications, including urethral stenosis, vaginal stenosis, tumor necrosis, urethrovaginal fistulae, and sepsis, were common.

With the newer techniques of megavoltage radiation and with refinement of interstitial therapy using radium, radon, gold, or iridium, results of therapy (for distal one-third urethral tumors) may be comparable to those of surgery (Delclos, 1982; Prempree et al., 1984). Antoniades (1969) suggested the combination of sur-

gery and interstitial radium therapy (5500–6000 rads) for distal neoplasms and the use of brachytherapy for residual disease following inadequate surgery. Taggart et al. (1972) cured seven of 11 females treated by interstitial brachytherapy alone. Elkon et al. (1980) recently reported cure of five patients treated with radium brachytherapy either for the primary tumor or for local recurrence.

Delclos (1982) has proposed interstitial therapy to be the treatment of choice for small, well-differentiated lesions confined to the distal urethra, and suggested that it could be used in combination with surgery for tumors of larger volume. Iridium[192] using the after-loading technique has improved the radiation distribution and has decreased the morbidity (Prempree et al., 1984) (Fig. 31–3).

CHEMOTHERAPY

Chemotherapy for palliation or as an adjunct to surgery or radiation has not been explored to any significant degree to warrant conclusion (Skolnick et al., 1977). The affinity of various chemotherapeutic agents for other epithelioid carcinomas suggests that these tumors may be potentially responsive as well. (See chemotherapy, carcinoma of the male urethra.)

CARCINOMA ARISING IN A DIVERTICULUM OF THE FEMALE URETHRA

Urethral diverticula are not uncommon. In autopsy series the incidence ranges between 0.6 and 1.9 per cent, with the majority seen in blacks (Peters and Vaughan, 1965; Davis and Robinson, 1970). Most authors suggest an acquired etiologic factor for these (Peters and Vaughan, 1965; Tines et al., 1982). Recurrent infection or trauma to the paired paraurethral Bartholin glands (and ducts) with subsequent destruction and abscess formation may lead to rupture into the urethra with subsequent diverticulum formation. Others believe that *some* diverticula arise secondary to a congenital anomaly, i.e., from ectopic cloacal epithelium in the urethra or secondary to wolffian or müllerian duct remnants (Torres and Quattlebaum, 1972; Cea et al., 1977).

Carcinoma arising within a urethral diverticulum is extremely rare. The first case was documented in 1951, and to date there are 40 reports in the literature (Hamilton and Leach, 1951; Evans et al., 1981; Tesluk, 1981; Tines et al., 1982; Srinivas and Dow, 1983).

The distribution of tumor histologic type

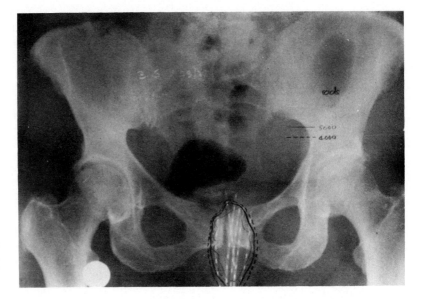

Figure 31–3. Anteroposterior view of pelvis showing iridium-192 implants with calculated dosimetry prior to surgery.

differs from that arising from the remainder of the urethra. This may reflect the paraurethral gland or ductal origin of these tumors. Adenocarcinoma is the most common type, occurring in 49 per cent of patients; transitional cell carcinoma occurs in 31 per cent, and squamous or epidermoid carcinoma is least frequent (18 per cent) (Tines et al., 1982).

Some advanced cases of urethral carcinoma may originate in a diverticulum, only to destroy the surrounding urethral architecture as they invade locally, such that their true origin is missed. This may be particularly true for adenocarcinoma (which is most frequent in the proximal urethra) and which may show histologic features of mesonephric duct origin (Graf et al., 1962; Cea et al., 1977; Tines et al., 1982).

The presenting complaints are not unlike those of carcinoma elsewhere in the urethra. Irritative urinary symptoms are common. Urethral discharge, recurrent urinary infections, spotting, or gross hematuria can occur in up to 80 per cent of patients. Obstructive voiding symptoms, stress urinary incontinence, or dysuria may also be presenting complaints. Symptoms can be present from a few weeks to several years. In general, most patients seek physician attention within 6 months (Tines et al., 1982).

Carcinoma within a diverticulum is suspected when an indurated suburethral mass is palpated in the anterior vaginal wall. Physical examination should include bimanual examination under anesthesia and palpation of the inguinal lymph nodes. Cystoscopic visualization of the tumor and biopsy confirm the diagnosis, and aid in defining the limits of the tumor within

the urethra. An intravenous pyelogram, chest film, and occasionally small and large bowel roentgenographic studies should be included in the investigation to determine site of tumor origin. Urethrography with double balloon catheter has also been utilized to evaluate the diverticulum and the tumor. As in other carcinomas of the urethra, sonography, CT scanning, and pedal lymphangiography may provide additional information regarding pelvic extension and regional nodal involvement (Dretler et al., 1972; Tines et al., 1982).

Excision of the diverticulum may be appropriate therapy for a small neoplasm; recurrences, however, are not infrequent (Evans et al., 1981). Local excision has also been combined with pre- or postoperative radiation or interstitial brachytherapy (Tines et al., 1982). For more extensive lesions, or for recurrent tumor, anterior exenteration following external-beam radiation is the treatment of choice (Reheis et al., 1981; Patanaphan et al., 1983).

OTHER URETHRAL MALIGNANCIES

Melanoma

Forty-five cases of primary melanoma arising in the female urethra have been accumulated in the literature (Katz and Grabstald, 1976; Ariel, 1981; Godec et al., 1981). Undoubtedly, many go unreported. Although melanoma is one of the rarer tumors of the female urethra (3–4 per cent), this location is the most common site of origin in the genitourinary tract. As is seen with other epithelial urethral neoplasms, the peak incidence occurs in the fifth and sixth decades of life. These lesions arise from the distal third of the urethra and frequently protrude through the meatus (Fig. 31–4). Presenting symptoms include dysuria, frequency, terminal hematuria, or the presence of a mass; some patients may be asymptomatic (Katz and Grabstald, 1976). There is one case of a melanoma developing on a caruncle (Rabon, 1964).

The prognosis is poor; diagnosis is usually late, recurrence is early, and widespread metastases are frequent. Five long-term survivors have been reported. Three underwent anterior exenteration; one patient was treated by local excision and bilateral lymphadenectomy, and the last had no therapy (DasGupta and Grabstald, 1965; Block and Hotchkiss, 1971; Katz and Grabstald, 1976).

Although it has been pointed out that these

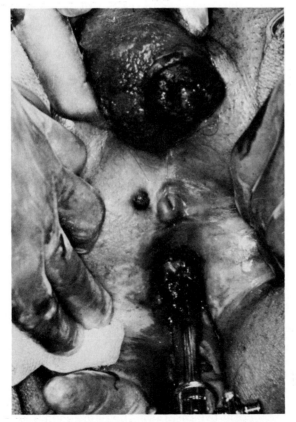

Figure 31–4. Melanoma of the female urethra.

tumors are relatively radioresistant, preoperative radiation therapy may be useful as a sterilization procedure to prevent viable tumor spill at the time of operation (Katz and Grabstald, 1976).

Melanomas may also metastasize to the urethra. Despite aggressive management, including anterior exenteration and bilateral inguinal lymphadenectomy, prognosis remains extremely unfavorable (DasGupta and Grabstald, 1965).

Mesenchymal Tumors

Of all mesenchymal tumors arising from the female urethra, the leiomyoma is the most common (16 cases) (Mooppan et al., 1979; Lake et al., 1981; Merrell and Brown, 1981). The peak incidence is in the third decade. Presenting symptoms commonly include a urethral mass, dypareunia, or urinary tract infection. These lesions arise from the circular fibers of the smooth muscle, which extend throughout the urethra and continue into the bladder. They can appear at any site in the urethra, but have a predilection for the proximal portion.

Simple surgical excision is the treatment of choice. Malignant transformation has not been reported, although there has been one instance of local recurrence (Mooppan et al., 1979).

Lipomas, lymphangiomas, and hemangioblastomas of the urethra are the subject of case reports (Das, 1981).

Malignant tumors of the urethral mesenchyme are extremely rare. Fibrosarcoma, leiomyosarcoma, myxosarcoma, spindle cell, round cell, or undesignated sarcomas have been described (McCrea, 1952; Roberts and Melicow 1977).

Secondary Malignant Tumors

Carcinoma of the bladder, vulva, vaginal cervix, and bowel may invade the urethra by direct extension. Metastases secondary to fundal and ovarian carcinoma are occasionally recognized in the suburethral area (Novak and Woodruff, 1979). Lymphoma choriocarcinoma and carcinoma of the lung involving the urethra have also been described (Roberts and Melicow, 1977; Novak and Woodruff, 1979).

Tumors of the Male Urethra

BENIGN URETHRAL LESIONS

Cysts

Congenital cysts of the urethra occur around the meatus and are rare. These parameatal cysts may develop as a result of obstruction of the urethral ducts (Shiraki, 1975). Retention cysts are best treated by excision. Recurrence is uncommon.

Angiomata

Small angiomatous lesions can frequently involve the urethral meatus. Usually, they are of no clinical significance. On rare occasions, if extensive hemangiomas develop in the urethra, surgical excision or grafting may be required (Begley, 1960; Manuel et al., 1977; Roberts and Devine, 1983).

Urethral Polyps

Urethral polyps are relatively unusual lesions but have been reported more frequently recently (Gunther et al., 1979; Kearney et al., 1979; Kimche and Lask, 1982). The polyps are usually located in the posterior urethra, arising from the floor in the region of the verumontanum (DeWolf and Fraley, 1973). Very occasionally they may be found in the anterior urethra (Foster et al., 1980). These lesions are usually discovered in the young child, but may occur in the adult or in the neonate (Nellans and Stein, 1975; Rao et al., 1981). Symptoms include urinary obstruction, infection, hematuria, or enuresis.

On histologic examination, they consist of a stalk composed of connective tissue, vessels, and smooth muscle, covered by transitional cell urothelium.

Surgical removal is the treatment of choice. Transurethral resection may be performed in older children and in adults. Both suprapubic excision and transurethral resection have been used in children (DeWolf and Fraley, 1973). Recurrences are rare after complete excision.

Benign Meatal, Parameatal, and Perimeatal Papillary Urethral Tumors

Papillary meatal excrescences include transitional cell papillomas, squamous papillomas, inflammatory polyps, and condylomata acuminata (Huvos and Grabstald, 1973). These are usually localized to the perimeatal area and fossa navicularis but occasionally may involve the entire urethra.

The peak occurrence for all these lesions is in the second to fourth decades. On gross appearance the lesions are quite similar. On histologic examination they are also similar, being composed of a proliferation of stratified squamous mucosa with papillomatosis and hyperkeratosis.

The transitional cell papilloma has a less abundant epithelium and a better defined and more highly vascularized connective tissue stalk than does the condyloma acuminatum. Leukocyte infiltration of the stalk is also substantially less. These transitional cell papillomas are seen more frequently in the older patient, and on occasion may be associated with papillomas of the proximal urethra and bladder.

Squamous metaplasia of the epithelial covering of these papillary excrescences has resulted in the descriptive term "squamous papilloma" or "inflammatory polyp." These may be histologically indistinguishable from the papillary excrescences at the meatus of the female urethra, and have been described as the male equivalent of the female caruncle (Huvos and Grabstald, 1973).

Symptoms are usually nonspecific and may include hematuria, urethral irritation, itching, or discharge. Most excrescences are visible upon eversion of the urethral meatus (Fig. 31–5). Local excision with light fulguration of the base (occasionally requiring adjunctive meatotomy) is usually adequate treatment. Intraurethral instillation of chemotherapeutic agents has occasionally been tried for more extensive urethral involvement (see later) (Huvos and Grabstald, 1973).

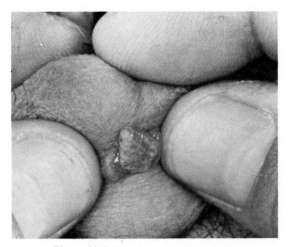

Figure 31–5. Urethral meatal papilloma.

Intraurethral Condylomata Acuminata

Condylomata acuminata are papillary excrescences occurring characteristically on the moist mucocutaneous regions of the external genitalia and are purportedly caused by a papova virus (Powell, 1978). The peak incidence and age distribution for both sexes have been described. (See female urethra, condylomata acuminata.)

In the male, the incidence of genital condylomata spreading to the urethra ranges between 0.5 and 5 per cent (Wein and Benson, 1977). Eighty per cent will be within 3 cm of the urethral meatus (Debenedictis et al., 1977). Anterior intraurethral lesions have been described in the absence of penile involvement; however, involvement of the proximal urethra without prior or concurrent involvement of the anterior urethra is rare. This warrants a high index of suspicion for concomitant urethral carcinoma (Morrow et al., 1952).

The gross and histologic characteristics of these papillary excrescences have also been described previously.

Symptoms of parameatal involvement may include a visible lesion at the meatus, urethral discharge, hematuria, or urethral irritation. On physical examination, everting the meatus will often disclose their presence. Pyuria, hematuria, or persistent urethral irritation may suggest more proximal intraurethral involvement.

The single, small, parameatal lesion can be controlled by excision and light fulguration of its base. This is best performed prior to investigative endoscopy to prevent the possibility of proximal intraurethral seeding (Dretler and Klein, 1975).

Many methods are available to treat more extensive intraurethral condylomata. Endoscopic excision with light fulguration of the base has been the most widely utilized; however, repeated fulguration has led to scarring and eventual stricture formation. Podophyllin (Kaplan, 1942), colchicine (a podophyllin-like drug), and chloropactin (oxychlorosene) have been employed to treat intraurethral condylomata as well (Scott and Stell, 1961; Gigax and Robinson, 1971). These agents cause severe irritation to normal skin, particularly to the urethral mucosa, and their use should be discouraged. Intraurethral administration of thiotepa is also generally unsuccessful (Halverstadt and Parry, 1969). Bacille Calmette-Guerin (BCG) or the administration of autogenous vaccine has been suggested in order to assist host immunodefense mechanisms against recurrent condyloma formation (Ablin and Curtis, 1975).

5-Fluorouracil (Efudex) cream or suppositories may be used to eradicate intraurethral condylomata alone or as an adjunct to surgery (Dretler and Kline, 1975; Bringel and de Andrade Arruda, 1981). This agent may carry the advantage of selectively destroying condyloma without injuring normal mucosa. Early recurrence, however, is not infrequent (Danoff et al., 1981). Radiation has also been used (with success), but this leads to extensive stricture formation (Morrow et al., 1952; Danoff et al., 1981).

Recently, laser energy has been proclaimed as a safe and effective method to eradicate urethral condylomata (Fuselier et al., 1980; Rosemberg et al., 1981). The benefits of laser therapy over conventional cauterization are that the extent and depth of the cauterized tissue can be regulated with great accuracy and that damage to the surrounding tissue is minimized. Bleeding and pain are limited by photocoagulation of superficial vessels and nerves, and healing is rapid with minimal fibrosis. Recurrence with this technique is approximately 13 per cent. This is comparable to other methods (Rosemberg et al., 1982).

Intravesical extension of urethral condylomata is infrequent. Rarely, the disease may carpet the bladder and become life-threatening secondary to ureteral obstruction or sepsis. On occasion, it may be difficult to distinguish extensive intravesical condylomata from squamous cell carcinoma of the bladder.

The uncomplicated small bladder or proximal urethral lesions are usually best treated by transurethral resection or intraurethral chemotherapy or both (Petterson et al., 1976). Extremely rarely, cystoprostatectomy, urethrectomy, and urinary diversion have been required for extensive, recurrent condylomata involving the entire urethra and bladder (Bissada et al., 1974).

Nephrogenic Adenoma

The nephrogenic adenoma is a rare urothelial lesion seen in the bladders of male patients. Forty-four cases have been accumulated in the literature. Infrequently, these lesions may involve or present primarily in the prostatic urethra. On histologic examination, they are composed of epithelial tubules in the lamina propria that are lined by a single layer of columnar cells and resemble portions of the renal nephron (Berger et al., 1981).

Their cause is unknown. Most authors consider them to be a metaplastic response to injury, since they frequently arise in association with trauma or a history of chronic infection (Berger et al., 1981; Bhagavan et al., 1981). On cystoscopic examination, these lesions can be confused with carcinoma in situ or papillary transitional cell carcinoma.

Transurethral excision is required for diagnostic and therapeutic purposes. Their malignant potential is not known (Bhagavan et al., 1981).

CARCINOMA OF THE MALE URETHRA

Incidence

Malignant tumors arising from the male urethra are rare. Since the first case cited by Thiaudierre in 1834, approximately 600 cases have been accumulated. Again, most go unreported (Kreutzmann and Colloff, 1939; Lower and Hausfeld, 1947; Hotchkiss and Amelar, 1952; Dean, 1956; Howe et al., 1963; King, 1964; Mandler and Pool, 1966; Grabstald et al., 1966; Kaplan et al., 1967; Guinn and Ayala, 1970; Mullin et al., 1974; Melicow and Roberts, 1978; Bracken et al., 1980). In spite of the greater length and complexity of the male urethra (Fig. 31–6), and the predisposition of other genitourinary tumors to occur more frequently in males, urethral carcinoma is two to four times more prevalent in the female (Grabstald, 1973).

No one institution has accumulated or

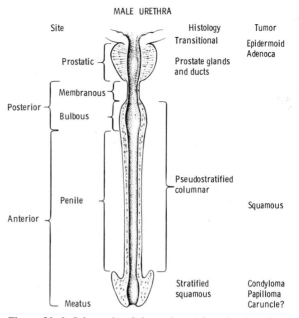

Figure 31–6. Schematic of the male urethra showing pleomorphism of the normal epithelium as well as the prevalent tumor types.

treated a sufficient number of patients to outline a definitive plan of treatment. Information concerning diagnosis, treatment, and survival, therefore, comes from the cumulative analysis of small series and case reports. Patients harboring a primary neoplasm of the urethra most frequently present in the late fifth or early sixth decade of life; there is no apparent racial predisposition.

Anatomy and Histology

The average male urethra is 21 cm in length and is divided into prostatic, membranous, bulbar, and penile or pendulous portions. The term "posterior" urethra usually refers to the prostatic and bulbomembranous portions, whereas the "anterior" urethra refers to those portions distal to the mid-bulb (Fig. 31–6).

On histologic examination, this conduit is seen to be composed of a mucous membrane supported by a connective tissue and vascular stroma. These structures are enclosed by the vascular corpus spongiosum. As the urethral mucosa progresses from the level of the bladder neck to the external meatus, it alters its histologic characteristics. Transitional cells line the prostatic and membranous portions of the urethra, whereas stratified or pseudostratified columnar epithelium lines the bulbar and pendulous portions. The fossa navicularis and meatus are covered by stratified squamous epithelium.

In the submucosa of the anterior urethra are numerous glands of Littre whose ducts communicate with the urethral lumen. Posteriorly, paired Cowper's glands lie inferolateral to the urethra as it passes within the urogenital diaphragm. The ducts of these glands communicate anteriorly with the bulb. As in the female urethra, the varied histopathologic characteristics of the neoplasms that arise here generally reflect this epithelioglandular distribution.

The lymphatic drainage of the urethra has been well documented (Hand, 1970). The penile urethra is drained by the lymphatics accompanying those of the glans penis. These empty into a plexus distal to the symphysis pubis, which flows directly into the deep inguinal and external iliac lymphatic chains. The bulbar, membranous, and prostatic urethra drain into three lymphatic channels. One extends along the dorsal vein of the penis beneath the infrapubic ligament through to the external iliac nodes; another along the pudendal artery to the obturator and internal iliac nodes; and the third to the presacral lymphatic chain. A urethral neoplasm arising distally may spread regionally to involve the inguinal lymph nodes first, while a proximal lesion drains directly into the pelvis. Crossover of lymphatic involvement is not infrequent and is dependent upon location and extent of the tumor and whether the neoplasm has obstructed the primary (regional) lymphatic channels.

Histopathology

Approximately 50 to 75 per cent of these neoplasms originate in the bulbar or bulbomembranous portions. The majority of the rest arise from the anterior urethra, and most are located at the meatus of the fossa navicularis (Grabstald, 1973; Ray et al., 1977).

The most common histologic types are squamous cell carcinoma (78 per cent) followed by transitional cell carcinoma (15 per cent). Adenocarcinoma of the urethra is much less common (4 per cent) and arises primarily in the bulbomembranous portion.

Occasionally, a urethral neoplasm may exhibit more than one histologic feature, and infrequently may be undifferentiated (less than 1 per cent) (Sullivan and Grabstald, 1978).

Primary melanoma is rare (2–3 per cent). The most common site of origin for these pigmented lesions is the meatus or navicular fossa.

Transitional cell carcinoma arising from the prostatic ducts will be discussed separately.

Etiology

The frequent history or associated finding of urethral inflammation, urinary infection, or trauma in patients presenting with carcinoma of the urethra has been considered by many investigators to contribute to the neoplastic process. The prevalence of stricture disease and neoplasms both occurring most frequently in the bulb and bulbomembranous portions of the urethra suggests chronic irritation to be the major predisposing factor. In a classic review of 232 patients (Kaplan et al., 1967), a history of venereal disease, stricture, or significant trauma was noted in 79 per cent of patients. Not all series have confirmed this high incidence of associated or predisposing inflammation. Mandler and Pool (1966) have argued that the original diagnosis of stricture may be erroneous and that the symptoms possibly represent early unrecognized carcinoma.

Other factors may also be operative in the development of a urethral neoplasm. Exogenous or endogenous carcinogens that initiate urothelial neoplasms elsewhere could conceivably be considered factors responsible for primary urethral neoplasms as well. In this case, a neoplasm in the upper tracts or in the bladder could, but would not necessarily, be an associated finding (see later).

There are several reports in the literature regarding the development of a urethral carcinoma after urethroplasty for stricture disease. In these cases, the successful management of the stricture did not prevent the later development of de novo neoplasm, suggesting that those factors responsible for the stricture were also later responsible for tumor induction (Colapinto and Evans, 1977; Williams and Ashken, 1980).

Natural History

In the male, carcinoma of the urethra is initially a locally destructive lesion. In the proximal urethra, the neoplasm may invade the urogenital diaphragm, rectum, prostate, and bladder neck by direct invasion or by surface extension. These neoplasms may also progress centrifugally with invasion of the corporal bodies and the perineum (Fig. 31–7). Scrotal thickening, fibrosis, and induration can be secondary to reaction from urinary extravasation; how-

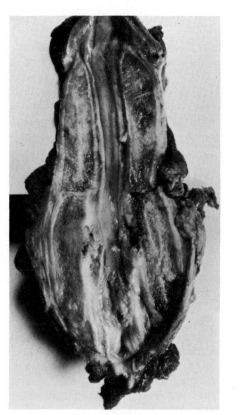

Figure 31–7. Urethral carcinoma invading the corporal bodies.

crease in the size and caliber of the stream, straining to urinate, dysuria, hematuria, urethral discharge, or occasionally a superimposed urinary tract infection. In one series, obstructive symptoms were noted in 47 per cent of patients, perineal mass in 39 per cent, periurethral abscess in 31 per cent, perineal fistula in 20 per cent, hematuria or urethral discharge in 22 per cent, and urinary retention in 10 per cent (Kaplan et al., 1967).

Large anterior lesions will characteristically present with a ventral periurethral mass or fistula, whereas a perineal mass, either fluctuant or solid, is more characteristic of a large bulbar or bulbomembranous neoplasm. Less common findings may include penile erosion, painful erections or priapism secondary to corporal body infiltration, and inguinal masses or necrosis secondary to regional lymph node metastases. Sexual impotence has also been reported (Raghavaiah, 1978).

Chronic suppuration may produce systemic symptoms such as anorexia, malaise, weight loss, or inanition. Uremia may develop as a result of chronic outlet obstruction.

The time interval between onset of symptoms to diagnosis of carcinoma is often long, ever, these signs most frequently signify invasion of the scrotum by the tumor (Fig. 31–8). Infiltration of the testis and the spermatic cord is rare (Kreutzmann and Colloff, 1939).

Metastases spread primarily to the regional inguinal or pelvic lymph node chains, depending on the site of tumor origin. The lymphatic drainage of the urethra has been described (Hand, 1970).

Clinically detectable distant metastases are rare at initial presentation (Ray et al., 1977; Riches and Cullen, 1951; Hopkins et al., 1984). Death is usually rapid and frequently results from local complications of the tumor, e.g., chronic infection, sepsis, inanition, or hemorrhage. At autopsy, distant metastases may be seen in about one third of patients.

Diagnosis

HISTORY

The most common symptoms for the patient harboring a urethral carcinoma relate to urinary obstruction or to incontinence secondary to overflow. Frequent complaints include a de-

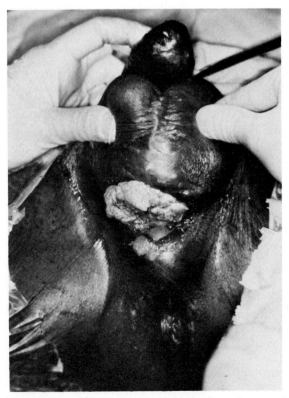

Figure 31–8. Urethral carcinoma invading the perineum and scrotum.

ranging from 2 to 33 months. As occurs in penile carcinoma, delay in presentation and recognition most frequently reflects failure of the patient to seek medical attention. Delay in recognition of an early neoplasm may also be physician-related, occurring only after a "stricture" has failed to respond to apparently adequate conservative therapy, or after local destructive changes such as urethral fistulization or development of a periurethral phlegmon have occurred. Profuse bleeding after gentle urethral dilatation may be characteristic of early carcinoma. Suspicion of urethral carcinoma in the patient harboring a stricture along with early endoscopic visualization of the urethra will reduce this chance of misdiagnosis.

PHYSICAL EXAMINATION

A careful physical examination follows the history in the patient suspected of harboring a urethral neoplasm. Examination of the penis is carried out in a systematic manner beginning distally and extending to the urogenital diaphragm. Palpation of the corpus spongiosum and corpora cavernosa for induration, presence of a mass, or both provides a rough estimate of the extent of periurethral invasion. The scrotum is invaginated to palpate the deep anterior urethra. Palpation of both inguinal areas identifies regional adenopathy.

LABORATORY STUDIES

Normochromic normocytic anemia and hypoalbuminemia can result from chronic infection. Outlet obstruction may cause azotemia. In several instances, hypercalcemia has been reported in the absence of osseous metastases. This has been attributed to the ectopic production of parathyroid hormone (PTH) by these tumors (Grabstald, 1973; Metcalfe et al., 1978; Saito, 1981).

RADIOLOGY

Retrograde urethrography may be helpful in both diagnosis and staging, although the presence of a luminal filling defect, obstruction, extravasation, or a fistulous tract is itself a nondiagnostic feature. Intravenous pyelography (IVP) may show lateral displacement of the ureters if retroperineal adenopathy is present. Bipedal lymphangiography may detect the presence of pelvic lymph node metastases, although the obturator and internal iliac chains are not routinely visualized by lymphangiography and therefore cannot be assessed with reliability. Computerized tomography (CT) may have potential value in detecting pelvic lymph node

metastases, although its reliability is as yet unknown.

Clinical evidence of distant metastases is unusual at the time of presentation, but may be seen in 10 to 14 per cent of patients (Kaplan et al., 1967; Ray et al., 1977). Routine chest films, whole lung tomography, computerized tomography, and radioisotope nuclear scans are usually negative.

BIOPSY AND EXAMINATION UNDER ANESTHESIA

Endoscopy and biopsy under anesthesia are mandatory for the diagnosis of a suspected urethral carcinoma. This may be obtained by a resectoscope loop, cupped biopsy forceps, or urethral curette. Open biopsy may be required to evaluate a palpable perineal mass, persistent granulation tissue, or a nonhealing perineal or scrotal abscess. This technique has been discouraged by those who suggest that it may result in a malignant urethral cutaneous fistula, which could compromise later therapy (Johnson, 1982). Urethral washings with cytologic examination may be helpful in detecting an early recurrent urethral neoplasm. For primary tumors, however, cytologic examination is more of academic interest than diagnostic value, since most lesions are relatively advanced at the time of diagnosis (Ray et al., 1977; Trott, 1971).

Bimanual examination under anesthesia permits evaluation of possible extension into the rectum, perineum, bladder base, or pelvis.

STAGING

There is no established or uniform staging system for classifying primary neoplasms of the male urethra. A staging system similar to that employed for bladder cancer was proposed by Ray et al. (1977). A modification of this system has been recently suggested by Levine (1980) in order to more closely correlate with the staging system used for carcinoma of the female urethra.

Stage 0 —In situ (limited to mucosa)
Stage A—Submucosal (not beyond submucosa)
Stage B—Into but not beyond the substance of the corpus spongiosum, or into but not beyond the prostate
Stage C—Direct extension into tissue beyond the corpus spongiosum (corpora cavernosa, muscle, fat, fascia, skin, direct skeletal involvement, or beyond the prostatic capsule
Stage D—Metastasis
   1. Inguinal lymph nodes
   2. Pelvic lymph nodes below the bifurcation of the aorta

3. Lymph nodes above the bifurcation of the aorta
4. Distant

DIFFERENTIAL DIAGNOSIS

The differential diagnosis of primary urethral carcinoma includes benign stricture disease with or without periurethral abscess, urethral extravasation, reaction to foreign body, calculous disease, tuberculosis, and syphilitic gumma.

Treatment

SURGICAL THERAPY: DISTAL URETHRAL NEOPLASMS

Treatment of the anterior carcinoma depends upon location of the cancer and its extent. Adequate therapy is directed toward removal of the entire neoplasm together with a 2-cm margin of normal tissue, and in general, distal tumors can be managed by partial penectomy or by total emasculation and perineal urethrostomy. Partial penectomy may be considered for the lesion that has not invaded the corporal bodies or when excision of the tumor allows the patient sufficient penile length to stand and direct his urinary stream. For more extensive tumor, total emasculation is usually required (Johnson, 1982).

Transurethral resection, fulguration, excisional biopsy, and segmental urethral excision with end-to-end anastomosis have each occasionally been employed in the patient with a low-grade superficial tumor. These techniques do not meet the criterion in cancer surgery for an adequate surgical margin, and tumor recurrence has been noted in several instances (Lower and Hausfeld, 1947; Flocks, 1956; Kaplan et al., 1967; Mullin et al., 1974; Konnak, 1980).

Local recurrence following adequate surgical amputation has been rare in the face of negative adenopathy, although tumors may recur in up to 20 per cent in patients who have previously required more radical amputation. Failure in these cases is a result of an unsuspected inadequate surgical margin or undetected regional nodal involvement (Kaplan et al., 1967; Ray et al., 1977; Bracken et al., 1980).

The 5-year survival for these patients is relatively good, and compares favorably with that in the female counterpart. Ray et al. (1977) reported a 66 per cent 5-year survival in 11 patients, and Kaplan et al. (1967) noted that more than half of their patients with an anterior neoplasm survived 5 years.

TREATMENT OF NODES

Clinical adenopathy with histologic evidence of metastases to the inguinal lymph nodes is not an infrequent finding in these patients. Bracken et al. (1980) found metastases in six of 11 patients with distal urethral tumors and clinical inguinal adenopathy. Ray et al. (1977) noted clinically enlarged inguinal nodes in four of nine patients with an anterior neoplasm. Inguinal node dissection or biopsy confirmed the presence of tumor. Hopkins et al. (1984) reported four of five patients to have palpable inguinal lymphadenopathy, and metastases were demonstrated in three by inguinal node biopsy or dissection. While the presence of inguinal lymph node metastases may worsen the patient's outcome, it is not uniformly poor. Interestingly, a surprising number of patients may survive for years after surgical extirpation of inguinal lymph nodes containing metastases (Kaplan et al., 1967; Ray et al., 1977; Bracken et al., 1980; Hopkins et al., 1983).

There are few data to support prophylactic lymphadenectomy. The incidence of subclinical metastases is not known, but, as in the female, diagnostic or therapeutic (unilateral or bilateral) inguinal lymph node dissection should probably be recommended only if nodes are palpable at the time of diagnosis or if delayed adenopathy appears following surgery (Johnson, 1982; Schellhammer, 1983).

SURGICAL THERAPY: PROXIMAL URETHRAL TUMORS

Neoplasms of the bulbar or bulbomembranous urethra may require total emasculation with en bloc cystoprostatectomy as the procedure of choice, although in many cases it is difficult to obtain an adequate margin and local recurrence is common, i.e., 40 to 60 per cent (Ray et al., 1977; Bracken et al., 1980; Schellhammer, 1983). To accomplish an adequate surgical margin, en bloc exenteration including resection of the inferior rami or pubic bone resection has been advocated as a single or staged procedure (Mackenzie and Whitmore, 1968; Bracken, 1982; Klein et al., 1983). The therapeutic benefit of this super-radical approach is currently unknown.

The 5-year survival for these patients has been uniformly poor. Kaplan et al. (1967) reported a 13 per cent 5-year survival rate for their patients, and a 21 per cent 5-year survival rate was seen by Ray et al. (1977), who noted that two of their three survivors had lesions that were either superficial or extending only into the corpus spongiosum. Others have confirmed this generally poor experience (Grabstald, 1973;

Sullivan and Grabstald, 1978; Bracken et al., 1980; Klein et al., 1983).

Up to one half of patients with bulbar or bulbomembranous urethral neoplasms may have disease too extensive for surgical removal. When anterior exenteration is to be undertaken, it is necessary *first* to examine the abdominal contents and pelvic lymph nodes. Documentation of visceral metastases or gross spread to the regional iliac or obturator lymph nodes obviates surgical removal. The prognosis for these patients is grave and only anecdotal long-term survivors have been reported (Guinn and Ayala, 1970).

Although the inguinal area is not a primary route for lymphatic drainage of these neoplasms, occasional metastases to this area have been documented and are usually indicative of extensive involvement of other nodes. The rare 5-year survivor has been seen after documentation of inguinal lymph nodes containing metastases.

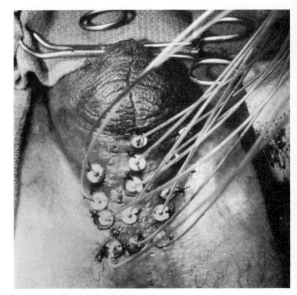

Figure 31–9. Brachytherapy (Ir-192) for a bulbar neoplasm.

RADIATION THERAPY

There are only a few cases of urethral carcinoma treated successfully by radiation therapy alone (Guinn and Alaya, 1970; Raghavaiah, 1978). In most series, patients have received external-beam therapy of 5000 to 7000 rads for palliation (Mandler and Pool, 1966; Bracken et al., 1980). Kaplan et al. (1967) reviewed 11 patients with distal urethral neoplasms who underwent radiation as primary therapy: three received radium implants and eight external-beam radiation. Of these, only two (one in each group) survived 5 years. They added one additional patient who survived 14 years with no evidence of carcinoma. In contrast, Raghavaiah (1978) reported four patients who were treated primarily with external-beam radiation. Two did well with complete disappearance of the tumor and one survived for 5 years.

In the same review by Kaplan et al. (1967) of 36 patients with bulbar or bulbomembranous neoplasms treated by radiation therapy alone, none survived 5 years. This has been the experience of others (Bracken et al., 1980).

An integrated approach using preoperative radiation of 2000 to 4000 rads followed by surgical removal is currently advocated in an attempt to decrease local recurrence (Sullivan and Grabstald, 1978; Bracken et al., 1980; Johnson, 1982). Follow-up is too short, however, to assign an advantage to this approach to survival. Some authors have utilized brachytherapy preoperatively or for controlling recurrence (Fig. 31–9) (Guinn and Ayala, 1970; Bracken et al., 1980; Hopkins et al., 1984).

CHEMOTHERAPY

Systemic chemotherapy has not been employed with any frequency in patients with carcinoma of the urethra. The response of other squamous cell neoplasms to adriamycin (Adr), bleomycin, methotrexate (MTX), or cis-diaminedichloroplatinum (DDP) suggests that urethral neoplasms may also respond to these agents. Reports, however, are anecdotal and inconclusive (Bolduan and Farah, 1981; Angel et al., 1981).

Topical chemotherapy using thiotepa or 5-fluorouracil has been employed to eradicate superficial papillary urethral neoplasms in combination with, or as an adjunct or alternative to, local surgery, and in select patients with prostatic urethral occurrence in association with superficial bladder tumors (Leissner and Johansson, 1980; Konnak, 1980). Thiotepa instillation for invasive urethral lesions has been unsuccessful (Cheng and Veenema, 1965).

TRANSITIONAL CELL CARCINOMA OF THE URETHRA IN ASSOCIATION WITH BLADDER NEOPLASMS

Preneoplastic and neoplastic changes of the urethra in association with, or following a prior history of, transitional cell tumors of the bladder may not be infrequent. Transitional metaplasia, carcinoma in situ, or frank neoplasia in the urethral remnant after cystoprostatectomy may occur in 4 to 14 per cent of males, and is particularly frequent in the patient with multicentric field disease (Cordonnier and Spjut, 1962; Johnson and Guinn, 1970; Schellhammer and Whitmore, 1976a; Raz et al., 1978). The fossa navicularis and urethral meatus are also highly susceptible to (transitional) neoplastic changes in spite of their lining of stratified squamous epithelium. In a series of 24 patients who developed a urethral recurrence after cystoprostatectomy, and in some instances subtotal urethrectomy, seven developed their tumor at the retained urethral meatus or navicular fossa (Schellhammer and Whitmore, 1976b). Therefore, while a proximal urethral recurrence may arise secondary to surface extension of tumor, or as a result of tumor cell implantation into the traumatized posterior urethra, an important factor that may be overlooked is the retained neoplastic potential of the *entire* urothelium to previous carcinogen exposure.

Cystoprostatectomy with en bloc total urethrectomy provides the greatest assurance of eliminating the potential for tumor formation in the functionless urethral remnant of the patient (with multifocal disease) at greatest risk (Schellhammer, 1983). For those patients with a single invasive tumor, a conservative approach has been favored by some authors who cite the low incidence of overt neoplasm (2.6–4 per cent) and the added time and potential morbidity of the procedure (Raz et al., 1978).

The diagnosis of a urethral recurrence may be heralded by bleeding, a urethral mass, and induration or pain in the perineum or urethral remnant. These signs and symptoms are frequently late manifestations and occur after the tumor has become relatively advanced. Schellhammer and Whitmore (1976a), in reviewing patients who developed recurrence following radical cystectomy, noted few long-term survivors.

Those patients not undergoing urethrectomy at the time of cystectomy should be followed closely. Intermittent cystoscopy or urography may be unreliable for detecting early neoplastic change. Urethral washing for cytologic examination is a readily applicable way of assessing early cellular abnormalities in the retained urethral remnant. In one series of 28 patients who had a positive or suspicious diagnosis by urethral washing, 23 were found to have either invasive carcinoma, carcinoma in situ, or metaplastic change in the surgical specimen. Only one of 37 other patients with negative cytologic results developed low-grade carcinoma (Wolinska et al., 1977).

Total urethrectomy, including the fossa navicularis and urethral meatus, should be ad-

equate therapy to prevent recurrence. If periurethral invasion has occurred, total emasculation may be required.

PRIMARY TRANSITIONAL CELL CARCINOMA OF THE PROSTATIC URETHRA

In the overwhelming majority of cases, a transitional cell carcinoma found in the prostatic urethra occurs with, or follows, a similar cancer elsewhere. Solitary or multiple papillary lesions in the prostate frequently coexist or follow urothelial tumors in the bladder, ureter, or renal pelvis. Not infrequently, these tumors may be noted following transurethral resection of a previous bladder tumor and this may reflect implantation of tumor cells in the prostate at the time of prior bladder resection (Grabstald, 1973; Seemayer et al., 1975). Rarely, a transitional cell carcinoma can arise primarily within the ducts or, to a lesser extent, the acini of the prostate gland.

Melicow and Hollowell (1952) were the first to allude to this tumor, citing three patients. Ortega et al. (1953) described similar findings in a case reported as Paget's disease of the urethra. Karpas and Moumgis (1969) argued that the "reserve" cells lying between the luminal epithelium and the basement membrane in the periurethral ducts were precursors of both transitional epithelial hyperplasia and frank neoplasia. Ullman and Ross (1967) reported on a series of cases in which the epithelium of the periurethral prostatic glands ranged from simple hyperplasia to definite carcinoma in situ, and suggested that this carcinoma in situ arising in the prostatic ducts may conceivably be the precursor to a more invasive prostatic cancer, as occurs in the bladder.

The clinical features of primary prostatic transitional cell carcinoma are similar to those of patients with other tumors of the prostate. The peak incidence occurs in the sixth decade and the presenting symptoms are usually those of obstruction, which may be rapid in progression. Gross hematuria occurs in 50 per cent of patients. Other symptoms may include urgency, frequency, and rectal pain (Johnson et al., 1972; Rhamy, et al., 1973a). On rectal examination, the prostate may be grossly enlarged and stony-hard. Not infrequently, the gland may appear to be enlarged and benign in consistency.

Anemia and azotemia may be present. Acid and alkaline phosphatase levels are usually normal but occasionally may be elevated. Some of these patients may have a coincident adenocarcinoma (Green et al., 1973).

Excretory urography reveals hydrone-phrosis in 20 per cent of cases. Osseous metastases are seen in 15 to 20 per cent of patients, but may be found only in those patients harboring an associated adenocarcinoma (Rhamy et al., 1973a).

On histologic examination, the majority of these cancers are of higher grade. For superficial lesions, transurethral resection is adequate, although 50 per cent of tumors may recur (Grabstald, 1973). For the more advanced lesion, orchiectomy or estrogen therapy offers no therapeutic benefit (Johnson et al., 1972; Grabstald, 1973; Rhamy et al., 1973a; Green et al., 1973).

External-beam radiation therapy alone or in conjunction with brachytherapy implants has not modified the poor prognosis for this tumor. Because of diffuse and extensive prostatic involvement in the majority of cases, radical prostatectomy is not indicated (Green et al., 1973; Rhamy et al., 1973a; Grabstald, 1973).

Currently, preoperative radiation combined with radical cystoprostatourethrectomy appears to be the most appropriate therapy, although follow-up statistics are lacking (Levine, 1980). Bilateral groin dissection has been suggested when inguinal lymph nodes are clinically palpable (Grabstald, 1973).

The prognosis for patients with invasive transitional cell carcinoma of the prostate is grave, with only a few patients surviving 5 years. Metastases appear in the brain and lung (Green et al., 1973). Overall, fewer than 100 cases have been reported in the literature.

COWPER'S GLAND ADENOCARCINOMA

This extremely rare neoplasm may invade the prostatic and bulbomembranous urethra, although it is conceivable that some patients with a diagnosis of Cowper's gland cancer may have prostatic carcinoma with extension (Bourque et al., 1970; Keen et al., 1970). Symptoms may include perineal pain, pain on defecation, constipation, irritative urinary symptoms, hematuria, hemospermia, or urinary obstruction. On physical examination, a perineal mass may be visualized, and on rectal palpation it is usually possible to separate the prostate behind the tumor.

Prompt radical cystoprostatourethrectomy is treatment of choice for patients with localized disease. Radiation therapy and chemotherapy have been used but have not altered the overall poor prognosis (Keen et al., 1970). Five-year survivors have not been reported.

CARCINOMA IN A DIVERTICULUM OF THE MALE URETHRA

There is one report of a urethral carcinoma associated with a urethral diverticulum. This patient had a history of gonococcal urethritis and had been previously treated for urethral stricture. Because this squamous cell carcinoma was seen both proximal and distal to the diverticulum, the focus or origin could not be proved (Allen and Nelson, 1978).

OTHER URETHRAL MALIGNANCIES

Melanoma

Primary melanoma of the male urethra is distinctly rare, as is metastatic melanoma (Grabstald, 1973). Fewer than 25 cases are reported. The peak incidence is seen in the sixth to seventh decades (Kokotas et al., 1981; Begun et al., 1984). Patients may present with symptoms of urinary irritation, obstruction, hematuria, and occasionally melanuria. While these tumors can arise in all anatomic sites in the urethra from the meatus to the prostatic urethra, the fossa navicularis and meatus are most frequently involved (Geelhoed and Myers, 1973; Kokotas et al., 1981; Begun et al., 1984).

The majority of reported cases have presented as clinical Stage I (i.e., a localized lesion without metastases to regional lymph nodes or other viscera) and treatment is primarily surgical. Because of the high incidence of local or regional recurrence, total penectomy in conjunction with cystoprostatectomy and bilateral ilioinguinal lymph node dissection may offer the best chance for cure (Bracken and Diokno, 1974). Few long-term survivors have been reported (Geelhoed and Myers, 1973; Kokotas et al., 1981). Radiation therapy and chemotherapy may be helpful adjuncts to surgery.

Sarcomas

Malignant tumors arising from the mesenchymal supporting tissue of the urethra are the subject of single case reports. Rhabdomyosarcoma, leiomyosarcoma, fibrosarcoma, lymphosarcoma, and myxosarcoma have been described (Bailey, 1932; Painter et al., 1968; Alabaster et al., 1981). These lesions can be found from infancy to the eighth decade. The patient may present with a penile mass, genital pain, or obstructive urinary symptoms. The proximity of the corporal bodies and the urethra often makes distinction between sarcomas originating in the penis and the urethra arbitrary. Treatment is surgical, usually partial or total penile amputation. The prognosis is poor.

Metastases

Urethral metastases are very rare and most frequently occur as extensions of, or simultaneous with, penile corporal involvement (Weitzner, 1971). The most frequent primaries metastasizing to the urethra are prostate (Iverson et al., 1972; Kotecha and Gentile, 1974), colon and rectum (Selikowitz ánd Olsson, 1973), and bladder. Involvement by other genitourinary primaries, such as the kidney (Abeshouse and Abeshouse, 1961), ureter, and testes (Weitzner, 1971) have also been reported. The most likely mechanisms of involvement are surface extension, direct cell implantation, or retrograde lymphatic and venous extension. Arterial seeding is also a possibility. The most frequent signs and symptoms include priapism, hematuria, obstruction, pain, urethral induration, or nodularity. Treatment is ineffective and survival is limited.

References

Abeshouse, B. S., and Abeshouse, G. A.: Metastatic tumors of the penis: A review of the literature and a report of two cases. J. Urol., 86:99, 1961.

Ablin, R. J., and Curtis, W. W.: Condylomata acuminata: Treatment by autogenous vaccine. Ill. Med. J., 147:343, 1975.

Ackerman, L. V.: Tumors of the male sex organs. In Dixon, F. J., and Moore, R. A. (Eds.): Atlas of Tumor Pathology. Section 8. Washington, D.C., Armed Forces Institute of Pathology, 1952, pp. 150–153.

Alabaster, A. M., Jordan, W. P., Jr., Soloway, M. S., Shippel, R. M., and Young, J. M.: Leiomyosarcoma of the bladder and subsequent urethral recurrence. J. Urol., 125:583, 1981.

Allen, R., and Nelson, R. P.: Primary urethral malignancy. Review of 22 cases. South. Med. J., 71:547, 1978.

Anderson, K. A., and McAninch, J. W.: Primary squamous cell carcinoma of anterior male urethra. Urology, 23:134, 1984.

Angel, J. R.., Kraus, S. D., McClung, T., Roth, J., and Dekernion, J. B.: Unusual case of urethral carcinoma. Urology, 18:74, 1981.

Antoniades, J.: Radiation therapy in carcinoma of the female urethra. Cancer, 24:70, 1969.

Ariel, I. M.: Malignant melanoma of the female genital system: A report of 48 patients and review of the literature. J. Surg. Oncol., 16:371, 1981.

Bailey, O. T.: Fibro-sarcoma of the male urethra. J. Urol., 32:109, 1932.

Baker, L. H., Al-Sarraf, M., and Opipari, M.: Combination chemotherapy (CHP) in patients with advanced urothelial cancers. (Meeting abstract.) Proc. Am. Assoc. Cancer Res., 21:429, 1980.

Begley, B. J.: Hemangioma of the male urethra: Treatment by Johanson–Denis Browne technique. J. Urol., 84:111, 1960.

Begun, F. P., Grossman, H. B., Diokno, A. C., and Sogani, P. C.: Malignant melanoma of the penis and male urethra. J. Urol., 132:123, 1984.

Berger, B. W., Bhagavan, S. B., Reiner, W., Engel, R., and Lepor, H.: Nephrogenic adenoma: Clinical features and therapeutic considerations. J. Urol., 126:824, 1981.

Bhagavan, B. S., Tiamson, E. M., Wenk, R. E., Berger, B. W., Hamamoto, G., and Eggleston, J. C.: Nephrogenic adenoma of the urinary bladder and urethra. Hum. Pathol., 12:907, 1981.

Bissada, N. K., Cole, A. T., and Fried, F. A.: Extensive condylomas acuminata of the entire male urethra and the bladder. J. Urol., 112:201, 1974.

Blath, R. A., and Boehm, F. H.: Carcinoma of the female urethra. Surg. Gynecol. Obstet., 136:574, 1973.

Block, N. L., and Hotchkiss, R. S.: Malignant melanoma of the female urethra: Report of a case with 5-year survival and review of the literature. J. Urol., 105:251, 1971.

Bolduan, J. P., and Farah, R. N.: Primary urethral neoplasms: Review of 30 cases. J. Urol., 125:198, 1981.

Bourque, J. L., Charghi, A., Gauthier, G. E., Drouin, G., and Charbonneau, J.: Primary carcinoma of Cowper's gland. J. Urol., 103:758, 1970.

Brack, C. B., and Dickson, R. J.: Carcinoma of the female urethra. Am. J. Roentgenol. Radium Ther. Nucl. Med., 79:472, 1958.

Bracken, R. B.: Exenterative surgery for posterior urethral cancer. Urology, 19:248, 1982.

Bracken, R. B., and Diokno, A. C.: Melanoma of the penis and the urethra: Two case reports and review of the literature. J. Urol., 111:198, 1974.

Bracken, R. B., Johnson, D. E., Miller, L. S., Ayala, A. G., Gomez, J. J., and Rutledge, F.: Primary carcinoma of the female urethra. J. Urol., 116:188, 1976.

Bracken, R. B., Henry, R., and Ordonez, N.: Primary carcinoma of the male urethra. South. Med. J., 73:1003, 1980.

Bracken, R. B., McDonald, M. W., and Johnson, D. E.: Cystectomy for superficial bladder cancer. Urology, 18:459, 1981.

Bringel, P. J. P., and de Andrade Arruda, R.: 5-Fluorouracil cream 5 per cent in the treatment of intraurethral condylomata. Br. J. Urol., 54:295, 1981.

Cantrell, B. B., Leifer, G., Deklerk, D. P., and Eggleston, J. C.: Papillary adenocarcinoma of the prostatic urethra with clear-cell appearance. Cancer, 48:2661, 1981.

Cea, P. C., Ward, J. N., Lavengood, R. W., Jr., and Gray, G. F.: Mesonephric adenocarcinomas in urethral diverticula. Urology, 10:58, 1977.

Cheng, S. F., and Veenema, R. J.: Topical application of Thiotepa to penile and urethral tumors. J. Urol., 94:159, 1965.

Chu, A. M.: Female urethral carcinoma. Radiology, 107:627, 1973.

Colapinto, V., and Evans, D. H.: Primary carcinoma of the male urethra developing after urethroplasty for stricture. J. Urol., 118:581, 1977.

Cordonnier, J. J., and Spjut, H. J.: Urethral occurrence of bladder carcinoma following cystectomy. J. Urol., 87:398, 1962.

Culp, O. S., Magid, M. A., and Kaplan, I. W.: Podophyllin treatment of condylomata acuminata. J. Urol., 51:655, 1944.

Danoff, D. S., Holden, S., Thompson, R. W., and David, R.: New treatment for extensive condylomata acuminata: External radiation therapy. Urology, 18:47, 1981.

Das, S. P.: Paraurethral cysts in women. J. Urol., 126:41, 1981.

DasGupta, T., and Grabstald, H.: Melanoma of the genitourinary tract. J. Urol., *93*:607, 1965.

Davis, B. L., and Robinson, J. G.: Diverticula of the female urethra: Assay of 120 cases. J. Urol., *104*:850, 1970.

Dean, A. L.: Carcinoma of the male and female urethra: Pathology and diagnosis. J. Urol., *75*:505, 1956.

Debenedictis, T. I., Marmar, T. L., and Praiss, D. E.: Intraurethral condylomas acuminata: Management and review of the literature. J. Urol., *118*:767, 1977.

Delclos, L.: Carcinoma of the female urethra. *In* Johnson, D. E., and Boileau, M. A. (Eds.): Genitourinary Tumors. Fundamental Principles and Surgical Techniques. New York, Grune & Stratton, 1982, pp. 275–286.

Desai, S., Libertino, J. A., and Zinman, L.: Primary carcinoma of the female urethra. J. Urol., *110*:693, 1973.

DeWolf, W. C., and Fraley, E. E.: Congenital urethral polyp in the infant: Case report and review of the literature. J. Urol., *109*:515, 1973.

Dobos, E. I., Downing, S. W., and Ashe, S. M. P.: Primary carcinoma originating in the Littre glands. Cancer, *7*:539, 1954.

Dretler, S. P., and Klein, L. A.: The eradication of intraurethral condylomata acuminata with 5-fluorouracil cream. J. Urol., *113*:195, 1975.

Dretler, S. P., Vermillion, C. D., and McCullough, D. L.: The roentgenographic diagnosis of female urethral diverticula. J. Urol., *107*:72, 1972.

Elkon, D., Kim, J., Huddleston, A. L., and Constable, W. C.: Primary carcinoma of the female urethra. South. Med. J., *73*:1439, 1980.

Ellendt, E. P., Martinez, P., Neiro, J. A., Silva, J., Gaomez Zarcajo, V. R., and Santamaria, L.: Leiomyoma of the female urethral and bladder neck. Eur. Urol., *1*:46, 1981.

Ende, N., Woods, L. P., and Shelley, H. S.: Carcinoma originating in ducts surrounding the prostatic urethra. Am. J. Clin. Pathol., *40*:183, 1963.

Evans, K. J., McCarthy, M. P., and Sands, J. P.: Adenocarcinoma of a female urethral diverticulum: Case report and review of the literature. J. Urol., *126*:124, 1981.

Fagan, G. E., and Hertig, A. T.: Carcinoma of the female urethra: Review of literature. Report of 8 cases. Obstet. Gynecol., *6*:1, 1955.

Flocks, R. H.: The treatment of urethral tumors. J. Urol., *75*:514, 1956.

Foster, R. S., Weigel, J. W., and Mantz, F. A.: Anterior urethral polyps. J. Urol., *124*:145, 1980.

Fuselier, H. A., Jr., McBurney, E. I., Brannan, W., and Randrup, E. R.: Treatment of condylomata acuminata with carbon dioxide laser. Urology, *15*:265, 1980.

Geelhoed, G. W., and Myers, G. H.: Primary melanoma of the male urethra. J. Urol., *109*:634, 1973.

Gigax, J. H., and Robinson, J. R.: The successful treatment of intraurethral condylomata acuminata with colchicine. J. Urol., *105*:809, 1971.

Gillenwater, J. Y., and Burros, H. M.: Unusual tumors of the female urethra. Obstet. Gynecol., *31*:617, 1968.

Godec, C. J., Cass, A. S., Hitchcock, C. R., and Hildreth, T. A.: Melanoma of the female urethra. J. Urol., *126*:553, 1981.

Gowing, N. F. C.: Urethral carcinoma associated with cancer of the bladder. Br. J. Urol., *32*:428, 1960.

Grabstald, H.: Tumors of the urethra in men and women. Cancer, *32*:1236, 1973.

Grabstald, H.: Resectoscopy loop for urethral biopsy following cystectomy in the male patient. J. Urol., *124*:605, 1980.

Grabstald, H.: Commentary: Urethral cancer. *In* Johnson,

D. E., and Boileau, M. A. (Eds.): Genitourinary Tumors. Fundamental Principles and Surgical Techniques. New York, Grune & Stratton, 1982, pp. 287–292.

Grabstald, H., Hilaris, B., Henschke, U. R., and Whitmore, W. F., Jr.: Cancer of the female urethra. JAMA, *197*:835, 1966.

Graf, E. C., Callahan, D. H., and Sozer, I.: A study of tumors of the female urethra. J. Urol., *88*:64, 1962.

Green, L. F., Mulcahy, J. J., Warren, M. M. W., and Dockerty, M. D.: Primary transitional cell carcinoma of the prostate. J. Urol., *110*:235, 1973.

Guinn, G. A., and Ayala, A. G.: Male urethral cancer. Report of 15 cases including a primary melanoma. J. Urol., *103*:176, 1970.

Gunther, I., Abrams, H. J., Sutton, A. P., and Buchbinder, M. I.: Fibroepithelial polyps of the verumontanum: A case report and review of the literature. J. Urol., *121*:525, 1979.

Halverstadt, D. B., and Parry, W. H.: Thiotepa in the management of intraurethral condylomata acuminata. J. Urol., *101*:729, 1969.

Hamilton, J. O., and Leach, W. B.: Adenocarcinoma arising in a diverticulum of the female urethra. Arch. Pathol., *51*:90, 1951.

Hand, J. R.: Surgery of penis and urethra. *In* Campbell, M. F., and Harrison, J. H. (Eds.): Urology. 3rd ed. Philadelphia, W. B. Saunders Co., 1970, pp. 2541–2647.

Hopkins, S. C., Vider, M., Nag, S., Tai, D. L., and Soloway, M. S.: Carcinoma of the female urethra: Reassessment of modes of therapy. J. Urol., *129*:568, 1983.

Hopkins, S. C., Nag, S. K., and Soloway, M. S.: Primary carcinoma of the male urethra. Urology, *23*:128, 1984.

Hotchkiss, R. S., and Amelar, R. D.: Primary carcinoma of the male urethra. Trans. Am. Assoc. Genitourin. Surg., *44*:177, 1952.

Hotchkiss, R. S., and Rouse, A. J.: Papillomatosis of the bladder and ureters, preceded by condyloma. J. Urol., *100*:723, 1968.

Howe, G. E., Prentiss, R. J., Mullenis, R. B., and Feeney, M. J.: Carcinoma of the urethra: Diagnosis and treatment. J. Urol., *89*:232, 1963.

Huvos, A. G., and Grabstald, H.: Urethral meatal and parameatal tumors in young men: A clinicopathologic and electron microscopic study. J. Urol., *110*:688, 1973.

Iversen, J., and Robins, R. E.: Mucosal malignant melanomas. Am. J. Surg., *139*:660, 1980.

Iverson, A. P., Blackard, C. E., and Schulberg, V. A.: Carcinoma of the prostate with urethral metastases. J. Urol., *108*:901, 1972.

Johnson, D. E.: Cancer of the female urethra: Overview. *In* Johnson, D. E., and Boileau, M. A. (Eds.): Genitourinary Tumors. Fundamental Principles and Surgical Techniques. New York, Grune & Stratton, 1982, pp. 267–274.

Johnson, D. E., and Guinn, G. A.: Surgical management of urethral carcinoma occurring after cystectomy. J. Urol., *103*:314, 1970.

Johnson, D. E., Hogan, J. M., and Ayala, A. G.: Transitional cell carcinoma of the prostate. A clinical and morphological study. Cancer, *29*:287, 1972.

Kamat, M. R., Kulkarni, J. N., and Dhumale, R. G.: Primary carcinoma of female urethra: Review of 20 cases. J. Surg. Oncol., *16*:105, 1981.

Kaplan, G. W., Bulkley, G. J., and Grayhack, J. T.: Carcinoma of the male urethra. J. Urol., *98*:365, 1967.

Kaplan, I. W.: Condylomata acuminata. New Orleans Med. Surg. J., *94*:388, 1941–42.

Karpas, C. M., and Moumgis, B.: Primary transitional cell

carcinoma of the prostate gland: Possible pathogenesis and relationship to reserve cell hyperplasia of prostatic periurethral ducts. J. Urol., 101:201, 1969.

Katz, J. I., and Grabstald, H.: Primary malignant melanoma of the female urethra. J. Urol., 116:454, 1976.

Kearney, G. P., Lebowitz, R. L., and Retik, A. B.: Obstructing polyps of the posterior urethra in boys: Embryology and management. J. Urol., 122:802, 1979.

Keen, M. R., Golden, R. L., Richardson, J. F., and Melicow, M. M.: Carcinoma of Cowper's gland treated with chemotherapy. J. Urol., 106:854, 1970.

Kimche, D., and Lask, D.: Congenital polyps of the prostatic urethra. J. Urol., 127:134, 1982.

King, L. R.: Carcinoma of the urethra in male patients. J. Urol., 91:555, 1964.

Kleiman, H., and Lancaster, Y.: Condyloma acuminata of the bladder. J. Urol., 88:52, 1962.

Klein, F. A., Whitmore, W. F., Jr., Herr, H. W., Morse, M. J., and Sogani, P. C.: Inferior pubic rami resection with en bloc radical excision for invasive proximal urethral carcinoma. Cancer, 51:1238, 1983.

Klotz, P. G.: Carcinoma of Skene's gland associated with urethral diverticulum: A case report. J. Urol., 112:487, 1974.

Kokotas, N. S., Kallis, E. G., and Fokitis, P. J.: Primary malignant melanoma of male urethra. Urology, 18:392, 1981.

Konnak, J. W.: Conservative management of low grade neoplasms of the male urethra: A preliminary report. J. Urol., 123:175, 1980.

Kotecha, N., and Gentile, R. L.: Carcinoma of prostate with urethral metastasis. Urology, 3:85, 1974.

Kreutzmann, H. A. R., and Colloff, B.: Primary carcinoma of the male urethra. Arch. Surg., 29:513, 1939.

Lake, M. H., Kossow, A. S., and Bokinsky, G.: Leiomyoma of the bladder and urethra. J. Urol., 126:742, 1981.

Leissner, K. H., and Johansson, S.: Topical application of 5-fluorouracil cream: A therapeutic alternative in the treatment of urothelial tumors of the distal urethra: A case report. Scand. J. Urol. Nephrol., 14:115, 1980.

Levine, R. L.: Urethral cancer. Cancer, 45 [Suppl.]:1965, 1980.

Lewis, H. Y., Wolf, P. L., and Pierce, J. M.: Condylomata acuminata of the bladder. J. Urol., 88:248, 1962.

Lower, W. E., and Hausfeld, K. F.: Primary carcinoma of the male urethra: Report of ten cases. J. Urol., 58:192, 1947.

Luc Man, L., and Vadas, G.: Transitional cloaegenic carcinoma of the urethra. Cancer, 31:1508, 1973.

Mackenzie, A. R., and Whitmore, W. F.: Resection of pubic rami for urologic cancer. J. Urol., 100:546, 1968.

Mandler, J. I., and Pool, T. L.: Primary carcinoma of the male urethra. J. Urol., 96:67, 1966.

Manuel, E. S., Seery, W. M., and Cole, A. T.: Capillary hemangioma of the male urethra: Case report with literature review. J. Urol., 117:804, 1977.

Marshall, F. C., Uson, A. C., and Melicow, M. M.: Neoplasms and caruncles of the female urethra. Surg. Gynecol. Obstet., 110:723, 1960.

Marshall, S., and Hirsch, K.: Carcinoma within urethral diverticula. Urology, 10:161, 1977.

McCrea, L. E.: Malignancy of the female urethra. Urol. Survey, 2:85, 1952.

Melicow, M. M., and Hollowell, J. W.: Intra-urothelial cancer. Carcinoma in situ, Bowen's disease of the urinary systems. Discussion of 30 cases. J. Urol., 68:763, 1952.

Melicow, M. M., and Roberts, T. W.: Pathology and natural history of urethral tumors in males. Review of 142 cases. Urology, 11:83, 1978.

Melicow, M. M., and Uson, A. C.: A spectrum of malignant

epithelial tumors of the prostate gland. J. Urol., 115:696, 1976.

Menville, J. G., and Counsellor, U. S.: Mucoid carcinoma of the female urethra. J. Urol., 33:76, 1935.

Merrell, R. W., and Brown, H. E.: Recurrent urethral leiomyoma presenting as stress incontinence. Urology, 18:588, 1981.

Metcalfe, J. B., Carey, T. C., and Barry, J. M.: Genitourinary malignancy and pseudohyperparathyroidism. J. Urol., 119:702, 1978.

Monaco, A. P., Murphy, G. B., and Dowling, W.: Primary cancer of the female urethra. Cancer, 11:1215, 1958.

Mooppan, M. M., Kim, H., and Wax, S. H.: Leiomyoma of the female urethra. J. Urol., 121:371, 1979.

Morrow, R. P., McDonald, J. R., and Emmett, J. L.: Condylomata acuminata of the urethra. J. Urol., 68:909, 1952.

Mostofi, F. K.: Testes, scrotum and penis. In Anderson, W. A. D., and Kissane, J. M. (Eds.): Pathology. 7th ed. St. Louis, C. V. Mosby Inc., 1977, pp. 1034–1035.

Mullin, E. M., Anderson, E. E., and Paulson, D. F.: Carcinoma of the male urethra. J. Urol., 112:610, 1974.

Murayama, T., Komatsu, H., Asano, M., Tahara, M., and Nakamura, T.: Mesonephric adenocarcinoma of the urethra in a woman: Report of a case. J. Urol., 120:500, 1978.

Nellans, R. E., and Stein, J. J.: Pedunculated polyp of posterior urethra. Urology, 6:474, 1975.

Novak, E. R., and Woodruff, J. D.: Diseases of the vulva. In Novak, E. R., and Woodruff, J. D. (Eds.): Novak's Gynecologic and Obstetric Pathology. 8th ed. Philadelphia, W. B. Saunders Co., 1979, pp. 1–58.

Ortega, L. G., Whitmore, W. F., Jr., and Murphy, A. I.: In situ carcinoma of the prostate with intra epithelial extension into the urethra and bladder: Paget's disease of the urethra and bladder. Cancer, 6:898, 1953.

Painter, M. R., O'Shaughnessy, E. J., Larson, P. H., and Ribbe, R. E.: Rhabdomyosarcoma of the male urethra. J. Urol., 99:455, 1968.

Patanaphan, V., Prempree, T., Sewchand, W., Hafiz, M. A., and Jaiwatana, J.: Adenocarcinoma arising in a female diverticulum. Urology, 22:259, 1983.

Peters, W. A., and Vaughan, E. O.: Urethral diverticulum in the female. Etiologic factors and postoperative results. Obstet. Gynecol., 92:106, 1965.

Peterson, D. T., Docketry, M. B., Utz, D. C., and Symmonds, R. E.: The peril of primary carcinoma of the urethra in women. J. Urol., 110:72, 1973.

Petterson, S., Hansson, G., and Blohme, I.: Condyloma acuminatum of the bladder. J. Urol., 115:535, 1976.

Pointon, R. C. S., and Poole-Wilson, D. S.: Primary carcinoma of the urethra. Br. J. Urol., 40:682, 1968.

Pompeius, R., and Ekroth, R.: A successfully treated case of condyloma acuminatum of the urethra and urinary bladder. Eur. Urol., 2:298, 1976.

Poole-Wilson, D. S., and Bernard, R. J.: Total cystectomy for bladder tumors. Br. J. Urol., 43:16, 1971.

Powell, I., Cartwright, H., and Jano, F.: Villous adenoma and adenocarcinoma of female urethra. Urology, 18:612, 1981.

Powell, L. C., Jr.: Condyloma acuminatum: Recent advances in development, carcinogenesis, and treatment. Clin. Obstet. Gynecol., 21:1061, 1978.

Prempree, T., Amornmarn, R., and Patanaphan, V.: Radiation therapy in primary carcinoma of the female urethra. II. An update on results. Cancer, 54:729, 1984.

Prempree, T., Wizenberg, M. J., and Scott, R. M.: Radiation treatment of primary carcinoma of the female urethra. Cancer, 42:1177, 1978.

Rabon, N. A.: Malignant melanoma developing in a urethral caruncle. I. Am. Med. Wo. Assoc., 19:855, 1964.

Raghavaiah, N. V.: Radiotherapy in the treatment of carcinoma of the male urethra. Cancer, *41*:1313, 1978.

Rao, P. L., Bhattacharya, N. C., Joshi, V. V., Pathak, I. C., and Mitra, S. K.: Posterior urethral polyp in a neonate. Postgrad. Med., *27*:125, 1981.

Ray, B., and Guinan, B. D.: Primary carcinoma of the urethra. *In* Javadpour, N. (Ed.): Principles and Management of Urologic Cancer. Baltimore, The Williams & Wilkins Co., 1979, pp. 445–473.

Ray, B., Canto, A. R., and Whitmore, W. F.: Experience with primary carcinoma of the male urethra. J. Urol., *117*:591, 1977.

Raz, S., McLorie, G., Johnson, S., and Skinner, D. G.: Management of the urethra in patients undergoing radical cystectomy for bladder carcinoma. J. Urol., *120*:298, 1978.

Reed, C. A. L.: Melanosarcoma of the female urethra. Urethrectomy: Recovery. Am. J. Obstet. Dis. Wo. Child., *34*:864, 1896.

Reheis, J. P., Goldstein, I. S., and Mogil, R. A.: Papillary adenocarcinoma arising in a urethral diverticulum accompanied by adenocarcinoma of the bladder: Case report and review of the literature. J. Urol., *126*:695, 1981.

Rhamy, R. K., Buchanan, R. D., and Spalding, M. J.: intraductal carcinoma of the prostate gland. J. Urol., *109*:457, 1973a.

Rhamy, R. K., Boldus, R. A., Allison, R. C., and Tapper, R. I.: Therapeutic modalities in adenocarcinoma of the female urethra. J. Urol., *109*:638, 1973b.

Richie, J. P., and Skinner, D. G.: Carcinoma in situ of the urethra associated with bladder carcinoma: The role of urethrectomy. J. Urol., *119*:80, 1978.

Riches, E. W., and Callen, T. H.: Carcinoma of the urethra. Br. J. Urol., *23*:209, 1951.

Roberts, J. W., and Devine, C. J., Jr.: Urethra hemangioma: Treatment by total excision and grafting. J. Urol., *129*:1053, 1983.

Roberts, T. W., and Melicow, M. M.: Pathology and natural history of urethral tumors in females. Review of 65 cases. Urology, *10*:583, 1977.

Rosemberg, S. K., Fuller, T., and Jacobs, H.: Rapid superpulse carbon dioxide laser treatment of urethral condylomata. Urology, *17*:149, 1981.

Rosemberg, S. K., Jacobs, H., and Fuller, T.: Some guidelines in the treatment of urethral condylomata with carbon dioxide laser. J. Urol., *127*:906, 1982.

Ruch, R. M., Frerichs, J. B., and Arneson, A. N.: Cancer of the female urethra. Cancer, *5*:748, 1952.

Saito, R.: Adenosquamous carcinoma of the male urethra with hypercalcemia. Hum. Pathol., *12*:383, 1981.

Schellhammer, P. F.: Urethral carcinoma. Semin. Urol., *1*:83, 1983.

Schellhammer, P. F., and Whitmore, W. F., Jr.: Transitional cell carcinoma of the urethra in men having cystectomy for bladder cancer. J. Urol., *115*:56, 1976a.

Schellhammer, P. F., and Whitmore, W. F., Jr.: Urethral meatal carcinoma following cystourethrectomy for bladder carcinoma. J. Urol., *115*:61, 1976b.

Scott, R., and Stell, R.: Intraurethral condylomata acuminata: Clorpactin as an adjunct to therapy. J. Urol., *86*:470, 1961.

Seemayer, T. A., Knaack, J., Thelmo, W. L., Wong, N., and Ahmed, M. N.: Further observation on carcinoma in situ of the urinary bladder: Silent but extensive intraprostatic involvement. Cancer, *36*:514, 1975.

Selikowitz, S. M., and Olsson, C. A.: Metastatic urethral obstruction. Arch. Surg., *107*:906, 1973.

Severino, L. J., Brockunier, A. Jr., and Davadian, M. M.: Adenocarcinoma of the urethra during pregnancy. Obstet. Gynecol., *50* [Suppl]: 22, 1977.

Sharpe, S.: A Critical Enquirey into the Present State of Surgery. London, J and R Tonson, 1750, pp. 1–68.

Shenasky, J. H., II, and Gillenwater, S. Y.: Management of transitional cell carcinoma of the prostate. J. Urol., *108*:462, 1972.

Shiraki, I. W.: Parameatal cysts of the glans penis: A report of nine cases. J. Urol., *114*:544, 1975.

Shuttleworth, K. E. D., and Lloyd-Davies, R. W.: Radical resection for tumors involving the posterior urethra. Br. J. Urol., *41*:739, 1969.

Silverman, M. L., Eyre, R. C., Zinman, L. A., and Corsson, A. W.: Mixed mucinous and papillary adenocarcinoma involving male urethra, probably originating in periurethral glands. Cancer, *47*:1398, 1981.

Skolnick, J. L., Anderson, W. H., Richman, A. C., and Conley, J. G.: Pulmonary metastases from urethral carcinoma. J. Ky. Med. Assoc., *75*:427, 1977.

Srinivas, U., and Dow, D.: Transitional cell carcinoma in a urethral diverticulum with a calculus. J. Urol., *129*:372, 1983.

Stadaas, J. O.: Pedunculated polyp of posterior urethra in children causing reflux and hydronephrosis. J. Pediatr. Surg., *8*:517, 1973.

Staubitz, W. J., Carden, L. M., Oberkircher, L. J., Lent, M. H., and Murphy, W. T.: Management of urethral carcinoma in the female. J. Urol., *73*:1045, 1955.

Sullivan, J., and Grabstald, H.: Management of carcinoma of the urethra. *In* Skinner, D. G., and deKernion, J. B. (Eds.): Genitourinary Cancer. Philadelphia, W. B. Saunders Co., 1978, pp. 419–429.

Taggart, C. G., Castro, J. R., and Rutledge, F. N.: Carcinoma of the female urethra. Am. J. Roentgenol. Radium. Ther. Nucl. Med., *114*:145, 1972.

Taylor, H. G., and Blom, J.: Transitional cell carcinoma of the prostate. Cancer, *51*:1800, 1983.

Tesluk, H.: Primary adenocarcinoma of female urethra associated with diverticula. Urology, *17*:197, 1981.

Tines, S. C., Bigongiari, L. R., and Weigel, J. W.: Carcinoma in diverticulum of the female urethra. AJR, *138*:582, 1982.

Torres, S. A., and Quattlebaum, R. B.: Carcinoma in a urethral diverticulum. South. Med. J., *65*:1374, 1972.

Trott, P. A.: Detection of urethral carcinoma using a soluble swab. Br. J. Surg., *58*:66, 1971.

Turner, A. G., and Hendry, W. F.: Primary carcinoma of the female urethra. Br. J. Urol., *52*:549, 1980.

Ullman, A. S., and Ross, O. A.: Hyperplasia, atypism and carcinoma in situ in prostatic periurethral glands. Am. J. Clin. Pathol., *47*:497, 1967.

Weimar, G. W., Milleman, L. A., Reiland, T. L., and Culp, D. A.: 5-Fluorouracil urethral suppositories for the eradication of condylomata acuminata. J. Urol., *120*:174, 1978.

Wein, A. J., and Benson, G. S.: Treatment of urethral condyloma acuminatum with 5-fluorouracil cream. Urology, *9*:413, 1977.

Weitzner, S.: Secondary carcinoma of the penis. Am. Surg., *37*:562, 1971.

Williams, G., and Ashken, M. H.: Urethral carcinoma following urethroplasty. J. R. Soc. Med., *73*:370, 1980.

Wolinska, W. H., Melamed, M. R., Schellhammer, P. F., and Whitmore, W. F., Jr.: Urethral cytology following cystectomy for bladder carcinoma. Am. J. Surg. Pathol., *1*:225, 1977.

Yagoda, A.: Chemotherapy of genitourinary tumors. Drug Ther., 19:94, 98, 102, 1980.

Zeigerman, J. H., and Gordon, S. F.: Cancer of the female urethra: A curable disease. Obstet. Gynecol., *36*:785, 1970.

CHAPTER 32

Carcinoma of the Prostate

WILLIAM J. CATALONA, M.D.
WILLIAM W. SCOTT, Ph.D., M.D., D.Sc.

EPIDEMIOLOGY

Incidence, Prevalence, Mortality

The *incidence* of a cancer is defined as the number of new cases reported per 100,000 population per year. In most developed countries, prostate cancer is one of the most common cancers occurring among males. In the National Cancer Institute Surveillance, Epidemiology and End Results (SEER) survey between 1973 and 1977, the incidence of prostate cancer in the United States was approximately 69 per 100,000 males per year (Young et al., 1981). Most epidemiologic surveys suggest that the incidence of prostate cancer has increased over the years, but this may be due in part to improved detection and reporting of prostate cancer cases.

The *prevalence* of a cancer is defined as the number of existing cases in the population at a point in time. The true prevalence of prostate cancer is unknown, but it is likely that if the incidental carcinomas found in simple prostatectomy specimens and at autopsy were counted (5 to 40 per cent in males over the age of 50), prostate cancer would be the most prevalent cancer in man.

The *mortality rate* of a cancer is defined as the number of cancer deaths caused per 100,000 population per year. The crude mortality rate for prostate cancer in the SEER study was 18.8 per 100,000 males per year (Young et al., 1981). Although only about one third of prostate cancers become clinically manifest during the patient's lifetime, because of the high prevalence of prostate cancer, the overall mortality associated with it is considerable. It was estimated that 24,100 men died from prostate cancer in the United States in 1983 (Silverberg and Lu-

bera, 1983). Prostate cancer ranks third among causes of cancer deaths in males after lung and colorectal cancer and accounts for approximately 10 per cent of all cancer deaths in American males (Silverberg and Lubera, 1983).

The mortality rate from prostate cancer also has increased over the years, but to a lesser extent than the incidence rate. This disparity between incidence and mortality rates has resulted in an apparent increase in the survival rate of prostate cancer patients that may be the result of better detection and reporting of prostate cancer cases as well as earlier and more effective treatment.

Etiology

Based upon epidemiologic observations, four factors have been suggested for the causation of prostate cancer: (1) genetic predisposition, (2) endogenous hormonal influences, (3) exposure to environmental chemical carcinogens, and (4) venereally transmitted infectious agents.

GENETIC FACTORS

Although several lines of evidence implicate genetic factors in the causation of prostate cancer, it is difficult to separate genetic factors from environmental factors and artifacts of reporting and classification.

Several studies (Woolf, 1960; Schuman et al., 1977) have reported a higher incidence of prostate cancer among relatives of prostate cancer patients; however, studies of HLA typing have not identified an association between any specific HLA haplotype and the occurrence of prostate cancer (Barry et al., 1980).

Significant national (Fig. 32–1) and racial (Fig. 32–2) differences in the incidence and mortality from prostate cancer have been reported (Hutchison, 1981). For instance, northern European and North American countries have relatively high rates; Latin American, South American, and southern European countries have intermediate rates; and eastern European and Far Eastern countries have relatively low rates (Wynder et al., 1971). Some of these differences may be attributable to differences in detection and reporting of prostate cancer cases.

The age-corrected incidence and mortality of prostate cancer among American blacks is nearly 50 per cent higher than among Caucasians (Blair and Fraumeni, 1978) (Fig. 32–2). It has been reported that American blacks develop prostate cancer at an earlier age than whites (Levine and Wilchinsky, 1979) and tend to present with a higher stage of disease. In contrast, American Indians, Orientals, and Hispanics have a significantly lower age-corrected incidence of prostate cancer than whites (Creagen and Fraumeni, 1972; Fraumeni and Mason, 1974; Menck et al., 1975).

In contrast to the striking racial and national differences in the incidence of clinically manifest prostate cancer, most studies suggest that the prevalence of incidental prostate cancer found at autopsy is similar among all races and in most countries (Hutchison, 1981). These results suggest that differences in the incidence of prostate cancers may exist only in the clinically manifest form of the disease. However, some studies (Breslow et al., 1977; Yatani et al., 1982) suggest that even latent prostate cancer is less prevalent among Orientals than among blacks or whites.

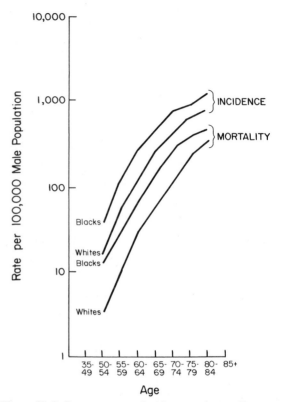

Figure 32–2. Prostate cancer incidence and mortality rates per 100,000 males for blacks and whites in the United States. (From Cutler, S. J., and Young, J. L., Jr.: Natl. Cancer Inst. Monogr., *41*:1975. Modified from Winkelstein and Ernster, 1981, and from Catalona, W. J.: Prostate Cancer. New York, Grune & Stratton, 1984. Used by permission.)

Differences in mortality from prostate cancer also have been reported among various religious groups, with Protestants having the highest mortality rate, Catholics having an intermediate rate, and Jews having the lowest rate (Winkelstein and Ernster, 1979).

HORMONAL FACTORS

Several observations suggest that hormonal factors may be etiologically important in the development of prostate cancer. These include: (1) the androgen dependence of most prostate cancers, (2) the fact that prostate cancer does not occur in eunuchs, (3) the fact that prostate cancer can be induced in Noble rats by the chronic administration of estrogen and androgen (Noble, 1977), and (4) the frequent histologic association of prostate cancer with areas of sclerotic prostatic atrophy (Moore, 1936).

Although some investigators have reported abnormalities of sex steroid metabolism in prostate cancer patients (lower androgen and higher estrogen levels), no consistent pattern of abnor-

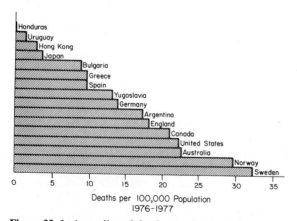

Figure 32–1. Age-adjusted death rates from prostate cancer per 100,000 males for selected countries. (From Silverberg, E., and Lubera, J. A.: CA, *33*:2, 1983; and from Catalona, W. J.: Prostate Cancer. New York, Grune & Stratton, 1984. Used by permission.)

mal steroid metabolism has been established (Zumoff et al., 1982).

Other indirect epidemiologic evidence suggesting a possible link between endocrine factors and prostate cancer includes reports of a significant correlation between the incidence of prostate cancer and breast cancer in different countries (Blair and Fraumeni, 1978), that fertile males have an increased incidence of prostate cancer (Armenian et al., 1975), and that patients with benign prostatic hyperplasia (BPH) are at an increased risk to develop prostate cancer (Armenian et al., 1974). All of these observations have been challenged (Wynder et al., 1971; Greenwald et al., 1974b; Winkelstein et al., 1977).

In regard to the relationship to BPH, Armenian and associates (1974) reported that patients having BPH were at an increased risk of developing prostate cancer as compared with age-matched controls. In contrast, Greenwald and associates (1974b) reported that BPH patients were not at an increased risk for prostate cancer. In Armenian's study, the diagnosis of BPH was made on clinical grounds alone in nearly one half of patients, whereas in Greenwald's study, it was made on histologic examination of a prostatectomy specimen in all patients. Thus, it is likely that more of Armenian's patients had occult prostate cancer that later became clinically manifest while most patients with occult prostate cancer were excluded from Greenwald's study. This suggests that patients having BPH are *not* at an increased risk to develop prostate cancer.

The weight of evidence suggests that the most important role of hormonal factors in the causation of prostate cancer may be a permissive one in which androgen is necessary to sustain the prostatic epithelium, but neoplastic transformation is induced by other mechanisms (Franks, 1973).

ENVIRONMENTAL FACTORS

Perhaps the most compelling evidence suggesting the etiologic importance of environmental factors in prostate cancer is the observation that migrants from low to high incidence areas maintain a low incidence of prostate cancer for one generation and then assume an intermediate incidence. This pattern has been reported in both Japanese (Dunn, 1975) and European (Staszewski and Haenszel, 1965) immigrants to the United States.

Minor regional variations in mortality from prostate cancer also have been reported within the United States (Blair and Fraumeni, 1978).

These differences in mortality could be due to genetic factors, environmental factors, or differences in mortality reporting.

A slightly higher mortality from prostate cancer has been reported among men living in urban environments, which appears to be more prominent among blacks. However, there is no significant correlation between socioeconomic status and the risk of developing prostate cancer (Blair and Fraumeni, 1978).

Several environmental factors have been identified from epidemiologic studies that suggest a possible etiologic role for chemical carcinogens or promoters in prostate cancer. These include exposure to automobile exhaust fumes, particulate air pollution, cadmium, fertilizer, and chemicals in the rubber, printing, painting, and shipfitting industries (Winkelstein and Ernster, 1979). It has been claimed that some of these epidemiologic studies have not been adequately controlled; therefore, the validity of these associations may be open to question. Several studies have demonstrated that prostate cancer is not associated with cigarette smoking (Wynder et al., 1971). Ingestion of a high-fat diet has been claimed to be associated with an increased risk of prostate cancer (Blair and Fraumeni, 1978).

INFECTIOUS AGENTS

An etiologic role for venereally transmitted infectious agents has been postulated for prostate cancer; however, epidemiologic, virologic, and immunologic studies have yielded conflicting results. Epidemiologic studies have suggested an increased risk for prostate cancer in association with an increasing number of sexual partners, prior history of venereal disease, frequency of sexual intercourse, use of prostitutes, extramarital sexual relationships, and an early age at onset of sexual activity (Steele et al., 1971; Schuman et al., 1977). In contrast, Rotkin's (1977) studies suggest that there is an increased risk for prostate cancer in association with repression of sexual activity, such as delayed onset, earlier peak, and premature cessation of sexual activity. Similarly, some studies have reported an increased risk among patients who were never married, and an even greater risk among those who fathered children (Schuman et al., 1977), but other studies (Wynder et al., 1971) have shown no significant correlation with marital status or the number of children. In fact, Ross and associates (1981) reported that Catholic priests had a slightly higher incidence of prostate cancer than controls. These conflicting results have not been satisfactorily resolved.

Studies of potential infectious agents similarly have yielded inconclusive results and do not make a strong case for an infectious cause of prostate cancer. Paulson and associates (1968) demonstrated that a DNA virus, SV-40, could induce neoplastic transformation of hamster prostate cells in vitro. Moreover, SV-40–neutralizing antibodies were reported in the serum of some prostate cancer patients. Nevertheless, there is no compelling evidence for a causal association between the SV-40 virus and human prostate cancer.

Centifano and associates (1973) demonstrated a herpes simplex type 2 virus by electron microscopy in a human prostate cancer. This virus could induce neoplastic transformation in vitro in hamster embryo cells. Herbert and associates (1976) reported that antibodies against herpes virus were present in 70 per cent of prostate cancer patients but also were present in 66 per cent of BPH patients. In contrast, Baker and associates (1981) reported that antibodies against herpes virus were more prevalent among prostate cancer patients than BPH patients.

Lang et al. (1974) demonstrated the presence of another DNA virus, cytomegalovirus (CMV), in human semen, and Sanford and associates (1977) isolated a strain of CMV that could induce neoplastic transformation of human cells in vitro. These transformed cells expressed CMV antigens. However, only 2 of 34 human prostate cancers tested expressed CMV antigens.

Evidence suggesting a possible role for RNA viruses also has been reported. Farnsworth (1973) reported that reverse transcriptase activity was present in human prostate cancer tissue, but this observation has not yet been confirmed. Dmochowski and associates (1975) reported C-type viral particles in three of 34 prostate cancers examined. Similarly, Ohtsuki and associates (1977) reported RNA virus-like particles in human prostate cancers. McCombs (1977) reported that RNA tumor virus core protein could be detected in both human BPH and prostate cancer tissue. Together, these reports provide little more than circumstantial evidence for a possible viral cause of prostate cancer.

Several epidemiologic studies have suggested a link between prostate cancer and venereal infections. Heshmat and associates (1975) compared the curve for prostate cancer deaths in Denmark with that of the incidence of gonorrhea and found that the curves matched well with a lag period of about 45 years. In contrast, Wynder and associates (1971) failed to confirm this association.

A high incidence of prostatitis in surgical specimens removed for prostate cancer has been reported (Wynder et al., 1971), while a significantly higher incidence of prostatic calculi has been found in prostate cancer patients than in controls. Nevertheless, it is undetermined whether prostatic calculi or infections play a significant etiologic role in prostate cancer.

PATHOLOGY

Classification of Prostate Cancers

The normal prostate is composed of acinar glands and their ducts arranged in a radial fashion within a fibromuscular stroma that contains blood vessels, lymphatics, and nerves. Normal prostatic acini are lined with a columnar epithelium two cell layers thick (Fig. 32–3). The peripheral prostatic ducts are lined with a single layer of cuboidal cells, whereas the central ducts are lined with a transitional cell epithelium that merges with the epithelium of the prostatic urethra.

The World Health Organization (WHO) classification of malignant tumors of the prostate gland is presented in Table 32–1. More than 95 per cent of prostate cancers are acinar adenocarcinomas (Halpert et al., 1963; Byar, 1972).

Acinar Adenocarcinoma

HISTOLOGIC DIAGNOSIS OF PROSTATE CANCER

Prostate cancers may exhibit a variety of abnormal histologic features, any of which may be absent and not all of which when present alone are sufficient to establish the diagnosis of prostate cancer. In a strict sense, the term "differentiation" refers to the degree of retention of the normal prostatic glandular pattern. The size and shape of the prostatic acini are almost always altered in prostate cancers and some cancers do not form acini. Generally, malignant acini tend to be small and closely packed with little interposed stroma between them. Some cancers may contain giant convoluted acini and tiny microacini. (Fig. 32–4A). Eosinophilic crystalloids are present within malignant acini in about one third of prostate cancers, particularly in well-differentiated tumors (Holmes, 1977). These crystalloids rarely appear in benign prostatic tissue.

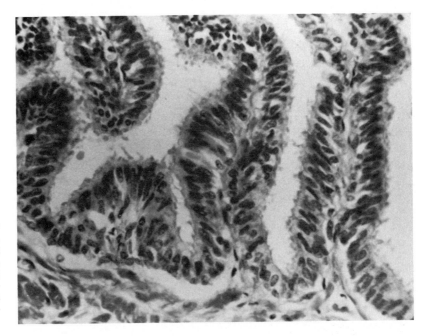

Figure 32–3. Normal prostatic acinar epithelium. (From Mostofi, F. K., et al.: Histological typing of prostate tumors. Geneva, World Health Organization, 1980; and from Catalona, W. J.: Prostate Cancer. New York, Grune & Stratton, 1984. Used by permission.)

The histologic architecture of the prostate frequently is disrupted in prostate cancer. Normally, the acini are distributed in a linear pattern radiating from the prostatic urethra. Malignant acini may grow in a random, irregular pattern, and in some cancers there may be little or no differentiation of epithelial cells into glands. Rather, the cancer cells diffusely infiltrate the prostatic stroma (Fig. 32–4*E* and *F*).

TABLE 32–1. World Health Organization Histologic Classification of Malignant Prostate Tumors

Epithelial
  Adenocarcinoma
    Small acinar
    Large acinar
    Cribriform
    Solid/trabecular
    Others (including endometrioid, papillary, papillary cystadenocarcinoma, mucinous, adenoid cystic)
  Transitional; cell carcinoma
  Squamous cell carcinoma
  Undifferentiated carcinoma
Nonepithelial
  Rhabdomyosarcoma
  Leiomyosarcoma
  Others (including fibrosarcoma, malignant fibrous histiocytoma)
Miscellaneous
  Carcinoid
  Carcinosarcoma
  Malignant melanoma
  Phyllode tumor

From Catalona, W. J.: Prostate Cancer New York, Grune & Stratton, 1984 (with permission).

The internal architecture of malignant acini also is deranged. Whereas normal acini are lined with columnar epithelium two cell layers thick, malignant acini usually are lined with only a single layer of low cuboidal epithelium (Fig. 32–4*A* and *C*) or may exhibit proliferation of the acinar epithelium to produce a cribriform pattern (Fig. 32–5). These abnormalities of the acinar epithelium alone are not sufficient to establish the diagnosis of cancer, since noncancerous prostatic tissues also may exhibit atypical acinar epithelial hyperplasia (Tannenbaum, 1974). The term "prostatic adenosis" has been used to describe these dysplastic glandular patterns (Brawn, 1982). Some pathologists have referred to acinar epithelial abnormalities in the absence of invasion of the stroma as carcinoma in situ, whereas other pathologists feel that they are early invasive cancers (Mostofi and Price, 1973). Brawn (1982) reported that patients having prostatic adenosis had the same likelihood of developing clinical manifestations of prostate cancer as patients having benign prostatic hyperplasia.

Prostate cancer cells commonly invade the perineural spaces of the prostate. Perineural invasion is an important criterion for establishing the diagnosis of cancer, but is not of prognostic significance (Rodin et al., 1967). Similarly, juxtaposition of cancer cells and striated muscle fibers within the prostate does not indicate that capsular penetration of the tumor has occurred and is not of prognostic significance

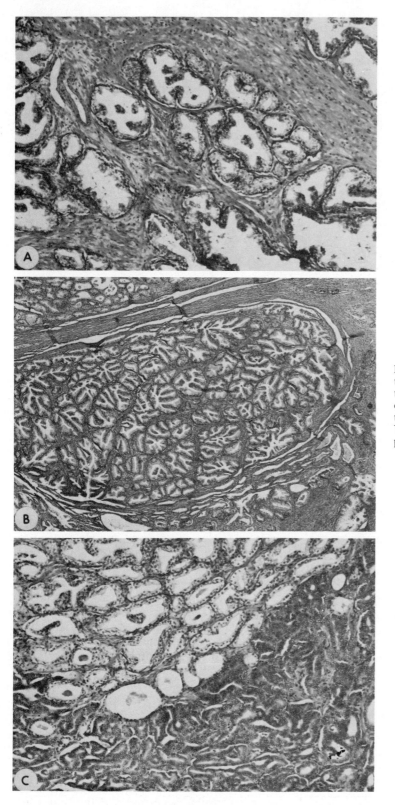

Figure 32–4. Different patterns of prostate cancer ranging from well differentiated to poorly differentiated, and all occurring in the same tumor. (From Catalona, W. J.: Prostate Cancer. New York, Grune & Stratton, 1984. Used by permission.)

Illustration continued on opposite page

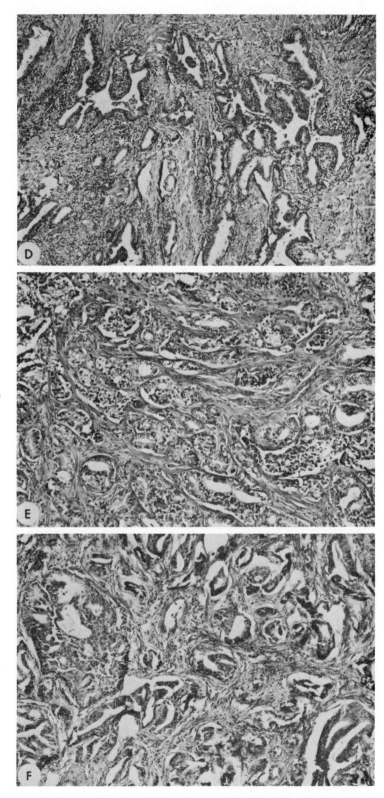

Figure 32–4 *(Continued)*

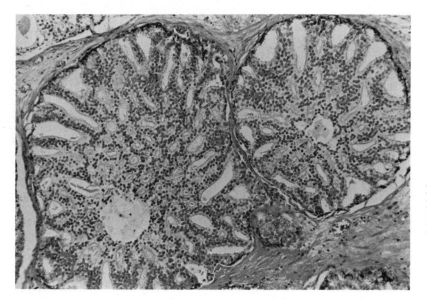

Figure 32–5. Cribriform pattern of prostate cancer. (From Mostofi, F. K., et al.: Histological typing of prostate tumors. Geneva, World Health Organization, 1980; and from Catalona, W. J.: Prostate Cancer. New York, Grune & Stratton, 1984. Used by permission.)

(Manley, 1966). However, the presence of cancer cells in endothelium-lined vascular or lymphatic spaces is an unfavorable prognostic sign (Mostofi and Price, 1973).

The term "anaplasia" refers to cytologic abnormalities of cancer cells including their nuclear characteristics and mitotic activity. Whereas normal prostatic epithelial cells are relatively uniform in size and have distinct cell borders, prostate cancer cells are pleomorphic with large nuclei, prominent eosinophilic nucleoli, and indistinct cell borders (Fig. 32–4*E* and *F*). Estrogen administration may produce squamous metaplasia of the prostatic ductal epithelium (Fig. 32–6).

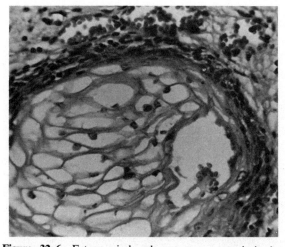

Figure 32–6. Estrogen-induced squamous metaplasia in prostate cancer. (From Mostofi, F. K., et al.: Histological typing of prostate tumors. Geneva, World Health Organization, 1980; and from Catalona, W. J.: Prostate Cancer. New York, Grune & Stratton, 1984. Used by permission.)

Histochemical studies are of limited value in prostate cancer patients. Immunohistochemical stains for prostatic acid phosphatase and prostate-specific antigen may be helpful in determining whether a tumor is of prostatic origin (Allhoff et al., 1983; Venable et al., 1983); however, falsely positive and falsely negative results have been reported using these techniques (Venable et al., 1983).

GRADING SYSTEMS

Most grading systems for prostate cancer are based on the appearance and arrangement of the malignant glands or the degree of anaplasia of the cancer cells, or both. Several different histologic features have independent prognostic importance. For example, the glandular pattern (Utz and Farrow, 1969; Gleason et al., 1974), the degree of nuclear anaplasia (Mostofi, 1976), and the distinctness of cell borders (Epstein and Fatti, 1976) are at least partially independent variables that correlate with cancer death rates. Moreover, because nearly 50 per cent of prostate cancers express more than one histologic pattern, it has been necessary to consider whether the assigned grade should be that of the predominant histologic pattern, the worst pattern, or the average pattern. Grading systems that attempt to take many or all of these variables into consideration involve a large number of possible combinations that makes grading complex. Accordingly, many pathologists simply grade prostate cancers as well, moderately, or poorly differentiated, claiming that simplified grading systems provide as much prognostic discrimination as more complex systems and are more reproducible.

The recent literature on prostate cancer contains frequent references to several different grading systems. The Gleason (1977) system considers only the degree of glandular differentiation and the relationship of the glands to the prostatic stroma under low-power magnification. Cellular anaplasia is not considered. The Gleason system includes five different histologic grades (Fig. 32–7). Because many tumors exhibit more than one grade, the predominant grade based on tumor area is called the primary grade and the less representative grade is called the secondary grade. Although there is a significant correlation between mortality rates and both the primary and secondary Gleason grades, mortality rates of patients having two different grades are intermediate between those of patients with homogeneous tumors of the two grades. Therefore, with the Gleason system, the primary and secondary grades are added together to obtain the Gleason histologic score. Homogeneous tumors are given the same primary and secondary grades to maintain uniformity. Accordingly, Gleason scores range from 2 to 10.

Gleason et al., (1974) also combined tumor score and tumor stage (Stage A = 1, B = 2, C = 3, D = 5) to yield a tumor category ranging from 3 to 15 that was more predictive of cancer mortality than either tumor score or tumor stage alone. The principal criticisms of the Gleason system are that it is of limited reproducibility when interpreted by the same individual at different points in time and between different individuals (Harada et al., 1977), and that while it has prognostic significance for groups of patients, it is not prognostically accurate for individual patients.

The Mostofi (1976) grading system takes cellular anaplasia into consideration as well as the glandular pattern and the relationship of the glands to the stroma. The Mostofi system groups tumors into three grades: Grade 1 tumors form glands and the cells exhibit only slight nuclear anaplasia; Grade 2 tumors also form glands, but there is moderate nuclear anaplasia; and Grade 3 tumors either do not form glands or form glands in which there is marked nuclear anaplasia. Mostofi and associates (Harada et al., 1977) claim that this grading system provides as good a prognostic index as the Gleason system.

The Gaeta grading system (Gaeta et al., 1980) also considers both the glandular pattern and cellular anaplasia. Tumors are grouped into four grades. The tumor is graded according to the worst elements present in at least one third of the specimen. This grading system also correlates well with cancer death rates.

The Mayo Clinic grading system (Utz and Farrow, 1969) considers acinar structure, cellular structure, nuclear characteristics, presence of nucleoli, cytoplasmic characteristics, mitotic activity, and the degree of invasiveness. Tumors are graded one to four, according to their predominant features. Pool and Thompson (1956) reported that the Mayo Clinic grading system correlated with patient survival.

The M.D. Anderson Hospital grading system (Brawn and associates, 1982) is based upon the percentage of the tumor that forms glands. Tumors are grouped into three major categories. Brawn and associates (1982) claimed that this system was more accurate in predicting patient survival than either the Gleason or Mostofi systems.

Diamond and associates (1982) used computer-assisted image analysis of histologic sections of prostate cancers to grade tumors based on nuclear roundness. Using this grading system in patients having clinical Stage B prostate cancers treated with radical prostatectomy, Diamond and associates (1982) could distinguish tumors with a high metastatic potential from those with a low metastatic potential without overlap and with greater accuracy than the Gleason system.

A theoretical limitation of grading prostate cancers based on needle biopsy specimens is that they may not be representative of the entire tumor (Catalona et al., 1982b; Lange and Narayan, 1983). In most instances, however, grading errors are of little clinical significance and

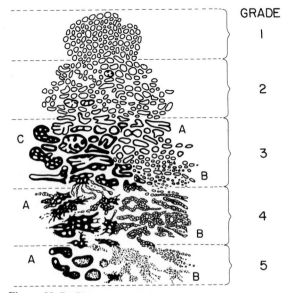

Figure 32–7. Gleason system for grading prostate cancer. (From Gleason, D. F.: *In* Tannenbaum, M. (Ed.): Urologic Pathology: The Prostate. Philadelphia, Lea & Febiger, 1977. Used by permission.)

do not materially reduce the prognostic significance of tumor grade (Catalona et al., 1982b).

Fine-needle aspiration biopsies of prostate cancers also can be graded in a meaningful fashion (Esposti, 1971). Fine-needle aspiration biopsies contain small tumor fragments as well as individual prostate cancer cells (Fig. 32–8). Grading of the cytologic aspirates is based on the appearance of the tumor fragments, the tendency of the tumor to dissociate into single cells, and the degree of anaplasia in individual cells. Generally, cancer cells are less cohesive and tend to have large nuclei with prominent nucleoli. Fine-needle aspiration biopsies of well-differentiated cancers show well-organized microadenomatous complexes with infrequent single cells exhibiting little nuclear pleomorphism and inconspicuous nucleoli. Moderately differentiated prostate cancers have more dissociated single cells that exhibit more nuclear pleomorphism. Poorly differentiated cancers are almost entirely dissociated into single cells that have pleomorphic nuclei with prominent nucleoli. Correlations between tumor grade on fine-needle aspiration biopsies and cutting needle biopsies have been good in Scandinavian series (Esposti, 1971) but less accurate in reports from other countries (Lin et al., 1979).

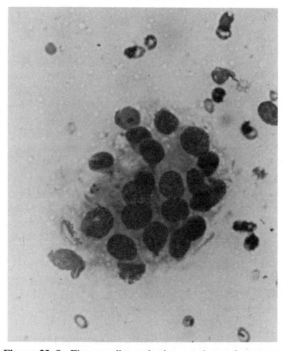

Figure 32–8. Fine needle aspiration cytology of prostate cancer. (From Catalona, W. J.: Prostate Cancer. New York, Grune & Stratton, 1984. Used by permission.)

Ductal Carcinomas

Ductal carcinomas account for less than 5 per cent of all prostate cancers. A spectrum of histologic changes occurs in prostatic ductal epithelium including atypia, hyperplasia, carcinoma in situ, papillary carcinoma, and invasive carcinoma. There are four types of intraductal carcinomas: (1) transitional cell carcinoma (including squamous cell carcinoma), (2) intraductal adenocarcinoma, (3) mixed ductal carcinoma, and (4) endometrioid carcinoma (Catalona et al., 1978). Mott (1979) postulated that squamous cell carcinomas are a metaplastic variant of transitional cell carcinoma. Clinically, transitional cell and squamous cell carcinomas behave similarly (Mostofi and Price, 1973). These tumors arise from the central prostatic ducts. Urinary cytologic examinations are frequently positive in patients having ductal carcinoma, and hematuria is a common presenting symptom. Acid phosphatase titers generally are normal (Johnson et al., 1972a; Greene et al., 1973), and these tumors do not respond to androgen-withdrawal therapy. Most reports suggest that transitional cell and squamous cell cancers behave aggressively, metastasizing to lymph nodes and lungs as nodular metastases and to bone as osteolytic metastases. The vast majority of patients afflicted ultimately succumb to cancer.

Cystoprostatectomy is the preferred treatment for patients having ductal carcinomas that are localized to the prostate (Wolfe and Lloyd-Davies, 1981); radiation therapy has yielded some favorable results in patients with clinical Stage C tumors (Kopelson et al., 1978). There is no known effective therapy for patients having distant metastases other than the standard chemotherapy for transitional and squamous cell carcinomas involving other sites.

Intraductal adenocarcinomas arise from the columnar epithelium of the peripheral prostatic ducts. These tumors may fill the prostatic ducts, producing the histologic pattern of comedocarcinoma. Some patients having intraductal carcinomas had elevated levels of acid phosphatase (Dube et al., 1973; Melicow and Uson, 1976), and although some patients may respond to hormonal therapy (Young and Lagios, 1973), most intraductal adenocarcinomas are not androgen-dependent (Dube et al., 1973; Rhamey et al., 1973). The prognosis for patients with intraductal adenocarcinoma is worse than that of patients with acinar adenocarcinoma.

Mixed ductal carcinomas contain either

mixtures of malignant ductal elements or mixtures of malignant ductal and acinar elements. These tumors exhibit the clinical properties of their constituent elements (Dube et al., 1973).

Endometrioid carcinomas are papillary tumors that arise in the prostatic urethra near the veru montanum. These tumors are histologically similar to endometrial carcinomas in women. Originally Melicow and Pachter (1967) postulated that they arose from müllerian ductal tissue. Accordingly, it was suggested that estrogen therapy was contraindicated and progesterone therapy was recommended (Melicow and Tannenbaum, 1971). More recent reports (Young and Lagios, 1973; Zaloudek et al., 1976) question the utricular origin of endometrioid tumors. These reports cite regression of endometrioid cancers following orchiectomy and provide histochemical evidence of acid phosphatase production in endometrioid cancer cells. Some patients with endometrioid tumors had elevated serum acid phosphatase titers. Moreover, ultrastructural studies reveal histologic similarities between normal prostatic tissues and endometrioid carcinomas. Accordingly, it is currently believed that endometrioid tumors are of prostatic ductal origin.

Generally, endometrioid carcinomas behave in a more indolent fashion than acinar carcinomas. Cystoprostatectomy is recommended for patients having tumors confined to the prostate. External-beam radiation therapy may be effective in some patients with Stage C disease. Androgen-withdrawal therapy may be beneficial in some patients with Stage D disease. Lanesky and associates (1979) reported on one patient who had a partial tumor regression in response to combination chemotherapy with 5-fluorouracil and doxorubicin.

Carcinosarcoma

Carcinosarcomas compose the remaining malignant epithelial tumors of the prostate. These tumors contain both malignant epithelial and mesenchymal elements, including chondrosarcoma, rhabdomyosarcoma, osteosarcoma, fibrosarcoma, or mixtures of these elements (Hamlin and Lund, 1967; Haddad and Reyes, 1970; Martin et al., 1979; Krastonova and Addonizio, 1981). In general, serum acid phosphatase levels are normal in patients with carcinosarcoma and endocrine therapy is without benefit. Often these tumors metastasize as nodular pulmonary metastases. Generally, the prog-

nosis is poor. Anterior pelvic exenteration offers the best chance for cure if the tumor is confined to the prostate. Radiation, hormonal, and endocrine therapy generally are ineffective.

The prostate may be secondarily involved by other tumors, especially lymphoreticular malignancies (Blank and Hodges, 1980). The most common solid tumors metastasizing to the prostate are lung cancer and malignant melanoma (Johnson et al., 1974).

PATTERNS OF DISSEMINATION

Prostate cancer spreads by direct local invasion and through vascular and lymphatic channels. Based on histopathologic studies of radical prostatectomy specimens, Byar and Mostofi (1972) postulated that prostate cancers have a multicentric origin, usually within the periphery of the gland. Because the prostatic capsule provides a barrier to invading cancer cells, prostate cancers spread first centrally, then penetrate the capsule and invade along the perivesicular sheath and bladder base, where the invading cancer may obstruct the ureters. Ureteral obstruction occurs in 10 to 35 per cent of prostate cancer patients (Michigan and Catalona, 1977; Kihl and Bratt, 1981), but direct extension to the rectum is rare (Winter, 1957). In some patients the urogenital diaphragm is invaded by the cancer, which renders the patient more vulnerable to urinary incontinence if transurethral resection of the prostate is performed.

The primary field of lymphatic drainage of the prostate includes the perivesical, hypogastric, obturator, presacral, and presciatic lymph nodes. The obturator nodes are the commonest site of involvement (Hilaris et al., 1974; McLaughlin et al., 1976). The secondary field of lymphatic drainage includes the inguinal, common iliac, and para-aortic nodes. The tertiary field includes the mediastinal and supraclavicular nodes. It is rare for juxtaregional lymph nodes to be involved in the absence of regional involvement.

Osseous metastases, which are present in about 85 per cent of patients dying of prostate cancer (Jacobs, 1983), are the commonest form of hematogenous metastases from prostate cancer. Osseous metastases have a predilection for the axial skeleton. The most frequent sites of skeletal involvement, in decreasing order of frequency, are the lumbar spine, proximal femur, pelvis, thoracic spine, ribs, sternum, skull, and humerus (Willis, 1973). In the past it was postulated that this distribution occurred because cancer cells were disseminated from the prostate through the vertebral venous plexus (Batson, 1940); however, recent studies suggest that tumors of nonprostatic origin produce the same distribution of osseous metastases (Dodds et al., 1981).

Osseous metastases involve the cancellous bone, altering the normal internal architecture with proliferating osteoblasts and new bone formation (Jacobs, 1983). These lesions frequently cause pain and may produce pathologic fractures. In the spine, metastases usually occur in the vertebral bodies and may cause spinal cord compression. Pathologic fractures in the femoral neck result in loss of ambulation and may require internal fixation.

The commonest sites of visceral metastases from prostate cancer are lung, liver, and adrenal gland, but virtually any organ may be involved. Pulmonary metastases, occurring in 25 to 38 per cent of patients dying of prostate cancer (Legge et al., 1971; Falkowski and O'Connor, 1981), often go unrecognized because they occur as microscopic nodules or lymphangitic infiltrates. These lesions can produce a cor pulmonale syndrome with respiratory insufficiency.

Central nervous system involvement in prostate cancer patients usually is secondary to osseous involvement. Metastases to the central nervous system usually occur in the meninges and may be clinically silent. Other neurologic manifestations of prostate cancer include organic brain syndrome, radiculopathy, and paraneoplastic syndromes (Campbell et al., 1981).

It has been speculated that prostate cancer disseminates first by invading into the periprostatic tissues, then by lymphatic embolization, and finally by hematogenous dissemination. However, the actual sequence of dissemination is unknown. While most patients having lymph node metastases also have local extraprostatic tumor extension, some exceptions to this pattern have been reported (Catalona and Stein, 1982a). Similarly, most patients having distant metastases also have lymph node metastases or local tumor extension (Varkarakis et al., 1975).

Whitmore (1973) postulated that prostate cancers may not progress in a steplike fashion from the prostate to the periprostatic tissues to the lymph nodes to distant sites (Fig. 32–9). Clinical evidence supports this hypothesis. Some cancers may metastasize directly to lymph nodes or other distant sites without the prior occurrence of direct local tumor extension.

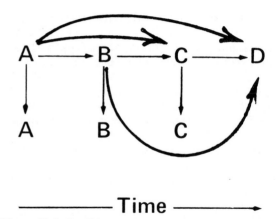

Figure 32–9. Possible patterns of progression of prostate cancer. (From Whitmore, W. F., Jr.: Cancer, *32*:1104, 1973. Used by permission.)

NATURAL HISTORY

The natural history of prostate cancer is variable and unpredictable. Some prostate cancers have a malignant potential so great that metastases occur before there are local signs or symptoms, whereas others are so indolent that they remain localized for the duration of the patient's life without producing symptoms. It is self-evident that the clinical evolution of cancers such as these will not be influenced by curative therapy. This has engendered in some clinicians a nihilistic view of prostate cancer in which it is considered that patients having biologically favorable tumors will fare well and patients having unfavorable tumors will not fare well, regardless of treatment. However, between these extremes of malignant potential may be a spectrum of prostate cancers, some of which have a significant malignant potential but may remain localized long enough to be influenced by curative therapy.

The natural history of a tumor is the result of host-tumor interactions. Attempts have been made to identify host and tumor characteristics that could be used to predict how the host-tumor interactions will affect the quality and duration of an individual patient's life. Considerably more is known about tumor factors than host factors in prostate cancer patients.

Three host factors—race, age, and immune competence—have been postulated to influence the natural history of prostate cancers. The incidence of prostate cancer is higher among American blacks as compared with whites, Orientals, and Hispanics, and prostate cancer tends to occur at an earlier age and is diagnosed in more advanced stages among blacks (Levine and Wilchinsky, 1979; Murphy et al., 1982). Several reports suggest that prostate cancer tends to behave more aggressively in blacks (Burbank and Fraumeni, 1972; Hutchison, 1975); however, most of these reports did not control for tumor stage, tumor grade, or treatment. The available controlled data reveal no striking differences in the behavior of clinically manifest prostate cancers among races when compared by stage, grade, and treatment (Levine and Wilchinsky, 1979).

There are conflicting opinions about whether prostate cancer is more lethal in young patients (Rosenberg, 1965; Tjaden et al., 1965; Byar and Mostofi, 1969; Johnson et al., 1972a; Cochran and Kadesky, 1981a). The results of the American College of Surgeons Survey (Huben et al., 1982; Murphy et al., 1982) revealed that patients under 50 years of age presented in more advanced stages of prostate cancer, principally because they had a lower incidence of incidentally discovered Stage A tumors. In this survey, the only significant difference was that patients under the age of 50 with Stage B tumors had a better survival rate than did Stage B patients over the age of 50. This higher survival rate may have been due to the fact that a greater proportion of younger patients were treated with radical prostatectomy. Otherwise, stage for stage and grade for grade, the prostate cancers behaved similarly among patients of all ages.

There are inconclusive data on the relationship between host immune competence and prognosis in prostate cancer patients. The available data suggest that in patients not receiving endocrine therapy and those whose tumors have relapsed after endocrine therapy, there is a correlation between immunocompetence and prognosis (Catalona et al., 1975).

Several tumor characteristics—growth rate, metastatic potential, and intrinsic responsiveness to treatment—have been postulated to influence the natural history of prostate cancers. Growth rate and metastatic potential are not completely independent variables. Tumors that have a high growth rate generally also have a high metastatic potential. Moreover, both of these variables also are partially linked to the tumor stage at the time of diagnosis.

Tumor grade reflects both the growth rate and the metastatic potential of a prostate cancer. The correlation between tumor grade and tumor stage has been examined as a potential means of predicting the natural history of prostate cancers in individual patients. For instance, it was suggested that the Gleason grade of a tumor may be used to identify patients having a high likelihood of having pelvic lymph node metastases (nearly 100 per cent in patients with Gleason 8–10) and those with a low likelihood (nearly zero per cent with Gleason 2–4) (Kramer et al., 1980; Paulson, 1980). However, subsequent studies (Smith and Middleton, 1982; Sagalowsky et al., 1982) have shown that in the vast majority of patients, Gleason grade alone is not sufficiently accurate to predict whether or not lymph node metastases are present. For example, Smith and Middleton (1982) reported that only about one third of patients having high Gleason grade tumors that were small (Stage B1) had lymph node metastases, whereas nearly one half of patients having low Gleason grade tumors that were large (Stage C) had nodal metastases.

Diamond and associates (1982) reported in a preliminary study that tumor grade as determined by computerized assessment of nuclear roundness provides a highly accurate prognosticator of subsequent treatment failure in patients having clinical Stage B prostate cancer who were treated with radical prostatectomy. Nonetheless, it remains to be demonstrated whether any morphologic feature of a tumor can provide an accurate estimate of the extent to which the tumor has realized its metastatic potential.

Tumor ploidy is another tumor characteristic that has been examined as a means of predicting the natural history of prostate cancers. Tavares and associates (1973) reported that patients having tumors with either a diploid or tetraploid karyotype had a favorable prognosis and a high response rate to endocrine therapy, whereas patients having triploid or hexaploid tumors had a worse prognosis and a lower response rate to endocrine therapy. However, in this study, no data on tumor grade or stage were provided. Therefore, it is not possible to determine whether tumor ploidy was an independent prognostic variable.

The ultimate clinical test of the metastatic potential of a prostate cancer is staging pelvic lymphadenectomy; however, even this test is of limited value. If no lymph node metastases are found, the presence of metastases in nodes not encompassed by the dissection or the presence of occult hematogenous metastases cannot be ruled out.

There are no known valid markers to determine the radiation sensitivity of a prostate cancer. It has been reported that undifferentiated tumors are more radiation-sensitive (McLoughlin et al., 1975), but in most series, patients having undifferentiated tumors responded poorly to radiation therapy. This is probably more a reflection of the biologic aggressiveness of high-grade tumors than their intrinsic lack of radiation sensitivity. It also has been postulated that tumors having lower levels of catalase activity may be more radiation-sensitive (McLoughlin et al., 1975), but this speculation has not been confirmed.

Measurement of nuclear androgen receptor content is predictive of the intrinsic responsiveness to androgen-withdrawal therapy in some prostate cancer patients. It is well established that for a target cell to be influenced by a steroid hormone, it must contain an intracellular receptor protein for that hormone. However, the mere presence of the receptor protein does not assure a response to the hormone. Clinical studies of prostate cancer patients (discussed further under Endocrine Therapy) have demonstrated that if dihydrotestosterone receptors are present in sufficient amounts in the tumor, a favorable response to androgen-withdrawal therapy will occur in most patients. If the receptor protein is absent or is present in only small quantities, a favorable clinical response will not occur (Trachtenberg and Walsh, 1982).

In order to evaluate the effectiveness of any treatment for prostate cancer, it is essential to know the natural history of each stage of the disease in untreated patients. Accurate information concerning the natural history of prostate cancers is not available. Nonetheless, it is useful to consider the reported cancer progression and cancer death rates for the various stages of prostate cancer in patients who either were not treated or were treated conservatively with endocrine therapy. It should be stressed, however, that these cancer progression and death rates represent crude estimates only and may have been influenced by tumor grade and the age and general medical condition of the patients.

In patients having clinical Stage A1 prostate cancer, approximately 8 per cent develop distant metastases and 2 per cent die of prostate cancer within 5 to 10 years (Correa et al., 1974; Heaney et al., 1977; Cantrell et al., 1981). Accordingly, older patients having Stage A1 prostate cancer do not require immediate treatment. This recommendation is less certain in younger patients who may be at risk for cancer progression longer

and in whom the first evidence of cancer progression may be distant metastases.

In patients having clinical Stage A2 tumors, approximately 30 per cent develop distant metastases and nearly 20 per cent die of prostate cancer within 5 to 10 years (Correa et al., 1974; Heaney et al., 1977; Cantrell et al., 1981). Accordingly, definitive treatment is indicated in most patients having Stage A2 tumors.

In patients with clinical Stage B1 tumors, approximately 35 per cent develop metastases within 5 years and 20 per cent die of prostate cancer (Cook and Watson, 1968; Chopp and Whitmore, 1980). Thus, definitive treatment also is appropriate in most patients having Stage B1 tumors.

In patients having clinical Stage B2 tumors, approximately 80 per cent develop distant metastases within 5 to 10 years and 70 per cent die of prostate cancer (Hanash et al., 1973). These patients also require definitive treatment.

In patients with clinical Stage C prostate cancer, more than 50 per cent develop distant metastases within 5 years and 75 per cent die of prostate cancer within 10 years (Blackard et al., 1973).

In patients having Stage D1 tumors, approximately 85 per cent develop distant metastases within 5 years (Kramer et al., 1981; Bagshaw, 1982; Grossman et al., 1982; Scardino et al., 1982) and the majority die of cancer within 3 years of developing metastases.

In patients having Stage D2 prostate cancer, approximately 50 per cent die of prostate cancer within 3 years, 80 per cent within 5 years, and 90 per cent within 10 years (Blackard et al., 1973). Patients having either an elevated acid phosphatase, 25 per cent or more involvement of the proximal femurs, or pulmonary metastases have an even worse prognosis (Hovsepian et al., 1979).

In patients having tumors that have relapsed after adequate endocrine therapy, approximately 90 per cent die of prostate cancer within 2 years (Slack et al., 1980). Most die during the first year.

DIAGNOSIS

Signs and Symptoms

Early in the course of disease, prostate cancer may produce no symptoms. The only clinical evidence of cancer may be induration in the prostate on digital rectal examination. Induration is present in most prostate cancers, although in some it may be subtle.

The normal prostate is the size of a chestnut and has the consistency of the tip of the nose. Prostate cancer usually has a hard consistency and may produce a discrete nodule or a uniformly firm consistency of the gland. In patients having extracapsular tumor extension, the margins may become obscured and the seminal vesicles, which normally are not palpable, may become firm, enlarged, and fixed.

A substantial proportion of prostate cancer patients have bladder outlet obstructive symptoms, and up to 25 per cent of patients who present with acute urinary retention may have prostate cancer (Emmett et al., 1961). Prostate cancer also may be coincidentally associated with obstructive benign hyperplasia with the cancer *not* being the major cause of bladder outlet obstruction. In many such cases, cancer is not detected on rectal examination but rather is discovered on examination of prostatic tissue removed for presumed benign hyperplasia.

Hematuria is an uncommon presenting symptom of prostate cancer. When it occurs, hematuria is usually associated with obstruction or infection, or both. The presenting signs and symptoms of prostate cancer in many patients are related to distant metastases. These include bone pain, weight loss, anemia, shortness of breath, lymphedema, neurologic symptoms, and lymphadenopathy.

Biopsy of the Prostate

Prostatic biopsy is indicated in all patients having clinical suspicion of prostate cancer. In patients who have obstructive symptoms without any palpable evidence of prostate cancer, blind needle biopsy of the prostate is a low-yield procedure (Catalona, 1980). Only 50 to 75 per cent of prostatic nodules are found to contain cancer on biopsy (Grayhack and Bockrath, 1981). The remainder contain benign hyperplasia, prostatic calculi, chronic prostatitis, postoperative fibrosis, or prostatic infarction.

CORE NEEDLE BIOPSY

Core needle biopsy of the prostate via the transperineal or transrectal route using a Tru-Cut or Vim-Silverman needle currently is the preferred means of establishing the diagnosis of prostate cancer. However, in the American College of Surgeons survey (Murphy et al., 1982), core needle biopsy was used to diagnose prostate cancer in only 23 per cent of patients (10 per cent perineal and 13 per cent rectal).

The advantages of transrectal biopsy are that it allows more accurate needle placement into a prostatic nodule and does not require anesthesia. The disadvantages are that it is associated with a higher incidence of septic complications (5–38 per cent) and bleeding from hemorrhoidal vessels (Table 32–2). Blood cultures are positive in up to 85 per cent of patients immediately following transrectal biopsy, but the incidence of clinically manifest infection is considerably less (Table 32–2). There is conflicting evidence about whether mechanical cleansing of the rectum before biopsy reduces the incidence of post-biopsy sepsis (Rees et al., 1980; Sharpe et al., 1982). However, it is prudent to administer prophylactic antibiotics before transrectal biopsy (Dowlen et al., 1974; Crawford et al., 1982). In general, core needle biopsy is a safe procedure with an acceptable complication rate. Implantation of tumor cells along the needle biopsy tract is rare (Burkholder and Kaufman, 1966; Blackard et al., 1971).

In many patients, prostatic needle biopsy can be performed as an outpatient procedure. In patients having small lesions, it is desirable to have sufficient anesthesia and sedation to allow several cores of tissue to be obtained if necessary. In general, however, it is desirable to obtain only enough cores to establish the diagnosis of cancer, since each pass of the needle carries a risk of infection and hemorrhage. Needle biopsies have a 10 per cent false negative rate (Zincke et al., 1973).

In performing transrectal biopsy (Fig. 32–10), the needle is inserted into the rectum along the volar aspect of the index finger. The needle tip is advanced until it abuts against the prostatic nodule. With the Vim-Silverman needle, the obturator is withdrawn and the cutting blades are inserted and advanced into the prostate. The outer sheath is then advanced over the cutting blades and twisted. The cutting blades are removed and the jaws are separated to remove the tissue. With the Tru-Cut needle, the procedure is similar but the cutting action is different.

Transperineal needle biopsy has a lower complication rate, but bimanual triangulation is required to place the needle into the prostatic nodule (Fig. 32–11). Advocates of transperineal biopsy claim that once the technique has been mastered, it is as accurate as the transrectal approach. In performing transperineal biopsy, the examining finger is inserted into the rectum and the region of induration is identified. The biopsy needle is inserted through the skin of the perineum and guided under bimanual control until the tip abuts against the prostatic nodule.

TABLE 32–2. COMPLICATIONS OF TRANSPERINEAL AND TRANSRECTAL BIOPSY OF THE PROSTATE

Reference	No. of Patients	Antibiotics	Infection (%)	Bleeding (%)	Retention (%)
Transperineal					
Catalona (1980)	71	Before and after	3	1	
Fortunoff (1962)	286	——	1	1	1
Kaufman et al. (1962)	656	——	0.1	1	
Parry (1960)	71	——	0	6	
Bianchi (1956)	82	0	0	0	
Transrectal					
Crawford et al. (1982)	23	Yes	17	——	——
	25	No	48		
Sharpe et al. (1982)	80	No	41	2	
Eaton (1981)	129	No	20	1	3
Bissada (1977)	306	Before and after	21		
		After only	37	2	11
		No	37		
Dowlen et al. (1974)	140	Yes	16	1	11
Barnes (1972)	217	——	6	2	——
Davison (1971)	173	Yes	27		
		No	35	——	——

Modified from Packer, M. G., Russo, P., and Fair, W. R.: Prophylactic antibiotics and Foley catheter usage in transperineal needle biopsy of the prostate. J. Urol. *131*:687, 1984 (with permission), and from Catalona, W. J.: Prostate Cancer. New York, Grune & Stratton, 1984 (with permission).

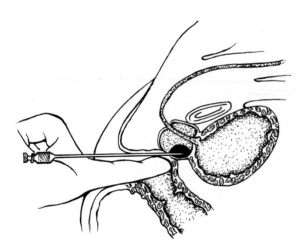

Figure 32–10. Technique of transrectal core needle biopsy of the prostate. (From Catalona, W. J.: Prostate Cancer. New York, Grune & Stratton, 1984. Used by permission.)

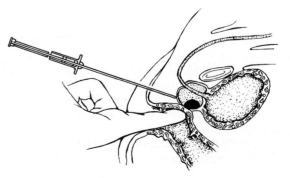

Figure 32–11. Technique of transperineal core needle biopsy of the prostate. (From Catalona, W. J.: Prostate Cancer. New York, Grune & Stratton, 1984. Used by permission.)

The biopsy is obtained in an identical fashion as for transrectal biopsy. The perineal skin need not be shaved and creation of a perineal stab wound is optional. Packer and associates (1983) reported that antibiotics are unnecessary in patients undergoing transperineal needle biopsy.

FINE-NEEDLE ASPIRATION BIOPSY

Fine-needle aspiration biopsy of the prostate is a cytologic technique that has been used extensively in Scandinavia (Esposti, 1971) and is gaining popularity elsewhere (Kaufman et al., 1982; Melograna et al., 1982). Aspiration biopsy can be performed as an outpatient procedure without anesthesia and the results can be available within hours. Aspirates are either air-dried and stained with May-Grünwald-Giemsa stain or fixed in alcohol and stained by the Papanicolaou method. The accuracy of aspiration biopsy in the Scandinavian series (Esposti, 1971) is comparable to that of core needle biopsy, but errors have been reported in up to 30 per cent of cases in some reports from other countries (Ackerman and Muller, 1977; Lin et al., 1979; Willems and Lowhagen, 1981; Melograna et al., 1982). False negative results may occur in patients having cytologically well differentiated carcinoma, and false positive results may occur in patients having granulomatous prostatitis or those in whom the seminal vesicles are inadvertently aspirated (Willems and Lowhagen, 1981). Aspiration biopsy has a considerably lower complication rate than core needle biopsy; febrile responses occur in less than 1 per cent of patients (Willems and Lowhagen, 1981).

Aspiration biopsy usually is performed with a Franzen needle (Fig. 32–12). The index finger is placed in the needle guide and a finger cot is placed over the examining finger and needle. The finger is then inserted into the rectum and the nodule is identified. A 22-gauge needle is passed through the needle guide and advanced into the nodule. Suction is applied and maintained while the needle tip is moved back and forth within the nodule. Suction is then released and the needle is withdrawn from the guide. The aspirate is then ejected onto a microscope slide and smeared.

OPEN PERINEAL BIOPSY

Open perineal biopsy of the prostate is performed infrequently because of the necessity of relying upon frozen sections and because of the risk of postoperative sexual impotency (Dahlin and Goodwin, 1957). This complication has been disputed (Culp, 1959).

TRANSURETHRAL BIOPSY

Traditionally, transurethral biopsy of the prostate has been considered inadequate for the diagnosis of early prostate cancer because prostate cancer tends to arise in the periphery of the gland. Hudson and associates (1954) reported that transurethral biopsy failed to detect nearly 50 per cent of prostate cancers found on open perineal biopsy. Transurethral biopsy is more reliable in patients having larger tumors (Denton et al., 1967; Bissada, 1977; Grayhack and Bockrath, 1981). In the American College of Surgeons survey, transurethral biopsy was the commonest means of establishing the diagnosis of prostate cancer, accounting for 58 per cent of cases (Murphy et al., 1982).

Cytologic Examination of Prostatic Secretions

Cytologic examination of expressed prostatic fluid reveals cancer cells in more than two thirds of prostate cancer patients (Frank and Scott, 1958; Sharifi et al., 1983). However, prostatic fluid cytologic examination generally is considered unreliable to establish or rule out the diagnosis of prostate cancer.

Screening for Prostate Cancer

The Veterans Administration Cooperative Urological Research Group (1967) reported that only about 25 per cent of prostate cancer patients had Stage A or B tumors at the time of diagnosis and that survival rates correlated inversely with advancing tumor stage. Although in the recent American College of Surgeons Survey 55 per cent of patients had Stage A or

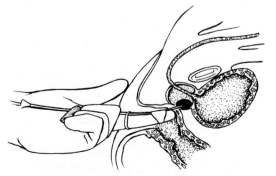

Figure 32–12. Franzen needle for fine needle aspiration of the prostate. (From Catalona, W. J.: Prostate Cancer. New York, Grune & Stratton, 1984. Used by permission.)

B tumors (Murphy et al., 1982), the early diagnosis of prostate cancer remains an important problem.

Mass screening for prostate cancer would require a screening test that is both highly sensitive for detecting early tumors and highly specific for prostate cancer (Galen and Gambino, 1978; Watson and Tang, 1980). No screening test currently available even approaches these requirements (Catalona and Menon, 1981). Rectal examination has only about 80 per cent sensitivity and 50 per cent specificity. Radioimmunoassay for serum prostatic acid phosphatase has only about 10 per cent sensitivity for early tumors and 90 per cent specificity.

STAGING

Whitmore-Jewett Staging System

The staging system most commonly used in the United States was introduced by Whitmore (1956) and modified by Jewett (1975) (Fig. 32–13). With this system, patients are grouped into four categories denoted by the letters A through D.

Stage A denotes tumors not suspected on digital rectal examination but detected on histologic examination of simple prostatectomy specimens. Approximately 10 per cent of patients who undergo prostatectomy for presumed benign hyperplasia are found to have prostate cancer (Bauer et al., 1960; Denton et al., 1965). The incidence of occult carcinoma increases to approximately 20 per cent (Denton et al., 1965) if step sections are examined. By definition, Stage A cancers are confined to the prostate gland and serum acid phosphatase titers are normal.

Jewett further subclassified Stage A prostate cancers according to whether the tumor was focal (Stage A1) or diffuse (Stage A2). Cantrell and associates (1981) determined that only 2 per cent of patients having less than 5 per cent cancer in the resected specimen had cancer progression during follow-up as compared with a cancer progression rate of 33 per cent among those having more than 5 per cent cancer in the specimen. Focal Stage A lesions that are other than well differentiated also are classified as Stage A2 (Jewett, 1975; Cantrell et al., 1981). Although this is contrary to most cancer staging schemes, it has a rationale in the biologic behavior of poorly differentiated focal Stage A prostate cancers. In general, most focal Stage A tumors are well differentiated (approximately

85 per cent), whereas most diffuse Stage A2 tumors are moderately or poorly differentiated (approximately 75 per cent).

In the Veterans Administration Cooperative Urological Research Group (VACURG) report (1967), only about 6 per cent of prostate cancer patients presented with Stage A disease. However, in recent reports (McMillen and Wettlaufer, 1976; Murphy et al., 1982), 37 to 53 per cent of patients presented with clinical Stage A disease.

Unsuspected lymph node metastases are found in only about 2 per cent of patients with clinical Stage A1 tumors and approximately 23 per cent with Stage A2 tumors (Donohue et al., 1981).

Stage B denotes tumors that are palpable on digital rectal examination and confined within the prostatic capsule. Serum acid phosphatase titers are normal in the majority of patients with Stage B tumors, although some have low-titer elevations of acid phosphatase despite normal bone scans and uninvolved lymph nodes on staging pelvic lymphadenectomy. These patients have been designated clinical Stage D0 (discussed later).

Stage B has also been subclassified into Stage B1 and B2, depending on whether there is focal or diffuse involvement of the prostate gland; however, the distinction between focal and diffuse involvement also is arbitrary. Some authors (Middleton and Smith, 1982) have designated Stage B1 as any nodule less than 2 cm in diameter and Stage B2 as any tumor more extensive than this that is confined within the prostatic capsule. Other authors (Catalona and Stein, 1982a) have designated Stage B1 as a tumor that is limited to less than one lobe of the prostate and Stage B2 as tumors in which there is induration of one or both lobes of the prostate.

In the VACURG study (1967), only 8 per cent of patients presented with Stage B disease; however, in more recent series (McMillen and Wettlaufer, 1976; Murphy et al., 1982), 22 to 26 per cent of patients presented with Stage B disease. Approximately 15 to 20 per cent of patients with clinical Stage B1 tumors have unsuspected pelvic lymph node metastases, whereas approximately 35 per cent with Stage B2 tumors have nodal involvement (Donohue et al., 1981).

Stage C denotes tumors that have extended beyond the prostatic capsule but have not produced distant metastases. Acid phosphatase titers are normal in most patients with Stage C tumors although, using radioimmunoassays, elevations of acid phosphatase titers have been reported in up to 35 per cent of patients with Stage C disease (Foti et al., 1977; Bruce et al., 1979; Fair et al., 1982). These patients also are designated as clinical Stage D0.

Stage C tumors are subclassified according to whether there is minimal extracapsular extension (Stage C1) or more extensive extracapsular tumor producing bladder outlet or ureteral obstruction (Stage C2).

In the VACURG studies (1967), 48 per cent of patients presented with clinical Stage C disease, while in more recent series (McMillen and Wettlaufer, 1976; Murphy et al., 1982), 9 to 15 per cent presented with Stage C disease. Overall, approximately 50 per cent of patients with clinical Stage C disease are found to have unsuspected pelvic lymph node metastases (Donohue et al., 1982).

Stage D denotes tumors that have metastasized distantly. Stage D is subclassified into four categories. Stage D0 denotes patients with clinically localized tumors having a normal bone scan but persistently elevated serum acid phosphatase titers (Whitesel et al., 1984). Stage D1 denotes patients presumed to have clinical Stage A, B, or C disease but who are found either at operation or by aspiration cytologic examination to have pelvic lymph node metastases. Stage D2 denotes patients having clinical evidence of distant metastases in bone or other distant organs. Stage D3 denotes patients with stage D2 prostate cancer who have relapsed after adequate endocrine therapy.

Serum acid phosphatase titers are elevated in all patients with stage D0 disease, in approximately 60 per cent of patients with Stage D1 disease, and in more than two thirds with clinical Stage D2 or D3 disease.

In the VACURG series (1967), 38 per cent of patients presented with Stage D disease. In more recent series (McMillen and Wettlaufer, 1976; Murphy et al., 1982), 10 to 28 per cent presented with Stage D disease. Most patients with Stage D disease have poorly differentiated tumors.

TNM Staging System

A tumor, node, metastasis (TNM) system has been adopted by the American Joint Committee for Cancer Staging and End Results Reporting (Fig. 32–13) (Wallace et al., 1975).

Stage T0a denotes a clinically occult tumor involving not more than three high-power fields or a needle biopsy being positive in only one lobe of the prostate. Stage T0b denotes a clinically occult tumor involving more than three high-power fields or needle biopsies being positive from both lobes of the prostate. Stage T1a denotes a 1 cm nodule confined to the prostate. Stage T1b denotes a tumor with induration larger than 1 cm but confined to one lobe of the prostate. Stage T1c denotes a tumor with induration involving both lobes of the prostate but being confined within the capsule. Stage T2 denotes a tumor that invades but does not penetrate the prostatic capsule. Stage T3 denotes a tumor that has penetrated the prostatic capsule and may involve seminal vesicles. Stage T4 denotes a tumor that is fixed to periprostatic tissues or invades adjacent viscera.

The TNM system also quantifies the extent of lymph node metastases.

N1 denotes a single homolateral regional lymph node metastases.

N2 denotes multiple or contralateral regional lymph node metastases.

N3 denotes bulky, fixed regional lymph node metastases.

N4 denotes widespread juxtaregional lymph node metastases.

The TNM system classifies distant metastases as either:

MX—minimum requirements to assess the presence of distant metastases cannot be met.

M0—no known distant metastases.

M1—distant metastases present.

Fisher and associates (1983) reported that stratification of patients according to the extent of nodal involvement yielded a striking correlation with tumor-free and overall survival. Only about one half of patients who had a single lymph node metastasis developed distant metastases within 5 years, whereas 83 per cent who had juxtaregional lymph node metastases developed distant metastases during the same interval. Similar results were reported by Paulson and associates (1980) and Prout and associates (1980). TNM stage grouping is shown in Table 32–3.

Chest Roentgenograph and Excretory Urogram

The chest roentgenograph and scout film of an excretory urogram provide radiographic screening for osseous metastases. Pulmonary metastases are present in approximately 25 per cent of patients dying of prostate cancer, but are recognized clinically in only about 10 per cent of patients because they appear as intersti-

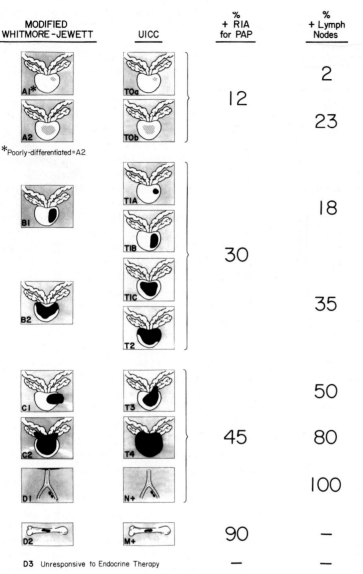

Figure 32–13. Whitmore-Jewett and UICC staging systems for prostate cancer. (From Catalona, W. J.: Prostate Cancer. New York, Grune & Stratton, 1984. Used by permission.)

tial streaking of the lung fields produced by lymphangitic or micronodular metastases.

Osseous metastases are most commonly osteoblastic, but also may be mixed osteoblastic-osteolytic or osteolytic (Fig. 32–14). Other abnormalities that may be found on excretory

urography in prostate cancer patients are distortion of the contours of the bladder, ureteral obstruction, and ureteral deviation from pelvic lymph node metastases.

Needle Biopsy of Prostate and Pelvic Lymph Nodes

In addition to establishing the diagnosis and histologic grade of a prostate cancer, needle biopsy also can be used as a means of staging the local lesion. Needle biopsies may reveal bilateral tumor involvement in patients in whom digital rectal examination suggests only unilateral involvement (Catalona and Stein, 1982a).

TABLE 32–3. Stage Grouping for TNM System

Stage A—T1a or b, T2a; N0, M0
Stage B—T2b, N0, M0
Stage C—T3, N0, M0
any T, N1, M0
Stage D—T4, N0, M0
any T, N2–3, M0
any T, any N, M1

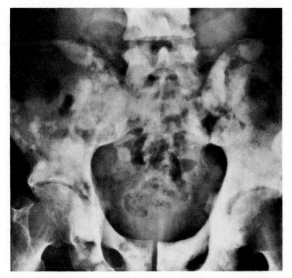

Figure 32–14. Mixed osteoblastic osteolytic metastases from prostate cancer. (From Catalona, W. J.: Prostate Cancer. New York, Grune & Stratton, 1984. Used by permission.)

Fine-needle aspiration biopsy of pelvic lymph nodes under radiographic or computerized tomographic control is a means of verifying (but not excluding) lymph node metastases.

Cystoscopy

Abnormalities produced by prostate cancer on cystoscopy include elevation of the bladder base and obstruction and rigidity of the prostatic urethra.

Bone Marrow Aspiration

Bone marrow aspiration has been evaluated as a means of detecting occult osseous metastases (Nelson et al., 1973); however, this technique has proved to be less sensitive than the bone scan. In contrast, bone marrow biopsy for radiographically equivocal lesions is a useful means of verifying osseous metastases but is inconclusive when tumor cells are not found in the aspirate.

Acid Phosphatase

In the normal prostate, acid phosphatase is produced in acinar cells and is secreted into the seminal fluid in the prostatic ductal system. Normally, little acid phosphatase is absorbed into the circulation. In the prostatic fluid, acid phosphatase levels are 500- to 1000-fold higher than in serum. In prostate cancer patients, elevations of serum acid phosphatase titers may occur because acid phosphatase produced by cancer cells that have lost their connection with the prostatic ductal system is absorbed directly into the circulation. Prostatic cancers are composed of a heterogeneous population of cells, some of which produce acid phosphatase and some of which do not (Allhoff et al., 1983). In general, prostate cancer tissue contains less acid phosphatase than does normal prostate or BPH tissue (Loor et al., 1981). Serum acid phosphatase titers also may be elevated because of compression of the prostatic ductal system, which causes back diffusion of acid phosphatase into the circulation. This mechanism also may be operative in patients with obstructive benign prostatic hyperplasia (Fleischmann et al., 1983). Acid phosphatase titers also may be elevated in patients having prostatitis (VanCangh et al., 1982) or prostatic infarction (Vihko and Kontturi, 1981).

Acid phosphatase was one of the earliest tumor markers and remains the most useful biochemical test for monitoring prostate cancer patients. Gutman and Gutman (1938) discovered that acid phosphatase titers were frequently elevated in the serum of patients having metastatic prostate cancer. In 1941, Huggins and Hodges demonstrated an abrupt decrease in serum acid phosphatase titers that correlated with clinical and radiographic evidence of tumor regression and the response to orchiectomy or estrogen administration in patients having Stage D prostate cancer.

Early in the studies of acid phosphatase, the limitations of colorimetric determinations became apparent. Nearly one third of patients with Stage D disease had normal acid phosphatase titers, whereas elevations of acid phosphatase were observed in patients with diseases other than prostate cancer including osteosarcoma, breast cancer, pancreatic cancer, Gaucher's disease, thromboembolic disease, and thrombocytopenia (Henneberry et al., 1979). Measurement of prostate-specific acid phosphatase was improved with the discovery that prostatic acid phosphatase is inhibitable by tartarate; however, it subsequently was discovered that some acid phosphatases of nonprostatic origin also are tartarate inhibitable (Abul-Fadl and King, 1949). Specificity was further improved with the discovery of substrates that are preferentially hydrolyzed by prostatic acid phosphatase. These include alpha-naphthol phosphate, beta-glycerophosphate, and, more recently, thymolphthalein monophosphate (Henneberry et al., 1979).

All enzymatic methods for measuring acid phosphatase exhibit some degree of nonspecificity. The best substrate for measuring the acid phosphatase isoenzyme of prostatic origin is thymolphthalein monophosphate (Roy et al., 1971). There are numerous isoenzymes of acid phosphatase that have different substrate specificities and different immunochemical properties (Yam et al., 1981; Vihko et al., 1982). The acid phosphatases of prostatic origin are primarily isoenzyme 2 and, to a lesser extent, isoenzyme 4. These are normally not detectable in human serum. Neutrophils contain some isoenzyme 2 and 4, and elevated serum levels of acid phosphatase have been reported in patients having granulocytic leukemia, polycythemia vera, and neutrophilia (Yam et al., 1981; Huber et al., 1982) as well as in patients having pancreatic carcinoma (Choe et al., 1978).

In the early 1970's, immunochemical methods, including radioimmunoassays (RIA) (Foti et al., 1975; Mahan and Doctor, 1979) and counterimmunoelectrophoresis (CIEP) (Chu et al., 1978), were developed for measuring prostatic acid phosphatase. An early report (Foti et al., 1977) suggested that RIA for prostatic acid phosphatase could be used as a screening test for early prostate cancer, identifying approximately 50 per cent of patients having intracapsular tumors with false positive results occurring in 4 to 11 per cent of various control patients. Subsequent studies have not confirmed this high sensitivity of RIA in patients with localized prostate cancer (Bruce et al., 1979; Pontes et al., 1981a; Fair et al., 1982; Huber et al., 1982). False positives also have been observed in patients with lipemic serum (Griffiths, 1980). In most studies, the incidence of elevated acid phosphatase in patients with intracapsular prostate cancer (10 per cent) is approximately the same as that in patients having benign prostatic hyperplasia. Thus, RIA and CIEP are not considered valuable screening tests for prostate cancer.

Early reports (Reynolds et al., 1973; Gursel et al., 1974) suggested that elevated acid phosphatase levels in bone marrow aspirates could identify patients having early metastatic disease. Subsequently, it was shown that enzymatic assays were unreliable for measuring prostatic acid phosphatase in bone marrow aspirates (Dias and Barnett, 1977). It was hoped that with the development of RIA, acid phosphatase titers in bone marrow could be measured more accurately; however, with most assays, the acid phosphatase titers in normal bone marrow are significantly higher than in the serum of the same subject (Bruce et al., 1979; Cooper et al., 1979; Huber et al., 1982). Although RIA is more specific for measuring prostatic acid phosphatase, there still appears to be some residual cross-reactivity with acid phosphatases of nonprostatic origin (Cooper et al., 1979; Pontes et al., 1979).

Bellville and associates (1981) reported that 36 per cent of patients having elevated bone marrow acid phosphatase titers developed distant metastases within 2 years as compared with only 3 per cent having normal acid phosphatase titers. In this study, serum acid phosphatase titers were not reported. Schellhammer and associates (1982) reported that serum acid phosphatase titers measured by CIEP were normal in only three of 55 patients having elevated bone marrow titers and concluded that bone marrow acid phosphatase added little to serum determinations. Similarly, Vihko and associates (1982a), using an RIA that was highly specific for prostatic acid phosphatase, reported that bone marrow acid phosphatase determinations were no more useful than serum determinations.

Interpretation of elevated acid phosphatase titers in individual patients is difficult because, theoretically, acid phosphatase can be elevated in patients having tumors that are confined within the prostate. An elevated acid phosphatase titer is neither necessary nor sufficient to establish the diagnosis of metastatic prostate cancer. Up to 40 per cent of patients having documented metastases have normal acid phosphatase titers. Nonetheless, the majority of patients having clinically localized prostate cancer with elevated acid phosphatases have occult metastases in lymph nodes, bone, or other organs (Pontes et al., 1981a; Whitesel et al., 1983).

There are fluctuations of acid phosphatase levels in both normal individuals and patients with prostate cancer. Using a colorimetric assay, Doe and Mellinger (1964) reported acid phosphatase secretion manifested a circadian variation with the highest point being reached at 2:00 P.M. and the lowest point occurring at 11:00 P.M. In contrast, Brenckman and associates (1981) and Nissenkorn and associates (1982), using immunochemical determination, reported marked random fluctuations in acid phosphatase titers that had no apparent circadian rhythm.

Digital rectal examination, urethral instrumentation, and prostatic resection can produce elevations of acid phosphatase that may persist for 24 to 48 hours (Pearson et al., 1983).

Current evidence suggests that although RIA and CIEP assays are more sensitive than enzymatic assays for measuring prostatic acid phosphatase, they yield more false positives when used to measure serum acid phosphatase titers. The RIA and CIEP also are more specific than enzymatic assays but yield some false positives due to cross-reactivity with acid phosphatases of nonprostatic origin. The heat lability of prostatic acid phosphatase generally is not a problem with RIA because it measures the antigenic activity of prostatic acid phosphatase; however, Huber and associates (1982) reported that freezing and thawing can have an effect on the amount of immunologically detectable acid phosphatase. Heat lability is a problem with CIEP and enzymatic assays because they measure the enzymatic activity of prostatic acid phosphatase, which is heat labile.

Neither RIA nor CIEP has proved valuable as a screening test for prostate cancer, and important treatment decisions should not be influenced by bone marrow acid phosphatase determinations alone. It has been reported that RIA may be more sensitive than enzymatic assays for following patients for tumor recurrence (Vihko et al., 1981), but in general, RIA offers no practical advantage over the more specific enzymatic determinations such as the thymolphthalein monophosphate determination (Roy et al., 1971). Moreover, RIA's are more expensive and time-consuming than enzymatic assays.

Alkaline Phosphatase

Alkaline phosphatase titers are elevated in patients with metastatic prostate cancer more frequently than are acid phosphatase titers. Alkaline phosphatase elevations are due to metabolic activity in bone surrounding metastatic lesions. As a tumor marker, alkaline phosphatase is less specific than acid phosphatase because alkaline phosphatase elevations also may occur in a variety of metabolic bone disorders and in patients having hepatobiliary disease. Alkaline phosphatase produced by bone can be distinguished from that produced in the liver in that the bone isoenzyme is heat labile. Normally, approximately 20 ± 5 per cent of serum alkaline phosphatase is of hepatic origin (heat stable). A characteristic flare response of alkaline phosphatase titers occurs following initiation of endocrine therapy in patients with metastatic prostate cancer (Huggins and Hodges, 1941). This is characterized by the titers rising transiently and then gradually declining toward normal in patients who have clinical remissions. Unlike acid phosphatase, alkaline phosphatase

titers do not fluctuate throughout the day (Brenckman et al., 1981).

Bone Scan

Bone scans are the most sensitive means of detecting osseous metastases (Schaffer and Pendergrass, 1976). Patients with metastatic prostate cancer may have abnormal bone scans with normal bone radiographs (Schaffer and Pendergrass, 1976). Falsely negative bone scans occur in less than 2 per cent of patients, and are due to the presence of widespread, symmetric metastases. The most useful radiopharmaceutical agent available for bone scanning is ^{99m} + technetium methylene diphosphonate, which has a high bone to soft tissue ratio and allows imaging 2 hours after injection of the isotope. Bone scanning isotopes are taken up in all areas of increased bone turnover, not just in metastatic lesions (Thrall et al., 1974). Bone scans are relatively nonspecific and should be

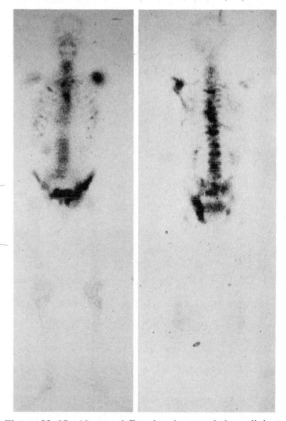

Figure 32–15. Abnormal ^{99m}technetium methylene diphosphonate bone scan in patient with metastatic prostate cancer. Note that metastatic lesions are multiple, are asymmetric, and involve the axial skeleton. The kidneys are visualized. (From Catalona, W. J.: Prostate Cancer. New York, Grune & Stratton, 1984. Used by permission.)

viewed along with bone radiographs. Characteristically, metastatic lesions involve the axial skeleton and are asymmetric and multiple (Fig. 32–15). Normally the kidneys are visualized on bone scans and the absence of visualization of the kidneys is a clue to a possibly falsely negative scan (Fig. 32–16). This occurs in patients having widespread metastases in whom virtually all of the isotope is taken up by the skeletal metastases and little remains to be excreted by the kidneys (Paulson et al., 1979).

The bone scan generally is performed before the skeletal survey because of its superior sensitivity. Detailed radiographic views are obtained to evaluate areas of increased isotope uptake. Bone scans also may be useful in evaluating the source of pain in patients with prostate cancer. Because of frequent occurrence of spinal involvement, pain produced by spinal cord or nerve root compression may radiate to distant sites. If a bone scan reveals the painful site to be free of metastases, palliative radiation therapy may be directed to the appropriate spinal level (Pollen et al., 1981b). Scans also have been used to assess the response of bone metastases to chemotherapy (Citrin et al., 1981b); changes in serial bone scans correlate with disease activity and have prognostic significance (Pollen et al., 1981a).

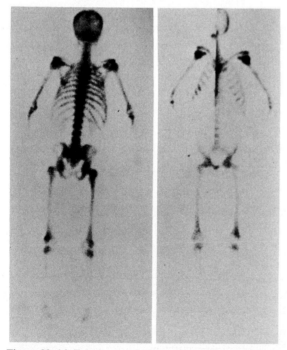

Figure 32–16. Falsely negative "super scan" in patient with diffuse, symmetric metastases. The kidneys are poorly visualized. (From Catalona, W. J.: Prostate Cancer. New York, Grune & Stratton, 1984. Used by permission.)

Skeletal Radiographs

Thirty to 50 per cent of bone must be replaced by tumor before it can be detected by routine radiographs (Lachman, 1955). Blastic metastases may be difficult to distinguish from a bone island that is a rest of cortical bone or from the sclerotic phase of Paget's disease. In Paget's disease, the serum alkaline phosphatase titers are elevated while acid phosphatase is normal.

Osteoblastic metastases may diminish or resolve completely following endocrine therapy. Osteolytic lesions may heal and recalcify, sometimes producing the appearance of enlarging osteoblastic metastases.

Lymph Node Evaluation

In a review of the literature, Donohue and associates (1981, 1982) reported that 2 per cent of patients with Stage A1, 23 per cent with Stage A2, 18 per cent with Stage B1, 35 per cent with Stage B2, and 46 per cent with Stage C tumors were found to have pelvic lymph node metastases (Table 32–4). The incidence of lymph node metastases correlates with tumor grade within each tumor substage. The commonest sites of metastatic involvement are the obturator, presacral, presciatic, hypogastric, and external iliac nodes. Patients with lymph node involvement have a guarded prognosis. Accordingly, lymph node staging should be performed in selected patients prior to definitive therapy.

TABLE 32–4. PERCENTAGE OF PATIENTS HAVING OCCULT LYMPH NODE METASTASES AS A FUNCTION OF TUMOR STAGE AND GRADE

Clinical Stage	Tumor Grade		
	WELL	MODERATE	POOR
A1	2	—	—
A2	5	23	50
B1	5	20	27
B2	28	27	38
C	18	42	68

Modified from Donohue, R. E., Mani, J. H., Whitesel, J. A., Mohr, S., Scanavino, D., Augspurger, R. R., Biber, R. J., Fauver, H. E., Wettlaufer, J. N., and Pfister, R. R.: Pelvic lymph node dissection: Guide to patient management in clinically locally confined adenocarcinoma of prostate. Urology, 20:559, 1982 (with permission); and from Catalona, W. J.: Prostate Cancer. New York, Grune & Stratton, 1984 (with permission).

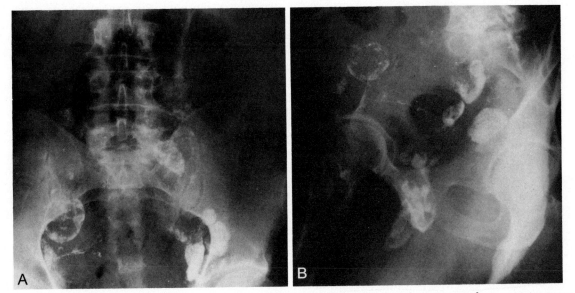

Figure 32–17. *A* and *B*, Abnormal lymphangiogram in a patient with pelvic lymph node metastases from prostate cancer. (From Catalona, W. J.: Prostate Cancer. New York, Grune & Stratton, 1984. Used by permission.)

Lymphangiography

Lymphangiography has been extensively evaluated as a nonsurgical means of staging the pelvic lymph nodes (Castellino et al., 1973). Lymph node metastases from prostate cancer distort the internal architecture of lymph nodes and appear as filling defects within them (Fig. 32–17). Lymphangiography has been used to determine radiation portals and has been combined with fine-needle aspiration of filling defects in lymph nodes as a means of documenting pelvic lymph node metastases. Fine-needle aspiration biopsies are positive in 50 to 90 per cent of patients having unequivocally positive or highly suspicious lymphangiograms, but in only 15 per cent of those having normal lymphangiograms (Efremidis, 1979; Correa et al., 1981; Dan et al., 1982; Wajsman et al., 1982; Von Eschenbach and Zornoza, 1982). False positive lymphangiograms occur in 5 to 10 per cent of patients. The principal limitation of lymphangiography is its lack of sensitivity. Lymphangiograms detect the presence of nodal metastases in only approximately 50 per cent of patients having them (Spellman et al., 1977; Grossman et al., 1980; Liebner et al., 1980; Hoekstra and Schroeder, 1981). Lymphangiography fails to detect metastases because the hypogastric and presacral nodes are not consistently visualized on bipedal lymphangiograms and because lymphangiograms cannot detect microscopic metastases.

Computerized Tomographic (CT) Scanning of Pelvic Lymph Nodes

Computerized tomography has been extensively evaluated as a means of staging pelvic lymph nodes (Redman, 1977; Levitt et al., 1978) (Fig. 32–18). CT scanning is unable to detect microscopic metastases and may produce false positive results owing to enlarged benign nodes, bowel loops that may be mistaken for enlarged lymph nodes, and confusion between blood vessels and lymph nodes. Most studies suggest that the sensitivity of CT scanning in detecting lymph

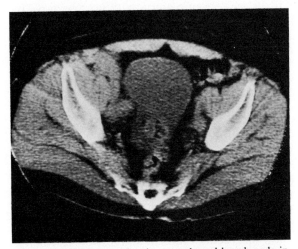

Figure 32–18. CT scan showing an enlarged lymph node in the right pelvis. (From Catalona, W. J.: Prostate Cancer. New York, Grune & Stratton, 1984. Used by permission.)

node metastases is only about 50 per cent and the false positive rate is approximately 10 per cent (Benson et al., 1981; Sawczuk et al., 1983; Weinerman et al., 1983). Fine-needle aspiration biopsy may also be performed under CT guidance.

Tumor Grade as a Predictor of Lymph Node Metastases

It has been suggested that the Gleason grade of a prostate cancer may identify patients in whom staging lymphadenectomy may be unnecessary because of a high likelihood of lymph node metastases (Gleason 8–10) or a low likelihood of lymph node metastases (Gleason 2–4) (Kramer et al., 1980; Paulson et al., 1980). Subsequent studies, however, demonstrated that Gleason grade alone could not predict accurately the presence or absence of pelvic lymph node metastases (Catalona et al., 1982b; Middleton and Smith, 1982; Olsson et al., 1982; Sagalowsky et al., 1982).

Pelvic Lymphadenectomy

Pelvic lymphadenectomy is the most accurate means of staging pelvic lymph nodes. Some authors have advocated performing pelvic lymphadenectomy as a separate staging procedure and waiting for permanent sections before making a treatment decision. Others have relied on frozen sections at the time of operation. Frozen sections are of limited value in detecting microscopic lymph node metastases. Falsely negative frozen sections have been reported in 8 to 19 per cent of patients with normal-appearing nodes, and frozen sections have failed to identify 20 to 40 per cent of patients having microscopic lymph node metastases (Saltzstein and McLaughlin, 1977; Fowler et al., 1981; Catalona and Stein, 1982; Middleton and Smith, 1982; Sadlowski et al., 1983). Most patients in whom frozen sections are falsely negative have only one or two microscopic metastases (Catalona and Stein, 1982b).

Staging pelvic lymphadenectomy has been associated with substantial morbidity (McCullough et al., 1977; Babcock and Grayhack, 1979; Herr, 1979; Lieskovsky et al., 1980). Postoperative complications occur in 20 to 35 per cent of patients and include wound infection (5–15 per cent), genital and lower extremity edema (5–10 per cent) and thromboembolic phenomena (5–10 per cent). When pelvic lymphadenectomy is combined with whole pelvis external-beam radiation therapy, up to 50 per cent of patients may have disabling genital or extremity edema (Freiha et al., 1979).

It has been reported (Paulson, 1980; Fisher et al., 1981) that limiting the node dissection to include only the lymph nodes medial to the external iliac vessels does not produce edema. It is claimed that this limited node dissection is as accurate as standard lymphadenectomy because the overall incidence of patients having positive nodes was similar to that of comparable patients previously staged with a standard pelvic lymphadenectomy (Brendler et al., 1980). However, studies in which the sites of lymph node metastases were specified have yielded conflicting results. Some reports suggest that a limited node dissection may fail to identify a substantial proportion of patients having lymph node metastases (McLaughlin et al., 1976; Golimbu et al., 1979; Fowler and Whitmore, 1981b). In the study of Fowler and Whitmore (1981b), 61 per cent of patients having a solitary lymph node metastasis had involvement of the obturator-hypogastric group, whereas 39 per cent had involvement of the external iliac nodes only. In contrast, in the series of Bruce and associates (1977), a limited pelvic lymphadenectomy would have detected 91 per cent of patients having nodal metastases. The extent to which a limited node dissection may underestimate the proportion of patients having lymph node metastases and the number of lymph nodes involved remains to be determined. Moreover, the inaccuracy of a limited node dissection must be weighed against the increased morbidity associated with more extensive dissections before the role of limited pelvic lymphadenectomy can be clearly defined.

Prophylactic anticoagulation has been recommended in patients undergoing staging pelvic lymphadenectomy. However, its role is controversial. Lieskovsky and associates (1980) reported a lower incidence of thromboembolic complications in patients receiving prophylactic warfarin sodium, while other authors have demonstrated no significant benefit from mini-dose heparin (Hindsley et al., 1980; Sogani et al., 1981). Moreover, an increased incidence of lymphocele formation has been reported in patients receiving mini-dose heparin (Catalona et al., 1980; Hindsley et al., 1980; Sogani et al., 1981).

Lymphoscintigraphy

Lymphoscintigraphy is a technique in which radiocolloids (^{99m}technetium phytate or ^{99m}technetium antimony sulfur colloid) are injected transrectally into the prostatic capsule or into the perianal tissues and scans are obtained to visualize the lymphatics (Gardiner et al., 1979; Stone et al., 1979; Whitmore et al., 1980; Ege, 1982). The limitations in resolution inherent in radionuclide imaging prevent lymphoscintigraphy from gaining widespread acceptance.

Repeat Circumferential Transurethral Resection of the Prostate

Repeat transurethral resection of the prostate has been advocated in patients having clinical Stage A1 prostate cancer to identify those who have more extensive residual cancer. In the initial study reported by McMillen and Wettlauffer (1976), approximately 25 per cent of patients with Stage A1 tumors were upstaged to Stage A2. However, in a follow-up study at the same institution, Bridges and associates (1983) reported that only 5 per cent of patients were upstaged to Stage A2 and there was no evidence that the upstaged patients fared worse than their counterparts who were not upstaged. Similar results were reported by Parfitt and associates (1981). Current evidence suggests that if the initial transurethral resection of the prostate is adequate, a repeat transurethral resection is unnecessary. Bridges and associates (1983) reported that needle biopsies performed at the time of repeat transurethral resection were positive in only 15 per cent of patients.

Prostatic Ultrasonography

Transrectal and transurethral ultrasonography have been evaluated as a means of diagnosing and staging the primary lesion of prostate cancer (Peeling et al., 1979; Resnick et al., 1980; Kohri et al., 1981). Prostate cancer produces focal, dense echo patterns that cannot be distinguished from prostatitis or prostatic calculi (Fig. 32–19). Therefore, ultrasonography is of most value as a means of following the response of the primary tumor to endocrine or radiation therapy (Carpentier et al., 1982). Transurethral ultrasonography also has been described as a means of evaluating the local extent of the primary tumor (Peeling et al., 1979; Resnick et al., 1980; Sekine et al., 1982).

Computerized Tomography of the Prostate

CT scans can demonstrate the prostate, bladder, and seminal vesicles and their relation-

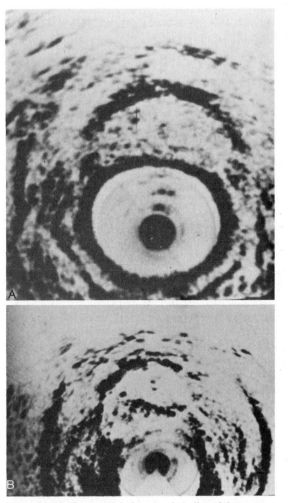

Figure 32–19. Transrectal ultrasound studies of the prostate. *A,* Benign prostatic hyperplasia with fine, diffuse internal echoes and preservation of periprostatic fat plane. *B,* Prostate cancer with dense internal echoes and loss of periprostatic fat planes. (From Catalona, W. J.: Prostate Cancer. New York, Grune & Stratton, 1984. Used by permission.)

ships to surrounding structures, but most studies have reported that CT is not accurate in determining extracapsular tumor spread. Moreover, urinary extravasation and hemorrhage following prostatic needle biopsy can mimic invasion of cancer through the prostatic capsule. CT scans also cannot provide accurate diagnostic information about the nature of the disease within the prostate gland. Accordingly, CT scanning has found its greatest use in estimating tumor volume in planning radiation therapy.

Nuclear Magnetic Resonance Scans of the Prostate

Nuclear magnetic resonance (NMR) scans can image the prostate and seminal vesicles;

however, insufficient experience is available to evaluate the practical applicability of NMR scanning.

Staging Errors in Clinically Localized Prostate Cancer

Considerable staging errors have been reported in patients having clinically localized prostate cancer (Catalona and Stein, 1982a; Thomas et al., 1982; Lange and Narayan, 1983). Understaging in terms of local tumor extension has been reported in 7 to 56 per cent of patients with clinical Stage A or B disease, and lymph node metastases have been reported in up to 60 per cent of patients having high-grade clinical Stage B2 tumors. Understaging is more likely to occur in patients having large tumors and those having poorly differentiated tumors.

Clinical overstaging of prostate cancer also has been reported (Turner and Belt, 1957; Byar and Mostofi, 1972). In these studies, approximately 30 per cent of patients judged by rectal examination to have early Stage C lesions were found to have tumor confined to the prostate on histologic examination of the radical prostatectomy specimen.

Indications for Staging Procedures

Staging procedures should be performed only on patients in whom treatment decisions will be influenced by the results of staging or to establish a baseline for future follow-up. Stage A1 prostate cancer patients in whom no immediate treatment is planned do not require further staging unless a baseline is desired. On the other hand, patients having clinical Stage A2 or B prostate cancer require further clinical evaluation to determine their candidacy for radical prostatectomy. This includes a general medical evaluation to determine whether there are disorders that would preclude a major operation. Routine chest radiographs provide a general evaluation of the cardiopulmonary status of the patient as well as screening for pulmonary metastases and osseous metastases in the upper axial skeleton. Excretory urography provides information about the urinary tract and also is a screening test for osseous metastases in the lower axial skeleton. CT and ultrasonic scans of the prostate have not proved to be sufficiently accurate to justify their routine use (Pilepich et al., 1980b). Serum acid phosphatase titers should be evaluated and, if abnormal, should be repeated. Bone scanning is the most sensitive means of detecting osseous metastases. Most patients having osseous metastases have multifocal, asymmetric areas of increased uptake in the axial skeleton. This pattern is virtually pathognomonic of metastatic prostate cancer but should be further evaluated with radiographs. If there are only one or two areas of increased isotope uptake, radiographs should be obtained and, if equivocal, needle biopsy confirmation should be sought.

Lymph node staging is necessary in patients considered to be potential candidates for radical prostatectomy. Nonsurgical means of evaluating pelvic lymph nodes (lymphangiography and CT) combined with needle aspiration biopsy are of limited sensitivity and also are invasive. The vast majority of patients having clinically localized prostate cancer have normal CT scans and lymphangiograms. Lymphangiography should be reserved for patients having high-grade, bulky primary tumors in whom the likelihood of pelvic lymph node metastases is high or for patients who are poor surgical risks. In such patients, aspiration biopsy of abnormal nodes should be performed in an attempt to document lymph node metastases and obviate the need for staging lymphadenectomy. Negative aspiration biopsies do not rule out lymph node metastases.

Staging pelvic lymphadenectomy is the most accurate means of identifying patients having lymph node metastases in whom the likelihood of cure by surgical excision is small. Pelvic lymphadenectomy generally is regarded as a staging procedure without proven therapeutic benefit and therefore may be limited to include only the nodes medial to the external iliac vessels. Frozen sections are of limited sensitivity but accuracy may be increased by careful histologic examination of the specimen.

In patients who are to be treated primarily with radiation therapy, the need for lymph node evaluation is less clear. Radiation therapy may be delivered to the prostate and pelvic lymph node–bearing areas without prior lymph node staging with the view that if the lymph nodes are negative, radiation therapy may be curative, and if they are positive, it will at least provide local control of the primary tumor. On the other hand, a limited lymph node dissection may be used as a means of identifying patients not having lymph node metastases who are more likely to be cured with radiation therapy. Lymph node status has not influenced the treatment of patients treated with interstitial ^{125}I or ^{192}Ir implantation therapy, whereas in patients treated with [198]Au implant therapy, lymph node status determines whether whole pelvis external-beam radiation also will be given. In patients having Stage D2 prostate cancer, lymph node evaluation is unnecessary because the results do not influence therapy.

RADICAL PROSTATECTOMY

Radical prostatectomy, popularized by Young (1905), was the first treatment for prostate cancer. Because many patients have local or distant tumor spread at the time of diagnosis, other treatment modalities have been developed. These newer treatments, including radiation therapy and endocrine therapy, have proved to be effective in some patients and consequently also have been used in patients with localized prostate cancer. However, because not all prostate cancers can be controlled with therapeutic doses of irradiation and because endocrine therapy is never curative, radical prostatectomy has continued to have an important role in the management of patients with localized prostate cancer.

Patient Selection

The most suitable candidates for radical prostatectomy are patients with tumors confined within the prostatic capsule. Some patients having seminal vesicle involvement (Stage C1) and some having minimal pelvic lymph node metastases (Stage D1) have enjoyed long-term, tumor-free survival following radical prostatectomy combined with pelvic lymphadenectomy. However, in patients with Stage C1 or D1 tumors, it is questionable whether the prospects for cure justify the morbidity and functional sacrifices that may be associated with radical prostatectomy.

CLINICAL STAGE A

There is a substantial difference in the biologic potential of Stage A1 and Stage A2 tumors. The vast majority of patients having Stage A1 tumors (especially older patients) do not require definitive treatment. However, it is noteworthy that young patients having Stage A1 tumors may have a considerably longer period of risk for cancer progression. The safety of expectant management of young patients with Stage A1 prostate cancer is not yet clearly established. Stamey (1982) suggested that the best evidence that Stage A1 tumors are not always latent is that the next stage, Stage A2, clearly is not latent. In some patients, the first clinical evidence of cancer progression may be distant metastases. Repeat transurethral resection does not provide a satisfactory solution to the problem of how best to treat young patients with Stage A1 disease. A properly performed nerve-sparing radical prostatectomy would be expected to leave the patient continent, sexually potent, and free of cancer, and may be considered a legitimate treatment option. However, radical prostatectomy may be therapeutic overkill in many patients with Stage A1 disease. Further information is needed to resolve this issue.

The efficacy of radical prostatectomy in controlling Stage A prostate cancer is unproved. The available data are presented in Table 32–5. Among these patients treated with radical prostatectomy for Stage A1 or A2 prostate cancer, only 10 per cent had cancer progression and only 1 per cent died of prostate cancer during follow-up. Although these patients represent a selected group of Stage A patients, the results suggest that radical prostatectomy may reduce cancer progression and cancer death rates in patients with Stage A2 disease. These results recently have been corroborated by Benson and associates (1984).

The argument against radical prostatectomy for Stage A prostate cancer is that nearly 25 per cent of patients having Stage A2 tumors have lymph node metastases and many also have poorly differentiated tumors. In either case, cure is unlikely. It also is claimed that secondary

TABLE 32–5. CANCER PROGRESSION AND MORTALITY RATES IN PATIENTS WITH STAGE A PROSTATE CANCER TREATED WITH RADICAL PROSTATECTOMY

Authors	No. of Patients	Cancer Progression No. (%)	Cancer Deaths No. (%)	Follow-up
Blackard et al. (1971)	24	2 (8)	1 (4)	1–9 yrs
Nichols et al. (1977)	33	3 (9)	0 (0)	0–25 yrs
Heaney et al. (1977)	8*	1 (13)	0 (0)	10 yrs—89%
Bass and Barrett (1980)	36†	4 (11)	0 (0)	
Total	101	10 (10%)	1 (1%)	0.5–12 yrs

*Number with stage A1 disease unknown.

†13 A1, 14 A2, 12 B.

Modified from Catalona, W. J., and Kelley, D. R.: Indications for total prostatectomy. AUA Update Series (Lesson 2) *3*:2, 1983 (with permission); and from Catalona, W. J.: Prostate Cancer, New York, Grune & Stratton, 1984 (with permission).

radical prostatectomy is technically unsatisfactory after a transurethral resection and may be associated with a higher complication rate. Radical prostatectomy is always more difficult to perform after an open prostatectomy; however, it usually is not more difficult after a transurethral resection.

Opinions are conflicting concerning the optimal interval between transurethral resection and radical prostatectomy. Nichols and coworkers (1977) reported that the complication rate was highest in patients who underwent radical prostatectomy before 6 weeks. In contrast, Bass and Barrett (1980) found that the interval was not of critical importance. Linder and associates (1983) reported that the incontinence rate was not higher among patients who had undergone prior transurethral resection of the prostate.

It has been claimed that transurethral resection may disseminate the cancer and thus preclude benefits from any form of local therapy. The clinical data bearing on this issue are conflicting (McGowan, 1980; Fowler et al., 1982; Scardino et al., 1982; Hanks et al., 1983) and do not warrent firm conclusions.

CLINICAL STAGE B

The long-term, tumor-free survival rates in patients with clinical Stage B prostate cancer treated with radical prostatectomy are unsurpassed by any other treatment. The most ideal candidates are patients having clinical Stage B1 disease, of whom approximately 90 per cent have tumors that are confined within the prostatic capsule (Elder et al., 1982) and only about 10 per cent of whom have pelvic lymph node metastases. In a review of the Johns Hopkins Hospital series, the 15-year tumor-free survival rate was 51 per cent (Walsh and Jewett, 1980). Stamey (1982) suggested that this survival rate is only an approximation, since several patients in this series were lost to follow-up. In a previous report of the Johns Hopkins series (Jewett et al., 1968), only 17 per cent of patients actually died of prostate cancer.

Excellent tumor-free survival results also were reported by Hodges and associates (1979) and by Cochran and Kadesky (1981b) (52 and 75 per cent 15-year tumor-free survival, respectively). Cochran and Kadesky's patients routinely received adjunctive estrogen therapy. These survival results are comparable to the expected survival of the general population not having prostate cancer (patients who are candidates for a major operation should have a life expectancy that is *better* than that of the general population).

Traditionally, patients having clinical Stage B2 disease have not been considered appropriate candidates for radical prostatectomy because most of them have seminal vesicle invasion (Walsh and Jewett, 1980; Elder et al., 1982). However, Elder and associates (1982) reported that the survival of patients having clinical Stage B2 tumors that were histologically confined to the prostate was comparable to that of patients having clinical Stage B1 tumors.

Middleton and Smith (1982) reported that pelvic lymph node status is an accurate predictor of local tumor extension in patients with clinical Stage B2 tumors (defined as a tumor larger than 2 cm). They found that the primary tumor was confined within the prostatic capsule in 86 per cent of patients not having pelvic lymph node metastases. Accordingly, they suggested that lymphadenectomy is a useful means of selecting patients with clinical Stage B2 disease for radical prostatectomy. Catalona and associates (1983), using a different definition of Stage B2 (tumor involving both lobes of the prostate), found that only 62 per cent of patients having uninvolved lymph nodes had tumors that were histologically confined within the prostatic capsule, but 90 per cent of these patients with uninvolved nodes also had uninvolved seminal vesicles. In Catalona's series (1983), 75 per cent of patients with lymph node metastases had local extracapsular tumor extension.

Prospective, randomized clinical trials of radical prostatectomy for Stages A and B prostate cancer have yielded conflicting results. The VACURG Study 2 (Byar et al., 1981) compared radical prostatectomy with placebo and concluded that there was no significant benefit from radical prostatectomy. This trial had many deficiencies that limit its current relevance. Among these are the inclusion of patients with Stage A1 tumors; the small size of the study group, which precluded detection of potentially important differences in survival; limited follow-up; excessive exclusions from the placebo group; and inadequate patient staging. Despite these deficiencies, the results revealed a 39 per cent reduction in the cancer progression rate in patients with Stage A tumors and a 59 per cent reduction in the cancer progression rate in patients with Stage B tumors, which approached, but did not achieve, statistical significance.

A prospective, randomized trial conducted by the Uro-Oncology Research Group (Paulson et al., 1982b) compared radical prostatectomy with external-beam radiation therapy in patients with Stage A2 or B prostate cancer. In this trial, patients were appropriately staged and tumors were graded using the Gleason system. Tumor grades were equally distributed between the two arms of the study. Using the time to first treatment failure as the end point, the tumor-free survival was significantly better in patients treated with radical prostatectomy.

CLINICAL STAGE C

In general, patients having clinical Stage C prostate cancer are not good candidates for radical prostatectomy, although some long-term, tumor-free survivals have been reported. Hodges and associates (1979) reported on seven Stage C patients who survived 15 years tumor-free. Schroeder and Belt (1975) reported that 11 per cent of Stage C patients treated with radical prostatectomy plus adjunctive estrogen therapy were tumor-free for 15 years. De Vere White and associates (1977) reported an overall 75 per cent 10-year survival in Stage C patients treated with radical prostatectomy and estrogens. Scott and Boyd (1969) reported on a series of Stage C patients whose tumors regressed on estrogen therapy, of whom 29 per cent survived 15 years after radical prostatectomy. An unanswered question in all series in which adjunctive hormonal therapy was given is how a group of comparable patients treated with hormonal therapy alone would have fared.

Adjunctive radiation therapy also has been used in conjunction with radical prostatectomy in Stage C patients. Flocks (1973) reported a 28 per cent 15-year survival rate in Stage C patients not having lymph node metastases following radical prostatectomy and adjunctive irradiation with interstitial colloidal [198]Au. Gill and associates (1980) reported on sandwich external-beam radiation therapy giving 3000 rads preoperatively and 4500 rads postoperatively. The follow-up in this series was insufficient to evaluate survival, but the postoperative complication rate was excessive. In contrast, Carson and associates (1980) reported that radical prostatectomy could be performed after radiation therapy with acceptable morbidity. Zincke and associates (1981) reported a 65 per cent 5-year, tumor-free survival in Stage C patients treated with radical prostatectomy, of whom 24 per cent received adjunctive hormonal or radiation therapy or both.

In most reported series of radical prostatectomy for Stage C disease, adjunctive therapy was used. Accordingly, it is impossible to determine to what extent favorable survival results are attributable to the radical prostatectomy or to the adjunctive therapy. It is unlikely that tumors that have extended through the prostatic capsule and infiltrated the periprostatic tissues can be cured by radical prostatectomy alone.

Tomlinson and associates (1977) reported that patients having Stage C tumors who were treated with radical prostatectomy had fewer problems with recurrent bladder outlet obstruction and bleeding (4 per cent) than patients treated conservatively (75 per cent); however, it is unclear whether the two patient groups were truly comparable. Gee and Cole (1980) reported that recurrent obstruction occurred in only 11 per cent of conservatively treated Stage C patients and Schroeder and Belt (1975) reported recurrent obstructive symptoms in 13 per cent treated with radical prostatectomy plus estrogens. Therefore, it is questionable whether radical prostatectomy is justified as prophylaxis against bladder outlet obstruction.

CLINICAL STAGE D1

A substantial proportion of patients having clinically localized prostate cancer are found to have unsuspected pelvic lymph node metastases. Distant metastases appear within 5 years in more than 85 per cent of patients with Stage D1 disease who receive no further treatment. In patients who are treated with external-beam radiation therapy, 85 per cent develop metastases within 5 years (Pilepich et al., 1980a; Bagshaw, 1982). Similarly, more than 75 per cent of Stage D1 patients treated with ^{125}I implantation therapy develop distant metastases within 5 years (de Vere White et al., 1982; Grossman et al., 1982) and 70 per cent treated with [198]Au implantation develop metastases (Scardino et al., 1982). Endocrine therapy significantly delays the appearance of distant metastases in Stage D1 patients. Meyers and associates (1983) reported that 88 per cent of Stage D1 patients not treated with endocrine therapy developed cancer progression within 5 years, whereas only 14 per cent treated with immediate endocrine therapy developed metastases during the same period. With all of these treatments, the primary tumor is left in situ. It is theoretically possible that in some instances, distant metastases may have derived from the primary tumor (after the lymphadenectomy) because the primary tumor was not controlled.

There are insufficient data on the efficacy of radical prostatectomy combined with pelvic lymphadenectomy to control Stage D1 disease. McCullough and Leadbetter (1972) reported that 24 per cent of their patients with lymph node metastases were tumor-free at follow-up, but only half had been followed for 5 years. Flocks (1973) reported that 13 per cent of patients having positive nodes survived for 15 years. Spaulding and Whitmore (1978) reported on one patient having nodal involvement who survived tumor-free for 10 years. Zincke and associates (1981, 1982) reported that the 5-year survival rate for patients having a single positive node was 95 per cent, whereas patients having multiple positive nodes had a 70 per cent 5-year survival rate; however, most of these patients also received adjunctive endocrine therapy. In an update of the Mayo Clinic Series, 41 per cent of patients having one to four positive nodes who were followed for at least 5 years had no evidence of cancer progression; however, all except one patient also received adjunctive endocrine therapy (Meyers et al., 1983). Schmidt and associates (1982) also reported on Stage D1 patients who were followed for a minimum of 5 years. One third of these patients were treated with radical prostatectomy. Overall only 36 per cent developed distant metastases within 5 years. Distant metastases occurred in only 14 per cent of patients having minimal lymph node metastases as compared with 47 per cent having more extensive nodal metastases. In this study, it was not stated how many patients also received adjunctive endocrine therapy. Morales and Golimbu (1980) reported that only 36 per cent of patients with Stage D1 prostate cancer treated with radical prostatectomy developed distant metastases within 2 to 7 years of follow-up. Taken together these studies suggest that patients with Stage D1 prostate cancer treated with radical prostatectomy and pelvic lymph-adenectomy may have a lower incidence of subsequent distant metastases than patients managed by treatments in which the prostate is left in situ. In contrast, Kramer and associates (1981) reported that the median time to treatment failure was the same in patients with Stage D1 prostate cancer who were treated with radical prostatectomy as in those treated with either delayed endocrine therapy or extended field radiation therapy.

The applicability of radical prostatectomy to patients with Stage D1 disease also is limited by the fact that most patients having lymph node metastases also have local extraprostatic tumor extension. Catalona and Stein (1982a) reported that only 25 per cent of patients with lymph node metastases had primary tumors that were histologically confined within the prostatic capsule. Further clinical data with long-term follow-up will be needed to determine whether radical prostatectomy is justified in patients with pelvic lymph node metastases.

Technique of Radical Prostatectomy

Currently, radical prostatectomy is most commonly performed either as a one-stage procedure through a retropubic approach or as a two-stage procedure including a staging pelvic lymphadenectomy through an abdominal incision followed by a total prostatectomy through a perineal incision. The details of these operations are presented in Chapter 76. The retropubic approach offers the advantage of one operation through one incision and the availability of a technique to preserve sexual potency (Walsh et al., 1983). The disadvantage of the retropubic approach is that the surgeon must rely on frozen section examination of the pelvic lymph nodes. The advantage of the perineal approach is that permanent sections of the pelvic lymph nodes are available before deciding whether to proceed with total prostatectomy, and the vesicourethral anastomosis is somewhat easier to perform from the perineal approach.

Complications of Radical Prostatectomy

The reported operative mortality associated with radical prostatectomy ranges up to 5 per cent (Culp, 1968; Jewett et al., 1968; Kopecky et al., 1970; Boxer et al., 1977; Nichols et al., 1977; Cochran and Kadesky, 1981b; Middleton, 1981); however, several authors have reported mortality rates of less than 1 per cent (Kopecky et al., 1970; Boxer et al., 1977; Middleton, 1981).

Incontinence rates have ranged from 2 to 57 per cent (Culp, 1968; Jewett et al., 1968; Kopecky et al., 1970; Boxer et al., 1977; Nichols et al., 1977; Kraus and Persky, 1981; Middleton, 1981; Linder et al., 1983). In experienced hands, virtually all patients should remain continent. The key to preserving continence is to avoid damage to the external sphincter mechanism of the urogenital diaphragm during the dissection.

Stricture at the vesicourethral anastomosis occurs in 2 to 23 per cent of patients (Culp, 1968; Jewett et al., 1968; Kopecky et al., 1970; Boxer et al., 1977; Nichols et al., 1977; Bass and Barrett, 1980; Middleton, 1981; Zincke et al., 1982; Linder et al., 1983). Kopecky and associates (1970) reported that anastomotic strictures were more common in patients in whom Vest sutures were used than in those who had a direct anastomosis. In experienced hands, the incidence of anastomotic stricture is less than 10 per cent. The key to avoiding anastomotic stricture is to approximate the bladder mucosa to the urethral mucosa and not close the bladder neck too tightly.

Rectal injury has been reported in up to 7 per cent of patients (Culp, 1968; Jewett et al., 1968; Nichols et al., 1977; Bass and Barrett, 1980; Middleton, 1981; Linder et al., 1983). In many instances, the rectal injury has been closed primarily (Culp, 1968; Jewett et al., 1968; Middleton, 1981); however, a diverting colostomy in addition to primary closure may be the most prudent measure.

Other complications of radical prostatectomy include thromboembolic phenomena, lymphocele, lymphedema, and wound infection. These occur in less than 10 per cent of patients. Mini-dose heparin has been used in an attempt to prevent thromboembolic complications; however, its efficacy has not been established and an increased incidence of lymphocele formation has been reported in patients receiving mini-dose heparin (Catalona et al., 1980; Hindsley et al., 1980; Sogani et al., 1981). Therefore, mini-dose heparin should be reserved for high-risk patients.

Erectile impotency has been reported in up to 90 per cent of patients following radical prostatectomy (Culp, 1968; Jewett et al., 1968; Zincke et al., 1982). Finkle and Taylor (1981) reported that 43 per cent of patients maintained potency following radical perineal prostatectomy. Damage to the parasympathetic innervation to the corpora cavernosa is responsible for postoperative impotence (Walsh and Donker, 1982). Walsh and associates (1983) developed a modification of retropubic prostatectomy that preserves sexual potency in the majority of patients. Sexual potency also may be restored with a penile prosthesis (Furlow, 1978; Kaufman et al., 1981).

Local Tumor Recurrences

Local tumor recurrences following radical prostatectomy have been reported in 4 to 22 per cent of patients, varying with the stage of the primary tumor (Turner and Belt, 1957; Flocks, 1973; Schroeder and Belt, 1975; Nichols et al., 1977; Bass and Barrett, 1980). Recurrences may not become clinically apparent for many years. Some surgeons routinely leave a button of apical prostatic tissue to facilitate the vesicourethral anastomosis. This is inadvisable, as Byar and

Mostofi (1972) reported that 75 per cent of radical prostatectomy specimens had cancer in the first or second sections taken from the prostatic apex.

Local recurrences also may occur from tumor extension into the periprostatic tissues. If local extension is present, postoperative radiation therapy to the prostatic bed and periprostatic tissues may be given (Ray et al., 1975; Taylor, 1977; Lange et al., 1983). Adjunctive radiation therapy should be delayed until there is complete wound healing. Preliminary observations suggest that adjunctive radiation therapy may be more effective if given before there is clinical evidence of local tumor recurrence (Ray et al., 1975; Taylor, 1977).

Exenterative Surgery

The results of cystoprostatectomy or total pelvic exenteration have been disappointing when there is tumor invasion of the bladder or rectum or pelvic lymph node metastasis. A 40 per cent 10-year survival rate was reported by McCullough and Leadbetter (1972) in patients having high-grade, endocrine-refractory tumors treated with exenterative surgery; however, only one of their long-term survivors had positive nodes. Spaulding and Whitmore (1978) reported a 22 per cent tumor-free, 5-year survival rate in patients treated with exenterative surgery. Two of their survivors had nodal involvement; however, no patient with bladder or rectal involvement survived tumor-free.

The most appropriate candidates for exenterative surgery are patients without evidence of metastases who have failed conventional endocrine therapy and radiation therapy.

RADIATION THERAPY

Radiation therapy was first used in the treatment of prostate cancer in the early 1900's, initially with intraurethral radium and subsequently with intracavitary and interstitial radium as well as implantation of radon seeds. In the 1920's and 1930's, external-beam orthovoltage radiation therapy was used; however, the tumor dose was severely limited by radiation damage produced in normal tissues. With the development of megavoltage external-beam radiation in the 1950's and 1960's generated by cobalt units and linear accellerators, interest in curative radiation therapy for prostate cancer was revived.

In the 1970's, modern interstitial radiation therapy using ^{125}I (iodine) seeds, ^{198}Au (gold) seeds, or ^{192}Ir (iridium) implants was developed.

External-Beam Radiation Therapy
(Figs. 32–20 to 32–22)

External-beam radiation therapy is the most thoroughly evaluated form of radiation therapy for prostate cancer, yet the information on long-term survival results is limited. Results of radiation therapy can be considered in terms of local tumor control, overall patient survival, and tumor-free survival. Many reports provide information about local tumor control and overall survival; however, in most studies, the follow-up is limited. Overall survival figures have been calculated using a variety of statistical techniques. In many instances, standard errors of the projected survival percentages either are not presented or are large. Not all studies report the tumor-free survival, which is an important index of the curative potential of any treatment. Moreover, most authors group patients with Stages A and B prostate cancer together, and only a few authors report survival figures for patients with Stage D1 disease.

LOCAL TUMOR CONTROL

Local tumor control by radiation therapy often is vaguely defined. It is not always clearly stated whether local failure indicates failure of the local lesion to regress completely or subse-

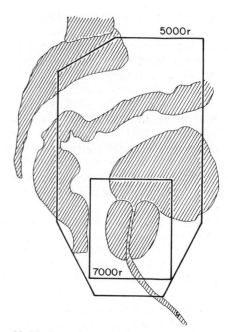

Figure 32–21. Lateral portals for external beam radiation therapy for prostate cancer. (From Bagshaw, M. A.: *In* Murphy, G. P. (Ed.): Prostatic Cancer. Littleton, Mass., PSG Publishing Co., 1979; and from Catalona, W. J.: Prostate Cancer. New York, Grune & Stratton, 1984. Used by permission.)

quent occurrence of clinical symptoms. Local tumor control has been reported to be achieved in 80 to 90 per cent of patients having Stage A or B prostate cancer (Neglia et al., 1977, 1980; Perez et al., 1977; Leibel et al., 1980). In Neglia's series (1977), there was a correlation between clinical substage and local control rates. In most series, local tumor control has not been documented histologically by needle biopsies.

TREATMENT FAILURES

Treatment failures following radiation therapy are classified as distant metastases only, local failure only, and both distant metastases and local failure. In most series, treatment failures occur in 20 to 35 per cent of patients. One half to two thirds of treatment failures are manifested by distant metastases only, whereas about 10 per cent have local failures only, and 25 to 30 per cent have both local failure and distant metastases. Tumor regression does not become clinically apparent until after completion of radiation therapy. Some tumor regression can be appreciated by 6 months in 80 per cent of patients (Leibel et al., 1980). Liebel and associates (1980) reported complete regression occurred in 27 per cent of Stage B patients by 6 months and in 74 per cent by 18 months.

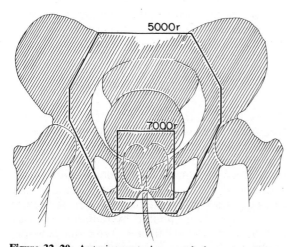

Figure 32–20. Anterior-posterior portals for external beam radiation therapy for prostate cancer. (From Bagshaw, M. A.: *In* Murphy, G. P. (Ed.): Prostatic Cancer. Littleton, Mass., PSG Publishing Co., 1979; and from Catalona, W. J.: Prostate Cancer. New York, Grune & Stratton, 1984. Used by permission.)

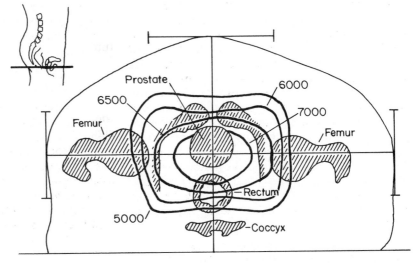

Figure 32–22. Cross-sectional distribution of radiation dose for external beam radiation therapy at the level of the prostate. (From Bagshaw, M. A.: *In* Murphy, G. P. (Ed.): Prostatic Cancer. Littleton, Mass., PSG Publishing Co., 1979; and from Catalona, W. J.: Prostate Cancer. New York, Grune & Stratton, 1984. Used by permission.)

Approximately 70 per cent of all treatment failures occur within 24 months (Ray et al., 1973). Local tumor control also correlates with tumor grade, occurring more commonly in low-grade tumors than in high-grade tumors (Perez et al., 1977; Lupu et al., 1982).

OVERALL SURVIVAL

The Stanford University series (Bagshaw, 1979, 1982) is the largest series with long-term follow-up. The projected overall survival for clinical Stages A and B combined was 78 ± 4.8 per cent at 5 years, 57 ± 6.4 per cent at 10 years, and 39 ± 8.4 per cent at 15 years. However, only 16 surviving patients had been followed for 15 years (Bagshaw, 1982). Stamey (1982) suggested that although the actuarial survival for 15 years was approximately 40 per cent, considering the 77 patients at risk for 15 years only 16 were alive, yielding a direct survival rate of only 21 per cent. Cupps and associates (1980) reported a correlation between tumor stage and 5-year survival, and McGowan (1977) reported a correlation between substage and 5-year survival.

In the Stanford series (Bagshaw, 1982), the overall actuarial survival for patients with clinical Stage C tumors was 59 ± 6 per cent at 5 years, 40 ± 6.8 per cent at 10 years, and 30 ± 7.4 per cent at 15 years, but only 8 patients were eligible for 15-year follow-up. Neglia and associates (1977) reported a correlation between survival and tumor substage within clinical Stage C. The highest survival rate reported for patients with Stage C disease was reported by Cupps and associates (1980) with an actuarial 5-year survival rate of 75 per cent and 10-year survival rate of 63 per cent.

Patients having Stage D1 disease have a substantially worse prognosis. Bagshaw (1982) reported the overall 5-year survival for patients with lymph node metastases was only 58 per cent.

TUMOR-FREE SURVIVAL

Tumor-free survival is of more importance because it reflects not only the quality of life but also the efficacy of radiation therapy in controlling prostate cancer. The most favorable 5-year tumor-free survival reported for patients with Stage B tumors is 80 per cent reported by Pilepich and associates (1980a). McGowan (1980) reported a correlation between tumor substage and tumor-free survival, with 70 per cent of patients with Stage B1 tumors being tumor-free for 5 years as compared with 39 per cent of patients with Stage B2 tumors. The most favorable 5-year tumor-free survival rate in Stage C was reported by Pilepich and associates (1980a) (56 per cent). In the Stanford series (Pistenma et al., 1979), only 8 per cent of patients having bladder invasion remained tumor-free and only 14 per cent having both pelvic and para-aortic lymph node metastases remained tumor-free. In the tabulation of the Stanford University series by Pistenma and associates (1979), only 39 per cent of patients having positive nodes remained tumor-free for 2 years. In Pilepich's series (1980a), no patient with tumor involvement of the bladder, rectum, pelvic side wall, or ureter survived more than 3 years.

Most studies suggest that a delay of radiation therapy has an adverse effect on prognosis (Ray et al., 1973; Cantril et al., 1974; Perez et al., 1977). Most studies also suggest that endocrine therapy in association with radiation therapy either has no effect or has an adverse effect on survival (Ray et al., 1973; Perez et al., 1974, 1977; van der Werf-Messing et al., 1976). In these studies, however, endocrine therapy was usually given because of symptomatic metastases. Neglia (1977), in a prospective study, administered estrogens to one group of patients following radiation therapy and treated a control group with radiation therapy only. The 5-year survival of patients treated with radiation plus estrogens was less than that in patients treated with radiotherapy alone. These results may have been influenced by the fact that a 5 mg dose of diethylstilbestrol used is associated with an increased cardiovascular death rate.

LYMPH NODE IRRADIATION AND EXTENDED FIELD RADIATION THERAPY

Only about 5000 rads can be safely delivered to the pelvic lymph node–bearing areas because of the limited tolerance of bowel to radiation (Fig. 32–23). This dose would be expected to sterilize only small primary tumors, but theoretically may be sufficient to control microscopic lymph node metastases. Studies examining the effect of extended field radiation therapy suggest that it is without therapeutic benefit (Hilaris et al., 1974; Bagshaw, 1979; Pistenma et al., 1979; Batata et al., 1980). Paulson and associates (1982a) reported that extended field radiation therapy in patients with positive nodes produced a slight delay in the appearance of distant metastases but did not improve overall 5-year survival rates. Smith and associates (1983) reported that 76 per cent of patients who received pelvic irradiation for positive nodes developed distant metastases within 5 years and only 10 per cent remained free of either local recurrence or distant metastases for 5 years.

EFFECT OF PRIOR TRANSURETHRAL RESECTION

McGowan (1980) reported that the 5-year tumor-free survival of patients with Stage B or C prostate cancer who had undergone a prior transurethral resection was significantly less than that of those who had not. Similarly, Hanks and associates (1983) reported that patients in whom the diagnosis of prostate cancer was made on the basis of a transurethral prostatectomy had a significantly higher recurrence rate at 3 years than those in whom cancer was diagnosed by needle biopsy. The death rate also was significantly higher in patients who had undergone transurethral resection. These results suggest that transurethral resection may disseminate prostate cancer. Hanks reported that the survival differences could not be explained by differences between groups in tumor volume or tumor grade. Fowler and associates (1982) found that patients who had undergone transurethral resection had a higher incidence of lymph node metastases than their counterparts who had not undergone transurethral resection and that survival rates were worse in patients with positive nodes; however, there was no significant survival difference between the patients who had undergone transurethral resection and those who had undergone needle biopsy if the patients were stratified according to tumor grade and lymph node status. Similarly, Hoffman and associates (1983) found that if

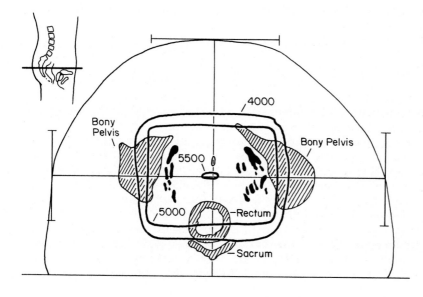

Figure 32–23. Cross-sectional distribution of radiation dose for external beam radiation therapy at the level of the pelvic lymph nodes. (From Bagshaw, M. A.: *In* Murphy, G. P. (Ed.): Prostatic Cancer. Littleton, Mass., PSG Publishing Co., 1979; and from Catalona, W. J.: Prostate Cancer. New York, Grune & Stratton, 1984. Used by permission.)

patients were stratified according to tumor stage, tumor grade, and degree of obstructive symptoms, no significant differences in survival or recurrence rates were observed between patients whose cancer was diagnosed by transurethral resection and those diagnosed by needle biopsy.

Because of the concern that transurethral resection may disseminate prostate cancer, it has been recommended that patients presenting with symptoms of vesical outlet obstruction who do not have documented metastases should not be subjected to transurethral resection. Gibbons and associates (1979) reported that only 10 per cent of patients with Stage C disease presenting with obstructive symptoms required transurethral resection after external-beam radiation therapy.

EXTERNAL–BEAM RADIATION THERAPY SALVAGE AFTER RADICAL PROSTATECTOMY

External-beam radiation therapy to the prostatic bed and periprostatic tissues can be delivered safely in patients who have either positive margins or local tumor recurrence after radical prostatectomy (Dykhuizen, 1968; Ray et al., 1975; Taylor, 1977; Neglia et al., 1977; Lange et al., 1983). Several authors have suggested that the results of salvage radiation therapy are better if the patient is treated within 4 months of radical prostatectomy than if treatment is delayed until there is palpable evidence of tumor recurrence; however, the clinical data presented are not sufficient to prove this claim (Ray et al., 1975; Taylor, 1977). Moreover, Jewett (1970) reported that capsular penetration in the absence of seminal vesicle invasion was not associated with a higher incidence of treatment failure. Radiation therapy in patients having lymph node metastases appears to be futile (Smith et al., 1983).

COMPLICATIONS OF EXTERNAL–BEAM RADIATION THERAPY

The complications of external-beam radiation therapy for prostate cancer involve the gastrointestinal and urinary tracts. Acute gastrointestinal side effects occur in 30 to 40 per cent of patients and usually develop during the fourth week of therapy (Loh et al., 1971; McGowan et al., 1977; Neglia et al., 1977; Perez et al., 1977; Bagshaw, 1979; Leibel et al., 1980). Gastrointestinal side effects consist of diarrhea, rectal discomfort, and tenesmus. These side effects should be managed by the administration of antidiarrheal agents and low-residue diets. Acute rectal symptoms sufficient to cause tem-

porary interruption of therapy occur in only about 5 per cent of patients. Chronic gastrointestinal complications occur in about 12 per cent of patients and consist of chronic diarrhea, rectal ulcers, strictures, and fistulae. Surgical intervention is required in less than 1 per cent of patients.

Urinary side effects include urinary frequency, dysuria, and microscopic or gross hematuria. Therapy must be interrupted for urinary side effects in only about 5 per cent of patients. Chronic urinary tract symptoms persist in about 10 per cent of patients. Among these are urethral stricture occurring in 4 to 8 per cent of patients (Ray et al., 1973; Perez et al., 1977; Gibbons et al., 1979; Leibel et al., 1980). Perez and associates (1974) reported that 8 per cent of patients who were continent of urine before radiation therapy became incontinent afterward. All had undergone prior transurethral resection of the prostate. To minimize the complications of radiation therapy, it is advisable to delay initiation of therapy until 4 weeks after transurethral resection or 6 weeks after open surgery. Patients having inflammatory bowel disease or diabetes mellitus with severe vascular complications generally are not good candidates for radiation therapy.

Lymphedema of the genitalia or lower extremities or both occurs infrequently in patients receiving whole pelvis radiation in the absence of tumor recurrence (Hill et al., 1974; Pistenma et al., 1979). Cutaneous complications are uncommon with the use of high-energy radiation sources except for erythema that may occur in the intergluteal folds. Loss of sexual potency has been reported in approximately 40 per cent of patients following external-beam radiation therapy (Ray et al., 1975; McGowan 1977; Perez et al., 1977; Leibel et al., 1980). Sexual impotency is probably caused by radiation injury to small vessels with secondary ischemic damage to the pelvic parasympathetic nerves as well as injury to larger vessels resulting in reduced penile blood pressure (Chapter 13).

Interstitial Radiation Therapy

[125]IODINE IMPLANTATION THERAPY

[125]Iodine (^{125}I) implantation therapy for prostate cancer was developed in the early 1970's (Whitmore et al., 1972). Initially, ^{125}I therapy was used in patients having Stages A, B, C, or D1 prostate cancer. It became apparent that patients with Stage A tumors who had

undergone transurethral resection of the prostate were unsuitable for ^{125}I implantation therapy because the remaining shell of prostatic tissue would not hold the seeds. It also became apparent that ^{125}I implantation therapy was ineffective in controlling either bulky Stage B or Stage C lesions. Moreover, patients having Stage D1 tumors generally have not fared well following ^{125}I implantation therapy, although a few patients have enjoyed long-term, tumor-free survival (Fisher et al., 1983). [125]I implantation therapy also has been used to treat tumor recurrences following definitive external-beam radiation therapy (Goffinet et al., 1980). The complication rate was excessively high when high-intensity seeds were implanted into large tumor volumes, and the tumor-free survival rates do not justify ^{125}I implantation in patients who have failed external-beam radiation therapy. Thus, applicability of ^{125}I implantation therapy is limited to patients having small Stage B tumors.

[125]I is a relatively low-energy isotope (27 KeV). Its half-value layer in tissue is only 1.7 cm. Accordingly, normal tissues surrounding the prostate are spared excessive dosages of radiation and ^{125}I is relatively safe for medical personnel and family members. [125]I emits pure gamma irradiation and has a half-life of about 60 days. Therefore, ^{125}I delivers therapeutic doses of irradiation over a period of approximately 1 year. This long half-life is disadvantageous if supplemental external-beam radiation therapy is needed. The complications of external-beam radiation therapy following ^{125}I implantation are excessive (Ross et al., 1982; de Vere White et al., 1982). Theoretically, ^{125}I implantation should deliver a radiation dose of approximately 18,000 rads to the periphery and 25,000 rads to the center of the prostate over 1 year. This is radiobiologically equivalent to 7000 rads delivered in 7 weeks.

[125]I implantation requires great care in achieving uniform distribution of seeds. Herr and Whitmore (1982) reported that the local failure rate was significantly higher in patients in whom there was an inhomogeneous distribution of seeds. The operation for ^{125}I implantation involves an extraperitoneal pelvic lymphadenectomy. Following the lymphadenectomy, the endopelvic fascia is incised on both sides of the prostate and the prostate is partially mobilized. With an index finger in the rectum, the radiation therapist places hollow 17-gauge needles about 1 cm apart into the prostate (Fig. 32–24). Computer analysis of postoperative radiographs is used to calculate the dose distribution.

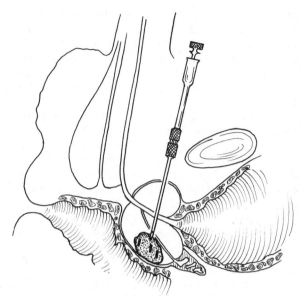

Figure 32–24. Technique for interstitial implantation therapy for prostate cancer. (From Catalona, W. J.: Prostate Cancer. New York, Grune & Stratton, 1984. Used by permission.)

Shipley and associates (1980) delivered 1050 rads external-beam radiation therapy to the pelvis before ^{125}I implantation to prevent metastases occurring from the implantation procedure. Kumar and Bartone (1981) have performed percutaneous transperineal ^{125}I implantation of the prostate using a template to obtain a more uniform distribution of seeds.

There are only limited data available on the efficacy of ^{125}I implantation therapy in the treatment of prostate cancer (Whitmore, 1980; Grossman et al., 1982). The available results are from the first 100 patients having Stage B or C tumors treated at the Memorial Sloan-Kettering Cancer Center who have been followed for 5 to 9 years. The overall survival of these patients was favorable, but the tumor-free survival was disappointing. Nearly two thirds of patients had clinical evidence of treatment failure within 5 years of treatment. Of these, 11 per cent had local recurrence only, 19 per cent had distant metastases only, and 32 per cent had both local recurrence and distant metastases. The overall 5-year survival rate for patients with Stage B disease was 87 per cent, but the tumor-free survival was only 64 per cent. For patients with Stage C tumors, the overall survival was 50 per cent, but the tumor-free survival was only 11 per cent. In Whitmore's analysis (1980), patients with Stage B tumors were divided into three substages based on the size of the tumor nodule. If these data are converted into more conventional substaging, with Stage B1 representing tumors involving one lobe of the prostate or less and B2 representing involvement of both lobes, the 5-year tumor-free survival rate for patients with B1 disease was only 62 per cent (as compared with 80 per cent in the Johns Hopkins radical prostatectomy series [Elder et al., 1982] and 70 per cent in the series of McGowan [1980] treated with external-beam radiation therapy). In patients having tumor involving both lobes of the prostate, the 5-year tumor-free survival rate was only 20 per cent (as compared with 60 per cent in the Johns Hopkins radical prostatectomy series [Elder et al., 1982] and 38 per cent from the series of McGowan and associates [1980] treated with external-beam radiation therapy). Grossman and associates (1982) reported an update of the Memorial Sloan-Kettering series in which the determinate 5-year tumor-free survival rate was 66 per cent for clinical Stage B1, 30 per cent for clinical Stage B2, and 21 per cent for Stage C.

Fisher and associates (1983) reported on 124 patients in the Memorial Sloan-Kettering series who had lymph node metastases. In this analysis, patients were stratified according to number and location of nodal metastases. There was a significant correlation between the N-stage of the patients and the subsequent appearance of distant metastases. Only 48 per cent of patients having a single positive node developed distant metastases during follow-up as compared with 69 per cent having two or three positive nodes and 93 per cent having positive juxtaregional nodes. The most favorable group included seven patients having low-grade, low T-stage primary tumors and only a single positive lymph node in which only 14 per cent developed distant metastases during follow-up.

The relatively poor tumor-free survival rate in the Memorial Sloan-Kettering experience may be influenced by the fact that only one half of the patients were staged with bone scans and nearly one quarter had elevated serum acid phosphatase titers. On the other hand, the relatively good overall survival rates may be influenced by the fact that patients who exhibited evidence of treatment failure were placed on endocrine therapy.

Whitmore (1980) reported that palpable tumor regression occurred in 57 per cent of patients treated with ^{125}I implantation and regression continued for as long as 3 years in some patients. Poor local tumor control was noted in patients who had large tumors, those who had undergone a prior transurethral resection, and those who had a split pattern of seeds

on postimplantation radiographs. Prostatic needle biopsies were reported positive in 33 to 50 per cent of patients 12 to 18 months following ^{125}I implantation (Lytton et al., 1979; Schellhammer et al., 1980; Kandzari et al., 1982, 1983). Kandzari and associates (1982) reported that approximately one half of the patients with positive biopsies had a higher histologic grade of cancer than was observed in the original tumor. However, in this series, the overall cancer death rate was only 4 per cent with a follow-up of 1 to 8 years. Lytton and associates found no significant correlation between positive biopsies and early treatment failure. More time is required for needle biopsy reports to be meaningful following ^{125}I implantation because the radiation dose is delivered over the course of approximately 1 year.

The complications of ^{125}I implantation therapy were reviewed by Fowler and associates (1979). Intraoperative complications occurred in 6 per cent of patients. Early postoperative complications occurred in 23 per cent of patients. Mini-dose heparin in a dose of 3000 units given subcutaneously every 12 hours did not reduce the incidence of thromboembolic complications. Fatal pulmonary emboli occurred in less than 1 per cent of patients. Acute urinary tract symptoms occurred in 50 per cent of the patients but usually cleared by the time of discharge from the hospital. Late complications occurred in 28 per cent of patients and included persistent voiding symptoms in 12 per cent, lower extremity or genital edema in 3 per cent, and rectal symptoms in 3 per cent. Three per cent of patients became incontinent following ^{125}I implantation. Loss of sexual potency occurred in the early postoperative period in 7 per cent of patients and another 3 per cent became impotent later. Ejaculatory disturbances occurred frequently. Similar complication rates were reported by Herr (1979), Lytton and associates (1979), Shipley and associates (1980), and Cumes and associates (1981). Mouli and associates (1983) reported on four patients who developed prostatorectal fistulae following ^{125}I implantation. Two had undergone transurethral resection prior to ^{125}I implantation and another underwent transurethral resection after implantation. Excessive postoperative complications were reported in patients who received supplemental external-beam radiation therapy after ^{125}I implantation therapy (Ross et al., 1982; de Vere White et al., 1982). Two patients in each of these series required diverting colostomy for rectal ulceration.

[125]I implantation therapy also has been used to treat tumor recurrences after external-beam

radiation therapy (Goffinet et al., 1980; Cumes et al., 1981). Although clinical control was attained in 11 of 14 patients treated, serious complications occurred in patients treated with high-intensity ^{125}I seeds implanted into large tumor volumes.

[198]Au COMBINED WITH EXTERNAL–BEAM RADIATION THERAPY AND PELVIC LYMPHADENECTOMY

Combined interstitial [198]gold ([198]Au) and external-beam radiation therapy offers the advantage of delivering a concentrated dose of radiation to the prostate that can be safely supplemented with external-beam irradiation without a marked increase in complications. This form of interstitial therapy has wider applicability than ^{125}I implantation therapy. Patients having Stages A2, B, and C1 tumors are appropriate candidates.

[198]Au is a high-energy isotope that emits both beta and gamma irradiation. Its half-value layer in tissue is 4.5 cm; therefore, precise localization of the seeds is not crucial. [198]Au has a short half-life (2.7 days), and 3 weeks after implantation the irradiation is essentially exhausted. This short half-life allows supplemental external-beam therapy to be given with the possibility of interrupting therapy if acute toxic effects develop. [198]Au creates more of a radiation protection hazard for hospital staff and is inconvenient to use because of its short shelf life. Pelvic lymphadenectomy is routinely performed before [198]Au implantation. Following the lymphadenectomy, 6 to 10 seeds are implanted as a booster dose to the prostate, attempting to cluster the seeds in the area of palpable tumor. [198]Au implants deliver approximately 3000 rads to the prostate and immediate periprostatic tissues over a period of about 3 weeks. Supplemental external-beam radiation therapy is given if the regional lymph nodes are free of metastases. Patients having nodal metastases are treated with adjunctive chemotherapy.

The results of combined interstitial [198]Au and external-beam radiation therapy were reported by Scardino and associates (1982). [198]Au therapy had little impact on cancer progression in patients with Stage A2 disease, of whom none remained tumor-free for 10 years. Accordingly, it has been recommended that patients with Stage A2 tumors should receive adjunctive chemotherapy. The overall survival results in patients with Stage B tumors are comparable to those achieved with other treatment modalities, but the 5-year tumor-free survival for a Stage B1 (71 per cent) was less than that achieved with radical prostatectomy (80 per cent in a Johns Hopkins series [Elder et al., 1982]) but better than that achieved with ^{125}I implantation therapy (62 per cent in the Memorial Sloan-Kettering series [Whitmore, 1980]). For Stage B2, the 5-year tumor-free survival rate of 59 per cent was equivalent to that achieved with radical prostatectomy and better than that achieved with ^{125}I implantation or external-beam radiation therapy (McGowan, 1980; Whitmore, 1980; Elder et al., 1982). In patients with Stage C1 tumors, the 5-year tumor-free survival rate was 46 per cent, which is comparable to that achieved with external-beam therapy alone (McGowan, 1980), and the 10-year tumor-free survival was 40 per cent, which is superior to that achieved with external-beam radiation therapy (McGowan, 1980). The 5-year tumor-free survival rate in patients with Stage D1 tumors was only 30 per cent, and no patient having Stage D1 disease survived tumor-free for 10 years. These results are similar to those observed with external-beam radiation therapy and ^{125}I implantation therapy.

Local tumor control was achieved in 94 per cent of patients treated with combined [198]Au and external-beam therapy, but needle biopsies remained positive in 39 per cent (Scardino et al., 1982). Any histologic changes suspicious for residual cancer were associated with the 40 to 50 per cent distant metastasis rate within 2 to 14 years. Patients having negative needle biopsies had a 20 per cent incidence of distant metastasis (Wheeler and Scardino, 1983). Approximately 12 per cent of patients experienced acute proctitis following [198]Au therapy. Persistent proctitis occurred in about 4 per cent of patients. Symptoms of acute bladder irritability occurred in 14 per cent of patients and persisted in 3 per cent. Sexual impotency occurred in approximately 30 per cent of patients. Less than 1 per cent of patients had lower extremity or genital edema, 2 per cent had lymphoceles, and thromboembolic complications occurred in 10 per cent of patients. Thromboembolic complications were not reduced with the use of prophylactic mini-dose heparin; accordingly, its use was abandoned (Scardino et al., 1982).

INTERSTITIAL ^{192}Ir IMPLANTATION THERAPY

Interstitial implantation using radioactive iridium (^{192}Ir) wires was developed in France (Court and Chassagne, 1977). [192]Ir is a gamma emitter with a half-life of 75 days; the half-value layer in tissue is 6 cm. With this technique, hollow needles containing empty plastic tubes are inserted into the prostate through the perineum at the time of pelvic lymphadenectomy. In the postoperative period, ^{192}Ir wires are loaded into the needles. This results in the delivery of 6000 to 7000 rads at a low-dose rate over approximately 6 days. Miller (1979) reported on the results of treatment with ^{192}Ir in 14 patients who also received 2000 rads of external-beam radiation therapy in 10 fractions before ^{192}Ir implantation. Major complications occurred in three patients, two of whom required colostomy. No comment was made concerning the efficacy of treatment. Tansey and associates (1983) reported on 40 patients treated with ^{192}Ir implantation followed by external-beam radiation. The ^{192}Ir seeds were inserted postoperatively to give 3000 to 3500 rads over 40 to 50 hours. Postoperatively, patients not having nodal metastases received 4000 rads to the prostate. Patients having nodal metastases received 4000 rads to the whole pelvis and 1000 rads to the pelvic nodes with the prostate, rectum, and bladder being shielded. Follow-up was insufficient to evaluate the efficacy of this treatment; however, no early local failures were noted. One patient developed urinary incontinence, and although the vast majority retained sexual potency, several had a decrease in the quality of erections. Post-implantation biopsies were negative in 15 of 16 patients.

Post-Irradiation Prostate Biopsies

Digital rectal examination is of limited reliability in determining the tumor response to radiation therapy, particularly if the primary tumor regresses only partially or remains unchanged. Because of the slow rate of regression of prostate cancer after radiation therapy, biopsies obtained before 1 year are not meaningful; however, after 1 year, between 35 per cent and 67 per cent of patients have positive biopsies (Grout et al., 1971; Rhamy et al., 1972; Mollenkamp et al., 1975; Sewell et al., 1975; Cox and Stoeffel, 1977; Nachtsheim et al., 1978; Bagshaw, 1979; Leach et al., 1982). Cox and Stoeffel (1977) suggested that the incidence of positive post-irradiation biopsies continues to decline for 3 years, after which about 20 per cent of patients have positive biopsies. In contrast, Kiesling et al. (1980) reported that positive biopsies more than 1 year after radiation therapy were likely to remain positive. In Kiesling's study, 62 per cent of patients who initially had negative biopsies subsequently were found to have positive biopsies, whereas only 25 per cent

who initially had positive biopsies subsequently converted to negative.

There are conflicting opinions about the significance of positive biopsies following radiation therapy. It has been stated that cancer cells remaining after radiation therapy may have lost their capacity to divide and metastasize (Kagan et al., 1977), and several authors (Cox and Stoeffel, 1977; Kagan et al., 1977; Lytton et al., 1979; Leach et al., 1982) have reported no significant correlation between biopsy results and prognosis. However, there is accumulating evidence that patients having positive biopsies more than 1 year after radiation therapy have a significantly increased risk of developing distant metastases (Perez et al., 1974; Cosgrove and Kaempf, 1976; Kurth et al., 1977; Kiesling et al., 1980; Scardino et al., 1982; Freiha, 1983). Scardino and associates (1982) reported that 59 per cent of patients had positive biopsies more than 1 year after radiation therapy and all developed distant metastases within 10 years. Of patients having negative biopsies, the 10-year tumor-free survival was 77 per cent. Similarly, Freiha (1983) reported that 61 per cent of patients had positive biopsies 18 months following external-beam radiation therapy and 84 per cent of patients with positive biopsies had either local or distant cancer progression within 5 to 11 years, as compared with a cancer progression rate of 25 per cent in patients having negative biopsies.

Herr and Whitmore (1982) suggested that needle biopsy should not be performed routinely after radiation therapy because a negative biopsy does not rule out residual cancer and a positive biopsy does not prove biologically significant tumor, but rather creates anxiety for both the patient and the physician.

Palliative Radiation Therapy

EXTERNAL-BEAM THERAPY FOR SKELETAL METASTASES

Radiation therapy in doses of 3000 to 3500 rads given in approximately 10 treatments is effective in palliating pain from skeletal metastases. Prophylactic radiation therapy to minimally symptomatic or asymptomatic lesions in weight-bearing areas such as the femoral neck or spine is advisable to prevent the occurrence of disabling pathologic fractures. Benson and associates (1982) reported that complete pain relief was achieved in 42 per cent of patients and partial pain relief was achieved in 35 per cent.

INTRAVENOUS ³²P THERAPY FOR SKELETAL METASTASES

Intravenous ^{32}P was used as a means of palliative radiation therapy in patients having widespread osseous metastases because the isotope is deposited in metastatic lesions in bone. A major drawback to this form of therapy was the severe hematologic toxicity that invariably occurred. Although favorable results were reported (Donati et al., 1966), the therapeutic benefits did not justify the toxicity. Consequently, intravenous ^{32}P therapy generally has been abandoned.

HEMIBODY IRRADIATION FOR OSSEOUS METASTASES

Low-dose hemibody or whole body irradiation has been used as palliative therapy for patients having widespread endocrine-refractory metastatic prostate cancer (Epstein et al., 1979; Keen, 1980; Rowland et al., 1981). The patient is irradiated in two large fields, first the upper body above the umbilicus and then the lower body. The radiation dose to the upper half of the body is only about 600 rads and the dose to the lower half of the body is usually 800 to 1000 rads. The reduced dose is given to the upper half of the body to prevent radiation pneumonitis. The interval between irradiation of the upper and lower halves of the body generally is 4 to 6 weeks.

Patients usually are hospitalized for hemibody irradiation. Severe nausea and vomiting occurs immediately following treatment and lasts for 3 to 6 hours. Other side effects include leukopenia and thrombocytopenia, which last for 4 to 6 weeks. The irradiated marrow is repopulated by stem cells from the nonirradiated marrow. Keen (1980) reported 70 per cent of patients treated with hemibody irradiation had partial pain relief and 29 per cent had complete relief. The onset of pain relief is rapid, occurring within 12 to 24 hours after treatment. The mean duration of response is about 5 months.

EXTERNAL–BEAM RADIATION THERAPY FOR URETERAL OBSTRUCTION

Radiation therapy in doses of 5000 to 6000 rads usually is effective in relieving ureteral obstruction from prostate cancer (Carlton et al., 1972; Megalli et al., 1974; Michigan and Catalona, 1977). Resolution of ureteral obstruction may require weeks to months; accordingly, percutaneous nephrostomy may be required in pa-

tients having bilateral obstruction. Palliative radiation therapy (4000 to 5000 rads) also is effective in controlling bleeding and rectal or urinary obstructive symptoms (Kraus et al., 1972).

PRE–ESTROGEN BREAST IRRADIATION

Approximately 70 per cent of patients treated with therapeutic doses of estrogen develop gynecomastia (Gagnon et al., 1979). Irradiation of the breasts before estrogen administration can prevent the development of gynecomastia. However, irradiation given either simultaneously with or after estrogen administration will not completely inhibit or reverse gynecomastia. Radiation should be given at least 2 days before estrogen therapy is started. Single doses of 800, 1000, and 1250 rads have proved to be effective, but the interval between single-dose irradiation and estrogen administration was 2 weeks. Single-dose irradiation also produces more skin changes in the breast. Gagnon and associates (1979) reported that 300 rads per day given on alternate days for a total dose of 1200 rads was uniformly effective in preventing gynecomastia. If emergency estrogen therapy is required, it has been recommended to use a single dose of 800 rads in 1 day. In patients having painful gynecomastia, breast irradiation with 1000 rads will relieve the pain but will not induce the regression of gynecomastia.

PREOPERATIVE RADIATION THERAPY

Preoperative radiation therapy followed by radical prostatectomy has been evaluated by Gill (1980) and Carson (1980) and their associates. In Carson's series, no increased complications were reported; however, in Gill's series, there was an unacceptably high incidence of postoperative complications. Preoperative radiation therapy is not ideally suited for radical prostatectomy because radical prostatectomy requires reconstruction of the lower urinary tract. Preoperative radiation therapy may impair healing or function and may induce stricture formation.

ENDOCRINE THERAPY

Physiologic Rationale

Prostatic cells are dependent upon androgen to carry out their normal metabolic functions. The biologic activity of androgens in the prostate is dependent upon their conversion to dihydrotestosterone (DHT) within the prostatic cell (Fig. 32–25). Testosterone is the major circulating androgen, 90 per cent of which is produced by the testes. Approximately 57 per cent of circulating testosterone is bound to sex steroid–binding globulin and 40 per cent is bound to albumin. Approximately 3 per cent of circulating testosterone remains unbound, which is the functionally active form of the hormone. Unbound testosterone diffuses passively through the prostatic cell membrane into the cytoplasm where it is converted to DHT by the 5-alpha reductase enzyme (Fig. 32–25). After conversion, DHT binds to a specific receptor protein in the cytoplasm, and the DHT-receptor complex is translocated into the cell nucleus. In the nucleus, the DHT-receptor complex binds to acceptor sites on the DNA of nuclear chromatin, activating the DNA to produce messenger RNA, which in turn codes for proteins that are important for the metabolic functions of the prostatic cell (Walsh, 1975). In the absence of androgen, the prostate undergoes atrophy. Physiologic concentrations of adrenal androgens alone are not sufficient to sustain the prostate.

Prostate cancers are composed of a heterogeneous population of cells that differ in their androgen requirements. Some cells require nearly physiologic levels of androgen for their maintenance, while others may thrive in the virtual absence of androgen. Tumors that are composed largely of androgen-dependent cells respond well to androgen-withdrawal therapy, whereas those that are composed largely of androgen-independent cells do not.

Androgen production by the testes and the adrenal glands is regulated by the hypothalamic-pituitary axis through two separate negative feedback mechanisms (Fig. 32–26). Testosterone secretion by the testes is stimulated by

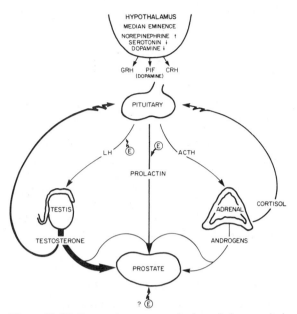

Figure 32–26. Interactions among the hypothalamus, pituitary, testes, adrenals, and prostate. Estrogen administration inhibits LH release and stimulates prolactin release. Adrenal androgen secretion is stimulated by ACTH; the feedback signal is cortisol. (From Catalona, W. J.: Prostate Cancer. New York, Grune & Stratton, 1984. Used by permission.)

luteinizing hormone (LH) released from the anterior pituitary upon stimulation by LH-releasing hormone (LHRH) from the anterior hypothalamus. LHRH is secreted into the hypothalamic-pituitary portal venous system and transported to the anterior pituitary where it stimulates LH and FSH (follicle-stimulating hormone) release. Testosterone is a mediator of negative feedback for LH secretion in males; however, estrogens also are potent inhibitors of LH secretion. Inhibition of LH secretion is believed to be the principal mechanism of action of estrogen therapy for prostate cancer.

Estrogens also produce an increase in circulating levels of sex steroid–binding globulin. In the presence of increased binding globulin, the total amount of free testosterone is reduced. Thus, estrogens further decrease the *functional* circulating levels of testosterone. In many men after the age of 60, testosterone levels decline and estradiol levels increase (Zumoff, 1982).

Androgen secretion by the adrenal (androstenedione and dehydroepiandrosterone) is stimulated by adrenocorticotropic hormone (ACTH) released from the anterior pituitary upon stimulation by corticotropic-releasing factor (CRF) from the hypothalamus (Fig. 32–26). Adrenal androgens do not mediate negative feedback on ACTH secretion; rather, cortisol is

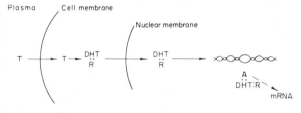

Figure 32–25. Testosterone (T) diffuses across the cell membrane and is converted by 5-d(alpha)-reductase to dihydrotestosterone (DHT). DHT binds to the cytosol receptor (R) and the DHT-R complex is translocated to the cell nucleus, where it binds to acceptor (A) sites on the DNA of nuclear chromatin. This stimulates the synthesis of messenger RNA (mRNA), which codes for proteins that are necessary for normal prostatic cell function. (From Walsh, P. C.: Urol. Clin. North Am., 2:125, 1975. Used by permission.)

the feedback signal. Adrenal androgens are relatively weakly androgenic as compared with testosterone or dihydrotestosterone (Table 32–6) and are bound almost exclusively to albumin.

Prolactin is another pituitary factor that influences androgen metabolism in the prostate (Grayhack, 1963). Prolactin increases the uptake and utilization of androgen by prostatic cells. Pituitary prolactin secretion normally is tonically inhibited by prolactin inhibitory factor (PIF) (dopamine) produced in the hypothalamus (Fig. 32–26). Estrogens are potent inhibitors of PIF; therefore, estrogens increase prolactin release and theoretically may enhance utilization of androgens by prostatic cells.

Mechanism of Endocrine Control of Prostate Cancer

The main objective of endocrine therapy for prostate cancer is to stop androgenic stimulation of the tumor. This may be accomplished by ablation of endocrine sources, by suppression of pituitary LH release, or by inhibition of androgen synthesis, androgen action, or androgen synergism.

ABLATION OF ENDOCRINE SOURCES

Orchiectomy. Bilateral orchiectomy reduces circulating testosterone levels from approximately 500 ng per dl to about 50 ng per dl (Young and Kent, 1968; Robinson and Thomas, 1971; Mackler, 1972; Shearer et al., 1973). Circulating testosterone levels remain low following castration (Young and Kent, 1968; Shearer et al., 1973; Walsh and Siiteri, 1975). This reduction in circulating androgen levels effectively arrests the metabolism of the androgen-dependent population of prostate cancer cells and induces a clinical remission in the majority of patients treated (Trachtenberg and Walsh, 1982).

Subcapsular orchiectomy has been decried because of the possibility of incomplete removal of Leydig cells (O'Connor et al., 1963). Recent studies have demonstrated, however, that testosterone levels are reduced to the castrate range following subcapsular orchiectomy and remain low even after HCG stimulation (Clark and Houghton, 1977; Senge et al., 1978). Favorable clinical responses occur in the vast majority of patients treated with subcapsular orchiectomy.

Adrenalectomy. The rationale for adrenalectomy is the elimination of adrenal androgens that may stimulate prostate cancer cells. Early studies measuring urinary 17-ketosteroids suggested that adrenal androgen secretion increased following orchiectomy. It was believed that increased levels of adrenal androgens were responsible for reactivation of prostate cancer (Huggins and Scott, 1945). However, more recent studies have shown that plasma adrenal androgen levels remain normal in patients who have undergone orchiectomy for prostate cancer (Walsh and Siiteri, 1975; Vermeulen et al., 1982). Moreover, because adrenal androgens alone are not sufficient to sustain normal prostatic epithelial cells, which are highly androgen-dependent, it is not surprising that removal of adrenal androgens has little effect on the growth of the predominantly androgen-independent prostate cancer cells that remain after orchiectomy or estrogen administration.

Hypophysectomy. Hypophysectomy removes the source of ACTH, which stimulates adrenal androgen secretion, and also the source of prolactin.

SUPPRESSION OF PITUITARY LH RELEASE

Estrogens. Estrogens have numerous influences on androgen metabolism. Estrogens suppress pituitary LH secretion, increase levels of sex steroid–binding globulin, reduce testosterone steroidogenesis in the testis, increase pitui-

TABLE 32–6. MAJOR CIRCULATING ANDROGENS

Source	Androgen	Amount Produced per Day (mg)	Relative Potency
Testis	Testosterone	6.6	100
Testis and peripheral tissues	Dihydrotestosterone	0.3	181
Adrenal	Androstenedione	1.4	39
Adrenal	Dehydroepiandrosterone	29	15

Modified from Coffey, D.S.: The biochemistry and physiology of the prostate and seminal vesicles. *In* Harrison, J. H., Gittes, R. F., Perlmutter, A. D., Stamey, T. A., and Walsh, P. C. (Eds.): Campbell's Urology. Philadelphia, W. B. Saunders Co., 1978, pp. 161–202 (with permission); and from Catalona, W. J.: Prostate Cancer, New York, Grune & Stratton, 1984 (with permission).

tary prolactin secretion, and, in very high concentrations, decrease DNA synthesis in prostate cancer cells.

The principal salutary effect of estrogens appears to be suppression of pituitary LH secretion. The most commonly used estrogen preparation is diethylstilbestrol (DES). DES in doses of less than 1 mg per day does not significantly suppress plasma testosterone levels, while a 1 mg daily dose may suppress testosterone levels incompletely and unreliably in some patients (Shearer et al., 1973; Prout et al., 1976). However, the vast majority of patients taking 1 mg of DES daily have testosterone levels suppressed to or near the castrate range (Beck et al., 1978). Moreover, dramatic clinical remissions can be achieved without complete suppression of testosterone levels. DES in the dose of 1 mg daily is not associated with an increased risk of cardiovascular complications or deaths. DES in doses of 3 mg to 5 mg daily suppresses plasma testosterone to castrate levels, but both of these doses are associated with an increased incidence of cardiovascular complications and deaths (VACURG, 1967; Glashan and Robinson, 1981). Higher doses of DES do not further suppress plasma testosterone levels. It is possible that a 2 mg daily dose of DES may be ideal for prostate cancer patients, but clinical studies using a daily 2 mg dose of DES have not been reported. The dose range in which estrogens are effective without producing excessive cardiovascular toxic effects is narrow.

Other estrogenic preparations also suppress plasma testosterone levels into the castrate range, but do not offer any significant advantage over DES. Chlorotrianisene (TACE) is a weak estrogen that is claimed to be clinically effective, but does not suppress pituitary LH and produces only a slight reduction in serum testosterone levels (Baker et al., 1973; Shearer et al., 1973; Baba et al., 1982). Estradurin in doses of 40 to 80 mg administered intramuscularly monthly also has been shown not to produce significant suppression of plasma testosterone levels (Lukkarinen et al., 1981).

Plasma testosterone levels return to normal within 6 months after withdrawal of estrogen therapy in patients who have been treated for less than 3 years. However, testosterone levels have been reported to remain low after estrogen withdrawal in patients who have been treated for longer than 3 years (Tomic et al., 1983). This observation has not yet been confirmed.

In experimental animals, estrogens have the paradoxical effect of acting synergistically with androgens in stimulating prostatic growth (Walsh and Wilson, 1976; Menon and Walsh, 1979). In high concentrations, estrogens reduce testicular steroidogenesis (Yanihara and Troen, 1972) and may directly influence the metabolism of prostate cells (Huggins and Clark, 1940; Schenken et al., 1942; Farnsworth, 1969; Harper et al., 1970).

Progestins. Progestins exhibit numerous therapeutically desirable features, including the capacity to bind to the DHT receptor and function as an antiandrogen, to block the 5-alpha reductase enzyme, thus inhibiting the conversion of testosterone to DHT, and to exert feedback inhibition of pituitary LH release (Geller et al., 1978). However, clinical studies have demonstrated that after 6 months an escape phenomenon occurs in which testosterone levels gradually return to normal (Geller et al., 1978). This can be prevented by the administration of low-dose DES (0.1 mg daily), which by itself is insufficient to suppress plasma testosterone. This low dose of DES is not associated with thromboembolic complications or fluid retention. A progestin frequently used in the treatment of prostate cancer is megestrol acetate.

Gonadotropin-Releasing Hormone Agonists and Antagonists. Gonadotropin-releasing hormone (GRH) agonists are synthetic peptides that have a structure similar to that of native GRH, but have been modified at positions 6 and 10 on the polypeptide chain (Corbin, 1982). Administration of these compounds in pulses stimulates the release of LH and FSH from the anterior pituitary, but prolonged chronic administration blocks gonadotropin release and thus achieves a pharmacologic hypophysectomy that is selective for gonadotropins. These agents must be administered by intranasal insufflation or subcutaneous injection. GRH agonists produce an initial increase in plasma testosterone levels that persists for approximately 2 weeks before plasma testosterone is suppressed into the castrate range. The initial increase in testosterone levels may stimulate tumor growth. Accordingly, it is advisable to administer estrogens or antiandrogens during the first 2 weeks of GRH agonist therapy.

GRH antagonists compete with LHRH at the level of the pituitary receptor, preempting the ability of LHRH to bind to the receptor and precluding its stimulation of LH and FSH secretion (Corbin, 1982). GRH antagonists therefore do not stimulate testosterone secretion. A direct effect of GRH antagonists on prostate cancer cells also has been postulated, but has not been clearly established. GRH agonists and antagonists are advantageous because they do not produce gynecomastia or cardiovascular side effects.

INHIBITION OF ANDROGEN

Synthesis. Testosterone is synthesized from cholesterol and acetate by a series of biochemical reactions that involve five enzymes (Walsh, 1975). Enzymatic inhibitors, including aminoglutethimide, spironolactone, cyanoketone, and medrogestone, interfere with the synthesis of testosterone.

Action. In order to exert their actions on the prostate cancer cells, androgens must bind to the intracellular cytoplasmic receptor protein. Accordingly, the action of androgens can be inhibited by agents that compete with DHT for binding to the receptor protein. Such agents are called antiandrogens and include cyproterone acetate, flutamide, and medrogestone (Walsh, 1975). It was hoped that antiandrogens would not produce gynecomastia; however, gynecomastia has developed in some patients. Cyproterone acetate is a progestational antiandrogen that also inhibits pituitary LH secretion and testosterone synthesis. Flutamide is a nonsteroidal antiandrogen that does not inhibit testosterone synthesis or LH secretion. Megestrol acetate is the only antiandrogen that is approved for use in the United States.

Synergism. Agents that inhibit prolactin release from the pituitary block the synergistic effects between prolactin and androgens in prostate cancer cells. Levodopa increases the dopamine concentration in the hypothalamus, and dopamine inhibits prolactin secretion by the pituitary. Bromoergocryptine stimulates dopamine receptors in the pituitary and thus effectively enhances the inhibitory effects of dopamine on prolactin secretion.

Clinical Studies of Endocrine Therapy

Huggins and Hodges (1941) reported that castration or estrogen administration in patients with metastatic prostate cancer induced regression of the cancer. This was usually associated with a decrease in serum acid phosphatase and an alkaline phosphatase "flare phenomenon" in which the serum alkaline phosphatase levels initially increased and then subsequently declined toward normal. Testosterone administration in orchiectomized patients resulted in stimulation of cancer growth and an increase in acid phosphatase levels. Huggins noted that orchiectomy often was more effective than estrogen

administration and that favorable responses occurred more frequently in patients having normal-sized testes and those having well-differentiated tumors.

Early clinical trials following the introduction of endocrine therapy suggested that endocrine therapy prolonged patient survival; however, these studies were limited by the fact that they were retrospective and the patient groups were not strictly comparable (Nesbit and Plumb, 1946; Vest and Frazier, 1946; Nesbit and Baum, 1950). Another major limitation was that the controls were not treated concurrently but rather were treated in the prehormonal era (also the preantibiotic era) when the expected survival of the general population was less. Nonetheless, the results of these early studies were accepted and there was widespread use of endocrine therapy for all stages of prostate cancer until the results of the Veterans Administration Cooperative Urological Research Group study (VACURG) were published (1967).

The VACURG clinical trials are the most comprehensive studies of endocrine therapy for prostate cancer available. In VACURG Study 1 (1967), patients with Stage C or D tumors were randomized to receive either placebo, 5 mg of DES daily, orchiectomy plus placebo, or orchiectomy plus 5 mg of DES daily (Table 32–7). Survival curves constructed for the cause of death revealed that patients who received 5 mg of DES had a significantly higher cardiovascular death rate and a correspondingly lower death rate from prostate cancer. This finding was unexpected, since it was believed at the time that estrogens had a salutary effect on cardiovascular disease (Coronary Drug Project Research Group, 1970). However, the previous data of Nesbit and Baum (1950) also had revealed that patients treated with DES had a higher percentage of deaths not due to cancer and a worse overall survival rate than patients treated with orchiectomy.

Another surprising finding of VACURG Study 1 was that the overall survival rate of patients treated with placebo was not significantly worse than that of patients treated with endocrine therapy. However, 70 per cent of patients with Stage C disease and all patients with Stage D disease were switched from placebo to endocrine therapy when they exhibited evidence of cancer progression (Blackard et al., 1973). The final results were tabulated according to the initial treatment assigned. Accordingly, the results of VACURG Study 1 demonstrated that delayed endocrine therapy was as effective as early endocrine therapy in terms of overall patient survival (Blackard et al., 1973).

TABLE 32–7. DEATHS BY STAGE, TREATMENT, AND CAUSE IN VACURG PROSTATE STUDY 1

	Stage A		Stage B		Stage C				Stage D			
	Px + P	Px + E	Px + P	Px + E	P	E	O + P	O + E	P	E	O + P	O + E
Number of patients	60	60	85	94	262	265	266	257	223	211	203	216
Cause of death												
Cancer of prostate	3	2	8	2	46	18	35	25	105	82	97	82
Cardiovascular causes	20	25	25	32	88	112	95	108	55	76	56	59
Other	7	10	9	12	43	50	54	48	29	23	29	40
Total deaths	30	37	42	46	177	180	184	181	189	181	182	181

Px = Radical prostatectomy; P = placebo; E = 5.0 mg diethylstilbestrol daily; O = orchiectomy.
Modified from Byar, D. P.: The Veterans Administration Cooperative Urological Research Group's studies of cancer of the prostate. Cancer, *32*:1126, 1973 (with permission).

VACURG Study 2 attempted to determine whether lower doses of DES were as effective as the 5 mg dose in controlling cancer progression without causing the excessive cardiovascular complications and deaths. Patients with Stage C or D tumors were randomized to receive either placebo, 0.2 mg DES daily, 1 mg DES daily, or 5 mg DES daily. In patients having Stage C or D tumors, 1 mg DES daily was as effective as 5 mg and significantly more effective than 0.2 mg or placebo in preventing cancer deaths and was not associated with an increased incidence of cardiovascular deaths (Table 32–8) (Bailar et al., 1970). Glashan and Robinson (1981) also demonstrated in a prospective study that a 3 mg daily dose of DES was associated with a significantly higher incidence of cardiovascular complications and deaths than orchiectomy. VACURG Study 2 also demonstrated that both 1 and 5 mg of DES significantly retarded the rate of progression from Stage C to Stage D disease.

VACURG Study 3 (Byar, 1973) attempted to determine whether oral estrogens or progestins offered any advantage over 1 mg of DES in patients with Stage C or D tumors. The results showed no significant advantage of any of these agents over 1 mg of DES daily in terms of overall survival or cancer mortality (Blackard, 1975).

A number of misconceptions have arisen from the VACURG studies. One misconception is the notion that endocrine therapy does not prolong patient survival. The results of VACURG Study 1 showed only that *delayed* endocrine therapy was as effective as *early* endocrine therapy in terms of overall patient survival. The data from VACURG Study 2 suggest that endocrine therapy does, in fact, prolong survival in patients with Stage D tumors. Unlike VACURG Study 1, in which all patients were switched from placebo to endocrine therapy when there was evidence of cancer progression, with the realization that estrogens could be harmful, in VACURG Study 2 there was less of a tendency to switch treatments. Accordingly, in VACURG Study 2, many patients who had cancer progression were maintained on placebo. The results of VACURG Study 2 revealed that only 19 per cent of patients assigned to placebo were alive at the time the results were tabulated as compared with 44 and 45 per cent respectively of patients receiving 1 or 5 mg of DES (Byar, 1973). This suggests, in a concurrent trial, that endocrine therapy does improve the survival of patients having Stage D tumors.

TABLE 32–8. DEATHS BY STAGE, TREATMENT, AND CAUSE IN VACURG PROSTATE STUDY 2

	Stage C				Stage D			
		DIETHYLSTILBESTROL				DIETHYLSTILBESTROL		
	PLACEBO	*0.2 mg daily*	*1.0 mg daily*	*5.0 mg daily*	PLACEBO	*0.2 mg daily*	*1.0 mg daily*	*5.0 mg daily*
Number of patients	75	73	73	73	53	52	55	54
Cause of death								
Cancer of prostate	11	9	3	3	21	28	17	14
Cardiovascular causes	15	14	18	31	10	7	10	10
Other	11	19	14	7	9	1	4	7
Total deaths	37	42	35	41	40	36	31	31

Modified from Byar, D. P.: The Veterans Administration Cooperative Urological Research Group's studies of cancer of the prostate. Cancer, *32*:1126, 1973 (with permission).

In a study designed to minimize the influence of general medical advances on patient survival, Lepor and associates (1982) compared the survival of patients with Stage C or D tumors treated late in the prehormonal era (1937–1940) with a similar group treated with hormonal therapy early in the hormonal era between 1942 and 1943. The median survival was longer in patients treated with hormonal therapy than in those treated in the prehormonal era, but the authors could not exclude the possibility that the difference was not due to a general increased longevity in the posthormonal era.

Another misconception that has arisen from the VACURG trials is the notion that estrogen therapy is more effective than orchiectomy in reducing prostate cancer deaths (Blackard et al., 1973). This notion is based on analysis of cancer deaths in VACURG Study 1, in which the estrogen-treated patients had the lowest percentage of cancer deaths. However, because estrogen-treated patients had an excessive number of cardiovascular deaths, most occurring during the first year, it is likely that many of these patients would have died of prostate cancer if they had not died of cardiovascular causes first. In fact, in Nesbit and Baum's analysis (1950), the 5-year survival of patients having Stage D tumors was 10 per cent for those treated with 1 to 5 mg of DES, 22 per cent for those treated with orchiectomy alone, and 20 per cent for those treated with both. These results suggest that orchiectomy was the most effective treatment and that administration of 1 to 5 mg of DES to orchiectomized patients did not further enhance survival.

The weight of evidence suggests that estrogen therapy and orchiectomy are equivalent and there is little to be gained from using both together. Orchiectomy may be preferred because it is a safer and a more certain means of achieving complete suppression of plasma testosterone. With estrogen therapy there also is concern about patient compliance, since estrogens may produce nausea, fluid retention, and gynecomastia. Moreover, Beck and associates (1978) reported that suppressed testosterone levels could return to within the normal range within 12 hours of neglecting to take a daily 1 mg dose of DES.

The thromboembolic and cardiovascular complications associated with estrogen therapy are related to fluid retention, suppression of plasma levels of antithrombin III into the hypercoagulable range (Dobbs et al., 1980; Varenhorst et al., 1981; Buller et al., 1982), increased platelet aggregation (Eisen et al., 1975; Koiso et al., 1982), and changes in serum lipids and triglycerides (Kontturi and Sotaniemi, 1971).

The timing of endocrine therapy in prostate cancer patients is not crucial. In sexually active, asymptomatic patients, delayed endocrine therapy is appropriate, whereas in patients who are not sexually active, early endocrine therapy may be used. Pre-estrogen breast irradiation should be given before starting treatment. Patients having symptomatic metastases including pain, neurologic symptoms, ureteral obstruction, vesical outlet obstruction, weight loss, anemia, edema, or shortness of breath should be treated immediately.

Although most patients manifest some response to endocrine therapy, the response is clinically significant in only about 80 per cent. In the National Prostatic Cancer Project (NPCP) study (Murphy et al., 1983) in which the response criteria used for cytotoxic chemotherapy were used, only 41 per cent of patients treated with endocrine therapy qualified as exhibiting objective tumor regression while 40 per cent remained objectively stable.

There is a remarkable variability of survival in patients treated with endocrine therapy for prostate cancer. In the VACURG studies (Jordan et al., 1977), 10 per cent survived longer than 10 years, 10 per cent survived less than 6 months, and 50 per cent survived less than 3 years. Reiner and associates (1979) reported that 16 per cent of patients treated with endocrine therapy survived longer than 10 years; however, using standard clinical parameters such as tumor grade and acid phosphatase levels, they could not identify those patients destined to have prolonged favorable responses.

Biochemical assays have been developed attempting to predict endocrine responsiveness in prostate cancer patients. In general, a prerequisite for steroid hormone effects on target tissues is the presence of an intracellular receptor protein for the hormone in the target tissue. For instance, in breast cancer patients it is well established that the response to endocrine therapy correlates with the presence of intracellular estrogen receptors in the tumor. The relationship between intracellular DHT receptor content of prostate cancer and response to endocrine therapy has been examined by several investigators (De Voogt and Dingjan, 1978; Krieg et al., 1978; Mobbs et al., 1978; Ekman et al., 1979; Martelli et al., 1980; Trachtenberg and Walsh, 1982). These studies have yielded somewhat conflicting results. In the most complete study available, Trachtenberg and Walsh

(1982) reported no significant correlation between *total* or *cytosol* androgen receptor content and either duration of response or survival. However, there was a significant correlation between *nuclear* DHT receptor content and both duration of response and duration of survival. In this study, a high nuclear DHT receptor content was necessary for a prolonged favorable response to endocrine therapy but was not sufficient to predict a prolonged response in all patients; i.e., patients having low DHT receptor values could be predicted to have no response or brief responses, whereas only about one half of those with tumors having a high DHT receptor content had prolonged responses.

Studies of estrogen receptors and progesterone receptors in prostate cancer patients also have yielded conflicting results. Young and associates (1979) reported a correlation between estrogen receptor content and the response to hormonal therapy, whereas Wagner (1978), Eckman and associates (1979), and Karr and associates (1979) found no such correlation.

PRIMARY ENDOCRINE THERAPY FOR LOCALIZED PROSTATE CANCER

Barnes and associates (1976, 1979) reported the most favorable results of primary endocrine therapy in patients with Stage A or B prostate cancer. In this series, the 15-year survival rate was 33 per cent but only 21 per cent had no clinical evidence of metastases. Barnes and associates (1979) also compared the survival of patients under 70 years old and those over 70 years old with that of the general population. Patients over 70 years of age survived nearly as long as expected with primary endocrine therapy, but those under 70 had a diminished survival with respect to the general population. In this series, no significant survival difference was observed between patients treated with immediate endocrine therapy and those treated with delayed therapy.

Clinical Studies of LHRH Agonists

Preliminary studies using LHRH agonists have documented suppression of plasma testosterone levels, tumor shrinkage, pain relief, decrease in acid and alkaline phosphatase levels, reduction in symptoms of bladder outlet obstruction, and decrease in metastatic lesions on bone scan (Warner et al., 1981; Corbin, 1982; Faure et al., 1982; and Tolis et al., 1982).

Smith and associates (1983) reported the preliminary results of clinical trials using the LHRH agonist Leuprolide. In this study, using the NPCP response criteria, 70 per cent of previously untreated patients had complete or partial objective responses and 27 per cent had stable disease. In addition, 30 per cent of patients who had relapsed after prior endocrine therapy had subjective improvement and 4 per cent had objective responses. Toxic effects included only hot flashes.

Labrie and associates (1983) have claimed that virtually 100 per cent of patients respond favorably to treatment with a LHRH agonist in combination with an antiandrogen; however, this high response rate has not yet been confirmed. Further studies will be required to evaluate this therapeutic regimen.

CLINICAL STUDIES OF SECONDARY ENDOCRINE THERAPY FOR RELAPSE AFTER PRIMARY ENDOCRINE THERAPY

In general, the results of secondary endocrine therapy in patients who have relapsed after adequate primary endocrine therapy have been disappointing. The most likely reason for this is that androgen-dependent cells have been suppressed by primary endocrine therapy and the remaining androgen-independent cells cannot be suppressed by further minor reductions in circulating androgen levels. However, in patients who have been treated with oral estrogens, testosterone suppression may be incomplete, particularly in those treated with TACE or Estradurin, which do not suppress testosterone levels into the castrate range. O'Connor and Sokol (1959) demonstrated that many patients treated with TACE subsequently benefited from orchiectomy.

Crossover Endocrine Therapy

Nesbit and Baum (1950) reported that 36 per cent of patients whose primary endocrine therapy was estrogen administration responded to subsequent orchiectomy, whereas only 17 per cent of those whose primary therapy was orchiectomy responded to estrogens. They pointed out that often secondary responses were subjective and did not represent true regression of the cancer. Other authors have reported similar results (Brendler and Prout, 1962; Bjorn et al., 1979; Stone et al., 1980). In contrast, Klugo and associates (1981) reported that more than 10 per cent of orchiectomized patients had testosterone levels in excess of 100 ng per dl and that administration of estrogens to some of these patients further lowered the plasma testosterone levels and induced clinical remissions. Although estrogen administration to orchiectomized patients may lower circulating levels of free testosterone by increasing the concentration of sex steroid–binding globulin, there is little objective evidence that administration of estrogens to orchiectomized patients results in clinical benefits. Significant decreases in total plasma testosterone levels in orchiectomized patients receiving estrogens have not been documented in other studies (Vermeulen et al., 1982).

High-Dose Diethylstilbestrol Diphosphate (Stilphostrol)

Diethylstilbestrol diphosphate (Stilphostrol) is a water-soluble estrogen that usually is given by intravenous infusion in high doses. Rohlf and Flocks (1969) reported that 75 per cent of patients who had relapsed after adequate endocrine therapy benefited from Stilphostrol infusion. Flocks and associates (1955) reported that only one of 66 patients treated with Stilphostrol had objective regression of metastases. Hawtrey and associates (1974) reported favorable responses in paraparetic and paraplegic patients treated with Stilphostrol, but many had not received prior endocrine therapy and most having favorable responses also were treated with laminectomy or orchiectomy or both. Susan and associates (1976) and Band and associates (1973) reported favorable responses in patients after endocrine therapy. Objective responses included reduction in prostatic size, decrease in hydronephrosis, and reduction in bone pain.

Adrenalectomy

Brendler (1973) and Bhanalaph and associates (1974) reviewed the clinical trials of adrenalectomy in prostate cancer patients. In these reviews, subjective improvement of symptoms was reported in approximately 50 per cent of patients, but objective tumor regression occurred in less than 6 per cent. Subjective and objective response rates were higher in the series of Mahoney and Harrison (1972); however, the criteria for objective improvement were not specified. Mahoney and Harrison (1972) found no correlation between the response to medical adrenal suppression and the subsequent response to adrenalectomy. Currently, adrenalectomy is not recommended for prostate cancer patients.

Medical Adrenalectomy with Aminoglutethimide or Spironolactone. Aminoglutethimide is an enzyme inhibitor that blocks the production of androgens as well as aldosterone and cortisol in the adrenal cortex. Robinson (1980) reported 30 per cent complete pain relief and 35 per cent partial pain relief in patients treated with aminoglutethimide plus cortisone and fludrocortisone acetate. Sanford and asso-

ciates (1976) reported a 39 per cent response rate in patients treated with aminoglutethimide plus dexamethasone with or without fludrocortisone acetate. Worgul and associates (1983), in an update of Sanford's series using the NPCP response criteria, reported that 4 per cent of patients had complete responses, 16 per cent had partial objective responses, and 24 per cent remained objectively stable. Taken together, these studies suggest that aminoglutethimide plus hydrocortisone induces favorable responses in approximately one third of patients who have relapsed after primary endocrine therapy; however, it has not been determined whether the favorable responses were due primarily to aminoglutethimide or to the hydrocortisone, which also inhibits adrenal androgen secretion through feedback inhibition of pituitary ACTH release. Sanford and associates (1976) suggested that aminoglutethimide is preferable to glucocorticoids for adrenal suppression because glucocorticoids produce Cushing's syndrome, which is not rapidly reversible.

Spironolactone, another inhibitor of testosterone synthesis, was shown by Walsh and Siiteri (1975) to suppress adrenal secretion of testosterone, androstenedione, and dehydroepiandrosterone in castrated prostate cancer patients. Baba and associates (1978) reported in a small series a 20 per cent subjective response rate in prostatic cancer patients treated with spironolactone.

Hypophysectomy

In a review of the literature on hypophysectomy through 1971, Brendler (1973) reported a 63 per cent subjective response rate and a 33 per cent objective response rate. Pituitary ablation in these series was accomplished by either open surgical removal, transsphenoidial implantation of [90]yttrium, or cryodestruction under stereotactic control. Other authors have performed pituitary ablation by stereotactically controlled injection of alcohol (Levin et al., 1978; Fitzpatrick et al., 1980). Silverberg (1977) reviewed the Stanford University experience with open transsphenoidal hypophysectomy and reported that 70 per cent had subjective improvement and 29 per cent had objective responses. The overall mean survival of the patients was only 6 months. No factors could be identified that would predict a favorable response preoperatively. Taken together, clinical studies of hypophysectomy suggest that the subjective clinical response rate may be somewhat higher than that associated with adrenalectomy, but objective responses are uncommon and prolongation of survival does not appear to result.

Hypophysectomy currently is not recommended for prostate cancer patients.

Medical Hypophysectomy using Glucocorticoids. Glucocorticoids have been used to suppress pituitary ACTH secretion, which results in decreased adrenal androgen secretion. The overall treatment results are comparable to those of surgical adrenalectomy, but in many instances striking subjective benefits may result from glucocorticoid administration. Valk and Owens (1954) reported subjective improvement in 40 per cent and objective improvement in 25 per cent. Mahoney and Harrison (1972) and Miller and Hinman (1954) reported more than 80 per cent of patients had subjective responses, while Miller and Hinman reported that 60 per cent had objective improvement.

Prolactin Inhibitors. Clinical trials of prolactin inhibitors including levodopa (Sadoughi et al., 1974; Plumpton and Morales, 1975; Farnsworth and Gonder, 1977) and 2-bromo-alpha-ergocryptine (Coune and Smith, 1975; Jacobi et al., 1978) have been conducted. Although some favorable responses have been reported (Sadoughi et al., 1974; Farnsworth and Gonder, 1977), beneficial results have not been documented in all studies. In general, prolactin inhibitors have not been clinically effective in the treatment of patients who have relapsed after adequate primary endocrine therapy.

Clinical Studies of Antiandrogens

Two antiandrogens, cyproterone acetate and flutamide, have been evaluated in clinical trials. Cyproterone acetate was evaluated by Scott and Schirmer (1966), Smith and associates (1973), Wein and Murphy (1973), and Tvetor and associates (1979). Flutamide was evaluated by Stoilar and Albert (1974), Sogani and associates (1975), Jacobo and associates (1976), and Narayana and associates (1981). These studies demonstrated that antiandrogen therapy is equally as effective as standard endocrine therapy in untreated patients but offers no significant benefits to hormonally refractory patients. Gynecomastia has been reported to occur in patients treated with cyproterone acetate or flutamide, although sexual potency was preserved in most patients treated with flutamide.

Clinical Studies of Antiestrogens

Human prostate cancers contain estrogen receptors and it has been speculated that estrogens may exert direct effects on prostate cancer cells. Tamoxifen is a nonsteroidal antiestrogen that binds specifically to estrogen receptors. Its efficacy in the treatment of breast cancer is well established. Tamoxifen was evaluated in prostate cancer patients by Glick and associates (1980, 1982). Using the NPCP response criteria in endocrine refractory patients, 5 per cent had partial objective responses, 8 per cent remained stable, and 87 per cent had cancer progression. Using standard Phase 2 criteria for patients having measurable lesions, only 10 per cent remained stable while 90 per cent had cancer progression. The authors concluded that this low response rate did not justify further clinical trials with tamoxifen for prostate cancer patients.

Clinical Studies of Testosterone Administration

Fowler and Whitmore (1982) reviewed the literature up to 1982 on testosterone administration in prostate cancer patients. Adverse responses occurred in 93 per cent of patients. In 7 per cent of patients, death was reported to have resulted from testosterone administration.

In a previous report of the Memorial Sloan-Kettering Cancer Center experience, Fowler and Whitmore (1981a) reported that adverse responses were more common in patients who had relapsed after endocrine therapy than in those who were in remission or those previously untreated. In this series, testosterone caused apparent irreversible cancer progression in 15 per cent of patients, which included the development of paraplegia and four deaths occurring within 2 weeks of testosterone administration. In the remainder of patients, the adverse effects were reversed when testosterone therapy was discontinued. A small proportion of patients exhibited symptomatic benefits from testosterone administration, but the authors speculated that favorable responses may have been due to placebo or anabolic effects. No patient experienced objective tumor regression.

Prostate cancer cells of patients who have relapsed after endocrine therapy may retain the capacity to be stimulated by androgens. This is consistent with the observation that many prostate cancers retain androgen receptors despite the fact the patient has relapsed. In general, favorable responses to testosterone administration have occurred in patients who have not been previously treated with androgen-withdrawal therapy. Tumors in these patients already may be nearly maximally stimulated by physiologic levels of androgens, and administration of exogenous androgen may not make a significant difference in the tumor growth rate but may produce favorable anabolic or placebo effects. Testosterone therapy is not recommended in patients with hormonally refractory metastatic prostate cancer.

CHEMOTHERAPY

Because most patients having metastatic prostate cancer respond favorably to endocrine therapy and those who relapse frequently are debilitated and have limited bone marrow reserve, cytotoxic chemotherapy has played a limited role in the treatment of of effective chemotherapy regimens for other solid tumors, large-scale clinical trials of chemotherapy for prostate cancer were initiated in the early 1970's. The most detailed studies of chemotherapy for prostate cancer have been conducted by the National Prostatic Cancer Project (NPCP) (Gibbons et al., 1981).

Prostate cancer poses special problems in interpreting the response to chemotherapy (Yagoda, 1973; Berry et al., 1979; Slack et al., 1980; Torti and Carter, 1980; Citrin et al., 1981a; Menon and Catalona, 1981). The variable natural history of prostate cancer is one factor that makes it difficult to evaluate the response. For instance, in the VACURG studies, 10 per cent of Stage D prostate cancer patients treated with endocrine therapy died within 6 months while 10 per cent lived longer than 10 years (Bayard et al., 1974). In these studies (Bayard et al., 1974; Byar et al., 1974), patients were categorized into different risk groups according to their signs and symptoms. The 5-year survival rates in the different risk groups ranged from 15 to 65 per cent. In general, elderly patients who had anemia, were bedridden, and had extensive osseous metastases or elevated acid or alkaline phosphatase levels had a worse prognosis. Survival appeared to be more a function of the presenting signs and symptoms than the treatment used, suggesting that the natural history of the tumor may be more important in determining the final outcome than the treatment selected.

It has been reported that patients not subjected to orchiectomy have less favorable responses to chemotherapy than those who have been orchiectomized (Yagoda, 1973; Schmidt et al., 1976; Berry et al., 1979; Herr, 1982b; Straus et al., 1982). In some chemotherapy protocols (e.g., the NPCP trials), estrogen therapy was discontinued before chemotherapy was initi-

ated. Because tumors that have relapsed after androgen-withdrawal therapy may be stimulated by androgens, cessation of estrogen therapy in patients who have not been orchiectomized may result in the return of plasma testosterone levels to normal with consequent stimulation of the tumor, producing inferior response rates (Yagoda et al., 1979). For this reason, patients who have relapsed after estrogen therapy should be maintained on estrogens during chemotherapy or be subjected to orchiectomy before starting chemotherapy.

To evaluate accurately the response to chemotherapy, patients must be stratified according to signs and symptoms of prognostic importance. Groups of patients being compared must be matched as closely as possible for prognostic factors. Although randomization theoretically should produce an equal distribution of prognostic variables, this cannot be taken for granted. An unequal distribution of prognostic variables was observed in some prospective, randomized trials (Schmidt et al., 1976; Loening et al., 1981).

The relationship between changes in acid phosphatase levels and the response to therapy is not always clearcut. Some patients may have tumor progression without an increase in acid phosphatase levels, whereas others may have tumor regression without a decrease in acid phosphatase. Moreover, significant diurnal variations in acid phosphatase levels occur in prostate cancer patients. Accordingly, arbitrary measures of change in acid phosphatase levels may not always be clinically significant. Some investigators have not considered an increase in acid phosphatase alone to be an indication of cancer progression (NPCP, Berry et al., 1979), whereas others feel that an increase in acid phosphatase should be considered as evidence of progression (Citrin et al., 1981a; Smalley et al., 1981).

Roentgenographic changes also are inaccurate in determining the response to chemotherapy. Radiographs are relatively insensitive in detecting and measuring bony metastases. Osteolytic lesions may respond favorably with new bone formation and may give the false impression of being enlarging osteoblastic metastases.

It is likely that many of the reported differences in treatment results derive from the fact that different response criteria were used. This was illustrated by Yagoda and associates (1979) in an analysis of patients treated with cis-platinum. They evaluated a group of patients using the response criteria of the Memorial Sloan-

Kettering Cancer Center (MSKCC), NPCP, Eastern Cooperative Oncology Group (ECOG), Mayo Clinic, and Duke University. Whereas 84 per cent of patients were considered to have cancer progression by MSKCC criteria, 72 per cent would have been classified as having cancer progression by NPCP criteria, 68 per cent by Mayo Clinic criteria, 60 per cent by ECOG criteria, and 59 per cent by Duke University criteria. Thus, there was a 30 per cent discrepancy in response rates in the same group of patients, depending upon the response criteria used.

The inclusion of stable disease as a favorable response to chemotherapy is based on the fact that most patients selected for cytotoxic chemotherapy have progressive cancer before the institution of chemotherapy. Accordingly, it is argued that stable disease represents a clinically meaningful cessation of cancer progression. The NPCP trials revealed that patients having stable disease have survival rates that were similar to those of patients having partial cancer regression and significantly better than those of patients exhibiting cancer progression (Slack et al., 1980). However, the validity of considering stable disease as a favorable response to therapy has been questioned (Yagoda et al., 1979; Citrin and Hogan, 1982). Patients having slowly growing tumors may require more time to exhibit the necessary criteria for cancer progression, but may have tumors that are progressing nonetheless. These patients are predetermined to have a longer survival (Herr, 1982b). If stable disease is indicative of a favorable response to therapy, clinical trials in which a significant proportion of patients treated with chemotherapy had stable disease should reveal a survival advantage of patients treated with chemotherapy; however, such is not the case.

The need for concurrent controls in clinical chemotherapy trials is illustrated in the NPCP protocols evaluating cyclophosphamide as a single agent. In NPCP protocol 100 (Scott et al., 1976), 7 per cent of cyclophosphamide-treated patients had partial cancer regression and 39 per cent had stable disease. This was significantly superior to the results observed in the standard therapy arm in which there were no partial regressions and 19 per cent had stable disease. However, in NPCP protocol 300 (Schmidt et al., 1979) in a group of comparable patients treated with the same cyclophosphamide regimen, no patient had cancer regression and only 25 per cent had stable disease. Thus, comparable patients treated with the same chemotherapy regimen at different points in time had different response rates.

A final important consideration in evaluating the response to chemotherapy is that a sufficient number of patients must be studied to ensure that the probability of missing a clinically meaningful response to therapy is less than 10 per cent.

The response rates observed in clinical trials of single agents have been reviewed by Catalona (1984) and are summarized in Table 32–9. These results indicate that some single agents have modest activity in prostate cancer patients. Most notable among these are cyclophosphamide, 5-fluorouracil, doxorubicin, imidazole carboxamide (DTIC), estramustine phosphate, and meth-

TABLE 32–9. SINGLE-AGENT CHEMOTHERAPY FOR PROSTATE CANCER

Agent	Objective Tumor Regression[†] (%)	Stable Disease[†] (%)	Duration of Response (mos)	Duration of Survival (mos)
Adriamycin	13–27	25–68	3	6
5-Fluorouracil	5–25	12–40	3–10	2–9
Cyclophosphamide	0–7	26–58	3–7	4–20
CCNU or MeCCNU	4–40	20–26	4–6	9–10
Cis-platinum	0–43	4–21	2–16	5–12
Imidazole carboxamide	3	19	5	9
Estramustine phosphate*	0–6	18–32	7–11	9–10
Hydroxyurea	8–22	8–40	3–19	2–13
Melphalan	0–7	0–75	2–6	2–6
Prednimustine	0–13	13	7	9
Procarbazine	0	9	9	7
Vincristine	3	12	5	9
Methotrexate	6	36	8	8

*Based on NPCP trials only.
†Response criteria used were not uniform; therefore, the response rates are not directly comparable.
From Catalona, W. J.: Prostate Cancer. New York, Grune & Stratton, 1984 (with permission).

otrexate. Subsequent studies have tested single agents in combination (Table 32–10). However, in controlled trials, combination chemotherapy has not yet proved to be superior to single-agent chemotherapy. More recently, cytotoxic chemotherapy has been used in conjunction with endocrine therapy in patients with early metastatic prostate cancer (reviewed by Elder and Catalona, 1984) and as an adjunct to radical surgery or radiation therapy (Gibbons et al., 1981). The preliminary results of these studies suggest that modest benefits may accrue from such adjunctive therapy (de Vere White et al., 1982; Murphy et al., 1983).

In general, the results of cytotoxic chemotherapy for prostate cancer have been disappointing. Overall, using the generally accepted Phase 2 response criteria, objective evidence of cancer regression has occurred in only 10 to 15 per cent of patients (median duration is approximately 6 months), and the survival rates of patients treated with cytotoxic chemotherapy (approximately 8 months) have not been significantly superior to those of patients treated with standard palliative therapy. Currently, several long-term, large-scale protocols of chemotherapy for prostate cancer are under way (Gibbons et al., 1981), but will require years before the results can be fully evaluated.

Intra-arterial infusion chemotherapy with 5-fluorouracil followed by radiation therapy was initially reported by Nevin and associates (1973). More recently, Scardino and Lehane (1982) performed hypogastric artery infusions with cis-platinum. Objective evidence of tumor regression occurred in a significant proportion of patients. Complications included skin necrosis and toxic neuritis.

Androgen priming of prostate cancer patients prior to chemotherapy has been evaluated as a possible means of rendering prostate cancer cells more susceptible to the toxic effects of chemotherapeutic drugs (Suarez et al., 1982), but the results have not been appreciably superior to those expected with chemotherapy alone. Androgen priming produced increased bone pain in many patients and spinal cord compression in one. The preliminary results suggest that the risks of androgen-priming therapy outweigh the benefits.

Immunotherapy and Cryotherapy

Evidence is lacking that human prostate cancers express tumor-specific antigens capable of inducing immunologic responses in the host (Catalona et al., 1982a). Brannen and associates

TABLE 32–10. COMBINATION CHEMOTHERAPY FOR PROSTATE CANCER

Agent	Objective Tumor Regression* (%)	Stable Disease* (%)	Approximate Duration of Response (mos)	Approximate Duration of Survival (mos)
5FU + Nitrogen mustard	42	—	—	—
5FU + Cytoxan	8–17	5–13	8	7
Cytoxan + Adriamycin	0–32	18–25	7.4–13	11
Adriamycin + DDP	6–50	29	0–24	7–18+
Estramustine + Prednismustine	2	11	7	9
Vincristine + Estramustine	0	24	3	7
DDP + Estramustine	0	33	3	7
Cytoxan, Adriamycin, 5FU	0–17	50–69	2–13	3–20
Cytoxan, Methotrexate, 5FU	7–15	20–47	3–5	8
Adriamycin, Mitomycin C, 5FU	50	—	7	—
Cytoxan, DDP, Prednisone	0	45	—	—
Cytoxan, DDP, Adriamycin	24	24	6	—
Adriamycin, BCNU, Cytoxan	26	15	5	7–13
Estramustine, Cytoxan, 5FU, DDP	39	—	10	—
Cytoxan, Methotrexate, 5FU, Vincristine, Prednisone	32	6	13	2–24
Vincristine, Melphalan, Methotrexate, 5FU, Prednisone	24	48	7	—
Vincristine, Bleomycin, Methotrexate, 5FU, Prednisone	13	—	—	4

*Response criteria used were not uniform; therefore, the response rates are not directly comparable.
From Catalona, W. J.: Prostate Cancer. New York, Grune & Stratton, 1984 (with permission).

(1975) reported positive skin test responses to tumor extracts in prostate cancer patients, but these observations have not been tested in subsequent studies. Studies based on in vitro cell-mediated cytotoxicity assays (Avis et al., 1975; Okabe et al., 1979) suggest that prostate cancer cells express antigens, but these antigens also are expressed on benign prostatic hyperplastic tissue and other adult tissues as well. Studies of in vitro leukocyte adherence inhibition suggest that leukocytes from prostate cancer patients recognize antigens in tumor extracts of prostate cancers, but antigen recognition is neither uniform nor tumor-specific (Ablin et al., 1976; Evans and Bowen, 1977; Kaneti et al., 1981).

Cell-mediated immunologic responsiveness as measured by skin test responses and in vitro lymphocyte proliferative responses is impaired in many prostate cancer patients. Moreover, circulating plasma factors capable of inhibiting in vitro immunologic responses have been demonstrated in prostate cancer patients (McLaughlin et al., 1974; Catalona et al., 1974). Suppressor lymphocytes in lymph nodes of prostate cancer patients were demonstrated by Herr (1980). These suppressor cells have the capacity to block lymphocyte proliferative responses to histocompatibility antigens. Information on antibody production of prostate cancer patients is limited. Ablin and associates (1972) postulated that blocking antibodies may be present in the plasma of prostate cancer patients. Whitmore and Gittes (1977) reported that the prostate was an immunologically privileged site for cell-mediated immune responses but not for humoral immune responses. The significance of impaired host immunologic responsiveness in prostate cancer patients is uncertain.

Cryosurgery

Based on animal studies suggesting that cryodestruction of the prostate produced antiprostate antibodies (Gonder et al., 1964), cryotherapy of human prostate cancer was initiated in the early 1970's. Early studies by Soanes and associates (1970) and Gursel and associates (1972) suggested a systemic therapeutic benefit may result from cryosurgery. Other investigators were unable to demonstrate objective evidence that cryotherapy induced an immune response in the host (Flocks et al., 1972; Schmidt, 1973; Milleman et al., 1980). O'Donoghue and associates (1975) reported that 75 per cent of patients treated with cryotherapy for prostate cancer experienced significant pain relief, but

only one patient had objective evidence of tumor regression. In this study, there was a 14 per cent incidence of urethrocutaneous fistula. Bonney and associates (1982) reported that the 5-year survival and cancer death rates were comparable in patients treated with cryosurgery or radical prostatectomy and the results of cryosurgery were superior to those achieved with other palliative therapeutic measures. In this study, adjunctive endocrine therapy was used in patients in all treatment groups, and the use of endocrine therapy may have obscured early differences between treatments. Bonney and associates (1983) also reported that cryosurgery eliminated palpable evidence of the primary tumor in two thirds of patients; however, local recurrences occurred in at least 41 per cent of patients. In this study also, many patients received concomitant endocrine therapy.

Specific Active Immunotherapy

Anecdotal trials of specific active immunotherapy in prostate cancer patients have been reported (Czajowski et al., 1967; Rothauge, 1983), but these trials do not permit definitive conclusions to be drawn.

Nonspecific Active Immunotherapy

Early studies of nonspecific active immunotherapy of prostate cancer also include anecdotal reports that do not warrant firm conclusions (Johnston, 1962; Nauts, 1973; Stehlin, 1979; Zamora et al., 1979; Nakagami et al., 1980).

Merrin and associates (1975) reported on immunotherapy with intraprostatic injections of BCG (bacille Calmette-Guerin). More than two thirds of patients were reported to have a 50 per cent decrease in the size of the local tumor but no objective regression of metastases was observed. Robinson and associates (1976, 1977) reported on two uncontrolled clinical trials of intraprostatic BCG. These authors also reported an improvement in voiding symptoms in two thirds of patients, but all patients died within 2 years. In these studies, some of the complications of intraprostatic BCG therapy were severe, including the development of rectoprostatic fistula, widespread granulomas, and fever.

Brosman (1977) reported on a randomized trial of intradermal BCG injections in patients with hormonally refractory prostate cancer. No significant survival advantage was detected in the BCG-treated patients. Guinan and associates (1982a,b) also used intradermal BCG therapy in a prospective randomized trial. The survival of the BCG-treated patients was significantly longer than that of control patients, and it was reported that the BCG-treated patients had significantly fewer infections. The morbidity associated with intradermal BCG was reported to be minimal.

Only anecdotal reports are available on the use of interferon in prostate cancer patients (Murphy, 1981; Madajewicz et al., 1982). The results of interferon therapy are too preliminary to warrant definitive conclusions.

In general, the accumulated data on immunotherapy for prostate cancer suggest that modulation of the host immune system does not provide significant therapeutic benefits to prostate cancer patients, and the morbidity associated with some immunotherapy regimens is considerable.

TREATMENT OPTIONS STAGE-BY-STAGE

Stage A1

The vast majority of patients (particularly older patients) having Stage A1 prostate cancer do not require immediate treatment and may be followed at appropriate (3-month) intervals. Patients with Stage A1 disease who are managed expectantly do not need lymph node staging. Those patients with Stage A1 disease who manifest clinical evidence of local cancer progression should be treated with radical prostatectomy, radiation therapy, or endocrine therapy, depending upon their general medical condition, life expectancy, and preference of treatment options.

The main concern about expectant management in patients with Stage A1 prostate cancer is that cancer progression may proceed directly from Stage A1 to Stage D without passing through Stages B or C. This is especially true in young patients who may be at risk for cancer progression for long periods of time. Patients under the age of 60 should be informed that long-term data on cancer progression rates in young patients are not yet available and there may be a higher risk of cancer progression with longer follow-up. Radical prostatectomy and radiation therapy are legitimate treatment options for young patients. Endocrine therapy also is an option for older patients with Stage A1 tumors who desire immediate treatment.

Stage A2

Most patients having Stage A2 prostate cancer should receive immediate definitive treatment with either radical prostatectomy or radiation therapy. Patients having Stage A2 prostate cancer in whom radical prostatectomy is planned should undergo staging pelvic lymphadenectomy. In general, external-beam radiation therapy is well tolerated in patients with Stage A2 prostate cancer if it is delayed until the resected prostatic fossa is completely healed. Interstitial radiation therapy with ^{125}I generally is not recommended for patients with Stage A2 tumors because the resected prostate does not retain the ^{125}I seeds. In contrast, interstitial radiation with ^{198}Au is not contraindicated in patients who have undergone prior transurethral resection because this technique employs fewer seeds with a tissue penetration that is considerably greater than that of ^{125}I. The capacity of interstitial radiation therapy with ^{192}Ir to control Stage A2 prostate cancer has not been determined.

Stage B1

Patients having clinical Stage B1 prostate cancer should be treated with radical prostatectomy if they are acceptable surgical risks and have a life expectancy of at least 10 years. External-beam radiation therapy may be used in patients with Stage B1 prostate cancer who are not suitable candidates for radical prostatectomy. Staging pelvic lymphadenectomy should be performed prior to radical prostatectomy, but is optional in patients to be treated with external-beam radiation therapy and should be limited in scope when performed.

Stage B2

Radical prostatectomy is a legitimate treatment option in patients having clinical Stage B2 prostate cancer in whom there is no evidence of pelvic lymph node metastases. Patients having tumor at the surgical margins or found to have extracapsular tumor extension may be either managed expectantly or treated with external-beam radiation therapy to the prostatic bed beginning 2 to 6 months after radical prostatectomy. In patients who are not acceptable surgical risks for radical prostatectomy, external-beam radiation therapy, ^{125}I implantation, and ^{198}Au implantation may be legitimate options. Staging pelvic lymphadenectomy is optional in patients to be treated with external-beam radiation therapy.

Stage C

Patients with Stage C prostate cancer are probably best treated with radiation therapy. Staging pelvic lymphadenectomy is optional in patients in whom external-beam radiation therapy is planned and should be limited in scope when performed. Patients having Stage C tumors producing ureteral obstruction should be treated preferentially with radiation therapy. Endocrine therapy also is a legitimate option in patients with Stage C disease and has been shown to delay the onset of distant metastases. However, early endocrine therapy does not prolong overall patient survival.

Stage D0

The treatment options for patients with stage D0 tumors (elevated acid phosphatase only) include (1) no immediate treatment; (2) staging pelvic lymphadenectomy to determine whether the patient has true Stage D0 disease (localized cancer with elevated acid phosphatase), Stage D1 disease (lymph node metastases completely resected with normalization of acid phosphatase), or occult Stage D2 disease (lymph nodes do not contain metastases or acid phosphatase remains elevated postoperatively, or both); (3) whole pelvis or extended field external-beam radiation therapy; (4) endocrine therapy; and (5) cytotoxic chemotherapy. In patients who are acceptable surgical risks, staging pelvic lymphadenectomy is recommended. Depending on the findings, patients should then be treated according to the surgical stage determined. In patients who are not acceptable surgical risks, external-beam radiation therapy offers the theoretical possibility for cure. Alternatively, endocrine therapy may be used.

Stage D1

Overall, only about 10 to 20 per cent of patients having nodal metastases enjoy long-term, tumor-free survival. Most long-term survivors have only minimal nodal involvement. In such patients, radical prostatectomy or radiation therapy, or both, may be considered legitimate options, although the prospects for cure are poor. Radical prostatectomy may control the primary tumor better than radiation therapy if the tumor is confined within the limits of resection. In patients having more extensive lymph node involvement, pelvic or extended field radiation therapy has not proved to be of significant benefit. These patients should be treated with endocrine therapy. If the patient is sexually active, delayed endocrine therapy is more appropriate. Early endocrine therapy may be used if the patient is not sexually active or desires early treatment. Orchiectomy is the preferred form of endocrine therapy. Alternatively, 1 mg of diethylstilbestrol daily with pre-estrogen breast irradiation (900 to 1500 rads over 2 or 3 days) may be used.

Adjunctive combination chemotherapy with cyclophosphamide and doxorubicin has been reported to decrease the incidence or delay the appearance of distant metastases in patients having Stage D1 disease (de Vere White et al., 1982). Patients should be made aware of this treatment option. In patients having bladder outlet obstruction, either endocrine therapy or transurethral resection of the prostate are legitimate options. Both endocrine therapy and radiation therapy are effective for the treatment of ureteral obstruction in patients with Stage D1 disease.

Stage D2

Endocrine therapy probably prolongs survival in most patients having Stage D2 prostate cancer; however, early endocrine therapy offers no significant survival advantage over delayed endocrine therapy. As mentioned previously, the sexual activity of the patient may determine whether early or delayed endocrine therapy is used. Patients having symptomatic metastases including bone pain, neurologic symptoms, edema, anemia, weight loss, dyspnea, bladder outlet obstruction, or ureteral obstruction should be treated with immediate endocrine therapy. Orchiectomy is the preferred form of endocrine therapy because it obviates concerns about patient compliance, cardiovascular side effects, or gynecomastia. Gonadotropin-releasing hormone agonists or antagonists may play an important future role in determining the endocrine sensitivity of the tumor and as a continuing therapeutic agent. The disadvantage of either estrogen therapy or gonadotropin-releasing hormone therapy is that it is a daily reminder to the patient that he has cancer.

Stage D3

The median survival of patients having Stage D3 prostate cancer (relapse after endocrine therapy) is less than 1 year. In these patients, localized external-beam radiation therapy should be used for palliation of painful skeletal metastases. Hemibody or whole body radiation therapy also is effective for diffuse, painful metastases. Prophylactic irradiation may be given to vertebral or femoral neck metastases to prevent disabling pathologic fractures.

Secondary endocrine therapy with diethylstilbestrol diphosphate, antiandrogens, aminoglutethimide, adrenalectomy, or hypophysectomy is beneficial in only a small proportion of patients; however, significant palliation may be achieved with the administration of glucocorticoids.

Cytotoxic chemotherapy induces objective tumor regression in only a small proportion of prostate cancer patients. Single agents that have some activity are cyclophosphamide, methotrexate, and doxorubicin; however, cyclophosphamide and methotrexate are not well tolerated in patients who have received prior radiation therapy, and doxorubicin is poorly tolerated in patients having underlying cardiac disease.

Combination chemotherapy with the three-drug regimen of doxorubicin, mitomycin C, and 5-fluorouracil (DMF) (Logothetis et al., 1982) or the five-drug combination of cyclophosphamide, methotrexate, 5-fluorouracil, vincristine, and prednisone (COMP–F) (Paulson et al., 1981) has been reported to produce good response rates in studies that have not yet been confirmed. In controlled studies, combination chemotherapy has not proved to be significantly more effective than single-agent therapy.

Patients who respond to cytotoxic chemotherapy have a greater survival expectancy than those who do not respond; however, the overall survival of patients treated with chemotherapy is not significantly superior to that of patients not treated with chemotherapy. Until more effective chemotherapeutic agents are available, the use of cytotoxic chemotherapy should be reserved for patients who have failed to respond to other less toxic forms of therapy or for patients who wish to participate in an experimental chemotherapy protocol.

In patients having Stage D3 prostate cancer with ureteral obstruction, either external-beam radiation therapy, internal ureteral stents, or percutaneous nephrostomy may be used to relieve ureteral obstruction. Ureteral reimplantation into the dome of the bladder also is an option in selected patients who are able to void satisfactorily. Ureteral reimplantation obviates the need for internal stents or external collecting devices. Bladder outlet obstruction may be man-aged in these patients with transurethral resection.

Spinal cord compression should be treated with the administration of high-dose corticosteroids (dexamethasone, 6 mg every 4 hours) and decompressive laminectomy if the lesion is localized. If the lesion is diffuse or the patient is not a suitable candidate for an operation, external-beam radiation therapy may be effective.

Control of pain may be achieved by administration of oral narcotics or Brompton's cocktail. More recently, long-term epidural catheters for the administration of morphine have been used successfully in some patients.

There are numerous treatment options for patients having each stage of prostatic cancer, and it is not desirable to make categorical treatment recommendations. Treatment plans should be tailored to needs of the individual patient. Although no treatment is uniformly effective, the judicious selection of the available treatment options can minimize the mortality and morbidity associated with prostatic cancer.

References

Ablin, R. J., Gonder, M. J., and Soanes, W. A.: Levels of C'3 in the serum of patients with benign and malignant diseases of the prostate. Neoplasma, *19*:61, 1972.

Ablin, R. J., Bhatti, R. A., Guinan, P. D., and Bruns, G. R.: Evaluation of cellular immunologic responsiveness in the clinical management of patients with prostatic cancer. IV. Leukocyte adherence inhibition. Urol. Int., *31*:459, 1976.

Abul-Fadl, M. A. M., and King, E. J.: Properties of the acid phosphatases of erythrocytes and of the human prostate gland. Biochem. J., *45*:51, 1949.

Ackermann, R., and Muller, H.-A.: Retrospective analysis of 645 simultaneous perineal punch biopsies and transrectal aspiration biopsies for diagnosis of prostatic carcinoma. Eur. Urol., *3*:29, 1977.

Allhoff, E. P., Proppe, K. H., Chapman, C. M., Lin, C.-W., and Prout, G. R., Jr.: Evaluation of prostate specific acid phosphatase and prostate specific antigen in identification of prostatic cancer. J. Urol., *129*:315, 1983.

Armenian, H. K., Lilienfeld, A. M., Diamond, E. L., and Bross, I. J. D.: Relation between benign prostatic hyperplasia and cancer of the prostate: A prospective and retrospective study. Lancet, *2*:115, 1974.

Armenian, H. K., Lilienfeld, A. M., Diamond, E. L., and Bross, I. D. J.: Epidemiologic characteristics of patients with prostatic neoplasms. Am. J. Epidemiol., *102*:47, 1975.

Avis, F., Avis, I, Cole, A. T., Freid, F., and Haughton, G.: Antigenic cross reactivity between benign prostatic hyperplasia and adenocarcinoma of the prostate. Urology, *5*:122, 1975.

Baba, S., Murai, M., Jitsukawa, S., Hata, M., and Tazaki, H.: Antiandrogenic effects of spironolactone: Hormonal and ultrastructural studies in dogs and men. J. Urol., *119*:375, 1978.

Baba, S., Janetschek, G., Pollow, K., Hahn, K., and Jacobi, G. H.: The effects of chlorotrianisene (T_{ace}) on kinetics of ^{3}H-testosterone metabolism in patients with carcinoma of the prostate. Br. J. Urol., 1982.

Babcock, J. R., and Grayhack, J. T.: Morbidity of pelvic lymphadenectomy. Urology, 13:483, 1979.

Bagshaw, M. A.: Perspectives on radiation treatment of prostate cancer: History and current focus. In Murphy, G. P. (Ed.).: Prostatic Cancer. Littleton, MA, PSG Publishing Company, Inc., 1979, pp. 151–174.

Bagshaw, M. A.: Radiation therapy of prostatic carcinoma. In Crawford, E. D., and Borden, T. A. (Eds.).: Genitourinary Cancer Surgery. Philadelphia, Lea & Febiger, 1982, pp. 405–411.

Bailar, J. C., Byar, D. P., and the Veterans Administration Cooperative Urological Research Group: Estrogen treatment for cancer of the prostate. Early results with 3 doses of diethylstilbestrol and placebo. Cancer, 26:257, 1970.

Baker, H. W., Burger, H. G., de Kretser, D. M., Hudson, B., and Straffon, W. G.: Effects of synthetic oral estrogens in normal men and patients with prostatic carcinoma: Lack of gonadotrophin suppression by chlorotrianisene. Clin. Endocrinol., 2:297, 1973.

Baker, L. H., Mebust, W. K., Chin, T. D. Y., Chapman, A. L., Hinthorn, D., and Towle, D.: The relationship of herpesvirus to carcinoma of the prostate. J. Urol., 125:370, 1981.

Band, P. R., Banerjee, T. K., Patwardhan, V. C., and Eid, T. C.: High-dose diethylstilbestrol diphosphate therapy of prostatic cancer after failure of standard doses of estrogens. Can. Med. Assoc. J., 109:697, 1973.

Barnes, R., Hirst, A., and Rosenquist, R.: Early carcinoma of the prostate: Comparison of stages A and B. J. Urol., 115:404, 1976.

Barnes, R., Hadley, H., Axford, P., and Kronholm, S.: Conservative treatment of early carcinoma of prostate. Comparison of patients less than seventy with those over seventy years of age. Urology, 14:359, 1979.

Barnes, R. W., and Ninan, C. A.: Carcinoma of the prostate: biopsy and conservative therapy. J. Urol., 108:897, 1972.

Barry, J. M., Goldstein, A., and Hubbard, M.: Human leukocyte A and B antigens in patients with prostatic adenocarcinoma. J. Urol., 124:847, 1980.

Bass, R. B., Jr., and Barrett, D. M.: Radical retropubic prostatectomy after transurethral prostatic resection. J. Urol., 124:495, 1980.

Batata, M. A., Hilaris, B. S., Chu, F. C. H., Whitmore, W. F., Jr., Song, H. S., Kim, Y., Horowitz, B., and Song, K. S.: Radiation therapy in adenocarcinoma of the prostate with pelvic lymph node involvement on lymphadenectomy. Int. J. Rad. Oncol. Biol. Phys., 6:149, 1980.

Batson, O. V.: The function of the vertebral veins and their role in the spread of metastases. Ann. Surg., 112:138, 1940.

Bauer, W. C., McGavran, M. H., and Carlin, M. R.: Unsuspected carcinoma of the prostate in suprapubic prostatectomy specimens: A clinicopathological study of 55 consecutive cases. Cancer, 13:370, 1960.

Bayard, S., Greenberg, R., Showalter, D., and Byar, D.: Comparison of treatments for prostatic cancer using an exponential type life model relating survival to concomitant information. Cancer Chemother. Rep., 58:845, 1974.

Beck, P. H., McAninch, J. W., Goebel, J. L., and Stutzman, R. E.: Plasma testosterone in patients receiving diethylstilbestrol. Urology, 11:157, 1978.

Belville, W. D., Mahan, D. E., Sepulveda, R. A., Bruce, A. W., and Miller, C. F.: Bone marrow acid phosphatase by radioimmunoassay: 3 years of experience. J. Urol., 125:809, 1981.

Benson, K. H., Watson, R. A., Spring, D. B., and Agee, R. E.: The value of computerized tomography in evaluation of pelvic lymph nodes. J. Urol., 126:63, 1981.

Benson, R. C., Jr., Hasan, S. M., Jones, A. G., and Schlise, S.: External beam radiotherapy for palliation of pain from metastatic carcinoma of the prostate. J. Urol., 127:69, 1982.

Benson, R. C., Jr., Tomera, K. M., Zincke, H., Fleming, T. R., and Utz, D. C.: Bilateral pelvic lymphadenectomy and radical retropubic prostatectomy for adenocarcinoma confined to the prostate. J. Urol., 131:1103, 1984.

Berry, W. R., Laszlo, J., Cox, E., Walker, A., and Paulson, D.: Prognostic factors in metastatic and hormonally unresponsive carcinoma of the prostate. Cancer, 44:763, 1979.

Bhanalaph, T., Varkarakis, M. J., and Murphy, G. P.: Current status of bilateral adrenalectomy for advanced prostatic carcinoma. Ann. Surg., 179:17, 1974.

Bianchi, F.: Practical advantages of the perineal biopsy of the prostate. J. Urol., 76:645, 1956.

Bissada, N. K.: Accuracy of transurethral resection of the prostate versus transrectal needle biopsy in the diagnosis of prostatic carcinoma. J. Urol., 118:61, 1977.

Bjorn, G. L., Gray, C. P., and Strauss, E.: Orchiectomy after presumed estrogen failure in treatment of carcinoma of the prostate. West. J. Med., 130:363, 1979.

Blackard, C. E.: The Veterans Administration Cooperative Urological Research Group: Studies of carcinoma of the prostate: A review. Cancer Chemother. Rep., 59:225, 1975.

Blackard, C. E., Soucheray, J. A., and Gleason, D. F.: Prostatic needle biopsy with perineal extension of adenocarcinoma. J. Urol., 106:401, 1971.

Blackard, C. E., Byar, D. P., Jordan, W. P., Jr., and the Veterans Administration Cooperative Urological Research Group: Orchiectomy for advanced prostatic carcinoma: A reevaluation. Urology, 1:553, 1973.

Blair, A., and Fraumeni, J. F., Jr.: Geographic patterns of prostate cancer in the United States. J. Natl. Cancer Inst., 61:1379, 1978.

Blank, B., and Hodges, C. V.: Leukemic infiltration of the prostate: A case report. J. Urol., 123:789, 1980.

Bonney, W. W., Platz, C. E., Fallon, B., Rose, E. F., Gerber, W. L., Sall, J. C., Hawtrey, C. E., Schmidt, J. D., Loening, S. A., Culp, D. A., and Narayana, A. S.: Cryosurgery in prostatic cancer: Survival. Urology, 19:37, 1982.

Bonney, W. W., Fallon, B., Gerber, W. L., Hawtrey, C. E., Loening, S. A., Narayana, A. S., Platz, C. E., Rose, E. F., Sall, J. C., Schmidt, J. D., and Culp, D. A.: Cryosurgery in prostatic cancer: Elimination of the local lesion. Urology, 22:8, 1983.

Boxer, R. J., Kaufman, J. J., and Goodwin, W. E.: Radical prostatectomy for carcinoma of the prostate 1951–1976. A review of 329 patients. J. Urol., 117:208, 1977.

Brannen, G. E., Gomolka, D. M., and Coffey, D. S.: Specificity of cell membrane antigens in prostatic carcinoma. Cancer Chemother. Rep., 59:127, 1975.

Brawn, P. N.: Adenosis of the prostate: A dysplastic lesion that can be confused with prostate adenocarcinoma. Cancer, 49:826, 1982.

Brawn, P. N., Ayala, A. G., Von Eschenbach, A. C., Hussey, D. H., and Johnson, D. E.: Histologic grading study of prostate adenocarcinoma: The development of a new system and comparison with other methods—a preliminary study. Cancer, 49:525, 1982.

Brenckman, W. D., Jr., Lastinger, L. B., and Sedor, F.: Unpredictable fluctuations in serum acid phosphatase activity in prostatic cancer. JAMA, 245:2501, 1981.

Brendler, C. B., Cleeve, L. K., Anderson, E. E., and Paulson, D. F.: Staging pelvic lymphadenectomy for carcinoma of the prostate: Risk versus benefit. J. Urol., 124:849, 1980.

Brendler, H.: Adrenalectomy and hypophysectomy for prostatic cancer. Urology, 2:99, 1973.

Brendler, H., and Prout, G., Jr.: A cooperative group study of prostatic cancer: Stilbestrol versus placebo in advanced progressive disease. Cancer Chemother. Rep., 16:323, 1962.

Breslow, N., Chan, C. W., Dhom, G., Drury, R. A. B., Franks, L. M., Gellei, B., Lee, Y. S., Lundberg, S., Sparke, B., Sternby, N. H., and Tulinius, H.: Latent carcinoma of prostate of autopsy in seven areas. Int. J. Cancer, 20:680, 1977.

Bridges, C. H., Belville, W. D., Insalaco, S. J., and Buck, A. S.: Stage A prostatic carcinoma and repeat transurethral resection: A reappraisal 5 years later. J. Urol., 129:307, 1983.

Brosman, S.: Nonspecific immunotherapy in GU cancer. *In* Crispen, R. G. (Ed.): Neoplasm Immunity: Solid Tumor Therapy. Philadelphia, Franklin Institute Press, 1977, pp. 97–107.

Bruce, A. W., O'Cleireachain, F., Morales, A., and Awad, S. A.: Carcinoma of the prostate: A critical look at staging. J. Urol., 117:319, 1977.

Bruce, A. W., Mahan, D. E., Morales, A., Clark, A. F., and Belville, W. D.: An objective look at acid phosphatase determinations: A comparison of biochemical and immunochemical methods. Br. J. Urol., 51:213, 1979.

Buller, H. R., Boon, T. A., Henny, C. P., Dabhoiwala, N. F., and Ten Cate, J. W.: Estrogen-induced deficiency and decrease in antithrombin III activity in patients with prostatic cancer. J. Urol., 128:72, 1982.

Burbank, F., and Fraumeni, J. F., Jr.: US cancer mortality: Nonwhite predominance. J. Natl. Cancer Inst., 49:649, 1972.

Burkholder, G. V., and Kaufman, J. J.: Local implantation of carcinoma of the prostate with percutaneous needle biopsy. J. Urol., 95:801, 1966.

Byar, D. P.: Survival of patients with incidentally found microscopic cancer of the prostate: Results of a clinical trial of conservative treatment. J. Urol., 108:908, 1972.

Byar, D. P.: The Veterans Administration Cooperative Urological Research Group's studies of cancer of the prostate. Cancer, 32:1126, 1973.

Byar, D. P., and Mostofi, F. K.: Cancer of the prostate in men less than 50 years old: An analysis of 51 cases. J. Urol., 102:726, 1969.

Byar, D. P., Mostofi, F. K., and the Veterans Administration Cooperative Urological Research Group: Carcinoma of the prostate: Prognostic evaluation of certain pathologic features in 208 radical prostatectomies. Examined by the step-section technique. Cancer, 30:5, 1972.

Byar, D. P., Huse, R., Bailar, J. C., III, and the Veterans Administration Cooperative Urological Research Group: An exponential model relating censored survival data and concomitant information for prostatic cancer patients. J. Natl. Cancer Inst., 52:321, 1974.

Byar, D. P., Corle, D. K., and the Veterans Administration Cooperative Urological Research Group: VACURG randomized trial of radical prostatectomy for stages I and II prostate cancer. Urology, 17 [Supp.]:7, 1981.

Campbell, J. R., Godsall, J. W., and Bloch, S.: Neurologic complications in prostatic carcinoma. Prostate, 2:417, 1981.

Cantrell, B. B., De Klerk, D. P., Eggleston, J. C., Boitnott, J. K., and Walsh, P. C.: Pathologic factors that influence prognosis in stage A prostatic cancer: The influence of extent versus grade. J. Urol., 125:516, 1981.

Cantril, S. T., Vaeth, J. M., Green, J. P., and Schroeder, A. F.: Radiation therapy for localized carcinoma of the prostate: Correlation with histopathological grading. Front. Radiat. Ther. Oncol., 9:274, 1974.

Carlton, C. E., Jr., Dawoud, F., Hudgins, P., and Scott, R., Jr.: Irradiation treatment of carcinoma of the prostate: A preliminary report based on 8 years of experience. J. Urol., 108:924, 1972.

Carpentier, P. J., Schroeder, F. H., and Blom, J. H. M.: Transrectal ultrasonography in the followup of prostatic carcinoma patients. J. Urol., 128:742, 1982.

Carson, C. C., III, Zincke, H., Utz, D. C., Cupps, R. E., and Farrow, G. M.: Radical prostatectomy after radiotherapy for prostatic cancer. J. Urol., 124:237, 1980.

Castellino, R. A., Ray, G., Blank, N., Govan, D., and Bagshaw, M.: Lymphangiography in prostatic carcinoma: Preliminary observations. JAMA, 223:877, 1973.

Catalona, W. J.: Yield from routine prostatic needle biopsy in patients more than 50 years old referred for urologic evaluation: A preliminary report. J. Urol., 124:844, 1980.

Catalona, W. J.: Prostate Cancer. New York, Grune & Stratton, 1984.

Catalona, W. J., and Menon, M.: New screening and diagnostic tests for prostate cancer and immunologic assessment. Urology, 17 [Suppl.]:61, 1981.

Catalona, W. J., and Stein, A. J.: Staging errors in clinically localized prostatic cancer. J. Urol., 127:452, 1982a.

Catalona, W. J., and Stein, A. J.: Accuracy of frozen section detection of lymph node metastases in prostatic carcinoma. J. Urol., 127:460, 1982b.

Catalona, W. J., Tarpley, J. L., Chretien, P. B., and Castle, J. R.: Lymphocyte stimulation in urologic cancer patients. J. Urol., 112:373, 1974.

Catalona, W. J., Smolev, J. K., and Harty, J. I.: Prognostic value of host immunocompetence in urologic cancer patients. J. Urol., 114:922, 1975.

Catalona, W. J., Kadmon, D., and Martin, S. A.: Surgical considerations in treatment of intraductal carcinoma of the prostate. J. Urol., 120:259, 1978.

Catalona, W. J., Kadmon, D., and Crane, D. B.: Effect of mini-dose heparin on lymphocele formation following extraperitoneal pelvic lymphadenectomy. J. Urol., 123:890, 1980.

Catalona, W. J., Ratliff, T. L., and McCool, R. E.: Immunology of Genitourinary Tumors. *In* Paulson, D. F. (Ed.): Genitourinary Cancer I. The Hague, Matinus Nijhoff Publishers, 1982a, pp. 169–214.

Catalona, W. J., Stein, A. J., and Fair, W. R.: Grading errors in prostatic needle biopsies: Relation to the accuracy of tumor grade in predicting pelvic lymph node metastases. J. Urol., 127:919, 1982b.

Catalona, W. J., Fleischmann, J., and Menon, M.: Pelvic lymph node status as predictor of extracapsular tumor extension in clinical stage B prostatic cancer. J. Urol., 129:327, 1983.

Centifano, Y. M., Kaufman, H. E., Zam, Z. S., et al.: Herpesvirus particles in prostatic carcinoma cells. J. Virol., 12:1608, 1973.

Choe, B.-K., Pontes, E. J., Rose, N. R., and Henderson, M. D.: Expression of human prostatic acid phosphatase in a pancreatic islet cell carcinoma. Invest. Urol., 15:312, 1978.

Chopp, R. T., and Whitmore, W. F.: Delayed treatment of prostatic carcinoma. American Urological Association Program Abstract #234, 1980.

Chu, T. M., Wang, M. C., Scott, W. W., Gibbons, R. P., Johnson, D. E., Schmidt, J. D., Loening, S. A., Prout, G. R., Jr., and Murphy, G. P.: Immunochemical detection of serum prostatic acid phosphatase: Methodology and clinical evaluation. Invest. Urol. *15*:319, 1978.

Citrin, D. L., and Hogan, T. F.: A phase II evaluation of adriamycin and cis-platinum in hormone resistant prostate cancer. Cancer, *50*:201, 1982.

Citrin, D. L., Cohen, A. I., Harbert, J., Schlise, S., Hougen, C., and Benson, R.: Systemic treatment of advanced prostate cancer: Development of a new system for defining response. J. Urol., *125*:224, 1981a.

Citrin, D. L., Hougen, C., Zweibel, W., Schlise, S., Pruitt, B., Ershler, W., Davis, T. E., Harberg, J., and Cohen, A. I.: The use of serial bone scans in assessing response of bone metastases to systemic treatment. Cancer, *47*:680, 1981b.

Clark, P., and Houghton, L.: Subcapsular orchidectomy for carcinoma of the prostate. Br. J. Urol., *49*:419, 1977.

Cochran, J. S., and Kadesky, M. C.: A private practice experience with adenocarcinoma of the prostate in men less than 50 years old. J. Urol., *125*:220, 1981a.

Cochran, J. S., and Kadesky, M. C.: Private practice experience with radical surgical treatment of cancer of prostate. Urology, *17*:547, 1981b.

Coffey, D. S.: The biochemistry and physiology of the prostate and seminal vesicles. *In* Harrison, J. H., Gittes, R. F., Perlmutter, A. D., Stamey, T. A., and Walsh, P. C. (Eds.): Campbell's Urology. Philadelphia, W. B. Saunders Co., 1978, pp. 161–202.

Cook, G. B., and Watson, F. R.: Twenty single nodules of prostate cancer not treated by total prostatectomy. J. Urol., *100*:672, 1968.

Cooper, J. F., Foti, A., and Herschman, H.: Combined serum and bone marrow radioimmunoassays for prostatic acid phosphatase. J. Urol., *122*:498, 1979.

Corbin, A.: From contraception to cancer: A review of the therapeutic applications of LHRH analogues as antitumor agents. Yale J. Biol. Med., *55*:27, 1982.

Coronary Drug Project Research Group: The Coronary Drug Project initial findings leading to modifications of its research protocol. JAMA, *214*:1303, 1970.

Correa, R. J., Jr., Anderson, R. G., Gibbons, R. P., and Mason, J. T.: Latent carcinoma of the prostate—Why the controversy? J. Urol., *111*:644, 1974.

Correa, R. J., Jr., Kidd, C. R., Burnett, L., Brannen, G. E., Gibbons, R. P., and Cummings, K. B.: Percutaneous pelvic lymph node aspiration in carcinoma of the prostate. J. Urol., *126*:190, 1981.

Cosgrove, M. D., and Kaempf, M. J.: Prostatic cancer revisited. J. Urol., *115*:79, 1976.

Coune, A., and Smith, P.: Clinical trial of 2-bromo-alpha-ergocryptine (NSC–169774) in human prostatic cancer. Cancer Chemother. Rep., *59*:209, 1975.

Court, B., and Chassagne, D.: Interstitial radiation therapy of cancer of the prostate using iridium 192 wires. Cancer Treat. Rep., *61*:329, 1977.

Cox, J. D., and Stoeffel, T. J.: The significance of needle biopsy after irradiation for stage C adenocarcinoma of the prostate. Cancer, *40*:156, 1977.

Crawford, E. D., Haynes, A. L., Story, M. W., and Borden, T. A.: Prevention of urinary tract infection and sepsis following transrectal prostatic biopsy. J. Urol., *127*:449, 1982.

Creagen, E. T., and Fraumeni, J. F., Jr.: Cancer mortality among American Indians, 1950–67. J. Natl. Cancer Inst., *49*:959, 1972.

Culp, O. S.: Significance and treatment of prostatic nodules. J. Mich. Med. Soc., *58*:585, 1959.

Culp, O. S.: Radical perineal prostatectomy: Its past, present and possible future. J. Urol., *98*:618, 1968.

Cumes, D. M., Goffinet, D. R., Martinez, A., and Stamey, T. A.: Complications of ^{125}iodine implantation and pelvic lymphadenectomy for prostatic cancer with special reference to patients who had failed external beam therapy as their initial mode of therapy. J. Urol., *126*:620, 1981.

Cupps, R. E., Utz, D. C., Fleming, T. R., Carson, C. C., Zincke, H., and Myers, R. P.: Definitive radiation therapy for prostatic carcinoma: Mayo Clinic experience. J. Urol., *124*:855, 1980.

Czajowski, N. P., Rosenblatt, M., Wolf, P. L., and Vazquez, J.: New method of active immunization of autologous human tumour tissue. Lancet, *2*:905, 1967.

Dahlen, C. P., and Goodwin, W. E.: Sexual potency after perineal biopsy. J. Urol., *77*:660, 1957.

Dan, S. J., Wulfsohn, M. A., Efremidis, S. C., Mitty, H. A., and Brendler, H.: Lymphography and percutaneous lymph node biopsy in clinically localized carcinoma of the prostate. J. Urol., *127*:695, 1982.

Davison, P., and Malament, M.: Urinary contamination as a result of transrectal biopsy of the prostate. J. Urol., *105*:545, 1971.

De Vere White, R., Paulson, D. F., and Glenn, J. F.: The clinical spectrum of prostate cancer. J. Urol., *117*:323, 1977.

De Vere White, R., Babaian, R. K., Feldman, M., Krane, R. J., and Olsson, C. A.: Adjunctive therapy with interstitial irradiation for prostate cancer. Urology, *19*:395, 1982.

De Voogt, H. J., and Dingjan, P.: Steroid receptors in human prostatic cancer. A preliminary evaluation. Urol. Res., *6*:151, 1978.

Denton, S. E., Choy, S. H., and Valk, W. L.: Occult prostatic carcinoma diagnosed by the step section technique of the surgical specimen. J. Urol., *93*:296, 1965.

Denton, S. E., Valk, W. L., Jacobson, J. M., and Kettunen, R. C.: Comparison of the perineal needle biopsy and the transurethral prostatectomy in the diagnosis of prostatic carcinoma: An analysis of 300 cases. J. Urol., *97*:127, 1967.

Diamond, D. A., Berry, S. J., Jewett, H. J., Eggleston, J. C., and Coffey, D. S.: A new method to assess metastatic potential of human prostate cancer: Relative nuclear roundness. J. Urol., *128*:729, 1982.

Dias, S. M., and Barnett, R. N.: Elevated bone marrow acid phosphatase: The problem of false positives. J. Urol., *117*:749, 1977.

Dmochowski, L., Maruyama, K., Ohtsuki, Y., et al.: Virologic and immunologic studies of human prostatic carcinoma. Cancer Chemother. Rep., *59*:17, 1975.

Dobbs, R. M., Barber, J. A., Weigel, J. W., and Bergin, J. E.: Clotting predisposition in carcinoma of the prostate. J. Urol., *123*:706, 1980.

Dodds, P. R., Caride, V. J., and Lytton, B.: The role of vertebral veins in the dissemination of prostatic carcinoma. J. Urol., *126*:753, 1981.

Doe, R. P., and Mellinger, G. T.: Circadian variation of serum acid phosphatase in prostatic cancer. Metabolism, *13*:445, 1964.

Donati, R. M., Ellis, H., and Gallagher, N. I.: Testosterone potentiated of ^{32}P therapy in prostatic carcinoma. Cancer, *19*:1088, 1966.

Donohue, R. E., Fauver, H. E., Whitesel, J. A., Augspurger, R. R., and Pfister, R. R.: Prostatic carcinoma: Influence of tumor grade on results of pelvic lymphadenectomy. Urology, *17*:435, 1981.

Donohue, R. E., Mani, J. H., Whitesel, J. A., Mohr, S., Scanavino, D., Augspurger, R. R., Biber, R. J., Fauver, H. E., Wettlaufer, J. N., and Pfister, R. R.: Pelvic lymph node dissection: Guide to patient management in clinically locally confined adenocarcinoma of prostate. Urology, *20*:559, 1982.

Dowlen, L. W., Block, N. L., and Politano, V. A.: Complications of transrectal biopsy of the prostate. South. Med. J., *67*:1453, 1974.

Dube, V. E., Farrow, G. M., and Greene, L. F.: Prostatic adenocarcinoma of ductal origin. Cancer, *32*:402, 1973.

Dunn, J. E.: Cancer epidemiology in populations of the United States—with emphasis on Hawaii and California and Japan. Cancer Res., *35*:3240, 1975.

Dykhuizen, R. F., Sargent, C. R., George, F. W., III, and Kurahara, S. S.: The use of cobalt 60 teletherapy in the treatment of prostatic carcinoma. J. Urol., *100*:333, 1968.

Eaton, A. C.: The safety of transrectal biopsy of the prostate as an out-patient investigation. Br. J. Urol., *53*:144, 1981.

Efremidis, S. C., Pagliarulo, A., Dan, S. J., Weber, H. N., Dillon, R. N., Nieburgs, H., and Mitty, H. A.: Postlymphangiography fine needle aspiration lymph node biopsy in staging carcinoma of the prostate: Preliminary report. J. Urol., *122*:495, 1979.

Ege, G. N.: Augmented iliopelvic lymphoscintigraphy: Application in the management of genitourinary malignancy. J. Urol., *127*:265, 1982.

Eisen, M., Napp, H. E., and Vock, R.: Thrombocyten-Aggregations-Hemming bei Oestrogen-behandelten Prostata-Carcinom-Patienten. Urologe, *14*:132, 1975.

Ekman, P., Snochowski, M., Dahlberg, E., and Gustafsson, J. A.: Steroid receptors in metastatic carcinoma of the human prostate. Eur. J. Cancer, *15*:257, 1979.

Elder, J. S., and Catalona, W. J.: Management of newly diagnosed metastatic carcinoma of the prostate. Urol. Clin. North Am., *2*:283, 1984.

Elder, J. S., Jewett, H. J., and Walsh, P. C.: Radical perineal prostatectomy for clinical stage B2 carcinoma of the prostate. J. Urol., *127*:704, 1982.

Emmett, J. L., Barber, K. W., Jr., and Jackman, R. J.: Transrectal biopsy to detect prostatic carcinoma: A review and report of 203 cases. Trans. Am. Assoc. Genitourin. Surg., *53*:460, 1961.

Epstein, L. M., Stewart, B. H., Antunez, A. R., Hewitt, C. B., Straffon, R. A., Montague, D. K., Dhaliwal, R. S., and Jelden, G.: Half and total body radiation for carcinoma of the prostate. J. Urol., *122*:330, 1979.

Epstein, N. A., and Fatti, L. P.: Prostatic carcinoma: Some morphological features affecting prognosis. Cancer, *37*:2455, 1976.

Esposti, P. L.: Cytologic malignancy grading of prostatic carcinoma by transrectal aspiration biopsy. Scand. J. Urol. Nephrol., *5*:199, 1971.

Evans, C. M., and Bowen, J. G.: Immunological tests in carcinoma of the prostate. Proc. R. Soc. Med., *70*:417, 1977.

Fair, W. R., Heston, W. D. W., Kadmon, D., Crane, D. B., Catalona, W. J., Ladenson, J. H., McDonald, J. M., Noll, B. W., and Harvey, G.: Prostatic cancer, acid phosphatase, creatine kinase-BB and race: A prospective study. J. Urol., *128*:735, 1982.

Falkowski, W. S., and O'Connor, V. J., Jr.: Long-term survivor of prostatic carcinoma with lung metastases. J. Urol., *125*:260, 1981.

Farnsworth, W. E.: A direct effect of estrogens on prostatic metabolism of testosterone. Invest. Urol., *6*:423, 1969.

Farnsworth, W. E.: Human prostatic reverse transcriptase and RNA-virus. Urol. Res., *1*:106, 1973.

Farnsworth, W. E., and Gonder, M. J.: Prolactin and prostate cancer. Urology, *10*:33, 1977.

Faure, N., Lemay, A., Belanger, A., and Labrie, F.: Inhibition of testicular steroidogenesis by chronic administration of a potent LHRH agonist, HOE 766, to patients with cancer of the prostate. J. Androl., *3*:43, 1982.

Finkle, A. L., and Taylor, S. P.: Sexual potency after radical prostatectomy. J. Urol., *125*:350, 1981.

Fisher, H., Herr, H., Sogani, P., and Whitmore, N. F., Jr.: Modified pelvic lymph node dissection in patients undergoing I-125 implantation for carcinoma of the prostate. American Urological Association Meeting Program Abstract #299, 1981.

Fisher, H., Kleinert, E., and Whitmore, W. F.: Stratification of node positive patients undergoing I-125 implantation: Effect on time to distant metastases. American Urological Association Meeting Program Abstract #302, 1983.

Fitzpatrick, J. M., Gardiner, R. A., Williams, J. P., Riddle P. R., and O'Donoghue, E. P. N.: Pituitary ablation in the relief of pain in advanced prostatic carcinoma. Br. J. Urol., *52*:301, 1980.

Fleischmann, J., Catalona, W. J., Fair, W. R., Heston, W. D. W., and Menon, M.: Lack of value of radioimmunoassay for prostatic acid phosphatase as a screening test for prostatic cancer in patients with obstructive prostatic hyperplasia. J. Urol., *129*:312, 1983.

Flocks, R. H.: The treatment of stage C prostatic cancer with special reference to combined surgical and radiation therapy. J. Urol., *109*:461, 1973.

Flocks, R. H., Marberger, H., Begley, B. J., and Prendergast, L. J.: Prostatic carcinoma: Treatment of advanced cases with intravenous diethystilbestrol diphosphate. J. Urol., *74*:549, 1955.

Flocks, R. H., Nelson, C. M. K., and Boatman, C. L.: Perineal cryosurgery for prostatic carcinoma. J. Urol., *108*:933, 1972.

Fortunoff, S.: Needle biopsy of the prostate: A review of 346 biopsies. J. Urol., *87*:159, 1962.

Foti, A. G., Herschman, H., and Cooper, J. F.: A solid-phase radioimmunoassay for human prostatic acid phosphatase. Cancer Res., *35*:2446, 1975.

Foti, A. G., Cooper, J. F., Herschman, H., and Malvaez, R. R.: Detection of prostatic cancer by solid-phase radioimmunoassay of serum prostatic acid phosphatase. N. Engl. J. Med., *297*:1357, 1977.

Fowler, J. E., Jr., and Whitmore, W. F., Jr.: The response of metastatic adenocarcinoma of the prostate to exogenous testosterone. J. Urol., *126*:372, 1981a.

Fowler, J. E., and Whitmore, W. F., Jr.: The incidence and extent of pelvic lymph node metastases in apparently localized prostatic cancer. Cancer, *47*:2941, 1981b.

Fowler, J. E., Jr., and Whitmore, W. F., Jr.: Considerations for the use of testosterone with systemic chemotherapy in prostatic cancer. Cancer, *49*:1373, 1982.

Fowler, J. E., Jr., Barzell, W., Hilaris, B. S., and Whitmore, W. F., Jr.: Complications of ¹²⁵iodine implantation and pelvic lymphadenectomy in the treatment of prostatic cancer. J. Urol., *121*:447, 1979.

Fowler, J. E., Torgerson, L., McLeod, D. G., and Stutzman, R. E.: Radical prostatectomy with pelvic lymphadenectomy: Observations on the accuracy of staging with lymph node frozen sections. J. Urol., *126*:618, 1981.

Fowler, J. E., Jr., Fisher, H. A. G., Kaiser, D. L., and

Whitmore, W. F., Jr.: Pelvic lymph node metastases and probability of survival without distant metastases in patients treated with 125-I implantation for localized prostatic cancer: Influence of pre-treatment transurethral resection of the prostate. American Urological Association Meeting Program Abstract #243, 1982.

Frank, I. N., and Scott, W. W.: The cytodiagnosis of prostatic carcinoma: A follow-up study. J. Urol., 79:983, 1958.

Franks, L. M.: Proceedings: Etiology, epidemiology and pathology of prostatic cancer. Cancer, 32:1092, 1973.

Fraumeni, J. F., Jr., and Mason, T. J.: Cancer mortality among Chinese-Americans, 1950–69. J. Natl. Cancer Inst., 52:659, 1974.

Freiha, F.: Carcinoma of the prostate: Results of postirradiation biopsy. American Urological Association Meeting Program Abstract #297, 1983.

Freiha, F. S., Pistenma, D. A., and Bagshaw, M. A.: Pelvic lymphadenectomy for staging prostatic carcinoma: Is it always necessary? J. Urol., 122:176, 1979.

Furlow, W. L.: Surgical management of impotence using the inflatage penile prosthesis: Experience with 103 patients. Br. J. Urol., 50:114, 1978.

Gaeta, J. F., Asirwatham, J. E., Miller, G., and Murphy, G. P.: Histologic grading of primary prostatic cancer: A new approach to an old problem. J. Urol., 123:689, 1980.

Gagnon, J. D., Moss, W. T., and Stevens, K. R.: Pre-estrogen breast irradiation for patients with carcinoma of the prostate: A critical review. J. Urol., 121:182, 1979.

Galen, R. S., and Gambino, S. R.: Beyond Normality: The Predictive Value and Efficiency of Medical Diagnosis. New York, Wiley, 1978.

Gardiner, R. A., Fitzpatrick, J. M., Constable, A. R., Cranage, R. W., O'Donoghue, E. P. N., and Wickham, J. E. A.: Improved techniques in radionuclide imaging of prostatic lymph nodes. Br. J. Urol., 51:561, 1979.

Gee, W. F., and Cole, J. R.: Symptomatic stage C carcinoma of prostate: Traditional therapy. Urology, 15:335, 1980.

Geller, J., Albert, J., and Yen, S. S. C.:Treatment of advanced cancer of prostate with megestrol acetate. Urology, 12:537, 1978.

Gibbons, R. P., Mason, J. T., Correa, R. J., Cummings, K. B., Taylor, W. J., Hafermann, M. D., and Richardson, R. G.: Carcinoma of the prostate: Local control with external beam radiation therapy. J. Urol., 121:310, 1979.

Gibbons, R. P., and Investigators, National Prostatic Cancer Project Cooperative Clinical Trials: Cooperative trial of single and combined agent protocols. Urology, 17[Suppl.]:48, 1981.

Gill, W. B., Schoenberg, H. W., Banno, J. J., Sutton, H. G., and Straus, F. H.: Sandwich radiotherapy (3,000 and 4,500 rads) around radical retropubic prostatectomy for stage C prostatic carcinoma. Urology, 16:470, 1980.

Glashan, R. W., and Robinson, M. R. G.: Cardiovascular complications in the treatment of prostatic carcinoma. Br. J. Urol., 53:624, 1981.

Gleason, D. F., and the Veterans Administration Cooperative Urological Research Group: Histologic grading and clinical staging of prostatic carcinoma. In Tannenbaum, M. (Ed.): Urologic Pathology: The Prostate. Philadelphia, Lea & Febiger, 1977, pp. 171–197.

Gleason, D. F., Mellinger, G. T., and the Veterans Administration Cooperative Urological Research Group: Prediction of prognosis for prostatic adenocarcinoma by combined histological grading and clinical staging. J. Urol., 111:58, 1974.

Glick, J. H., Wein, A., Padavic, K., Negendank, W., Harris, D., and Brodovsky, H.: Tamoxifen in refractory metastatic carcinoma of the prostate. Cancer Treat. Rep., 64:813, 1980.

Glick, J. H., Wein, A., Padavic, K., Negendank, W., Harris, D., and Brodovsky, H.: Phase II trial of tamoxifen in metastatic carcinoma of the prostate. Cancer, 49:1367, 1982.

Goffinet, D. R., Martinez, A., Freiha, F., Pooler, D. M., Pistenma, D. A., Cumes, D., and Bagshaw, M. A.: 125Iodine prostate implants for recurrent carcinomas after external beam irradiation: Preliminary results. Cancer, 45:2717, 1980.

Golimbu, M., Morales, P., Al-Askari, S., and Brown, J.: Extended pelvic lymphadenectomy for prostatic cancer. J. Urol., 121:617, 1979.

Golimbu, M., Glasser, J., Schinella, R., and Morales, P.: Stage A prostate cancer from pathologist's viewpoint. Urology, 18:134, 1981.

Gonder, M. H., Soanes, W. A., and Smith, V.: Experimental prostate cryosurgery. Invest. Urol., 1:610, 1964.

Grayhack, J. T.: Pituitary factors influencing growth of the prostate. Workshops on the biology of the prostate and related tissues. Natl. Cancer Inst. Monogr., 12:189, 1963.

Grayhack, J. T., and Bockrath, J. M.: Diagnosis of carcinoma of prostate. Urology, 17 [Suppl.]:54, 1981.

Greene, L. F., Mulcahy, J. J., Warren, M. M., and Dockerty, M. B.: Primary transitional cell carcinoma of the prostate. J. Urol., 110:235, 1973.

Greenwald, P., Damon, A., Kirmss, V., and Polan, A. K.: Physical and demographic features of men before developing cancer of the prostate. J. Natl. Cancer Inst., 53:341, 1974a.

Greenwald, P., Kirmss, V., Polan, A. K., and Dick, V. S.: Cancer of the prostate among men with benign prostatic hyperplasia. J. Natl. Cancer Inst., 53:335, 1974b.

Griffiths, J. C.: Prostate-specific acid phosphatase: Reevaluation of radioimmunoassay in diagnosing prostatic disease. Clin. Chem., 26:433, 1980.

Grossman, H. B., Batata, H., Hilaris, B., and Whitmore, W. F., Jr.: 125-I implantation for carcinoma of the prostate: Further followup of first 100 cases. Urology, 20:591, 1982.

Grout, D. C., Grayhack, J. T., Moss, W., and Holland, J. M.: Radiation therapy in the treatment of carcinoma of the prostate. J. Urol., 105:411, 1971.

Guinan, P., Toronchi, E., Crispin, R., Mouli, K., and Shaw, M.: BCG immunotherapy in advanced prostate cancer. In Terry, W. D., and Rosenberg, S. A. (Eds.): Immunotherapy of Human Cancer. New York, Excerpta Medica, 1982a, pp. 323–327.

Guinan, P., Toronchi, E., Shaw, M., Crispin, R., and Sharifi, R.: Bacillus Calmette-Guerin (BCG) adjuvant therapy in stage D prostate cancer. Urology, 20:401, 1982b.

Gursel, E. O., Roberts, M., and Veenema, R. J.: Regression of prostatic cancer following sequential cryotherapy to the prostate. J. Urol., 108:928, 1972.

Gursel, E. O., Rezvan, M., Sy, F. A., and Veenema, R. J.: Comparative evaluation of bone marrow acid phosphatase and bone scanning in staging of prostatic cancer. J. Urol., 111:53, 1974.

Gutman, A. B., and Gutman, E. B.: "Acid" phosphatase occurring in the serum of patients with metastasing carcinoma of prostate gland. J. Clin. Invest., 17:473, 1938.

Haddad, J. R., and Reynes, E. C.: Carcinosarcoma of the prostate with metastases of both elements: Case report. J. Urol., *103*:80, 1970.

Halpert, B., Sheehan, E. E., Schmalhorst, W. R., and Scott, R., Jr.: Carcinoma of the prostate: A survey of 5000 autopsies. Cancer, *16*:737, 1963.

Hamlin, W. B., and Lund, P. K.: Carcinosarcoma of the prostate: A case report. J. Urol., *97*:518, 1967.

Hanash, K. A., Utz, D. C., Cook, E. N., Taylor, W. F., and Titus, J. L.: Carcinoma of the prostate: A 15 year followup. J. Urol., *107*:450, 1973.

Hanks, G. E., Leibel, S., and Kramer, S.: The dissemination of cancer by transurethral resection of locally advanced prostate cancer. J. Urol., *129*:309, 1983.

Harada, M., Mostofi, F. K., Corle, D. K., Byar, D. P., and Trump, B. F.: Preliminary studies of histologic prognosis in cancer of the prostate. Cancer Treat. Rep., *61*:223, 1977.

Harper, M. E., Fahmy, A. R., Pierrepoint, C. G., and Griffiths, K.: The effect of some stilbestrol compounds on DNA polymerase from human prostatic tissues. Steroids, *15*:89, 1970.

Hawtrey, C. E., Welch, M. J., Jr., Schmidt, J. D., Culp, D. A., Flocks, R. H.: Paraplegia and paraparesis due to prostatic cancer. Urology, *4*:431, 1974.

Heaney, J. A., Chang, H. C., Daly, J. J., and Prout, G. R., Jr.: Prognosis of clinically undiagnosed prostatic carcinoma and influence of endocrine therapy. J. Urol., *118*:283, 1977.

Henneberry, M. O., Engel, G., and Grayhack, J. T.: Acid phosphatase. Urol. Clin. North Am., *6*:629, 1979.

Herbert, J. T., Birkhoff, J. D., Feorino, P. M., and Caldwell, G. G.: Herpes simplex virus type 2 and cancer of the prostate. J. Urol., *116*:611, 1976.

Herr, H. W.: Complications of pelvic lymphadenectomy and retropubic prostatic ^{125}I implantation. Urology, *14*:226, 1979.

Herr, H. W.: Suppressor cells in immunodepressed bladder and prostate cancer patients. J. Urol., *123*:635, 1980.

Herr, H. W.: Pelvic lymphadenectomy and iodine-125 implantation. *In* Johnson, D. E., and Boileau, M. A. (Eds.): Genitourinary Tumors: Fundamental Principles and Surgical Techniques. New York, Grune & Stratton, 1982a, pp. 63–73.

Herr, H. W.: Cyclophosphamide, methotrexate and 5-fluorouracil combination chemotherapy versus chloroethyl-cyclohexy-nitrosurea in the treatment of metastatic prostatic cancer. J. Urol., *127*:462, 1982b.

Herr, H. W., and Whitmore, W. F., Jr.: Significance of prostatic biopsies after radiation therapy for carcinoma of the prostate. Prostate, *3*:339, 1982.

Heshmat, M. Y., Kovi, J., Herson, J., Jones, G. W., and Jackson, M. A.: Epidemiologic association between gonorrhea and prostatic carcinoma. Urology, *6*:457, 1975.

Hilaris, B. S., Whitmore, W. F., Jr., Batata, M. A., and Grabstald, H.: Radiation therapy and pelvic node dissection in the management of cancer of the prostate. Am. J. Roentgenol., *121*:832, 1974.

Hill, D. R., Crews, Q. E., Jr., and Walsh, P. C.: Prostate carcinoma: Radiation treatment of the primary and regional lymphatics. Cancer, *34*:156, 1974.

Hindsley, J. P., Sanfelippo, C. J., Fowler, J. E., and Whitmore, W. F., Jr.: Mini-dose heparin therapy in pelvic lymphadenectomy and ^{125}I implantation for localized prostatic cancer. Urology, *15*:272, 1980.

Hodges, C. V., Pearse, H. D., and Stille, L.: Radical prostatectomy for carcinoma: 30-year experience and 15-year survivals. J. Urol., *122*:180, 1979.

Hoekstra, W. J., and Schroeder, F. H.: The role of lymph-angiography in the staging of prostatic cancer. Prostate, *2*:433, 1981.

Hoffman, G. S., Scardino, P. T., and Carlton, C. E., Jr.: The effect of TURP on survival and dissemination in prostatic cancer. American Urological Association Meeting Program Abstract #416, 1983.

Holmes, E. J.: Crystalloids of prostatic carcinoma: Relationship to Bence-Jones crystals. Cancer, *39*:2073, 1977.

Hovsepian, J. A., Byar, D. P., and the Veterans Administration Cooperative Urological Research Group: Quantitative radiology for staging and prognosis of patients with advanced prostatic carcinoma: Correlations with other pretreatment characteristics. Urology, *14*:145, 1979.

Huben, R., Mettlin, C., Natarajan, N., Smart, C. R., Pontes, E., and Murphy, G. P.: Carcinoma of prostate in men less than fifty years old: Data from American College of Surgeons' National Survey. Urology, *20*:585, 1982.

Huber, P. R., Scholer, A., Linder, E., Hagmaier, V., Vogt, H., Christen, P., Eppenberger, U., and Rutishauser, G.: Measurement of prostatic acid phosphatase in serum and bone marrow: Radioimmunoassay and enzymatic measurement compared. Clin. Chem., *28*:2044, 1982.

Hudson, P. B., Finkle, A. L., Trufilio, A., and Wolan, C. T.: Prostatic cancer. IX. Value of transurethral biopsy in search of early prostatic carcinoma. Surgery, *35*:897, 1954.

Huggins, C., and Clark, P. J.: Quantitative studies of prostatic secretion. II. The effect of castration and of estrogen injection on the normal and on the hyperplastic prostatic glands of dogs. J. Exp. Med., *72*:747, 1940.

Huggins, C., and Hodges, C. V.: Studies on prostatic cancer; effect of castration, of estrogen and of androgen injection on serum phosphatases in metastatic carcinoma of the prostate. Cancer Res., *1*:293, 1941.

Huggins, C., and Scott, W. W.: Bilateral adrenalectomy in prostatic cancer. Clinical features and urinary excretion of 17-ketosteroids and estrogen. Ann. Surg., *122*:1031, 1945.

Hutchison, G. B.: Etiology and prevention of prostatic cancer. Cancer Chemother. Rep., *59*:57, 1975.

Hutchison, G. B.: Incidence and etiology of prostate cancer. Urology, *17* [Suppl.]:4, 1981.

Jacobi, G. H., Sinterhauf, K., Kurth, K. H., and Altwein, J. E.: Bromocryptine and prostatic carcinoma: Plasma kinetics production and tissue uptake of ^{3}H-testosterone in vivo. J. Urol., *119*:240, 1978.

Jacobo, E., Schmidt, J. D., Weinstein, S. H., and Flocks, R. H.: Comparison of flutamide (SCH–13521) and diethylstilbestrol in untreated advanced prostatic cancer. Urology, *8*:231, 1976.

Jacobs, S. C.: Spread of prostatic cancer to bone. Urology, *21*:337, 1983.

Jewett, H. J.: The case for radical perineal prostatectomy. J. Urol., *103*:195, 1970.

Jewett, H. J.: The present status of radical prostatectomy for stages A and B prostatic cancer. Urol. Clin. North Am., *2*:105, 1975.

Jewett, H. J., Bridge, R. W., Gray, G. F., Jr., and Shelley, W. M.: The palpable nodule of prostatic cancer. Results 15 years after radical excision. JAMA, *203*:115, 1968.

Johnson, D. E., Hogan, J. M., and Ayala, A. G.: Transitional cell carcinoma of the prostate. A clinical morphological study. Cancer, *29*:287, 1972a.

Johnson, D. E., Lanieri, J. P., Jr., and Ayala, A. G.: Prostatic adenocarcinoma occurring in men under 50 years of age. J. Surg. Oncol., *4*:207, 1972b.

Johnson, D. E., Chalbaud, R., and Ayala, A. G.: Secondary tumors of the prostate. J. Urol., *112*:507, 1974.

Johnston, B. J.: Clinical effects of Coley's toxin. I. A controlled study. Cancer Chemother. Rep., *21*:19, 1962.

Jordan, W. P., Jr., Blackard, C. E., and Byar, D. P.: Reconsideration of orchiectomy in the treatment of advanced prostatic carcinoma. South. Med. J., *70*:1411, 1977.

Kagan, A. R., Gordon, J., Cooper, J. F., Gilbert, H., Nussbaum, H., and Chan, P.: A clinical appraisal of post-irradiation biopsy in prostatic cancer. Cancer, *39*:637, 1977.

Kandzari, S. J., Belis, J. A., Kim, J. C., Gnepp, D. R., and Riley, R. S.: Clinical results of early stage prostatic cancer treated by pelvic lymphadenectomy and ^{125}iodine implants. J. Urol., *127*:923, 1982.

Kandzari, S. J., Belis, J. A., and Riley, R. S.: Post-radiation biopsy and histological effects in early stage prostatic cancer treated with ^{125}iodine implants. American Urological Association Meeting Program Abstract #296, 1983.

Kaneti, J., Thomson, D. M. P., and Reid, E. C.: Prostaglandin E2 affects the tumor immune response in prostatic carcinoma. J. Urol., *126*:65, 1981.

Karr, J. P., Wajsman, Z., Madajewecz, S., Kirdani, R. Y., Murphy, G. P., and Sandberg, A. A.: Steroid hormone receptors in the prostate. J. Urol., *122*:170, 1979.

Kaufman, J. J., and Schultz, J. I.: Needle biopsy of the prostate: A re-evaluation. J. Urol., *87*:164, 1962.

Kaufman, J. J., Boxer, R. J., Boxer, B., and Quinn, M. C.: Physical and psychological results of penile prosthesis: A statistical survey. J. Urol., *126*:173, 1981.

Kaufman, J. J., Ljung, B. M., Walther, P., and Waisman, J.: Aspiration biopsy of prostate. Urology, *19*:587, 1982.

Keen, C. W.: Half body radiotherapy in the management of metastatic carcinoma of the prostate. J. Urol., *123*:713, 1980.

Kiesling, V. J., McAninch, J. W., Goebel, J. L., and Agee, R. E.: External beam radiotherapy for adenocarcinoma of the prostate: A clinical followup. J. Urol., *124*:851, 1980.

Kihl, B., and Bratt, C.-G.: Reimplantation of the ureter in prostatic carcinoma associated with bilateral ureteric obstruction. Br. J. Urol., *53*:349, 1981.

Klugo, R. C., Farah, R. N., and Cerny, J. C.: Bilateral orchiectomy for carcinoma of prostate. Response to serum testosterone and clinical response to subsequent estrogen therapy. Urology, *17*:49, 1981.

Kohri, K., Kaneko, S., Akiyama, T., Yachiku, S., and Kurita, T.: Ultrasonic evaluation of prostatic carcinoma. Urology, *17*:214, 1981.

Koiso, K., Akima, H., and Niijima, T.: Prevention of platelet aggregation in patients with prostatic cancer during estrogen therapy. Urology, *19*:579, 1982.

Kontturi, M., and Sotaniemi, E.: Thromboembolism during estrogen therapy of prostatic cancer. Report on two cases. Scand. J. Urol. Nephrol., *5*:108, 1971.

Kopecky, A. A., Laskowski, T. Z., and Scott, R., Jr.: Radical retropubic prostatectomy in the treatment of prostatic carcinoma. J. Urol., *103*:641, 1970.

Kopelson, G., Harisiadis, L., Romas, N. A., Veenema, R. J., and Tannenbaum, M.: Periurethral prostatic duct carcinoma: Clinical features and treatment results. Cancer, *42*:2894, 1978.

Kramer, S. A., Spahr, J., Brendler, C. B., Glenn, J. F., and Paulson, D. F.: Experience with Gleason's histopathologic grading in prostatic cancer. J. Urol., *124*:223, 1980.

Kramer, S. A., Cline, W. A., Jr., Farnham, R., Carson,

C. C., Cox, E. B., Hinshaw, W., and Paulson, D. F.: Prognosis of patients with stage D1 prostatic adenocarcinoma. J. Urol., *125*:817, 1981.

Krastanova, L. J., and Addonizio, J. C.: Carcinosarcoma of prostate. Urology, *18*:85, 1981.

Kraus, C. T., and Persky, L.: Radical perineal prostatectomy in patients over age of seventy. Urology, *18*:368, 1981.

Kraus, P. A., Lytton, B., Weiss, R. M., and Prosnitz, L. R.: Radiation therapy for local palliative treatment of prostatic cancer. J. Urol., *108*:612, 1972.

Krieg, M., Grobe, I., Boigt, K. D., Altenahr, E., and Klosterhalfen, H.: Human prostatic carcinoma: significant differences in its androgen binding and metabolism compared to the human benign prostatic hypertrophy. Acta Endocrinol., *88*:397, 1978.

Kumar, P. P., and Bartone, F. F.: Transperineal percutaneous I-125 implant of prostate. Urology, *17*:238, 1981.

Kurth, K. H., Altwein, J. E., Skoluda, D., and Hohenfellner, R.: Followup of irradiated prostatic carcinoma by aspiration biopsy. J. Urol., *117*:615, 1977.

Labrie, F.: Novel hormone mix unveiled to stay prostatic cancer spread. Urol. Times, August 1983, p. 1.

Lachman, E.: Osteoporosis—The potentialities and limitations of its roentgenologic diagnosis. Am. J. Roentgenol. Radium Ther. Nucl. Med., *74*:712, 1955.

Lanesky, J., Opipari, M. I., and McKenzie, M.: Multiple primary prostate cancer. Urology, *13*:667, 1979.

Lang, D. J., Kummer, J. F., and Hartley, D. P.: Cytomegalovirus in semen: Persistence and demonstration in extracellular fluids. N. Engl. J. Med., *291*:121, 1974.

Lange, P. H., and Narayan, P.: Understaging and undergrading of prostate cancer: Argument for postoperative radiation as adjuvant therapy. Urology, *21*:113, 1983.

Lange, P. H., Moon, T. D., Haselow, R. E., Medini, E., and Rao, Y.: Radiation therapy after radical prostatectomy. American Urological Association Meeting Program Abstract #300, 1983.

Leach, G. E., Cooper, J. F., Kagan, A. R., Snyder, R., and Forsythe, A.: Radiotherapy for prostatic carcinoma: Post-irradiation prostatic biopsy and recurrence patterns with long-term followup. J. Urol., *128*:505, 1982.

Legge, D. A., Good, C. A., and Ludwig, J.: Roentgenologic features of pulmonary carcinomatosis from carcinoma of the prostate. Am. J. Roentgenol., *111*:360, 1971.

Leibel, S. A., Pino, Y., Torres, J. L., and Order, S. E.: Improved quality of life following radical radiation therapy for early stage carcinoma of the prostate. Urol. Clin. North Am., 7:593, 1980.

Lepor, H., Ross, A., and Walsh, P. C.: The influence of hormonal therapy on survival of men with advanced prostatic cancer. J. Urol., *128*:335, 1982.

Levin, A. B., Benson, R. C., Jr., Katz, J., and Nilsson, T.: Chemical hypophysectomy for relief of bone pain in carcinoma of the prostate. J. Urol., *119*:517, 1978.

Levine, R. L., and Wilchinsky, M.: Adenocarcinoma of the prostate: A comparison of the disease in blacks versus whites. J. Urol., *121*:761, 1979.

Levitt, R. G., Sagel, S. S., Stanley, R. J., and Evens, R. G.: Computed tomography of the pelvis. Semin. Roentgenol., *13*:193, 1978.

Liebner, E. J., Stefani, S., and the Uro-Oncology Research Group: An evaluation of lymphography with nodal biopsy in localized carcinoma of the prostate. Cancer, *45*:728, 1980.

Lieskovsky, G., Skinner, D. G., and Weisenburger, T.: Pelvic lymphadenectomy in the management of carcinoma of the prostate. J. Urol., *124*:635, 1980.

Lin, B. P., Davies, W. E., and Harmata, P. A.: Prostatic aspiration cytology. Pathology, *11*:607, 1979.

Linder, A., deKernion, J. B., Smith, R. B., and Katske, F. A.: Risk of urinary incontinence following radical prostatectomy. J. Urol., *129*:1007, 1983.

Loening, S. A., Scott, W. W., deKernion, J., Gibbons, R. P., Johnson, D. E., Pontes, J. E., Prout, G. R., Schmidt, J. D., Soloway, M. S., Chu, T. M., Gaeta, J. F., Slack, N. H., and Murphy, G. P.: A comparison of hydroxyurea, methyl-chloroethyl-cyclohexy-nitrosourea and cyclophosphamide in patients with advanced carcinoma of the prostate. J. Urol., *125*:812, 1981.

Logothetis, C. J., von Eschenbach, A. C., Samuels, M. L., Trindade, A., and Johnson, D. E.: Doxorubicin, mitomycin, and 5-FU (DMF) in the treatment of hormone-resistant stage D prostate cancer: A preliminary report. Cancer Treat. Rep., *66*:57, 1982.

Loh, E. S., Brown, H. E., and Beiler, D. D.: Radiotherapy of carcinoma of the prostate: Preliminary report. J. Urol., *106*:906, 1971.

Loor, R., Wang, M. C., Valenzuela, L., and Chu, T. M.: Expression of prostatic acid phosphatase in human prostate cancer. Cancer Letters, *14*:63, 1981.

Lukkarinen, O., Hammond, G. L., Kontturi, M., and Vihko, R.: Long-term effects of endocrine treatment on serum pituitary hormones in advanced prostatic carcinoma patients. Scand. J. Urol. Nephrol., *15*:207, 1981.

Lupu, A. N., Petrovich, Z., Corvalan, J., Katske, F. A., and Kaufman, J. J.: Teletherapy for stage C adenocarcinoma of the prostate. J. Urol., *128*:75, 1982.

Lytton, B., Collins, J. T., Weiss, R. M., Schiff, M., Jr., McGuire, E. J., and Livolsi, V.: Results of biopsy after early stage prostatic cancer treatment by implantation of ^{125}I seeds. J. Urol., *121*:306, 1979.

Mackler, M. A., Liberti, J. P., Smith, M. J. V., Koontz, W. W., Jr., and Prout, G. R., Jr.: The effect of orchiectomy and various doses of stilbestrol on plasma testosterone levels in patients with carcinoma of the prostate. Invest. Urol., *9*:423, 1972.

Madajewicz, S., Creaven, P., Ozer, H., O'Malley, J., Grossmayer, B., Pontes, E., Mittelman, A., Soloman, J., and Ferraresi, R.: A phase I study of rising doses of recombinant DNA alpha-2 interferon from *E. coli*. (Abstract.) Third International Congress for Interferon Research, 1982.

Mahan, D. E., and Doctor, B. P.: A radioimmune assay for human prostatic acid phosphatase-levels in prostatic disease. Clin. Biochem., *12*:10, 1979.

Mahoney, E. M., and Harrison, J. H.: Bilateral adrenalectomy for palliative treatment of prostate cancer. J. Urol., *108*:936, 1972.

Manley, C. B., Jr.: The striated muscle of the prostate. J. Urol., *95*:234, 1966.

Martelli, A., Soli, M., Bercovich, E., Prodi, G., Grilli, S., De Giovanni, C., and Galli, M. C.: Correlation between clinical response to antiandrogenic therapy and occurrence of receptors in human prostatic cancer. Urology, *16*:245, 1980.

Martin, S. A., Fowler, M., Catalona, W. J., and Boyarsky, S.: Carcinosarcoma of the prostate: Report of a case with ultrastructural observations. J. Urol., *122*:709, 1979.

McCombs, R. M.: Role of oncornaviruses in carcinoma of the prostate. Cancer Treat. Rep., *61*:131, 1977.

McCullough, D. L., and Leadbetter, W. F.: Radical pelvic surgery for locally extensive carcinoma of the prostate. J. Urol., *108*:939, 1972.

McCullough, D. L., McLaughlin, A. P., and Gittes, R. F.: Morbidity of pelvic lymphadenectomy and radical pros-

tatectomy for prostatic cancer. J. Urol., *117*:206, 1977.

McGowan, D. G.: Radiation therapy in the management of localized carcinoma of the prostate: A preliminary report. Cancer, *39*:98, 1977.

McGowan, D. G.: The adverse influence of prior transurethral resection on prognosis in carcinoma of the prostate treated by radiation therapy. Int. J. Rad. Oncol. Biol. Phys., *6*:1121, 1980.

McLaughlin, A. P., III, and Brooks, J. D.: A plasma factor inhibiting lymphocyte reactivity in urologic cancer patients. J. Urol., *112*:366, 1974.

McLaughlin, A. P., III, Kessler, W. O., Triman, K., and Gittes, R. F.: Immunologic competence in patients with urologic cancer. J. Urol., *111*:233, 1974.

McLaughlin, A. P., Saltzstein, S. L., McCullough, D. L., and Gittes, R. F.: Prostatic carcinoma: Incidence and location of unsuspected lymphatic metastases. J. Urol., *115*:89, 1976.

McLoughlin, M., Hazra, T., Schirmer, H. K. A., and Scott, W. W.: Telecobalt therapy for prostatic cancer: Rationale, results, and future considerations. J. Urol., *113*:378, 1975.

McMillen, S. M., and Wettlaufer, J. N.: The role of repeat transurethral biopsy in stage A carcinoma of the prostate. J. Urol., *116*:759, 1976.

Megalli, M. R., Gursel, E. O., Demirag, H., Veenema, R. J., and Guttman, R. L.: External radiotherapy in uretral obstruction secondary to locally invasive prostatic cancer. Urology, *3*:562, 1974.

Melicow, M. M., and Pachter, M. R.: Endometrial carcinoma of prostatic utricle (uterus masculinus). Cancer, *20*:1715, 1967.

Melicow, M. M., and Tannenbaum, M.: Endometrial carcinoma of uterus masculinus (prostatic utricle). Report of 6 cases. J. Urol., *106*:892, 1971.

Melicow, M. M., and Uson, A. C.: A spectrum of malignant epithelial tumors of the prostate gland. J. Urol., *115*:696, 1976.

Melograna, F., Oertel, Y. C., and Kwart, A. M.: Prospective controlled assessment of fine-needle prostatic aspiration. Urology, *19*:47, 1982.

Menck, H. R., Henderson, B. E., Pike, M. C., Mack, T., Martin, S. P., and SooHoo, J.: Cancer incidence in the Mexican-American. J. Natl. Cancer Inst., *55*:531, 1975.

Menon, M., and Catalona, W. J.: Interpreting response to treatment in advanced prostatic cancer. Rev. Endocr.-Rel. Cancer, *10*:11, 1981.

Menon, M., and Walsh, P. C.: Hormonal therapy for prostatic cancer. *In* Murphy, G. P. (Ed.): Prostate Cancer. Littleton, MA, PSG Publishing Company, Inc., 1979, pp. 175–200.

Merrin, C., Han, T., Klein, E., Wajsman, Z., and Murphy, G. P.: Immunotherapy of prostatic carcinoma with Bacillus Calmette-Guerin. Cancer Chemother. Rep., *59*:157, 1975.

Meyers, R. P., Zincke, H., Flemming, T. R., Farrow, G. M., Furlow, W. L., and Utz, D. C.: Hormonal treatment at time of radical retropubic prostatectomy for stage D1 prostate cancer. J. Urol., *130*:99, 1983.

Michigan, S., and Catalona, W. J.: Ureteral obstruction from prostatic carcinoma: Response to endocrine and radiation therapy. J. Urol., *118*:733, 1977.

Middleton, A. W., Jr.: Pelvic lymphadenectomy with modified radical retropubic prostatectomy as a single operation: Technique used and results in 50 consecutive cases. J. Urol., *125*:353, 1981.

Middleton, R. G., and Smith, J. A., Jr.: Radical prostatectomy for stage B2 prostatic cancer. J. Urol., *127*:702, 1982.

Milleman, L. A., Weissman, W. D., and Culp, D. A.:

Serum protein, enzyme and immunoglobulin responses following perineal cryosurgery for carcinoma of the prostate. J. Urol., *123*:710, 1980.

Miller, G. M., and Hinman, F., Jr.: Cortisone treatment in advanced carcinoma of the prostate. J. Urol., *72*:485, 1954.

Miller, L. S.: After-loading transperineal iridium-192 wire implantation of the prostate. Radiology, *131*:527, 1979.

Mobbs, B. G., Johnson, I. E., Connolly, J. G., and Clark, A. F.: Androgen receptor assay in human benign and malignant prostatic tumour cytosol using protamine sulphate precipitation. J. Steroid Biochem., *9*:289, 1978.

Mollenkamp, J. S., Cooper, J. F., and Kagan, A. R.: Clinical experience with supervoltage radiotherapy in carcinoma of the prostate: A preliminary report. J. Urol., *113*:374, 1975.

Moore, R. A.: The evolution and involution of the prostate gland. Am. J. Pathol., *12*:599, 1936.

Morales, P., and Golimbu, M.: The therapeutic role of pelvic lymphadenectomy in prostatic cancer. Urol. Clin. North Am., 7:623, 1980.

Mostofi, F. K.: Problems of grading carcinoma of prostate. Semin. Oncol., *3*:161, 1976.

Mostofi, F. K., and Price, E. B.: Tumors of the male genital system. *In*: Atlas on Tumor Pathology. Series 2. Fasc. 8. Washington, DC, Armed Forces Institute of Pathology, 1973, pp. 196–219.

Mott, L. J. M.: Squamous cell carcinoma of the prostate: Report of 2 cases and review of the literature. J. Urol., *121*:833, 1979.

Mouli, K., Sharifi, R., Ray, P., Baumbartner, G., and Guinan, P.: Prostatorectal fistula associated with 125-iodine seed radiotherapy. J. Urol., *129*:387, 1983.

Murphy, G. P.: Current report on the interferon program at Roswell Park Memorial Institute. J. Surg. Oncol., *17*:99, 1981.

Murphy, G. P., Natarajan, N., Pontes, J. E., Schmitz, R. L., Smart, C. R., Schmidt, J. D., and Mettlin, C.: The national survey of prostate cancer in the United States by the American College of Surgeons. J. Urol., *127*:928, 1982.

Murphy, G. P., Beckley, S., Brady, M. F., Chu, T. M., deKernion, J. B., Dhabuwala, C., Gaeta, J. F., Gibbons, R. P., Loening, S. A., McKiel, C. F., McLeod, D. G., Pontes, J. E., Prout, G. R., Scardino, P. T., Schlegel, J. U., Schmidt, J. D., Scott, W. W., Slack, N. H., and Soloway, M. S.: Treatment of newly diagnosed metastatic prostate cancer patients with chemotherapy agents in combination with hormones versus hormones alone. Cancer, *51*:1264, 1983.

Nachtsheim, D. A., Jr., McAninch, J. W., Stutzman, R. E., and Goebel, J. L.: Latent residual tumor following external radiotherapy for prostate adenocarcinoma. J. Urol., *120*:312, 1978.

Nakagami, Y., Chin, H., Tannowa, K., Matsumoto, K., and Kawai, H.: Adjuvant immunotherapy with a *S. pyogenes* preparation (OK432) in urogenital cancer patients. Urology, *17*:386, 1980.

Narayana, A. S., Loening, S. A., and Culp, D. A.: Flutamide in the treatment of metastatic carcinoma of the prostate. Br. J. Urol., *53*:152, 1981.

Nauts, H. C.: Enhancement of natural resistance to renal cancer: Beneficial effects of concurrent infections and immunotherapy with bacterial vaccines. Monograph No. 12. New York, New York Cancer Research Institute, 1973.

Neglia, W. J., Hussey, D. H., and Johnson, D. E.: Megavoltage radiation therapy for carcinoma of the prostate. Int. J. Rad. Oncol. Biol. Phys., *2*:873, 1977.

Nelson, C. M. K., Boatman, D. L., and Flocks, R. H.:

Bone marrow examination in carcinoma of the prostate. J. Urol., *109*:667, 1973.

Nesbit, R. M., and Baum, W. C.: Endocrine control of prostatic carcinoma. Clinical and statistical survey of 1818 cases. JAMA, *143*:1317, 1950.

Nesbit, R. M., and Plumb, R. T.: Prostatic carcinoma: A follow-up on 795 patients treated prior to endocrine era and comparison of survival rates between these and patients treated by endocrine therapy. Surgery, *20*:263, 1946.

Nevin, J. E., Melnick, I., Baggerly, J. T., Hoffman, A., Landes, R. R., and Easley, C.: The continuous arterial infusion of 5-fluorouracil as a therapeutic adjunct in the treatment of advanced carcinoma of the bladder and prostate: A preliminary report. Cancer, *31*:138, 1973.

Nichols, R. T., Barry, J. M., and Hodges, C. V.: The morbidity of radical prostatectomy for multifocal stage I prostatic adenocarcinoma. J. Urol., *117*:83, 1977.

Nissenkorn, I., Mickey, D. D., Miller, D. B., and Soloway, M. S.: Circadian and day-to-day variation of prostatic acid phosphatase. J. Urol., *127*:1122, 1982.

Noble, R. L.: The development of prostatic adenocarcinoma in Nb rats following prolonged sex hormone administration. Cancer Res., *37*:1929, 1977.

O'Connor, V. J., and Sokol, K. J.: Secondary regression in carcinoma of the prostate after orchiectomy. Presented at the American Urologic Association Meeting, 1959.

O'Connor, V. J., Chiang, S. P., and Grayhack, J. T.: Is subcapsular orchiectomy a definitive procedure? Studies of hormone excretion before and after orchiectomy. J. Urol., *89*:236, 1963.

O'Donoghue, E. P. N., Milleman, L. A., Flocks, R. H., Culp, D. A., and Bonney, W. W.: Cryosurgery for carcinoma of prostate. Urology, *5*:308, 1975.

Ohtsuki, Y., Seman, G., Dmochowski, L., Bowen, J. M., and Johnson, D. E.: Brief communication: Virus-like particles in a case of human prostate carcinoma. J. Natl. Cancer Inst., *58*:1493, 1977.

Okabe, T., Ackermann, R., Wirth, M., and Frohmuller, H. G. W.: Cell-mediated cytotoxicity in patients with cancer of the prostate. J. Urol., *122*:628, 1979.

Olsson, C. A., Tannenbaum, M., Babayan, R., O'Brien, M., and De Vere White, R.: Prediction of pelvic lymph node metastases in adenocarcinoma of the prostate. American Urological Association Meeting Program Abstract #237, 1982.

Packer, M. G., Russo, P., and Fair, W. R.: Prophylactic antibiotics and Foley catheter usage in transperineal needle biopsy of the prostate. J. Urol., *131*:687, 1984.

Parfitt, H. E., Smith, J. A., Jr., and Middleton, R. G.: Evaluation and staging of stage A1 adenocarcinoma of the prostate. American Urological Association Meeting Program Abstract #182, 1981.

Parry, W. L., and Finelli, J. F.: Biopsy of prostate. J. Urol., *84*:643, 1960.

Paulson, D. F.: The prognostic role of lymphadenectomy in adenocarcinoma of the prostate. Urol. Clin. North Am., 7:615, 1980.

Paulson, D. F., Rabson, A. S., and Fraley, E. E.: Viral neoplastic transformation of hamster prostate tissue in vitro. Science, *159*:200, 1968.

Paulson, D. F., and the Uro-Oncology Research Group: The impact of current staging procedures in assessing disease extent of prostatic adenocarcinoma. J. Urol., *121*:300, 1979.

Paulson, D. F., Piserchia, P. V., and Gardner, W.: Predictors of lymphatic spread in prostatic adenocarcinoma: Uro-Oncology Research Group Study. J. Urol., *123*:697, 1980.

Paulson, D. F., Walker, R. A., Berry, W. R., Cox, E. B.,

and Hinshaw, W.: Vincristine, bleomycin, methotrexate, 5-fluorouracil, and prednisone in metastatic, hormonally unresponsive prostatic adenocarcinoma. Urology, *17*:443, 1981.

Paulson, D. F., Cline, W. A., Jr., Koefoot, R. B., Jr., Hinshaw, W., Stephani, S., and the Uro-Oncology Research Group: Extended field radiation therapy versus delayed hormonal therapy in node positive prostatic adenocarcinoma. J. Urol., *127*:935, 1982a.

Paulson, D. F., Lin, G. H., Hinshaw, W., Stephani, S., and the Uro-Oncology Research Group: Radical surgery versus radiotherapy for adenocarcinoma of the prostate. J. Urol., *128*:502, 1982b.

Pearson, J. C., Dombrovskis, S., Dreyer, J., and Williams, R. D.: Radioimmunoassay of serum acid phosphatase after prostatic massage. Urology, *21*:37, 1983.

Peeling, W. B., Griffiths, G. J., Evans, K. T., and Roberts, E. E.: Diagnosis and staging of prostatic cancer by transrectal ultrasonography: A preliminary study. Br. J. Urol., *51*:565, 1979.

Perez, C. A., Ackerman, L. V., Silber, I., and Royce, R. K.: Radiation therapy in the treatment of localized carcinoma of the prostate. Preliminary report using 22-MeV photons. Cancer, *34*:1059, 1974.

Perez, C. A., Bauer, W., Garza, R., and Royce, R. K.: Radiation therapy in the definitive treatment of localized carcinoma of the prostate. Cancer, *40*:1425, 1977.

Perez, C. A., Walz, M. D., Zivnuska, F. R., Pilepich, M., Prasad, K., and Bauer, W.: Irradiation of carcinoma of the prostate localized to the pelvis: Analysis of tumor response and prognosis. Int. J. Rad. Oncol. Biol. Phys., *6*:555, 1980.

Pilepich, M. V., Perez, C. A., and Bauer, W.: Prognostic parameters in radiotherapeutic management of localized carcinoma of the prostate. J. Urol., *124*:485, 1980a.

Pilepich, M. V., Perez, C. A., and Prasad, S.: Computed tomography in definitive radiotherapy of prostatic carcinoma. Int. J. Rad. Oncol. Biol. Phys., *6*:923, 1980b.

Pistenma, D. A., Bagshaw, M. A., and Freiha, F. S.: Extended-field radiation therapy for prostatic adenocarcinoma: Status report of a limited prospective trial. *In* Johnson, D. E., and Samuels, M. L. (Eds.): Cancer of the Genitourinary Tract. New York, Raven Press, 1979, pp. 229–247.

Plumpton, K., and Morales, A.: Letter to the Editor: Levodopa in cancer of the prostate. J. Urol., *114*:482, 1975.

Pollen, J. J., Gerber, K., Ashburn, W. L., and Schmidt, J. D.: Nuclear bone imaging in metastatic cancer of the prostate. Cancer, *47*:2585, 1981a.

Pollen, J. J., Gerber, K., Ashburn, W. L., and Schmidt, J. D.: The value of nuclear bone imaging in advanced prostatic cancer. J. Urol., *125*:222, 1981b.

Pontes, J. E., Choe, B., Rose, N. R., and Pierce, J. M., Jr.: Reliability of bone marrow acid phosphatase as a parameter of metastatic prostatic cancer. J. Urol., *122*:178, 1979.

Pontes, J. E., Choe, B. K., Rose, N. R., Ercole, C., and Pierce, J. M., Jr.: Clinical evaluation of immunological methods for detection of serum prostatic acid phosphatase. J. Urol., *126*:363, 1981a.

Pontes, J. E., Rose, N. R., Ercole, C., and Pierce, J. M., Jr.: Immunofluorescence for prostatic acid phosphatase: Clinical applications. J. Urol., *126*:187, 1981b.

Pool, T. L., and Thompson, G. J.: Conservative treatment of carcinoma of the prostate. JAMA, *160*:833, 1956.

Prout, G. R., Jr., Irwin, R. J., Jr., Kliman, B., Daly, J. J., MacLaughlin, R. A., and Griffin, P. P.: Prostatic cancer and SCH-13521: II. Histological alterations and the pituitary gonadal axis. J. Urol., *113*:834, 1975.

Prout, G. R., Jr., Kliman, B., Daly, J. J., MacLaughlin, R. A., Griffin, P. P., and Young, H. H., II: Endocrine changes after diethylstilbestrol therapy. Effects on prostatic neoplasm and pituitary-gonadal axis. Urology, *7*:148, 1976.

Prout, G. R., Jr., Heaney, J. A., Griffin, P. P., Daly, J. J., and Shipley, W. U.: Nodal involvement as a prognostic indicator in patients with prostatic carcinoma. J. Urol., *124*:226, 1980.

Ray, G. R., Cassady, R., and Bagshaw, M. A.: Definitive radiation therapy of carcinoma of the prostate: A report on 15 years of experience. Radiology, *106*:407, 1973.

Ray, G. R., Cassady, J. R., and Bagshaw, M. A.: External-beam megavoltage radiation therapy in the treatment of post-radical prostatectomy residual or recurrent tumors: Preliminary results. J. Urol., *114*:98, 1975.

Redman, H. C.: Computed tomography of the pelvis. Radiol. Clin. North Am., *15*:441, 1977.

Rees, M., Ashby, E. C., Pocock, R. D., and Dowding, C. H.: Povidone-iodine antisepsis for transrectal prostatic biopsy. Br. Med. J., *281*:650, 1980.

Reiner, W. G., Scott, W. W., Eggleston, J. C., and Walsh, P. C.: Long-term survival after hormonal therapy for stage D prostatic cancer. J. Urol., *122*:183, 1979.

Resnick, M. I., Willard, J. W., and Boyce, W. H.: Transrectal ultrasonography in the evaluation of patients with prostatic carcinoma. J. Urol., *124*:482, 1980.

Reynolds, R. D., Greenberg, B. R., Martin, N. D., Lucas, R. N., Gaffney, C. N., and Hawn, L.: Usefulness of bone marrow serum acid phosphatase in staging carcinoma of the prostate. Cancer, *32*:181, 1973.

Rhamy, R. K., Wilson, S. K., and Caldwell, W. L.: Biopsy-proved tumor following definitive irradiation for resectable carcinoma of the prostate. J. Urol., *107*:627, 1972.

Rhamy, R. K., Buchanan, R. D., and Spalding, M. J.: Intraductal carcinoma of the prostate gland. J. Urol., *109*:457, 1973.

Robinson, M. R. G.: Aminoglutethimide: Medical adrenalectomy in the management of carcinoma of the prostate. A review after 6 years. Br. J. Urol., *52*:328, 1980.

Robinson, M. R. G., and Thomas, B. S.: Effect of hormonal therapy on plasma testosterone levels in prostatic carcinoma. Br. Med. J., *4*:391, 1971.

Robinson, M. R. G., Rigby, C. C., Pugh, R. C. B., and Dumonde, D: C.: Prostate carcinoma: Intratumor BCG immunotherapy. Natl. Cancer Inst. Monogr., *49*:351, 1976.

Robinson, M. R. G., Rigby, C. C., Pugh, R. C. B., and Dumonde, D. C.: Adjuvant immunotherapy with BCG in carcinoma of the prostate. Br. J. Urol., *49*:221, 1977.

Rodin, A. E., Larson, D. L., and Roberts, D. K.: Nature of the perineural space invaded by prostatic carcinoma. Cancer, *20*:1772, 1967.

Rohlf, P. L., and Flocks, R. H.: Stilphosterol therapy in 100 cases of prostatic carcinoma. J. Iowa Med. Soc., *59*:1096, 1969.

Rosenberg, S. E.: Is carcinoma of the prostate less serious in older men? J. Am. Geriatr. Soc., *13*:791, 1965.

Ross, G., Jr., Borkon, W. D., Landry, L. J., Edwards, M. F., Weinstein, S. H., and Abadir, R.: Preliminary observations on the results of combined ¹²⁵iodine seed implantation and external irradiation for carcinoma of the prostate. J. Urol., *127*:699, 1982.

Ross, R. K., Deapen, D. M., Casagrande, J. T., Paganini-Hill, A., and Henderson, B. E.: A cohort study of mortality from cancer of the prostate in Catholic priests. Br. J. Cancer, *43*:233, 1981.

Rothauge, C. F.: BCG adjuvant therapy in stage D prostatic carcinoma. Urology, *21*:211, 1983.

Rotkin, I. D.: Studies in the epidemiology of prostatic cancer: Expanded sampling. Cancer Treat. Rep., *61*:173, 1977.

Rowland, C. G., Bullimore, J. A., Smith, P. J. B., and Roberts, J. B. M.: Half-body irradiation in the treatment of metastatic prostatic carcinoma. Br. J. Urol., *53*:628, 1981.

Roy, A. V., Brower, M. E., and Hayden, J. E.: Sodium thymolphthalein monophosphate: A new acid phosphatase substrate with greater specificity for the prostatic enzyme in serum. Clin. Chem., *17*:1093, 1971.

Sadlowski, R. W., Donohue, D. J., Richman, A. V., Sharpe, J. R., and Finney, R. P.: Accuracy of frozen section diagnosis in pelvic lymph node staging biopsies for adenocarcinoma of the prostate. J. Urol., *129*:324, 1983.

Sadoughi, N., Razvi, M., Bush, I., Ablin, R., and Guinan, P.: Cancer of prostate. Relief of bone pain with levodopa. Urology, *4*:107, 1974.

Sagalowsky, A. I., Milam, H., Reveley, L. R., and Silva, F. G.: Prediction of lymphatic metastases by Gleason histologic grading in prostatic cancer. J. Urol., *128*:951, 1982.

Saltzstein, S. L., and McLaughlin, A. P.: Clinicopathologic features of unsuspected regional lymph node metastases in prostatic adenocarcinoma. Cancer, *40*:1212, 1977.

Sanford, E. J., Drago, J. R., Rohner, T. J., Jr., Santen, R., and Lipton, A.: Aminoglutethimide medical adrenalectomy for advanced prostatic carcinoma. J. Urol., *115*:170, 1976.

Sanford, E. J., Geder, L., Laychock, A., Rohner, T. J., Jr., and Rapp, F.: Evidence for the association of cytomegalovirus with carcinoma of the prostate. J. Urol., *118*:789, 1977.

Sawczuk, I. S., De Vere White, R., Gold, R. P., and Olsson, C. A.: Sensitivity of computed tomography in evaluation of pelvic lymph node metastases from carcinoma of bladder and prostate. Urology, *21*:81, 1983.

Scardino, P. T., and Lehane, D.: Intermittent arterial infusion chemotherapy for advanced, hormonally resistant, radiorecurrent carcinoma of the prostate. American Urological Association Meeting Program Abstract #222, 1982.

Scardino, P. T., Guerriero, W. G., and Carlton, C. E., Jr.: Surgical staging and combined therapy with radioactive gold grain implantation and external irradiation. *In* Johnson, D. E., and Boileau, M. A. (Eds.): Genitourinary Tumors: Fundamental Principles and Surgical Techniques. New York, Grune & Stratton, 1982, pp. 75–90.

Schaffer, D. L., and Pendergrass, H. P.: Comparison of enzyme, clinical, radiographic and radionuclide methods of detecting bone metastases from carcinoma of the prostate. Radiology, *121*:431, 1976.

Schellhammer, P. F., Ladaga, L. E., and El-Mahdi, A.: Histological characteristics of prostatic biopsies after ^{125}iodine implantation. J. Urol., *123*:700, 1980.

Schellhammer, P. F., Warden, S. S., Wright, G. L., and Sieg, S.: Bone marrow acid phosphatase by counterimmune electrophoresis: Pre-treatment and post-treatment correlations. J. Urol., *127*:66, 1982.

Schenken, J. R., Burns, E. L., and Kahle, P. J.: The effect of diethylstilbestrol and diethylstilbestrol-disproprinate on carcinoma of the prostate gland. II. Cytological changes following treatment. J. Urol., *48*:99, 1942.

Schmidt, J. D.: Cryosurgical prostatectomy. Cancer, *32*:1141, 1973.

Schmidt, J. D. Johnson, D. E., Scott, W. W., Gibbons, R. P., Prout, G. R., Murphy, G. P., and the National Prostatic Cancer Project: Chemotherapy of advanced prostatic cancer. Urology, *7*:602, 1976.

Schmidt, J. D., Scott, W. W., Gibbons, R. P., Johnson, D. E., Prout, G. R., Loening, S. A., Soloway, M. S., Chu, T. M., Gaeta, J. F., Slack, N. H., Saroff, J., and Murphy, G. P.: Comparison of procarbazine, imidazole-carboxamide and cyclophosphamide in relapsing patients with advanced carcinoma of the prostate. J. Urol., *121*:185, 1979.

Schmidt, J. D., McLaughlin, A. P., III, Saltzstein, S. L., and Garcia-Reyes, R.: Risk factors for the development of distant metastases in patients undergoing pelvic lymphadenectomy for prostatic cancer. Am. J. Surg., *144*:131, 1982.

Schroeder, F. H., and Belt, E.: Carcinoma of the prostate: A study of 213 patients with stage C tumors treated by total perineal prostatectomy. J. Urol., *114*:257, 1975.

Schuman, L. M., Mandel, J., Blackard, C., Bauer, H., Scarlett, J., and McHugh, R.: Epidemiologic study of prostatic cancer: Preliminary report. Cancer Treat. Rep., *61*:181, 1977.

Scott, W. W., and Boyd, H. L.: Combined hormone control therapy and radical prostatectomy in the treatment of selected cases of advanced carcinoma of the prostate: A retrospective study based upon 25 years of experience. J. Urol., *101*:86, 1969.

Scott, W. W., and Schirmer, H. K. A.: A new oral progestational steroid effective in treating prostatic cancer. Trans. Am. Assoc. Genitourin. Surg., *58*:54, 1966.

Scott, W. W., Gibbons, R. P., Johnson, D. E., Prout, G. R., Schmidt, J. D., Saroff, J., and Murphy, G. P.: The continued evaluation of the effects of chemotherapy in patients with advanced carcinoma of the prostate. J. Urol., *116*:211, 1976.

Sekine, H., Oka, K., and Takehara, Y.: Transrectal longitudinal ultrasonotomography of the prostate by electronic linear scanning. J. Urol., *127*:62, 1982.

Senge, T., Hulshoff, T., Tunn, V., Schenck, B., and Neumann, F.: Testosterone Konzentration in Serum nach Subcapsulär Orchiectomie. Urologe, *17*:382, 1978.

Sewell, R. A., Braren, V., Wilson, S. K., and Rhamy, R. K.: Extended biopsy followup after full course radiation for resectable prostatic carcinoma. J. Urol., *113*:371, 1975.

Sharifi, R., Shaw, M., Ray, V., Rhee, H., Nagubadi, S., and Guinan, P.: Evaluation of cytologic techniques for diagnosis of prostate cancer. Urology, *21*:417, 1983.

Sharpe, J. R., Sadlowski, R. W., Finney, R. P., Branch, W. T., and Hanna, J. E.: Urinary tract infection after transrectal needle biopsy of the prostate. J. Urol., *127*:255, 1982.

Shearer, R. J., Hendry, W. F., Sommerville, I. F., and Ferguson, J. D.: Plasma testosterone: An accurate monitor of hormone treatment in prostatic cancer. Br. J. Urol., *45*:668, 1973.

Shipley, W. U., Kopelson, G., Novack, D. H., Ling, C. C., Dretler, S. P., and Prout, G. R., Jr.: Preoperative irradiation, lymphadenectomy and ^{125}iodine implant for patients with localized prostatic carcinoma: A correlation of implant dosimetry with clinical results. J. Urol., *124*:639, 1980.

Silverberg, G. D.: Hypophysectomy in the treatment of disseminated prostate carcinoma. Cancer, *39*:1727, 1977.

Silverberg, E., and Lubera, J. A.: A review of American Cancer Society estimates of cancer cases and deaths. CA, *33*:2, 1983.

Slack, N. H., Mittelman, A., Brady, M. F., Murphy, G. P., and Investigators in the National Prostatic Cancer

Project: The importance of the stable category for chemotherapy treatment patients with advanced and relapsing prostate cancer. Cancer, 46:2393, 1980.

Smalley, R. V., Bartolucci, A. A., Hemstreet, G., and Hester, M.: A phase II evaluation of a 3-drug combination of cyclophosphamide, doxorubicin and 5-fluorouracil and of 5-fluorouracil in patients with advanced bladder carcinoma or stage D prostatic carcinoma. J. Urol., 125:191, 1981.

Smith, J. A., Jr., and Middleton, R. G.: Pelvic lymph node metastasis from prostatic cancer: Influence of tumor grade and stage. American Urological Association Program Abstract #238, 1982.

Smith, J. A., Jr.: Clinical effects of a new GnRh analog in prostate cancer. American Urological Association Meeting Program Abstract #426, 1983.

Smith, J. A., Jr., Harris, T. H., and Middleton, R. G.: Clinical effects of external irradiation on patients with lymph node metastases from prostatic cancer. American Urological Association Meeting Program Abstract #301, 1983.

Smith, R. B., Walsh, P. C., and Goodwin, E. W.: Cyproterone acetate in the treatment of advanced carcinoma of the prostate. J. Urol., 110:106, 1973.

Soanes, W. A., Ablin, R. J., and Gonder, M. J.: Remission of metastatic lesions following cryosurgery in prostate cancer. J. Urol., 104:154, 1970.

Sogani, P. C., and Whitmore, W. F., Jr.: Experience with flutamide in previously untreated patients with advanced prostatic cancer. J. Urol., 122:640, 1979.

Sogani, P. C., Ray, B., and Whitmore, W. F., Jr.: Advanced prostatic carcinoma: Flutamide therapy after conventional endocrine treatment. Urology, 6:164, 1975.

Sogani, P. C., Watson, R. C., and Whitmore, W. F., Jr.: Lymphocele after pelvic lymphadenectomy for urologic cancer. Urology, 17:39, 1981.

Spaulding, J. T., and Whitmore, W. F., Jr.: Extended total excision of prostatic adenocarcinoma. J. Urol., 120:188, 1978.

Spellman, M. C., Castellino, R. A., Ray, G. R., Pistenma, D. A., and Bagshaw, M. A.: An evaluation of lymphography in localized carcinoma of the prostate. Radiology, 125:637, 1977.

Stamey, T. A.: Cancer of the prostate. An analysis of some important contributions and dilemmas. Monogr. Urol., 3:67, 1982.

Staszewski, J., and Haenszel, W.: Cancer mortality among the Polish-born in the United States. J. Natl. Cancer Inst., 35:291, 1965.

Steele, R., Lees, R. E. M., Kraus, A. S., and Rao, C.: Sexual factors in the epidemiology of cancer of the prostate. J. Chronic Dis., 24:29, 1971.

Stehlin, J.: Holistic oncology and nude mouse. JAMA, 241:1321, 1979.

Stoilar, B., and Albert, D. J.: SCH-13521 in the treatment of advanced carcinoma of the prostate. J. Urol., 111:803, 1974.

Stone, A. R., Merrick, M. V., and Chisholm, G. D.: Prostatic lymphoscintigraphy. Br. J. Urol., 51:556, 1979.

Stone, A. R., Hargreave, T. B., and Chisholm, G. D.: The diagnosis of oestrogen escape and the role of secondary orchiectomy in prostatic cancer. Br. J. Urol., 52:535, 1980.

Straus, M. J., Fleit, J. P., and Engelking, C.: Treatment of advanced prostate cancer with cyclophosphamide, doxorubicin, and methotrexate. Cancer Treat. Rep., 66:1797, 1982.

Suarez, A. J., Lamm, D. L., Radwin, H. M., Sarosdy, M., Clark, G., and Osborne, C. K.: Androgen priming and cytotoxic chemotherapy in advanced prostatic cancer. Cancer Chemother. Pharmacol., 8:261, 1982.

Susan, L. P., Roth, R. B., and Adkins, W. C.: Regression of prostatic cancer metastasis by high doses of diethylstilbestrol diphosphate. Urology, 7:598, 1976.

Tannenbaum, M.: Atypical epithelial hyperplasia or carcinoma of prostate gland: The surgical pathologist at an impasse? Urology, 4:758, 1974.

Tansey, L. A., Shanberg, A. M., Syed, A. M., and Puthawala, A.: Treatment of prostatic carcinoma by pelvic lymphadenectomy, temporary iridium-192 implant, and external irradiation. Urology, 21:594, 1983.

Tavares, A. S., Costa, J., and Maia, J. C.: Correlation between ploidy and prognosis in prostatic carcinoma. J. Urol., 109:676, 1973.

Taylor, W. J.: Radiation oncology: Cancer of the prostate. Cancer, 39:856, 1977.

Thomas, R., Lewis, R. W., Sarma, D. P., Coker, G. B., Rao, M. K., and Roberts, J. A.: Aid to accurate clinical staging—histopathologic grading in prostatic cancer. J. Urol., 128:726, 1982.

Thrall, J. H., Ghaed, N., Geslien, G. E., Pinsky, S. M., and Johnson, M. C.: Pitfalls in Tc^{99m} polyphosphate skeletal imaging. Am. J. Roentgenol. Radium Ther. Nucl. Med., 121:739, 1974.

Tjaden, H. B., Culp, D. A., and Flocks, R. H.: Clinical adenocarcinoma of the prostate in patients under 50 years of age. J. Urol., 93:618, 1965.

Tolis, G., Ackman, D., Stellos, A., Mehta, A., Labrie, F., Fazekas, A. T. A., Comaru-Schally, A. M., and Schally, A. V.: Tumor growth inhibition in patients with prostatic carcinoma treated with luteinizing hormone-releasing hormone agonists. Proc. Natl. Acad. Sci. USA, 79:1658, 1982.

Tomic, R., Bergman, B., and Damber, J.-E.: Testicular endocrine function after withdrawal of oestrogen treatment in patients with carcinoma of the prostate. Br. J. Urol., 55:42, 1983.

Tomlinson, R. L., Currie, D. P., and Boyce, W. H.: Radical prostatectomy: Palliation for stage C carcinoma of the prostate. J. Urol., 117:85, 1977.

Torti, F. M., and Carter, S. K.: The chemotherapy of prostatic adenocarcinoma. Ann. Intern. Med., 92:681, 1980.

Trachtenberg, J., and Walsh, P. C.: Correlation of prostatic nuclear androgen receptor content with duration of response and survival following hormonal therapy in advanced prostatic cancer. J. Urol., 127:466, 1982.

Turner, R. D., and Belt, E.: A study of 229 consecutive cases of total perineal prostatectomy for cancer of the prostate. J. Urol., 77:62, 1957.

Tvetor, K. J., Attramadal, A., Hannestad, R., and Otnes, B.: A morphological study of the effect of cyproterone acetate on human prostatic carcinoma. Scand. J. Urol. Nephrol., 13:237, 1979.

Utz, D. C., and Farrow, G. M.: Pathologic differentiation and prognosis of prostatic carcinoma. JAMA, 209:1701, 1969.

Valk, W. L., and Owens, R. H.: Endocrine inhibition as related to carcinoma of the prostate. J. Urol., 72:516, 1954.

Van Cangh, P. J., Opsomer, R., and DeNayer, P. H.: Serum prostatic acid phosphatase determination in prostatic diseases: A critical comparison of an enzymatic and a radioimmunologic assay. J. Urol., 128:1212, 1982.

van der Werf-Messing, B., Sourek-Zikova, V., and Blonk,

D. I.: Localized advanced carcinoma of the prostate: Radiation therapy versus hormonal therapy. Int. J. Rad. Oncol. Biol. Phys., *1*:1043, 1976.

Varenhorst, E., Wallentin, L., and Risberg, B.: Clotting predisposition in carcinoma of the prostate. (Letter.) J. Urol., *126*:419, 1981.

Varkarakis, M. J., Murphy, G. P., Nelson, C. M. K., Chehval, M., Moore, R. H., and Flocks, R. H.: Lymph node involvement in prostatic carcinoma. Urol. Clin. North Am., *2*:197, 1975.

Venable, D. D., Hastings, D., and Misra, R. P.: Unusual metastatic patterns of prostate adenocarcinoma. J. Urol., *130*:980, 1983.

Vermeulen, A., Schelfhout, W., and De Sy, W.: Plasma androgen levels after subcapsular orchiectomy or estrogen treatment for prostatic carcinoma. Prostate, *3*:115, 1982.

Vest, S. A., and Frazier, T. H.: Survival following castration for prostatic cancer. J. Urol., *56*:97, 1946.

Veterans Administration Cooperative Urological Research Group: Treatment and survival of patients with cancer of the prostate. Surg. Gynecol. Obstet., *124*:1011, 1967.

Vihko, P., and Kontturi, M.: Transient high serum prostate-specific acid phosphatase measured by radioimmunoassay in prostatic infarction. Scand. J. Urol. Nephrol., *15*:213, 1981.

Vihko, P., Lukkarinen, O., Kontturi, M., and Vihko, R.: Effectiveness of radioimmunoassay of human prostate-specific acid phosphatase in the diagnosis and follow-up of therapy in prostatic carcinoma. Cancer Res., *41*:1180, 1981.

Vihko, P., Kontturi, M., Lukkarinen, O., and Vihko, R.: Radioimmunoassayable prostate-specific acid phosphatase in peripheral and bone marrow sera compared in diagnosis of prostatic cancer patients. J. Urol., *128*:739, 1982a.

Vihko, P., Jokipalo, A., Tenhunen, R., Alfthan, O., and Oravisto, K. J.: Comparison of radioimmunological and conventional acid phosphatase assays in the serum of prostatic cancer patients. Scand. J. Urol. Nephrol., *16*:105, 1982b.

Von Eschenbach, A. C., and Zornoza, J.: Fine-needle percutaneous biopsy: A useful evaluation of lymph node metastasis from prostate cancer. Urology, *20*:589, 1982.

Wagner, R. K.: Extracellular and intracellular steroid binding proteins: Properties, discrimination, assay and clinical application. Acta Endocrinol., 88[Suppl.]:3, 1978.

Wajsman, Z., Gamarra, M., Park, J. J., Beckley, S., and Pontes, J. E.: Transabdominal fine needle aspiration of retroperitoneal lymph nodes in staging of genitourinary tract cancer (correlation with lymphography and lymph node dissection findings). J. Urol., *128*:1238, 1982.

Wallace, D. M., Chisholm, G. D., and Hendry, W. F.: TNM classification for urological tumors (UICC)–1974. Br. J. Urol., *47*:1, 1975.

Walsh, P. C.: Physiologic basis for hormonal therapy in carcinoma of the prostate. Urol. Clin. North Am., *2*:125, 1975.

Walsh, P. C., and Donker, P. J.: Impotence following radical prostatectomy: Insight into etiology and prevention. J. Urol., *128*:492, 1982.

Walsh, P. C., and Jewett, H. J.: Radical surgery for prostatic cancer. Cancer, *45*:1906, 1980.

Walsh, P. C., and Siiteri, P. K.: Suppression of plasma androgens by spironolactone in castrated men with carcinoma of the prostate. J. Urol., *114*:254, 1975.

Walsh, P. C., and Wilson, J. D.: The induction of prostatic

hypertrophy in the dog with androstanediol. J. Clin. Invest., *57*:1093, 1976.

Walsh, P. C., Lepor, H., and Eggleston, J. C.: Radical prostatectomy with preservation of sexual function: Anatomical and pathological considerations. Prostate, *4*:473, 1983.

Warner, B. A., Santen, R. J., Demers, L. M., and Max, D. T.: [D-Leu[6] Des-Gly-NH$_2$[10], Pro-ethylamide[9]]—gonadotropin releasing hormone (Leuprolide): A "medical castration" for the treatment of prostatic carcinoma. Clin. Res., *29*:666A, 1981.

Watson, R. A., and Tang, D. B.: The predictive value of prostatic acid phosphatase as a screening test for prostatic cancer. N. Engl. J. Med., *303*:497, 1980.

Wein, A. J., and Murphy, J. J.: Experience in the treatment of prostatic carcinoma with cyproterone acetate. J. Urol., *109*:68, 1973.

Weinerman, P. M., Arger, P. H., Coleman, B. G., Pollack, H. M., Banner, M. P., and Wein, A. J.: Pelvic and bladder adenopathy from bladder and prostate carcinoma: Detection by rapid sequence computed tomography. Am. J. Radiol., *140*:95, 1983.

Wheeler, T. M., and Scardino, P. T.: Detailed pathologic review of prostate biopsy following irradiation for carcinoma of the prostate. American Urological Association Meeting Program Abstract #298, 1983.

Whitesel, J. A., Donohue, R. E., Mani, J. H., Fauver, H. E., Angspurger, R. R., Biber, R. J., Scanavino, D. J., and Pfister, R. R.: Acid phosphatase—its influence on pelvic lymph node dissection. J. Urol., *131*:70, 1984.

Whitmore, W. F., Jr.: Hormone therapy in prostatic cancer. Am. J. Med., *21*:697, 1956.

Whitmore, W. F., Jr.: The natural history of prostatic cancer. Cancer, *32*:1104, 1973.

Whitmore, W. F., Jr.: Interstitial radiation therapy for carcinoma of the prostate. Prostate, *1*:157, 1980.

Whitmore, W. F., and Gittes, R. F.: Studies on prostate and testis as immunologically privileged sites. Cancer Treat. Rep., *61*:217, 1977.

Whitmore, W. F., Jr., Hilaris, B., and Grabstald, H.: Retropubic implantation of iodine 125 in the treatment of prostatic cancer. J. Urol., *108*:918, 1972.

Whitmore, W. F., Blute, R. D., Kaplan, W. D., and Gittes, R. F.: Radiocolloid scintigraphic mapping of the lymphatic drainage of the prostate. J. Urol., *124*:62, 1980.

Willems, J. S., and Lowhagen, T.: Transrectal fine-needle aspiration biopsy for cytologic diagnosis and grading of prostatic carcinoma. Prostate, *2*:381, 1981.

Willis, R. A.: Secondary tumours of bones. *In*: The Spread of Tumours in the Human Body. 3rd ed. London, Butterworth & Co., 1973, pp. 229–250.

Winkelstein, W., Jr., and Ernster, V. L.: Epidemiology and etiology. *In* Murphy, G. P. (Ed.): Prostatic Cancer. Littleton, MA, P.S.G. Publishing Company, Inc., 1979, pp. 1–17.

Winkelstein, W., Jr., Sacks, S. T., Ernster, V. L., and Selvin, S.: Correlations of incidence rates for selected cancers in the nine areas of the Third National Cancer Survey. Am. J. Epidemiol., *105*:407, 1977.

Winter, C. C.: The problem of rectal involvement by prostatic cancer. Surg. Gynecol. Obstet., *105*:136, 1957.

Wolfe, J. H. N., and Lloyd-Davies, R. W.: The management of transitional cell carcinoma in the prostate. Br. J. Urol., *53*:253, 1981.

Woolf, C. M.: An investigation of the familial aspects of carcinoma of the prostate. Cancer, *13*:739, 1960.

Worgul, T. J., Santen, R. J., Samojlik, E., Veldhuis, J. D., Lipton, A., Harvey, H. A., Drago, J. R., and Rohner, T. J.: Clinical and biochemical effect of aminoglutethimide in the treatment of advanced prostatic cancer. J. Urol., *129*:51, 1983.

Wynder, E. L., Mabuchi, K., and Whitmore, W. F., Jr.: Epidemiology of cancer of the prostate. Cancer, *28*:344, 1971.

Yagoda, A.: Non-hormonal cytotoxic agents in the treatment of prostatic adenocarcinoma. Cancer, *32*:1131, 1973.

Yagoda, A., Watson, R. C., Natale, R. B., Barzell, W., Sogani, P., Grabstald, H., and Whitmore, W. F.: A critical analysis of response criteria in patients with prostatic cancer treated with cis-diaminedichloride platinum II. Cancer, *44*:1553, 1979.

Yam, L. T., Janckila, A. J., Li, C.-Y., and Lam, W. K. W.: The presence of "prostatic" acid phosphatase in human neutrophils. Invest. Urol., *19*:34, 1981.

Yanihara, T., and Troen, P.: Studies of the human testis. III. Effect of estrogen on testosterone formation in human testis in vitro. J. Clin. Endocrinol. Metab., *34*:968, 1972.

Yatani, R., Chigusa, I., Akazaki, K., Stemmerman, G. N., Welsh, R. A., and Correa, P.: Geographic pathology of latent prostatic carcinoma. Int. J. Cancer, *29*:611, 1982.

Young, B. W., and Lagios, M. D.: Endometrial (papillary) carcinoma of the prostatic utricle—response to orchiectomy: A case report. Cancer, *32*:1293, 1973.

Young, H. H.: The early diagnosis and radical cure of carcinoma of the prostate. Being a study of 40 cases and presentation of a radical operation which was carried out in 4 cases. Bull. Johns Hopkins Hosp., *16*:315, 1905.

Young, H. H., II, and Kent, J. R.: Plasma testosterone levels in patients with prostatic carcinoma before and after treatment. J. Urol., *99*:788, 1968.

Young, J. D., Jr., Suresh, M. S., and Bashirelahi, N.: The role of estrogen, androgen and progestogen receptors in the management of carcinoma of the prostate. Trans. Am. Assoc. Genitourin. Surg., *71*:23, 1979.

Young, J. L., Jr., Percy, C. L., Asire, A. J., et al.: Cancer incidence and mortality in the United States, 1973–77. Natl. Cancer Inst. Monogr., *57*:1, 1981.

Zaloudek, C., Williams, J. W., and Kempson, R. L.: "Endometrial" adenocarcinoma of the prostate: A distinctive tumor of probable prostatic duct origin. Cancer, *37*:2255, 1976.

Zamora, S., Bhatti, R. A., Ablin, R. J., Rao, R., Baumgartner, G., and Guinan, P. D.: In vitro stimulation of tumor-associated immunity in prostatic cancer by levamisole. Cell. Mol. Biol., *25*:57, 1979.

Zincke, H., Campbell, J. T., Utz, D. C., Farrow, G. M., and Anderson, M. J.: Confidence in the negative transrectal needle biopsy. Surg. Gynecol. Obstet., *136*:78, 1973.

Zincke, H., Fleming, T. R., Furlow, W. L., Myers, R. P., and Utz, D. C.: Radical retropubic prostatectomy and pelvic lymphadenectomy for high-stage cancer of the prostate. Cancer, *47*:1901, 1981.

Zincke, H., Utz, D. C., Myers, R. P., Farrow, G. M., Patterson, D. E., and Furlow, W. L.: Bilateral pelvic lymphadenectomy and radical retropubic prostatectomy for adenocarcinoma of prostate with regional lymph node involvement. Urology, *19*:238, 1982.

Zumoff, B., Levin, J., Strain, G. W., Rosenfeld, R. S., O'Connor, J., Freed, S. Z., Kream, J., Whitmore, W. S., Fukushima, D. K., and Hellman, L.: Abnormal levels of plasma hormones in men with prostate cancer: Evidence toward a "two-disease" theory. Prostate, *3*:579, 1982.

CHAPTER 33

Neoplasms of the Testis

MICHAEL J. MORSE, M.D.
WILLET F. WHITMORE, M.D.

Although rare, testis tumors have evoked widespread interest among tumor biologists, pathologists, and clinicians, for a variety of reasons. Not least of these is the dramatic improvement in survival witnessed over the last decade for those patients suffering from advanced testicular cancer. Integrated programs combining effective multidrug regimens, refined diagnostic techniques, and improved surgical and radiotherapeutic skills have been credited with the marked reduction in patient mortality from nearly 50 per cent prior to 1970 to approximately 10 per cent or less today. Testis tumors are the most common solid tumor in young adult males and have now become the most curable cancer, overall, in all age groups. Despite these astonishingly favorable developments, clinical researchers have begun to explore the possibility of reducing the therapeutic burden in selected subsets of patients. These potential changes in treatment philosophy, while somewhat controversial, are based upon sound observations relative to the natural history of this disease and upon extrapolations from clinical trials.

Several characteristics in the natural behavior of testis tumors favor successful therapeutic manipulation. These features include: (1) origin from germ cells, which are highly sensitive to irradiation and a wide variety of chemotherapeutic agents; (2) capability for differentiation, spontaneous or induced, into a histologically benign counterpart; (3) predictable and systematic pattern of spread from the primary tumor to metastatic sites; (4) rapid rate of growth; (5) frequent production of biologic marker substances; and (6) occurrence in otherwise healthy young males capable of tolerating the rigors of multimodal therapy.

Experimental results in the histopathology, immunocytochemistry, and cytogenetics of tumor models (experimental animal and human) demonstrate parallels between ontogeny (normal cell cycle kinetics) and oncogenesis (malregulated differentiation). Based on current hypotheses it can be speculated that uncommitted primordial cells that fail to follow normal genetic regulation do so because of specifically timed internal or external influences. The expression of tumor-indexing marker substances, cell surface antigens, and morphologic characteristics represent phenotypic manifestations of deviant primordial stem cells.

This chapter attempts a review and summation of the tremendous and ever increasing volume of clinical information on testicular neoplasms, no doubt subject to the prejudices of the authors. The text is divided into sections on (1) classification and histogenesis, (2) adult germ cell tumors, and (3) non–germ cell tumors.

CLASSIFICATION AND HISTOGENESIS

Histologic Classification of Testicular Tumors

The normal testis is composed of seminiferous tubules, arranged in 200 to 300 lobules, and collecting tubuli recti arranged in a loose stromal network encased by a dense fibrous coat, the tunica albuginea. The tubuli recti coalesce in the mediastinum of the testis to form the rete testis, which merges into the efferent ductules, the latter traversing the testis proper to enter the globus major of the epididymis. The seminiferous tubules contain two cell populations—the sustentacular cells of Sertoli and the germ cells. The "supporting" Sertoli cells line the basement membrane of the seminiferous tubules and envelop the germ cells as they pass through various stages of spermatogenesis. Within the testicular interstitium the androgen-producing (interstitial) cells of Leydig are arranged in clusters. Primary neoplasms of the testis may arise from any cell component and are conveniently divided into "germinal" and "nongerminal" tumors. Germinal tumors account for 90 to 95 per cent and nongerminal for 5 to 10 per cent of all primary testicular neoplasms. The latter category includes neoplasms arising from gonadal stroma, mesenchymal structures, and ducts, in addition to other miscellaneous lesions. While metastasis to the testis is uncommon, testis involvement by neoplasms of the reticuloendothelial system is by no means rare.

Histologic classifications, grading systems, and staging evaluations have traditionally provided a major clinical basis for therapeutic decisions. Morphologic descriptions provide standardized means of identifying a given tumor and, in conjunction with past clinical experience, of estimating its potential for local growth or distant metastases, or both. Clinical and surgical staging indicates the extent to which a given tumor's potential has been realized at the time of evaluation. Although histologic and staging systems play important roles in treatment selection, grading schema have not been uniformly employed. Freidman and Moore (1946) provided one of the first generally accepted histologic classifications; this system, later modified by Dixon and Moore (1952) and Mostofi (1973), has become the North American standard classification. Teilum (1959) suggested the incorporation of the endodermal sinus tumor (infantile embryonal type) in the germ cell category (Pierce, 1975). Mostofi and Price (1973) subdivided teratomas into mature and immature varieties and coined the term "polyembryoma." The British Testicular Tumour Panel (Pugh and Cameron, 1976) formalized the English version of testicular tumor nomenclature. The World Health Organization (Mostofi and Sobin, 1977) modified the earlier system of Mostofi and Price (1973) by including the term "yolk sac" and by subdividing the embryonal carcinoma with teratoma category. The commonly used histologic classifications are summarized and compared in Tables 33–1 and 33–2.

Tumorigenesis in Humans

Somatic (non–germ cell) neoplasms display widespread heterogeneity in terms of histologic pattern, growth potential, and metastatic behav-

TABLE 33–1. HISTOLOGIC CLASSIFICATION OF TESTICULAR NEOPLASMS

I. Primary neoplasms
  A. Germinal neoplasms (demonstrating one or more of the following components)
    1. Seminoma
      a. Classic (typical) seminoma
      b. Anaplastic seminoma
      c. Spermatocytic seminoma
    2. Embryonal carcinoma
    3. Teratoma (with or without malignant transformation)
      a. Mature
      b. Immature
    4. Choriocarcinoma
    5. Yolk sac tumor (endodermal sinus tumor; embryonal adenocarcinoma of the prepubertal testis)
  B. Nongerminal neoplasms
    1. Specialized gonadal stromal neoplasms
      a. Leydig cell tumor
      b. Other gonadal stromal tumor
    2. Gonadoblastoma
    3. Miscellaneous neoplasms
      a. Adenocarcinoma of the rete testis
      b. Mesenchymal neoplasms
      c. Carcinoid
      d. Adrenal rest "tumor"
II. Secondary neoplasms
  A. Reticuloendothelial neoplasms
  B. Metastases
III. Paratesticular neoplasms
  A. Adenomatoid
  B. Cystadenoma of epididymis
  C. Mesenchymal neoplasms
  D. Mesothelioma
  E. Metastases

ior but resemble their cellular origins both morphologically and functionally. Germ cell tumors are unique in that they represent a diverse group of tumors with or without features resembling the mature spermatogonia. Primitive germ cells and their malignant counterparts (embryonal carcinoma cells) retain the ability to differentiate into more mature forms, presumably under the influence of predisposing genetic and alterable environmental factors. Anaplastic embryonal carcinoma cells closely resemble those of the early-stage embryo (morula). Trophoblastic and yolk sac elements (extraembryonic tissues) and teratomas (intraembryonic tissues) are representative of more advanced stages of embryogenesis. The more mature extraembryonic forms appear morphologically less anaplastic and often produce oncofetal substances such as human chorionic gonadotropin and alpha-fetoprotein (see further on).

Although all somatic cells may possess similar genetic machinery (DNA content), it appears that certain developmental capabilities are forfeited during early embryogenesis. It has

TABLE 33–2. GERM CELL NOMENCLATURE

Friedman and Moore (1946)	Mostofi and Price (1973)	British (Pugh, 1976)	Mostofi and Sobin (1977)
Seminoma	Seminoma ("typical") Spermatocytic Anaplastic	Seminoma Spermatocytic —	Seminoma Spermatocytic
Teratoma	Teratoma Mature Immature With malignant transformation	Teratoma differentiated (TD)	Teratoma Mature Immature With malignant transformation
Teratocarcinoma	Embryonal carcinoma with teratoma	Malignant teratoma —intermediate (MTI)	Embryonal carcinoma and teratoma
Embryonal carcinoma	Embryonal carcinoma—adult Polyembryoma	Malignant teratoma —undifferentiated (MTU)	Embryonal carcinoma (adult type)
Chorioepithelioma	Choriocarcinoma with or without embryonal carcinoma and/or teratoma	Malignant teratoma —trophoblastic (MTT)	Choriocarcinoma with or without embryonal carcinoma and/or teratoma
—	Embryonal carcinoma (juvenile type)	Yolk sac tumor	Yolk sac tumor (endodermal sinus tumor)

been suggested that when a cell is committed to one of the three germ layers (mesoderm, ectoderm, entoderm) during embryonic development, the potential for re-expression of primitive elements is lost. In the early uncommitted phases of development, the primordial germ cell (embryonal carcinoma) possesses an unlimited capacity to differentiate into tissues that resemble germ cells (seminoma) or into cells that resemble other cell types—extraembryonic (choriocarcinoma, yolk sac tumor) or intraembryonic (teratoma) forms (Fig. 33–1). There is no evidence, animal or human, that committed germ cell tumors can dedifferentiate back into more primitive states and re-express primitive

capabilities. A teratoma or yolk sac tumor presumably will not revert to a malignant embryonal carcinoma, although all three elements may be found within the same tumor. The malignant, uncommitted germ cells can still respond to organizer or inducer influences and are still capable of differentiating into benign somatic elements. Although the situation is not analogous, it is commonly acknowledged that nongerminal prostate cancers also remain responsive to organizer substances (hormones).

Differentiation in germ cell and non–germ cell tumors is perceived as a one-way path. Oncogenesis is a deviation from this process, which may result in the reactivation of uncom-

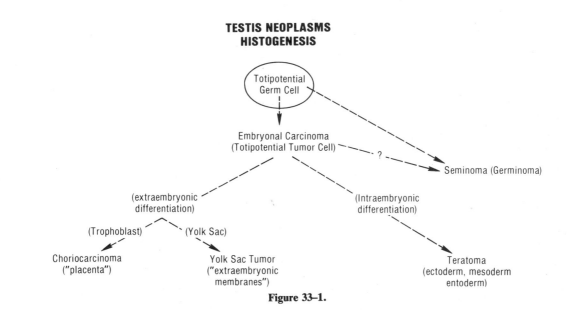

TESTIS NEOPLASMS HISTOGENESIS

Figure 33–1.

mitted cellular behavior. One remedy to onco-genesis may be the reinduction of differentia-tion. Strickland and Mahdavi (1978) and Speers (1982) successfully induced differentiation in murine teratocarcinomas using retinoids; unfor-tunately, Bosl (1984) was unable to do likewise in humans (see further on).

Histogenesis

Teilum's (1971) modified version of the Dixon and Moore classification is widely ac-cepted in North America for its simplicity and theoretical foundations. Primitive totipotential germ cells are thought to undergo malignant transformation, for as yet unexplained reasons. These transformed cells are recognized as em-bryonal carcinoma that can differentiate along germ cell lines (to seminoma) or along pathways to embryonic tissues ("extraembryonic" or "in-traembryonic" elements). If the embryonal cells become committed to intraembryonic develop-ment, somatic germ cell layers form as a tera-toma with either mature or immature elements. The combination of embryonal carcinoma and teratoma is readily appreciated as a transfor-mation state; there are some lines of evidence suggesting that anaplastic seminoma represents a similar transition state to the "typical" variant. Typical seminoma, which resembles seminifer-ous epithelium, is probably not capable of fur-ther neoplastic transformation. Extraembryonic differentiation results in the formation of yolk sac tumors or choriocarcinoma. The former may elaborate alpha fetoproteins, which are also produced by the normal fetal yolk sac. Pierce (1975) has shown that if embryonal carcinoma proceeds toward choriocarcinoma, cytotropho-blastic elements develop prior to those of the syncytiotrophoblast. Human chorionic gonado-tropins are produced in great quantities by the normal placenta and choriocarcinomas. The clinical observation that many embryonal car-cinomas and some seminomas also produce tro-phoblastic-mediated human chorionic gonado-tropins is consistent with either a germ cell or an embryonic origin.

ANIMAL MODELS

Epidemiologic data in humans and experi-mental studies in animals have demonstrated that genetic and environmental factors are im-portant in the development of germ cell and non–germ cell neoplasms. Although various in-fluences are known to participate in human germ cell tumorigenesis, the importance of precisely timed relationships has been better defined in animals. The exact origin of germ cell tumors has been questioned. It would be logical to assume that the source of these tumors is the primordial germ cell, since nearly all arise in the testis or ovary. This logic, however, does not explain the occasional occurrence of mor-phologically and functionally similar extrago-nadal germinal tumors. Observation of the latter has been one of the main arguments favoring "misplaced embryonic cells" as the most logical source of all germ cell tumors. This theory holds that during ontogeny, multipotential embryonic cells are sequestered in various locations (in-cluding the gonad), where they may subse-quently give rise to "germ cell" tumors. Reviews by Damjanov and Solter (1976) and Jewett (1977) offer some relevant information on this topic and indicate interesting parallels between experimental animal models and human disease.

Stevens (1967, 1968) developed and suc-cessfully manipulated a testicular teratoma line in a strain of the 129 mouse. The original congenital Stevens' model tumors arose spon-taneously within the seminiferous tubules of testis in 12-day-old embryos. The majority of the tumors developed as teratomas that spon-taneously stopped growing. More primitive-ap-pearing embryonal cells occasionally persisted; if these were implanted within the peritoneal cavity, yolk sac tumors and "embryoid bodies" were produced. Stevens also found microscopic teratomas in the genital ridges of 129 strain mice. If on the eleventh or twelfth day of gestation, the embryonic genital ridge was trans-planted into the scrotum of an adult mouse, an 80 per cent rate of tumor production was ob-tained. The grafts failed if ridge transplantation was attempted to other sites outside the scro-tum. In a strain (A/He) with a very low rate of incidence of spontaneous tumors, genital ridge transplantation was equally successful. In an-other strain bred with no germ cells in the genital ridge, transplantation failed to produce tumors. These observations indicate the impor-tance of genetic predisposition, environmental factors, and timing sequences in oncogenesis, while lending support to the germ cell origin of testis tumors.

Damjanov and Solter (1976) observed that transplantation of very early stage (day 1 to 7) mouse embryos from some strains (C3H, A, CBA) to extrauterine sites resulted in the pro-duction of rapidly growing teratocarcinomas. These could be retransplanted in vivo or culti-vated in vitro. After the eighth day of gestation, however, transplantation resulted in the production of a teratoma only. The teratomas were composed of mature somatic elements with slow growth rates, and they were not transplantable. These experiments provide evidence favoring the concept of the misplaced embryo as the origin of germinal tumors.

Primordial germ cells, early embryos, and embryonal carcinoma cells share similar characteristics, including (1) pluripotency, (2) ultrastructural appearance, (3) alkaline phosphatase content, (4) formation of embryoid bodies, and (5) surface antigens. During the process of differentiation these features become altered. Artz and Jacob (1974) noted that some cell surface antigens remain unchanged, whereas others, notably histocompatibility antigens, do not make their appearance until primitive elements have matured into adult forms. It is hoped that monoclonal antibody techniques will clarify these differentiation antigens and perhaps find therapeutic value (Fradet et al., 1983).

ADULT GERM CELL TUMORS

Epidemiology

INCIDENCE

Approximately 5000 new cases and 1000 deaths related to testicular cancer are reported in the United States annually (Silverberg, 1983). Estimates indicate that for American white males the lifetime probability of developing testicular cancer is approximately 0.2 per cent, or 1 in 500 (Zdeb, 1977). The average annual age-adjusted incidence rate for American males from 1969 to 1971 was 3.7 per 100,000—nearly twice the rate of 2.0 per 100,000 from 1937 to 1939. The average rate among American black males is 0.9 per 100,000, unchanged in the last 40 years. During the 40-year period from 1936 to 1976 the age-adjusted mortality in the United States showed little variation, but the rates between the ages of 15 and 29 years increased significantly (46 to 100 per cent); the trends remained stable or decreased in the 30 to 59 and over 60 age groups, respectively (Petersen and Lee, 1972; Schottenfeld et al., 1980).

Similar trends have been noted in Denmark, where the age-adjusted incidence rose from 3.4 to 6.4 per 100,000 between 1945 and 1970 (Clemmesen, 1974). Data compiled by Muir and Nectoux (1979) indicate considerable variability in the worldwide incidence of adult germ cell tumors. The average annual rate (age-adjusted) is highest in Scandinavia (Denmark, adjusted) is highest in Scandinavia (Denmark, Norway), Switzerland, Germany, and New Zealand; is intermediate in the United States and Great Britain; and is low in Africa and Asia. In data collected by Clemmesen (1974) the age-adjusted rate rose from 3.2 to 6.7 per 100,000 in Copenhagen between 1943 and 1967. Prevalence rates in Copenhagen were double those of rural Denmark during the same period.

AGE

Peak incidences of testicular tumors occur in late adolescence to early adulthood (20 to 40 years), in late adulthood (over 60 years), and in infancy (0 to 10 years). Overall the highest incidence is noted in young adults, making these neoplasms the most common solid tumors of men between 20 and 34 years of age in the United States and Great Britain. Seminoma is rare below the age of 10 and above the age of 60, but it is the most common histologic type overall with a peak incidence between the ages of 35 and 39 years. Spermatocytic seminoma (approximately 10 per cent of seminomas) occurs most often in patients over the age of 50 years. Embryonal carcinoma and teratocarcinoma occur predominantly between the ages of 25 and 35 years. Choriocarcinoma (1 to 2 per cent of germ cell tumors) occurs more often in the 20- to 30-year age group. Yolk sac tumors are the predominant lesions of infancy and childhood but are frequently found in combination with other germ cell elements in young adults. Histologically benign pure teratoma occurs most often in the pediatric age group but frequently appears in combination with other elements in adulthood. Malignant testicular lymphomas are predominantly tumors of men over 50 years of age.

RACIAL FACTORS

Variable incidence rates are noted between different ethnic groups within a given geographic region. The incidence of testicular tumors in the American black is approximately one-third that in the American white but 10 times that in his African counterpart. In Israel, Jews have at least an eightfold higher incidence of testis tumors in comparison with non-Jewish countrymen. In Hawaii, the incidence among Filipino/Japanese sectors is approximately one-tenth that of the Chinese/Caucasian/native Hawaiian populations.

Graham and Gibson (1972) presented data indicating a higher incidence among professional men. Mack and Henderson (1980) noted higher incidence rates in upper and middle socioeconomic classes of whites in Los Angeles County.

Although similar trends have been noted in American blacks (Ross et al., 1979), the rate is still less than one-third that of whites of comparable social status.

GENETIC FACTORS

Although a relatively higher incidence of testicular tumors has been reported in twins, brothers, and family members, the evidence for a predominant genetic influence is not overwhelming (Johnson, 1976). In nearly 7000 sets of twins from the Danish Twin Registry, Harvald and Hauge (1963) found no higher incidence of cancer in twins than was expected in the general population. Muller (1962) reported that there was a familial history of malignant disease in approximately 16 per cent of cases. The 2 to 3 per cent incidence of bilateral tumors may suggest the potential importance of genetic (or congenital) factors.

LATERALITY AND BILATERALITY

Testicular neoplasms appear to be slightly more common in the right testis than in the left, similar to the slightly greater incidence of right-sided cryptorchidism. Approximately 2 to 3 per cent of testicular tumors are bilateral, occurring either simultaneously or successively. If secondary testicular tumors (specifically reticuloendothelial malignancies, discussed later) are excluded, the incidence of bilateral tumors is between 1 and 2.8 per cent of all cases of germinal neoplasms (Sokal et al., 1980). Similar rather than different histology in the two testes predominates with bilateral tumors. Bach et al. (1983) tabulated the histology in 337 cases of bilateral testicular tumors. Bilateral seminoma was the most common histologic type (48 per cent); bilateral similar nonseminomas were found in 15 per cent; germinal tumors with different histology were present in 15 per cent; and nongerminal tumors with similar histology

occurred in 22 per cent. A history of cryptorchidism (uni- or bilateral) in nearly half these men is consistent with observations that bilateral dysgenesis occurs frequently in unilateral maldescent (Sohval, 1956; Weissbach and Ibach, 1975). Long-term surveillance of patients with a history of cryptorchidism or previous orchiectomy for a germ cell tumor is mandatory.

FREQUENCY OF HISTOLOGIC TYPES

Germinal tumors constitute between 90 and 95 per cent of all primary testicular malignancies. Variability in the reported frequency of histologic types may reflect true differences in the incidence of such tumors. It is possible, however, that such variations merely reflect demographic differences, variance of histologic interpretations, or other unquantified selection factors. From Table 33–3 the overall incidence rates have been tabulated as follows: seminoma, 40 per cent; embryonal carcinoma, 20 to 25 per cent; teratocarcinoma, 25 to 30 per cent; teratoma, 5 to 10 per cent; and pure choriocarcinoma, 1 per cent. When combined histologic patterns (more than one histologic pattern) are considered as a separate entity, the frequency approximates: seminoma, 30 per cent; embryonal carcinoma, 30 per cent; teratoma, 10 per cent; teratocarcinoma, 25 per cent; choriocarcinoma, 1 per cent; and combined patterns (e.g., seminoma plus embryonal carcinoma, embryonal carcinoma plus choriocarcinoma), 15 per cent (Mostofi, 1973).

Etiology

Experimental and clinical evidence supports the importance of congenital factors in the etiology of germ cell tumors. During development the primordial germ cell may be altered by environmental factors, resulting in disturbed

TABLE 33–3. FREQUENCY OF HISTOLOGIC TYPES

Author	Total Cases	Seminoma	Embryonal	Terato-carcinoma	Teratoma	Chorio-carcinoma
Dixon and Moore (1953)*	866	325	174	281	76	10
Melicow et al. (1955)	100	55	23	17	5	—
Patton et al. (1960)	556	206	177	149	14	10
Vechinski et al. (1965)*	104	47	36	9	8	4
Kurohara et al. (1968)†	366	205	85	68	4	4
Total (Average %)	1992	838 (42)	495 (25)	524 (26)	107 (5)	28 (1)

*Categorized according to predominant pattern.

†Forty-eight additional patients with mixed histologic patterns not included.

differentiation. The germ cell is conceivably detained from normal development by cryptorchidism, gonadal dysgenesis, or hereditary predisposition, or by chemical carcinogens, trauma, or orchitis. The teratocarcinoma tumor model (Stevens, 1968) suggests the crucial influence of temporal relationships on normal versus abnormal differentiation.

CONGENITAL CAUSES

Cryptorchidism. LeComete (1851) is credited with the initial observation that testicular maldescent and tumor formation are interrelated. Pooled data from several large series indicate that approximately 7 to 10 per cent of patients with testicular tumors have a prior history of cryptorchidism (Table 33–4) (Whitaker, 1970). Mostofi (1973) lists five possible, but unquantified, factors that may play a causative role in the cryptorchid/malignant testis: abnormal germ cell morphology, elevated temperature, interference with blood supply, endocrine dysfunction, and gonadal dysgenesis.

The exact incidence of cryptorchidism is unknown, as much of the relevant information on testicular maldescent includes data on patients with retractile testes. From accumulated series Scorer and Farrington (1971) estimate that approximately 4.3 per cent of neonates, 0.8 per cent of infants and children, and 0.7 per cent of adult males over the age of 18 years (army selectees) harbor a truly cryptorchid testis. In reviewing more than 7000 cases of testicular tumor, Gilbert and Hamilton (1940) found a history of cryptorchidism in 840 men (12 per cent). Based on the observed incidence of cryptorchidism in military inductees (0.23 per cent, roughly 1 in 500), they calculated the estimated risk of tumorigenesis in a man with a history of maldescent to be 48 times that of men with normally descended testes. More recent epidemiologic studies have reported the relative risk of testicular cancer in patients with cryptorchidism to be much lower, 3 to 14 times the normal expected incidence (Henderson et al. 1979; Morrison, 1976; Mostofi, 1979, 1983; Schottenfeld et al., 1980).

Between 5 and 10 per cent of patients with a history of cryptorchidism develop malignancy in the contralateral, normally descended gonad. This observation is consistent with the findings of Berthelsen and Skakkebaek (1982). They have provided biopsy data in 250 patients with testis cancer relative to the contralateral testis. Carcinoma in situ (CIS) was found in 13 (5.2 per cent), representing one third of patients with atrophy of the remaining testis and one fifth of patients with a history of cryptorchidism. Two of the patients (10 per cent) with contralateral CIS subsequently developed a second testis cancer. Campbell (1942) noted that roughly 25 per cent of patients with bilateral cryptorchidism and a history of testis cancer were subject to the risk of a second germ cell tumor.

Campbell (1942) indicated that nearly half of patients with malignancy associated with cryptorchidism have impalpable abdominal testes. Although the anatomic position (inguinal versus abdominal) may play a role in determining the degree of gonadal damage (and the risk of subsequent tumor formation), the relative influence upon the cryptorchid testis may depend largely upon the observer (Gilbert, 1940).

Ultrastructural abnormalities of the spermatogonia and Sertoli cells are readily apparent in the cryptorchid testis by the age of 3 years. Cellular degeneration is followed by progressive fibrosis, destruction of the basement membrane, and deposition of myelin and lipids (Mengel et

TABLE 33–4. TESTICULAR TUMORS AND CRYPTORCHIDISM

Series	Total Patients	Patients with Cryptorchidism	Patients with Tumor in Contralateral Scrotal Testis
Schwartz and Reed (1956)	167	15	3
Thurzo and Pinter (1961)	139	9	3
Field (1962)	135	9	2
Hope-Stone et al. (1963)	282	17	2
Collins and Pugh (1964)	995	58	9
Johnson et al. (1968)	147	12	3
Gehring et al. (1973)	529	37	7
Mostofi and Price (1973)	2000	72	—
Cameron and Pugh (1976)	1812	123	—
Batata et al. (1982)	1152	137	13
Total	7358	489 (6.6%)	42

al., 1982). Consideration of these histologic changes and other social factors has favored the practice of early orchiopexy. Such a philosophy, however, has not completely prevented tumor formation in the testis (Martin, 1979; Batata et al., 1982).

ACQUIRED CAUSES

Trauma. Although trauma is considered a contributing factor in zinc- or copper-induced fowl teratomas, there is little to suggest a cause and effect relationship in humans (Michalowsky, 1928; Bagg, 1936; Carleton, 1953). Horseback riding has been implicated by Sobin as a cause of testicular tumors in Afghanistan (Mostofi and Price, 1973), but most investigators conclude that trauma to the enlarged testis is an event that prompts medical evaluation rather than being a causative factor.

Hormones. Sex hormone fluctuations may contribute to the development of testicular tumors in experimental animals and humans. The administration of estrogen to pregnant mice may cause maldescent and dysgenesis of the testis in the offspring (Nomura and Kanzak, 1977). Similar findings have been noted in the male offspring of women exposed to diethylstilbestrol (Cosgrove et al., 1977) or oral contraceptives (Rothman and Louik, 1978). Exogenous estrogen administration has also been linked to the induction of Leydig cell tumors (see further on). Recent epidemiologic studies found relative risk rates ranging from 2.8 to 5.3 per cent for testicular tumor in the male progeny of diethylstilbestrol-treated mothers (Henderson et al., 1983; Schottenfeld et al., 1980).

Atrophy. Nonspecific or mumps-associated atrophy of the testis has been suggested as a potential causative factor in testicular cancer. Gilbert (1944) collected 80 cases of testicular tumor occurring in patients with a history of nonspecific atrophy and 24 additional cases related to a previous history of mumps orchitis among 5500 cases of testicular tumors. Although a causative role for atrophy remains speculative, it is tempting to invoke local hormonal imbalance as a possible cause for malignant transformation.

Pathogenesis and Natural History

Local growth characteristics and patterns of spread have been well defined by the clinical observation of patients with germinal testicular tumors. Following malignant transformation, intratubular carcinoma in situ (CIS) extends be-

yond the basement membrane and may eventually replace most of the testicular parenchyma. Local involvement of the epididymis or spermatic cord is hindered by the tunica albuginea, and seemingly, as a consequence, lymphatic or hematogenous spread may occur first. Approximately half of patients with nonseminomatous tumors present with disseminated disease (Bosl et al., 1981). Involvement of the epididymis or cord may lead to pelvic and inguinal lymph node metastasis, whereas tumors confined to the testis proper are usually spread to retroperitoneal nodes. Hematogenous spread to lung, bone, or liver is occasioned either by direct vascular invasion or indirectly from previously established lymphatic metastasis, by way of the thoracic duct and subclavian veins or other lymphaticovenous communications. The natural history of germinal testis tumors has been the subject of numerous treatises and appears sufficiently well defined to permit the following generalizations (Whitmore, 1968; Barzell and Whitmore, 1978):

1. Complete spontaneous regressions are rare.

2. All germinal testis tumors in adults should be regarded as malignant. Although the infantile teratoma may be regarded as "benign," teratoma of the adult testis may be associated with vascular invasion microscopically and a definite mortality risk in patients treated with orchiectomy alone (as high as 29 per cent, according to Mostofi and Price, 1973). Clinical experience has shown that retroperitoneal teratoma in the adult, whether resulting from maturation of embryonal carcinoma or from regression of the embryonal carcinoma component of a teratocarcinoma (spontaneous or induced), may be accompanied by unrelenting local growth and ultimate fatality (Hong et al., 1977).

3. The tunica albuginea is a natural barrier to expansile local growth. Extension through this dense membrane occurs at the testicular mediastinum, where the blood vessels, lymphatics, nerves, and efferent tubules exit the testis proper. Local involvement of the epididymis or spermatic cord occurs in 10 to 15 per cent of cases and increases the risks of lymphatic or blood-borne metastasis.

4. Lymphatic metastasis is common to all forms of germinal testis tumors, although pure choriocarcinoma almost uniformly disseminates by means of vascular invasion as well. The spermatic cord contains four to eight lymphatic channels that traverse the inguinal canal and retroperitoneal space. As the spermatic vessels cross ventral to the ureter, these lymphatics fan

out medially and drain into the retroperitoneal lymph node chain. The primary drainage of the right testis is usually located within the group of lymph nodes in the interaortocaval region at the level of the second vertebral body; the first echelon of nodes draining the left testis is located in the para-aortic region in the compartment bounded by the left ureter, the left renal vein, the aorta, and the origin of the inferior mesenteric artery. Subsequent cephalad drainage is to the cisterna chyli, thoracic duct, and supraclavicular nodes (usually left), but retrograde spread may occur to common, external, and inguinal lymph nodes. Although the thoracic duct–subclavian vein juncture is the major site of communication, other lymphaticovenous communications may be occasioned by massive retroperitoneal lymph node deposits. Furthermore, it has been demonstrated by spermatic lymphangiography that testicular lymphatics can rarely communicate directly with the thoracic duct, bypassing the retroperitoneal nodes. Lymphatics of the epididymis drain into the external iliac chain, affording locally extensive testicular tumors access to pelvic lymph nodes. Inguinal node metastasis may result from scrotal involvement by the primary tumor, prior inguinal or scrotal surgery, or retrograde lymphatic spread secondary to massive retroperitoneal lymph node deposits.

5. Extranodal distant metastasis results from either direct vascular invasion or tumor emboli from lymphatic metastasis via major thoracoabdominal channels or minor lymphaticovenous communications. Most, but not all, blood-borne metastasis occurs following lymph node involvement. This is of obvious practical importance in treatment and prognosis. Despite surgical excision of negative retroperitoneal lymph nodes, the distant failure rate is approximately 5 per cent (Whitmore, 1968, 1973). In programs reserving further treatment following inguinal orchiectomy for clinical Stage A nonseminoma patients, approximately 20 per cent will fail, most with retroperitoneal lymph node metastasis (80 per cent of failures) and the remainder with extralymphatic distant metastasis (20 per cent of failures) independent of retroperitoneal deposits (Peckham, 1983; Sogani, 1984).

Primary and secondary deposits of nongerminal tumors frequently vary histologically. Pure seminomas, however, rarely metastasize as another form of germinal tumor; nonseminomas rarely metastasize as pure seminomas unless the primary lesion has combined histology containing seminomatous elements (Ray et

al., 1974). Although the clinical incidence of nonseminomatous metastasis from an apparently pure seminoma is less than 10 per cent, 30 to 45 per cent of patients dying from apparently pure seminoma harbor nonseminomatous metastases (Bredael et al., 1982).

With the exception of seminoma, the growth rate among germ cell tumors tends to be high. Doubling times calculated on the basis of serial chest radiographs usually range from 10 to 30 days. Alterations in the production of tumor marker substances (B-hCG, AFP, LDH) are in keeping with rapid metabolic activity and growth. The anticipated rapid demise of patients failing treatment has been confirmed by clinical observation: 85 per cent of patients dying from germ cell tumors do so within 2 years and the majority of the remainder within 3 years. Because of a sometimes indolent course, seminoma may recur from 2 to 10 years following apparently successful initial management.

Because of the short natural history of germinal tumors, it has become customary to regard 2-year survival as an end point for judging the effectiveness of therapy. With the evolution of multimodal therapy, "surviving" patients may not be actually "cured" of their neoplasm, and a disease-free interval of 5 years may be a more appropriate yardstick for assessing curability.

CLINICAL MANIFESTATIONS

Survival in patients with germ cell tumors is directly related to the stage at presentation (tumor burden) and to the effectiveness of subsequent treatment. Patients presenting with advanced metastatic disease have a much poorer prognosis than do those with disease confined to the testis. Delay in diagnosis is the result of patient-related factors (ignorance, denial, fear) and physician-related bias (misdiagnosis). Despite the voluminous literature emphasizing the importance of early diagnosis, 40 to 50 per cent of patients still present with metastatic disease (Bosl et al., 1981). Physician-related causes remain prevalent factors in delayed treatment, emphasizing the need for continuing medical as well as lay education programs.

SYMPTOMS

The usual presentation in the patient with a testicular tumor is a nodule or painless swelling or altered consistency of the testis noted incidentally by the patient, who usually describes it as a "lump" or "swelling" or "hardness" of the testis. Less commonly, the patient may note a dull ache or heavy sensation in the lower abdomen, inguinal area, or scrotum that he may or may not associate with an abnormality in the testis. Occasionally, patients will complain that a previously small atrophic testis has enlarged to the size of the normal contralateral testis. Acute pain is relatively uncommon unless the symptoms are the same as those of epididymitis or epididymo-orchitis, an unfortunate presentation that occurs in roughly 10 per cent of patients. Such a misdiagnosis often delays appropriate treatment. Rarely, infertility may be the presenting complaint (Collins and Pugh, 1964; Skakkebaek, 1972).

In approximately 10 per cent of patients the presenting manifestations may be due to metastases, including a neck mass (supraclavicular lymph node metastasis); respiratory symptoms, such as cough or dyspnea (pulmonary metastasis); gastrointestinal disturbances, such as anorexia, nausea, vomiting, or hemorrhage (retroduodenal metastasis); lumbar back pain (bulky retroperitoneal disease involving the psoas muscle or nerve roots); bone pain (skeletal metastasis); central and peripheral nervous system manifestations (cerebral, spinal cord, or peripheral root involvement); unilateral or bilateral lower extremity swelling (iliac or caval venous obstruction or thrombosis).

Gynecomastia, seen in about 5 per cent of patients with testicular germ cell tumors, may be regarded as a systemic endocrine manifestation of these neoplasms. Gynecomastia may or may not be associated with elevated levels of human chorionic gonadotropin (hCG), human chorionic somatomammotropin (hCS), prolactin, estrogens, or androgens (see further on). Relationships between gynecomastia, the morphologic characteristics of the primary tumor, and endocrine abnormalities remain incompletely defined.

PHYSICAL EXAMINATION

A complete physical examination is essential in the assessment of patients with a suspected testicular tumor. Bimanual examination of the scrotal contents, beginning with the normal contralateral testis, is a logical starting point. This maneuver provides a baseline for appreciation of relative size, contour, and consistency in the suspect gonad. Usually a testicular tumor is a firm, relatively nontender mass located within the tunica albuginea. As such, the epididymis is usually separable from the lesion and there is no involvement of the cord, scrotal investments, or skin. A tumor can be small (and accompanied by distant spread) or large (with disease locally confined). In general,

seminoma tends to expand within the testis proper as a painless, rubbery enlargement, whereas embryonal carcinoma or teratocarcinoma characteristically produces an irregular, rather than a discrete, mass surrounded by normal testicular parenchyma.

Even when a testicular tumor attains large size, it tends to remain ovoid, being limited by the tough investing tunica. Spread to the epididymis or cord occurs infrequently (10 to 15 per cent of cases) and may be associated with a more advanced stage of disease. Although uncommon, a hydrocele may accompany (and camouflage) a testicular neoplasm. Rapid apparent growth of a testicular tumor may result from hemorrhage and necrosis, manifested clinically as acute pain, mimicking an inflammatory process, torsion, or incarcerated hernia. Rarely, a patient will present with acute abdominal pain from bleeding into an undescended testis or from a ruptured metastatic deposit.

Palpation of the abdomen may reveal evidence of nodal disease or visceral invasion. Examination of the thorax may disclose gynecomastia or the presence of respiratory tract involvement. Assessment of inguinal, supraclavicular, and scalene lymph nodes may reveal adenopathy. Neuromuscular findings or peripheral edema may herald involvement of the nervous and musculoskeletal systems.

Although the great majority of germinal tumors are clinically recognizable as being of testicular origin, in a few patients the primary tumor in the testis may be so small that it is clinically undetectable. Furthermore, extragonadal germ cell tumors, morphologically identical with those in the testis, may arise in the retroperitoneum, mediastinum, or brain.

DIFFERENTIAL DIAGNOSIS

An erroneous diagnosis is made upon initial examination in approximately one fourth of patients, resulting in a delay in treatment or an inappropriate surgical approach. Five to 15 per cent of patients with a testicular neoplasm are treated for epididymitis (or epididymo-orchitis) before a diagnosis of malignancy is made secondarily (Patton et al., 1959; Fergusson, 1962). Hydrocele, hernia, hematoma, spermatocele, and syphilitic gumma are rare problems in differential diagnosis. Distinction between acute or chronic epididymitis and a testicular neoplasm may be difficult. If a vigorous 2-week course of conservative management produces no clear evidence of improvement, exploration is indicated. Diagnosis may be aided by testicular ultrasonography or determination of serum tumor markers, or both.

Clinical Staging

Staging evaluations may be based on clinical assessment or surgical findings with pathologic examination and may provide specific and sometimes overlapping information. The history and physical findings have been discussed. Several variables influence the survival of patients with testicular germ cell tumors, and extent of the neoplasm is a principal consideration. Clinical staging attempts to define the extent of disease at the time of diagnosis, during the course of treatment, and at subsequent follow-up. The predictable mode of metastasis in patients with germ cell tumors and several recent technological advances, notably imaging techniques and biochemical marker assays, have made initial clinical evaluations remarkably accurate. Comparisons between treatments hinge equally upon the treatment and the definition of the stage treated. For testicular tumors the system proposed by Boden and Gibb (1951) has been the mainstay of clinical staging, although

refinement in staging methods and treatment has led to the development of many "substages." The staging systems suggested by various authors represent attempts to define therapeutically and prognostically significant subcategories. Differences among these staging systems (Table 33–5) make interinstitutional comparisons difficult and less meaningful.

IMAGING STUDIES

Ultrasonography. Immersion and high-resolution ultrasonography may aid in the clinical evaluation of scrotal masses (Leopold et al., 1979; Friedrich et al., 1981). Intrascrotal fluid collections are no barrier to the examination of the underlying testicular parenchyma by ultrasonography. In patients with palpably normal genitalia and evidence of extragonadal germ cell malignancy, sonography has been reported to be successful in identifying occult testicular neoplasms (Glazer et al., 1982). Unpublished data from Memorial Sloan-Kettering Cancer Center (MSKCC) indicate that in a selected group of

TABLE 33–5. CLINICAL STAGING SYSTEMS

Boden/Gibb Stage	MSKCC	Royal Marsden Hospital	M.D. Anderson Hospital	American Joint Committee

A (I)
Tumor confined to testis
	A	I	I	TX unknown status
				T0 no evidence
				  primary
				T1 confined to testis
				T2 beyond tunica
				T3 invades rete testis
				  or epididymis
				T4a invades cord
				T4b invades scrotum

B (II) Spread to regional nodes	B1 <5 cm	IIA <2 cm	IIA Neg LAG/Pos nodes*	NX unknown status N0 no nodes involved N1 1 homolateral node
	B2 >5 cm	IIB >2, <5 cm	IIB Pos LAG	N2 contralateral/ bilateral nodes

	B3 >10 cm
	  ("bulky")
		IIC >5 cm	N/A	N3 abdominal or fixed
				  groin masses
				N4 juxtaregional nodes

C (III)
Spread beyond retroperitoneal nodes
	C	III
		Supraclavicular (SCN)
		or mediastinal
		involvement
			IIIA SCN
			IIIB-1 gynecomastia
			IIIB-2
			minimal lung
			IIIB-3
			advanced lung
			IIIB-4
			advanced abdominal
			(any palpable mass)
			IIIB-5
			visceral spread
			(excluding lung)
				MX not assessed
				M0 no distant
				  metastasis found
				M1 distant metastasis
				  present

		IV Extralymphatic metastasis		

*Surgically determined

patients, gray-scale sonography was capable of identifying 32 of 33 malignant tumors, 3 of 3 benign epididymal cysts, and 2 otherwise undetected testicular neoplasms in patients previously thought to have primary retroperitoneal tumors. Sonographic examination complements the overall clinical picture, but a high index of suspicion, based on physical examination alone, should be the overriding factor in determining the advisability of inguinal exploration. Although less frequently utilized than computerized tomography (CT), abdominal ultrasound scanning appears to have approximated the sensitivity of CT in assessment of the retroperitoneum.

Radiographic Studies. Posteroanterior and lateral chest x-rays provide the minimal assessment of the lung parenchyma and mediastinal structures. Stereo projections, lung tomography, and chest CT scans provide more sensitive evaluations of the thorax, increasing the detection of pulmonary metastases.

Intravenous urogram (IVU), pedal lymphangiograms (LAG), ultrasonography (US), and abdominal CT scanning have been widely utilized in evaluating the retroperitoneal space for metastatic lymph node and soft tissue disease. Each examination has a specific role. The IVU defines renal abnormalities—congenital anomalies, obstruction, and ureteral deviations. The pedal LAG is capable of delineating the internal architecture of retroperitoneal lymph nodes, even of normal size. An ipsilateral LAG may be used in patients with nonseminomatous tumors to reveal crossover patterns and the specific features of ipsilateral lymphatic anatomy. A bilateral LAG performed in patients with testicular seminoma facilitates accurate planning of radiation therapy portals. Intraoperative radiographs after LAG help assess the adequacy of retroperitoneal lymph node dissection, while serial radiographs obtained in follow-up of patients treated by alternative means help monitor the effectiveness of therapy. A 24-hour film of the chest following injection of contrast material may provide information regarding mediastinal or supraclavicular lymph nodes.

Estimates of the overall accuracy of pedal lymphangiography in the evaluation of retroperitoneal lymph nodes, determined by radiographic-pathologic correlation, indicate a false negative rate of approximately 25 per cent and a false positive rate of less than 5 per cent (Hussey et al., 1977; Barzell and Whitmore, 1978; Peckham et al., 1982). The degree of accuracy for this or any other staging modality must be interpreted relative to the tumor burden being studied. For example, bulky retroperitoneal lymph node deposits may be detected by physical examination, IVU, pedal LAG, abdominal US, or abdominal CT scan with 100 per cent accuracy!

Computerized Tomography. Lymph nodes in the upper para-aortic regions above the cisterna chyli or in the porta hepatis, mesentery, and renal hilum are not opacified following pedal injection of lymphangiographic contrast. With the use of conventional LAG, tumor size is estimated from the displacement of adjacent structures. Abdominal CT scans identify small (<2 cm) lymph node deposits (variable with slice thickness) and deposits in the upper para-aortic regions not seen with LAG. Abdominal CT provides a generally accurate three-dimensional estimate of tumor size, extension to adjacent soft tissue structures, and involvement of regional viscera. Few series make valid comparisons between the results obtained by conventional staging methods and those obtained following the development of CT. At the Royal Marsden Hospital the addition of CT study of the chest and abdomen in patients with germ cell tumors reduced the clinical understaging error by 22 per cent (Husband et al., 1981).

Steady improvements in diagnostic imaging techniques, such as lymphangiography, computed tomography, and ultrasonography, have revolutionized the management of patients with germ cell tumors. Positron emission tomography (PET) and nuclear magnetic resonance (NMR) imaging, currently under development, will permit exploration of certain physicochemical properties of neoplastic tissue; whether these methods will be capable of detecting tumor burdens less than 10 mm in diameter (10^9 cells) or of quantifying tumor viability is uncertain, however. The identification and quantification of specific tumor marker substances produced by the majority of germ cell neoplasms may surpass the resolution of diagnostic imaging methods currently available and under development.

TUMOR MARKERS

Germinal testis tumors are among a select group of neoplasms identified as producing so-called marker proteins that are relatively specific and readily measurable in minute quantities using highly sensitive radioimmunoassay (RIA) technology. Applied to the study of body fluids and tissue sections these biochemical markers theoretically may be capable of detecting small tumor burdens (10^5 cells) that are not detectable by currently available imaging techniques (Bagshawe and Searle, 1977). The study of biochemical marker substances, particularly alpha-feto-protein (AFP) and human chorionic gonadotropin (hCG), is clinically useful in the diagnosis, staging, and monitoring of treatment response in patients with germ cell neoplasms and may be useful as a prognostic index (Table 33–6). Germ cell tumor markers belong to two main classes: (1) oncofetal substances associated with embryonic development (alpha-fetoprotein and human chorionic gonadotropin), and (2) certain cellular enzymes, such as lactic acid dehydrogenase (LDH) and placental alkaline phosphatase (PALP).

The production by germ cell tumors of oncofetal substances provides evidence that oncogenesis and ontogenesis are closely related. Alpha-fetoprotein is a dominant serum protein of the early embryo, and human chorionic gonadotropin is a secretory product of the placenta. During normal maturation of the fetus both products fall to barely detectable levels soon after birth. The production of AFP and hCG by trophoblastic and syncytiotrophoblastic cells, respectively, within germ cell neoplasms implies the re-expression of repressed genes (presumably lost during differentiation) or malignant transformation of a pluripotential cell that has retained the ability to differentiate into cells capable of producing oncofetal proteins (Abelev et al., 1974; Uriel, 1979).

Alpha-Fetoprotein (AFP). Alpha-fetoprotein is a single-chain glycoprotein (molecular weight approximately 70,000) first demonstrated by Bergstrand and Czar (1954) in normal human fetal serum. In the fetus, AFP is a major serum binding protein produced by the fetal yolk sac, liver, and gastrointestinal tract. The highest concentrations noted during the twelfth to fourteenth weeks of gestation gradually decline so that 1 year following birth, AFP is detectable only at low levels (<40 ng/ml). In 1963 Abelev et al. detected AFP in mouse embryos and in the sera of mice with chemically induced liver tumors. Further investigation led to the discovery of elevated levels in humans with hepatomas and testis tumors. The metabolic half-life of AFP in humans is between 4 and 6 days, a fact useful in evaluating treatment response (see further on).

After the first 6 weeks of postnatal life an elevated AFP may be detected in association with a number of malignancies (testis, liver, pancreas, stomach, lung), normal pregnancy, benign liver disease, ataxia telangiectasia, and tyrosinemia. In endodermal sinus (or yolk sac) tumors, immunofluorescent methods indicate that the epithelial lining of the cysts and tubules is the site of the synthesis of AFP (Teilum, 1975). Alpha-fetoprotein may be produced by pure embryonal carcinoma, teratocarcinoma, yolk sac tumor, or combined tumors but not by pure choriocarcinoma or pure seminoma (Javadpour, 1980a and b). Taken together, these observations indicate that yolk sac elements are not always recognizable by conventional light microscopy in individuals with elevated serum AFP due to germ cell tumors. Binding studies with lectins have shown that AFP produced in the fetal liver has a different molecular structure from that produced in yolk sac tumors, a characteristic that may discriminate benign from malignant liver disease (Ruoslahti et al., 1978).

TABLE 33–6. BIOCHEMICAL AND BIOLOGIC CHARACTERISTICS OF ALPHA-FETOPROTEIN (AFP) AND HUMAN CHORIONIC GONADOTROPIN (hCG)

	AFP	hCG
Structure	Glycoprotein Alpha-1 globulin Single-chain	Glycoprotein Double-chain (alpha and beta)
Molecular weight	70,000	38,000
Half-life	4–6 days	24 hours
Fetal source	Yolk sac, liver, GI tract	Placenta
Malignant tumor sources	Testis, liver, pancreas, lung	Testis, pancreas, lung, breast, kidney, bladder
Benign causes	Ataxia telangiectasia, tyrosinemia	Marijuana(?) LH elevation (Cross reaction)
Source	Trophoblastic mononuclear cells	Syncytiotrophoblastic multinucleated giant cells
Histology		
Seminoma	−	+
Teratoma	−	−
Embryonal	+	+
Choriocarcinoma	−	+

Human Chorionic Gonadotropin (hCG). This glycoprotein (molecular weight 38,000) is composed of alpha and beta polypeptide chains and is normally produced by trophoblastic tissue. Pituitary hormones (luteinizing hormone, follicle stimulating hormone, thyroid stimulating hormone) possess alpha subunits closely resembling that of hCG. The beta subunit of hCG is structurally and antigenically distinct from that of the pituitary hormones and allows the production of specific antibodies against the purified β-hCG subunit used in RIA techniques (Vaitukaitis, 1979).

During pregnancy, hCG is secreted by the placenta for the maintenance of the corpus luteum. Zondek (1930) was the first to demonstrate that hCG is detectable in the sera of some patients with germ cell tumors. An elevated hCG may also be demonstrated in various other malignancies (liver, pancreas, stomach, lung, breast, kidney, bladder) and perhaps in marijuana smokers. In germ cell tumors, syncytiotrophoblastic cells have been found responsible for the production of hCG. Some of the RIA techniques for hCG variously cross-react with luteinizing hormone, and accordingly, caution should be exercised with patients whose LH may be physiologically elevated (e.g., postcastration).

The serum half-life of hCG is between 24 and 36 hours, but the individual subunits are cleared much more rapidly (20 minutes for the alpha subunit and 45 minutes for the beta subunit). All patients with choriocarcinoma and 40 to 60 per cent of patients with embryonal carcinoma are expected to have elevated serum levels of hCG. Approximately 5 to 10 per cent of patients with "pure" seminoma have detectable levels of hCG (usually below the level of 500 ng/ml), apparently produced by the syncytiotrophoblast-like giant cells occurring in some seminomas.

CLINICAL APPLICATIONS OF AFP AND hCG. Among patients with nonseminomatous testis tumors, approximately 50 to 70 per cent have elevated levels of AFP and approximately 40 to 60 per cent have elevated levels of hCG when sensitive RIA techniques are used. If both markers are measured simultaneously, approximately 90 per cent of patients will have elevations of one or both marker substances (Barzell and Whitmore, 1979; Fraley et al., 1979; Javadpour, 1980a; Bosl et al., 1981). These values are derived from patient populations comprising clinical Stages I, II, and III tumors. In patients with clinical Stage I tumors only, the incidence of positive markers is lower.

CLINICAL STAGING ACCURACY. The overall sensitivity of any test or marker will vary with the amount of tumor burden. Determinations of AFP and hCG, in concert with other staging modalities, have helped reduce the understaging error in germ cell tumors to a level of 10 to 15 per cent. Expressed another way, approximately 10 to 15 per cent of patients with nonseminomatous germ cell tumors can be expected to have normal marker levels even at advanced stages of disease. Although large numbers of patients with clinical Stage I nonseminoma have not had markers drawn before orchiectomy, data from the University of Minnesota suggest that roughly two thirds will have elevated levels of AFP or hCG, or both (Lange and Raghavan, 1983). Up to 90 per cent of such patients are expected to produce marker substances in the presence of advanced disease.

Following orchiectomy, persistent elevation of one or both markers suggests residual tumor, and while a rapid normalization of previously elevated marker(s) conceivably represents elimination of tumor, this is not categorically the case. In patients with disease clinically confined to the testis (clinical Stage I) approximately 20 per cent will develop metastatic disease while under surveillance despite negative tumor markers immediately following inguinal orchiectomy (see further on). Similarly, a persistent marker elevation following a technically satisfactory retroperitoneal lymph node dissection indicates the presence of residual disease (Stage III), whereas normal values do not categorically exclude the possibility of future recurrence.

MONITORING THERAPEUTIC RESPONSE. The rate of tumor marker decline relative to expected marker half-life following treatment has been proposed as a prognostic index. Patients whose values decline according to negative half-lives following treatment appear more likely to be disease-free than those whose marker decline is slower or whose markers never return to normal levels (Thompson and Haddow, 1979; Lange and Raghavan, 1983). Serial determinations of AFP and hCG closely reflect the effectiveness of therapy in patients with testicular tumors. The rate of marker decline following treatment (surgery, irradiation, chemotherapy) is proportional to the decrease in tumor burden and viability. Following apparently successful treatment, serologic relapse may precede clinical detection by an appreciable but unquantified interval. Alternative therapy may be initiated when minimal tumor burden is thereby perceived.

Following treatment of metastatic disease

with irradiation, systemic drugs, or surgery, persistent marker elevation indicates an incomplete response. Because of a therapeutic lag following irradiation or chemotherapy, definition of the "expected" rate of decline and subsequent normalization of markers remains somewhat uncertain; no clear end point of tumor destruction can be identified. Such an end point has been precisely defined for surgery, in that serum markers should fall immediately according to half-life, if such a procedure eradicates the tumor. Nevertheless, marker determinations do act as guidelines following primary chemotherapy or irradiation. Clinical experience has shown that if a patient with advanced disease fails to achieve normalization of tumor markers following aggressive combination chemotherapy, attempts at surgical excision almost uniformly fail. Normalization of marker levels after treatment cannot be equated with the absence of residual disease. Between 20 and 30 per cent of patients receiving combined systemic chemotherapy for bulky metastatic disease, and subsequently subjected to retroperitoneal lymph node dissection, will have viable tumor confirmed histologically despite normal preoperative tumor marker levels. Similarly, failure to achieve normal levels of AFP and β-hCG following definitive irradiation indicates persistent tumor.

HISTOLOGIC DIAGNOSIS. Classification of germ cell neoplasms according to morphologic appearance is invaluable in treatment selection. The broad distinction between seminomas and nonseminomas has been particularly important in determining management strategies for retroperitoneal lymph node metastasis. In that germ cell tumors arise from pluripotential cells, a variety of elements may inhabit a given primary tumor or its secondary metastatic sites. Ray et al. (1974) noted that in the majority of patients (71 of 75, or 95 per cent), a primary tumor containing embryonal carcinoma and seminoma either metastasized as pure embryonal carcinoma or combined with other elements but rarely metastasized as pure seminoma (2 of 75, or 3 per cent). Heterogeneity among germ cell neoplasms is an expected consequence of their pluripotential origin. Biochemical marker "probes" can provide a means of delineating tumor heterogeneity, which may be useful in treatment selection.

Relative to seminoma, the detection of an elevated AFP or hCG value strongly suggests the presence of a nonseminomatous element. Step sections of the primary tumor may further define the source of the marker abnormality.

Metastatic disease accompanied by an elevated serum AFP from a pure seminoma in all probability indicates a nonseminomatous element, and treatment plans should be restructured to include such a possibility. Parenthetically, 30 to 45 per cent of patients dying with seminoma are found to have elements of nonseminomatous histology at autopsy. It is generally accepted that between 5 and 10 per cent of patients with "pure" seminoma will have mild elevation of hCG because of the presence of syncytiotrophoblastic giant cell forms. If step sections of the primary tumor fail to disclose nonseminomatous elements, conventional therapy is justified. Current clinical evidence has indicated that hCG levels as high as 500 ng/ml may be found in association with a pure seminoma, although such an occurrence is rare.

PROGNOSTIC VALUE. Heterogeneity within nonseminomatous tumors is indicated by differences in marker levels and may parallel differences in growth rate, metastatic potential, and response to therapy and survival. The identification of factors associated with a poor prognosis or high risk provides a basis for altering therapeutic guidelines. Analyses concerning the prognostic implications of elevated marker values are conflicting. The degree of AFP or hCG elevation does appear directly proportional to the amount of tumor burden (stage and number of metastatic sites). The importance attached to the elevation of one tumor marker or another is not readily appreciated unless all potential variables are subjected to multivariate analysis. In studying interrelationships between tumor histology, tumor markers, tumor burden, and number of metastatic sites, Bosl et al. (1983) identified elevation of hCG and/or LDH and number of metastatic sites as the most important prognostic factors in determining survival in patients with germ cell tumors. Elevation of either tumor marker associated with multiple sites of metastasis implies a high risk of treatment failure despite the use of aggressive multidrug chemotherapy regimens.

TUMOR LOCALIZATION

Javadpour (1979) has utilized venous sampling techniques and the known half-life of the hCG subunits (alpha, 20 minutes; beta, 45 minutes) to determine the site responsible for persistent hCG elevations. Lange and Raghavan (1983) have explored the possibility of using marker-labeled radionuclide staging techniques for identifying the site of tumor persistence or recurrence. Inherent technical considerations limit the practicality of these procedures for everyday use.

Lactic Acid Dehydrogenase (LDH). Lactic acid dehydrogenase is a ubiquitous cellular enzyme (molecular weight 134,000) with particularly high levels detectable in smooth, cardiac, and skeletal muscles, liver, kidney, and brain. Elevation of serum LDH or one of its isoenzymes (LDH I–IV) has been reported useful in monitoring the treatment of germ cell tumors. Because of its low specificity (high false positive rate), serum LDH levels must be correlated with other clinical findings in making therapeutic decisions.

In evaluating experience with serum LDH as a tumor marker for nonseminomatous germ cell tumors, Boyle and Samuels (1977) reported a direct relationship between tumor burden and LDH levels. Increased LDH values were noted in 7 of 92 (8 per cent) patients with Stage I disease, 15 of 42 (32 per cent) with Stage II, and 57 of 70 (81 per cent) with Stage III. Recurrence rates in patients with Stages I and II disease were higher—15 of 22 (77 per cent) if pretreatment LDH values were elevated —than in those with normal levels—42 of 112 (40 per cent). The first fraction (LDH-I) as determined by agar-gel electrophoresis was responsible for LDH elevation in 25 of 29 patients studied. Skinner and Scardino (1980) found that an elevated LDH may be the sole biochemical abnormality in as many as 10 per cent of patients with persistent or recurrent nonseminomatous tumors. Serum LDH may be even more useful as a marker substance in the surveillance of patients with advanced seminoma. In reviewing their experience in patients with advanced "pure" seminoma, Stanton et al. (1983) found elevation of LDH in 21 of 26 patients (81 per cent).

Placental Alkaline Phosphatase (PLAP) and Gamma-glutamyl Transpeptidase (GGT). Placental alkaline phosphatase is a fetal isoenzyme structurally different from adult alkaline phosphatase. Small studies using recently developed enzyme-linked immunoabsorbent assays indicate that as many as 40 per cent of patients with advanced disease have elevated levels of PLAP (Javadpour, 1983). Gamma-glutamyl transpeptidase (GGT) is a hepatocellular enzyme frequently elevated in benign or neoplastic diseases of the liver. Its presence has been documented in humans in the early placenta, normal testis, and seminal fluid and in sacrococcygeal teratocarcinoma and testicular seminoma (Krishnaswamy et al., 1977). Javadpour (1983) found that one third of patients with active seminomas had elevated levels of GGT. Although the individual sensitivity of PLAP and GGT is low, simultaneous determinations revealed elevation of one or both in 24 of 30 patients (80 per cent) considered to have active disease.

Treatment

Principal treatment strategies for patients with germ cell tumor of the testis have evolved from conceptions of tumor natural history, clinical staging (assessment of the extent of disease), and effectiveness of treatment (alteration of natural history). Analysis of tumor histology and of the frequency and pattern of spread indicates some predictable features of germ cell neoplasms. Pathologic stage is a function of disease progression, and clinical staging is application of the methods available for assessment of pathologic stage. Selection of treatment alternatives is dependent upon the relative advantages and disadvantages of different regimens. Multimodal therapy has been largely credited with recent treatment successes, but the current accuracy of clinical staging, the ability to recognize failure early, and the high probability of successful treatment of such failures have prompted investigations aimed at reducing the therapeutic burden.

Each of the major treatment alternatives— surgery, irradiation and chemotherapy—has a particular but imperfectly defined role in the management of testicular tumors. As a means of establishing local control, inguinal or "radical" orchiectomy is clearly preferred. Such a procedure provides histologic diagnosis and local staging information (P-category); controls the neoplasm locally with virtually 100 per cent effectiveness, the rare exception usually being attributable to iatrogenic influence; results in the cure of patients with tumor confined to the testis; and is accomplished with minimal morbidity and virtually no mortality. Surgical excision of a retained spermatic cord remnant or of the "contaminated" scrotum is recommended following scrotal violation or tumor spillage, although additional irradiation of groin and ipsilateral hemiscrotum will suffice when pure seminoma is diagnosed. Because more than half of patients with testicular tumors present with metastatic disease, further treatment following orchiectomy is usual.

Clinical staging in addition to treatment of the retroperitoneal lymph nodes is a logical next step if no evidence of disease is detected in supradiaphragmatic or extralymphatic sites. It is now generally acknowledged that the majority of patients with large retroperitoneal metastatic deposits are best managed by chemotherapy initially. For smaller metastatic deposits, surgical excision or radiation therapy has been employed with acceptable but imperfect results. The choice of one method or the other appears to be dictated largely by the experience (and bias) of the centers treating relatively large numbers of patients.

NATURAL HISTORY

Certain aspects of the natural history of testis tumors have been detailed (see earlier). The success of treatment may be at least partially attributed to several more or less unique features in the natural history of germ cell neoplasms. These include (1) a germ cell origin, which is associated with responsiveness to irradiation and a wide range of chemotherapeutic agents; (2) remission, spontaneous or induced, into a histologically benign counterpart; (3) a generally predictable and systematic pattern of spread from the primary tumor site; (4) a rapid growth rate, which favors responses to chemotherapy or irradiation and which quickly identifies treatment successes and failures; (5) the frequent production of tumor marker substances; and (6) usual occurrence in otherwise healthy young adults capable of tolerating vigorous treatment regimens.

Histologic diagnosis is a major factor in the natural history of testicular neoplasms. Between 65 and 85 per cent of all seminomas are clinically confined to the testis, whereas 60 to 70 per cent of nonseminomas present with recognizable metastatic disease. Both the relatively low rate of spread and radiosensitivity have made radiation therapy the most widely accepted form of treatment for seminomas following inguinal orchiectomy. Radiation therapy, principally in Europe, and surgical excision, in North America, have been employed in the management of regional lymph node metastasis from nonseminomas. Each method has advantages and disadvantages relative to accuracy of clinical staging, perceived treatment successes and failures, and side effects.

SEMINOMA

Inguinal orchiectomy followed by therapeutic or adjuvant radiation therapy has been the established treatment for patients with pure seminomas. Although the role of irradiation is unquestioned, it has become apparent that survival in patients with nonseminomatous tumors now parallels or exceeds that of patients with seminomas when compared stage for stage. Recent analyses of treatment failures have exposed a number of controversial issues in the management of patients with seminomatous tumors. A reappraisal of the salient features in the natural history, staging, and treatment of these neoplasms underscores an obligation to explore integrated therapeutic regimens in some clinical settings and a reduction of treatment burden in others.

Natural History

Large series and collective reviews indicate that seminomas account for approximately 40 per cent (range 27 to 71 per cent) of all germ cell testicular tumors. Conventional treatment, consisting of inguinal orchiectomy and radiation therapy, has consistently yielded overall survival rates of greater than 85 per cent. Approximately 75 per cent of patients with seminomas present with Stage I disease, and in this group greater than 90 per cent survival is anticipated. Historical accounts indicate that patients treated by orchiectomy alone for pure seminoma clinically confined to the testis have enjoyed a 5-year survival of roughly 65 per cent (Whitmore, 1968).

Autopsy studies in patients dying with seminoma reveal that liver and lung involvement is common (roughly 75 per cent) and that bone and brain metastases are not unusual (approximately 50 per cent and 25 per cent, respectively). Roughly one third of patients with histologically pure seminoma of the testes who ultimately die of the disease are found to harbor nonseminomatous elements in metastatic sites (Dixon and Moore, 1953; Johnson, 1976; Bredael et al., 1982).

Staging

Staging evaluation by physical examination, radiographic studies, and biochemical marker determinations indicates that approximately 75 per cent of seminomas are confined to the testis at the time of clinical presentation. Between 10 and 15 per cent will harbor metastatic disease in regional retroperitoneal lymph nodes and no more than 5 to 10 per cent will have advanced to juxtaregional lymph node or visceral metastases. Data on the incidence of retroperitoneal lymph node involvement in clinical Stage I seminoma are sparse but suggest that roughly 15 per cent of patients with negative history, physical examination, and IVP have nodal metastasis documented by retroperitoneal lymphadenectomy (Whitmore, 1968). Owing to the recognized effectiveness of radiation therapy, improved staging methods, and a favorable natural history, few advocate lymph node dissection in patients with Stage I seminoma.

Following inguinal orchiectomy, determination of serum tumor markers may provide additional clinicopathologic information relative to treatment selection for patients with "pure" seminomas. Although no ideal tumor marker exists for seminoma, determination of AFP and hCG supplements the histologic characterization of all germ cell tumors. An elevated AFP virtually excludes a diagnosis of pure seminoma, in that step sectioning of the primary tumor or histologic examination of secondary deposits almost uniformly discloses nonseminomatous elements. An elevated hCG level occurs in 5 to 10 per cent of pure seminomas, although levels over 1000 ng/ml have not been reported (Javadpour, 1978). Syncytiotrophoblastic giant cell elements responsible for the production of β-hCG have been detected by immunoperoxidase techniques. A specific predictive value of an elevated β-hCG value has not been noted, and such patients apparently enjoy an excellent prognosis following orchiectomy and radiation therapy (Javadpour, 1978; Mauch et al., 1979; Peckham et al., 1981).

The system of Boden and Gibb (1951) has been modified through the years as clinical staging procedures have become more precise and have been more precisely correlated with treatment results. For the most part, extent of disease has been defined by three clinical stages: Stage I, tumor confined to the testis +/− epididymis and/or spermatic cord; Stage II, metastasis present in retroperitoneal lymph nodes only; and Stage III, spread beyond retroperitoneal lymph nodes. Currently, most workers subdivide Stage II into II-A (nonbulky retroperitoneal deposits) and II-B (palpable or radiographically bulky [>10 cm diameter] retroperitoneal disease). Others distinguish between supradiaphragmatic lymph node metastasis (Stage III) and visceral involvement (Stage IV). Table 33–7 offers a comparison between various staging systems in common use.

Histology

Three subtypes of pure seminomas have been described: "classic," anaplastic, and spermatocytic. The histologic and biochemical properties, natural history, and response to therapy of these subtypes have been characterized.

TYPICAL SEMINOMA

Typical or classic seminoma accounts for 82 to 85 per cent of all seminomas, occurring most commonly in the fourth decade but not uncommonly in the fifth and sixth decades. Seminoma rarely, if ever, occurs in the adolescent or infantile population but may occur in patients over the age of 60 years. Histologically, it is composed of islands or sheets of relatively large cells with clear cytoplasm and densely staining nuclei. Syncytiotrophoblastic elements occur in 10 to 15 per cent and lymphocytic infiltration in approximately 20 per cent. The incidence of syncytiotrophoblastic elements corresponds to the frequency of β-hCG production. The slower growth rate of seminomas may be inferred from the observation that treatment failures may become evident 2 to 10 years following apparently adequate irradiation of metastatic sites.

TABLE 33–7. COMPARISON OF CLINICAL STAGING SYSTEMS IN SEMINOMA

Clinical Extent of Disease	Walter Reed (Maier and Sulak, 1973)	M.D. Anderson (Doornbos et al., 1975)	Royal Marsden (Peckham et al., 1982)	UCLA (Crawford et al., 1983)
Testis/Cord	I-A (II−B=I-A but positive RPLND)	I	I	I
Retroperitoneal nodes	II	II-A <10 cm II-B >10 cm	II-A <2 cm II-B 2–5 cm II-C >5 cm	II-A <2 cm II-B 2–10 cm II-C >10 cm
Nodes above diaphragm	III	III	III	III
Viscera	III	III	IV	III

ANAPLASTIC SEMINOMA

This accounts for between 5 and 10 per cent of all seminomas and has an age distribution similar to that of the typical subtype. Despite its rarity, discrimination of the anaplastic seminoma is noteworthy, since up to 30 per cent of patients dying with seminoma have an anaplastic morphology. A number of features suggest that the anaplastic seminoma is a more aggressive and potentially more lethal variant of the typical seminoma. These characteristics include (1) greater mitotic activity, (2) a higher rate of local invasion, (3) an increased rate of metastatic spread, and (4) a higher rate of tumor marker production (β-hCG).

Histologically, anaplastic seminoma is typified by increased mitotic activity (three or more mitoses per high-power field), nuclear pleomorphism, and cellular anaplasia (Mostofi, 1973). Morphologically, histiocytic lymphoma and embryonal carcinoma may closely resemble anaplastic seminoma. Relative to the rate of metastasis, Percapio et al. (1979) noted in a series of 77 patients with anaplastic seminoma that 19 (25 per cent) had clinical evidence of Stage II disease. Shulman et al. (1983) reported a similar incidence of metastatic disease (29 per cent), a relatively high rate of extragonadal extension (46 per cent), and an unexpectedly high rate (36 per cent) of elevated β-hCG in 14 patients with anaplastic seminoma.

The less favorable results of treatment for patients with anaplastic seminoma may merely reflect a greater metastatic potential; there is no difference from classic seminoma when patients are treated appropriately and compared stage for stage. Analyses of treatment results indicate that inguinal orchiectomy plus radiation therapy is equally effective in controlling anaplastic and classic seminoma.

SPERMATOCYTIC SEMINOMA

This lesion is composed of cells varying in size with deeply pigmented cytoplasm and rounded nuclei containing characteristic filamentous chromatin. The cells closely resemble different phases of maturing spermatogonia. Spermatocytic seminoma accounts for 2 to 12 per cent of all seminomas, and nearly half occur in males over the age of 50 years. Bilateral tumors have been reported, but no cases have occurred in conjunction with cryptorchidism. The association of spermatocytic seminoma with other nonseminomatous tumors is rare.

The metastatic potential of spermatocytic seminoma is extremely low, and prognosis is accordingly favorable. Reviews by Thackray and Crane (1976), Weitzner (1976), Rossai (1969), and Mostofi and Price (1973) document no cases of metastatic disease. When histologic and staging evaluations have confirmed the diagnosis and the fact that disease is limited to the testis, treatment beyond inguinal orchiectomy appears unwarranted.

Treatment

The natural history and radiosensitivity of seminoma favor megavoltage irradiation in relatively modest amounts as the treatment of choice in the vast majority of patients following inguinal orchiectomy. Since the staging error may be 15 to 25 per cent for Stage I seminoma, any treatment (or lack of it) should produce a cure in 75 per cent of patients, or better. The overall effectiveness of radiation therapy is confirmed, however, in that 2500 to 3500 rad delivered over a 3-week period to the periaortic and ipsilateral inguinopelvic lymph nodes results in 5-year survival rates of 90 to 95 per cent. In Stage II disease, 5-year survival rates of roughly 80 per cent are anticipated following therapeutic retroperitoneal irradiation with or without additional treatment of the mediastinum. Deposits in supradiaphragmatic nodes or distant sites and bulky abdominal disease respond less favorably to primary radiation therapy, which by itself yields survival rates as low as 20 to 30 per cent. Recent evidence indicates that seminoma is exquisitely sensitive to various chemotherapy regimens, particularly platinum-based ones, with response rates of 60 to 100 per cent being reported.

In Stage I and limited-volume Stage II seminoma, irradiation of the periaortic and inguinopelvic lymphatics is delivered through anterior and posterior parallel-opposing fields. The periaortic field usually extends from the body of the tenth or eleventh thoracic vertebra to the sacrococcygeal junction vertically, and between the renal hila horizontally. The pelvic portal stretches from the fourth lumbar vertebra to the inguinal ligament, which includes the orchiectomy scar, and may be extended to include a retained spermatic cord remnant, contaminated scrotum, or the groin. Metastatic deposits larger than 5 cm in diameter have been electively treated with additional doses of 1000 to 2000 rad to focal portals or, alternatively, with chemotherapy. Elective supradiaphragmatic irradiation for Stage I neoplasms is not recommended. Although controversy persists

TABLE 33–8. RADIATION THERAPY IN CLINICAL STAGES I AND II SEMINOMA (DISEASE-FREE SURVIVAL)

Author	Stage I		Stage II		YEARS FOLLOW-UP (A/C)*
	No. PATIENTS	SURVIVAL (%)	No. PATIENTS	SURVIVAL (%)	
Maier and Sulak (1973)	284	97	34	91	5 (A)
Earle et al. (1973)	71	100	27	85	5 (A)
Peckham and McElwain (1974)	78	98	27	93	4 (A)
Doornbos et al. (1975)	79	94	48	77	3 (C)
Blandy (1976)	98	93	35	71	5 (A)
van der Werf–Messing (1976)	91	100	67	85	5 (A)
Batata et al. (1979)	227	88	53	62	5 (C)
Dosoretz et al. (1981)	135	97	18	92	5 (A)
Thomas et al. (1982)	338	94	86	74	5 (A)

*A = actuarial survival. C = crude survival.

regarding prophylactic treatment of the mediastinum in Stage II seminoma, current evidence favors its omission.

Patients with Stages I and II seminoma enjoy 5-year survival rates of approximately 95 per cent (88 to 100 per cent) and 78 per cent (62 to 93 per cent), respectively (Table 33–8). Analyses of treatment failure in those with Stage I disease indicate roughly equal relapse rates in the abdomen or pelvis, mediastinum or supraclavicular nodes, and visceral or multiple sites (Thomas et al., 1982). The majority of failures in Stage II occur in patients with bulky retroperitoneal metastasis. Survival in those with Stage II-A disease treated with orchiectomy and radiation therapy is approximately 87 per cent, only slightly less than rates achieved in Stage I (Doornbos et al., 1975; Thomas et al., 1982). Roughly three quarters of those with Stage II disease are designated as II-A (< 10 cm in diameter). Many radiotherapists recommend prophylactic irradiation of the mediastinum in the presence of retroperitoneal metastasis; recent data suggest, however, that relapse rates are not materially influenced by such additional treatment. Although a randomized series has not addressed this issue, no patient with II-A disease reported from the Massachusetts General and Princess Margaret Hospitals failed in sites above the diaphragm following primary abdominal irradiation (Dosoretz et al., 1981; Thomas et al., 1982).

The overall disease-free survival in patients with Stage II-B (> 10 cm in diameter) disease treated with abdominal irradiation is approximately 50 per cent (20 to 75 per cent). Treatment failure occurs with equal frequency in the abdomen or distant sites, whether or not elective mediastinal irradiation is administered. Whereas most patients who experience relapse in supradiaphragmatic sites may be salvaged with appropriate radiation therapy, a significant number die of disease. With the notable exception of the recent report by Green et al. (1983), results of irradiation in the treatment of bulky abdominal deposits have been disappointing (Table 33–9). Green et al. (1983) noted excellent responses to radiation therapy in 17 of 18 patients with metastatic disease greater than 6 cm in diameter, although five were lost to follow-up within 2 years. Considerably lower response rates to irradiation have been observed by others, prompting the use of multidrug regimens that incorporate cis-platinum, bleomycin, and vinblastine as primary therapy of bulky seminoma following orchiectomy. Preliminary re-

TABLE 33–9. RADIATION THERAPY IN CLINICAL STAGES II-B AND III SEMINOMA (DISEASE-FREE SURVIVAL)

Author	Stage II-B		Stage III	
	No. PATIENTS	SURVIVAL (%)	No. PATIENTS	SURVIVAL (%)
Maier and Sulak (1973)	—	—	18	17
Doornbos et al. (1975)	22	61	14	21
Blandy (1976)	—	—	17	12
van der Werf–Messing (1976)	21	75	30	43
Smith (1978)	7	29	14	14
Batata et al. (1979)	—	—	24	42
Dosoretz et al. (1981)	7	43	9	44
Thomas et al. (1982)	46	48	20	32
Green et al. (1983)	18	94*	—	—

*5/18 lost to follow-up < 2 years

sults indicate higher survival rates in patients treated with chemotherapy than in those treated with radiation therapy alone (Table 33–10). Response rates to chemotherapy are higher in individuals who received no prior radiation therapy, an argument for employing the former as primary therapy following orchiectomy.

Similarly disappointing results have been documented in Stage III seminoma following radiation therapy, with 5-year survival rates as low as 20 to 30 per cent (Smith, 1978; Caldwell et al., 1980). Experience with single-drug treatment of metastatic seminoma has identified the activity of alkylating agents, such as phenylalanine mustard, chlorambucil, and cyclophosphamide (Yagoda and Vugrin, 1979). Recent evidence indicates that seminomas are even more sensitive than nonseminomas to platinum-based chemotherapy regimens. Since approximately one third of patients dying with seminoma harbor relatively radioresistant but chemosensitive nonseminomatous elements at autopsy, initial combination chemotherapy of disseminated seminoma appears appropriate. Over 90 per cent of patients who present with Stage III disease or recurrent disease following radiation therapy will achieve a complete response to chemotherapy alone, and approximately 90 per cent of the responders have remained free of disease during short-term follow-up of 17 to 48 months (see Table 33–10).

Following inguinal orchiectomy the role of surgical excision is limited. It has been suggested that retroperitoneal lymph node dissection may be preferable for patients with anaplastic seminoma or an elevated β-hCG, but at present clear evidence for such an approach is lacking. Surgery does play an occasional role in the management of patients with renal anomalies (horseshoe or ipsilateral pelvic kidney), in those with a second testicular primary tumor, or in those who fail or cannot tolerate irradiation and systemic chemotherapy. Surgical excision of residual masses following chemocytoreduction of bulky metastatic seminoma confers no clear therapeutic advantage over chemotherapy alone (Morse et al., 1983).

Irradiation and chemotherapy are highly effective against seminomatous testis tumors. The usually favorable natural history of seminomas portends a minimal therapeutic burden, justifying radiation therapy as the mainstay of treatment following orchiectomy in most patients. Platinum-based chemotherapy regimens are currently favored as initial treatment for advanced seminomas, whereas surgery is reserved for treatment failures and other selected and rare situations. While the question of surveillance following orchiectomy only in Stage I seminoma is currently being studied (Oliver, 1984), the excellent results and acceptable toxicity of low-dose retroperitoneal irradiation make this the recommended treatment.

NONSEMINOMA

Tumors designated as "nonseminoma" (NSGCTT) include those that are histologically composed of embryonal carcinoma, teratoma, choriocarcinoma, and yolk sac elements alone or in various combinations. Tumors containing both seminomatous and nonseminomatous elements are generally regarded as nonseminomas, a consideration that may have practical bearing upon treatment selection. Aside from morphologic differences, distinctions between seminoma and nonseminoma are made relative to natural behavior, clinical staging, and treatment strategies.

Natural History

Clinical evidence is strong that nonseminomas follow a potentially less favorable natural history than do pure seminomas. Depending to

TABLE 33–10. PRIMARY CHEMOTHERAPY FOR ADVANCED SEMINOMA

Author	Regimen	No. Patients	Prior Irradiation No. (%)	CR + PR	NED	Follow-up (mos.)
Einhorn and Williams (1980)	PVB (A)	19	13 (68)	12 + 7	11 (58)	19
Vugrin et al. (1981)*	DDP + Cy	9	6 (67)	5 + 4	7 (78)	19
Morse et al. (1983)*	VAB VI	22	8 (38)	9 + 10	17 (77)	17
Wajsman et al. (1983)	DDP + VBPr/ VP-16	12	4 (33)	12	12 (100)	—
Crawford et al. (1983)†	VAC	16	1 (7)	15	15 (94)	48

*Both series contain patients with extragonadal primary tumors and patients who received additional surgery +/− radiation therapy.

†15/16 patients received radiation therapy following chemotherapy.

some degree upon referral patterns and staging criteria, 50 to 70 per cent of patients with nonseminoma, but only 20 to 30 per cent of those with seminoma, will present with metastatic disease at the time of diagnosis. The first echelon of spread for all germ cell tumors is most commonly the retroperitoneal lymph nodes. Evidence for this generalization stems from post-mortem and clinical experiences. Autopsy studies indicate that roughly three quarters of patients dying with germ cell tumors have a concomitant or prior history of retroperitoneal nodal and parenchymal metastases despite therapeutic retroperitoneal irradiation or lymphadenectomy. After retroperitoneal lymph nodes, lung metastasis is the next most common site of spread. This observation is evident from autopsy studies and from the follow-up of patients after lymph node dissection, in that lung metastasis represents the most frequently recognized site of treatment failure regardless of lymph node status. Next in frequency of spread are liver, brain, bone, and kidney, although almost any site may be involved. Table 33–11 illustrates the MSKCC experience relative to the sites and frequency of metastatic disease in 144 patients dying with disseminated testis cancer (16 with seminomas, 128 with nonseminomas).

Currently, overall cure rates in patients with nonseminoma or seminoma appear similar. Following surgical excision or irradiation of clinically negative nodes, survival is roughly equivalent (90 to 95 per cent or greater). Retroperitoneal lymph node dissection (RPLND) is not currently utilized as a treatment for Stage II seminoma, largely owing to the demonstrated success of irradiation. In selected patients with limited nodal disease from NSGCTT, surgical excision and radiation therapy are comparably effective, whereas selected patients with more advanced nodal metastasis appear to be more favorably treated by surgery. Both seminoma and nonseminoma are exquisitely sensitive to a wide range of chemotherapy agents (see further on). Consideration of the latter has minimized, to some extent, differences in treatment philosophy espoused by surgical and radiation oncologists.

Clinical Staging

The natural history and frequency of disease dissemination favor the accurate clinical staging of nonseminomatous tumors. The rapid development of precise imaging techniques and tumor-indexing substances frequently produced by nonseminomas also foster staging accuracy (see earlier). The principal differences between staging systems for seminomas and nonseminomas relate to the roles of surgical lymph node sampling and serum tumor markers. The staging system of Boden and Gibb has been modified to identify subsets of patients with different extent of metastasis (see Table 33–12). For most purposes in this discussion, the simple stratification proposed by Boden and Gibb will suffice.

Histology

Embryonal carcinoma is generally discovered as a small, rounded but irregular mass invading the tunica vaginalis and not infrequently involving contiguous cord structures. The cut surface reveals a variegated, grayish white, fleshy tumor, often with areas of necrosis or hemorrhage and a poorly defined capsule. The typical histologic appearance is that of distinctly malignant epithelioid cells arranged in glands or tubules. The cell borders are usually indistinct, the cytoplasm pale or vacuolated, and the nuclei rounded with coarse chromatin and one or more large nucleoli. Pleomorphism, mitotic figures, and giant cells are features common to these highly malignant tumors.

Pure choriocarcinoma may occur as a palpable nodule, the size depending upon the extent of local hemorrhage. Patients with pure choriocarcinoma may present with evidence of advanced distant metastasis and what seems a paradoxically small intratesticular lesion that may not distort the normal testicular size or shape. Central hemorrhage with viable grayish white tumor at the periphery may be seen on the cut surface if the lesion can be demonstrated

TABLE 33–11. Most Common Sites and Frequency of Distant Metastasis (Excluding Lymph Nodes)

Site	Number of Patients	Per Cent
Lungs	129/144	89
Liver	106/144	73
Brain	38/120	31
Bone	43/144	30
Kidney	43/144	30
Adrenal	42/144	29
GI tract	39/144	27
Spleen	19/144	13
Vena cava	16/144	11

Modified from Bredael J. J., et al.: Cancer, *50*:548, 1982.

grossly. Microscopically, two distinct and appropriately oriented cell types must be demonstrated to satisfy the histologic diagnosis of choriocarcinoma—syncytiotrophoblasts and cytotrophoblasts. The syncytiotrophoblasts may be large multinucleated cells containing abundant, often vacuolated, eosinophilic cytoplasm and large, hyperchromatic, irregular nuclei. Less commonly, the syncytial elements may be spindle-shaped and contain one large dark-staining nucleus. The cytotrophoblasts are closely packed, intermediate-sized, uniform cells with a distinct cell border, clear cytoplasm, and a single vesicular nucleus.

Teratoma contains more than one germ cell layer in various stages of maturation and differentiation. "Mature" elements resemble benign structures derived from normal ectoderm, entoderm, and mesoderm. "Immature" teratoma consists of undifferentiated primitive tissues from each of the three germ cell layers. Grossly the tumors are usually large, lobulated, and nonhomogeneous in consistency. The cut surface may reveal variably sized cysts containing gelatinous, mucinous, or hyalinized material interspersed with islands of solid tissue often containing cartilage or bone. Histologically the cysts may be lined by squamous, cuboidal, columnar, or transitional epithelium; the solid component may contain any combination of cartilage; bone; intestinal, pancreatic, or liver tissue; smooth or skeletal muscle; and neural or connective tissue elements. On rare occasions, malignant changes may be recognized in such differentiated tissues, justifying the designation "malignant teratoma."

Yolk sac tumor is the most common testis tumor of infants and children. In adults it occurs most frequently in combination with other histologic types and is presumably responsible for the production of AFP. The terms *entodermal sinus tumor, adenocarcinoma of the infantile testis, juvenile embryonal carcinoma,* and *orchioblastoma* are used synonymously. In its pure form the lesion has a homogeneous yellowish, mucinous appearance. Microscopically the tumor is composed of epithelioid cells that form glandular and ductal structures arranged in columns, papillary projections, or solid islands within a primitive mesenchymal stroma. The individual epithelial tumor cells may be columnar, cuboidal, or flat, with poorly defined cell borders and vacuolated cytoplasm containing glycogen and fat. The large, irregularly shaped nuclei contain one or more prominent nucleoli and variable amounts of chromatin. Embryoid bodies, a common finding in yolk sac tumors,

resemble 1- to 2-week-old embryos. These ovoid structures, commonly measuring less than 1 mm in diameter, consist of a cavity surrounded by loose mesenchyme containing syncytiotrophoblasts and cytotrophoblasts.

In classifying over 6000 testis tumors, Mostofi (1973) found that in roughly 40 per cent, more than one histologic pattern was identified. Because of its frequent occurrence (24 per cent of testis tumors), the combination of teratoma and embryonal carcinoma, termed "teratocarcinoma," is usually classified as a specific entity. Teratocarcinomas are frequently large and frequently disseminated. Metastatic deposits associated with teratomas usually contain embryonal carcinoma (80 per cent) and, less frequently, teratoma or choriocarcinoma. The bisected tumor exhibits cysts, typical of teratoma, within a solid, sometimes hemorrhagic stroma containing embryonal elements.

The pluripotential nature of germ cell tumors, and in particular nonseminomatous tumors, is evident from the varied histologic patterns of metastasis, over half of which display different morphologies in primary versus metastatic sites, although pure choriocarcinoma invariably spreads unaltered. While post-mortem studies indicate that 30 to 45 per cent of patients dying with seminoma harbor nonseminomatous metastases, the converse is rarely documented (see earlier).

Treatment

World War II greatly influenced the treatment of germ cell testis tumors by exposing a large number of patients to the collaborative efforts of surgeons, radiation therapists, and pathologists in referral centers. Among these centers were the Walter Reed Army Hospital in the United States and the Royal Marsden and London Hospitals in the United Kingdom. The early experiences of Lewis (1948) and Kimbrough and Cook (1953) fostered inguinal orchiectomy plus retroperitoneal lymphadenectomy as the preferred locoregional treatment for patients with testis tumors in North America. Oncologists in Europe, conversely, have utilized radiation therapy as the primary means for sterilizing nodal deposits, reserving surgical excision for residual tumor masses. While controversy still exists over the preferred treatment for nodal metastasis, surgeons and radiotherapists agree that the advent of effective chemotherapy has minimized important differences in their respective treatment philosophies. The role of inguinal orchiectomy remains unchallenged. This procedure is accomplished with little morbidity and no mortality, while providing (1) histologic diagnosis and pathologic P-category, (2) local control with virtual 100 per cent effectiveness, and (3) cure of some patients by such means alone (Whitmore, 1970).

The accuracy of clinical staging, widely accepted as the most important determinant in treatment selection, is dependent upon the extent and volume of tumor burden as well as sensitivity and specificity of available staging techniques. Three characteristics of NSGCTT favorably influence clinical staging accuracy and subsequent treatment following orchiectomy: (1) With the exception of pure choriocarcinoma, these tumors generally spread to the retroperitoneal lymph nodes before disseminating to other less assessable sites, such as liver, bone, and brain. (2) The most common site of metastasis following spread to the retroperitoneum is the lung, conveniently monitored by plain radiographs. (3) Frequent production of β-hCG or AFP, or both, is measurable in the serum.

STAGE I (TUMOR CONFINED TO THE TESTIS)

Disease control, morbidity and mortality of treatment, quality of life following treatment, cost effectiveness, treatment availability, and patient compliance should be considered in evaluating the results of any treatment. Of these parameters, only the ability to control the disease and the morbidity and mortality of treatment can be quantified from the data available.

Surgical Treatment. Anatomic studies at the turn of the century by Most (1898) and Cuneo (1901) and later work by Jamieson and Dobson (1910) and Rouviere (1938) demonstrated the primary lymphatic drainage of the testis in the retroperitoneum. Since that time, surgeons and radiotherapists have concentrated upon regional control after establishing local control by orchiectomy. This is an important consideration in that approximately 75 per cent of patients present with disease clinically limited either to the testis (35 per cent) or to the testis plus retroperitoneal lymph nodes (40 per cent). A thorough excision with pathologic examination of the retroperitoneal lymph nodes remains the epitome of staging. Despite the increasing accuracy of noninvasive staging techniques, comparisons between clinical and pathologic categories indicate that 10 to 20 per cent of patients with clinical Stage I disease are understaged. Among patients with pathologically confirmed Stage I disease, 80 to 100 per cent are cured (Table 33–12).

Roughly 90 per cent of patients who relapse will do so within the first 2 years after diagnosis. In patients surgically staged, approximately 10 to 15 per cent will experience recurrent disease, most frequently in the chest. This suggests either a surgical or pathologic error or a hematogenous spread that preceded lymphatic dissemination. Retroperitoneal recurrences have been clinically recognized in less than 5 per cent of patients with previously negative lymph node dissections. (Such a low rate of local recurrence may in part reflect the lack of relevant autopsy data.) The majority of relapsing patients can be saved by additional treatment. Chemotherapy for systemic or locoregional recurrence, reserving surgical excision for persistent disease, is an appropriate strategy. A 3-year disease-free survival was observed in 165 of 167 (99 per cent) patients assembled from three different institutions and

TABLE 33–12. Two- to Five-Year Survival after Orchiectomy and RPLND in Pathologic Stage I NSGCTT

Author	NED (Number)	(Per Cent)	Years Follow-Up
Whitmore (1970)	50/58	86	5
Walsh et al. (1971)	24/25	96	3
Bradfield et al. (1973)	28/40	70	3
Staubitz et al. (1974)	42/45	93	3
Johnson et al. (1976)	65/72	90	5
Skinner (1976)*	39/43	91	2
Donohue et al. (1978)	27/30	90	3
Fraley et al. (1979)	28/28	100	2
Bredael et al. (1983)†	126/138	91	3
Total	429/479	*Average* 90	

*Adjuvant actinomycin D
†30 patients received adjuvant chemotherapy

treated by RPLND, which was followed by adjuvant or salvage chemotherapy (Skinner, 1983).

Verification of Stage I status is important in that such patients may be followed expectantly if kept under close surveillance. Regardless of stage, all patients who have completed treatment should be followed at monthly intervals during the first year and at bimonthly intervals during the second year. The need for long-term surveillance is emphasized by reports indicating that late relapses, although rare, do occur. Such a phenomenon may become more prevalent in the future, since current treatments may be "responsible" for delaying an otherwise early relapse (Terebelo et al., 1983).

Retroperitoneal lymph node dissection (RPLND) is a major operative procedure, lasting generally between 3 and 6 hours, with negligible mortality and acceptably low morbidity. Reports from major institutions indicate that the mortality rate in patients with Stage I and nonbulky Stage II disease is less than 1 per cent. Morbidity rates ranging from 5 to 35 per cent have been reported, the more common complications being wound infection, atelectasis, pneumonitis, and ileus. Less frequently, lymphocele, chylous ascites, thrombophlebitis, pulmonary embolism, wound dehiscence, pancreatitis, enterocutaneous fistula, and vascular injury have been reported (Whitmore, 1982a and b) (see chapter 83).

A major drawback of retroperitoneal lymphadenectomy is the disruption of normal seminal emission, which results from the interruption of sympathetic nerve pathways to the ejaculatory ducts and seminal vesicles. The precise frequency of this complication remains poorly documented, but it seems likely (75 per cent) following the usual surgical excision; modifications in surgical technique may reduce this side effect. Erectile function, ejaculatory sensation, and orgasm are not disturbed by surgery, but fertility is lost. Sympathomimetic drugs have occasionally restored seminal emission following surgery, while preoperative semen cryopreservation offers another but uncertain alternative (Bracken and Johnson, 1976; Kedia et al., 1977). The argument against surgery posed by the resultant loss of seminal emission appears somewhat weakened by recent studies of gonadal function in men with testis tumors following unilateral orchiectomy (Berthelsen and Skakkebaek, 1983). Impaired gonadal function was ascribed not only to orchiectomy but also to pre-existing defects of spermatogenesis in the remaining testis and to elevated hCG levels.

Clinical stage and histology did not independently influence semen or hormonal analyses or morphology of the non–tumor bearing testis.

Radiation Therapy. Megavoltage irradiation has been available since the 1950's and in common use since the 1960's, by which time RPLND had already become established, especially in the United States. As a form of treatment for Stages I and II seminoma, radiation therapy has been adopted worldwide. Irradiation of the retroperitoneum in patients with clinical Stage I NSGCTT remains accepted practice in many treatment centers outside North America. The main objections to the use of retroperitoneal lymph node irradiation have been the inaccuracy of clinical staging of the retroperitoneal lymph nodes; the resultant lack of survival data that could be reasonably compared with surgical data; and the concern that, in the event of postirradiation relapse, the prior irradiation might preclude adequate chemotherapy or surgical excision. Modern staging techniques have reduced the falsely negative staging error in clinical Stage I to approximately 20 per cent. In patients with clinical Stage I disease subjected to RPLND, 10 to 15 per cent will harbor undetected nodal metastasis and another 5 to 10 per cent will relapse following surgery, almost always in extranodal sites. The tumoricidal dose for NSGCTT ranges between 4000 and 5000 rad, far in excess of that required to sterilize seminoma. A dose of 4000 to 4500 rad delivered in 4 to 5 weeks to the para-aortic and ipsilateral pelvic lymph nodes is the recommended radiation standard in clinical Stage I NSGCTT. The long-term complications of para-aortic irradiation include radiation enteritis, bowel obstruction, and bone marrow suppression, with a reported frequency of between 5 and 10 per cent. Secondary malignancy has been reported following abdominal radiation therapy for Hodgkin's disease, but such reports following treatment for testis tumors are anecdotal.

The overall success rate of radiation therapy in the treatment of clinical Stage I NSGCTT in terms of 5-year survival is between 80 and 95 per cent when chemotherapy is used to treat relapses (Table 33–13). Relapse rates following radiation therapy for clinical Stage I are as high as 24 per cent (14/59), 3 per cent within the irradiated volume and 21 per cent outside (Raghavan et al., 1982). Allowing for the falsely negative staging error of approximately 10 to 20 per cent, these figures compare favorably with those obtained by surgical excision of the retroperitoneal nodes.

Surveillance. In patients whose disease is

TABLE 33–13. SURVIVAL AFTER ORCHIECTOMY AND RADIOTHERAPY
FOR CLINICAL STAGES I AND II NSGCTT (2–5 YEARS)

Author	Stage I	Stage II	Total
Battermann et al. (1973)	24/30 (80%)	6/19 (32%)	30/49 (61%)
Tyrrell and Peckham (1976)	73/88 (84%)	14/29 (48%)	87/117 (74%)
van der Werf–Messing (1976)*	26/29 (90%)	16/35 (46%)	42/64 (66%)
Maier and Mittemeyer (1977)	25/29 (86%)	9/11 (82%)	34/40 (85%)
Peckham et al. (1981)†	37/39 (95%)	17/21 (81%)	54/60 (90%)
Blandy et al. (1983)	125/162 (77%)	—	125/162 (77%)
Total	310/377 (82%)	62/115 (54%)	372/492 (76%)

*Extrapolated from actuarial tables.

†Includes patients treated successfully for relapse and patients in Stage II treated primarily with preirradiation chemotherapy.

truly confined to the testis, orchiectomy alone should yield survival results equal to therapeutic strategies that also incorporate treatment of the para-aortic region. In such cases, surgical removal or irradiation of pathologically negative lymph nodes is obviously unnecessary. Approximately 10 per cent of patients with surgical Stage I and 20 per cent of patients with clinical Stage I disease, respectively, relapse following RPLND or radiation therapy. Clinical experience has shown that chemotherapy can salvage up to 90 per cent of the latter group. The overall results of treatment in clinical Stage I NSGCTT are thus approaching 100 per cent with either retroperitoneal lymphadenectomy or retroperitoneal irradiation as initial treatment. An appropriate consideration is to attempt a reduction of the therapeutic burden while maintaining these excellent results. The factors that support the feasibility of studying this question include the following: (1) RPLND or irradiation constitutes a therapeutic risk; (2) current clinical staging methods are 80 to 90 per cent accurate in identifying metastatic disease; (3) the natural history of NSGCTT favors early detection of failures if surveillance is appropriate; and (4) available multimodal therapy is highly effective in controlling metastasis.

Practices of case selection and surveillance in reported series have varied, but the following policies were instituted in the MSKCC trial: (1) Only those patients with negative physical examination, chest x-ray, pedal lymphangiogram (LAG), abdominal and pelvic computed tomography (CT), intravenous pyelogram, and post-orchiectomy serum markers (hCG, AFP, LDH) are entered; (2) patients with a prior history of contralateral testis tumor or previous ipsilateral inguinal or scrotal surgery are excluded; (3) patients with a scrotal violation or tumor involving the spermatic cord are excluded; and

(4) only patients capable of monthly follow-up are eligible. Physical examination, chest x-ray, and serum tumor markers are repeated monthly during the first year and bimonthly during the second year of follow-up. Abdominal CT scans are obtained at 3-month intervals during the first year and at 6-month intervals during the second year. Plain abdominal films are used to monitor the initial LAG, which is repeated during the sixth month of surveillance.

The results of four reported studies are shown in Table 33–14. Median duration of follow-up is short, ranging from 10 to 23 months, but the preliminary results indicate that 80 per cent of patients require no further treatment following orchiectomy alone in properly selected cases of Stage I NSGCTT. In those patients relapsing during surveillance, 40 of 41 were salvaged with appropriate therapy. The majority of patients relapsing do so within the first year of follow-up; most frequently, patients relapse in the retroperitoneal lymph nodes and the remainder develop lung metastasis. The report of Sturgeon et al. (1983) indicates an alarmingly high relapse rate of 40 per cent; to what extent this can be attributed to selection factors remains unquantified. From the early MSKCC experience, it has become evident that retroperitoneal CT scans should be carried out more frequently during the initial year of follow-up than was called for in the original protocol.

The overall preliminary data from these selected series are encouraging. Of 194 patients entered on protocol, 153 remain NED (no evidence of disease) following orchiectomy alone, and 40 of 41 relapsed patients have achieved complete remission with appropriate further therapy. The short duration of follow-up and the relatively small numbers of patients, however, expose such results to rightful criticism. It is currently inadvisable to pursue such man-

TABLE 33–14. ORCHIECTOMY ALONE FOR STAGE I NONSEMINOMATOUS GERM CELL TUMORS

Author	Total No. Patients	Patients NED	Median Follow-up (mos.)	Patients Relapsing	Complete Remission	Median Duration CR (mos.)
Peckham (1983)	84	68 (81%)	22	16 (19%)	16/16	21
Sturgeon (1983)	20	12 (60%)	14	8 (40%)	8/8	—
Sogani (1984)	59	47 (80%)	23	12 (20%)	11/12	11
Johnson (1984)	31	26 (84%)	10	5 (16%)	5/5	15
Total	194	153 (80%)		41 (20%)	40/41 (98%)	

agement outside the conditions of a carefully planned clinical trial.

STAGE II (SPREAD TO RETROPERITONEAL LYMPH NODES)

Surgical Treatment. The potential advantages of retroperitoneal lymph node dissection in the treatment of testis cancer stem from the fact that retroperitoneal deposits are usually the first and frequently the sole evidence of extragonadal spread. Such therapy is capable of eradicating resectable disease in over half of patients with Stage II tumors. Analysis of different surgical experiences reveals that several uncontrolled variables exist. These include the clinical staging accuracy, the extent and quality of node dissection, the criteria of surgical resectability, the pathologic examination of surgical specimen, and the use of adjuvant or "salvage" (for recurrent disease) chemotherapy. The failure to analyze treatment results in terms of clinical stage invalidates comparisons between surgical and radiotherapy series.

A variety of surgical approaches to retroperitoneal lymphadenectomy have been explored. Thoracoabdominal and midline transperitoneal exposures are in common use today. The usual distribution of nodal metastasis as determined by anatomic studies, surgical exploration, and lymphangiography extends from the superior border of the renal vessels around the aorta and vena cava to either ureter laterally and along the common iliac vessels to just beyond their bifurcations. The extent of lymph node dissection is individualized from the following considerations: (1) serum tumor marker levels after orchiectomy, (2) lymphangiographic or abdominal CT interpretations, and (3) findings at laparotomy. Positive markers following orchiectomy or positive radiographic studies indicate the need for a complete bilateral lymphadenectomy. Clinical experience has shown that surgical exploration alone is more than 90 per cent accurate in assessing the presence or absence of lymph node metastasis. When suspicious lymph nodes are encountered at laparotomy, a complete bilateral lymphadenectomy is recommended. Suprarenal nodal metastasis occurs infrequently in the absence of advanced infrarenal disease. Routine suprahilar lymph node dissection in the absence of palpable metastasis in this region has not demonstrably improved local control rates. When serum markers, lymphangiogram and CT scan, and laparotomy are collectively negative, a modified bilateral dissection may be performed.

Since first popularized by Lewis (1948), RPLND has been used with varying success to treat regional metastasis from testis cancer. Selected results from recent experiences, summarized in Table 33–15, indicate that surgical excision can cure roughly half of patients with

TABLE 33–15. TWO- TO FIVE-YEAR SURVIVAL AFTER ORCHIECTOMY AND RPLND IN PATHOLOGIC STAGE II

Author	NED		Years of Follow-up
	NUMBER	PER CENT	
Whitmore (1970)	18/41	44	5
Bradfield et al. (1973)	11/34	32	3
Skinner (1976)*	28/36	78	2
Donohue (1977)	24/28	86	3
Hussey (1979)	16/41	39	3
Fraley et al. (1979)	21/26	81	2
Staubitz (1979)	15/27	56	3
Total	133/233	*Average* 57	

*Adjuvant chemotherapy

TABLE 33–16. PATHOLOGIC STAGING OF NSGCTT

Stage	Description of Retroperitoneal Nodes
I	Negative
II	Positive
N-1	Microscopic involvement
N-2	Nodes grossly involved
A	< 5 nodes involved with none > 2 cm diameter
B	> 5 nodes involved and/or nodes > 2 cm diameter
N-3	Extranodal extension (gross or microscopic), resectable
N-4	Incompletely resected/unresectable disease

spread limited to retroperitoneal lymph nodes. The data generally exclude those with unresectable tumors and include a few who may have received some form of adjuvant chemotherapy. Although the results are to some degree biased by such factors, RPLND is certainly capable of controlling regional node metastasis in selected patients. The majority of surgical series furnish little information relating the frequency of relapse and curability to the size, number, site, or histology of the nodal metastasis. Surgicopathologic correlation according to criteria in Table 33–16 may provide some relevant data.

The high relapse and unresectability rates in patients with bulky retroperitoneal disease, coupled with the demonstrated effectiveness of multidrug regimens in treating disseminated cancer, prompted the use of chemotherapy as initial therapy for those with advanced nodal or pulmonary metastases during the mid-1970's. Almost simultaneously, advances in clinical staging identified patients who might benefit from such a strategy. Because chemotherapy was so effective in treating disseminated disease, it appeared prudent to redefine the role of surgery following primary chemotherapy. This question was approached by systematically administering combination-drug therapy and then

subjecting patients to surgical excision of residual disease, if such were judged feasible. The results from different institutions using varying drug combinations and techniques of lymphadenectomy indicated that chemotherapy is capable of sterilizing bulky disease, with resultant tumor necrosis or fibrosis, in roughly one third of cases. Another one third, however, harbored residual malignant elements and the remainder, teratoma (Table 33–17). Survival was excellent in patients with necrotic or fibrosed tumor and in those with teratoma or completely resected viable cancer. Complete resection was rarely feasible in patients with persistently elevated serum markers following chemotherapy. Negative post-treatment serum markers did not exclude the possible existence of a histologically viable cancer.

The recognition of teratoma within surgically excised residual masses following combination chemotherapy for advanced disease is a relatively recent phenomenon (Merrin et al., 1975; Hong et al., 1977). The surgical removal of benign "mature" or "immature" teratoma should be accomplished for five reasons: (1) preoperative studies cannot rule out the possibility of residual malignancy; (2) pathologic examination may not detect small malignant foci within an apparently benign mass; (3) expansion of benign solid and cystic teratomatous elements may compromise vital organ function; (4) teratoma may exist as or degenerate into a malignant sarcomatous form; and (5) chemotherapy and radiation therapy are ineffective against benign or malignant teratoma.

Roughly one third of patients with advanced NSGCTT who have normal serum tumor markers following preoperative cytoreductive chemotherapy have a malignant component within the excised residual tissues (Einhorn et al., 1981a; Vugrin et al., 1981d). Although pathologic techniques vary, it is unlikely that step-sectioning is routine in the assessment of

TABLE 33–17. PATHOLOGIC EXAMINATION OF SURGICAL SPECIMENS FOLLOWING PRIMARY CHEMOTHERAPY

Author	Total Patients	Surgical Resections	Unresectable	Fibrosis	Teratoma	Carcinoma
Einhorn et al. (1981)	57	62		15	25	22
Vugrin et al. (1981)	48*	37	11	18	8	11
Bracken et al. (1983)	45†	45		22	10	12
Total	150	144		55/143 (38%)	43/143 (30%)	45/143 (31%)

*Includes nine patients with elevated serum tumor markers prior to surgery.

†Includes 22 patients with apparent complete response to chemotherapy; patients with elevated markers after chemotherapy excluded; one patient had neurofibroma (= excluded from denominator).

all resected material, implying that a malignant element may be missed by sampling error. Logothetis et al. (1982) described the "growing teratoma syndrome" after observing the enlargement of teratomatous deposits during or following chemotherapy. While the early recognition and resection of teratoma have been accompanied by an excellent prognosis, untreated disease may possess a lethal potential by virtue of continued local growth or from putative subsequent malignant transformation of histologically benign components. These considerations, together with the inability of current radiographic techniques to distinguish between teratoma and carcinoma and the uncertain natural history of untreated teratoma, warrant surgical resection of residual masses following chemocytoreduction. Although irradiation may have favorable effects in such a setting, relevant pathologic data are wanting.

Surgical excision of residual nodal tissue or extranodal masses following treatment with multidrug chemotherapy is recommended. Irradiation of radiographically defined residual sites is an alternative approach. If chemotherapy is given initially for pulmonary metastasis alone (when pretreatment studies fail to demonstrate significant retroperitoneal disease) and there is no serologic or radiographic evidence of neoplasm after therapy, surveillance without RPLND may be undertaken but with an apparently substantial risk.

Radiation Therapy. The value of retroperitoneal irradiation in the management of clinical Stage II NSGCTT remains controversial. Several factors invalidate comparisons between most surgical and radiation series, including: (1) the lack of well-designed randomized studies; (2) differences in histologic and staging classifications; (3) uncertain influences of prior therapy or pretreatment selection; and (4) unquantified influences of therapy administered for relapses. Radiation therapy series are unfavorably influenced by the inclusion of patients with surgically unresectable nodal deposits. Contemporary surgical and radiation series are both prejudiced by the frequent administration of adjuvant chemotherapy. The marked effectiveness of multidrug regimens negates some of the biases between such series and overrides the therapeutic value of either approach.

Acknowledging the limitations of such comparisons, it seems apparent that megavoltage irradiation is capable of controlling retroperitoneal metastasis in roughly one half of patients with Stage II NSGCTT (see Table 33–13). In reviewing their experience at the Royal Marsden

Hospital, Tyrrell and Peckham (1976) noted that small nodal volumes (<2 cm) responded favorably to radiation therapy, with 12 of 14 (86 per cent) patients maintaining disease-free status; patients with larger metastasis (>2 cm) relapsed frequently, however, with only 5 of 15 remaining disease-free. The majority of relapses (12 of 15, or 80 per cent) occurred within the irradiated volume. In another study, Klein and Maier (1977) appraised the effect of radiation therapy by pathologic examination of lymph nodes excised from patients in clinical Stage II after preoperative irradiation. Of 49 patients subjected to RPLND after receiving 2500 to 3000 rad in 3 weeks before surgery, 26 (53 per cent) harbored persistent tumor; in 57 not given preoperative radiotherapy, 52 (91 per cent) had positive retroperitoneal nodes. Hussey (1981) collected data that circumstantially confirmed the salutary effect of retroperitoneal irradiation on limited nodal disease. He also reviewed the results of preoperative irradiation with RPLND and concluded that integrated treatment was superior to either primary radiotherapy or lymphadenectomy alone in disease control.

The evolution of effective multidrug regimens has changed the attitudes of both radiation and surgical oncologists. Many radiotherapists now recommend the use of chemotherapy as initial treatment for (1) nodal metastasis clinically judged larger than 2 cm in diameter, (2) supradiaphragmatic node involvement, and (3) extralymphatic spread. Supplementary irradiation is then delivered to initially large nodal deposits, with surgical excision being reserved for selected patients with residual masses (Peckham, 1979). The main drawback of such an approach is that if relapse occurs following radiation therapy for small-volume disease or following an integrated scheme, the effectiveness of chemotherapy may be undermined by cumulative myelosuppression. Furthermore, surgical treatment of focally persistent disease may be complicated by prior irradiation.

STAGE III

Primary Chemotherapy. Testis cancer has become the most curable solid tumor in man, largely owing to the development of effective combination chemotherapy programs during the last two decades. Multidrug regimens incorporating cisplatin now cure, sometimes with the help of adjuvant surgery, 70 to 80 per cent of patients with Stage III disease. Despite these impressive results, one current approach among medical oncologists is to explore even more aggressive treatments for high-risk patients and to reduce the therapeutic burden of established programs for low-risk individuals. A retrospective account of chemotherapeutic successes and failures provides logical direction for the development of such future treatment strategies.

Li et al. (1960), drawing on experience with combined drug therapy for tuberculosis, reported three complete remissions (CR) in 23 patients treated with their own "triple therapy" (chlorambucil, methotrexate, and actinomycin D) for disseminated testis cancer. MacKenzie (1966) subsequently reviewed the MSKCC experience in 154 patients with advanced disease and concluded that actinomycin D was effective treatment for metastatic NSGCTT, whether given alone or in combination with other agents. Vinblastine and bleomycin entered clinical trials in the late 1960's. Samuels and Howe (1970) reported four CR's in 21 patients with advanced disease using vinblastine either alone or with melphalan. The European Organization for Research on the Treatment of Cancer (EORTC) in 1970 and Yagoda et al. in 1972 reported the activity of bleomycin in NSGCTT. In 1972, investigators at MSKCC inaugurated the combination of vinblastine, actinomycin D, and bleomycin (VAB-1), later reporting partial remission (PR) in 19 per cent and CR in 19 per cent (Wittes et al., 1976).

The report by Higby et al. (1974), indicating the activity of cisplatin, heralded the arrival of the single most important drug yet identified against NSGCTT. The potential for nephrotoxicity and ototoxicity initially limited the use of cis–platinum, although Higby et al. reported that doses of 20 mg/m^2 could be given safely with adequate hydration. Hayes et al. (1977) were to note later that doses of 120 mg/m^2 could be administered with concomitant hydration and mannitol-induced diuresis. In 1974, VAB-2, which added cisplatin to VAB-1 (vinblastine, actinomycin D, bleomycin by continuous infusion), and the Indiana University PVB regimen (cisplatin, vinblastine, bleomycin, bacillus Calmette-Guérin by scarification) were launched. Both the VAB-2 and the PVB programs incorporated 2-year periods of "maintenance" therapy in patients who had fully responded to the induction phases of the regimen. In a preliminary report by Einhorn and Donohue (1977a), 16 CR's and 4 PR's were noted in 21 patients treated with PVB; Cheng et al. (1978) reported 50 per cent CR and 34 per cent PR rates with VAB-2 in patients followed for at least 2 years. Both schedules were complicated by moderately severe but tolerable side effects, most notably myelosuppression. Following the completion of VAB-2 chemotherapy, a number of patients were subjected to second-look surgical procedures in efforts to salvage some of the clinical PR's, establishing the utility of such efforts.

The 50 per cent relapse rate in patients achieving CR with VAB-2 led investigators at MSKCC in 1975 to inaugurate the VAB-3 regimen. In addition to an increased dose of cisplatin, the VAB-3 regimen added cyclophosphamide to the induction phase and Adriamycin to the maintenance schedule, based on reports by Buckner et al. (1974) and Monfardini et al. (1972), respectively. The overall CR rate with VAB-3, regardless of prior treatment status, was 61 per cent, but the durable CR rate was only 44 per cent. VAB-3 involved two major inductions, spaced 5 to 6 months apart; in 1976, VAB-4 was initiated in an effort to reduce relapse rates by introducing a third induction at 16 weeks. In 41 evaluable patients, the VAB-4 combination resulted in a CR rate of 80 per cent (61 per cent from chemotherapy alone and 20 per cent from chemotherapy plus additional surgery for clinical PR's); 5 of 33 (15 per cent) CR's relapsed during follow-up (Vugrin et al., 1981a). A more intensive and complicated regimen (VAB-5) was initiated in 1977 for individuals with poor prognostic features, such as bulky (>5 cm in diameter) retroperitoneal metastasis; liver, brain, or multiple sites of involvement; very high elevations of serum tumor markers; and failure of prior chemotherapy. A disappointing CR rate of 47 per cent, severe toxicity, and poor patient acceptance reported by Vugrin et al. (1983) led to the abandonment of this regimen.

The VAB-6 regimen initiated at MSKCC in 1979 and the PVB programs developed at Indiana University between 1974 and 1980 have both involved frequent early cisplatin-containing inductions (Table 33–18). Scarification with BCG was dropped from the original PVB regimen soon after the trial began. In analyzing the results of the first PVB protocol (1974 to 1976), Williams and Einhorn (1983) noted that 27 of 47 (57 per cent) patients remained alive with no evidence of disease (NED) 5 or more years after therapy. The major toxicity of this regimen (two drug-related deaths) was attributed to myelosuppression from high-dose vinblastine (0.4 mg/kg). To study the efficacy of reduced vinblastine dosages (1976 to 1978), patients were randomized to receive (1) the original PVB (0.4 mg/kg vinblastine); (2) PVB with reduced vinblastine (0.3 mg/kg); or (3) PVB (vinblastine 0.2 mg/kg) plus Adriamycin (50 mg/m^2). The overall CR rates with chemotherapy (with or without surgery) in each of the three arms were comparable (88 per cent, 78 per cent, and 80 per cent, respectively). The 25 per cent reduction in vinblastine produced less hematologic toxicity and no drug-related fatalities, while the addition of Adriamycin had no impact upon response rates (Williams and Einhorn, 1983).

The VAB-6 regimen, initiated in 1978, shortened the interval between inductions and omitted Adriamycin and chlorambucil. Sequential studies comparing 1 year of maintenance therapy with no maintenance therapy and a randomized study comparing maintenance and no maintenance have revealed no advantages to maintenance regimens. Preliminary results of the first MSKCC study indicated an overall (chemotherapy plus surgery) CR rate of 92 per cent, and a later report noted that only 9 per cent achieving CR relapsed (Vugrin et al., 1981b, 1983). Overall, 80 per cent of those entering treatment remain NED with a median follow-up of 3 years or more.

Maintenance Chemotherapy. The role of PVB maintenance therapy following CR (achieved by chemotherapy with or without surgery) was studied by the Southeastern Cancer Study Group between 1978 and 1980, and results were published by Einhorn et al. (1981b). The second phase of the VAB-6 program, which addressed the issue of maintenance prophylaxis in nonrandomized studies, was completed in 1980; the randomized protocol was not completed, as patients refused either the concept of randomization or the allocated treatment.

In the PVB study, 25 per cent of those randomized to receive maintenance vinblastine (0.3 mg/kg monthly for 21 months) refused therapy but 58 accepted, and 55 patients were followed without additional treatment. In both groups the relapse rates and overall disease-free status in those who initially reached CR were almost identical, roughly 8 per cent and 96 per cent, respectively (Einhorn et al., 1981b). The VAB-6 trials confirmed that relapse following successful induction, with or without surgery and with or without maintenance, was uncommon (10 per cent) and that 90 per cent of those achieving CR remained NED (Vugrin et al., 1983). The overall CR rates with PVB and VAB-6 were comparable, approximately 80 per cent and 90 per cent, respectively, and both studies indicated that maintenance chemotherapy was unnecessary.

Adjuvant Chemotherapy. At present, patients with Stage I or II NSGCTT are treated primarily by surgical excision or radiation therapy, but clinical experience indicates that roughly 10 to 50 per cent of patients will ultimately relapse. The established efficacy of chemotherapy for disseminated disease supports the use of adjuvant regimens. The excellent survival of patients with surgical Stage I disease without additional treatment indicates that adjuvant chemotherapy is generally unnecessary. Such therapy logically can be reserved for relapse (10 to 15 per cent), in which case a 90 per cent CR from chemotherapy would be anticipated.

The overall relapse rate in Stage II, despite surgery or radiation therapy, is approximately 50 per cent, a setting that invites prophylaxis. In analyzing early experience with adjuvant chemotherapy with "mini-VAB" following RPLND, Vugrin et al. (1979) recorded no relapses in 33 patients with Stage II/N-1 or II/N-2A, whereas 10 of 29 (34 per cent) patients with Stage II/N-2B or II/N-3 relapsed within 2 years of follow-up. The highest rate of relapse was noted in the N-3 category, in which 7 of 13 (54 per cent) failed. Adjuvant "mini-VAB" therapy consisted of a modified and less toxic form of VAB-1 (vinblastine, actinomycin D, bleomycin, chlorambucil). Skinner and Scardino (1980) found that the relapse rate following RPLND and actinomycin D alone in resectable Stage II/N-2B or II/N-3 was only 14 per cent. Cisplatin-based regimens (VAB-3, VAB-6, PVB) have been found to be effective in maintaining CR rates of greater than 95 per cent in patients with

TABLE 33–18. CHEMOTHERAPY FOR ADVANCED TESTIS CANCER

	PVB[*]	**VAB-6**[†]
Vinblastine	0.3 mg/kg every 3 weeks	4 mg/m^2, day 1
Actinomycin D		1 mg/m^2, day 1
Cyclophosphamide		600 mg/m^2, day 1
Bleomycin	30 units weekly × 12 weeks	30 units, day 1 + 20 units/day × 3 days by continuous infusion
Cisplatin	20 mg/m^2/day × 5 days	120 mg/m^2, day 4
	Repeat vinblastine and cisplatin × 3–4 cycles	Repeat × 3 cycles, omitting bleomycin from third cycle

[*]Einhorn and Williams (1980)
[†]Vugrin et al. (1981b)

Stage II/N-2B or II/N-3 (Vugrin et al., 1981c, 1982; Einhorn et al., 1981b).

As an alternative to adjuvant chemotherapy, Williams et al. (1980a) proposed surveillance following surgical excision of Stage II disease, reserving additional treatment for those who relapsed. All patients studied apparently achieved CR with chemotherapy if and when failure occurred.

Since not all patients will fail and since a high salvage rate with chemotherapy can be anticipated, a "wait and see" attitude may be justified. The risks of intensive adjuvant chemotherapy in all Stage II patients must be weighed against the prospects of salvaging those who relapse with appropriate chemotherapy if adjuvant therapy is not employed. The Intergroup Testicular Cancer Study Group (ITCSG) is currently conducting a randomized trial in which patients with positive nodes and no other evidence of disease either do or do not receive adjuvant chemotherapy following primary RPLND. Although the early results indicate no significant overall differences between the two approaches when protocol violations are excluded, a formal report of the results should be available soon (DeWys, 1984).

Salvage Chemotherapy. Roughly 10 to 20 per cent of patients with disseminated germ cell tumors will fail initial induction chemotherapy, and a similar number achieving CR will experience later treatment failure. Treatment results for the majority of patients who relapse following, or progress during, "optimal" combination therapy are controversial and, in the main, disappointing.

The activity of VP-16-213 (etoposide), a synthetic podophyllotoxin, in the treatment of germ cell tumors was reported by Fitzharris et al. in 1979 after preliminary communications by Newlands and Bagshawe and Cavalli et al. (1977). Williams et al. (1980b) reported responses in 29 of 33 previously treated patients (14 CR's, 15 PR's) when VP-16-213 was used alone or in combination with cisplatin and/or bleomycin and Adriamycin, supporting the combined use of VP-16-213 and cisplatin for "salvage" chemotherapy. Reports by others, however, who combined VP-16-213 and cisplatin with or without Adriamycin were less encouraging (Mortimer et al., 1982; Lederman et al., 1983). Bosl et al. (1984) treated 23 patients with VP-16-213 (100 mg/m² × 5 days) and cisplatin (20 mg/m² × 5 days): No responses and two deaths were reported among 14 patients who had not previously achieved a complete response to cisplatin-based therapy. From this and other reports it seems that although the combination is active, CR's in patients previously refractory to other cisplatin regimens are infrequent.

With the lack of new and effective agents, therapy is currently at a standstill. Phase II trials recently conducted at MSKCC indicate few responders in patients with cisplatin-resistant disease treated with a variety of single agents: vindesine—three PR's/19 patients; 1,2-diaminocyclohexane platinum (DACCP)—0/9; cis-retinoic acid—0/15; methylglyoxal bis-guanylhydrazone 0/7 (Bosl, 1984). Explorations of superdoses of cisplatin given in conjunction with 3 per cent saline are in progress in a number of centers. The prevalent climate clearly favors the continued search for active pharmacologic agents and a renewed interest in the biology of human and animal model systems.

Other Considerations. Life-threatening infectious complications remain a most serious potential sequel of multidrug chemotherapy regimens, although the vast majority can be successfully treated if recognized early. Gastrointestinal disturbances, stomatitis, and alopecia are universally short-lived and tolerable. Vascular complications from vinblastine, cisplatin nephrotoxicity and ototoxicity, and bleomycin pneumonitis are potential hazards. The possible long-term effects of chemotherapy upon virtually all body systems await evaluation.

Therapeutic prospects depend largely upon the development of new methods for those with resistant disease and a reduction in the therapeutic burden for those with little risk of failure. Clinical variables, such as histology, serum tumor markers, and extent of disease, have been used as predictive indices to define patient populations who will do well with standard therapy in contrast to those who will not. Patients with pure choriocarcinoma or metastatic malignant teratoma (sarcomatous teratoma) do poorly despite aggressive multimodal therapy. When tumor markers are analyzed exclusively for their predictive value, the data, even from a single institution, may appear conflicting (Bosl et al., 1983; Vugrin et al., 1983). Univariate analyses from the M.D. Anderson, Indiana University, and Royal Marsden Hospitals have indicated the direct relationship between tumor volume and response to chemotherapy (Samuels et al., 1976; Einhorn and Donohue, 1977b; Juttner and McElwain, 1981). Such data are clearly meaningful in predicting the outcome of therapy but do not consider interdependent relationships between individual variables. A recent MSKCC multivariate analysis of several prognostic factors defined the relative value of each clinical parameter. Serum levels of LDH and hCG and the number of metastatic sites were found to be statistically important prognostic indices, whereas serum values of AFP and CEA, histopathology, prior treatment history, and size of metastases were not. From these data, a mathematical model for predicting treatment response was constructed and tested at two separate institutions in patients with advanced disease. The model prospectively differentiated between good- and poor-risk patient subsets who received either PVB or VAB-6 chemotherapy. The purpose of such an exercise is to identify individuals in whom lesser treatment strategies may be "safe and sure," as opposed to certain others in whom current therapy is unlikely to be effective. In the latter group, different and more aggressive approaches are warranted from the outset of treatment; in the former group, explorations involving reductions of therapeutic burden may be justified.

EXTRAGONADAL TUMORS

Primary tumors of extragonadal origin are rare, with fewer than 1000 cases described in the literature. Distinction between a primary extragonadal germ cell tumor (EGT) and metastatic disease from an undetected testis primary tumor may be difficult but has obviously important clinical implications. Surgical and autopsy series have confirmed the absence of a "burned-out" testicular primary lesion in a number of cases, laying to rest some of the skepticism surrounding the diagnosis of EGT in the past (Luna and Valenzuela-Tamariz, 1976; Prym, 1927). More recently, testicular ultrasonography has emerged as a sensitive technique for the detection of tiny neoplasms a few millimeters in size within the clinically "normal" testis. Although the exact incidence of EGT's is unknown, clinical data suggest that roughly 3 to 5 per cent of all germ cell tumors are of extragonadal origin.

The most common sites of origin are, in decreasing order of frequency, the mediastinum, retroperitoneum, sacrococcygeal region, and pineal gland, although many unusual sources have also been reported. Two schools of thought exist as to the origin of these neoplasms: (1) displacement of primitive germ cells during early embryonic migration from the yolk sac entoderm; and (2) persistence of pluripotential cells in sequestered primitive rests during early somatic development. The theory of misplaced germ cells holds that during ontogeny, migration through the retroperitoneum is misdirected cephalad to the mediastinum and pineal gland or caudad to the sacrococcygeal region, rather than to the genital ridges. The alternative hypothesis maintains that primitive pluripotential cells may be dislocated during early embryogenesis (blastema or morula phase). A germ cell rest in the third brachial cleft, for example, could result in a mediastinal tumor, which, interestingly, often resembles a thymoma histologically.

Males are predominantly affected, although a female predominance has been noted with sacrococcygeal lesions. With the exception of sacrococcygeal tumors in the newborn, these tumors generally lack encapsulation, unlike their testicular counterparts, and tend to invade or envelop contiguous structures. The majority of adults with EGT's present with advanced local disease and distant metastases. These tumors most commonly spread to regional lymph nodes, lung, liver, and bone. Histologically, all germ cell types are represented, with pure seminoma accounting for roughly half the tumors in the mediastinum and retroperitoneum. In general, sacrococcygeal tumors of the newborn and young adult are functionally and histologically benign, whereas tumors discovered during infancy prove malignant in about half the cases.

Extragonadal germ cell tumors may reach a large size with no or relatively few symptoms. Diagnosis of mediastinal EGT is most commonly established during the third decade, with or without signs and symptoms of chest pain, cough, or dyspnea. Patients with primary retroperitoneal tumors may present with abdominal or back pain, a palpable mass, vascular obstruction, or other vague constitutional symptoms. Sacrococcygeal tumors are most often diagnosed in the neonate (1 in 40,000 births) and less frequently during infancy or adulthood, with findings of a palpable mass, skin discoloration or hairy nevus, or bowel or urinary obstruction. Tumors of the pineal gland occur in children and young adults, producing symptoms of increased intracranial pressure (headache, visual impairment), oculomotor dysfunction (diplopia, ptosis), hearing loss, hypopituitarism (abnormal menses), and hypothalamic disturbances (diabetes insipidus).

Complete local excision of mediastinal or retroperitoneal tumors is rarely feasible because of frequent local extension and high rates of metastatic disease. In reviewing 30 cases of primary mediastinal tumors, Martini et al. (1974) found only 4 of 30 patients who presented with no evidence of metastasis. Three of these four had pure seminoma. In the ten patients with pure seminoma, only four were long-term survivors following surgery or radiotherapy. Of 20 patients with elements of embryonal carcinoma, only one was alive at 20 months following surgery, radiotherapy, and chemotherapy. Sterchi et al. (1975) reviewed 108 patients with mediastinal seminoma, finding a 5-year survival rate of 58 per cent following primary radiation therapy or surgery. The recent MSKCC experience with 21 cases of extragonadal seminoma was reviewed by Jain et al. (1984). In 11 patients treated with primary cisplatin-based chemotherapy, only one died of metastatic disease, with the remainder disease-free at 19+ to 46+ months' follow-up. Patients with primary retroperitoneal seminoma appear equally responsive to intensive chemotherapy regimens (Stanton et al., 1983). In contrast, patients with nonseminomatous EGT have done poorly despite surgery, radiotherapy, and chemotherapy (Recondo and Libshitz, 1978; Reynolds, 1979). Disappointingly, only 2 of 18 patients treated at MSKCC with successive VAB protocols have achieved CR. While Garnick et al. (1983) reported similar results, those of Hainsworth et al. (1982), using the PVB regimen, were superior. The reason for this apparent discrepancy remains unclear.

Wide local excision is the treatment of choice for sacrococcygeal tumors, in that the majority are benign. Limited experience renders uncertain the advisability of adjunctive irradiation or chemotherapy for malignant tumors. Radical excisions for pineal tumors have been disappointing from the standpoints of local control and operative morbidity. Such procedures have been largely abandoned in favor of primary radiation therapy, although a cerebrospinal fluid shunt may be required (Cole, 1971).

OTHER TESTIS NEOPLASMS

Under the designation "other testis neoplasms" are included a heterogeneous group of tumors of relatively infrequent occurrence. Together, they constitute between 5 and 10 per cent of all testis tumors.

Sex Cord–Mesenchyme Tumors (Gonadal Stromal Tumors; Sex Cord–Stromal Tumors)

Both semantic and histogenetic uncertainties have contributed to the continuing difficulties in the classification of such lesions. Distinguishing between hyperplasia and benign and malignant tumors has added to the problems of classification. Teilum (1946, 1971) was principally responsible for calling attention to this group of tumors and for emphasizing the comparative pathology of the analogous ovarian and testicular neoplasms. The cell type, architecture, and degree of differentiation of these tumors may closely duplicate the supporting tissues in the gonads of either sex. In the testis, the microscopic appearance may be that of undifferentiated gonadal stroma, a Sertoli cell tumor in germ cell–free seminiferous tubules, or a Leydig cell tumor. More rarely, tumors that are apparently composed of granulosa cells or theca cells occur.

INTERSTITIAL CELL LESIONS (LEYDIG CELL TUMORS)

Varying degrees of apparent focal or diffuse interstitial cell hyperplasia may be noted with a variety of conditions associated with seminiferous tubule atrophy. To what extent these represent absolute or relative increases in interstitial cells may be difficult to assess. Interstitial cell tumors, the most common of the sex cord–mesenchyme lesions, make up between 1 and 3 per cent of all testis tumors. Although the majority have been recognized in males between the ages of 20 and 60 years, approximately one fourth have been reported before puberty.

The etiology of Leydig cell tumors is unknown. In contrast to germ cell tumors, there appears to be no association with cryptorchidism. The experimental production of Leydig cell tumors in mice following chronic estrogen administration or following intrasplenic testicular autografting is consistent with a hormonal basis.

The lesions are generally small, yellow to brown, and well circumscribed, and rarely exhibit hemorrhage or necrosis. Microscopically, the tumors consist of relatively uniform, polyhedral, closely packed cells with round and slightly eccentric nuclei and eosinophilic granular cytoplasm with lipoid vacuoles, brownish pigmentation, and occasional characteristic inclusions known as Reinke crystals. Pleomorphism with large and bizarre cell forms may occur, and mitotic figures may or may not be identified. None of these features appears to be consistently related to malignant potential. Furthermore, limited observations suggest that ultrastructural features will not categorically distinguish between normal and neoplastic Leydig cells, whether benign or malignant.

Approximately 10 per cent of interstitial cell tumors are malignant, but there are no consistently reliable histologic criteria for making this judgment. Large size, extensive necrosis, gross or microscopic evidence of infiltration, invasion of blood vessels, and excessive mitotic activity are all features that suggest the possibility of malignancy, but metastasis is generally regarded as the only reliable criterion of malignancy. Like other testis tumors, malignant lesions may involve retroperitoneal lymph nodes, lung, and bone. Of importance is the observation that malignancy is nonexistent in the prepubertal age group.

Clinical Presentation. In the prepubertal cases (average age 5 years), presenting manifestations are usually those of isosexual precocity with prominent external genitalia, mature masculine voice, and pubic hair growth. Hormonal assays in such patients have been few and generally incomplete or have been carried out by antiquated techniques. An increased testosterone production is usually demonstrable, and urinary 17-ketosteroid output may or may not be elevated. Virilizing types of congenital adrenocortical hyperplasia may also produce the endocrine signs and symptoms of interstitial cell tumors, so that differential tests must be carried out to clarify the diagnosis. Such tests include estimation of urinary 17-hydroxy- and 17-ketosteroid levels as well as plasma cortisol before and after ACTH stimulation and dexamethasone suppression. Since interstitial cell carcinomas have been shown to possess 21-hydroxylase activity and to be capable of forming cortisol and hydroxylating steroids at the 11-beta position, it is clear that interstitial cell tumors may possess some of the same functional activities as adrenocortical tissue. The similar embryologic origin of interstitial cells and adrenocortical cells and the occurrence of adrenal rests in the testis complicate interpretation. The paradox of the tumor's arising in the interstitial cells of a prepubertal testis and behaving metabolically like its adult counterpart, in conjunction with cells in the normal prepubertal testis containing enzymes capable of producing testosterone, explains the occurrence of spermatogenesis in the seminiferous tubules immediately adjacent to the tumor and the absence of spermatogenesis in tubules more remote from the tumor.

In adults, the majority of reported cases have shown manifestations of endocrine imbalance, although some do not. The endocrinologic manifestations may precede the palpable testis mass, which is the most common presenting feature. In the remaining adult cases, symptoms of a feminizing nature, such as impotence, decreased libido, and gynecomastia, may occur. The slow progression of these neoplasms is suggested by the long duration of gynecomastia, which may precede recognition of the testicular mass. In contrast to the situation with adult germ cell tumors, the duration of gynecomastia with adult interstitial cell tumors has ranged from 6 months to 10 years and averages more than 3 years. Elevation of urinary and plasma estrogens in association with this tumor is relatively common. Lockhart et al. (1976) reported a nonfunctioning interstitial cell tumor of the testis of a malignant type in which there was neither clinical nor chemical manifestation of endocrinopathy. Hormonal disturbance, therefore, is not an essential feature. In cases in which a testicular swelling is not clinically apparent, Gabrilove (1975) performed selective venous catheterization and measurement of the testicular venous effluent to assess gynecomastia of obscure etiology. Measurement of AFP and the beta subunit of hCG may be helpful in differential diagnosis. Other considerations in the differential diagnosis include feminizing adrenocortical disorders, Klinefelter's syndrome, and other feminizing testicular disorders.

Treatment. Radical inguinal orchiectomy is the initial procedure of choice. With documentation of Leydig cell tumor, endocrinologic studies and further clinical staging evaluations are indicated. In the event of histopathologic suspicion of malignancy, lymphangiogram, CT scan, or ultrasound (alone or in combination) of the retroperitoneum is indicated to seek retroperitoneal adenopathy. As with germ cell tumors of the adult testis, spread to the lung, liver, or supradiaphragmatic lymph nodes is possible. The potential production of hormones by metastatic tumor invites exploration of these substances as markers for metastatic disease, but data are lacking. Urinary estrogens, androgens, corticoids, and pregnanediol have each demonstrated abnormalities on the basis of the metabolic activity of different interstitial cell tumors. Retroperitoneal lymph node dissection has been recommended as routine in patients whose interstitial cell tumors appear histologically or biochemically malignant. Total experience with any form of therapy, however, is limited by the small number of patients who have been treated, although the existing data suggest the relative radioresistance of this tumor. Ortho-para-prime-DDD has been utilized with evidence of benefit in some patients (Azer and Braumstein, 1981; Tamoney and Noriega,

1969). A variety of chemotherapeutic agents, including *cis*-platinum, vinblastine, bleomycin, cyclophosphamide, doxorubicin, and vincristine, have been utilized in various combination regimens without convincing benefit, but experience is very limited. Experimental evidence of estrogen receptors in various mouse Leydig cell tumor lines provides an experimental basis for trials of endocrine therapy (Sato et al., 1978). In addition, inhibition of mitochondrial protein synthesis with concomitant arrest of in vivo growth of solid Leydig cell tumors in rats by oxytetracycline has been reported (Van den Bogert et al., 1983).

The prognosis for Leydig cell tumors is good because of their generally benign nature. The persistence of virilizing and feminizing features following orchiectomy is not necessarily an indication of malignancy, since these changes are to some extent irreversible. As might be anticipated from the characterization of malignancy, i.e., metastasis, the average survival time from surgery for patients with a malignant Leydig cell tumor is approximately 3 years.

SERTOLI CELL TUMORS (ANDROBLASTOMA; GONADAL STROMAL TUMOR; SERTOLI CELL–MESENCHYME TUMOR)

Nodules of immature seminiferous tubules with lumina lined by undifferentiated cells are found not infrequently in cryptorchid testes and in roughly one fourth of patients with testicular feminization. Such lesions were formerly considered tubular adenomas, but it seems probable that they are not neoplastic, and malignant change appears not to have been reported.

True Sertoli cell–mesenchyme tumors constitute less than 1 per cent of all testicular tumors and may occur in any age group, including infancy. Although rare in humans, they are the most common testicular tumor in dogs. The majority of Sertoli cell tumors are benign, but approximately 10 per cent have proved malignant on the basis of the currently accepted criterion of malignancy—the demonstration of metastasis. As with Leydig cell tumors, definitive histologic criteria of malignancy remain to be established.

The etiology of these tumors has not been determined. The majority have arisen in apparently normal intrascrotal testes, although occurrence in maldescended or cryptorchid testes has been reported.

Grossly, these tumors vary in size from 1 cm to more than 20 cm. The cut surface is usually gray-white to creamy yellow, with a uniform consistency interrupted by cystic change

that becomes increasingly evident with increasing tumor size. The benign lesions are usually well circumscribed, whereas the malignant lesions tend to be larger and less well demarcated. Invasion of paratesticular structures may occur and is suggestive of malignancy.

The precise origin of these tumors remains somewhat uncertain, although derivation from the primitive gonadal mesenchyme is suspected. A diversity of microscopic appearances is evident not only between tumors but also between different areas within the same tumor. The essential diagnostic features include epithelial elements resembling Sertoli cells and varying amounts of stroma. The amount and organization of these two components have led to various attempts to subclassify the tumors. The epithelial element, on the one hand, may be arranged in tubules with or without lumina and lined by radially arranged cells in one or multiple layers; on the other hand, the epithelial cells may form columns or sheets of trabeculae growing between stromal elements. The stromal elements may be scant, or the tumor may be largely composed of stroma resembling a fibroma but containing strands of epithelial cells. Secretory material forming Call-Exner–like bodies are occasionally seen within tubules, the morphologic appearance resembling that of granulosa cell tumors. Furthermore, the stromal elements may be sufficiently well differentiated to be recognizable as Leydig cells. The enormous potential for variation both in stromal and epithelial components and in degrees of differentiation accounts for the wide range of morphologic appearances described for these lesions and contributes to the difficulty in their classification.

Although large size, poor tumor demarcation, invasion of adjacent structures, blood vessel and lymphatic invasion, and increased mitotic activity are all suggestive of a malignant potential, as with Leydig cell tumors, the designation of malignancy can be made with certainty only in the presence of metastasis.

The presenting signs and symptoms are those of a testicular mass with or without pain and with or without gynecomastia. Although the lesions have been reported in all age groups, approximately one third of the recorded patients have been 12 years of age or less. About one third of the patients have had gynecomastia. Gynecomastia in the presence of a testis tumor in the prepubertal age group is an important finding in differential diagnosis, since feminization in boys with Leydig cell tumors is always superimposed on virilism.

Studies of the endocrinologic activity of these tumors have been uncommon. Gynecomastia is presumably a consequence of estrogen production, but whether or not the Sertoli cells or the stromal elements are responsible for estrogen production remains to some extent uncertain. Gabrilove et al. (1980) reported an elevated plasma testosterone value in association with some virilizing features in a young patient with Sertoli cell tumor.

Radical orchiectomy is the initial procedure of choice and will, of course, be curative in the 90 per cent of cases that are benign. In the small proportion of patients in whom malignancy has been demonstrated by the presence of metastasis, retroperitoneal lymph node involvement has been common, and retroperitoneal lymph node dissection has been performed with apparent therapeutic success (Rosvoli and Woodward, 1968). The course of the disease, even in patients with metastasis, may be protracted compared with that of patients with metastatic germ cell tumors. Lung and bone metastasis may occur and warrants the inclusion of chest films and bone scans in the staging evaluation. The value of radiation therapy and chemotherapy in the management of patients with this disease is uncertain. Although hormone production is a potential marker for follow-up in patients with apparently malignant tumors, clinical evidence on this point is lacking.

Gonadoblastoma (Tumors of Dysgenetic Gonads; Mixed Germ Cell Tumor; Gonadocytoma)

These rare tumors, occurring almost exclusively in patients with some form of gonadal dysgenesis, constitute approximately 0.5 per cent of all testis neoplasms and occur in all age groups from infancy to beyond 70 years, although the majority have occurred in individuals under 30 years of age.

Grossly, the lesions may be unilateral or bilateral and may vary in size from microscopic to greater than 20 cm in diameter. Aggressive growth may replace and obscure the nature of the gonad from which the tumor arose, and lesions weighing more than 1000 gm have been reported. The tumors generally are round, with a smooth and slightly lobulated surface, and vary from soft and fleshy to firm or hard in consistency. Calcified areas are frequent and probably reflect the extensive spontaneous retrogressive changes common with these lesions. The cut surface is grayish white to yellow but

may vary considerably, depending upon the histologic makeup of the tumor.

Although gonadoblastomas are currently regarded as neoplasms, the possibility that they represent hamartomas or nodular hyperplasia in response to pituitary gonadotrophins has been suggested. First clearly described by Scully (1953), the tumors consist of three elements: Sertoli cells, interstitial tissue, and germ cells, the proportions of which show considerable variation. In about half such tumors, germ cell overgrowth, with the evolution of what is readily recognized as seminoma, or germ cell element(s) with histologic features of embryonal carcinoma, teratoma, choriocarcinoma, or yolk sac tumor may occur. Throughout the tubules, characteristic Call-Exner bodies may be identified, consisting of PAS-positive material similar to that seen in the basement membrane of the tubules.

The clinical manifestations of patients with this tumor are the consequence of three factors: (1) the usual concurrence of gonadal dysgenesis with resultant abnormalities in the external genitalia and gonads; (2) the presence of germ cells with malignant potential; and (3) the endocrine function of the gonadal stromal components of the tumor, usually with the production of androgen. Although interstitial cells may not be evident by light microscopy, a steroidogenic potential of the tumor may exist. Furthermore, demonstration of Leydig cells in the tumor does not necessarily dictate virilism, either because the resultant steroids may be biologically inactive or because the end-organs may be defective. The usual appearance is that of solid tubules of varying size containing germ cells in close association with Sertoli cells and of mature interstitial cells evident between the tubules.

The germ cells of gonadoblastoma are similar to those of seminoma, and if germ cell proliferation occurs, it may progress from an in situ stage to invasive germinoma (seminoma), referred to as gonadoblastoma with germinoma (seminoma).

Approximately four fifths of patients with gonadoblastoma are phenotypic females, usually presenting with primary amenorrhea and sometimes with a lower abdominal mass. The remainder are phenotypic males, almost always presenting with cryptorchidism, hypospadias, and some female internal genitalia. However, gonadoblastoma has been described in an anatomically normal male (Talerman, 1972). In the phenotypic females the breasts are small, the internal genitalia hypoplastic, and the gonads usually of the streak type. Sex chromatin is negative, and the chromosome analysis usually shows XY or XO or XO/XY patterns. Virilization in the phenotypic female usually manifests as hypertrophy of the clitoris. In the phenotypic male, gynecomastia may occasionally be present, and there is usually hypospadias, some female internal genitalia, and dysgenetic testes usually located in the abdomen or inguinal region; sex chromatin is negative and the chromosome pattern is XY or XO/XY.

In general, 90 per cent of patients with gonadal dysgenesis and gonadoblastoma are chromatin-negative and over half have an XY karyotype, with the remainder demonstrating mosaicism. The external sex organs of patients with gonadoblastoma show a wide range of appearances ranging from normal to completely ambiguous. The secondary sex organs usually consist of a hypoplastic uterus and two normal or slightly hypoplastic fallopian tubes. Male internal sex organs, such as epididymis, vas deferens, and prostate, are found sometimes in phenotypic virilized females and always in phenotypic male pseudohermaphrodites.

Treatment. Radical orchiectomy is the first step in therapy, and the high incidence of bilaterality (50 per cent) argues for contralateral gonadectomy when gonadal dysgenesis is present. The prognosis is excellent for patients with gonadoblastoma or gonadoblastoma with germinoma. In the presence of seminoma or other germ cell tumor types, clinical staging employing the techniques used for the staging of germ cell tumors of the adult testis may be indicated, although experience is too limited to justify categorical recommendations. As with germ cell tumors of the adult testis, therapy may logically be based upon tumor histology and the results of clinical staging.

Neoplasms of Mesenchymal Origin

A variety of neoplasms derived from mesenchymal elements may arise on the tunica albuginea or, more rarely, within the testis. Included are benign fibroma, angioma, neurofibroma, and leiomyoma. Occurring as painless masses, they are of concern chiefly because of the possibility of a malignant tumor. Differential diagnosis includes abnormalities of the testicular appendages, fibrous pseudotumors, adenomatoid tumors, and non-neoplastic cystic lesions. Varying from minute "shot-like" lesions on the surface of the testis to masses of several centimeters, the reported lesions have been variously treated by local excision or orchiectomy.

Malignant mesothelioma may arise from any site on the mesothelial membrane—pleura, peritoneum, pericardium, or tunica vaginalis. Fewer than 20 cases involving the tunica vaginalis have been reported. The lesion occurs in patients from 21 to 78 years of age, and the usual presentation is with a hydrocele. Radical orchiectomy is indicated for local control, but local recurrence and abdominal and pulmonary metastases may ensue. Limited experience suggests that surgery and irradiation may be of some value in controlling intra-abdominal metastasis. The value of chemotherapy remains to be defined, although doxorubicin appears active.

Miscellaneous Primary Non–Germ Cell Tumors

The testis may be the primary site of a number of tumors of unrelated histogenesis and varied pathologic type, including the following.

EPIDERMOID CYST

Representing an estimated 1 per cent of testis tumors (Shah et al., 1981), approximately half occur in the third decade and most of the remainder between the second and fourth decades. Grossly, these lesions present as round, sharply circumscribed, firm, and encapsulated intratesticular nodules; the cut surface reveals a grayish white to yellowish, cheesy, amorphous mass. Microscopically, the wall is composed of dense fibrous tissue lined by stratified squamous keratinized epithelium, desquamations from which, with degeneration and microcalcification, make up the amorphous interior.

Although the histogenesis remains uncertain, a common thesis is that the tumor represents a monolayer teratoma. Such a histogenesis is circumstantially supported by the age and racial incidences of such tumors and by the occasional association with cryptorchidism. This histogenesis, in turn, supports the use of radical orchiectomy as the usual treatment, since the possibility of other germ cell elements in association with such lesions can be excluded only by careful microscopic examination. Nevertheless, the clinical behavior of these tumors has been consistently benign; apparently, no instance of associated, clinically unrecognized but microscopically confirmed germ cell tumor has been reported. Rare instances of bilaterality have been reported (as with germ cell tumors) (Forrest and Whitmore, 1984). Testicular ultrasonography may demonstrate a well-circumscribed lesion with a solid central core and may aid in the distinction from a germ cell tumor. Although most have been managed by radical orchiectomy, local excision in a small number of patients appears to have been equally successful. The weakness in the latter approach stems from uncertainty in clinical diagnosis and the potential risks of spillage of a germ cell tumor.

ADENOCARCINOMA OF THE RETE TESTIS

These rare but highly malignant tumors occur uniformly in adults, over a wide age range (20 to 80 years). Jacobellis et al. (1981) reported only the nineteenth case. The usual presentation is a painless scrotal mass, commonly with an associated hydrocele. Pathologic evaluation reveals a multicystic papillary adenocarcinoma composed of small cuboidal cells with elongated nuclei and scanty cytoplasm, presumably arising from the rete tubules of the testicular mediastinum. Despite radical orchiectomy, half the patients die within 1 year from the time of diagnosis. Metastasis has occurred in inguinal and retroperitoneal lymph nodes, lungs, bone, and liver. The observation that retroperitoneal deposits may represent the sole site of metastasis supports the rationale of retroperitoneal lymphadenectomy in the absence of distant metastasis. Irradiation and chemotherapy with methotrexate, 5-fluorouracil, actinomycin D, or cyclophosphamide in the treatment of metastasis have been of limited, if any, benefit.

ADRENAL REST TUMORS

The association of bilateral testis tumors with congenital adrenal hyperplasia and the remission of both endocrine manifestations and tumors following appropriate corticoid treatment call attention to these unusual lesions. Whether they represent neoplasms or hyperplasia and whether they derive from "normal" adrenal rests or from abnormal interstitial cells remain uncertain in some cases. Kirkland et al. (1977) suggested that luteinizing hormones (LH) may contribute to the growth of these tumors, since (1) high serum LH may be seen in association with incomplete suppression of adrenal steroid secretion, and (2) there is evidence of gonadotrophin secretion with testicular tumors in some patients with congenital adrenal hyperplasia (CAH). Nevertheless, these tumors are primarily dependent upon ACTH for growth and steroid secretion; the most likely circumstance is that they arise from the adrenal cortical rests that may occur normally in the testis but that are abnormally stimulated in the syndrome of CAH. Recognition of CAH and appropriate medical treatment may obviate surgical treatment of the testis "tumors."

ADENOMATOID TUMORS (ANGIOMATOID TUMORS OF THE ENDOTHELIUM; ADENOFIBROMA; MESOTHELIOMA; LYMPHANGIOMA; ADENOFIBROMYOMA; ADENOMA)

These lesions are characteristically small benign tumors peculiar to the genital tract of males and females. They consist of a fibrous stroma in which disoriented spaces of epithelial cells occur, resembling endothelium, epithelium, or mesothelium. Histogenesis remains debatable; although the lesion occurs primarily in the epididymis in the male, occasional instances of tumor confined to the testis have been reported.

CARCINOID

Carcinoid is uncommon outside the gastrointestinal tract. Nearly 150 cases of carcinoid in the ovary have been recorded as well as 23 in the testis, 17 of which were primary and 6 metastatic (Talerman et al., 1978). On gross pathologic examination the tumors have been circumscribed and limited to the testis, with diameters ranging up to 8 cm. Microscopically, the tumors are composed of islands, nests, or discrete masses of round, oval, or polygonal cells separated by fibrous strands and exhibiting a solid acinar structure. Although most of the reported cases have been pure carcinoids, a few have arisen in association with teratoma. In primary ovarian carcinoids, the majority have arisen in association with teratoma. The histogenesis of these tumors remains uncertain, but one-sided development of a teratoma or origin from argentaffin or enterochromaffin cells within the gonad are the alternatives. A slow, progressive, painless testicular enlargement is the most frequent presentation. Although minimal symptoms suggestive of carcinoid syndrome were noted in one patient, estimations of serum serotonin and 5-hydroxyindoleacetic acid have not been performed preoperatively. Treatment has been inguinal orchiectomy, which apparently has been curative in patients with primary testicular carcinoid. In contrast, patients with metastatic carcinoid to the testis have a poor prognosis.

Secondary Tumors of the Testis

LYMPHOMA

Testicular involvement by lymphoma may be (1) a manifestation of primary extranodal disease, (2) the initial manifestation of clinically occult nodal disease, or (3) a later manifestation of disseminated nodal lymphoma. Accounting for about 5 per cent of all testis tumors, these lesions constitute the most common secondary neoplasms of the testis and the most frequent of all testis tumors in patients over 50 years of age. The median age of occurrence is approximately 60 years. Primary lymphoma of the testis may occur in children, eight cases in patients ranging from 2 to 12 years of age having been reviewed by Weitzner and Gropp (1976).

Grossly, the testis is diffusely enlarged, usually to a diameter of 4 to 5 cm or more, bulging with a granular gray to light tan to pink solid tumor. Foci of hemorrhage and necrosis may be evident, and there may be gross extension to the epididymis or cord. Microscopically, all varieties of reticuloendothelial neoplasms, including Hodgkin's disease, have been described in the testis. However, the vast majority are diffuse; of these, most are histiocytic (74 per cent), according to the Rappaport classification, or large noncleaved (70 per cent), according to the Lukes and Collins classification. Diffuse replacement of the normal architecture is the rule, with focal sparing of the seminiferous tubules.

Malignant lymphoma confined to the testis at the time of clinical onset of disease is rare compared with the frequency with which the gonadal mass represents the initial clinical manifestation of occult or apparent nodal disease. However, when lymph node disease is limited to the regional nodes it is possible that the neoplasm arose in the gonad and metastasized to the regional nodes. The pattern of dissemination of testicular lymphomas is similar to that of testicular germ cell tumors. In autopsy cases a pattern of pulmonary nodules not contiguous to the mediastinum or hilum strongly suggests a propensity of testicular lymphomas to spread by the hematogenous route, consistent with the observation of vascular invasion not infrequently seen in patients with testicular lymphoma.

A poor prognosis may be anticipated when there is evidence of generalized disease within a year after diagnosis. As with lymphomas elsewhere, patients with poorly differentiated lymphocytic types tend to survive longer than those with the histiocytic type. Disease-free survivals of 60 months or longer in patients with testicular lymphoma treated by orchiectomy alone provide strong circumstantial evidence that a true primary testicular lymphoma occurs occasionally. However, even patients whose disease seems to be limited to the gonads after clinical and surgical staging may still have a short survival time. On the other hand, patients who have no clinical evidence of systemic spread 1 year after therapy have a high probability of cure. Whether the long-term survival following orchiectomy alone is a reflection of a cured primary testicular tumor or of a spontaneous regression or prolonged remission of a generalized disease remains debatable.

A common clinical presentation is a painless enlargement of the testis, although about one fourth of the patients present with generalized constitutional symptoms, including weight loss, weakness, and anorexia. Bilateral tumors occur in almost half the patients, simultaneously in roughly 10 per cent, and metachronously in the remainder.

Investigation may include a complete blood count, peripheral smears, bone marrow studies, chest x-ray, bone scan, CT scan or intravenous pyelogram, lymphogram, and liver and spleen scans. There appears to be a high probability of generalized disease if para-aortic nodes are involved, indicating the importance of retroperitoneal staging. Although radical orchiectomy provides the diagnosis and initial treatment, once the diagnosis of lymphoma has been established, referral to a medical oncologist is advisable for staging evaluation and decisions regarding further treatment.

Survival is poor with bilateral disease and poor in patients presenting with lymphoma at other sites and later experiencing a testicular relapse, but among patients with disease apparently confined to the testis, Turner et al. (1981) reported 8 of 14 to be alive and well for 7 to 87 months (mean 2.5 years).

LEUKEMIC INFILTRATION OF THE TESTIS

The testicle appears to be a prime initial site of relapse in male children with acute lymphocytic leukemia. Stoffel (1975) reported an 8 per cent incidence of extramedullary involvement of the testis in children with acute leukemia, the majority of patients being in complete remission at the time of testicular enlargement. The interval from testicular involvement to death ranges from 5 to 27 months, with a median of 9 months. Kuo (1976) reported seven children who developed testicular swelling during bone marrow remission in whom needle biopsy was used to confirm leukemic infiltration.

The leukemic infiltration occurs mainly in the interstitial spaces, with destruction of the tubules by infiltration in advanced cases. Enlargement is bilateral in 50 per cent of cases and is commonly associated with scrotal discoloration. Testicular irradiation with doses of 1200 rad over 6 to 8 days is clinically successful in local control. Because of the frequency of bilateral involvement microscopically, bilateral irradiation seems advisable even with apparent unilateral involvement. Almost all patients can be expected to develop subsequent marrow relapse, despite control of testicular involvement by irradiation, unless effective systemic chemotherapy is given.

Biopsy is essential to the diagnosis, orchiectomy is probably unwarranted, and the treatment of choice is testicular irradiation with 2000 rad in ten fractions plus reinstitution of adjunctive chemotherapy in those children off chemotherapy, or reinduction therapy for children who relapse in the testis while on chemotherapy. The prognosis of male children who undergo such a bout of testicular infiltration is guarded.

METASTATIC TUMORS

Approximately 200 cases of metastatic carcinoma to the testis have been reported. In the vast majority it is discovered incidentally at autopsy in patients dying of widespread metastatic disease. In rare circumstances a metastatic focus in the testis may be the presenting feature of an occult neoplasm or the first evidence of a recurrent, previously diagnosed and treated neoplasm.

The usual pathologic feature of secondary testicular cancers is the microscopic demonstration of neoplastic cells in the interstitium, with relative sparing of the tubules. The route of dissemination to the testis may be hematogenous, lymphatic, or by direct invasion from contiguous masses. Renal adenocarcinoma may involve the testis via the spermatic vessels; rarely, dropped metastasis from a diffuse intra-abdominal malignancy can involve the cord and testis via a patent processus vaginalis. Retrograde extension through the vas deferens presumably may be a source as well. The common primary sources in decreasing order of frequency are prostate, lung, gastrointestinal tract, melanoma, and kidney. A relatively high incidence of prostatic lesions reflects in part the frequency with which carcinoma of the prostate occurs and the use of orchiectomy in its treatment. Metastatic tumors to the testis occur later in life, usually in the sixth or seventh decade, in contrast to primary testicular tumors. Metastasis has been bilateral in a small proportion of cases. Approximately 2.5 per cent of lymphomas are found in the testis in metastatic fashion.

References

Classification and Staging

Abelev, G. I.: Alpha-fetoprotein as a marker of embryo-specific differentiation in normal and tumor tissue. Transplant. Rev., 20:3, 1974.

Abelev, G. I., Perova, S. D., Kramkova, N. I., Postnikova, Z. A., and Irlin, I. S.: Production of embryonal alpha I globulin by transplantable mouse hepatomas. Transplantation, 1:174, 1963.

Artz, K., and Jacob, R.: Absence of serologically detectable H2 on primitive teratocarcinoma cells in culture. Transplantation, 17:632, 1974.

Bach, D. W., Weissbech, L., and Hartlapp, J. H.: Bilateral testicular tumors. J. Oncol., 129:989, 1983.

Bagg, H. J.: Experimental production of teratoma testis in the fowl. Am. J. Cancer, 26:69, 1936.

Bagshawe, K. D., and Searle, F.: Tumour markers. In Marks, C. N., and Hales, C. N. (Eds.): Essays in Medical Biochemistry. Vol. 3. London, Biochemical Society, 1977, pp. 25–74.

Bartone, F. F., and Schmidt, M. A.: Cryptorchidism: incidence of chromosomal anomalies in 50 cases. J. Urol., 127:1105, 1982.

Barzell, W. E., and Whitmore, W. F., Jr.: Tumors of the testis. In Harrison, J. H., et al. (Eds.): Campbell's Urology. 4th ed. Philadelphia, W. B. Saunders Co., 1978.

Barzell, W. E., and Whitmore, W. F., Jr.: Clinical significance of biological markers. Memorial Hospital experience. Semin. Oncol., 6:48, 1979.

Batata, M. A., Chu, F. C. H., Hilaris, B. S., Whitmore, W. F., Jr., and Golbey, R. B.: Testicular cancer in cryptorchids. Cancer, 49:1023, 1982.

Bergstrand, C. G., and Czar, B.: Demonstration of new protein from carcinoma of the colon. J. Urol., 72:712, 1954.

Berthelsen, J. G., Skakkebaek, N. E., Sorensen, B. C., and Mogensen, P.: Screening for carcinoma in situ of the contralateral testis in patients with germinal testicular cancer. Br. Med. J., 285:1683, 1982.

Boden, G., and Gibb, R.: Radiotherapy and testicular neoplasms. Lancet, 2:1195, 1951.

Bosl, G. J.: Personal communication, 1984.

Bosl, G. J., Geller, N. L., Cirrincione, C., et al.: Multivariate analysis of prognostic variables in patients with metastatic testicular cancer. Cancer Res., 43:3403, 1983.

Bosl, G. J., Vogelzang, N. J., Goldman, A., Fraley, E. E., Lange, P. H., Levitt, S. H., and Kennedy, B. J.: Impact of delay in diagnosis on clinical stage of testicular cancer. Lancet, 2:970, 1981.

Boyle, L. E., and Samuels, M. L.: Serum LDH activity and isoenzyme patterns in nonseminomatous germinal (NSG) testis tumors. Proc. Am. Soc. Clin. Oncol., 18:278, 1977.

Bredael, J. J., Vugrin, D., and Whitmore, W. F., Jr.: Autopsy findings in 154 patients with germ cell tumors of the testis. Cancer, 50:548, 1982.

Campbell, H. E.: Incidence of malignant growth of the undescended testicle. Arch. Surg., 44:353, 1942.

Carleton, R. L., Freidman, N. B., and Bomge, E. J.: Experimental teratomas of the testis. Cancer, 6:464, 1953.

Clemmesen, J.: Statistical studies in malignant neoplasms. Acta Pathol. Microbiol. Scand. (Suppl.), 247:1, 1974.

Collins, D. H., and Pugh, R. C. B.: Classification and frequency of testicular tumors. Br. J. Urol. (Suppl.), 36:1, 1964.

Cosgrove, M. D., Benton, B., and Henderson, B. E.: Male genitourinary abnormalities and maternal diethylstilbestrol. J. Urol., *117*:220, 1977.

Damjanov, I., and Solter, D.: Animal model: embryo-derived teratomas and teratocarcinomas in mice. Am. J. Pathol., *83*:241, 1976.

Dixon, F. J., and Moore, R. A.: Tumors of the Male Sex Organs. Armed Forces Institute of Pathology. Fascicle 32. Washington, D.C., 1952, pp. 48–103.

Dixon, F. J., and Moore, R. A.: Clinicopathologic study. Cancer, *6*:427, 1953.

Fergusson, J. D.: Tumours of the testis. Br. J. Urol., *34*:407, 1962.

Field, T. E.: Malignancy and the ectopic testicle in army patients. J. R. Army Med. Corps, *108*:189, 1962.

Fradet, Y., Houghton, A. N., Bosl, G. J., Bronson, D., and Whitmore, W. F., Jr.: Cell surface antigens of human teratocarcinoma cell lines identified with monoclonal antibodies. Cold Spring Harbor Symposium on Cell Proliferation. Teratocarcinoma. Stem Cells *10*:591, 1983.

Fraley, E. E., Lange, P. H., and Kennedy, B. J.: Germ-cell testicular cancer in adults. N. Engl. J. Med., *301*:1370, 1420, 1979.

Freidman, N. B., and Moore, R. A.: Tumors of the testis. A report on 922 cases. Milit. Surg., *99*:573, 1946.

Friedrich, M., Claussen, C. D., and Felix, R.: Immersion ultrasound of testicular pathology. Radiography, *141*:235, 1981.

Gehring, G. G., Rodriquez, F. R., and Woodhead, D. M.: Malignant degeneration of cryptorchid testis following orchiopexy. Transactions of the 52nd Annual Meeting of the American Urological Association, 1973, pp. 30–40.

Gilbert, J. B.: Tumors of the testis following mumps orchitis: Case report and review of 24 cases. J. Urol., *51*:296, 1944.

Gilbert, J. B., and Hamilton, J. B.: Studies in malignant testis tumors; incidence and nature of tumors in ectopic testis. Surg. Gynecol. Obstet., *71*:731, 1940.

Glazer, H. S., Lee, J. K. T., Melson, G. L., and McClennan, B. C.: Sonographic detection of occult testicular neoplasms. Am. J. Radiol., *138*:673, 1982.

Graham, S., and Gibson, R.: Social epidemiology of cancer of the testis. Cancer, *29*:1243, 1972.

Harvald, B., and Hauge, M.: Heredity of cancer elucidated by a study of unselected twins. JAMA, *186*:749, 1963.

Henderson, B. E., Benton, B., Jing, J., Hu, M. C., and Pike, M. C.: Risk factors for cancer of the testis in young men. Int. J. Cancer, *23*:598, 1979.

Henderson, B. E., Ross, R. K., Pike, M. C., and Depue, R. H.: Epidemiology of testis cancer. *In* Skinner, D. G. (Ed.): Urological Cancer. New York, Grune & Stratton, 1983, pp. 237–250.

Hong, W. K., Wittes, R. E., Hajdu, S. T., Cvitkovic, E., Whitmore, W. F., Jr., and Golbey, R. B.: The evolution of mature teratoma from malignant testicular tumors. Cancer, *40*:2987, 1977.

Hope-Stone, H. F., Blandy, J. P., and Dayan, A. N.: Treatment of tumors of the testis. Br. Med. J., *1*:984, 1963.

Husband, J. E., Barrett, A., and Peckham, M. J.: Evaluation of computed tomography in the management of testicular teratoma. Br. J. Urol., *53*:179, 1981.

Hussey, D. H., Luk, K. H., and Johnson, D. E.: The role of radiation therapy in the treatment of germinal cell tumors of the testis other than pure seminoma. Radiology, *123*:175, 1977.

Jacobson, G. K., Henriksen, O. B., and van der Masse, H.

V.: Carcinoma in situ of testicular tissue adjacent to malignant germ cell tumors. Cancer, *47*:2660, 1981.

Javadpour, N.: Multiple biochemical tumor markers in seminoma. Cancer, *52*:887, 1983.

Javadpour, N.: The value of biologic markers in diagnosis and treatment of testicular cancer. Semin. Oncol., *6*:37, 1979.

Javadpour, N.: The role of biologic tumour markers in testicular cancer. Cancer, *45*:1755, 1980*a*.

Javadpour, N.: Significance of elevated serum alpha-feto-proteins (AFP) in seminoma. Cancer, *45*:2166, 1980*b*.

Jewett, M. A. S.: Biology of testicular tumors. Urol. Clin. North Am., *4*:495, 1977.

Johnson, D. E.: Epidemiology of testicular tumors. *In* Johnson, D. E. (Ed.): Testicular Tumors. 2nd ed. Flushing, N.Y., Medical Examination Publishing Co., 1976, pp. 37–46.

Johnson, D. E., Appelt, G., Samuels, M. C., and Luna, M.: Metastases from testicular carcinoma. Urology, *8*:234, 1976.

Johnson, D. E., Woodhead, D. M., Pohl, D. R., and Robison, J. R.: Cryptorchism and testicular tumorigenesis. Surgery, *63*:919, 1968.

Krishnaswamy, P. R., Tate, S., and Meister, A.: Gamma-glutamyl transpeptidase of human seminal fluid. Life Science, *20*:681, 1977.

Kurohara, S. S., Badib, A. O., Webster, J. H., Martin, L. S. J., and Woodruff, M. W.: Prognostic factors in the common testis tumors. Am. J. Roentgenol., *103*:827, 1968.

Kurohara, S. S., George, F. W., III, Dykhuisen, R. F., and Leary, M. L.: Testicular tumors: Analysis of 196 cases treated in the U.S. Naval Hospital, San Diego. Cancer, *20*:1089, 1967.

Lange, P. H., and Raghavan, D.: Clinical application of tumor markers in testicular cancer. *In* Donohue, J. P. (Ed.): Testes Tumor. Baltimore, The Williams & Wilkins Co., 1983, pp. 111–130.

LeComete (1851). Quoted by Grove, J. S.: The cryptorchid problem. J. Urol., *71*:735, 1954.

Leopold, G. R., Woo, V. L., Scheible, F. W., Nachtsheim, D., and Gosink, B. B.: High resolution ultrasonography of scrotal pathology. Radiography, *131*:719, 1979.

Mack, T. M., and Henderson, B. E.: Cancer Registries for General and Special Uses. *In* US-USSR Monograph, NIH Publ. No. 80-2044, 1980, pp. 57–61.

Martin, D. C.: Germinal cell tumors of the testis after orchiopexy. J. Urol., *121*:422, 1979.

Mauch, P., Weichselbaum, R., and Botnick, L.: The significance of positive chorionic gonadotropins in apparently pure seminoma of the testis. Int. J. Radiol. Oncol. Biol. Phys., *5*:887, 1979.

Melicow, M. M.: Classification of tumors of testis: Clinical and pathological study based on 105 primary and 13 secondary cases in adults, and 3 primary and 4 secondary cases in children. J. Urol., *73*:547, 1955.

Mengel, W., Wronecki, K., Schroeder, J., and Zimmermann, F. A.: Histopathology of the cryptorchid testis. Urol. Clin. North Am., *9*:331, 1982.

Michalowsky, I.: Eine Experimentelle Erzeugung Teratioder Geschwulste der Hoden Beim Hahn. Zweite Mitteilung. Virchows Arch (Pathol. Anat.), *267*:27, 1928.

Morrison, A. S.: Some social and medical characteristics of Army men with testicular cancer. Am. J. Epidemiol., *104*:511, 1976.

Mostofi, F. K.: Testicular tumors. Epidemiologic, etiologic and pathologic features. Cancer, *32*:1186, 1973.

Mostofi, F. K., and Price, E. B.: Tumors of the male genital system. Atlas of Tumor Pathology, Second Series. Fascicle 8. Washington, D.C., Armed Forces Institute of Pathology, 1973.

Mostofi, F. K., and Sobin, L. H.: International Histological Classification of Tumors of Testes (No 16). Geneva, World Health Organization, 1977.

Muir, C. S., and Nectoux, J.: National Cancer Institute Monograph, 53:157, 1979.

Muller, K.: Cancer Testis Thesis. Copenhagen, Munksgaard, 1962.

Nomura, T., and Kanzak, T.: Induction of urogenital anomalies and some tumor in the progeny of mice receiving diethylstilbestrol during pregnancy. Cancer Res., 37:1099, 1977.

Patton, J. F., and Mallis, N.: Tumors of the testis. J. Urol., 81:457, 1959.

Patton, J. F., Hewitt, C. B., and Mallis, N.: The diagnosis and treatment of tumors of the testis. JAMA, 171:2194, 1959.

Patton, J. F., Sietzman, D. N., and Zone, R. A.: Diagnosis and treatment of testicular tumors. Am. J. Surg., 99:525, 1960.

Peckham, M. J.: Testicular tumours, investigation and staging: General aspects and staging classifications. In Peckham, M. J. (Ed.): The Management of Testicular Tumours. Chicago, Year Book Medical Publishers, 1982, pp. 89–101.

Peckham, M. J., Barrett, A., McElwain, T. J., Hendry, W. F., and Raghavan, D.: Nonseminoma germ cell tumours (malignant teratoma) of the testis: Results of treatment and an analysis of prognostic factors. Br. J. Urol., 53:162, 1981.

Petersen, G. R., and Lee, J. A. H.: Secular trends of malignant tumors of the testis in white men. J. Natl. Cancer Inst., 49:339, 1972.

Pierce, G. B.: Teratocarcinoma: introduction and perspectives. In Sherman, M. I., and Solter, D. (Eds.): Teratomas and Differentiation. New York, Academic Press, 1975, pp. 3–12.

Pugh, R. C. B., and Cameron, K.: Teratoma. In Pugh, R. C. B. (Ed.): Pathology of the Testis. Oxford, Blackwell Scientific Publications, 1976, pp. 199–244.

Ray, B., Hajou, S. I., and Whitmore, W. F., Jr.: Distribution of retroperitoneal lymph node metastases in testicular germinal tumors. Cancer, 33:340, 1974.

Ross, R. K., McCurtis, J. W., Henderson, B. F., et al.: Descriptive epidemiology of testicular and prostatic cancer in Los Angeles. Br. J. Cancer, 39:284, 1979.

Rothman, K. J., and Louik, C.: Oral contraceptives and birth defects. N. Engl. J. Med., 299:522, 1978.

Ruoslahti, E., Engvall, E., Pekkala, A., and Seppala, M.: Developmental changes in carbohydrate moiety of human alpha-fetoprotein. Int. J. Cancer, 22:515, 1978.

Schottenfeld, D., Warshauer, M. E., Sherlock, S., Zauber, A. G., Leder, M., and Payne, R.: The epidemiology of testicular cancer in young adults. Am. J. Epidemiol., 112:232, 1980.

Schwartz, J. W., and Reed, J. F., Jr.: The pathology of cryptorchidism. J. Urol., 76:429, 1956.

Scorer, C. C., and Farrington, G. H.: Congenital Deformities of the Testis and Epididymis. Chapter 2. New York, Appleton-Century-Crofts, 1971.

Silverberg, E.: Cancer statistics. Ca. 33:9, 1983.

Skakkebaek, N. E.: Carcinoma in situ of the testis. Lancet, 2:516, 1972.

Sohval, A. R.: Testicular dysgenesis in relation to neoplasm of the testicle. J. Urol., 75:285, 1956.

Sokal, M., Peckham, M. J., and Hendry, W. F.: Bilateral

germ cell tumours of the testis. Br. J. Urol., 53:158, 1980.

Speers, W. C.: Conversion of malignant murine embryonal carcinomas to benign teratomas by chemical induction of differentiation in vivo. Cancer Res., 42:1843, 1982.

Stanton, G. F., Bosl, G. J., Vugrin, D., Whitmore, W. F., Myers, W. P. L. M., and Golbey, R. B.: Treatment of patients with advanced seminoma with cyclophosphamide, bleomycin, actinomycin D, vinblastine and cisplatin (VAB-6) (Abstract C-551). Proc. Am. Soc. Clin. Oncol., 2:1, 1983.

Stevens, L. C.: Origin of testicular teratomas from primordial germ cells in mice. J. Natl. Cancer Inst., 38:549, 1967.

Stevens, L. C.: The development of teratomas from intratesticular grafts of tubal mouse eggs. J. Embryol. Exp. Morphol., 20:329, 1968.

Strickland, S., and Mahdavi, V.: The induction of differentiation in teratocarcinoma stem cells by retinoic acid. Cell, 15:393, 1978.

Teilum, G.: Endodermal sinus tumors of ovary and testis: comparative morphogenesis of so-called mesonephroma ovarie (Schiller) and extraembryonic structure of rat placenta. Cancer, 12:1092, 1959.

Teilum, G.: Special Tumors of Ovary and Testis. Comparative Pathology and Histological Classification. Philadelphia, J. B. Lippincott Co., 1971.

Teilum, G., Albrechtsen, R., and Norgaard-Pederson, B.: The histogenetic embryologic basis for re-appearance of alpha-feto-protein in endodermal sinus tumors (yolk sac tumors) and teratoma. Acta Pathol. Microbiol. Scand., 83:80, 1975.

Thackray, A. C., and Crane, W. A. J.: Seminoma. In Pugh, R. C. B. (Ed.): Pathology of the Testis. Oxford, Blackwell Scientific Publications, 1976.

Thompson, D. K., and Haddow, J. E.: Serial monitoring of serum alpha-fetoprotein and chorionic gonadotropin in males with germ cell tumors. Cancer, 43:1820, 1979.

Thurzo, R., and Pinter, J.: Cryptorchidism and malignancy in men and animals. Urol. Int., 11:216, 1961.

Uriel, J.: Retrodifferentiation and the fetal patterns of gene expression in cancer. Adv. Cancer Res., 29:127, 1979.

Vaitukaitis, J. L.: Human chorionic gonadotropin: a hormone secreted for many reasons. N. Engl. J. Med., 301:324, 1979.

Vechinski, T. O., Jaeschke, W. H., and Vermund, H.: Testicular tumors: an analysis of 112 consecutive cases. Am. J. Roentgenol., 95:494, 1965.

Weissbach, L., and Ibach, B.: Neue Aspekte zur Bedeutung und Behandlung von Hodendescensusstorungen. Klin. Paediatr., 187:289, 1975.

Whitaker, R. H.: Management of the undescended testis. Br. J. Hosp. Med., 4:25, 1970.

Whitmore, W. F., Jr.: The treatment of germinal tumors of the testis. In Proceedings of the Sixth National Cancer Conference. Philadelphia, J. B. Lippincott Co., 1968, pp. 347–355.

Whitmore, W. F., Jr.: Germinal tumors of the testis. In Proceedings of the Seventh National Cancer Conference. Philadelphia, J. B. Lippincott Co., 1973, pp. 485–499.

World Health Organization: Laboratory Manual for the Examination of Human Semen and Semen-Cervical Mucus Interaction. Singapore, Press Concern, 1980.

Zdeb, M. S.: The probability of developing cancer. Am. J. Epidemiol., 106:6, 1977.

Zondek, B.: Versuch Einer Biologischen (Hormonalen) Diagnostik Beim Malignen Hodentumor. Chirurg, 2:1072, 1930.

Seminoma

Batata, M. A., Chu, F. C. H., Hilaris, B. S., Unal, A., Whitmore, W. F., Jr., Grabstald, H., and Golbey, R. B.: Radiation therapy role in testicular germinomas. Adv. Med. Oncol., *6*:279, 1979.

Blandy, J. P.: Urology, Vol. 2, Oxford, Blackwell Scientific Publications, 1976, p. 1203.

Caldwell, W. L., Kademian, M. T., Frias, Z., and Davis, T. E.: The Management of Testicular Seminoma, 1979. Cancer, *45*:1768, 1980.

Crawford, E. D., Smith, R. B., and deKernion, J. B.: Treatment of advanced seminoma with pre-radiation therapy. J. Urol., *129*:752, 1983.

Doornbos, J. F., Hussey, D. H., and Johnson, D. E.: Radiotherapy for pure seminoma of the testis. Radiology, *116*:401, 1975.

Dosoretz, D. E., Shipley, W. U., Blitzer, P. H., Gilbert, S., Prat, J., Parkhurst, E., and Wang, C. C.: Megavoltage irradiation for pure testicular seminoma: results and patterns of failure. Cancer, *48*:2184, 1981.

Earle, J. D., Bagshaw, M. A., and Kaplan, H. S.: Supervoltage radiation therapy of the testicular tumors. Am. J. Roentgenol., *117*:653, 1973.

Einhorn, L. H.: Radiotherapy in seminoma—more is not better. Int. J. Radiat. Oncol. Biol. Phys., *8*:309, 1981.

Einhorn, L. H., and Williams, S. D.: Chemotherapy of disseminated seminoma. Cancer Clin. Trials, *3*:307, 1980.

Green, N., Broth, E., George, F. W., Kaplan, R., Lombardo, L., Skaist, L., Weinstein, E., and Petrovich, Z.: Radiation therapy in bulky seminoma. Urology, *21*:467, 1983.

Javadpour, N., McIntire, K. R., and Waldmann, T. A.: Human chorionic gonadotropin (hCG) and alpha-fetoprotein (AFP) in sera and tumor cells of patients with testicular seminoma. Cancer, *42*:2768, 1978.

Johnson, D. E., Appelt, G., Samuels, M. L., and Luna, M.: Metastases from testicular carcinoma: Study of 78 autopsied cases. Urology, *8*:234, 1976.

Johnson, D. E., Gomez, J. J., and Ayala, A. G.: Anaplastic seminoma. J. Urol., *114*:80, 1975.

Maier, J. G., and Sulak, M. H.: Radiation therapy in malignant testis tumors. Part I: Seminoma. Cancer, *32*:1212, 1973.

Maier, J. G., Mittemeyer, B. T., and Sulak, M. H.: Treatment and prognosis in seminoma of the testis. J. Urol., *99*:72, 1968.

Mendenhall, W. L., Williams, S. D., Einhorn, L. H., and Donohue, J. P.: Disseminated seminoma: re-evaluation of treatment protocols. J. Urol., *126*:493, 1981.

Morse, M. J., Herr, H. W., Sogani, P. C., Bosl, G. J., and Whitmore, W. F., Jr.: Surgical exploration of metastatic seminoma following VAB-6 chemotherapy (Abstract C-559). Proc. Am. Soc. Clin. Oncol., *2*:143, 1983.

Oliver, R. T.: Surveillance for stage I seminoma and single agent cis-platin for metastatic seminoma (Abstract C-636). Proc. Am. Soc. Clin. Oncol., *3*:162, 1984.

Peckham, M. J., and McElwain, T. J.: Radiotherapy of testicular tumors. Proc. R. Soc. Med., *67*:300, 1974.

Percarpio, B., Clements, J. C., McLeod, D. G., Sorgen, S. D., and Cardinale, F. S.: Anaplastic seminoma. An analysis of 77 patients. Cancer, *43*:2510, 1979.

Rossai, J., Silber, I., and Khodadoust, K.: Spermatocytic seminoma. Clinicopathologic study of six cases and review of the literature. Cancer, *24*:92, 1969.

Shulman, Y., Ware, S., Al-Askari, S., and Morales, P.: Anaplastic seminoma. Urology, *21*:379, 1983.

Smith, R. B.: Management of testicular seminoma. *In* Skinner, D. G., and deKernion, J. B. (Eds.): Genitourinary Cancer. Philadelphia, W. B. Saunders Co., 1978, pp. 460–469.

Thomas, G. M., and Herman, J. G.: The role of radiation in the management of seminoma. *In* Kurth, K. H., et al. (Eds.): Progress and Controversies in Oncological Urology. New York, Alan R. Liss, 1984, pp. 91–102.

Thomas, G. M., Rider, W. D., Dembo, A. J., Cummings, B. J., Gospodarowicz, M., Hawkins, M. B., Herman, J. G., and Keen, C. W.: Seminoma of the testis: Results of treatment and patterns of failure after radiation therapy. Int. J. Radiat. Oncol. Biol. Phys., *8*:165, 1982.

van der Werf–Messing, B.: Radiotherapeutic treatment of testicular tumors. Int. J. Radiat. Oncol. Biol. Phys., *1*:235, 1976.

Vugrin, D., Whitmore, W. F., Jr., and Batata, M.: Chemotherapy of disseminated seminoma with combination of cis-diamminedichloroplatinum (II) and cyclophosphamide. Cancer Clin. Trials, *4*:423, 1981.

Wajsman, Z., Beckley, S. A., and Pintes, J. E.: Changing concepts in the treatment of advanced seminomatous tumors. J. Urol., *129*:303, 1983.

Weitzner, S.: Spermatocytic seminoma. Urology, *7*:646, 1976.

Yagoda, A., and Vugrin, D.: Theoretical considerations in the treatment of seminoma. Semin. Oncol., *6*:74, 1979.

Nonseminoma

Battermann, J. J., Delemarre, J. F. M., Hart, A. A. M., et al.: Testicular tumors: a retrospective study. Arch. Chir. Neerl., *25*:457, 1973.

Bech, P. H., and Stutzman, R. E.: Complications of retroperitoneal lymphadenectomy for nonseminomatous tumor of the testis. Urology, *13*:244, 1979.

Berthelson, J. G., and Skakkebaek, N. E.: Gonadal function in men with testis tumor. Fertil. Steril., *39*:68, 1983.

Blandy, J. P., Oliver, R. T. D., and Hope-Stone, H. F.: A British approach to the management of patients with testicular tumors. Testes Tumors, *7*:207, 1983.

Bosl, G. J., Geller, N., Cirrincione, C., Nisselbaum, J., Vugrin, D., Whitmore, W. F., Jr., and Golbey, R. B.: Serum tumor markers in patients with metastatic germ cell tumors of the testis. Am. J. Med., *75*:29, 1983*a*.

Bosl, G. J., Geller, N., Cirrincione, C., Hadju, S., Whitmore, W. F., Jr., Nisselbaum, J., Vugrin, D., and Golbey, R. B.: Interrelationships of histopathology and other clinical variables in patients with germ cell tumors of the testis. Cancer, *51*:2121, 1983*b*.

Bosl, G. J., Geller, N. L., Cirrincione, C., Vogelzang, N. J., Kennedy, B. J., Whitmore, W. F., Jr., Vugrin, D., Scher, H., Nisselbaum, J., and Golbey, R. B.: Multivariate analysis of prognostic variables in patients with metastatic testicular cancer. Cancer Res., *43*:3403, 1983*c*.

Bosl, G. J., Yagoda, A., Whitmore, W. F., Jr., Sogani, P., Herr, H., Vugrin, D., Dukeman, M., and Golbey, R.: VP-16-213 and cisplatinum in the treatment of patients with refractory germ cell tumor. Am. J. Clin. Oncol., *7*:327, 1984.

Bracken, R. B., and Johnson, D. E.: Sexual function and fecundity after treatment of testicular tumors. Urology, *12*:35, 1976.

Bracken, R. B., Johnson, D. E., Frazier, O. H., Logothetis, C. J., Trindade, A., and Samuels, M. L.: The role of surgery following chemotherapy in stage III germ cell neoplasms. J. Urol., *129*:39, 1983.

Bradfield, J. S., Hagen, R. O., and Ytredal, D. O.: Carcinoma of the testis: an analysis of 104 cases with germinal tumors of the testis other than seminoma. Cancer, *31*:633, 1973.

Bredael, J. J., Vugrin, D., and Whitmore, W. F., Jr.: Autopsy findings in 154 patients with germ cell tumors of the testis. Cancer, *50*:548, 1982.

Bredael, J. J., Vugrin, D., and Whitmore, W. F., Jr.: Recurrences in surgical stage I non-seminomatous germ cell tumors of the testis. J. Urol., *130*:476, 1983.

Buckner, C. D., Clift, R. A., Fefer, A., et al.: High-dose cyclophosphamide (NSC-26271) for the treatment of metastatic testicular neoplasms. Cancer Chemother. Rep., *58*:709, 1974.

Cavalli, F., Sonntag, R. W., and Brunner, K. W.: Epipodophyllotoxin derivative (VP16-213) in treatment of solid tumors. Lancet, 2:362, 1977.

Cheng, E., Cvitkovic, E., Wittes, R. E., and Golbey, R. B.: Germ cell tumors. VAB II in metastatic testicular cancer. Cancer, *42*:2162, 1978.

Clinical Screening Co-operative of the European Organization for Research on the Treatment of Cancer: Study of clinical efficiency of bleomycin. Br. Med. J., 2:643, 1970.

Cuneo, B.: Note sur les lymphatiques du testicle. Bull. Soc. Anat. (Paris), *76*:105, 1901.

DeWys, W.: Testicular Cancer Intergroup Study. Personal communication, 1984.

Donohue, J. P.: Retroperitoneal lymphadenectomy. Urol Clin. North Am., *4*:517, 1977.

Donohue, J. P., Einhorn, L. H., and Perez, J. M.: Improved management of non-seminomatous testis tumors. Cancer, *42*:2903, 1978.

Einhorn, L. H., and Donohue, J. P.: Cis-diaminedichloroplatinum, vinblastine, and bleomycin combination chemotherapy in disseminated testicular cancer. Ann. Intern. Med., *87*:293, 1977*a*.

Einhorn, L. H., and Donohue, J. P.: Improved chemotherapy in disseminated testicular cancer. J. Urol., *117*:65, 1977*b*.

Einhorn, L. H., and Donohue, J. P.: Improved chemotherapy in disseminated testicular cancer. J. Urol., *305*:727, 1981.

Einhorn, L. H., and Williams, S. D.: The management of disseminated testicular cancer. In Einhorn, L. H. (Ed.): Testicular Tumors. New York, Masson Publishing Co., 1980, pp. 117–149.

Einhorn, L. H., Williams, S. D., Mandebaum, I., and Donohue, J. P.: Surgical resection in disseminated testicular cancer following chemotherapeutic cytoreduction. Cancer, *48*:904, 1981*a*.

Einhorn, L. H., Williams, S. D., Turner, S., Troner, M., and Greco, F. A.: The role of maintenance therapy in disseminated testicular cancer. Proc. Am. Soc. Clin. Oncol., *22*:474, 1981*b*.

Fitzharris, B. M., Kaye, S. B., Saverymuttu, S., Newlands, E. S., Barrett, A., Peckham, M. J., and McElwain, T. J.: VP16-213 as a single agent in advanced testicular tumors. Eur. J. Cancer, *16*:1193, 1979.

Fraley, E. E., Lange, P. H., and Kennedy, B. J.: Germ-cell testicular cancer in adults (Part I). N. Engl. J. Med., *301*:1370, 1979*a*.

Fraley, E. E., Lange, P. H., and Kennedy, B. J.: Germ-cell testicular cancer in adults (Part II). N. Engl. J. Med., *301*:1420, 1979*b*.

Glatstein, E.: Radiotherapy in the management of nonseminomatous testicular carcinoma. Cancer Treat. Rep., *63*:1649, 1979.

Hayes, D. M., Cvitkovic, E., Golbey, R. B., Scheiner, E., Helson, L., and Krakoff, I. H.: High dose cis-platinum

diammine dichloride. Amelioration of renal toxicity by mannitol diuresis. Cancer, *39*:1372, 1977.

Higby, D. J., Wallace, H. J., Albert, D. J., and Holland, J. K.: Diaminodichloroplatinum: A Phase I study showing responses in testicular and other tumors. Cancer, *33*:1219, 1974.

Hong, W. K., Wittes, R. E., Hajdu, S. T., Cvitkovic, E., Whitmore, W. F., Jr., and Golbey, R. B.: The evolution of mature teratoma from malignant testicular tumors. Cancer, *40*:2987, 1977.

Hussey, D. H.: Experience with preoperative radiotherapy and lymphadenectomy for germinal cell tumors of the testis other than pure seminoma. In Johnson, D. E., and Samuels, M. L. (Eds.): Cancer of the Genitourinary Tract. New York, Raven Press, 1979, pp. 149–172.

Hussey, D. H.: A comparison of treatment methods for germinal cell tumors of the testis other than pure seminoma. Radiology, *139*:181, 1981.

Jain, K. K., Bosl, G. J., Vugrin, D., Whitmore, W. F., Jr., and Golbey, R. B.: The treatment of extragonadal seminoma. J. Clin. Oncol., 2:280, 1984.

Jamieson, J. K., and Dobson, J. F.: The lymphatics of the testicle. Lancet, *1*:493, 1910.

Johnson, D. E., Bracken, R. B., and Blight, E. M.: Prognosis for pathologic Stage I non-seminomatous germ cell tumors of the testis managed by retroperitoneal lymphadenectomy. J. Urol., *116*:63, 1976.

Johnson, D. E., Lo, R. K., von Eschenbach, A. C., and Swanson, D. A.: Surveillance alone for patients with clinical Stage I nonseminomatous germ cell tumors of the testis: Preliminary results. J. Urol., *131*:491, 1984.

Juttner, C. A., and McElwain, T. J.: Chemotherapy of testicular teratoma. In Peckham, M. J. (Ed.): The Management of Testicular Tumours. Chicago, Year Book Medical Publishers, 1981, pp. 202–217.

Kedia, K. R., Markland, C., and Fraley, E. E.: Sexual function after high retroperitoneal lymphadenectomy. Urol. Clin. North Am., *4*:523, 1977.

Kimbrough, J. C., and Cook, F. E., Jr.: Carcinoma of the testis. JAMA, *153*:1436, 1953.

Klein, K. A., and Maier, J. G.: Positive nodes and treatment failures in testicular tumors. Int. J. Radiat. Oncol. Biol. Phys., 2:1229, 1977.

Koops, H. S., Oldhoff, J., Sleijfer, D. Th., Oosterhuis, J. W., and Homan van der Heide, J. N.: The role of surgery after remission-induction chemotherapy in nonseminoma Stage III testicular tumors. In Kurth, K. H., et al. (Eds.): Progress and Controversies in Oncological Urology. New York, Alan R. Liss, 1984, pp. 233–238.

Lederman, G. S., Garnick, M. B., Ritchie, J. P., and Canellos, G. P.: VP-16-213 and cis-platinum as secondary therapy in patients with refractory testicular and extragonadal germ cell cancer (Abstract 576). Proc. Am. Assoc. Cancer Res., *24*:146, 1983.

Lewis, L. G.: Testis tumor: report on 250 cases. J. Urol., *59*:763, 1948.

Li, M. C., Whitmore, W. F., Jr., Golbey, R., and Grabstald, H.: Effects of combined drug therapy on metastatic cancer of the testis. JAMA, *174*:1291, 1960.

Logothetis, C. J., Samuels, M. C., Trindade, A., and Johnson, D. E.: The growing teratoma syndrome. Cancer, *50*:1629, 1982.

MacKenzie, A. R.: The chemotherapy of metastatic seminoma. J. Urol., *96*:790, 1966.

Maier, J. G., and Mittemeyer, B. T.: Carcinoma of the testis. Cancer, *39*:981, 1977.

Merrin, C., Baumastner, G., and Wajsman, Z.: Benign

transformation of testicular carcinoma by chemotherapy. Lancet, 2:43, 1975.

Monfardini, S., Basetta, E., Musumeci, R., and Bonadonna, G.: Clinical use of Adriamycin in advanced testicular cancer. J. Urol., 108:293, 1972.

Mortimer, J., Bukowski, R. M., Montie, J., Hewlett, J. S., and Livingston, R. B.: VP-16-213 cisplatinum, and Adriamycin salvage therapy of refractory and/or recurrent nonseminomatous germ cell neoplasms. Cancer Chemother. Pharmacol., 61:99, 1984.

Most, H.: Uber Malique Loden ges Chwulste Und Ihrematastasin. Arch. Pathol. Anat., 154:1898.

Mostofi, F. K.: Proceedings: Testicular tumors. Epidemiologic, etiologic, and pathologic features. Cancer, 32:1186, 1973.

Newlands, E. S., and Bagshawe, K. D.: Epipodophyllin derivative (VP16-213) in malignant teratomas and choriocarcinomas. Lancet, 2:87, 1977.

Peckham, M. J.: An appraisal of the role of radiation therapy in the management of nonseminomatous germ-cell tumors of the testis in the era of effective chemotherapy. Cancer Treat. Rep., 63:1653, 1979.

Peckham, M. J., Barrett, A., McElwain, T. J., Hendry, W. F., and Raghavan, D.: Non-seminoma germ cell tumours (malignant teratoma) of the testis. Br. J. Urol., 53:162, 1981.

Peckham, M. J., Barrett, A., Horwich, A., and Hendry, W. F.: Orchiectomy alone for Stage I testicular non-seminoma. Br. J. Urol., 55:754, 1983.

Peckham, M. J., Hendry, W., McElwain, T. J., and Calman, P. M. M.: The multimodality management of testicular teratomas. In Salmon, S. E., and Jones, S. E. (Eds.): Adjuvant Therapy of Cancer. Amsterdam, North-Holland, 1977, pp. 305–320.

Raghavan, D., Peckham, M. J., Heyderman, E., Tobias, J. S., and Austin, D. E.: Prognostic factors in clinical Stage I non-seminomatous germ-cell tumours of the testis. Br. J. Cancer, 45:167, 1982.

Reynolds, T. F., Vugrin, D., Cvitkovic, E., Cheng, E., Braum, D. W., O'Hehir, M. A., Dukeman, M. E., Whitmore, W. F., Jr., and Golbey, R. B.: VAB-3 combination chemotherapy of metastatic testicular cancer. Cancer, 48:888, 1981.

Rouviere, H.: Anatomy of the Human Lymphatic System (Translated by M. J. Tobias). Ann Arbor, Mich., Edwards Bros., 1938.

Sago, A. L., Ball, T. P., and Novick, D. E.: Complication of retroperitoneal lymphadenectomy. Urology, 13:241, 1979.

Samuels, M. L., and Howe, C. D.: Vinblastine in the management of testicular cancer. Cancer, 25:1009, 1970.

Samuels, M. L., Holoye, P. Y., and Johnson, D. E.: Bleomycin combination chemotherapy in the management of testicular neoplasia. Cancer, 36:318, 1975.

Samuels, M. L., Lanzoti, V. J., Holoye, P. Y., Boyle, L. E., Smith, T. L., and Johnson, D. E.: Combination chemotherapy in germinal tumors. Cancer Treat. Rep., 3:185, 1976.

Scher, H., Bosl, G. J., Geller, N., Cirrincione, C., Whitmore, W. F., Jr., and Golbey, R. B.: Long-term follow-up of patients with testicular germ cell tumors achieving complete remission after chemotherapy (CT) alone or CT plus surgery (Abstract 621). Proc. Am. Assoc. Cancer Res., 24:157, 1983.

Skinner, D. G.: Surgical management of germ cell tumors of the testis. In Skinner, D. G. (Ed.): Urological Cancer. New York, Grune & Stratton, 1983, pp. 301–314.

Skinner, D. G.: Nonseminomatous testis tumors: a plan of management based on 96 patients to improve survival in all stages by combined therapeutic modalities. J. Urol., 115:65, 1976.

Skinner, D. G., and Scardino, P. T.: Relevance of biochemical tumor markers and lymphadenectomy in management of non-seminomatous testis tumors: current perspective. J. Urol., 123:378, 1980.

Sogani, P. C., Whitmore, W. F., Jr., Herr, H. W., Bosl, G. J., Golbey, R. B., Watson, R. C., and DeCasse, J.: Orchiectomy alone in the treatment of clinical Stage I non-seminomatous germ cell tumor of the testis. J. Urol., 2:267, 1984.

Staubitz, W. J.: Surgical treatment of nonseminomatous germinal testis tumors. In Johnson, D. E., and Samuels, M. C. (Eds.): Cancer of the Genitourinary Tract. New York, Raven Press, 1979, pp. 135–138.

Staubitz, W. J., Early, K. S., Magoss, I. V., and Murphy, G. P.: Surgical management of testis tumor. J. Urol., 111:205, 1974.

Sturgeon, J. F., Herman, J. G., Jewett, M. A., Alison, R. E., Gospodarowicz, M. K., and Comisarow, R.: A policy of surveillance alone after orchidectomy for clinical Stage I non-seminomatous testis tumors (Abstract C-558). Proc. Am. Soc. Clin. Oncol., 2:142, 1983.

Terebelo, H. R., Taylor, H. G., Brown, A., Martin, N., Stutz, F. H., Blom, J., and Geier, L.: Late relapse of testicular cancer. J. Clin. Oncol., 1:566, 1983.

Tyrrell, C. J., and Peckham, M. J.: The response of lymph node metastasis of testicular teratoma to radiation therapy. Br. J. Urol., 48:363, 1976.

van der Werf–Messing, B.: Radiotherapeutic treatment of testicular tumors. Int. J. Radiat. Oncol. Biol. Phys., 1:235, 1976.

Vugrin, D., Cvitkovic, E., and Whitmore, W. F., Jr.: Adjuvant chemotherapy in resected non-seminomatous germ cell tumors of testis: Stage I and II. Semin. Oncol., 6:94, 1979.

Vugrin, D., Cvitkovic, E., Whitmore, W. F., Jr., Cheng, E., and Golbey, R. B.: VAB-4 combination chemotherapy in the treatment of metastatic testis tumors. Cancer, 47:833, 1981a.

Vugrin, D., Freidman, A., and Whitmore, W. F., Jr.: Correlation of serum tumor markers in advanced germ cell tumors with responses to chemotherapy and surgery. Cancer, 53:1440, 1984.

Vugrin, D., Herr, H., Whitmore, W. F., Jr., Sogani, P. C., and Golbey, R. B.: VAB-6 combination chemotherapy in disseminated cancer of the testis. Ann. Intern. Med., 95:59, 1981b.

Vugrin, D., Whitmore, W. F., Jr., Cvitkovic, E., Grabstald, H., Sogani, P., Barzell, W., and Golbey, R. B.: Adjuvant chemotherapy combination of vinblastine, actinomycin D, bleomycin, and chlorambucil following retroperitoneal lymph node dissection for Stage II testis tumor. Cancer, 47:840, 1981c.

Vugrin, D., Whitmore, W. F., Jr., and Golbey, R. B.: VAB-5 combination chemotherapy in prognostically poor risk patients with germ cell tumors. Cancer, 51:1072, 1983.

Vugrin, D., Whitmore, W. F., Jr., Sogani, P. C., Bains, M., Herr, H., and Golbey, R. B.: Combined chemotherapy and surgery in treatment of advanced germ-cell tumors. Cancer, 47:2228, 1981d.

Vugrin, D., Whitmore, W. F., Jr., Cvitkovic, E., Grabstald, H., Sogani, P. C., and Golbey, R. B.: Adjuvant chemotherapy with VAB-3 of Stage II-B testicular tumor. Cancer, 48:233, 1981e.

Vugrin, D., Whitmore, W. F., Jr., Herr, H., Sogani, P. C., and Golbey, R. B.: Adjuvant vinblastine, actinomycin D, bleomycin, cyclophosphamide and cis-platinum chemotherapy regimen with and without maintenance in patients with resected Stage II-B testis cancer. J. Urol., *128*:715, 1982.

Vugrin, D., Whitmore, W. F., Jr., and Golbey, R. B.: VAB-6 combination chemotherapy without maintenance in treatment of disseminated cancer of the testis. Cancer, *51*:211, 1983.

Walsh, P. C., Kaufman, J. J., Coulson, W. F., and Goodwin, W. E.: Retroperitoneal lymphadenectomy for testicular tumors. JAMA, *217*:309, 1971.

Whitmore, W. F., Jr.: Surgical treatment of clinical stage I nonseminomatous germ cell tumours of the testis. Cancer Treat. Rep., *66*:5, 1982.

Whitmore, W. F., Jr.: Germinal tumors of the testes. *In* Proceedings of the Sixth National Cancer Conference. Philadelphia, J. B. Lippincott Co., 1970, pp. 219–221.

Whitmore, W. F., Jr.: Surgical treatment of adult germinal testis tumors. Semin. Oncol., *6*:55, 1979.

Williams, S. D., and Einhorn, L. H.: Chemotherapy of disseminated testicular cancer. *In* Donohue, J. P. (Ed.): Testis Tumors. Baltimore, The Williams & Wilkins Co., 1983, pp. 252–264.

Williams, S. D., Einhorn, L. H., and Donohue, J. P.: High cure rate I or II testicular cancer with or without adjuvant therapy (Abstract C-407). Proc. Am. Assoc. Cancer Res. Am. Soc. Clin. Oncol., *21*:1, 1980*a*.

Williams, S. D., Einhorn, L. H., Greco, F. A., Oldham, R., and Fletcher, R.: VP-16-213 salvage therapy for refractory germinal neoplasms. Cancer, *46*:2154, 1980*b*.

Wittes, R. E., Yagoda, A., Silvay, O., Magill, G. B., Whitmore, W. F., Jr., Krakoff, I. H., and Golbey, R. B.: Chemotherapy of germ cell tumors of the testis. Cancer, *37*:637, 1976.

Yagoda, A., Mukherji, B., Young, C., Etcubanas, E., LaMonte, C., Smith, J. R., Tan, C. T. C., and Krakoff, I. H.: Bleomycin, an antitumor antibiotic. Ann. Intern. Med., *77*:861, 1972.

Extragonadal Tumors

Beattie, E. J., Jr.: Mediastinal germ cell tumors (surgery). Semin. Oncol., *6*:109, 1979.

Cole, H.: Tumours in the region of the pineal. Clin. Radiol., *22*:110, 1971.

Garnick, M. B., Canellos, G. P., and Richie, J. P.: Treatment and surgical staging of testicular and primary extragonadal germ cell cancer. JAMA, *250*:1733, 1983.

Hainsworth, J. D., Einhorn, L. H., Williams, S. D., Stewart, M., and Greco, F. A.: Advanced extragonadal germ cell tumors. Successful treatment with combination chemotherapy. Ann. Intern. Med., *97*:7, 1982.

Jain, K. K., Bosl, G. J., Bains, M. S., Whitmore, W. F., Jr., and Golbey, R. B.: The treatment of extragonadal seminoma. J. Clin. Oncol., *2*:820, 1984.

Johnson, D. E., Laneri, J. P., Mountain, C. F., and Luna, M.: Extragonadal germ cell tumors. Surgery, *73*:85, 1973.

Luna, M. A., and Valenzuela-Tamariz, J.: Germ cell tumors of the mediastinum: Post-mortem findings. Am. J. Clin. Pathol., *65*:450, 1976.

Martini, N., Golbey, R. B., Hajdu, S. I., Whitmore, W. F., and Beattie, E. J.: Primary mediastinal germ cell tumors. Cancer, *33*:763, 1974.

Prym, P.: Spontanheilung eines Bosartigen, Wahrscheinlich Chorion-epithelio-matosen Gewachs im Hoden. Virchows Arch., *265*:239, 1927.

Recondo, J., and Libshitz, H. I.: Mediastinal extragonadal germ cell tumors. Urology, *11*:369, 1978.

Reynolds, T. F., Yagoda, A., Vugrin, D., and Golbey, R. B.: Chemotherapy of mediastinal germ cell tumors. Semin. Oncol., *6*:113, 1979.

Stanton, G. F., Bosl, G. J., Vugrin, D., Whitmore, W. F., Jr., Myers, W. P. L. M., and Golbey, R. B.: Treatment of patients with advanced seminoma with cyclophosphamide, bleomycin, actinomycin D, vinblastine and cisplatin (VAB-6) (Abstract C-551). Proc. Am. Soc. Clin. Oncol., *2*:141, 1983.

Sterchi, M., and Cordell, A. R.: Seminoma of the anterior mediastinum. Ann. Thorac. Surg., *19*:371, 1975.

Utz, D. C., and Buscemi, M. F.: Extragonadal testicular tumors. J. Urol., *105*:271, 1971.

Nongerminal Tumors

Sex Cord–Mesenchyme Tumors

Akdas, A., Remzi, D., and Finci, R.: Bilateral interstitial cell tumour of testes. Br. J. Urol., *55*:123, 1983.

Azer, P. C., and Braumstein, G. D.: Malignant Leydig cell tumor. Cancer, *47*:1251, 1981.

Caldamone, A. A., Altebarmakian, V., Frank, I. N., and Linke, C. A.: Leydig cell tumor of testis. Urology, *14*:39, 1979.

Campbell, C. M., and Middleton, A. W., Jr.: Malignant gonadal stromal tumor: Case report and review of the literature. J. Urol., *125*:257, 1981.

Davis, S., DiMartino, N. A., and Schneider, G.: Malignant interstitial cell carcinoma of the testis. Cancer, *47*:425, 1981.

Feldman, P. S., Kovacs, K., Horvath, E., and Andelson, G. L.: Malignant Leydig cell tumor. Cancer, *49*:714, 1982.

Gabrilove, J. L., Freiberg, E. K., Leiter, E., and Nicolis, G. L.: Feminizing and non-feminizing Sertoli cell tumors. J. Urol., *124*:757, 1980.

Gabrilove, J. L., Nicolis, G. L., Mitty, H. A., and Sohval, A. R.: Feminizing interstitial cell tumor of the testis: personal observations and a review of the literature. Cancer, *35*:1184, 1975.

Klippel, K. F., Jonas, U., Hohenfellner, R., and Walther, D.: Interstitial cell tumor of the testis: A delicate problem. Urology, *14*:79, 1979.

Lockhart, J. L., Dalton, D. L., Vollmer, R. T., and Glenn, J. F.: Nonfunctioning interstitial cell carcinoma of the testis. Urology, *8*:392, 1976.

Marshall, F. F., Kerr, W. S., Jr., Kliman, B., and Scully, R. E.: Sex cord–stromal (gonadal stromal) tumors of the testis: A report of 5 cases. J. Urol., *117*:180, 1977.

Mostofi, F. K., Theiss, E. A., and Ashley, J. B.: Tumors of specialized gonadal stroma in human male patients. Cancer, *12*:946, 1959.

Ober, W. B., Kabakow, B., and Hecht, H.: Malignant interstitial cell tumor of the testis: a problem in endocrine oncology. N.Y. Acad. Med., *52*:561, 1976.

Rosvoll, R. V., and Woodart, J. R.: Malignant Sertoli cell tumor of the testis. Cancer, *22*:8, 1968.

Sato, B., Huseby, R. A., and Samuels, L. T.: Characterization of estrogen receptors in various mouse Leydig cell tumor lines. Cancer Res., *38*:2842, 1978.

Sohral, A. R., Churg, J., Suzuki, Y., Katz, N., and Gabrilove, J. L.: Electron microscopy of a feminizing Leydig cell tumor of the testis. Human Pathol., *8*:621, 1977.

Talerman, A.: Malignant Sertoli cell tumor of the testis. Cancer, *28*:446, 1971.

Tamoney, H. J., Jr., and Noriega, A.: Malignant interstitial cell tumor of the testis. Cancer, *24*:547, 1969.

Teilum, G.: Arrhenoblastoma-androblastoma: Homologous ovarian and testicular tumors. Acta Pathol. Microbiol. Scand., *23*:252, 1946.

Teilum, G.: Special Tumors of Ovary and Testis and Related Extragonadal Lesions. Philadelphia, J. B. Lippincott Co., 1971.

Van den Bogert, C., Dontje, B. H. J., and Kroon, A. M.: Arrest in in vivo growth of a solid Leydig cell tumor by prolonged inhibition of mitochondrial protein synthesis. Cancer Res., *43*:2247, 1983.

Gonadoblastoma

Bolen, J. W.: Mixed germ cell–sex cord stromal tumor. Am. J. Clin. Pathol., *75*:565, 1981.

Garvin, J. A., Pratt-Thomas, H. R., Spector, M., Spicer, S. S., and Williamson, H. O.: Gonadoblastoma: histologic, ultrastructural, and histochemical observations in five cases. Am. J. Obstet. Gynecol., *125*:459, 1976.

Hart, W. R., and Burkons, D. M.: Germ cell neoplasms arising in gonadoblastomas. Cancer, *43*:669, 1979.

Ishida, T., Tagatz, G. E., and Okagaki, T.: Gonadoblastoma. Cancer, *37*:1770, 1976.

Melicow, M. M.: Tumors of dysgenetic gonads in intersexes: case reports and discussion regarding their places in gonadal oncology. Bull. N.Y. Acad. Med., *42*:3, 1966.

Scully, R. E.: Gonadoblastoma. Cancer, *25*:1340, 1970.

Scully, R. E.: Gonadoblastoma. A gonadal tumor related to the dysgerminoma (seminoma) and capable of sex-hormone production. Cancer, *6*:455, 1953.

Talerman, A.: A distinctive gonadal neoplasm related to gonadoblastoma. Cancer, *30*:1219, 1972.

Neoplasms of Mesenchymal Origin

Berdjis, C. C., and Mostofi, F. K.: Carcinoid tumors of the testis. J. Urol., *118*:777, 1977.

Kadir, R. G., Block, M. B., Katz, F. H., and Hofeldt, F. D.: "Masked" 21-hydroxylase deficiency of the adrenal presenting with gynecomastia and bilateral testicular masses. Am. J. Med., *62*:278, 1977.

Newell, M. E., Lippe, B. M., and Ehrlich, R. M.: Testis tumors associated with continuing diagnostic and therapeutic dilemmas. J. Urol., *117*:256, 1977.

Sullivan, J. L., Packer, J. T., and Bryant, M.: Primary malignant carcinoid of the testis. Arch. Pathol. Lab. Med., *105*:515, 1981.

Miscellaneous Primary Non–Germ Cell Tumors

Albert, P. S., and Mininberg, D. T.: Leiomyoma of the tunica albuginea. J. Urol., *107*:869, 1972.

Antman, K., Cohen, S., Dimitrov, N. Y., Green, M., and Muggia, F.: Malignant mesothelioma of the tunica vaginalis testis. J. Clin. Oncol., *2*:447, 1984.

Belville, W. D., Insalaco, S. J., Dresner, M. L., and Buck, A. S.: Benign testis tumors. J. Urol., *128*:1198, 1982.

Black, W. C., Benitez, R. E., Buesing, O. R., and Hojnoski, W.: Bizarre adenomatoid tumor of testicular tunics. Cancer, *17*:1472, 1964.

Bonard, M., and Boillat, J. J.: Epidermoid cysts of testis. Cancer, *47*:577, 1981.

Cricco, C. F., Jr., and Buck, A. S.: Hemangioendothelioma of the testis: second reported case. J. Urol., *123*:131, 1980.

Forrest, J. B., and Whitmore, W. F., Jr.: Bilateral synchronous epidermoid cysts. World J. Urol., *2*:76, 1984.

Gilchrist, K. W., and Benson, R. C., Jr.: Multifocal fibrous pseudotumor of testicular tunics. Urology, *4*:285, 1979.

Goldstein, A. M. B., Mendez, R., Vargas, A., and Terry, R.: Epidermoid cysts of testis. Urology, *15*:186, 1980.

Jacobellis, U., Ricco, R., and Ruotolo, G.: Adenocarcinoma of the rete testis 21 years after orchiopexy: case report and review of the literature. J. Urol., *125*:429, 1981.

Jimenez, R. M., and Matsuda, G. T.: Cysts of the tunica albuginea. Report of four cases and review of the literature. J. Urol., *114*:730, 1975.

Kirkland, R. T., Kirkland, J. L., Keenan, B. S., Bongiov-

anni, A. M., Rosenberg, H. S., and Clayton, G. W.: Bilateral testicular tumors in congenital adrenal hyperplasia. J. Clin. Endocrinol. Metab., *44*:367, 1977.

Lewis, H. Y., and Pierce, J. M., Jr.: Multiple fibromas of the tunica vaginalis. J. Urol., *87*:142, 1962.

Lirolsi, V. A., and Schiff, M.: Myxoid neurofibroma of the testis. J. Urol., *118*:341, 1977.

Lowenthal, S. B., Goldstein, A. M. B., and Terry, R.: Cholesterol granuloma of tunica vaginalis simulating testicular tumor. Urology, *18*:89, 1981.

Mennemeyer, R. P., and Mason, J. T.: Non-neoplastic cystic lesions of the tunica albuginea: an electron microscopic and clinical study of 2 cases. J. Urol., *121*:373, 1979.

Nistal, M., Paniagua, R., Regadera, J., and Abaurrea, M. A.: Testicular capillary haemangioma. Br. J. Urol., *54*:433, 1983.

Shah, K. H., Maxted, W. C., and Chun, B.: Epidermoid cysts of the testis. Cancer, *47*:577, 1981.

Talerman, A., Gratama, S., Miranda, S., and Okagaka, T.: Primary carcinoid tumor of the testis. Cancer, *42*:2696, 1978.

Vogelzang, N. J., Schultz, S. M., Iannucci, A. M., and Kennedy, B. J.: Malignant mesothelioma. Cancer, *53*:377, 1984.

Warner, K. E., Noyes, D. T., and Ross, J. S.: Cysts of the tunica albuginea testis: a report of 3 cases with a review of the literature. J. Urol., *132*:131, 1984.

Secondary Tumors of the Testis

Askin, R. R., Colby, T. V., and MacKintosh, F. R.: Testicular lymphomas. Cancer, *48*:2095, 1981.

Braren, V., Lukens, J. N., Stroup, S. L., Bolin, M. G., and Rhamy, R. K.: Testicular infiltrate in childhood acute lymphocytic leukemia. Urology, *16*:370, 1980.

Buskirk, S. J., Evans, R. G., Banks, P. M., O'Connell, M. J., and Earle, J. D.: Primary lymphoma of the testis. Int. J. Radiat. Oncol. Biol. Phys., *8*:1699, 1982.

Cricco, R. P., and Kandzari, S. J.: Secondary testicular tumors. J. Urol., *118*:489, 1977.

Hanash, K. A., Carney, J. A., and Kelalis, P. P.: Metastatic tumors to testicles: routes of metastasis. J. Urol., *102*:465, 1969.

Haupt, H. M., Mann, R. B., Trump, D. L., and Abeloff, M. D.: Metastatic carcinoma involving the testis. Cancer, *54*:709, 1984.

Johnson, D. E., Jackson, L., and Ayala, A. G.: Secondary carcinoma of the testis. South. Med. J., *64*:1128, 1971.

Kuo, T. T., Tschang, T. P., and Chu, J. Y.: Testicular relapse in childhood acute lymphocytic leukemia during bone marrow remission. Cancer, *38*:2604, 1976.

Paladugu, R. R., Bearman, R. M., and Rapaport, H.: Malignant lymphoma with primary manifestation in the gonad. Cancer, *45*:561, 1980.

Scheinman, L. J.: Reticulum cell sarcoma of testis. Urology, *10*:469, 1977.

Stoffel, T. J., Nesbit, M. E., and Levitt, S. H.: Extramedullary involvement of the testis in childhood leukemia. Cancer, *35*:1203, 1975.

Sussman, E. B., Hajdu, S. I., Lieberman, P. H., and Whitmore, W. F., Jr.: Malignant lymphoma of the testis: a clinicopathologic study of 37 cases. J. Urol., *118*:1004, 1977.

Talerman, A.: A primary malignant lymphoma of the testis. J. Urol., *118*:783, 1977.

Turner, R. R., Colby, T. V., and MacKintosh, F. R.: Testicular lymphomas. Cancer, *48*:2095, 1981.

Weitzner, S., and Gropp, A.: A primary reticulum cell sarcoma of testis in a 12-year old. Cancer, *37*:935, 1976.

Werth, V., Yu, G., and Marshall, F.: Non-lymphomatous metastatic tumor of the testis. J. Urol., *127*:142, 1982.

CHAPTER 34

Tumors of the Penis

PAUL F. SCHELLHAMMER, M.D.
HARRY GRABSTALD, M.D.

Coverage of the subject of abnormal penile growths must include discussion of benign tumors of the penis as well as penile cancer. Some penile lesions are strictly benign, some are premalignant or at least possess the potential for malignancy, and some are malignant but are of a histologic origin other than squamous cell penile carcinoma. A brief initial description of these lesions will serve to establish their anatomic, etiologic, and histologic relationship to squamous cell carcinoma of the penis.

BENIGN LESIONS

Congenital inclusion cysts have been reported to occur in the penoscrotal raphe (Cole and Helwig, 1976). Acquired inclusion cysts subsequent to trauma or circumcision are more common. Retention cysts arise from the sebaceous glands located on the mucosal surface of

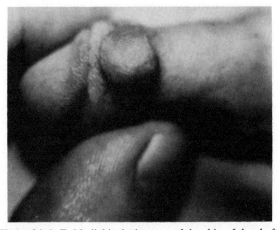

Figure 34–1. Epithelial inclusion cyst of the skin of the shaft just proximal to the coronal sulcus. It was removed by enucleation.

the prepuce and on the skin of the shaft (Fig. 34–1). Sebaceous glands are not found on the glans penis. Retention cysts may also occur in the parameatal area as a result of urethral gland obstruction (Shiraki, 1975).

Cutaneous nevi occurring on the skin of the penis must be distinguished from malignant melanoma by biopsy (see further on) (Figure 34–2).

Benign tumors of the supporting structures include angiomas, fibromas, neuromas, lipomas, and myomas and are discussed further under the section of sarcomas of the penis. Angiomas are usually superficial. They appear as punctate reddish macules or papules that occur most frequently on the coronal aspect of the glans and resemble the small angiokeratomas found on the scrotum.

Penile masses and deformities, or pseudotumors, may be secondary to self-administered injections or foreign body implants (Nitidandhaprabhas, 1975). Testosterone in oil (Zalar et al., 1969) and other common oils (Engelman et al., 1974) have been placed on or injected into the penis, producing a destructive lipogranulomatous process that may grossly mimic carcinoma. Endogenous lipoid degeneration may at times produce a similar inflammatory response (Smetana and Bernhard, 1950).

Hirsutoid papillomas, pearly penile papules, or coronal papillae are common and normal findings on the glans penis. They consist of linear, curved, or irregular rows of conical or globular excrescences that are arranged along the coronal sulcus and vary in color from white to yellow to red. When larger than usual they may be confused with small condylomata acuminata. No active treatment is necessary, and no association with infection or malignancy is reported (Tanenbaum and Becker, 1965).

Occasionally, phlebitis (Grossman et al.,

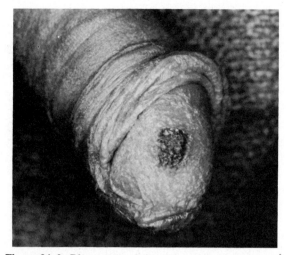

Figure 34–2. Blue nevus of the glans penis. (Courtesy of Dr. Peter Scardino.)

1965), lymphangitis (Ball and Pickett, 1975; Nickel and Plumb, 1962), or angitis (Rubenstein and Wolff, 1964) may produce subcutaneous penile nodules or cords.

When a diagnosis is in question, all benign lesions are best treated with local excision and careful histologic diagnosis to rule out malignancy.

DERMATOLOGIC LESIONS

CUTANEOUS HORNS

The cutaneous horn rarely occurs on the penis. This lesion is characterized by an overgrowth and a cornification of the epithelium, forming a solid protuberance. On microscopic examination there is extreme hyperkeratosis, dyskeratosis, and acanthosis. This process usually develops over a pre-existing skin condition (i.e., wart, nevus, area of trauma, or malignant change) and may enlarge quite rapidly. Treatment consists of surgical excision to include a margin of normal tissue around the base of the lesion. Since this growth may be stimulated by an underlying carcinoma, careful histologic study of the base and close follow-up of the scar are necessary (Hassan et al., 1967; Pressman et al., 1962).

BALANITIS XEROTICA OBLITERANS

The most frequent manifestation of balanitis xerotica obliterans is a white patch on the prepuce or on the glans that extends to and around the urethral meatus and occasionally into the fossa navicularis. The meatus itself may appear white, indurated, and edematous. The lesions may be multiple, involving a large portion of the glans and the prepuce, and may assume a mosaic appearance. Glandular erosions, fissures, and meatal stenosis may occur. Symptoms consist of pain, discharge, pruritus, local penile discomfort, painful erections, and urinary obstruction (Bainbridge et al., 1971).

The lesion occurs in both circumcised and uncircumcised males, but it is more frequent in the latter (Bainbridge et al., 1971). It is most common in the middle-aged male but has been reported in children (McKay et al., 1975). The histologic characteristics of the lesion are similar to those of lichen sclerosus et atrophicus found on other cutaneous surfaces (Laymon and Freeman, 1944). The character of the lesion is confirmed by biopsy, which shows an atrophic epidermis with loss of rete pegs, homogenization of the collagen on the upper third of the dermis, and a zone of lymphocytic and histocytic infiltration.

Treatment is directed at relief of meatal stenosis by meatotomy, urethral dilatation, or the local application of topical steroids (Poynter and Levy, 1967). Well-localized lesions on the glans may be treated with a corticosteroid injection (Poynter and Levy, 1967). Surgical excision has also been employed (Rheinschild and Olsen, 1970). Since there are rare reports of malignant degeneration (Laymon and Freeman, 1944; Rheinschild and Olsen, 1970), the lesions require periodic examination and follow-up biopsy if there is a change in their clinical appearance.

LEUKOPLAKIA

Leukoplakia is a descriptive term that implies a sharply defined white cutaneous plaque that may be hypertrophic or atrophic. It may be associated with a number of entities. The lesion may present with local irritative symptoms. Histologic examination is necessary to determine the presence of malignancy. On histologic examination, hyperkeratosis, parakeratosis, and hypertrophy of the rete pegs with dermal edema and lymphocytic infiltration are seen. Treatment is aimed at elimination of the sources of chronic irritation. Circumcision is warranted in the uncircumcised patient. Both surgical excision and radiation have been employed in the treatment of leukoplakia. Since leukoplakia may coexist with or may antecede the occurrence of carcinoma (Hanash et al., 1970; Reece and Koontz, 1975), close follow-up of the excision scar and periodic biopsy of lesions that have not been completely excised are necessary to detect early evidence of malignant degeneration.

CONDYLOMA ACUMINATUM

Condylomata acuminata are typically soft, friable, reddish, cyanotic papillary lesions, which are also termed "venereal warts" or "genital warts." They have a predilection for the moist glabrous areas of the body and the mucocutaneous surfaces of the genital and perineal areas. Condylomata may occur singularly on a narrow pedicle or in a grapelike cluster on a sessile broad base. Condylomata acuminata rarely occur prior to puberty (Copulsky et al. 1975; Redman and Meacham, 1973). In the male, condylomata occur most commonly on the prepuce, the penile shaft, and the glans. The lesions, single or multiple, are apt to recur in the same area or different areas after treatment. Careful inspection may reveal intrameatal lesions, and approximately 5 per cent of patients with condylomata acuminata will demonstrate urethral involvement that may extend as far proximally as the prostatic urethra (Culp et al., 1944). Bladder involvement, though rare, has been reported, and adequate treatment presents a formidable task (Bissada et al., 1974; Kleiman and Lancaster, 1962).

Evidence is convincing that the lesion is caused by a filterable papovavirus (Kovi et al., 1974; Oriel and Almeida, 1970) that is transmissible and autoinoculable (Barrett et al., 1954; Oriel and Almeida, 1970).

The appearance of condylomata acuminata on histologic study is that of an undulating outer layer of keratinized tissue covering papillary fronds that are supported by connective tissue stroma. The epithelial pegs consist of well-ordered rows of squamous cells. A dermal lymphocytic infiltrate is normally present. Caution must be exercised in the interpretation of microscopic abnormalities of condylomata acuminata in the patient who has received treatment with podophyllin. This agent, which effects cell division, can induce histologic changes consistent with carcinoma (King and Sullivan, 1947). Therefore, preliminary biopsy for definitive histologic identification of lesions that appear to be condylomata acuminata, but that are large or atypical, is advisable prior to podophyllin therapy.

Since the reported success in 1944 of podophyllin in the treatment of condylomata acuminata among army recruits (Culp et al., 1944), this agent has been commonly used to eradicate the lesion. Care must be taken to supervise therapy carefully, since normal skin is also disrupted by podophyllin (King and Sullivan, 1947). Circumcision is advisable to remove preputial lesions, to gain exposure for treatment, and to permit patient and physician to watch for recurrences. Fulguration and local excision of large bulky lesions may be advisable in expediting treatment and avoiding large areas of maceration and secondary infection.

Recently 5-fluorouracil in a 5 per cent base Efudex cream instilled via a nozzle tip has been effective for complete eradication of urethral lesions and carries the advantage of selectively destroying the condyloma without injuring normal mucosa (Bissada et al., 1974; Dretler and Klein, 1975; Coetzee, 1977; Boxer and Skinner, 1977). Scrotal skin must still be protected from the cream, however. The application of 5-fluorouracil cream to lesions of the meatus, glans, and prepuce is an alternative to podophyllin or surgical excision and provides a method for retreatment of recurrent lesions. Local application of 0.1 per cent bleomycin has also proved effective (Ichikawa et al., 1969).

Condylomata acuminata have been diagnosed prior to the appearance of squamous cell carcinoma of the penis, have been found in close proximity to squamous cell carcinoma, and have on histologic examination contained changes consistent with malignancy (Beggs and Spratt, 1961; Dawson et al., 1965; Gursel et al., 1973; Kovi et al., 1974; Rhatigan et al., 1972). Malignant transformation of condyloma to squamous cell carcinoma has been reported (Coetzee, 1977; Boxer and Skinner, 1977; Pereira, 1982). Condylomata acuminata located in the perianal area and the oral cavity have undergone malignant degeneration (Siegel, 1962). Certainly the number of patients with condylomata acuminata who subsequently develop carcinoma of the penis is quite small, however. The suggestion that the presence of condylomata acuminata may identify the host with greater susceptibility to development of carcinoma is worthy of consideration (Rhatigan et al., 1972).

BUSCHKE-LOWENSTEIN TUMOR (VERRUCOUS CARCINOMA, GIANT CONDYLOMA ACUMINATUM)

The characteristics of the Buschke-Lowenstein tumor were recognized by Buschke in 1925, and later by Lowenstein in 1939 in the United States (Lowenstein, 1939; Buschke and Lowenstein, 1925). A histologically identical lesion termed "verrucous carcinoma" was described as occurring in the oral cavity (Ackerman, 1948). Because of its large size and its resemblance to condyloma acuminata, the term "giant condyloma" has also been used to identify this lesion. Frequently it is grossly indistinguishable from squamous cell carcinoma. It may originally present as a small localized papillary growth, which over a period of time develops into a large necrotic exophytic lesion that may cover and destroy much of the penis. Urethral erosion and fistulization occur. This progressive growth, associated with discharge, odor, and bleeding, prompts the patient to seek medical attention.

The true incidence of the Buschke-Lowenstein tumor is unknown but is undoubtedly higher than reported, since many are labeled low-grade squamous cell carcinoma of the penis. Retrospective analyses of series of penile carcinoma have revealed a number of verrucous cancers or giant condylomata included under the category of low-grade squamous cell carcinoma (Davies, 1965; Hanash et al., 1970).

As in the case of condyloma acuminatum, the etiology may be viral (Dawson et al., 1965). The Buschke-Lowenstein tumor differs from condyloma acuminatum in that the latter, no matter how large, remains superficial, sparing adjacent tissue. The former tumor displaces, penetrates, and destroys adjacent structures by compression. Apart from this unrestrained local growth, it shows no signs of malignancy on histologic examination. On microscopic examination the tumor forms a luxuriant mass composed of broad, rounded rete pegs, which often extends far into the underlying tissue. The pegs are composed of well-differentiated squamous cells that show no cellular anaplasia. These epithelial pegs are characteristically surrounded by a dense band of acute and chronic inflammatory cells.

Lymph node metastases are rare with verrucous carcinoma (Ackerman, 1948; Davies 1965), and their presence probably reflects malignant degeneration in the primary lesion. Malignant alterations are known to evolve in verrucous carcinoma of the larynx, the oral cavity, and the female genital area (Davies, 1965; Dawson et al., 1965).

Excisional biopsy or multiple deep biopsies are necessary to distinguish the lesion from true penile carcinoma. Once the diagnosis has been established treatment consists of excision, sparing as much of the penis as possible. Large lesions, however, may require total amputation. Owing to the high frequency of recurrence after surgery, close follow-up is required. Treatment with podophyllin has proved unsuccessful, probably owing to its inability to penetrate the thick layer of stratum corneum that is characteristic of the tumor. Topical administration of 5-fluorouracil has also been reported to be unsuccessful (Bruns et al., 1975). The specificity of bleomycin for squamous cell lesions and its success in the treatment of both benign and malignant cutaneous lesions suggest that in the future it may prove useful as a primary or adjunctive mode of therapy for verrucous carcinoma (Misma and Matunalea, 1972). At present, however, topical chemotherapy has no place in the treatment of any large exophytic penile cancer. Radiation therapy is not advised. It is ineffective and has been associated with rapid malignant changes when directed at verrucous carcinoma in other locations (Kraus and Perez-Mesa, 1966; Lepow and Leffler, 1960; Proffitt et al., 1970).

NONSQUAMOUS MALIGNANCY OF THE PENIS

Melanoma and basal cell carcinoma rarely occur on the penis. Malignancies arising from the supporting structures of the penis are also quite rare and include any combination of tumors of smooth or striated muscle or of fibrous, fatty, or vascular tissue. Information regarding appropriate treatment of these malignancies is derived from the review of single case reports and small series.

MELANOMA

Fewer than 40 cases of melanoma of the penis have been reported. Of 1200 melanomas treated at Memorial-Sloan Kettering Cancer Center, only 2 were of penile origin (Das Gupta and Grabstald, 1965). At the M.D. Anderson Cancer Treatment Center, less than 1 per cent of all primary penile carcinomas were malignant melanomas (Johnson and Ayala, 1973). Melanoma presents as a blue-black to reddish-brown pigmented papule, plaque, or ulceration on the glans penis; less frequently it is found on the prepuce. Definitive diagnosis is accomplished by histologic examination of biopsy specimens, which reveals atypical junctional cell activity with displacement of pigmented cells into the dermis. Distant metastatic spread has been present in 60 per cent of patients studied (Abeshouse, 1958; Johnson et al., 1973). Hematogenous metastases occur via the vascular structures of the corporal bodies; lymphatic spread to the regional ilioinguinal nodes occurs by lymphatic permeation.

Surgery is the primary mode of treatment, with radiotherapy and chemotherapy being of only adjunctive or palliative benefit. For Stage I melanoma (localized lesion without metastases) and Stage II melanoma (metastases confined to one regional area), adequate excision of the primary tumor by partial or total penile amputation together with en bloc bilateral ilio-inguinal node dissection offers the greatest prospects for cure (Bracken and Diokno, 1974; Johnson et al., 1973). However, the prognosis with this neoplasm is poor, with few reported 5-year survivors (Reid, 1957; Wheelock and Clark, 1943), owing to the frequency of metastases occurring beyond the confines of surgical resection.

BASAL CELL CARCINOMA

The rarity of basal cell carcinoma of the penis contrasts with the frequency of this lesion in other cutaneous surfaces. Treatment is by local excision (Hall et al., 1968).

SARCOMAS

Primary mesenchymal tumors of the penis are very rare. A thorough review of 46 such tumors from the Armed Forces Institute of Pathology revealed an equal number of benign and malignant lesions (Dehner and Smith, 1970). The patients ranged in age from newborn to the eighth decade of life, and the presenting symptoms, that is, subcutaneous mass, penile pain and enlargement, priapism, and urinary obstructive symptoms, were the same for both benign and malignant lesions. A sarcoma has been reported to "masquerade" as a Peyronie plaque (Moore et al., 1975). Malignant lesions were found more frequently on the proximal shaft; benign lesions were more often located distally. The most common malignant lesions were those of vascular origin (hemangioendothelioma), followed in frequency by those of neural, myogenic, and fibrous origin (Ashley and Edwards, 1957).

Sarcomas have been classified as superficial when they arise from the integumentary supporting structures and as deep when they arise from the corporal body supporting structures (Pratt and Ross, 1969). Wide local surface excision and partial penile amputation for the superficial tumors have been suggested, reserving total penile amputation for tumors of deep corporal origin. Local recurrences are characteristic of sarcomas (Dehner and Smith, 1970): to avoid them, a total amputation even for superficial malignancies of any cell type should be considered. Regional metastases are rare; therefore, unless adenopathy is palpable, node dissections are not recommended (Hutcheson et al., 1969). Distant metastases have also been unusual (Dehner and Smith, 1970), and this fact encourages aggressive local treatment in anti-cipation of cure. Radiation therapy and chemotherapy have not been used extensively enough to comment upon their efficacy.

PAGET DISEASE

Paget disease of the penis is extremely rare. Less than 15 cases have been reported (Mitsudo et al., 1981). It appears grossly as an erythematous, eczematoid, well-demarcated area that cannot be clinically distinguished from erythroplasia of Querat, Bowen disease, or, therefore, carcinoma in situ of the penis. Clinical presentation includes local discomfort, pruritus, and occasionally a serosanguineous discharge. On microscopic examination, identification is clearly made by the presence of large, round or oval, clear-staining hydropic cells with hypochromatic nuclei, the "Paget cell." Paget disease may often herald a deeply seated carcinoma with "Paget cells" moving through ducts or lymphatics to the epidermal surface. In the penis, a sweat gland carcinoma may be the primary neoplasm (Mitsudo et al., 1981). Complete local surgical excision of the skin and subcutaneous tissue is the recomended form of therapy. If inguinal adenopathy is present, radical node dissection is advised (Hagan et al., 1975). Careful observation for recurrence at the margins is necessary.

LYMPHORETICULAR MALIGNANCY

Primary lymphoreticular malignancy rarely occurs on the penis (Dehner and Smith, 1970). Leukemia may infiltrate the corpora, resulting in priapism (Pochedly et al., 1974).

Kaposi sarcoma, usually a cutaneous manifestation of a generalized lymphoreticular disorder, may produce genital lesions. Kaposi sarcoma appears initially on the penile shaft or the glans as a small elevated painful papule or ulcer with bluish discoloration. Occasionally, bleeding will occur. On histologic examination the tumors are vasoformative with endothelial proliferation and spindle cell formation. The lesions are amenable to local excision and are radiosensitive. A combination of surgical excision and postoperative radiotherapy has been effective in eradication of the majority of lesions (Summers et al., 1972). Chemotherapy alone may be effective (Scott and Voight, 1966). A review from Memorial-Sloan Kettering Cancer Center suggests that radiotherapy alone be used for the treatment of these lesions (Linker et al., 1975). Since Kaposi sarcoma is a manifestation of a generalized disease, and multiple occurrences at other sites (cutaneous and visceral) are common, local conservative therapy for ths lesion when it appears on the genitals is appropriate.

METASTASES

Metastatic lesions to the penis are unusual. Approximately 200 cases have been reported in the literature. Their infrequency is somewhat puzzling when one considers the rich blood and lymphatic supply to the organ and its proximity to the bladder, the prostate, and the rectum—areas frequently involved with neoplasm. It is from these three organs that the majority of metastatic penile lesions originate (Abeshouse, 1958). Renal and respiratory neoplasms have also metastasized to the penis. The most likely routes of spread are by direct extension, retrograde venous and lymphatic transport, or arterial embolism.

The most frequent sign of penile metastases is priapism; penile swelling, nodularity, or ulceration have also been reported (Abeshouse and Abeshouse, 1961; McCrea and Tobias, 1958; Weitzner, 1971). Urinary obstruction and hematuria may occur. The most common histologic feature of penile invasion by metastatic lesions is the replacement of one or both corpora cavernosa, a ready explanation for the frequent finding of priapism. Solitary cutaneous, preputial, and glanular deposits are less common.

The differential diagnosis includes idiopathic priapism, venereal or other infectious ulcerations, tuberculosis, Peyronie plaque, and primary, benign, or malignant tumors.

Penile metastases represent an advanced form of virulent disease and usually present rather rapidly after recognition and treatment of the primary lesion (Abeshouse and Abeshouse, 1961; Hayes and Young, 1967). On rare occasions, a long period may elapse between the treatment of the primary lesion and the appearance of penile metastases (Abeshouse and Abeshouse, 1961). Because of the association of a penile metastatic lesion with advanced disease, survival after its presentation is limited, and the majority of patients die within 1 year. Successful treatment may occasionally be possible in the case of solitary nodules or localized distal penile involvement if complete excision by partial amputation succeeds in removing the entire area of malignant infiltration (Spaulding and Whitmore, 1978). A poor prospect for surgical cure exists if proximal corporal invasion is present. Treatment with radiation therapy has been generally unsuccessful, and chemotherapy has not been employed in sufficient cases to warrant definitive recommendations.

CARCINOMA OF THE PENIS

CARCINOMA IN SITU (ERYTHROPLASIA OF QUEYRAT, BOWEN DISEASE)

Carcinoma in situ of the penis is discussed, and appropriately so, under the heading of carcinoma of the penis. However, it is an entity that urologists and dermatologists refer to as erythroplasia of Queyrat. This lesion has not routinely been identified as carcinoma of the penis. The terms "erythroplasia of Queyrat" and "Bowen disease" have served to separate carcinoma in situ from the mainstream of thinking and reporting of penile carcinoma. Its epidemiology and natural history parallel that of early carcinoma of the penis. So as not to depart totally from convention, its characteristics are summarized under one heading rather than being interdispersed in the main body of the discussion on squamous cell carcinoma of the penis.

The erythroplasia described originally by Queyrat in 1911 (Queyrat, 1911) consists of a red, velvety, well-marginated lesion found on the glans penis and, less frequently, on the prepuce (Fig. 34–3A and B). It invariably is found in the uncircumcised male. It occasionally is superficially ulcerative and associated with discharge and pain. On histologic examination, the normal mucosa is replaced by atypical hyperplastic cells characterized by disorientation, vacuolation, multiple hyperchromatic nuclei, and mitotic figures at all levels. The epithelial rete extends into the submucosa and appears elongated, broadened, and bulbous; the submucosa shows capillary proliferation and ectasia with a surrounding inflammatory infiltrate usually rich in plasma cells. These microscopic features distinguish it from chronic localized balanitis and the benign dermatosis that it may grossly resemble.

Intraepithelial neoplasm of the skin associated with a high occurrence of subsequent internal malignancy was described as a distinct entity by Bowen in 1912 (Bowen, 1912). Erythroplasia of Queyrat and Bowen disease occurring on the penis appear similar on histologic examination (Graham and Helwig, 1973). They are both characterized by the noninvasive epithelial cellular changes of carcinoma in situ. Visceral malignancy is not associated with erythroplasia of Queyrat. A recent study compares and distinguishes the two entities (Graham and Helwig, 1973); both are best characterized as carcinoma in situ of the penis.

Treatment requires proper identification of

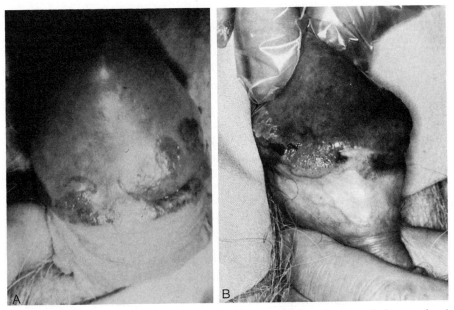

Figure 34–3. *A* and *B,* Erythroplasia of Queyrat characterized by superficial erythematous lesions on the glans penis and coronal sulcus.

malignancy. Therefore, biopsies should be multiple and of adequate depth to detect invasion. When lesions are small and noninvasive, local excision that spares penile anatomic structure and function is adequate. If a lesion is preputial, circumcision will suffice. Fulguration is occasionally successful but often is associated with recurrences. Radiation therapy has been successful in eradicating the lesion. Appropriately delivered and planned radiation results in minimal morbidity (Kelley et al., 1974; Grabstald and Kelley, 1980). Topical 5-fluorouracil has been used with good success and there are few complications (Goette, 1974; Graham and Helwig, 1973; Hueser and Pugh, 1969; Lewis and Bendl, 1971). Five percent 5-fluorouracil base cream causes denudation and dissolution of areas involved with malignant and premalignant changes while preserving normal skin. Cosmetic results are excellent. Recurrences are easily treated with repeated application. Systemic absorption of 5-fluourouracil is minimal (Dillaha et al., 1965). Isolated reports of the use of CO_2 laser therapy (Rosenberg, 1980) and liquid nitrogen cryosurgery (Sonnex et al., 1982; Madej and Meyza, 1982) have described both excellent control of disease and cosmetic outcome.

INVASIVE CARCINOMA OF THE PENIS

Incidence. Penile carcinoma constitutes less than 1 per cent of all malignancies among the United States male population—an incidence of 1 to 2 cases per 100,000 per annum. It is most commonly diagnosed during the sixth and seventh decades of life; in two studies the mean age was 58 years (Gursel et al., 1973) and 55 years (Derrick et al., 1973). It is not rare, however, among males in the fourth and fifth decades of life. Twenty-two per cent of patients in one large series were younger than 40 years of age (Dean, 1935). Carcinoma of the penis has been reported in children (Kini, 1944). No identifiable racial predisposition has been encountered in some series (Beggs and Spratt, 1961); others have found an increased incidence in the black population (Johnson et al., 1973). Rather than showing genetic predilection the proportionally greater frequency among blacks may be a reflection of the greater number of uncircumcised black males (Schrek and Lenowitz, 1947).

Etiology. The incidence of carcinoma of the penis varies markedly with the hygienic standards and the cultural and religious practices of different countries. Circumcision has been well established as a prophylactic measure that virtually eliminates the occurrence of penile carcinoma. Its development among the uncircumcised has been attributed to the chronic irritative effects of smegma, a by-product of bacterial action on desquamated cells that are retained within the preputial sac. This chronic irritation and exposure are accentuated by the presence of phimosis, which most large series report to occur in 25 to 75 per cent of patients presenting with carcinoma of the penis. Although definite evidence that smegma is a carcinogen is lacking (Reddy and Baruah, 1963), it nevertheless must be suspect (Plaut and Kohn-Speyer, 1947; Pratt-Thomas et al., 1956). It is certainly of interest that though carcinoma of the scrotum has been clearly identified as being associated with chemical irritants that act as carcinogens (i.e., coal, dust, tar, paraffin), a relationship between carcinoma of the penis and these chemicals does not exist, though its exposure must be identical to that of the scrotum.

Carcinoma of the penis is almost unknown among the Jewish population, among whom neonatal circumcision is customary. When it does occur, the rarity warrants comment (Licklider, 1961). In the United States, where neonatal circumcision is frequent, penile carcinoma composes less than 1 per cent of malignancies in the male. This figure is in marked contrast to the incidence of carcinoma of the penis among the uncircumcised African tribes (Dodge, 1965) and the uncircumcised Asian population, among whom it composes 10 to 20 per cent of all malignancies in the male. In Paraguay, penile carcinoma is the most common genitourinary malignancy (Lynch and Krush, 1969). In India, carcinoma of the penis is extremely rare among the neonatally circumcised Jewish population; it is somewhat more frequent among Moslems who practice prepubertal circumcision; and it is quite common among the uncircumcised Christian and Hindu population (Paymaster and Gangadharan, 1967). Data from most large series reveal that the tumor, though rarely developing in the neonatally circumcised, is more frequent when circumcision is delayed until puberty (Frew et al., 1967; Gursel et al., 1973; Johnson et al., 1973). Adult circumcision offers little or no protection against the future appearance of penile carcinoma (Thomas and Small, 1963). Some period of exposure to smegma, however, brief, may account for the decreased effectiveness of pubertal circumcision and the negligible protective effect of adult circumcision.

Publications periodically will decry routine neonatal circumcision as a form of aesthetic and sexual mutilation (Morgan, 1965; Preston, 1970). The debate about whether or not to circumcise has become associated with an almost hysterical outcry against the "mutilating operation of circumcision." One should not confuse facts—the extreme rarity of cancer in the circumcised—with opinion. It is also well to emphasize that circumcision may not be as important in countries in which good hygiene is practical and soap and water are readily available. Any argument against circumcison must take into account the fact that penile carcinoma represents the only neoplasm for which there exists a predictable and simple means of prophylaxis that spares the organ at risk (Dagher et al., 1973).

Another etiologic factor of recent interest involves the association of penile carcinoma and cervical carcinoma and the possible relationship, therefore, to herpes infection. A three- to eightfold increase in incidence of cervical carcinoma among the sexual partners of patients with penile carcinoma has been documented in several series (Goldberg et al., 1979). However, this relationship has not been confirmed by others (Redd et al., 1977).

Although a history of trauma often predates the appearance of carcinoma of the penis, it is felt that this is coincidental rather than causal (Hanash et al., 1970). No consistent etiologic relationship of penile carcinoma to venereal disease (syphilis, granuloma inguinale, and chancroid) has been found, and any association of these diseases with penile carcinoma is probably coincidental (Schrek and Lenowitz, 1947).

Although the state of immune suppression among the renal transplant population is associated with a marked increase in squamous cell malignancies, only one case of penile cancer in a transplant recipient has been reported (Previte et al., 1979).

Natural History. Carcinoma of the penis usually begins with a small lesion that gradually extends to involve the entire glans, shaft, and corpora. The lesion may be papillary and exophytic or flat and ulcerative; if untreated, penile autoamputation may eventually occur. The rate of growth of the papillary and ulcerative lesions is quite similar, but the flat ulcerative tumor has a tendency to earlier nodal metastasis and is associated with poorer 5-year survival rates (Dean, 1935; Marcial et al., 1962). Lesions larger than 5 cm (Beggs and Spratt, 1961) and those extending to cover 75 per cent of the shaft (Staubitz et al., 1955) are also associated with an increased incidence of metastases and a decreased survival rate. However, a consistent relationship of lesion size to the presence of metastasis and to decreased survival has been questioned (Ekstrom and Edsmyr, 1958; Puras et al., 1978).

Buck's fascia acts as a temporary natural barrier protecting the corporal bodies from invasion of neoplasm. Penetration of Buck fascia and the tunica albuginea permits invasion of the vascular corpora and establishes the potential for vascular dissemination. Urethral and bladder involvement is rare (Riveros and Gorostiaga, 1962; Thomas and Small, 1963).

Metastases to the regional femoral and iliac nodes represent the earliest route of dissemination from penile carcinoma. A detailed description of lymphatic drainage of the penis is found in Chapter 82. Briefly, the lymphatics of the prepuce form a connecting network that joins with lymphatics from the skin of the shaft. These tributaries drain into the superficial inguinal nodes (the nodes above the fascia lata). The lymphatics of the glans join the lymphatics draining the corporal bodies, and they form a collar of connecting channels at the base of the penis that drain via the superficial or deep inguinal nodes (the nodes beneath the fascia lata) and from there to the pelvic nodes (external iliac, internal iliac, and obturator). There are multiple cross communications throughout all levels of drainage so that penile lymphatic drainage is bilateral to both inguinal areas.

Metastatic enlargement in the femoral regional nodes eventually leads to skin necrosis, chronic infection, and death from inanition, sepsis, or hemorrhage secondary to erosion into the femoral vessels. Clinically detectable distant metastatic lesions to the lung, liver, bone, or brain are uncommon and are reported as occurring in 1 to 10 per cent of large series (Begg and Spratt, 1961; Derrick et al., 1973; Puras et al., 1978; Johnson et al., 1973; Kossow et al., 1973; Riveros and Gorostiaga, 1962; Staubitz et al., 1955). Such metastases usually occur late in the course of disease after the local lesion has been treated. Distant metastases in the absence of regional node metastases are unusual.

Carcinoma of the penis is characterized by a relentless progressive course, causing death for the vast majority of untreated patients within 2 years (Beggs and Spratt, 1961; Derrick et al., 1973; Skinner et al., 1972). Rarely, long survival will occur even with advanced local disease and regional node metastases (Beggs and Spratt, 1961; Furlong and Uhle, 1953). No report of spontaneous remission of carcinoma of the penis is known. Five to 15 per cent of patients have been reported to subsequently develop a second primary neoplasm (Beggs and Spratt, 1961; Buddington et al., 1963; Gursel et al., 1973).

Modes of Presentation

SIGNS. Almost without exception the penile lesion itself calls attention to the possibility of carcinoma. It may appear as an area of induration or erythema, as a small bump, a pimple, a warty growth, or a more luxuriant exophytic lesion. Alternatively it may appear as a shallow-

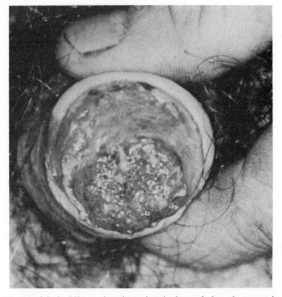

Figure 34–4. Ulcerating invasive lesion of the glans penis, obscuring meatus. Foreskin has been retracted.

based nonhealing erosion or a deeply excavating ulcer with elevated or rolled-in margins (Fig. 34–4). Phimosis may obscure a lesion and thus result in a prolonged period of neglect. Eventually, erosions through the prepuce, a foul preputial odor, and discharge with or without bleeding call attention to disease (Fig. 34–5).

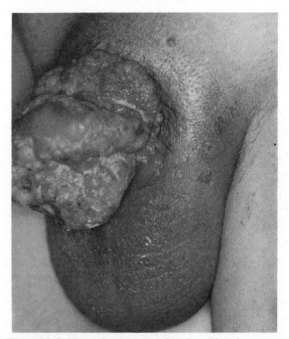

Figure 34–5. Ulcerating lesion perforating phimotic prepuce and associated with extensive purulence and secondary infection.

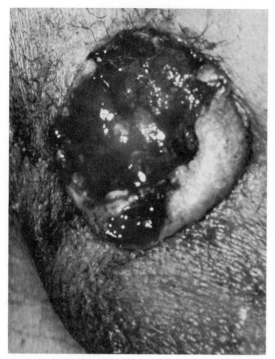

Figure 34–6. Ulcerating inguinal nodal metastasis from carcinoma of the penis.

Penile carcinoma is most frequent on the glans, the coronal sulcus, and the prepuce. It is less commonly found on the shaft or at the meatus. A possible explanation is that the shaft and the meatus—unlike the glans, coronal sulcus, and inner surface of the prepuce—are not constantly exposed to smegma and other irritants contained within the preputial sac.

Occasionally a mass, ulceration, necrosis, suppuration, and hemorrhage in the inguinal area resulting from nodal metastases present prior to a lesion concealed in the phimotic preputial sac (Fig. 34–6). Local corporal involvement rarely progresses to the stage at which urinary retention or urinary fistula are among the presenting signs, but these symptoms associated with autoamputation of the penis may occur (Fig. 34–7).

SYMPTOMS. Pain does not develop in proportion to the extent of the local destructive process and usually is not a presenting complaint. Weakness, weight loss, fatigue, and systemic malaise occur secondary to chronic suppuration. Occasionally, significant blood loss from the penile lesion or the nodal lesion, or both, occurs. Presenting symptoms referable to distant metastases are rare, since local and regional nodal disease are characteristically far advanced before distant metastases are detectable.

Diagnosis

DELAY. The time from the initiation of signs and symptoms to the time of presentation to a physician is usually long, considering the rather advanced condition of the lesions at presentation. Fifteen to 50 per cent of patients have been reported to delay medical care for more than 1 year (Buddington et al., 1963; Dean, 1935; Furlong and Uhle, 1953; Gursel et al., 1973; Hardner et al., 1972). Patients with carcinoma of the penis, more than patients with other types of carcinoma, delay seeking medical attention (Lynch and Krush, 1969). Possible explanations are multiple, namely, personal neglect, embarrassment, guilt, fear, and ignorance. No reason appears justified, however, since the penis is an organ handled and observed on a daily basis. Of even greater concern are

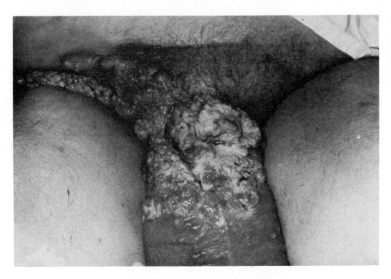

Figure 34–7. Extensive invasive carcinoma of the penis with autoamputation of the glans and shaft. Extensive inguinal nodal metastasis with ulceration and secondary infection. Multiple satellite lesions involving scrotal skin.

the estimates of the length of delay by the physician in initiating appropriate therapy (Lynch and Krush, 1969). According to some studies (Elstrom and Edsmyr, 1958; Johnson et al., 1973), the difference in survival rates between patients presenting early and those having delayed presentation is negligible. However, decreased survival rates associated with longer delay have been noted by others (Hardner et al., 1972). It appears logical that patients would have achieved better survival rates if they had been treated earlier.

EXAMINATION. At presentation the great majority of lesions are confined to the penis (Derrick et al., 1973; Johnson et al., 1973; Skinner et al., 1972). The penile lesion is assessed with regard to its size, location, fixation, and involvement of the corporal bodies. Inspection of the base of the penis and scrotum is necessary to rule out extension into these areas. Rectal and bimanual examination provides information regarding perineal body invasion or the presence of a pelvic mass. Careful bilateral palpation of the inguinal area for adenopathy is of extreme importance.

STAGING. Accurate assessment of the extent of the primary lesion and identification of regional and distant metastatic disease are necessary in directing appropriate initial therapy and assessing end results. However, clinical evaluation for the presence of inguinal metastases is

TABLE 34–1. TNM CLASSIFICATION OF PENILE CARCINOMA*

T = Primary Tumor
TIS Preinvasive carcinoma (carcinoma in situ)
T0   No evidence of primary tumor
T1   Tumor 2 cm or less in its largest dimension, strictly superficial or exophytic
T2   Tumor larger than 2 cm but not more than 5 cm in its largest dimension with minimal infiltration
T3   Tumor more than 5 cm in its largest dimension, or tumor of any size with deep infiltration, including into the urethra
T4   Tumor infiltrating neighboring structures
N = Regional Lymph Nodes
    The clinician may record whether palpable nodes are considered to contain growth.
N0   No palpable nodes
N1   Movable unilateral nodes
      $N1_a$ Nodes not considered to contain growth
      $N1_b$ Nodes considered to contain growth
N2   Movable bilateral nodes
      $N2_a$ Nodes not considered to contain growth
      $N2_b$ Nodes considered to contain growth
N3   Fixed nodes
M = Distant Metastases
M0 No evidence of distant metastases
M1 Distant metastases present

*From TNM Classification of Malignant Tumours, 2nd ed. Geneva, Imprimerie G. de Buren S.A., 1974.

TABLE 34–2. MINIMAL DIAGNOSTIC CRITERIA FOR CARCINOMA OF THE PENIS

T = Primary Tumor
    Clinical examination
    Incisional-excisional biopsy of lesion
N = Regional Lymph Nodes
    Clinical examination
    CAT scan or Cheba biopsy (or both)
    Superficial femoral node biopsy (optional but recommended)
    Lymphangiography (optional)
M = Distant Metastases
    Clinical examination
    Chest x-ray
    Biochemical determinations (liver functions, calcium
    CAT scan, bone scan (optional)

subject to significant inaccuracy. Furthermore, no universally accepted staging system for penile carcinoma exists (Baker and Watson, 1975). A TNM classification that is under consideration, along with diagnostic criteria, is listed in Tables 34–1 and 34–2. The most commonly employed classification, suggested by Jackson (1966), is listed in Table 34–3. Cross comparison of results among different series, specifically with regard to the characteristic of the initial primary lesion—that is, whether it be superficial, invasive, small, large, limited to the glans or involving other structures—and with regard to nodal metastases (solitary, multiple, superficial inguinal, deep inguinal, pelvic, unilateral, bilateral) is often quite impossible.

BIOPSY. Identifying carcinoma of the penis by microscope study of a biopsy specimen is mandatory prior to therapy. Biopsy may be a separate procedure from amputation. Enough tissue must be obtained to determine the depth of invasion if radiotherapy is to be considered (see further on). Frequently, a dorsal slit is necessary to gain adequate exposure of the lesion for appropriate biopsy. No harmful effects secondary to biopsy, that is, dissemination, are recognized. Biopsy with confirmation of tumor by frozen section while the patient is still anesthetized, and immediate surgical excision, with partial or total amputation (with full prior

TABLE 34–3. CLASSIFICATION FOR CARCINOMA OF THE PENIS

Stage I (A): Tumors confined to glans or prepuce, or both.
     II (B): Tumors extending onto shaft of penis.
    III (C): Tumors with inguinal metastasis that are operable.
    IV (D): Tumors involving adjacent structures, or tumors associated with inoperable inguinal metastasis or distant metastasis.

informed consent from the patient) would constitute an alternative means of diagnosis and simultaneous treatment.

HISTOLOGY. The vast majority of tumors of the penis are squamous cell carcinomas demonstrating keratinization, epithelial pearl formation, and various degrees of mitotic activity. The normal rete pegs are disrupted. Invasive lesions penetrate the basement membrane and surrounding structures.

GRADING. Most malignancies of the penis are low grade (Murrell and Williams, 1965; Staubitz et al., 1955). Lack of correlation between grade and survival has been noted by a number of investigators (Beggs and Spratt, 1961; Edwards and Sawyers, 1968; Hardner et al., 1972; Johnson et al., 1973; Kuruvilla et al., 1971; Staubitz et al., 1955). In contrast, other series have reported reduced survival rates among patients with anaplastic neoplasms (Ekstrom and Edsmyr, 1958; Frew et al., 1967; Puras et al., 1978; Hanash et al., 1970; Marcial et al., 1962). Patterns of growth have occasionally been a prognostic aid (Frew et al., 1967). A relationship between the degree of plasma cell, lymphocytic, or eosinophilic infiltrate and survival has not been found (Kuruvilla et al., 1971).

LABORATORY STUDIES. Laboratory evaluation in patients with penile carcinoma is usually normal. Anemia, leukocytosis, and hypoalbuminemia may be present in patients with long-term illness malnutrition and extensive suppuration at the area of the primary and inguinal metastatic sites. Azotemia may occur secondary to urethral or ureteral obstruction. Hypercalcemia in the absence of detectable osseous metastasis associated with penile carcinoma has been noted (Anderson and Glenn, 1965; Rudd et al., 1972). In a recent review from Memorial Sloan-Kettering Cancer Center (Sklaroff and Yagoda, 1982) 17 of 81 patients (20.9 per cent) with penile carcinoma were hypercalcemic; 16 of 17 patients (94 per cent) with clinical inguinal metastases were hypercalcemic. Hypercalcemia seems to be largely a function of bulk of the disease. It is often associated with inguinal metastases and may resolve with surgical removal of the inguinal nodes (Block et al., 1973). Parathormone-like substances may be produced by the tumor and metastases (Malakoff and Schmidt, 1975). Medical treatment includes saline hydration and administration of diuretics, steroids, calcitonin, and mithramycin (Lindeman and Papper, 1975).

RADIOLOGIC STUDIES. Metastases to lung, bone, and brain are rarely identified on x-ray examination or by scanning. Intravenous pyelography usually demonstrates normal findings unless there is massive retroperitoneal adenopathy. The role of lymphangiography is not well established because certain difficulties are inherent in the study. The filling of external iliac nodes might be suboptimal owing to the inflammatory or metastatic obstruction in the superficial and deep inguinal systems, and distinction between inflammatory and metastatic nodal changes is difficult in the inguinal area. The potential of lymphangiography would seem to lie in the identification of nodal abnormalities in the common iliac and para-aortic nodes. In patients with corporal invasion, inguinal adenopathy, or abnormalities on bimanual examination, computerized tomography of the abdomen and pelvis offers promise for the identification of pelvic or para-aortic adenopathy. Positive identification of tumor by Chiba needle aspiration of these nodes contraindicates any surgery other than that for palliation.

DIFFERENTIAL DIAGNOSIS. A number of penile lesions must be considered in the differential diagnosis of penile carcinoma. They include some already discussed, namely condyloma acuminatum, Buschke-Lowenstein tumor, and a number of inflammatory lesions, namely, chancre, chancroid, herpes, lymphopathia venereum, granuloma inguinale, and tuberculosis. These diseases can be identified by appropriate skin tests, tissue studies, serologic examinations, cultures, or specialized staining techniques. Minimal diagnostic criteria for carcinoma of the penis are outlined in Table 34–2.

Surgical Treatment

TREATMENT OF THE PRIMARY NEOPLASM. The infrequency of distant metastatic disease, the significant morbidity from untreated local regional disease, and the success of long-term palliation and survival even with advanced local and regional disease support aggressive local and regional therapy whenever possible. The desired goal in the treatment of the primary tumor is complete excision with adequate tumor-free margins. In certain selected cases of small lesions involving only the prepuce this may be accomplished by circumcision (Ekstrom and Edsmyr, 1958). Circumcision alone, however, is frequently followed by tumor recurrence (Gursel et al., 1973; Hardner et al., 1972; Marcial et al., 1962). A recent series documented a recurrence rate of 50 per cent (Narayana et al., 1982). For lesions involving the glans and the distal shaft, even when they are apparently superficial, partial amputation with a 2-cm margin proximal to the tumor is necessary to guard against local recurrences. Frozen section of the proximal margin is recommended for microscopic confirmation of a tumor-free margin of resection. Following this guideline, recurrent tumor at the line of resection is rare even with deep corporal invasion, since tumor spread is by embolic metastases and not by lymphatic permeation (Ekstrom and Edsmyr, 1958; De-Kernion et al., 1973; Hardner et al., 1972). In contrast, local wedge excision has been associated with recurrence rates that approach 50 per cent (Jensen, 1977). Adequate partial amputation in the absence of inguinal metastases can produce a 5-year survival rate of 70 to 80 per cent (Table 34–4). The residual penile stump is usually serviceable for upright micturition and sexual function.

If the proximal penile shaft is involved by malignancy to the extent that resection leaves a questionable 2-cm margin and a stump that prohibits upright voiding and is useless for sexual function, total penectomy is performed to ensure adequate margins and to allow more convenient micturition in a sitting position via perineal urethrostomy (Fig. 34–8). For the rare lesion of the skin of the penile shaft, removal of the skin and subcutaneous tissue may be adequate. We have treated a single patient in this manner with good results (Grabstald, 1970) (Fig. 34–9A and B).

A series of patients treated with the Nd:YAG laser has been reported, with excellent control of the primary lesion on 2- to 3-year follow-up (Hofstetter and Frank, 1983).

In more advanced tumors, in which the scrotal contents and inguinal nodes are involved; radical extirpation of the entire neoplasm may require hemipelvectomy or hemicorporectomy,

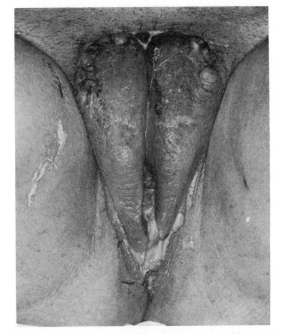

Figure 34–8. Appearance after total penectomy and partial scrotectomy and formation of perineal urethrostomy.

which in certain well-selected individuals merits consideration (Block et al., 1973) (Fig. 34–10).

PHALLIC RECONSTRUCTION. Such reconstruction following loss of the penis presents genitourinary surgery with one of its greatest reconstructive challenges. The anatomy and function of the erectile corpora cavernosa are unique and are not usually reproduced by the transfer of any other tissue in the human body. Early attempts at phallic reconstruction consisted of the "tube within a tube" concept, utilizing a tubed flap of abdominal skin for the

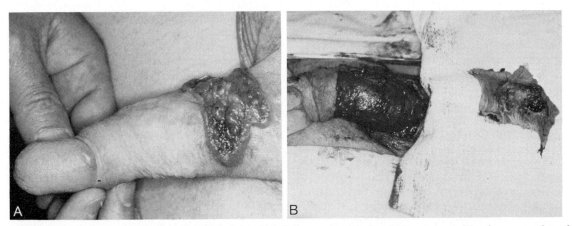

Figure 34–9. *A,* Erosive, but superficial, lesion of the skin of the proximal shaft, which was treated by sleeve resection of the skin and preservation of the penis. *B,* Postresection appearance, together with excised lesion and surrounding skin.

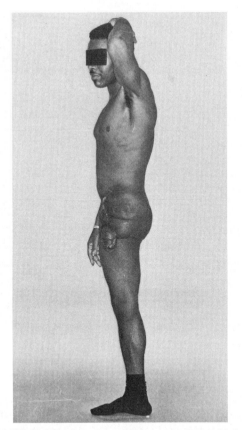

Figure 34–10. Hemicorporectomy in young male with invasive penile carcinoma with inguinal nodal metastasis but without evidence of positive juxtaregional nodes or distant metastasis.

urethra enclosed within another covering flap of abdominal skin. Such reconstructions often failed either because of the multiple procedures involved or because the phallus lacked sensation and had suboptimal aesthetic appearance.

Arterialized flaps (superficial groin flap) and myocutaneous flaps (gracilis, rectus femoris, and rectus abdominis) have been used with moderate success in phallic reconstruction. Although these local flaps decrease the number of reconstructive stages, they often lack sensation, tend to atrophy, and are dependent upon the consistency, texture, and hair distribution of the tissues in the lower abdomen, groin, perineum, and thighs.

Our unit has had a long involvement in phallic reconstruction. The close cooperation of urologists and plastic surgeons utilizing newer concepts in microsurgical reconstruction has produced improvements in the function and appearance of the neophallus. Ideally, phallic reconstruction should address the following requirements: (1) a one-stage microsurgical procedure, (2) creation of a competent urethra to achieve normal voiding, (3) restoration of a phallus that has the capability of both tactile and erogenous sensibility, (4) enough bulk to tolerate a prosthetic stiffener for successful vaginal penetration, and (5) aesthetic acceptance by the patient.

In an attempt to meet these five reconstructive criteria, we first embarked on a technique employing microneurovascular transfers. The urethra was constructed with a full-thickness graft and was then wrapped with a tubed free flap. Either a saphenous flap or a deltoid flap was used. Both of these flaps have an identifiable artery, vein, and sensory nerve. The donor arteries and veins were anastomosed to the deep inferior epigastric artery and vein. The sensory nerves were coapted to the ilioinguinal nerve in the recipient site. Despite acceptable appearance, there was not an adequate amount of tactile sensation and none that was erogenous in nature.

More recently the phallus has been reconstructed by tubing the skin overlying the rectus abdominis muscle to create a neourethra. The rectus abdominis skin muscle unit can be rotated into an acceptable phallic position based on its blood supply from the inferior epigastric artery and vein. This exposed skin muscle unit is then covered with a neurotized free flap (dorsalis pedis) to provide sensation to the shaft of the phallus. The superficial perineal nerve of the free flap is coapted to the recipient deep pudendal nerve. There are early indications that patients so treated have some return of erogenous sensation.

These recent advances in free tissue transfer have been utilized to help meet the criteria described for successful phallic reconstruction. The vascularized epithelial neourethra has less tendency for stricture formation than does a full-thickness skin graft, and it carries urine to the phallic tip. A potential for augmenting the neophallus with a prosthetic stiffener is enhanced by including rectus abdominis muscle bulk in the reconstruction. The aesthetic appearance of the phallus is improved over previous reconstructive attempts.

Using cooperation between the urologist and the plastic surgeon, the reconstruction of a neophallus is becoming more of a reality. Experience with microneurovascular tissue transfers has demonstrated that a successful one-stage phallic reconstruction is now possible.*

———————
*The authors gratefully acknowledge the contribution of David A. Gilbert, M.D., Associate Professor of Plastic Surgery, Eastern Virginia Medical School, for detailing these most recent advances in microneurovascular surgery.

TREATMENT OF INGUINAL NODES. The prognosis for patients with carcinoma of the penis is markedly worsened by the presence of inguinal metastases. This factor affects the prognosis much more than tumor grade, gross appearance, or morphologic and microscopic patterns of the tumor.

Controversial issues concerning the treatment of regional lymph nodes center around the timing and extent of surgery. Should lymphadenectomy be performed only for patients with palpable inguinal lymphadenopathy that is persistent after treatment of the primary penile lesion and a course of antibiotics in order to allow for subsidence of nodal enlargement secondary to inflammation, or should dissections also be performed on a prophylactic or adjunctive basis in patients with clinically negative inguinal examinations? Should adenectomy be performed bilaterally if only unilateral nodes are palpable or should node dissections be limited to the side of palpable adenopathy? Should lymphadenectomy be extended to the pelvic lymph nodes, unilaterally or bilaterally, or should it be restricted to the inguinal lymph node area? The rarity of penile carcinoma will make it impossible to conduct adequate prospective randomized trials to resolve these controversies surrounding the treatment of regional nodes. Based on historic and retrospective data accumulated from the literature, these questions will be discussed individually. Although guidelines can be developed from retrospective analysis, treatment must often be individualized according to the dictates of a particular case.

Should lymphadenectomy be performed in the presence of clinically palpable inguinal nodes after appropriate treatment of the primary lesion and subsidence of inflammation? This question can be answered in the affirmative. The recommendation for inguinal node dissection for patients having positive nodes at presentation is well substantiated. Evidence to support this statement is based on the following: Patients with penile carcinoma and inguinal metastases who do not undergo treatment rarely survive 2 years and almost never survive 5 years. No spontaneous regression of penile carcinoma has been reported. However, 20 to 50 per cent of patients with inguinal node metastases who are treated by inguinal lymphadenectomy achieve a 5-year disease-free survival (Table 34–4). It should be noted that palpable adenopathy at initial presentation does not inevitably indicate the presence of tumor. A false-positive rate of up to 50 per cent related to node enlargement caused by inflammation has been

reported (Table 34–4). However, the persistence of adenopathy after treatment of the primary tumor and a course of antibiotics or the appearance of adenopathy during follow-up, or both of these possibilities, is more likely due to metastasis than inflammatory reaction.

Should inguinal lymphadenectomy be routinely performed in patients with clinically negative groin examination at the time of presentation of the primary lesion? This question invites the greatest amount of controversy. After answering the question in the negative, it is important to discuss alternatives and make qualifications. As stated, inguinal adenectomy when nodes are positive for malignancy ranges between 20 and 50 per cent. A cure rate of this magnitude in the face of regional nodal metastases parallels the urologist's experience with testicular carcinoma in which retroperitoneal lymphadenectomy used alone results in cure in a significant number of patients with positive nodes. This is contrary to the experience with other common genitourinary malignancies— bladder, prostate, and renal—in which surgical cure is rarely achieved in the presence of nodal metastases. Why then is there any discussion concerning the wisdom of node dissection for treatment of a tumor when the potential for cure is substantial, especially in view of the fact that node dissections are frequently advocated in the treatment of urologic malignancies when evidence of their efficacy is marginal at best? The problem arises from the significant morbidity of inguinal node dissection in contrast to the limited morbidity of retroperitoneal and pelvic lymphadenectomy. Early complications of phlebitis, pulmonary embolism, wound infection, flap necrosis and late complications of lymphedema (Fig. 34–11) occur with disconcerting frequency after inguinal adenectomy. The admonition of Hippocrates, "primum non nocere" ("first, do no harm") deserves serious consideration and serves as a focal point for the following discussion of the role of prophylactic or adjunctive adenectomy in the absence of palpable adenopathy.

The incidence of metastases to the inguinal nodes has been reported in 2 to 25 per cent of patients presenting with penile carcinoma who have clinically negative inguinal examinations (see Table 34–4). A very large series reported a 38 per cent false-negative rate (Puras et al., 1978) on the basis of impalpable microinvolvement of the nodes or changes in the inguinal area, such as postsurgical induration, scar, or obesity, that make accurate examination impossible. The incidence of metastases to clinically

TABLE 34–4. CARCINOMA OF THE PENIS

SERIES, NUMBER OF PATIENTS (YEAR)	Clinical and Pathologic Characteristics of Inguinal Adenopathy			5-Year Survival Rates	
	PER CENT WITH PALPABLE NODES	PER CENT CLINICALLY FALSE-POSITIVE (NODES PALPABLE; HISTOLOGIC FINDINGS NEGATIVE)	PER CENT CLINICALLY FALSE-NEGATIVE (NODES NOT PALPABLE; HISTOLOGIC FINDINGS POSITIVE)	INGUINAL NODES NEGATIVE ON HISTOLOGIC OR REPEATED PHYSICAL EXAMINATION	INGUINAL NODES RESECTED AND POSITIVE ON HISTOLOGIC EXAMINATION OF ADENECTOMY SPECIMEN
Ekstrom et al., 229 (1958)	33%	48%	—	80%[a]	42%
Beggs et al., 88 (1961)	35%	36%	20%	72.5%	45%
Thomas et al., 190 (1968)	—	64%	20%	—	26%
Edwards et al., 77 (1968)	—	—	0%	68%	25%
Hanash et al., 169 (1970)	—	58%[b]	2%[b]	77%[c]	—
Kuruvilla et al., 153 (1971)	39%	63%	10%	69%	33%
Hardner et al., 100 (1972)	42%	41%[b]	16%[b]	—	—
Gursel et al., 64 (1973)	53%	60%[b]	—	58%	—
Skinner et al., 34 (1973)	29%	40%	—	75% (87%[d])	20% (50%[d])
DeKernion et al., 48 (1973)	54%	38%[b]	—	84%[e]	55%[e]
Derrick et al., 87 (1973)	29%	52%	—	53% (76%[d])	22% (55%[d])
Johnson et al., 153 (1973)	—	—	—	64.4%	21.8%
Kossow et al., 100 (1974)	51%	49%	25%	—	—
Flores et al., 500 (1976)	60%	47%	38%[b]	89%	47%[g] 29%[h]
Cabanas, 80 (1976)	96%	65%	100%	90%	70%[i] 50%[j] 20%[k]

[a]Majority of patients received prophylactic or preoperative radiotherapy to inguinal area.
[b]Histologic classification based on node biopsy, not node dissection.
[c]Corrected 5-yr survival; i.e., patients dying prior to 5 yr without evidence of disease are excluded.
[d]Patients dying free of cancer before 5 yr are considered surgical cures.
[e]Three-yr survival.
[f]Patients with palpable nodes judged benign.
[g]Positive findings in inguinofemoral nodes.
[h]Positive findings in inguinofemoral and pelvic nodes.
[i]Single inguinal node with positive findings.
[j]More than one inguinal node with positive findings.
[k]Three-yr survival with positive findings in inguinal and pelvic nodes.

normal nodes is based on information derived both from complete node dissections and limited lymph node biopsies. Since some patients subsequently developed positive nodes after initial selected biopsies were negative, and since the detection of metastases on pathologically submitted material is dependent upon the number of sections per node examined—that is, how hard the pathologist looks for tumor—these figures for false-negative clinical examinations represent a conservative estimate. The curative benefit of lymphadenectomy in the presence of grossly palpable nodes involved with tumor has already been established; therefore, it is logical to presume that a lymphadenectomy performed in the setting of microscopic nodal disease would confer an even greater survival advantage. However, it is difficult to justify submitting approximately 75 per cent or more of patients with negative clinical examinations and negative nodes to the morbidity of inguinal lymphadenectomy. Furthermore no apparent detrimental effect on 5-year survival rates has been documented among those patients with negative nodes initially who are carefully followed and later, upon clinical appearance of adenopathy, undergo node dissection. The 5-year survival rate in this group approaches that of patients presenting with metastatic adenopathy initially who are treated with node dissection (Baker et al., 1976). However, in both instances adenectomy is being undertaken in the presence of grossly palpable tumor, and this observation does not exclude the possibility that adenectomy for clinically imperceptible, that is, microscopic, disease might yield better results. Supporting information is not available, since series have not separately analyzed survival of patients with

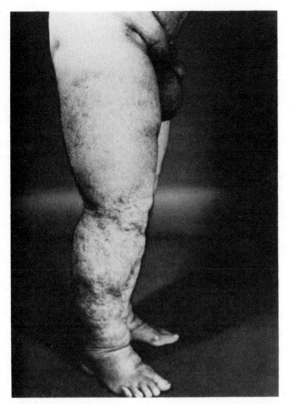

Figure 34–11. Extensive lymphedema with cutaneous changes secondary to recurrent lymphangitis and phlebitis.

clinically palpable nodes that are positive for neoplasm on histologic examination compared with survival of patients with clinically negative nodes that are positive for neoplasm on histologic examination. A recent large series, however, (Puras et al., 1978) has identified surgical removal of the primary tumor followed within 1 month by routine lymphadenectomy as the treatment protocol associated with the highest 5-year survival rate; another series (Cabanas, 1977) has reported much improved survival by employing early node biopsy, which, if positive, is followed by complete node dissection.

Therefore, in an attempt to identify patients with subclinical metastases and proceed directly with node dissection, the alternative of superficial node dissection or sentinel node biopsy has been proposed. Superficial node dissection involves removal of those nodes superficial to the fascia lata with progression to total lymphadenectomy—that is, removal also of those nodes deep to the fascia lata contained within the femoral triangle—if the superficial nodes are positive. The concept of sentinel node biopsy as described by Cabanas is predicated on his detailed penile lymphangiographic studis that have demonstrated consistent drainage of the penile

lymphatics into a "sentinel node" or group of nodes located superiomedial to the junction of the saphenous and femoral veins in the area of the superficial epigastric vein (Cabanas, 1977). When this sentinel node was negative for tumor, metastases to other ileoinguinal lymph nodes did not occur in his series. Metastases to this node indicated the need for a complete superficial and deep inguinal dissection. Cabanas' data are recent and are in the process of further clinical trial. Exceptions to his findings have been reported (Catalona, 1980). Superficial node dissection has been proposed for patients with no palpable adenopathy but with invasive corporal lesions that place them at high risk. If nodes are positive, a complete adenectomy is performed (DeKernion et al., 1973). Recently, a proposal has been made for routine ileoinguinal node dissection in medically suited patients with clinically negative nodes whose primary lesion is deeply invasive (Catalona, 1980).

Should inguinal lymphadenectomy be bilateral rather than unilateral for patients presenting with unilateral adenopathy at initial presentation of the primary tumor? The answer to this question is in the affirmative. The anatomic crossover of lymphatics of the penis is well established, and bilateral drainage is therefore the rule. Bilateral lymphadenectomy is recommended in patients presenting with palable adenopathy in conjunction with the primary lesion. Support for this procedure is based on the finding of contralateral metastases in greater than 50 per cent of patients so treated, even if the contralateral nodal region appears negative to clinical palpation (Ekstrom and Edsmyr, 1958).

Should bilateral inguinal lymphadenectomy be performed in patients who present with unilateral adenopathy sometime after the initial presentation in treatment of the primary tumor? The answer to this question would logically appear to be affirmative based on the data presented in the preceding paragraph. However, it is generally felt that a bilateral node dissection in this setting is not necessary. This recommendation of unilateral rather than bilateral node dissection with delayed unilateral adenopathy is supported by the elapsed disease-free observation on the normal side. If one assumes that nodal metastases will enlarge at the same rate, the clinical palpation of metastases, if present in both groins, should appear at approximately the same time. The absence of clinical adenopathy on one side dictates a higher probability of freedom from disease on that side (Ekstrom and Edsmyr, 1958).

Should pelvic lymphadenectomy be performed in patients with positive inguinal metastases? The therapeutic gain of extending nodal dissection to include the iliac nodes is undetermined. Information is limited regarding the frequency of pelvic node metastases in the presence of inguinal nodes positive for neoplasm and the frequency of iliac node metastases in the absence of tumor in the inguinal nodes. Iliac nodes have been found to be positive for tumor metastases in 15 of 45 patients (30 per cent) (Riveros and Gorostiaga, 1962), in 9 of 30 patients (29 per cent) with positive inguinal nodes (Puras et al., 1978), in 5 of 13 patients (35 per cent) at autopsy (Gursel et al., 1973) and in 2 of 4 patients having staging laparotomy (Uehling, 1973). Puras reported no instance of positive pelvic nodes in the absence of positive inguinal nodes. Survival of patients with positive iliac nodes is limited. For this reason specific recommendations against pelvic node dissection have appeared (Hanash et al., 1970). Until more information is available, a definitive statement about the advisability of pelvic node dissection is not possible. Yet, since involvement of pelvic nodes on microscopic examination may occur with some frequency, survival with positive pelvic nodes having been documented (Cabanas, 1977; DeKernion et al., 1973; Puras et al., 1980) (see Table 34–4), and since duration of survival has been lengthened after iliac node dissection (Hardner et al., 1972), performing the procedure in the young male who is a good surgical risk appears reasonable.

Information identifying the specific location at dissection (femoral, iliac, bilateral, unilateral) of nodes with positive findings or identifying the number of nodes involved with tumor or histologic examination is also unavailable. More accurate data relating the pattern and extent of nodal metastases to patient survival will aid in accurately defining the natural history of penile carcinoma.

On the basis of available information, a well-accepted plan of treatment of inguinal nodes is outlined as follows (Whitmore, 1970).

Stage A, B (TIS, T1–T4, N0, M0). Patients with penile neoplasms but no palpable adenopathy require periodic examination of the inguinal area after treatment of the primary tumor. The appearance of unilateral adenopathy provides indication for unilateral inguinal node dissection with added pelvic node dissection as determined by the patient's medical status. If adenopathy later presents in the opposite side of the groin, a similar procedure should be undertaken. Since most inguinal metastases have occurred within a 2- to 3-year period

following initial therapy (Beggs and Spratt, 1961; Derrick et al., 1973; Johnson et al., 1973), this period of risk must be closely supervised with examinations at 2- to 3-month intervals. The patient should be taught careful self-examination of the inguinal areas for early detection of metastases. Delayed appearance of inguinal metastases may occur; therefore, the patient should never be dismissed from close physical examination. Such a program requires close cooperation of the patient—a formidable responsibility in a group of patients who historically have demonstrated a lack of reliability by presenting rather late in the course of their original penile lesion. It may be anticipated that approximately 20 per cent of Stage A patients will develop inguinal metastases (Whitmore, 1970) (see Table 34–4).

Still undetermined is the improvement in survival that might accrue when lymphadenectomy is performed in patients with subclinical metastatic disease, and, therefore, superficial node dissection needs consideration (see earlier discussion).

Stage C (TIS, T1–T4, N1, N2, M0). Patients with penile carcinoma and initial palpable adenopathy require control of the primary tumor, followed by a re-evaluation of the inguinal nodes 2 to 6 weeks after infection is controlled and inflammatory adenopathy has resolved. Simultaneous bilateral radical ilioinguinal node dissections are recommended if either unilateral or bilateral adenopathy persists. If adenopathy is unilateral, metastases are anticipated in approximately 50 per cent of the clinically normal contralateral groins. The policy of unilateral node dissection for Stage A and Stage B lesions when unilateral adenopathy appears on follow-up examination and of routine initial bilateral dissections for Stage C neoplasms (even if only one inguinal area is clinically palpable) is supported by data from a large series (Ekstrom and Edsmyr, 1958) (see earlier discussion).

Stage D (TIS, T1–T4, N3 and M+). This category includes patients with distant metastases or inguinal adenopathy that is inoperable owing to invasion and fixation or to recurrence following surgery. Treatment is often limited to palliative chemotherapy or radiotherapy. In selected patients with fixed nodes but no distant metastases, radical hemipelvectomy or hemicorporectomy provides a surgical option. Prior staging laparotomy is necessary to exclude disease in the abdomen or in the high common iliac or para-aortic nodes.

Radiation Therapy

Evaluation of the overall success of radiation therapy in the treatment of primary lesions of carcinoma of the penis is made difficult by the lack of uniformity of radiation treatment within single series as well as among different series. Time schedules of treatment, total rad exposure, and the type of delivery system used—such as external beam therapy (Jackson, 1966), radium mold (Jackson, 1966), electron beam (Kelley et al., 1974), interstitial implants (Pierquin et al., 1971)—vary considerably. Assessment of the treatment of the inguinal area is hampered by the uncertainty arising from the lack of histologic confirmation of the presence or absence of nodal metastases. Information concerning the use of radiation therapy as a primary mode of treatment for penile carcinoma comes primarily from European countries where surgery is usually reserved for radiation failures.

DISADVANTAGES. Objections to radiation therapy in the treatment of primary lesions rest on a number of observations.

1. Squamous cell carcinoma is characteristically radioresistant, and the doses of radiation—6000 rads (Kelley et al., 1974)—necessary to sterilize deeply infiltrating penile tumors frequently result in urethral fistula, stenosis, and stricture, with or without penile necrosis, pain, and edema. These complications may require secondary penectomy (Duncan and Jackson, 1972).

2. Infection so frequently associated with penile carcinoma markedly decreases the effect of radiation therapy on the neoplasm and increases the incidence of damage to the radiosensitive penile tissue (low therapeutic index) (Murrell and Williams, 1965).

3. The lengthy treatment schedule of 3 to 6 weeks followed by several months of morbidity after the termination of treatment represents a formidable burden. This is especially so for the elderly group of patients for whom partial penectomy, in contrast, represents a relatively simple and expeditious procedure.

4. It is well accepted that if radiation therapy is to equal the success rate of initial surgical treatment, radiation failures (i.e., those patients without complete resolution of the treated lesion at 3 to 6 months post-therapy or those with evidence of recurrences) must be promptly treated with penectomy in order not to jeopardize survival. Therefore, careful follow-up of the patient to detect recurrence is mandatory. This may be a difficult task among a group of patients who have already demonstrated unreliability and neglect in seeking prompt attention for their original primary lesion. Furthermore, distinguishing postradiation ulcer, scar, and fibrosis from possible recurrent carcinoma represents a problem requiring repeated biopsy investigation.

Objections to the treatment of inguinal node metastases are that inguinal areas tolerate radiation poorly and are subject to skin maceration and ulceration. Infectious adenopathy will reduce the effectiveness of radiation therapy and magnify complications. The perilymphatic fat that frequently surrounds nodes may act as a protective barrier to the effective radiation treatment of intranodal metastatic deposits (Harlin, 1952).

ADVANTAGES. The sole advantage of initial radiation therapy over initial surgery rests on the preservation of penile anatomic structure and function—a consideration of importance among young patients. Surgical amputation must follow if radiation therapy fails. It should be noted that partial penectomy, though anatomically deforming, does not necessarily preclude upright micturition and satisfactory sexual function. Among elderly patients, preservation of an aesthetic anatomic structure and sexual function are of secondary importance.

INDICATIONS. Radiation therapy does warrant consideration in a select group of patients: (1) Young individuals presenting with small (2 to 3 cm), superficial, noninvasive lesions, carcinoma in situ, on the glans or coronal sulcus. These lesions may be treated primarily by radiation or radiation may be given after having failed a course of topical 5-fluorouracil cream. (2) Those patients refusing surgery as an initial form of therapy, and (3) patients with inoperable or distant metastases who express desire to retain the penis are also candidates. Prior to radiation therapy, circumcision (or at the very least a dorsal slit) is necessary to expose the lesion, to allow resolution of surface infection, and to prevent moist maceration and preputial edema.

RADIATION THERAPY OF PRIMARY LESION. When radiation therapy is employed as the initial treatment for penile carcinoma, control of the primary lesions occurs with much less frequency than when surgery is primarily employed (Table 34–5). Approximately half the lesions so treated will persist or recur when treatment is directed at all stages. Penile amputation is at times required owing to radiation injury to the penis. It has been generally accepted that a patient's prognosis is not altered if surgery is promptly performed when radiation fails to control the carcinoma (Murrell and Williams, 1965). Jackson (1966), however, did show that nodal metastases develop more frequently after or during a course of radiation

TABLE 34–5. Surgery Required after Radiation Therapy for Carcinoma of the Penis

Series (Year)	Number of Patients	Amputation for Recurrent or Persistent Disease, or Both*	Other Surgery	Total
Lederman et al. (1953)	48	35%	—	35%
Murrell et al. (1965)	92	48%	—	48%
Jackson et al. (1966)	58	51%	—	51%
Knudson et al. (1967)	145	62%	6%†	68%
Almgard et al. (1973)	33	52%	18%‡	70%
Englestadt (1948)	64	45%§	8%†	53%
Raynal (1977)	45	22%	8%†	30%
Salaverria (1979)	13	23%	—	23%
Haile et al. (1980)	20	10%	10%†	20%
Daly et al. (1982)	22	5%	10%†	15%

*Difference from 100% indicates cure from radiation alone.
†Penectomy for radiation complications.
‡Local excision or electrocoagulation of recurrent neoplasm.
§Includes seven radiation therapy failures not having further surgery.

therapy than after surgery, and this suggests the potential for metastases to occur during or following a course of unsuccessful radiation therapy.

Radiation therapy to selected, small, superficial lesions is quite successful. A 90 per cent rate of control of the primary tumor among 20 patients treated with megavoltage radiation has been reported (Duncan and Jackson, 1972). However, the dosages employed (5000 to 5700 rads over 3 weeks) produced a significant number of complications, that is, penile necrosis in 10 per cent of patients and urethral stricture in 30 per cent. The most successful series thus far employing radiation therapy is that reported from Memorial Sloan-Kettering Cancer Center (Kelley et al., 1974). Applying electron beam therapy, a 100 per cent success rate in controlling superficial lesions in 10 carefully selected patients was achieved clinically and confirmed histologically by negative biopsies of the lesion. A 5- to 10-year update on this series reported 9 patients tumor free. In one patient, carcinoma developed at another penile site suggesting a new primary tumor. Nine patients retained sexual function. The most common complication was urethral stricture in four patients (Grabstald and Kelley, 1980). A recent series from the M.D. Anderson Hospital and Tumor Institute also reports good control of smaller lesions without significant morbidity (Haile and Delclos, 1980), and similar success with well-selected cases has been reported from other centers (Raynal et al., 1977; Salaverria et al., 1979; Daly et al., 1982).

In summary, small superficial tumors will respond well to radiotherapy, and with careful planning complications can be minimized. The treatment of larger invasive malignancies is less

successful, may be associated with severe local complications, and theoretically may provide an interval during which metastatic dissemination may occur. Other untoward effects of radiation may include testicular damage and secondary neoplasia (Lederman, 1953). In the case of a sexually active young patient with an invasive lesion, surgical amputation followed by penile reconstruction (see earlier discussion) rather than primary radiation therapy should be considered.

RADIATION THERAPY TO THE INGUINAL NODES. Owing to the accuracy of clinical staging and the lack of the histologic studies of inguinal nodes, the adjunctive or therapeutic use of radiation in treatment is controversial. Even if metastases are documented by node biopsy, the efficacy of subsequent radiation is impossible to judge because all tumor may have been removed by the biopsy. In one series 70 per cent of nodal metastases involved a solitary node, and 5-year survival in this group was 70 per cent (Cabanas, 1977). Radiotherapy for inguinal metastases documented by histologic examination has been compared with surgery for the node-positive groin. There was a 50 per cent 5-year survival rate among the surgically treated group and a 25 per cent 5-year survival rate in the irradiated group (Staubitz et al., 1955). Other series report that radiation to the inguinal areas has not proved therapeutically effective (Murrell and Williams, 1965; Jenson, 1977). Several Scandinavian centers have delivered radiation therapy to inguinal nodes as well as to primary tumor in all cases of penile carcinoma; surgical adenectomy followed if palpable nodes persisted or appeared subsequently (Ekstrom and Edsmyr, 1958; Engelstad, 1948). In a series of 130 patients initially having clinically impalpable nodes, 18 subsequently developed palpable nodal disease requiring lymphadenectomy, and another 11 patients had metastases but no operation. Therefore 29 or 22 per cent of men who received prophylactic groin irradiation subsequently developed inguinal metastases (Ekstrom and Edsmyr, 1958). Murrell and Williams (1965) found that 3 of 11 patients (25 per cent) who received radiation therapy to the inguinal area without initially palpable nodes subsequently developed inguinal metastases. These percentages closely approximate the incidence of subclinical metastases that are encountered when node dissection is performed after inguinal examination is normal (see Table 34–5), and they suggest that radiation therapy did not alter the course of disease. Furthermore, the clinical evaluation of the groin postradiation is difficult, and the complications encountered with groin dissection postradiation can be significant.

Lastly, the 5-year survival rate in patients with prophylactically irradiated groins followed as necessary by lymphadenectomy differs little from patients having surgery alone. Although a large randomized controlled study might definitely answer the question of efficacy of radiation therapy for inguinal metastases, both microscopic and macroscopic, it is unlikely that such a study could be realized. Present information identifies surgical therapy of inguinal metastasis as superior to radiation therapy.

Radiation therapy may be considered in patients presenting with early inoperable fixed and ulcerative inguinal lymph nodes. Occasionally, radiation to these areas is well tolerated, may result in significant palliation, and may postpone local complications for prolonged periods (Furlong and Uhle, 1953; Staubitz et al., 1955; Vaeth et al., 1970). If a patient is a poor surgical risk or refuses surgery, a superficial node dissection to confirm positive nodes followed by radiation therapy presents an alternative treatment option.

In summary, radiation therapy to the inguinal area is not as effective therapeutically as lymph node dissection, but it may be useful if surgery can not be performed. Furthermore, palliation can at times be achieved for inoperable nodes. Our policy has been not to combine preoperative radiation therapy with inguinal lymphadenectomy, but others have advocated the combination (Ekstrom and Edsmyr, 1958; Engelstad, 1948).

Chemotherapy

Reports from Japan (Ichikawa et al., 1969) describe a substantial and reproducible response of penile and scrotal carcinoma using bleomycin. Ichikawa reports excellent response in six previously untreated patients with carcinoma of the penis. Reports from Uganda (Kyalwazi and Bhana, 1973) show complete or partial regression in the vast majority of patients. A review of 67 patients from the world literature who could be evaluated reveals a 73 per cent response rate to bleomycin (Blum et al., 1973). However, these promising results have not been confirmed in a study from Memorial Sloan-Kettering Cancer Center, where 13 patients with advanced diseases were treated. Only two responses were noted and these were short-lived.

Cis-platinum and methotrexate, also tested at Memorial Sloan-Kettering Cancer Center, have shown more activity than bleomycin. *Cis*-platinum produced objective response in three of nine patients (Sklaroff and Yagoda, 1979). Methotrexate given in high doses with folinic acid rescue produced a complete remission in one of three patients and low-dose methotrexate produced partial remission in two of five patients treated (Sklaroff and Yagoda, 1980). Methotrexate has been demonstrated to be effective in other series (Mills, 1972).

The rarity of penile carcinoma in the United States will make it difficult to accumulate sufficient numbers of patients to adequately test agents in Phase II disease oriented trials. This information will need to come from trials in South America and Asia. Such information will be of significant value in identifying agents to be used as adjuvants to surgery in patients with metastases in resected nodes and as a means of palliation in patients with locally inoperable tumors or distant metastases, or both.

References

Abeshouse, B. S.: Primary and secondary melanoma of the genitourinary tract. South. Med. J., *51*:994, 1958.

Abeshouse, B. S., and Abeshouse, G. A.: Metastatic tumors of the penis: A review of the literature and a report of two cases. J. Urol., *86*:99, 1961.

Ackerman, L. V.: Verrucous carcinoma of the oral cavity. Surgery, *23*:670, 1948.

Almgard, L. E., and Edsmyr, F.: Radiotherapy in treatment of patients with carcinoma of the penis. Scand. J. Urol. Nephrol., *7*:1, 1973.

Anderson, E. E., and Glenn, J. F.: Penile malignancy and hypercalcemia. JAMA, *192*:128, 1965.

Ashley, D. J. B., and Edwards, E. C.: Sarcoma of the penis: Leiomyosarcoma of the penis: Report of a case with a review of the literature on sarcoma of the penis. Br. J. Surg., *45*:170, 1957.

Bainbridge, D. R., Whitaker, R. H., and Shepheard, B. G. F.: Balanitis xerotica obliterans and urinary obstruction. Br. J. Urol., *43*:487, 1971.

Baker, B. H., and Watson, F. R.: Staging carcinoma of the penis. J. Surg. Oncol., *7*:243, 1975.

Baker, B. H., Spratt, J. S., Perez-Mesa, C., Watson, F. R., and Le Duc, R. J.: Carcinoma of the penis. J. Urol., *116*:458, 1976.

Ball, T. P., and Pickett, J. D.: Traumatic lymphangitis of penis. Urology, *6*:594, 1975.

Barrett, T. J., Silbar, J. D., and McGinley, J. P.: Genital warts—a venereal disease. JAMA, *154*:333, 1954.

Beggs, J. H., and Spratt, J. S.: Epidermoid carcinoma of the penis. J. Urol., *91*:166, 1961.

Bissada, N. K., Cole, A. T., and Fried, F. A.: Extensive condylomas acuminata of the entire male urethra and the bladder. J. Urol., *112*:201, 1974.

Block, N. L., Rosen, P., and Whitmore, W. F.: Hemipelvectomy for advanced penile cancer. J. Urol., *110*:703, 1973.

Blum, R. H., Carter, S. K., and Agre, K.: A clinical review of bleomycin—a new antineoplastic agent. Cancer, *31*:903, 1973.

Bowen, J.: Precancerous dermatoses: A review of two cases of chronic atypical epithelial proliferation. J. Cutan. Dis., *30*:241, 1912.

Boxer, R. J., and Skinner, D. G.: Condylomata acuminata and squamous cell carcinoma. Urology, *9*:72, 1977.

Bracken, R. B., and Diokno, A. C.: Melanoma of the penis and the urethra: 2 case reports and review of the literature. J. Urol., *111*:198, 1974.

Bruns, T. N. C., Lauvetz, R. J., Kerr, E. S., and Ross, G.: Buschke-Lowenstein giant condylomas: Pitfalls in management. Urology, *5*:773, 1975.

Buddington, W. T., Kickham, C. J. E., and Smith, W. E.: An assessment of malignant disease of the penis. J. Urol., *89*:442, 1963.

Buschke, A., and Lowenstein, L.: Uber carcinomahnliche condylomata acuminata des penis. Klin. Wochenschr., *4*:1726, 1925.

Cabanas, R.: An approach to the treatment of penile carcinoma. Cancer, *39*:456, 1977.

Catalona, W. J.: Role of lymphadenectomy in carcinoma of the penis. Urol. Clin. North Am., *7*:785, 1980.

Catalona, W. J., et al.: Effect of mini-dose heparin on lymphocele formation following extraperitoneal pelvic lymphadenectomy. J. Urol., *123*:890, 1980.

Coetzee, T.: Condyloma acuminatum. South Afr. J. Surg., *15*:75, 1977.

Cole, L. A., and Helwig, E. B.: Mucoid cysts of the penile skin. J. Urol., *115*:397, 1976.

Copulsky, J., Whitehead, E. D., and Orkin, L. A.: Condyloma acuminata in a three-year-old boy. Urology, *5*:372, 1975.

Culp, O. S., Magid, M. A., and Kaplan, I. W.: Podophyllin treatment of condylomata acuminata. J. Urol., *51*:655, 1944.

Dagher, R., Selzer, M. L., and Lapides, J.: Carcinoma of the penis and the anti-circumcision crusade. J. Urol., *110*:79, 1973.

Daly, N. J., Douchez, J., and Combes, P. F.: Treatment of carcinoma of the penis by iridium 192 wire implant. Int. J. Radiat. Oncol. Biol. Phys., *8*:1239, 1982.

Das Gupta, T., and Grabstald, H.: Melanoma of the genitourinary tract. J. Urol., *93*:607, 1965.

Davies, S. W.: Giant condyloma acuminata: Incidence among cases diagnosed as carcinoma of the penis. J. Clin. Pathol., *18*:142, 1965.

Dawson, D. F., Duckworth, J. K., Bernhardt, H., and Young, J. M.: Giant condyloma and verrucous carcinoma of the genital area. Arch. Pathol., *79*:225, 1965.

Dean, A. L.: Epithelioma of the penis. J. Urol., *33*:252, 1935.

Dehner, L. P., and Smith, B. H.: Soft tissue tumors of the penis. Cancer, *25*:1431, 1970.

DeKernion, J. B., Tynbery, P., Persky, L., and Fegen, J. P.: Carcinoma of the penis. Cancer, *32*:1256, 1973.

Derrick, F. C., Lynch, K. M., Kretkowski, R. C., and Yarbrough, W. J.: Epidermoid carcinoma of the penis: Computer analysis of 87 cases. J. Urol., *110*:303, 1973.

Dillaha, C. J., Jansen, T., Honeycutt, W. M., and Holt, G. A.: Further studies with topical 5-fluorouracil. Arch. Dermatol., *92*:410, 1965.

Dodge, O. G.: Carcinoma of the penis in East Africans. Br. J. Urol., *37*:223, 1965.

Dretler, S. P., and Klein, L. A.: The eradication of intraurethral condyloma acuminata with 5-fluorouracil cream. J. Urol., *113*:195, 1975.

Duncan, W., and Jackson, S. M.: The treatment of early cancer of the penis with megavoltage x-rays. Clin. Radiol., *23*:246, 1972.

Edwards, R. H., and Sawyers, J. L.: The management of carcinoma of the penis. South. Med. J., *61*:843, 1968.

Ekstrom, T., and Edsmyr, F.: Cancer of the penis: A clinical study of 229 cases. Acta. Chir. Scand., *115*:25, 1958.

Engelman, E. R., Herr, H. W., and Ravera, J.: Lipogranulomatosis of external genitalis. Urology, *3*:358, 1974.

Engelstad, R. B.: Treatment of cancer of the penis at the Norwegian Radium Hospital. Am. J. Roentgenol., *60*:801, 1948.

Frew, I. D. O., Jefferies, J. D., and Swiney, J.: Carcinoma of the penis. Br. J. Urol., *39*:398, 1967.

Furlong, J. H., and Uhle, C. A. W.: Cancer of penis: A report of eighty-eight cases. J. Urol., *60*:550, 1953.

Fuselier, H. A., Jr., McBurney, E. I., Brannan, W., and Randrup, E. R.: Treatment of condylomata acuminata with carbon dioxide laser. Urology, *15*:265, 1980.

Goette, D. K.: Erythroplasia of Queyrat. Arch. Dermatol., *110*:271, 1974.

Goldberg, H. M., Pell-Ilderton, R., Daw, E., and Saleh, N.: Concurrent squamous cell carcinoma of the cervix and penis in a married couple. Br. J. Obstet. Gynecol., *86*:585, 1979.

Grabstald, H.: Carcinoma of the penis involving skin of base. J. Urol., *104*:438, 1970.

Grabstald, H., and Kelley, C. D.: Radiation therapy of penile cancer. Urology, *15*:575, 1980.

Graham, J. H., and Helwig, E. B.: Erythroplasia of Queyrat. Cancer, *32*:1396, 1973.

Grossman, L. A., Kaplan, H. J., Grossman, M., and Ownby, F. D.: Thrombosis of the penis. Interesting facet of thromboangitis obliterans. JAMA, *192*:329, 1965.

Gursel, E. O., Georgountzos, C., Uson, A. C., Melicow, M. M., and Veenema, R. J.: Penile cancer. Urology, *1*:569, 1973.

Hagan, K. W., Braren, V., Viner, N. A., Page, D. L., and Rhamy, R. K.: Extramammary Paget's disease in the scrotal and inguinal areas. J. Urol., *114*:154, 1975.

Haile, K., and Delclos, L.: The place of radiation therapy in the treatment of carcinoma of the distal end of the penis. Cancer, *45*:1980, 1980.

Hall, T. C., Britt, D. B., and Woodhead, D. M.: Basal cell carcinoma of the penis. J. Urol., *99*:314, 1968.

Hanash, K. A., Furlow, W. L., Utz, D. C., and Harrison, E. G.: Carcinoma of the penis: a clinicopathologic study. J. Urol., *104*:291, 1970.

Hardner, G. J., Bhanalaph, T., Murphy, G. P., Albert, D. J., and Moore, R. H.: Carcinoma of the penis: Analysis of therapy in 100 consecutive cases. J. Urol., *108*:428, 1972.

Harlin, H. C.: Carcinoma of the penis. J. Urol., *67*:326, 1952.

Hassan, A. A., Orteza, A. M., and Milam, D. F.: Penile

horn: Review of literature with 3 case reports. J. Urol., *97*:315, 1967.

Hayes, W. T., and Young, J. M.: Metastatic carcinoma of the penis. J. Chronic Dis., *20*:891, 1967.

Hofstetter, A., and Frank, F.: Laser Use in Urology. In Dixon, J. A. (Ed.): Surgical Application of Lasers. Chicago, Yearbook Medical Publishers, 1983, pp. 146–162.

Hueser, J. N., and Pugh, R. P.: Erythroplasia of Queyrat treated with topical 5-fluorouracil. J. Urol., *102*:595, 1969.

Hutcheson, J. B., Wittaker, W. W., and Fronstin, M. H.: Leiomyosarcoma of the penis: Case report and review of literature. J. Urol., *101*:874, 1969.

Ichikawa, T., Nakano, I., and Hirokawa, I.: Bleomycin treatment of the tumors of penis and scrotum. J. Urol., *102*:699, 1969.

Jackson, S. M.: The treatment of carcinoma of the penis. Br. J. Surg., *53*:33, 1966.

Jensen, M. S.: Cancer of the penis in Denmark 1942 to 1962 (511 cases). Danish Med. Bull., *24*:66, 1977.

Johnson, D. E., and Ayala, A. G.: Primary melanoma of penis. Urology, *2*:174, 1973.

Johnson, D. E., Fuerst, D. E., and Ayala, A. G.: Carcinoma of the penis: Experience with 153 cases. Urology, *1*:404, 1973.

Kelley, C. D., Arthur, K., Rogoff, E., and Grabstald, H.: Radiation therapy of penile cancer. Urology, *4*:571, 1974.

King, L. S., and Sullivan, M.: Effects of podophyllin and of colchicine on normal skin, on condyloma acuminatum and on verruca vulgaris. Arch. Pathol., *43*:374, 1947.

Kini, M. G.: Cancer of the penis in a child, aged two years. Indian Med. Gaz., *79*:66, 1944.

Kleiman, H., and Lancaster, Y.: Condyloma acuminata of the bladder. J. Urol., *88*:52, 1962.

Knudsen, O. S., and Brennhovd, I. O.: Radiotherapy in the treatment of the primary tumor in penile cancer. Acta Chir. Scand., *133*:69, 1967.

Kossow, J. H., Hotchkiss, R. S., and Morales, P. A.: Carcinoma of penis treated surgically: Analysis of 100 cases. Urology, *2*:169, 1973.

Kovi, J., Tillman, R. L., and Lee, S. M.: Malignant transformation of condyloma acuminatum. Am. J. Clin. Pathol., *61*:702, 1974.

Kraus, F. T., and Perez-Mesa, C.: Verrucous carcinoma: Clinical and pathologic study of 105 cases involving oral cavity, larynx and genitalia. Cancer, *19*:26, 1966.

Kuruvilla, J. T., Garlick, F. H., and Mammen, K. E.: Results of surgical treatment of carcinoma of the penis. Aust. N.Z. J. Surg., *41*:157, 1971.

Kyalwazi, S. K., and Bhana, D.: Bleomycin in penile carcinoma. East Afr. Med. J. *50*:331, 1973.

Kyalwazi, S. K., Bhana, D., and Harrison, N. W.: Carcinoma of the penis and bleomycin chemotherapy in Uganda. Br. J. Urol., *46*:689, 1974.

Laymon, C. W., and Freeman, C.: Relationship of balanitis xerotica obliterans to lichen sclerosus et atrophicus. Arch. Dermat. Syph., *49*:57, 1944.

Lederman, M.: Radiotherapy of cancer of the penis. Br. J. Urol., *25*:224, 1953.

Lepow, H., and Leffler, N.: Giant condylomata acuminata (Buschke-Lowenstein tumor): Report of two cases. J. Urol., *83*:853, 1960.

Lewis, R. J., and Bendl, B. J.: Erythroplasia of Queyrat: Report of a patient successfully treated with topical 5-fluorouracil. Can. Med. Assoc. J., *104*:148, 1971.

Licklider, S.: Jewish penile carcinoma. J. Urol., *86*:98, 1961.

Linderman, R. D., and Papper, S.: Therapy of fluid and electrolyte disorders. Ann. Intern. Med., *82*:64, 1975.

Linker, D., Lieberman, P., and Grabstald, H.: Kaposi's sarcoma of genitourinary tract. Urology, *5*:684, 1975.

Lowenstein, L. W.: Carcinoma-like condylomata acuminata of the penis. Med. Clin. North Am., *5*:789, 1939.

Lynch, H. T., and Krush, A. J.: Delay factors in detection of cancer of the penis. Nebr. State Med. J., *54*:360, 1969.

Madej, G., and Meyza, J.: Cryosurgery of penile carcinoma. Oncology, *39*:350, 1982.

Malakoff, A. F., and Schmidt, J. D.: Metastatic carcinoma of penis complicated by hypercalcemia. Urology, *5*:510, 1975.

Marcial, V. A., Figueroa-Colon, J., Marcial-Rojas, R. A., and Colon, J. E.: Carcinoma of the penis. Radiology, *79*:209, 1962.

McCrea, L. W., and Tobias, G. L.: Metastatic disease of the penis. J. Urol., *80*:489, 1958.

McKay, D. L., Fuqua, F., and Weinberg, A. G.: Balanitis xerotica obliterans in children. J. Urol., *114*:773, 1975.

Mills, E. E. D.: Intermittent intravenous methotrexate in the treatment of advanced epidermoid carcinoma. S. Afr. Med. J., *46*:398, 1972.

Misma, Y., and Matunalea, M.: Effect of bleomycin on benign and malignant cutaneous tumors. Acta Derm. Venereol. (Stockh.), *52*:211, 1972.

Mitsudo, S., Nakanishi, I., and Koss, L. G.: Paget's disease of the penis and adjacent skin. Arch. Pathol. Lab. Med., *105*:518, 1981.

Moore, S. W., Wheeler, J. E., and Hefter, L. G.: Epithelioid sarcoma masquerading as Peyronie's disease. Cancer, *35*:1706, 1975.

Morgan, W. K. C.: The rape of the phallus. JAMA, *193*:223, 1965.

Murphy, G. P.: Tumors of the Penis and Male Urethra. In Devine, C. J., Jr., and Stecker, J. F., Jr. (Eds.): Urology in Practice. Boston, Little, Brown & Co., 1978, pp. 725–732.

Murrell, D. S., and Williams, J. L.: Radiotherapy in the treatment of carcinoma of the penis. Br. J. Urol, *37*:211, 1965.

Narayana, A. S., Olney, L. E., Loening, S. A., Weimar, G. W., and Culp, D. A.: Carcinoma of the penis: Analysis of 219 cases. Cancer, *49*:2185, 1982.

Nickel, W. R., and Plumb, R. T.: Nonvenereal sclerosing lymphangitis of penis. Arch. Dermatol., *86*:761, 1962.

Nitidandhaprabhas, P.: Artificial penile nodules: Case reports from Thailand. Br. J. Urol., *47*:463, 1975.

Oriel, J. D., and Almeida, J. D.: Demonstration of virus particles in human genital warts. Br. J. Vener. Dis., *46*:37, 1970.

Paymaster, J. C., and Gangadharan, P.: Cancer of the penis in India. J. Urol., *97*:110, 1967.

Pereira-Bringel, P. J., and de Andrade Arruda, R.: 5-Fluorouracil cream 5% in the treatment of intraurethral condylomata acuminata. Br. J. Urol., *54*:295, 1982.

Pierquin, B., Chassagne, D., and Cox, J. D.: Toward consistent local control of certain malignant tumors. Radiology, *99*:661, 1971.

Plaut, A., and Kohn-Speyer, A. C.: The carcinogenic action of smegma. Science, *105*:391, 1947.

Pochedly, C., Mehta, A., and Feingold, E.: Priapism with hyperacute stem-cell leukemia. N.Y. State J. Med., *75*:540, 1974.

Poynter, J. H., and Levy, J.: Balanitis xerotica obliterans: Effective treatment with topical and sublesional steroids. Br. J. Urol., *39*:420, 1967.

Pratt, R. M., and Ross, R. T. A.: Leiomyosarcoma of the penis. Br. J. Surg., *56*:870, 1969.

Pratt-Thomas, H. R., Heins, H. C., Latham, E., Dennis, E. J., and McIver, F. A.: The carcinogenic effect of human smegma: An experimental study. Cancer, *9*:671, 1956.

Pressman, D., Rolnick, D., and Turbow, B.: Penile horn. Am. J. Surg., *104*:640, 1962.

Preston, E. N.: Whither the foreskin? A consideration of routine neonatal circumcision. JAMA, *213*:1853, 1970.

Previte, S. R., Karian, S., Cho, S. I., and Austen, G., Jr.: Penile carcinoma in renal transplant recipient. Urology, *13*:298, 1979.

Proffitt, S. D., Spooner, T. R., and Kosek, J. C.: Origin of undifferentiated neoplasm from verrucous epidermal carcinoma of oral cavity following irradiation. Cancer, *26*:389, 1970.

Puras, A., Fortuno, R., Gonzalez-Flores, B., and Soto-longo, A.: Staging lymphadenectomy in the treatment of carcinoma of the penis. Proceedings of the Kimbrough Urological Seminar, *14*:15, 1980.

Puras, A., Gonzalez-Flores, B., et al.: Treatment of carcinoma of the penis. Proceedings of the Kimbrough Urological Seminar, *12*:143, 1978.

Queyrat, L.: Erythroplasie du gland. Soc. Franc. Dermatol. Syphilol., *22*:378, 1911.

Raynal, M., Chassagne, D., Baillet, F., and Pierquin, B.: Endocuritherapy of penis cancer. Recent Results Cancer Res., *60*:135, 1977.

Redd, C. R. R. M., et al.: A study of 80 patients with penile carcinoma combined with cervical biopsy study of their wives. Int. Surg., *62*:549, 1979.

Reddy, D. G., and Baruah, I. K. S. M.: Carcinogenic action of human smegma. Arch. Pathol., *75*:414, 1963.

Redman, J. F., and Meacham, K. R.: Condyloma acuminata of the urethral meatus in children. J. Pediatr. Surg., *8*:939, 1973.

Reece, R. W., and Koontz, W. W., Jr.: Leukoplakia of the urinary tract: A review. J. Urol., *114*:165, 1975.

Reid, J. D.: Melanosarcoma of the penis. Cancer, *10*:359, 1957.

Rosemberg, S. K., and Fuller, T. A.: Carbon dioxide rapid superpulsed laser treatment of erythroplasia of Queyrat. Urology, *16*:181, 1980.

Rhatigan, R. M., Jimenez, S., and Chopskie, E. J.: Condyloma acuminatum and carcinoma of the penis. South. Med. J., *65*:423, 1972.

Rheinschild, G. W., and Olsen, B. S.: Balanitis xerotica obliterans. J. Urol., *104*:860, 1970.

Riveros, M., and Gorostiaga, R.: Cancer of the penis. Arch. Surg., *85*:377, 1962.

Rubenstein, M., and Wolff, S. M.: Penile nodules as a major manifestation of subacute angitis. Arch. Intern. Med., *114*:449, 1964.

Rudd, F. V., Rott, R. K., Skoglund, R. W., and Ansell, J. S.: Tumor-induced hypercalcemia. J. Urol., *107*:986, 1972.

Salaverria, J. C., Hope-Stone, H. F., Paris, A. M. I., Molland, E. A., and Blandy, J. P.: Conservative treatment of carcinoma of the penis. Br. J. Urol., *51*:32, 1979.

Schrek, R., and Lenowitz, H.: Etiologic factors in carcinoma of the penis. Cancer Res., 7:180, 1947.

Scott, W. P., and Voight, J. A.: Kaposi's sarcoma. Cancer, *19*:557, 1966.

Shiraki, I. W.: Parameatal cysts of the glans penis: A report of nine cases. J. Urol., *114*:544, 1975.

Siegel, A.: Malignant transformation of condyloma acuminatum. Am. J. Surg., *103*:613, 1962.

Skinner, D. G., Leadbetter, W. F., and Kelley, S. B.: The surgical management of squamous cell carcinoma of the penis. J. Urol., *107*:273, 1972.

Sklaroff, R. B., and Yagoda, A.: Cis-diamminedichloride platinum II (DDP) in the treatment of penile carcinoma. Cancer, *44*:1563, 1979.

Sklaroff, R. B., and Yagoda, A.: Methotrexate in the treatment of penile carcinoma. Cancer, *45*:214, 1980.

Sklaroff, R. B., and Yagoda, A.: Penile cancer: Natural History and Therapy. *In* Chemotherapy and Urological Malignancy. New York, Springer-Verlag, 1982, pp. 98–105.

Smetana, H. F., and Bernhard, W.: Sclerosing lipogranuloma. Arch. Pathol., *50*:296, 1950.

Sonnex, T. S., Ralfs, I. G., Maria, P. D., and Dawber, R. P. R.: Treatment of erythroplasia of Queyrat with liquid nitrogen cryosurgery. Br. J. Urol., *106*:581, 1982.

Spaulding, J. T., and Grabstald, H.: In Walsh, Gittes, Perlmutter, and Stamey (Eds.): Campbell's Urology, 5th ed. Philadelphia: W. B. Saunders Co. In press.

Spaulding, J. T., and Whitmore, W. F., Jr.: Extended total excision of prostatic adenocarcinoma. J. Urol., *120*:188, 1978.

Staubitz, W. J., Melbourne, H. L., and Oberkircher, O. J.: Carcinoma of the penis. Cancer, *8*:371, 1955.

Summers, J. L., Wilkerson, J. E., and Wegryn, J. F.: Conservative therapy for Kaposi's sarcoma of the external genitalia. J. Urol., *108*:287, 1972.

Tannenbaum, M. H., and Becker, S. W.: Papillae of the corona of the glans penis. J. Urol., *93*:391, 1965.

Thomas, J. A., and Small, C. S.: Carcinoma of the penis in southern India. J. Urol., *160*:520, 1963.

Uehling, D. T.: Staging laparotomy for carcinoma of penis. J. Urol., *110*:213, 1973.

Vaeth, J. M., Green, J. P., and Lowry, R. O.: Radiation therapy of carcinoma of the penis. Am. J. Roentgenol. Rad. Ther. Nucl. Med., *108*:130, 1970.

Weitzner, S.: Secondary carcinoma in the penis: Report of three cases and literature review. Am. Surg., *37*:563, 1971.

Wheelock, M. C., and Clark, P. J.: Sarcoma of penis. J. Urol., *49*:478, 1943.

Whitmore, W. F.: Tumors of the Penis, Urethra, Scrotum, and Testes. *In* Campbell, M. F., and Harrison, H. H. (Eds.): Urology, 3rd ed. Philadelphia, W. B. Saunders Co., 1970, pp. 1190–1229.

Zalar, J. A., Knode, R. E., and Mir, J. A.: Lipogranuloma of the penis. J. Urol., *102*:75, 1969.

CHAPTER 35

Tumors of Testicular Adnexal Structures and Seminal Vesicles

GERALD P. MURPHY, M.D.
JOHN F. GAETA, M.D.

EPITHELIAL TUMORS OF TESTICULAR ADNEXA

Primary epithelial neoplasms of the testicular adnexal structures are very rare, although both the epididymis and the supporting structures of the testis are frequently involved by extensions from primary testicular (germinal) tumors. Most epithelial tumors of the epididymis described in the literature correspond to benign epithelial hyperplasias or adenomas, which because of their frequently cystic nature have been designated as cystadenomas, adenomas, or papillary cystadenomas. Sherrick (1956) described the first case in the literature, and about 20 cases have been the subjects of subsequent publications. Review of the latter indicates that at least one third of the cases are bilateral, and they are frequently part of the picture of von Hippel–Lindau disease. According to Mostofi and Price (1973), those cases in which the lesion is unilateral can be regarded as "forme fruste" of the disease complex. The tumor occurs most often in young adults and produces either mild local discomfort or no symptoms; when seen in the elderly, it is frequently an incidental finding in an orchidectomy specimen following ablative surgery.

In its typical form, the lesion is at least partially cystic, and its wall is studded by one or several nodules of epithelial cells arranged in small glands and papillary structures (Fig. 35–1). The latter form irregular projections on thin fibrous stalks. Most of these are made up of columnar and ciliated cells, many of which display a vacuolated or clear cytoplasm. This finding indicates the presence of abundant glycogen, which will be removed with diastase when the cells are stained with the periodic acid–Schiff (PAS) method. Meyer et al. (1964) also demonstrated the presence of abundant stainable lipid in the clear cells. Because of these cytologic and histochemical features, the histologic findings of the epididymal cystadenoma can be very similar if not identical to those of some renal cell adenocarcinomas of the kidney, thus posing a difficult problem in histologic distinction, especially since the latter are well known for the unpredictable character of their metastatic spread.

A review of the literature reveals that about 80 cases of epidermoid cysts of the testis have been reported, 85 per cent of which have been treated by orchiectomy. A recent report summarized this and described an enucleation of the cyst with preservation of the testis. This report was felt to be important, since the condition is most common in young adults, and the clinical course of the tumor, in these authors' opinion, is entirely benign (Rao, and Lorimer, 1982; Takihara et al., 1982; Cotter et al., 1984). On the other hand, a case of simple testicular cyst in a report of a cyst under the tunica albuginea has also recently been described. Cysts of the testis are apparently quite rare, and a recent report was able to collect only 12 cases.

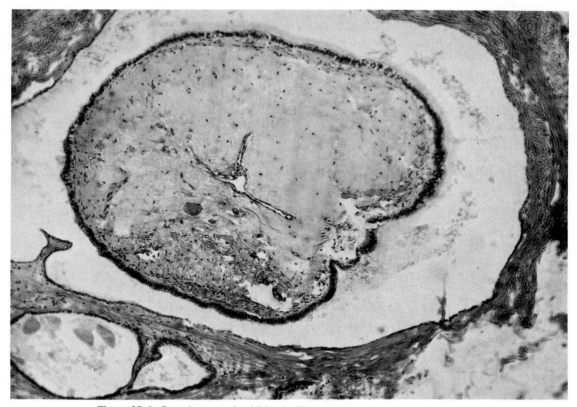

Figure 35–1. Cystadenoma of epididymis. Hematoxylin and eosin staining; × 90.

Of these 12 patients, 7 had simple cysts and 5 had associated cysts of the tunica albuginea (Takihara et al., 1982). Again, routine orchiectomy was performed and is described as a preferred approach. Other conditions associated with epididymal cysts have been reported. For example, a young man who presented with seminoma and epididymal cyst is believed to have developed these male genital tract abnormalities as a result of in utero exposure to diethylstilbestrol. This particular case may be a coincidental one and needs further follow-up, as it has been only briefly described (Conley et al., 1982). However, recently a papillary adenocarcinoma was reported. The tumor cells were examined by both regular and electron microscopic techniques. The tumor was localized in the rete testis and showed no involvement with the adjacent testicular parenchyma or the epididymis. The tumor cells manifested a transition from normal cells of the rete testis. The electron microscopic features of the tumor were also contrasted with those of the normal epithelial cells of the rete testis (Fukunaga et al., 1982).

The location and the cytologic features of these adenomas point to an origin in the epithelial lining of the epididymis or in the adjacent efferent ductules; since both structures have a mesonephric derivation, most authors believe that these lesions are of mesonephric origin (Easton and Claridge, 1964; Grant and Hoffman, 1963; Hill, 1962; Meyer et al., 1964: Mostofi and Price, 1973; Thompson, 1936). In fact, their papillary structure and general characterization show affinities to many of the mesonephric tumors of the female genital tract studied by Novak and associates (1954).

There are some descriptions in the literature of primary carcinomas of the epididymis (Thompson, 1936), but most of these are poorly documented, and the histologic findings indicate that many of them fall into the category of adenomatoid tumors (Fisher and Klieger, 1966), seminomas (Thompson, 1936), or embryonal carcinomas (Thompson, 1936). The case reported by Salm (1969) is probably the best illustration of what appears to be the malignant counterpart of a cystadenoma of the epididymis, as demonstrated by its initial location, papillary organization, and necrosis as well as by the presence of metastatic spread to the retroperitoneal area.

Primary carcinoma of rete testis has been reported in the literature (Schoen and Rush, 1959; Scully and Parham, 1948; Shillitoe, 1952; Willis, 1967), but its close anatomic proximity to the epididymal lesion and the histologic similarities pose the question as to whether the two can be differentiated with certainty (Fukunaga et al., 1982).

Cysts arising in the tunica albuginea are exceedingly rare. In a search of the literature, four cases have been noted in which that diagnosis was established and adequate information on clinical and pathologic aspects was given (Arcadi, 1952; Frater, 1929). These cysts generally appear in individuals in the fifth or sixth decade of life. The cysts can be asymptomatic and discovered incidentally; they can also be associated with testicular pain or swelling, as in two of the patients reported by Arcadi (1952). Cysts of the tunica albuginea are small, can be solitary, multiple, or multiloculated, and are characteristically located in the anterior and lateral aspects of the testis. The fibrous walls are widely connected to the tunica albuginea, and in some cases, the cystic lesions seem to be clearly invested by it. The cysts commonly contain a serous fluid and are lined by cuboidal epithelium. Epithelial inclusions in the cystic walls and in the albuginea have not been frequently described. The cause of these cysts is not known. It has been mentioned that trauma and subsequent hemorrhage into the albuginea could lead to cyst formation (Bullitt, 1900; Frater, 1929). It has also been maintained that these lesions are retention cysts secondary to trauma or infection. Arcadi (1952) regards infection as a possible etiologic factor, since he found evidence of testicular inflammation in two of his patients. The differential diagnosis of this rare lesion usually does not present a problem, since a high orchiectomy is commonly performed because of the suspicion of cancer being present.

Leiomyoma, the second most common tumor of the epididymis, is said to be frequently accompanied by hydrocele (Payan et al., 1967). Furthermore, these tumors of the testis and epididymis are generally painful. The diagnosis of "leiomyomatous proliferation of the epididymis" should be entertained in patients with hydrocele with dull scrotal pain. The presence of a slightly enlarged, firm, tender epididymis would support such a diagnosis. Resection of the epididymis (without the testis) appears to be possible in these patients.

Metastatic tumors of the epididymis are rare. In 1960, Brotherus reviewed five case reports (Derman, 1927; Henke and Lubarsch, 1925; Humphrey, 1944; Katzen, 1941; Lewis et al., 1944) and added two cases of his own. The primary tumor was in the kidney in two cases, in the stomach in three cases, and in the prostate in two cases.

Adenomatoid Tumors

Adenomatoid tumors are described as a separate group, since there is no universal agreement as to their exact cellular origin. The term "adenomatoid" was first applied to these lesions by Golden and Ash in 1945. Other designations include mesothelioma, adenofibroma, angiomatoid tumor, and lymphangioma. When diagnosed correctly, they account for approximately 30 per cent of all paratesticular tumors. In the male, they are located in the epididymis and in the spermatic cord; in the female, they have been described in the uterus, in the fallopian tube, and in the ovary. In our experience, they occur most often in individuals in the third or fourth decade of life, and they present clinically as a small, solid, asymptomatic mass, generally found on routine physical examination. They are generally rounded and discrete and usually lie anywhere in the epididymis, but they can be embedded in the testicular tunics. On sectioning, they appear uniformly white, yellow, or tan. Their histologic features are somewhat rich and variable, which perhaps helps to account for the multiple theories about their histogenesis.

On microscopic examination, the lesion is made up of two different elements: epithelium-like cells and fibrous stroma. The epithelium-like cells can be arranged in a variety of ways, the most characteristic being a framework of poorly delineated spaces, sometimes lined by flattened or cuboidal cells, sometimes lined by plump elements, in which case an epithelial or mesothelial origin is suggested (Fig. 35–2). In some cases, these epithelium-like cells can be traced to the intervening stroma, either in their glandular form or when arranged in a plexiform or elongated fashion, also indicating a possible transition to the mesenchymal substance or to smooth muscle elements. Some of the epithelial cells contain vacuoles, which according to some authors (Mostofi and Price, 1973) may be im-

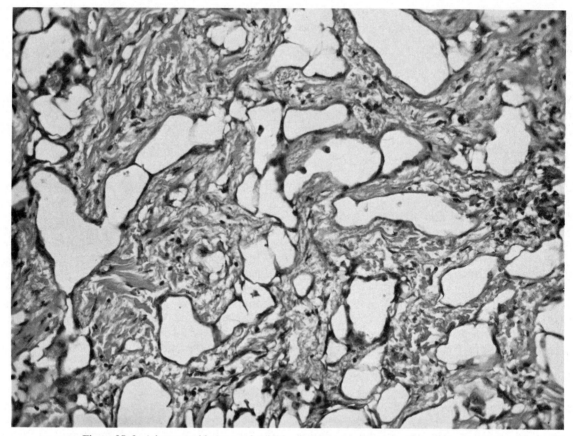

Figure 35–2. Adenomatoid tumor of epididymis. Hematoxylin and eosin staining; × 260.

plicated in the mechanism of their lumen formation. In our experience, histochemical stains have failed to identify the presence of secretory substance. At the cellular level, the nuclei show marked uniformity in size and in chromatin distribution, and we have never seen any evidence of mitotic activity. Miller and Lieberman (1968) reported a group of 12 adenomatoid tumors, calling attention to the presence of locally invasive features in 3 of them, although they were not able to find any clinical differences in the rest of the group. The literature does not contain a single well-documented case of metastasizing adenomatoid tumor, and none of the 12 cases in our records showed evidence of either recurrence or spread into the adjacent testis.

A multiplicity of explanations has been given to justify the origin of this strange tumor. Naegeli (1912) was the first to suggest an epithelial origin from vestiges of the müllerian duct, and although no definite proof was given, a significant number of authors have supported the concept (Codnere and Flynn, 1946; Jackson, 1958; Longo et al., 1951). Masson et al. (1942)

supported the concept of a mesothelial origin chiefly on histologic grounds, and although no further evidence was given, this resulted in the erroneous classification of true mesotheliomas of the tunica vaginalis and adenomatoid tumors into a single group. On this basis, several reports of adenomatoid tumors have appeared in the literature (Bàrbera and Rubino, 1957; Fajers, 1949; Kasdon, 1969), many of them under the designation of mesotheliomas.

Another view currently held is that the adenomatoid tumor is of endothelial origin and probably represents a special type of hemangioma or lymphangioma, even though the characteristic adenomatoid spaces of the lesion never show evidence of blood. A stronger view contradicting this theory is supported by the ultrastructural findings of Marcus and Lynn (1970), who failed to see any similarities when they compared the electron microscopic features of hemangiomas with those of a characteristic adenomatoid tumor. In fact, they found a closer morphologic similarity when they compared the tumor with pleural mesotheliomas, although they were not able to commit themselves unequivocally regarding the origin of the epididymal lesion.

That these tumors could be considered possibly malignant may be suggested by occasionally observed cellular atypia and by an invasive mode of growth, even around nerves and vessels, as well as by a dissemination of metastatic growths within the tunica vaginalis. The long history of such tumors and the paucity of mitoses, however, as well as the absence of distant metastases suggest a benign nature and a limited degree of malignancy. Treatment is thus mainly surgical (Söderström and Liedberg, 1966).

A more recent report (Aubert et al., 1983) has described five cases of adenomatoid tumors of the tunica vaginalis. These cases are of particular value since there is a follow-up period of at least 3 years in each instance. As stated, it is important that the exact histologic nature of the lesion, if possible, be determined at the time of operation, thus preventing the sometimes unnecessary excision of a gonad. As has been emphasized, these tumors are generally benign and can be treated with limited excision and conservation of the testis. However, there are a few malignant forms that have been described in the literature (Japko et al., 1982); hence the need for careful histologic evaluation. Ultrastructural studies of such tumors are also of value and have recently been described (Mucientes, 1983). Acid mucopolysaccharides have been found in the tubular structures of the tumor, and, thus, such findings support its mesothelial origin.

Mesothelioma

Since the tunica vaginalis represents a pinched-off portion of the celomic cavity, it can be the site of origin of a wide spectrum of mesothelial proliferative changes, ranging from well-localized "reactive" lesions to others better designated as mesothelial neoplasms on the basis of their size, their extension, and their invasive or metastasizing features. It is difficult to ascertain the incidence of mesothelioma of the testicular tunics. In our experience, the lesion is sometimes mistaken for an unusual form of embryonal carcinoma chiefly on the basis of a papillary pattern, with complete disregard for its characteristic lack of cellular anaplasia. On the other hand, our knowledge about this tumor is clouded even further by several literature reports of other tumors (adenomatoid) that are under the erroneous designation of mesothelioma (Fajers, 1949; Masson et al., 1942). Bàrbera and Rubino (1957) should be credited with the first article that dealt with a detailed description of the differences between mesothelioma and adenomatoid tumor, as well as the histogenetic reasons to support their separation.

Paratesticular mesothelioma can be encountered in practically any age group, including children. In its characteristic form, the tumor presents as a firm and painless scrotal mass, often associated with hydrocele. The orchiectomy specimen demonstrates a white, yellow, or brown, poorly demarcated lesion that is sometimes firm and frequently shaggy and friable. The microscopic picture (Figs. 35–3 and 35–4) consists of a combination of papillary and solid structures against a background of densely fibrous or delicate fibroconnective tissue. In our experience, small and well-localized mesotheliomas tend to be predominantly papillary, whereas their structural organization seems to become more solid and variegated as they attain a certain size. The tumor cells have a generous amount of cytoplasm and poorly defined cytoplasmic borders. The nuclei are often vesicular and frequently display a single small nucleolus. Mitotic activity is either occasional or totally absent. Characteristic papillae are slender when cut longitudinally, and they are frequently lined with a single row of neoplastic cells. It is not rare to see calcification scattered throughout these neoplastic structures in the form of psammoma bodies identical with those seen in other papillary neoplasms (thyroid, ovary, and so forth). Many solid mesotheliomas disclose small or sometimes extensive areas in which the tumor cells are spindle-shaped, resulting in a disturbing sarcomatous picture. This feature is probably devoid of any clinical significance, but if extensive, it can lead to an erroneous diagnosis of fibrosarcoma, leiomyosarcoma, or any other soft tissue sarcoma that can be encountered in this area.

It is difficult, if not impossible, to separate mesotheliomas into a benign group and a malignant group. If we define malignancy in terms of metastasizing potential, then approximately 15 per cent of testicular mesotheliomas have been documented to result in metastatic involvement of inguinal lymph nodes or abdominal structures (Kasdon, 1969). We believe they are all capable of local invasion, and in our experience, the likelihood of their metastasizing is related to their size at the time of initial orchiectomy. Cases of metastatic disease reported in the lit-

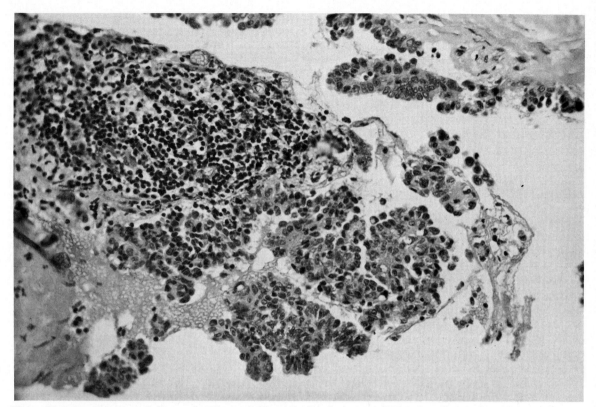

Figure 35–3. Papillary mesothelioma of tunica vaginalis testis. Small circumscribed lesion. Patient free of disease 8 years after excision. Hematoxylin and eosin staining; × 320.

erature indicate a significant size or the presence of multicentricity at the time of initial surgery. Conversely, it is also difficult to rely on isolated reports of their good prognosis, because some small lesions diagnosed as mesothelioma may be in actuality unusual instances of reactive mesothelial proliferation (Rao and Lorimer, 1982). Clinical management today usually consists of adequate surgical excision with follow-up examination, and biopsy if a metastatic focus is suspected (Hollands et al., 1982). Most recently, cases have been described in which conservative management failed and recurrence was observed (Antman et al., 1984). Limited experience with chemotherapy and radiotherapy has been studied without any conclusions being reached for such tumors. Staging procedures have included procedures similar to those used clinically in primary testis tumors, such as CAT scanning of the chest and abdomen and laparotomy, if necessary, for evaluation of intra-abdominal disease. This latter report describes 18 cases with malignant tumor, but these have also been reported elsewhere.

TUMORS OF THE SEMINAL VESICLE

A recent report described a fluctuant scrotal mass that measured 8 × 16 cm. At surgery, however, a hydrocele sac studded with multiple nodules was found (Chen et al., 1982). Following appropriate surgery the patient developed a tumor metastasizing widely and leading to his death 2½ years after the diagnosis. These authors reviewed the literature and found that they could describe only seven cases of malignant mesothelioma. They did, however, point out the histologic difference, in their opinion, between benign variance and the more malignant variety, which generally shows nuclear atypia, mitotic activity, invasion of the epididymis or spermatic cord, or lymphatic invasion as well as involvement of the fibrous tissue of the tunica (Hollands et al., 1982). It has always been the opinion of many that this rare tumor is best treated with orchiectomy via an inguinal approach with excision of the hemiscrotum at the earliest possible stage. This is, of course,

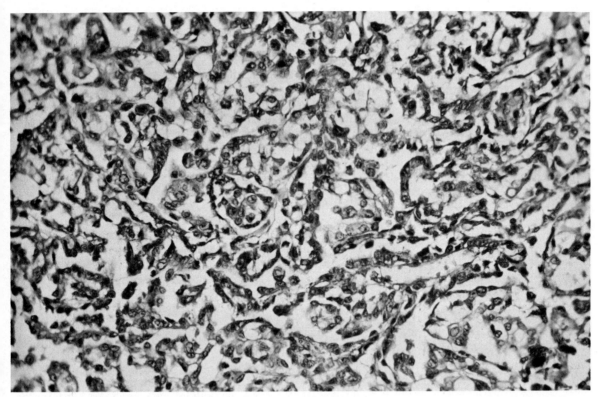

Figure 35–4. Papillary and solid mesothelioma of the tunica vaginalis testis. Patient died with abdominal involvement. Hematoxylin and eosin staining; × 320.

recommended only for malignant mesothelioma; it may in some instances require a two-stage procedure.

Anatomically, the seminal vesicles are bilateral outpouchings from the vas deferens; physiologically, they play an important role in the act of ejaculation. Histologically, however, they share many features with the prostate gland, not only because of the presence of similar glandular and fibromuscular components, but also because of their common response to testicular hormones.

Tumors of the seminal vesicles are rare, and because of their close anatomic and histologic relationship to the prostate gland, it is difficult and often impossible to verify the authenticity of those reported in the literature. Lazarus (1946) found 23 cases in his review of the subject and, being unable to differentiate between intrinsic tumors of the seminal vesicle and those arising from the prostate or from the retrovesical space, could accept only 7 cases as authentic.

Even with these limitations, there are only occasional accounts of primary mesenchymal tumors of the seminal vesicle. Buck and Shaw (1972) described two mesenchymal lesions in this location. One was large and encapsulated, which caused significant displacement of the urinary bladder, and was diagnosed as low-grade fibrosarcoma. The second case was an incidental finding characterized as a benign leiomyoma.

Primary carcinoma of the seminal vesicle is also a very rare tumor, but it shows some distinctive features that allow its separation from prostatic cancer. In its most characteristic form, it involves one or both seminal vesicles and only the peripheral portion of the adjacent prostate gland. The age distribution for individuals with this condition is also similar to that for those with carcinoma of the prostate, although it is even more rare than the latter in patients younger than 50 years of age.

On microscopic examination, carcinomas of the seminal vesicle tend to have a papillary configuration and a certain cystic character. In addition, we have seen more distinctive features of cellular anaplasia in these than are currently seen in prostatic cancer. Surgical therapy has usually involved an approach similar to a radical perineal or retropubic prostatectomy with the addition of the removal of the seminal vesicles in their entirety.

Cysts have been excised, aspirated, and even massaged. The diagnosis of a cystic lesion has been aided in selected cases by angiography, direct injection of contrast media into the lesion, and even ultrasonography. More experience has recently been described with ultrasound, particularly utilizing the transrectal approach, which seems to be superior to the alternative routes (Schuller and Walther, 1983). Histologic confirmation, however, remains advisable.

PARATESTICULAR TUMORS OF CONNECTIVE TISSUE AND MUSCLE

There are occasional reports of purely testicular mesenchymal tumors (one-sided teratomas) (Davis, 1962), but for the most part, the overwhelming majority of mesenchymal tumors in this area arise from paratesticular structures, although sometimes it may be difficult to determine whether the primary origin was the spermatic cord, the epididymis, or the tunica vaginalis.

Most series agree that rhabdomyosarcoma in its juvenile form probably accounts for approximately 40 per cent of all paratesticular tumors, benign and malignant. Leiomyosarcoma appears to be the second most common lesion in this area, followed by occasional occurrences of fibrosarcoma, liposarcoma, and undifferentiated mesenchymal tumors, which complete the spectrum of this group. Cooperative Study Groups have described some of their results with these tumors as well. One is dependent on this sort of accrual, as the rarity of the tumor makes certain conclusions on therapy still tentative. In a recent report (Kingston et al., 1983), four boys with primary paratesticular tumors were seen. There are now late relapses, defined as recurrence or tumor persistence 2 years after the diagnosis and treatment. This should be kept in mind for follow-up evaluation of such tumors.

RHABDOMYOSARCOMA

Paratesticular rhabdomyosarcoma occurs predominantly in children and adolescents and, with some exceptions, is most commonly seen during the first two decades of life. Most articles on this subject give credit to the work of Stout and Hill (1958), Horn and Enterline (1958), and Riopelle and Thériault (1956) for providing accurate accounts of this condition and for familiarizing pathologists with the numerous histologic variants of this tumor.

Clinically, this tumor usually presents as a large intrascrotal mass that compresses the testes and the epididymis, sometimes reaching the external inguinal ring; the location varies somewhat, depending on the exact point of origin. On gross inspection it can appear circumscribed, but on microscopic examination it often extends well beyond the margin seen by the naked eye. The cut surface is solid, grayish white, and firm, and is rarely hemorrhagic. Some patches of necrosis can be noted, especially around the central portion of the lesion.

The microscopic features of paratesticular rhabdomyosarcoma (Fig. 35–5) are largely characterized by pronounced variation from case to case and even within the same tumor, provided that a sufficient number of samples are obtained. Most of them show more than one pattern of the spectrum, ranging from totally undifferentiated mesenchymal elements to the distinctive features of skeletal muscle fibers. When the undifferentiated elements predominate, numerous samples may have to be studied before a diagnosis can be fully established. If no differentiating features are demonstrated, it is difficult to be certain of the myoblastic nature of the neoplasm. In fact, in some of the published series, totally anaplastic tumors are classified among the embryonal group (Horn and Enterline, 1958), whereas other authors prefer to designate this lesion as "undifferentiated malignant mesenchymal tumor" (Mostofi and Price, 1973). It is more characteristic, however, to find a combination of various patterns containing an admixture of cellular elements accurately described by Patton and Horn (1962), which include: (1) irregular, acidophilic cells with small budding extensions indicative of early rhabdomyosarcomatous differentiation; (2) broad, elongated, or ribbon-shaped cells, also displaying intense cytoplasmic acidophilia; (3) bizarre forms, often multinucleated and generally referred to as "tadpole" cells; and (4) any of the foregoing demonstrating a combination of myoblastic striations, some longitudinal, some in the cross pattern; these are generally accepted as the most, if not the only, objective demonstration of rhabdomyoblastic differentiation in a mesenchymal tumor. The latter is well demonstrated in well-fixed and thinly cut sections, either readily or after prolonged search. Phos-

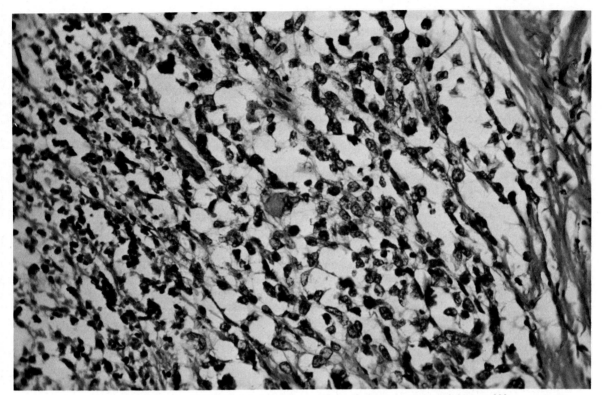

Figure 35–5. Paratesticular rhabdomyosarcoma. Hematoxylin and eosin staining; × 320.

photungstic acid and Masson staining techniques have gained wide acceptance as methods to enhance their identification.

Some paratesticular rhabdomyosarcomas are partially or predominantly arranged in an "alveolar" fashion identical with the distinctive pattern frequently seen in other locations that was first designated as "alveolar rhabdomyosarcoma" by Riopelle and Thériault (1956) and is currently accepted as a variant of embryonal rhabdomyosarcoma.

Riehle and Venkatachalam (1982) make the point that has often been made about other sarcomas, namely that electron microscopic diagnosis assisted more frequently in sorting out aberrations, variance, and, particularly, identification of the sarcoma in question. Electron microscopy has been successfully used to identify the cytoplasmic myofilaments and Z bands in a paratesticular rhabdomyosarcoma. This, of course, applies to paratesticular tumors as well.

To summarize, the main problems of rhabdomyosarcoma are (1) the distinction of undifferentiated examples from other small cell malignancies, especially soft tissue Ewing's sarcoma and lymphoma; (2) distinction of the spindle cell examples from fibrosarcoma, leiomyosarcoma, malignant fibrohistiocytoma, polyhistiocytoma, and other sarcoma; (3) recognition of the minimal criteria on small samples, such as needle biopsied specimens and frozen sections, which can be difficult; and (4) recognition of rhabdomyosarcoma in other uncommon sites as well as those of the genital tract. A recent report from the Royal Alexandra Hospital for Children (Bale et al., 1983) has provided considerable emphasis and experience in these precise areas. More experience is being gained in rhabdomyosarcoma in childhood. Particular comments may be made about the fact that survival is generally favorable in the paratesticular and genitourinary sites, compared with survival rates for other sites such as extremity, head and neck, trunk, or orbit.

Testicular and Paratesticular Tumor Management

The primary testicular or paratesticular tumor should be removed by inguinal orchiectomy with high ligation of the cord. Retroperitoneal exploration is then best performed through a long transperitoneal midline incision for careful evaluation of the renal hilar nodes on both sides, the para-aortic nodes, the iliac nodes, and the residual cord at the level of the internal ring.

The primary lymphatic drainage of the testis and the cord courses through lymphatics parallel to the testicular vessels; these intercommunicate with para-aortic nodes at the level of the renal vessels. The lower para-aortic and iliac nodes serve as a route of lymphatic spread when the primary spermatic lymphatics have become occluded by fibrosis or tumor (Burrington, 1969). Several papers discussing these tumors have recommended routine bilateral iliac and retroperitoneal lymph node dissection (Arlen et al., 1969; Burrington, 1969; Ghavimi et al., 1973; Hays et al., 1969; Johnson, 1975). Most recently, the fact that rhabdomyosarcoma is the most common malignant spermatic cord tumor has been reaffirmed. To date, 162 cases have been described and summarized (Sago and Novicki, 1982). A 5 year survival rate of 75 per cent, using multimodal treatment, remains the current goal. Current adjuvant therapy is as follows.

RADIOTHERAPY

Cobalt 60 teletherapy can be delivered in a total tumor dose of 4000 to 6000 rads over a period of 5 to 8 weeks through ports extending well beyond the known confines of the tumor. Dose and port size are determined by the primary site and extent of the tumor and by the age of the patient. Radiotherapy can be utilized for local tumors even when the tumor is generalized.

There are some reports of the management of these tumors that rely on primary excision, node resection, chemotherapy, and no radiotherapy, the rationale being that the radiotherapy might be harmful in the long term, and that results comparable with those of current management can be achieved without radiotherapy. This particular point remains to be proved, as more cases must be collected.

CHEMOTHERAPY

Chemotherapy with vincristine (1.5 mg per sq m), cyclophosphamide (300 mg per sq m), and dactinomycin (0.4 mg per sq m) was administered IV at weekly intervals for 6 weeks; then vincristine and cyclophosphamide were given every 2 weeks for 6 to 12 months (Pratt et al., 1972). This represents a variation from a previous schedule so as to provide more intensive chemotherapy early in the course of treatment (Pratt, 1969; Pratt et al., 1968). The 6-week course of dactinomycin was repeated at 3-month intervals. Chemotherapy was initiated concurrently with radiotherapy, immediately after histologic confirmation of diagnosis. Chemotherapy was administered for 6 months to patients with localized tumor and for 12 months to patients with regional or generalized tumor. Drug doses were adjusted to the biologic tolerance of each patient by the use of total white blood cell count as the primary guide (Pratt et al., 1972).

A report by Ghavimi et al. (1975) describes 29 children younger than 15 years of age with embryonal rhabdomyosarcoma who were treated according to a multidisciplinary protocol, which consisted of surgical removal of the tumor, if possible, followed by chemotherapy, and also by radiation therapy in patients with gross or microscopic residual disease. Radiation therapy was given in a dose in the 4500- to 7000-rad range. Additional new trials of chemotherapy consisted of cycles of sequential administration of dactinomycin, Adriamycin, vincristine, and cyclophosphamide, with obligatory periods of rest. The drug therapy was continued for 2 years. In addition, at the present time early phase II trials are also employing a method of intravenous administration of methyl-CCNU (Semustine) that appears promising.

A recent paper described, along with another series, the management following removal of the primary tumor with subsequent retroperitoneal lymphadenectomy. Because all of the lymph nodes were negative for tumor, the authors felt justified in dispensing with radiation therapy to that area, and postoperatively the patient was successfully treated with vincristine, actinomycin D, and cyclophosphamide, the so-called VAC regime, weekly for 13 weeks. The patient is now 9 years post surgery with no evidence of recurrent tumor. It is this type of approach that, as mentioned previously, may result, in selected instances, in dispensing with the use of radiotherapy (Sago and Novicki, 1982).

Tumor stage and site are now considered important prognostic indicators. Grosfeld et al. (1983) state that chemotherapy improves survival in Stage I (91 per cent) and in Stage II (86 per cent) and may shrink bulky Stage III tumors, allowing less radical procedures in certain selective sites, particularly the urinary tract. It is still true, however, that survival is poor in Stage III, with 35 per cent survival, and dismal in Stage IV, with 5.2 per cent survival, despite combined therapy. Relapses are generally fatal despite attempts at second-look resection, altered chemotherapy, and radiation (Grosfeld et al., 1983).

Leiomyosarcoma

Smooth muscle tumors of the spermatic cord and epididymis are rare, and their exact incidence is difficult to determine: first, because the clinical and histologic (Fig. 35–6) differences between benign smooth muscle tumors and malignant ones are very slight; and second, because some adenomatoid tumors are erroneously classified as leiomyomas, especially those that exhibit a significant component of smooth muscle (Wilson, 1949). In fact, as indicated by Stout and Hill (1958), "The whole field of tumors of the soft tissues and peripheral nerves is so complex, that errors in diagnosis are bound to occur, even if one has a large experience." Most cases of benign and malignant smooth muscle tumors described in the literature are in patients between the fifth and eighth decades of life.

Kyle (1966) reports that neoplasms of the spermatic cord are infrequent, and leiomyosarcomas of the spermatic cord are rare. Satter and colleagues in 1959 found 10 previously published cases involving the spermatic cord and epididymis. They also state that they found in the literature more than 200 cases of primary malignancies of the spermatic cord, the epididymis, and the testicular tunics.

According to Hinman and Gibson (1924), 90 per cent of extratesticular tumors occurring within the scrotum are found in the spermatic cord. Of the latter, 30 per cent are malignant, and 70 per cent are benign. Of the malignant variety, the majority are mesenchymal sarcomas, i.e., fibrosarcoma, myxosarcoma, liposarcoma, rhabdomyosarcoma, and leiomyosarcoma. There are more than 25 cases reported of leiomyosarcoma of the spermatic cord. Local invasion of the adjacent tissues was found in 5 of the 13 cases in which this detail was described. The first recurrence was usually local, in the scrotum or at the distal spermatic stump. This feature was described in six cases; in Thomp-

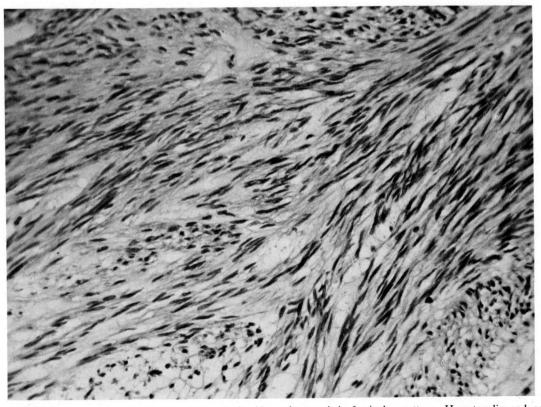

Figure 35–6. Leiomyosarcoma of paratesticular tunic. Note characteristic fascicular pattern. Hematoxylin and eosin staining; × 320.

son's case, it was only a local recurrence, followed by survival (Thompson, 1936). In his case the tumor was excised locally on three separate occasions.

Distant spread has been hematogenous in a large number of cases, i.e., in tumors of humerus, liver, ileum, and lung. Autopsies were not done in many cases, however, and the clinical finding of abdominally palpable masses probably represented metastatic disease in the para-aortic lymph nodes. The ratio of the number of cases in which hematogenous spread was known to have occurred to the number with known lymphatic spread is 6:2. These facts, at least, support the opinion of Strong (1942) and of others who believe that the spread is as frequently hematogenous as lymphatic. The importance of electron microscopy in the documentation of these particular tumors, as contrasted to light microscopy, has been emphasized (Gaffney et al., 1984).

The philosophy and planning of treatment have been greatly affected by the mode of spread. It is agreed that all cases of tumor of the spermatic cord should be explored, and the growth should be removed. A frozen section of the tumor should be studied. If it is benign, simple excision is all that is necessary. The standard therapy for leiomyosarcoma has been radical orchiectomy in which a high ligation of the cord is carried out. Owing to the high incidence of hematogenous spread, the surgeon should carry out early clamping of the cord to prevent escape of tumor cells. Double-draping techniques to prevent seeding of the tumor locally would seem important. The peritoneum should be opened and the retroperitoneal, para-aortic, and iliac nodes palpated for evidence of spread.

Because the series presented is still too small to be of statistical significance, only generalizations can be made about the rationale of deep radiation therapy and of radical retroperitoneal lymph node dissections.

The clinical course of ten patients with aggressive sarcoma of the spermatic cord has been presented, however (Malek et al., 1972). The importance of spermatic cord and testicular invasion, the favorable role of retroperitoneal lymphadenectomy, and the promising results of aggressive chemotherapy for the invasive tumors seem reasonable based on current results.

Electron microscopy is extremely helpful in the differentiation of the type of testicular sarcoma. Although at present management may not be radically changed, depending on the

histologic description there are differences as to whether a bilateral retroperitoneal node dissection or a thoracoabdominal one should be done, or, for that matter, as to the extent of dissection of the nodes. This exists not only for tumors of this variety but also for tumors in general (Hermanek and Sigel, 1982). In young persons the complications of node dissection have been minimal, although these obviously have to be considered as well as in adults (Waters et al., 1982). Particularly important for young individuals is a discussion with the parents concerning obvious difficulties with fertility in the future. This aspect has been addressed recently but chiefly in adult patients (Lipshultz, 1982). The additional use of tumor markers must be further explored in these entities, and experience at the present time is limited in contrast to what might be called adult testis tumors (Vugrin et al., 1982).

Miscellaneous Mesenchymal Tumors of the Spermatic Cord

Isolated cases of other mesenchymal tumors of the spermatic cord, including liposarcoma, lipoma, fibrosarcoma, and myxochondrosarcoma, have been recorded. Liposarcoma is probably the most significant one in this group on account of its greater frequency. Samellas (1964), in his review of 112 tumors of the spermatic cord, added one case of his own to three cases already reported, and Gowing and Morgan (1964) found two cases in their review of paratesticular tumors of connective tissue.

On histologic examination, liposarcomas of the spermatic cord and of the scrotal area show essentially the same features as those described in other soft tissue sites, although most of the recorded cases just mentioned were predominantly characterized as well differentiated. The Armed Forces Institute of Pathology collected 14 paratesticular liposarcomas that also appear to show this tendency to be well differentiated. In most cases, they appear as a discrete nodular mass, sometimes attaining a large size, frequently located near the spermatic cord and entirely separate from the testicle.

On histologic examination, they are characterized by the presence of a rather uniform pattern of interwoven bundles of long spindle-shaped cells with blunt-ended nuclei and with cytoplasmic myofibrils extending along their longitudinal axis. Leiomyoma is separated from leiomyosarcoma on the basis of occasional or absent mitotic figures and because of its uniform cellular arrangement. According to Stout and Hill (1958), approximately 70 per cent of those considered malignant on initial histologic examination either recur or metastasize, or both, regardless of their location. To our knowledge, those located in the spermatic cord and the epididymis appear to follow the same pattern of recurrence or spread; if the latter occurs, the lungs tend to be the favored site for vascular metastases. The clinical management of these malignant or benign lesions does not differ from that previously described.

Malignant neoplasms arising within the spermatic cord are uncommon, with 161 cases reported in the literature by 1969 (Arlen et al., 1969). Sporadic cases have continued to appear, but the cumulative number remains relatively small (Banowsky and Shultz, 1970; Bonzanini, 1974; Brenez, 1973; Datta et al., 1971; Duhart et al., 1970; Jenkins and Subbuswamy, 1972; Krawitt and Siegel, 1970; Malek et al., 1972; Weitzner, 1973). Although Banowsky and Shultz (1970) have described 19 histologic types of sarcoma originating from the spermatic cord and the tunics, none was classified as neurofibrosarcoma. Johnson and associates (1975) have described such a case.

Although Johnson could find no mention in the literature of a primary neurofibrosarcoma arising within the spermatic cord, it is doubtful that this tumor is rare. Instead, he believes it is more likely that many of these tumors have been mistaken for fibrosarcoma or liposarcoma. It is frequently impossible to classify a sarcoma as neurogenic in origin in spite of the light microscopic findings of nuclear palisading and of alternating cellular and loose myoid areas. Indeed, D'Agostino et al. (1963a and b) state that the only feature distinguishing a malignant neurilemoma from a fibrosarcoma is origin within a nerve trunk.

References

Antman, K., Cohen, S., Dimitrov, N. V., Green, M., and Mussia, F.: Malignant mesothelioma of the tunica vaginalis testis. J. Clin. Oncol., 2(5):447, 1984.

Arcadi, J. A.: Cysts of the tunica albuginea testis. J. Urol., 68:631, 1952.

Arlen, M., Grabstald, H., and Whitmore, W. F., Jr.: Malignant tumors of the spermatic cord. Cancer, 23:525, 1969.

Aubert, J., Touchard, G., Mazet, B., Dore, B., and Caron, J. J.: Adenomatoid tumor of the tunica vaginalis testis. Apropos of 5 cases. J. Urol. (Paris), 89(9):677, 1983.

Bale, P. M., Parsons, R. E., and Stevens, M. M.: Diagnosis and behavior of juvenile rhabdomyosarcoma. Hum. Pathol., 14(7):596, 1983.

Banowsky, L. H., and Shultz, G. N.: Sarcoma of the spermatic cord and tunics: Review of the literature, case report and discussion of the role of retroperitoneal lymph node dissection. J. Urol., 103:628, 1970.

Bàrbera, V., and Rubino, M.: Papillary mesothelioma of the tunica vaginalis. Cancer, 10:183, 1957.

Bonzanini, C.: Fibrosarcoma del funicolo spermatico. Minerva Chir., 29:156, 1974.

Brenez, J.: La résection endoscopique. Acta Urol. Belg., 41:61, 1973.

Brotherus, J. V.: Metastatic tumors of the epididymis and the spermatic cord. J. Urol., 83:171, 1960.

Buck, A. C., and Shaw, R. E.: Primary tumours of the retro-vesical region with special reference to mesenchymal tumours of the seminal vesicles. Br. J. Urol., 44:47, 1972.

Bullitt, J. B.: Cystic tumors of the testis and epididymis. Med. Rec. N. Y., 57:943, 1900.

Burrington, J. D.: Rhabdomyosarcoma of the paratesticular tissues in children. Report of eight cases. J. Pediatr. Surg., 4:503, 1969.

Chen, K. T. K., Arhelger, R. B., Flam, M. S., and Hanson, J. H.: Malignant mesothelioma of the tunica vaginalis testis. Urology, 20(3): 316, 1982.

Codnere, J. T., and Flynn, J. E.: Adenomatoid tumors of the epididymis: Report of three cases. J. Urol., 56:448, 1946.

Conley, G. R., Sant, G. R., and Mitcheson, H. D.: Seminoma and epididymal cysts in a young man with known diethylstilbestrol exposure in utero. Poster Session, American Urological Association, Annual Meeting, Kansas City, Mo., May 16–20, 1982.

Cotter, M., Lampert, I. A., and Salm, R.: Epidermoid cysts of testis. Clin. Oncol., 10:149, 1984.

D'Agostino, A. N., Soule, E. H., and Miller, R. H.: Primary malignant neoplasms of nerves (malignant neurilemomas) in patients without manifestations of multiple neurofibromatosis (von Recklinghausen's disease). Cancer, 16:1003, 1963a.

D'Agostino, A. N., Soule, E. H., and Miller, R. H.: Sarcomas of the peripheral nerves and somatic soft tissues associated with multiple neurofibromatosis (von Recklinghausen's disease). Cancer, 16:1015, 1963b.

Datta, N. S., Singh, S. M., and Bapna, B. C.: Liposarcoma of the spermatic cord: Report of a case and review of the literature. J. Urol., 106:888, 1971.

Davis, A. E., Jr.: Rhabdomyosarcoma of the testicle. J. Urol., 87:148, 1962.

Derman, G. L.: Ein primärer gelatinös-scirrhöser Nierenkrebs mit Metastasen in die Epididymis. Virchows Arch., 265:304, 1927.

Duhart, J. E., Padorno, E. A., and Fredotovich, N. M.: Sarcoma de cordón espermático. Rev. Argent. Urol. Nefrol., 39:160, 1970.

Easton, J. A., and Claridge, M.: Cystadenoma of the epididymis. Br. J. Urol., 36:416, 1964.

Fajers, C. M.: Mesotheliomas of the genital tract. A report of five new cases and a survey of the literature. Acta Pathol. Microbiol. Scand., 26:1, 1949.

Fisher, E. R., and Klieger, H.: Epididymal carcinoma (malignant adenomatoid tumor, mesonephric, mesodermal carcinoma of epididymis). J. Urol., 95:568, 1966.

Frater, K.: Cysts of the tunica albuginea (cysts of the testis). J. Urol., 21:135, 1929.

Fukunaga, M., Aizawa, S., Furusato, M., Akasaka, Y., and Machida, T.: Papillary adenocarcinoma of the rete testis. A case report. Cancer, 50(1): 134, 1982.

Gaffney, E. F., Harte, P. J., and Browne, H. J.: Paratesticular leiomyosarcoma: an ultrastructural study. J. Urol., *132*(1):133, 1984.

Ghavimi, E., Exelby, P. R., D'Angio, G. J., Cham, W., Lieberman, P. H., Tan, C., Miké, V., and Murphy, M. L.: Multidisciplinary treatment of embryonal rhabdomyosarcoma in children. Cancer, *35*:677, 1975.

Ghavimi, F., Exelby, P. R., D'Angio, G. J., Whitmore, W. F., Jr., Lieberman, P. H., Lewis, J. L., Jr., Miké, V., and Murphy, M. L.: Proceedings: Combination therapy of urogenital embryonal rhabdomyosarcoma in children. Cancer, *32*:1178, 1973.

Golden, A., and Ash, J. E.: Adenomatoid tumors of the genital tract. Am. J. Pathol., *21*:63, 1945.

Gowing, N. F., and Morgan, A. D.: Paratesticular tumors of connective tissue and muscle. Br. J. Urol., *36*(Suppl.):78, 1964.

Grant, S. M., and Hoffman, E. F.: Bilateral papillary adenomas of the epididymides. Arch. Pathol., *76*:620, 1963.

Grosfeld, J. L., Weber, T. R., Weetman, R. M., and Baener, R. L.: Rhabdomyosarcoma in childhood: analysis of survival in 98 cases. J. Pediatr. Surg., *18*(2):141, 1983.

Hays, D. M., Mirabal, V. O., Patel, H. R., Shore, N., and Woolley, M. M.: Rhabdomyosarcoma of the spermatic cord. Surgery, *65*:845, 1969.

Henke, F., and Lubarsch, O.: Handbuch der Speziellen Pathologischen, Anatomie und Histologie. Vol. 6, p. 666. Berlin, Julius Springer Verlag, 1925.

Hermanek, P., and Sigel, A.: Necessary extent of lymph node dissection in testicular tumours. A histopathological investigation. Eur. Urol., *8*(3): 135, 1982.

Hill, R. B., Jr.: Bilateral papillary, hyperplastic nodules of epididymis. J. Urol., *87*:155, 1962.

Hinman, F., and Gibson, T. E.: Tumors of the epididymis, spermatic cord and testicular tunics. A review of the literature and report of three new cases. Arch. Surg., *8*:100, 1924.

Hollands, M. J., Dottori, V., and Nash, A. G.: Malignant mesothelioma of the tunica vaginalis testis. Eur. Urol., *8*(2):121, 1982.

Horn, R. C., Jr., and Enterline, H. T.: Rhabdomyosarcoma: A clinicopathological study and classification of 39 cases. Cancer, *11*:181, 1958.

Humphrey, M. A.: Metastasis in the epididymis from cancer of the prostate: Case report. J. Urol., *51*:641, 1944.

Jackson, J. R.: The histogenesis of the "adenomatoid" tumor of the genital tract. Cancer, *11*:337, 1958.

Japko, L., Horta, A. A., Schreiber, K., Mitsudo, S., Karwa, G. L., Singh, G., and Koss, L. G.: Malignant mesothelioma of the tunica vaginalis testis: report of first case with preoperative diagnosis. Cancer, *49*(1):119, 1982.

Jenkins, D. G., and Subbuswamy, S. G.: Leiomyosarcoma of the spermatic cord. Br. J. Surg., *59*:408, 1972.

Johnson, D. E., Kaesler, K. E., Mackay, B. M., and Ayala, A. G.: Neurofibrosarcoma of spermatic cord. Urology, *5*:680, 1975.

Johnson, D. G.: Trends in surgery for childhood rhabdomyosarcoma. Cancer, *35*:916, 1975.

Kasdon, E. J.: Malignant mesothelioma of the tunica vaginalis propria testis. Report of two cases. Cancer, *23*:1144, 1969.

Katzen, P.: Metastatic carcinoma of the epididymis: Report of a case. J. Urol., *46*:734, 1941.

Kingston, J. E., McElwain, T. J., and Malpas, J. S.:

Childhood rhabdomyosarcoma: experience of the Children's Solid Tumor Group. Br. J. Cancer, *48*(2):195, 1983.

Krawitt, D. R., and Siegel, V.: Spermatic cord tumors: A case report. Mt. Sinai J. Med. N. Y., *37*:603, 1970.

Kyle, V. N.: Leiomyosarcoma of the spermatic cord: A review of the literature and report of an additional case. J. Urol., *96*:795, 1966.

Lazarus, J. A.: Primary malignant tumors of the retrovesical region with special reference to malignant tumors of the seminal vesicles: Report of a case of retrovesical sarcoma. J. Urol., *55*:190, 1946.

Lewis, L. G., Goodwin, W. E., and Randall, W. S.: Carcinoma of the spermatic cord and epididymis extension from primary carcinoma of the stomach. J. Urol., *51*:75, 1944.

Lipshultz, L. I.: Management of infertility following treatment for testicular carcinoma. Cancer Bull., *34*(1): 31, 1982.

Longo, V. J., McDonald, J. R., and Thompson, G. J.: Primary neoplasms of the epididymis. Special reference to adenomatoid tumors. JAMA, *147*:937, 1951.

Malek, R. S., Utz, D. C., and Farrow, G. M.: Malignant tumors of the spermatic cord. Cancer, *29*:1108, 1972.

Marcus, J. B., and Lynn, J. A.: Ultrastructural comparison of an adenomatoid tumor, lymphangioma, hemangioma, and mesothelioma. Cancer, *25*:171, 1970.

Masson, P., Riopelle, J. L., and Simard, L. C.: Le mésothéliome bénin de la sphère génitale. Rev. Can. Biol., *1*:720, 1942.

Meyer, J. S., Roth, L. M., and Silverman, J. L.: Papillary cystadenomas of the epididymis and spermatic cord. Cancer, *17*:1241, 1964.

Miller, F., and Lieberman, M. K.: Local invasion in adenomatoid tumors. Cancer, *21*:933, 1968.

Mostofi, F. K., and Price, E. B., Jr.: Tumors of male genital system. *In* Atlas of Tumor Pathology, Series 2, Fasc. 8. Washington, D. C., Armed Forces Institute of Pathology, 1973.

Mucientes, F.: Adenomatoid tumor of the epididymis. Ultrastructural study of three cases. Pathol. Res. Pract., *176*(2–4):258, 1983.

Naegeli, T.: Ein Mischtumor des Samenstranges. Virchows Arch., *208*:364, 1912.

Novak, E., Woodruff, J. D., and Novak, E. R.: Probable mesonephric origin of certain female genital tumors. Am. J. Obstet. Gynecol., *68*:1222, 1954.

Patton, R. B., and Horn, R. C., Jr.: Rhabdomyosarcoma: Clinical and pathological features and comparison with human fetal and embryonal skeletal muscle. Surgery, *52*:572, 1962.

Payan, H. M., Mendoza, C., Jr., and Ceraldi, A.: Diffuse leiomyomatous proliferation in the epididymis. A cause of pain in hydrocele. Arch. Surg., *94*:427, 1967.

Pratt, C. B.: Response of childhood rhabdomyosarcoma to combination chemotherapy. J. Pediatr., *74*:791, 1969.

Pratt, C. B., Hustu, H. O., Fleming, I. D., and Pinkel, D.: Coordinated treatment of childhood rhabdomyosarcoma with surgery, radiotherapy, and combination chemotherapy. Cancer Res., *32*:606, 1972.

Pratt, C. B., James, D. H., Jr., Holton, C. P., and Pinkel D.: Combination therapy including vincristine (NSC-67574) for malignant solid tumors in children. Cancer Chemother. Rep., *52*:489, 1968.

Rao, K. G., and Lorimer, A.: Epidermoid cyst of testis. Benign intratesticular tumor. Urology, *19*(6):662, 1982.

Riehle, R. A., and Venkatachalam, H.: Electron microscopy in diagnosis of adult paratesticular rhabdomyosarcoma. Urology, *19*(6):658, 1982.

Riopelle, J. L., and Thériault, J. P.: Sur une forme meconnue de sarcome des parties molles: le rhabdomyosarcome alvéolaire. Ann. Anat. Pathol. (Paris), *1*:88, 1956.

Sago, A. L., and Novicki, D. E.: Rhabdomyosarcoma of spermatic cord. *19*(6):606, 1982.

Salm, R.: Papillary carcinoma of the epididymis. J. Pathol., *97*:253, 1969.

Samellas, W.: Malignant neoplasms of spermatic cord. Liposarcoma. N. Y. State J. Med., *64*:1213, 1964.

Satter, E. J., Heidner, F. C., II, and Wear, J. B.: Primary sarcoma of the spermatic cord and epididymis. J. Urol., *82*:148, 1959.

Schoen, S. S., and Rush, B. F., Jr.: Adenocarcinoma of the rete testis. J. Urol., *82*:356, 1959.

Schuller, J., and Walther, V.: Transrectal ultrasound tomography with an electronic line scanner. Ultraschal. Med., *4*(1):7–12, 1983.

Scully, R. E., and Parham, A. R.: Testicular tumors. II. Interstitial cell and miscellaneous neoplasms. Arch. Pathol., *46*:229, 1948.

Sherrick, J. C.: Papillary cystadenoma of the epididymis. Cancer, *9*:403, 1956.

Shillitoe, A. J.: Carcinoma of the rete testis. J. Pathol. (Bacteriol.), *64*:650, 1952.

Sóderström, J., and Liedberg, C. F.: Malignant "adenomatoid" tumour of the epididymis. Acta Pathol. Microbiol. Scand., *67*:165, 1966.

Stout, A. P., and Hill, W. T.: Leiomyosarcoma of the superficial soft tissues. Cancer, *11*:844, 1958.

Strong, G. H.: Lipomyxoma of the spermatic cord: Case report and review of literature. J. Urol., *48*:527, 1942.

Takihara, H., Valvo, J. R., Tokuhara, M., and Cockett, A. T. K., Intratesticular cysts. Urology, *20*(1): 80, 1982.

Thompson, G. J.: Tumors of the spermatic cord, epididymis, and testicular tunics. Review of literature and report of forty-one additional cases. Surg. Gynecol. Obstet., *62*:712, 1936.

Vugrin, D., Whitmore, W. F., Nisselbaum, J., and Watson, R. C.: Correlation of serum tumor markers and lymphangiograpy with degrees of nodal involvement in surgical Stage II testis cancer. J. Urol. *127*(4): 683, 1982.

Waters, W. B., Garnick, M. B., and Richie, J. P.: Complications of retroperitoneal lymphadenectomy in the management of nonseminomatous tumors of the testis. Surg. Gynecol. Obstet., *154*(4): 501, 1982.

Weitzner, S.: Leiomyosarcoma of spermatic cord and retroperitoneal lymph node dissection. Am. Surg., *39*:352, 1973.

Willis, R. A.: Pathology of Tumors. 4th ed., pp. 585, 593, 967. New York, Appleton-century-Crofts, 1967.

Wilson, W. W.: Adenomatoid leiomyoma of the epididymis. Br. J. Surg., *37*:240, 1949.

EMBRYOLOGY AND ANOMALIES OF THE GENITOURINARY TRACT

CHAPTER 36

Genetic Determinants of Urologic Disease

LESTER WEISS, M.D.

The reduction in the number of patients seen with infectious diseases has contributed to a relative increase in the number of patients who have either genetic disorders or congenital abnormalities. Significant congenital malformations are recognized during the newborn period in 3 to 5 per cent of live-born infants. An equal number of malformations are identified later in life. Single-gene defects are present in more than 1 per cent of all newborns, although many of these are not diagnosed in the neonatal period. Congenital abnormalities of the genitourinary tract are among the more common and more important birth defects. Unfortunately, many of these malformations are not diagnosed in the neonatal period because they are overlooked in the standard "inspection and palpation" physical examination. This is in marked contrast to the striking visibility in the newborn period of "surface" defects, such as cleft palate, clubfoot, and cutaneous abnormalities.

The rapid expansion of medical genetics during the past 25 years has included a corresponding increase in knowledge of the genetics of urologic disorders and malformations. Although genetic counseling may be the primary responsibility of someone other than the urologic surgeon, his authority on genitourinary tract disorders is often recognized as encompassing genetics by families seeking such information. Realization that a certain condition may be genetic can result in ascertaining malformations in other family members before irreparable damage has been done.

The urologist will be treating patients having genetic disorders that can result from (1) chromosome abnormalities, (2) single-gene defects (mendelian inheritance), or (3) the interaction of genes with environmental factors or other genes.

CHROMOSOME ABNORMALITIES

A number of technical advances in the late 1950's resulted in the explosion during the 1960's of knowledge of chromosomes and their relationship to human disease (Hamerton, 1971; (Schinzel, 1984). In 1960, the 46 human chromosomes could be arranged in groups and some individual chromosomes identified. Clinical syndromes associated with abnormalities of chromosome number or large structural abnormalities were defined.

It was usually mitotic metaphase chromosomes that were examined. A metaphase chromosome consists of two chromatids joined at the primary constriction, the centromere. Chromosomes were classified morphologically as metacentric, submetacentric, or acrocentric, according to the position of the centromere (Fig. 36–1). The short arm of the chromosome was designated "p" and the long arm "q." The acrocentric chromosomes often have "satellites" attached to the short arm with a slender stalk.

Based on these morphologic features a standard nomenclature was developed. The chromosomes of the human karyotype were classified in groups designated by letters A through G and individual pairs (in decreasing order of size) by arabic numerals 1 to 22, plus X and Y. The chromosomes 1 to 22 are "auto-

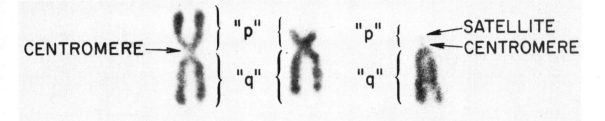

Figure 36–1. Human metacentric, submetacentric, and acrocentric chromosomes.

somes," and the X and Y are the "sex chromosomes." Only chromosomes 1, 2, 3, 16, 17, 18, and Y could be identified with certainty with the early standard techniques (Fig. 36–2). In 1970 Caspersson and his associates published the results of their studies of human chromosomes stained with quinacrine mustard (Q-banding) and examined by fluorescence microscopy. They demonstrated that each of the individual chromosomes could be identified by a series of light and dark bands within each chromosome.

The 22 autosome pairs and the two sex chromosomes can today be identified by any of several banding techniques. The autosomes are numbered in decreasing order of size, and the sex chromosomes are designated X and Y, respectively (Paris Conference, 1971). The light and dark bands divide the long and short arms into regions and bands that are designated by arabic numerals. The addition, loss, or rearrangement of relatively small portions of chromosomes can be detected. Figures 36–3 and 36–4 are karyotypes from a normal male and a

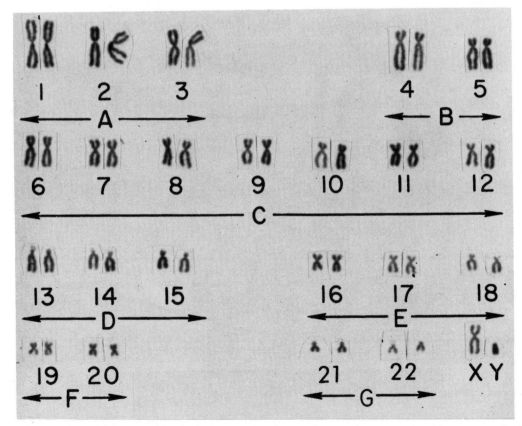

Figure 36–2. Normal male karyotype, 46,XY.

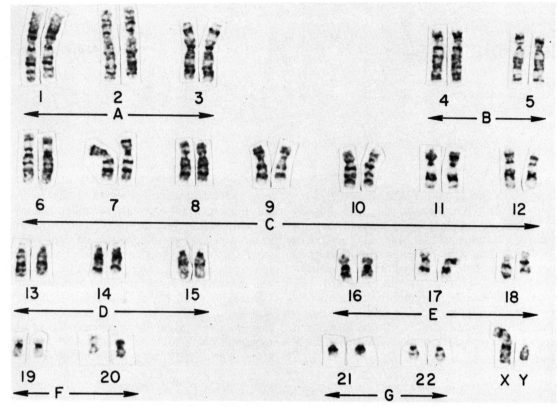

Figure 36–3. Normal male karyotype, 46,XY. G-banding technique.

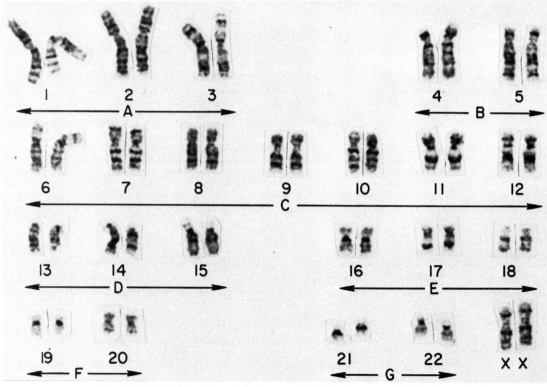

Figure 36–4. Normal female karyotype, 46,XX. G-banding technique.

normal female, respectively, banded with the G-banding obtained by treatment of the slide with trypsin prior to staining by the Giemsa method. Approximately 150 bands can be identified in routine chromosome preparations. A newer technique that is available in a number of centers involves the examination of prometaphase chromosomes. In prometaphase preparations, between 1000 and 1500 bands can be identified. The addition or loss of material from an autosome usually results in a syndrome of multiple congenital malformations. Genitourinary tract abnormalities are frequently seen as part of these syndromes.

Chromosome abnormalities can involve the autosomes or the sex chromosomes. There are both numerical and structural abnormalities. The structural abnormalities are further subdivided into deletions, duplications, and rearrangements. Rearrangements can be translocations or inversions and may be either familial or de novo.

The first autosomal trisomic syndrome, Down syndrome (mongolism), was described in 1959 by Lejune and his colleagues. Patients with Down syndrome have an extra No. 21 chromosome (trisomy 21). According to the standard nomenclature, it is written 47,XY,+21. The total chromosome number is expressed first; the sex chromosome constitution, second; and finally, any addition or loss of chromosome material. Down syndrome is often associated with cryptorchidism, penile and scrotal underdevelopment, and hypospadias. There is apparently no increased risk of kidney or collecting system abnormalities (Egli and Stalder, 1973). Most often, Down syndrome is sporadic and associated with increased maternal age. However, approximately 5 per cent of these patients have a chromosome rearrangement known as a translocation. When this translocation is present in a "carrier" parent, the risk of a subsequent child's being born with Down syndrome is usually 1 chance in 7 but can be as high as 100 per cent.

The trisomy 18 syndrome (Edwards et al., 1960; Warkany et al., 1966) is due to an extra No. 18 chromosome (46,XX,+18) (Fig. 36–5). While this multiple malformation syndrome often results in death within the first year of life, a number of affected children live into the middle years of childhood or adolescence. Children with trisomy 18 have characteristic facies, mental retardation, growth failure, congenital heart disease, and skeletal abnormalities. Malformations of the kidney and collecting system are also common and can result in recurrent urinary tract infections (Fig. 36–6). An awareness of the high frequency of urinary tract

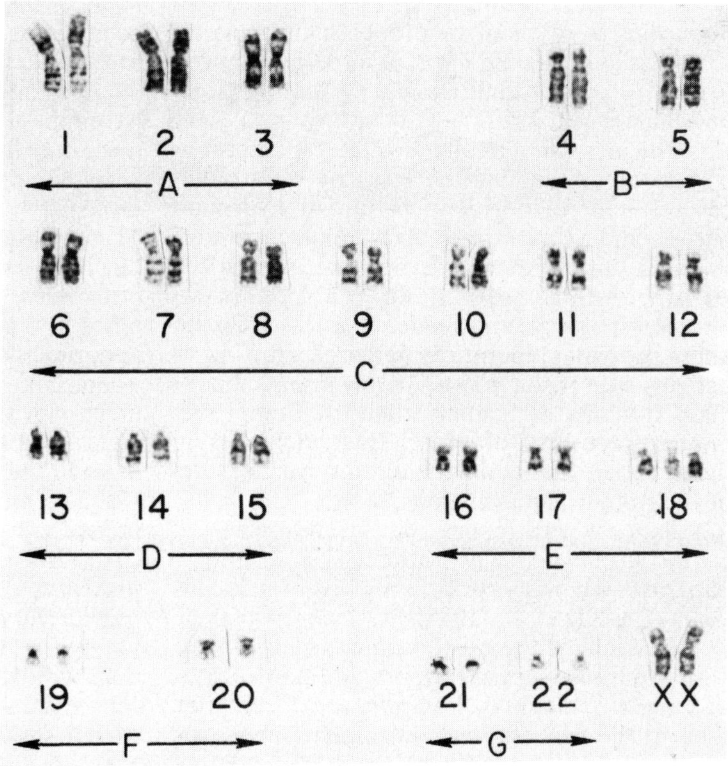

Figure 36–5. Karyotype from a patient with trisomy 18 syndrome, 47,XX,+18. Note three No. 18 chromosomes. G-banding technique.

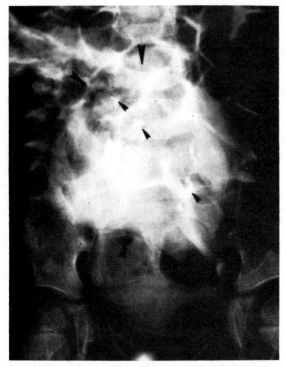

Figure 36–6. Bilateral fused ectopic kidneys ("cake" kidney) in a patient with trisomy 18. Supine film from an excretory urogram made during late nephrographic and early excretory phase shows the rounded contours of the solitary fused renal mass (large arrows) and partial filling of some of the calyces (small arrows). (Courtesy of Dr. W. A. Reynolds.)

anomalies is essential to proper management. These children should have an intravenous pyelogram as part of their clinical evaluation (Egli and Stalder, 1973).

The increasing frequency with which obstetricians are examining the fetus by ultrasound has resulted in the identification of hydronephrosis and urinary tract obstruction in utero. Prenatal surgical therapy is being attempted on an experimental basis. Before an attempt at intrauterine surgery is made, it is essential to know the karyotype of the fetus because most patients with trisomy 13 or 18 have renal anomalies. It would be inappropriate to attempt the in utero correction of urinary tract anomalies in those patients who would not survive because of their other malformations.

Patients with trisomy of chromosome No. 8 have urinary tract abnormalities and, unlike patients with trisomy 18, may live for many years (Cassidy et al., 1975).

A decreased life expectancy is less likely with syndromes caused by the addition or loss of smaller amounts of chromosome material than in the trisomy syndromes. Therefore, re-

current infections due to urologic abnormalities become a much more significant problem. For example, the "cat-eye syndrome" is due to an extra segment derived from a No. 22 chromosome in the karyotype (Egli and Stalder, 1973; Freedom and Gerald, 1973). Children with this duplication of chromosome material commonly have obstructive uropathies and other abnormalities of the urinary tract.

Rearrangements of chromosome material can be the result of inversions or translocations. As long as a familial translocation involves no loss or gain of chromosome material, it has no phenotypic affect. These rearrangements occur in approximately 1 in 250 individuals (Van Dyke et al., 1983). The carrier of these balanced familial rearrangements are at increased risk of having offspring with an unbalanced karyotype with additional or missing chromosome material and, therefore, of having multiple malformations. When a chromosome rearrangement is de novo, that is, occurring in the gamete that formed the individual, there is a 5 to 15 per cent risk of mental retardation or multiple congenital malformations, or both.

Structural or numerical abnormalities of the sex chromosomes are extremely common, and most urologists will see patients with the resulting syndromes. Approximately 1 in every 400 live-born infants has an abnormal sex chromosome constitution (Robinson and Puck, 1967). Most of these individuals have normal external genitalia in the newborn period and are therefore not detected until later in life.

Patients with Klinefelter syndrome may have mild to moderate retardation, but many of these individuals have normal intelligence and are first diagnosed when they appear in the urologist's office, complaining of infertility. These patients have a normal male phenotype but have small, firm testes after puberty. They often have poor muscle tone in addition to infertility, and a higher incidence of behavioral abnormalities is associated with this syndrome. There is at least anecdotal evidence that treatment with testosterone results in both improvement in muscle tone and strength and improvement in the behavioral sphere (Smith, 1975).

The most common karyotype found in patients with Klinefelter syndrome is 47,XXY (Fig. 36–7). Mosaicism, which refers to the presence, in one individual, of some cells with one karyotype and others with a different karyotype, is not uncommon. For example, a patient with Klinefelter syndrome may have some cells with a 47,XXY karyotype and other cells with a 48,XXXY karyotype. Any postpubertal

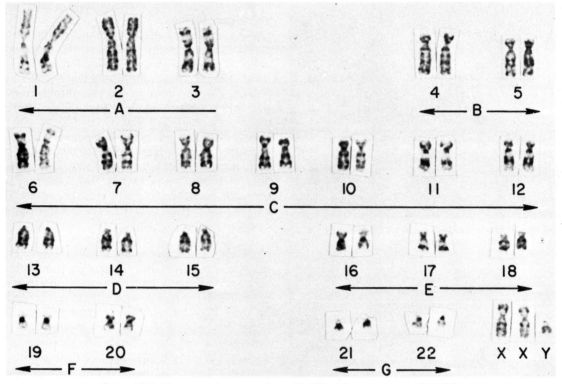

Figure 36–7. Karyotype from a patient with Klinefelter syndrome, 47,XXY.

male with hypogonadism should undergo testing with a buccal smear or karyotyping, or both, as part of his evaluation.

The buccal smear is a simple technique for determining the number of X chromosomes present in the karyotype of an individual. Professor Murray Barr (Barr and Bertram, 1949)

found that the nuclei of cells from normal females had a densely staining chromatin mass adjacent to the nuclear membrane that was not present in the nuclei of cells from normal males (Fig. 36–8A). The dark-staining chromatin mass is sometimes called the Barr body but more properly is the X chromatin body. This dark-

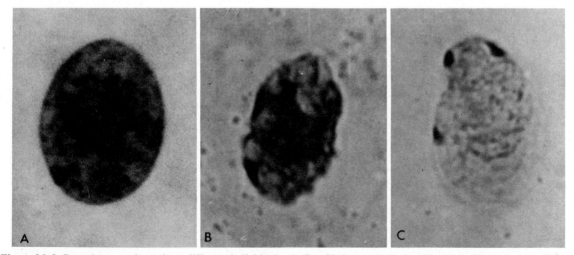

Figure 36–8. Buccal smears from three different individuals. *A,* One X chromatin body adjacent to the nuclear membrane from a normal female, 46,XX. *B,* Two X chromatin bodies in a buccal epithelial cell nucleus from a patient with Klinefelter syndrome, 48,XXXY. *C,* Three chromatin bodies from a patient with Klinefelter syndrome, 49,XXXXY.

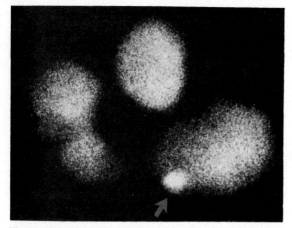

Figure 36–9. The brilliantly fluorescent F body in the nucleus of a polymorphonuclear leukocyte.

staining X chromatin body in the normal female represents the X chromosome that is inactivated (Ohno and Makino, 1961). When there are more than two X chromosomes present, all except one are inactivated. This is a means of dosage compensation so that the active chromosome material is the same in males and females. Therefore, the number of X chromosomes is one more than the number of X chromatin bodies. In Figure 36–8*B*, two X chromatin bodies can be seen. Therefore, this cell has three X chromosomes. The karyotype could be either 48,XXXY or 47,XXX. Figure 36–8*C* is from a patient with a 49,XXXXY karyotype. After the development of the Q-banding technique it was found that the Y chromosome in most males has a brillant fluorescent region at the distal end of the long arm. This fluorescent region can be seen in interphase nuclei and is called the Y chromatin body, or sometimes the F body (Fig. 36–9). Patients with Klinefelter syndrome have one or more X chromatin bodies plus a Y chromatin body in their interphase nuclei.

Patients with Turner syndrome have a variety of karyotypes (Ferguson-Smith, 1965). They may be 45,X; or they may exhibit mosaicism such as 45,X/46,XX; or they may have a structural abnormality of one of the X chromosomes, such as a deletion or a ring. This syndrome may be detected in the newborn because of lymphedema and webbing of the neck; during childhood because of short stature; or during adolescence, when the patients may present with primary amenorrhea and failure to develop secondary sex characteristics. Some individuals with mosaic Turner syndrome may have secondary amenorrhea, and a few have even been fertile.

More than half the patients with Turner syndrome have abnormalities of the kidneys or collecting system (Egli and Stalder, 1973; Hortling, 1955). These abnormalities include horseshoe kidney, ectopic kidney, duplication of the collecting system, and hypoplastic kidney, which can result in renal hypertension. All patients with Turner syndrome should have an intravenous pyelogram or renal ultrasound examination as part of their evaluation, so that abnormalities of the kidney and collecting system can be detected early and damage secondary to infection or hypertension can be minimized.

Individuals with the mosaic karyotype 45,X/46,XY have a variable phenotype. They may be clinically indistinguishable from patients with 45,X Turner syndrome; they may present in the newborn period with ambiguous genitalia; or they may be completely masculinized. Patients with a 45,X/46/XY karyotype often have testicular remnants as part of the dysgenetic gonads. These gonads should be surgically removed because of a high risk of gonadoblastoma (Taylor et al., 1966). If the patient is raised as a female and the gonads are not removed before adolescence, it is possible that the testicular remnant may produce testosterone and virilization.

Infertile males with 46,XX karyotypes have been described. They are phenotypically normal males with small, soft testes. Some of these XX males have a translocation of a small portion of the Y chromosome to one of the two X chromosomes (Fig. 36–10) (Magenis et al., 1982).

Abnormalities of the sex chromosomes that result in abnormal sex differentiation will be discussed in detail in Chapter 41.

It is known that there is an excess of retarded males compared with retarded females. Approximately half of this excess can be accounted for by the "fragile X syndrome." Many of these retarded males have enlarged testes

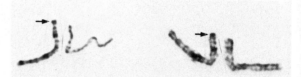

Figure 36–10. Karyotype from an XX male demonstrating the translocation of a small part of a Y to an X chromosome. (Courtesy of Dr. D. L. Van Dyke.)

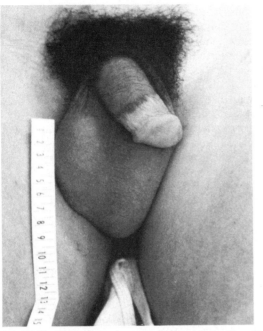

Figure 36–11. The enlarged testes of a retarded male with the fragile X syndrome.

and may therefore be referred to a urologist (Fig. 36–11). If peripheral blood lymphocytes are cultured in a folate-deficient medium, a break can be seen in the distal end of the long arm of one X chromosome (Fig. 36–12). This is an X-linked cause of mental retardation and can be prenatally diagnosed by amniocentesis.

There is an ever-increasing interest in the cytogenetics of solid tumors and in the relationship between congenital malformations and malignancies. The increased risk of leukemia in Down syndrome is well documented. Less well known is the increased risk of Wilms' tumor in patients with trisomy 18. The relationship be-

tween Wilms' tumor, aniridia, and other congenital malformations was described by Miller and coworkers in 1964. A distinct chromosome abnormality (an interstitial deletion in the short arm of chromosome 11) is associated with the aniridia–Wilms' tumor syndrome. Chromosome abnormalities are reported in familial renal cell carcinomas.

SINGLE-GENE DEFECTS— MENDELIAN INHERITANCE

Single-gene defects can result in structural or functional abnormalities, or both, of the urinary or reproductive system. Metabolic disorders can also result in significant derangement of renal function, even to the degree that nephrectomy and renal transplantation are required. Mendelian characteristics can be transmitted in any of four simple patterns: autosomal dominant, autosomal recessive, X-linked recessive, or X-linked dominant (Thompson and Thompson, 1980).

Autosomal Dominant Inheritance

A trait or gene is said to be dominant when it is expressed in the phenotype, whether the individual is homozygous or heterozygous for that gene. An individual is homozygous when both members of a pair of genes are identical. When two different alleles are present, the individual is said to be heterozygous. Figure 36–13 is the pedigree of a family in which the dominant gene for adult polycystic disease is segregating. A number of characteristics of autosomal dominant inheritance are exemplified by the pedigree.

1. The abnormality appears in each carrier. There is no "skipping" of generations.

2. An affected person, will, on the average, transmit the gene to half his children. That is,

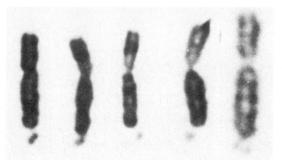

Figure 36–12. X chromosomes from a retarded male with the fragile X syndrome demonstrating the fragile site at Xq23. (Courtesy of Dr. D. L. Van Dyke.)

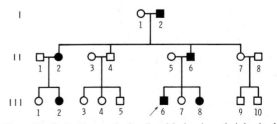

Figure 36–13. Pedigree of a family with dominantly inherited adult polycystic disease of the kidneys.

with each pregnancy, there is a 50 per cent risk that the offspring will be affected.

3. Unaffected individuals do not transmit the trait to their children.

4. The sex of an individual does not influence the likelihood of having or transmitting the trait. That is, males and females are affected in equal numbers, and the trait can be transmitted by either sex to male and female offspring.

Exceptions to this transmission of autosomal dominant traits occur. Sometimes the *expression* of an autosomal dominant gene may be influenced by the sex of an individual in such a way that the severity of the disorder is greater in one sex than in the other. Hereditary nephritis with deafness (Alport syndrome) is one example of such a sex-influenced autosomal dominant trait (Cohen et al., 1961). In this disorder the male may have much more severe renal disease, often leading to renal failure, whereas an affected female may exhibit only microscopic hematuria.

In some pedigrees, for reasons that are not always clear, a gene may have reduced "penetrance." That is, an individual may not have phenotypic manifestations of a gene, even though he carries that dominant gene. Under these circumstances the carrier may transmit the gene to his offspring, in whom it might be fully expressed. Reduced penetrance may occur in families with tuberous sclerosis and von Hippel–Lindau syndrome.

Some of the disorders with which the urologist may be concerned that are inherited as autosomal dominant traits are listed below (McKusick, 1983).

Adult polycystic disease
Benign familial hematuria
Ehlers-Danlos syndrome
Hereditary nephritis with deafness (Alport syndrome)
Hyperparathyroidism
Medullary sponge kidney
Renal tubular acidosis
Tuberous sclerosis
von Hippel–Lindau syndrome
Ureteral reflux (in some families)
Cryptorchidism (in some families)
Hypospadias (in some families)

When an individual has a disorder suspected of being inherited in an autosomal dominant fashion, appropriate family studies should be undertaken. These studies should extend, whenever possible, at least to grandparents and cousins. In many instances the course or com-

plications of a disease can be altered by appropriate management. Adult polycystic kidney disease accounts for approximately 10 per cent of the patients treated for end-stage renal disease. This is a severe burden on the family and society. In a study of 22 patients with end-stage renal disease due to adult polycystic kidney disease, only 23 per cent knew that their disorder was hereditary at the time of diagnosis. In only 18 per cent was genetic counseling proposed. Diagnostic studies of children at risk were rarely suggested. The diagnosis can be made by ultrasound examination before the patients reach their middle 20's and the information used for making reproductive decisions (Sahney et al., 1982).

Autosomal Recessive Inheritance

A trait that is transmitted by an autosomal recessive gene is expressed only in the individual who is homozygous for the abnormal gene. Recessive traits usually appear in the siblings of the propositus but not in other family members. An exception to this occurs when there is extensive inbreeding. Figure 36–14 is the pedigree of a family with cystic disease of the kidney and congenital hepatic fibrosis (Weiss et al., 1974). The disorder in the siblings of the proband was discovered by family studies only after the exact nature of the disease in the proband was elucidated. The higher than expected frequency of affected individuals in this pedigree is due to a combination of factors. The inclusion of the individual who brought the family to the attention of the investigator (the proband or propositus) in the calculation of the frequency among siblings results in a falsely high number of affected individuals. This is known as "bias of

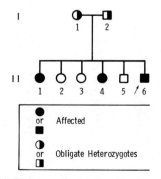

Figure 36–14. Pedigree of a family with recessively inherited polycystic disease of the kidneys and congenital hepatic fibrosis.

ascertainment." Furthermore, in a small pedigree, chance alone can result in a higher than expected number of affected members. The expected ratio of normal-to-affected siblings is 3 to 1. Families in which there are autosomal recessive conditions have the following characteristics:

1. Males are as likely to be affected as females.

2. The parents of an affected child often have common ancestors.

3. The trait typically appears in siblings of affected individuals but not in their parents, offspring, or other relatives.

4. An average of one of four siblings of the propositus will be affected.

The parents of an affected child may ask for genetic counseling, or a sibling may inquire regarding his genetic risk.

When the disorder is transmitted by an autosomal recessive gene, the chance with each pregnancy of the parents' having another affected child is one in four, or 25 per cent. There is a one in four chance of the child's being homozygous normal, a one in four chance of his being affected, and a one in two chance of his being an unaffected carrier of the abnormal gene. If an unaffected sibling inquires about the genetic prognosis (the risk of having an affected child), the risk can be calculated. The chance of an unaffected sibling's being a carrier is two chances in three. If he does not marry a "blood" relative, the chance of his marrying a carrier depends on the frequency of carriers in the population. For most of the rare conditions under consideration, the carrier rate is often 1 per cent or less. The chance of a sibling's being a carrier and also marrying a carrier is the product of the individual risks, or $2/3 \times 1/100$. If the parents are both carriers, the chance (with each pregnancy) of having an affected child is one in four; therefore, the risk that a sibling will have an affected child is $2/3 \times 1/100 \times 1/4$, or approximately 1 chance in 600.

A few of the autosomal recessive disorders that the urologist may encounter are listed below (McKusick, 1983).

Disorders affecting the urinary system:

Polycystic disease of the kidney and liver
Juvenile nephronophthisis
Sickle cell anemia
Sickle cell trait (can cause hematuria)
Alcaptonuria
Cystinosis
Hyperoxaluria
Renal tubular acidosis
Renal dysplasia with retinal aplasia

Disorders affecting the reproductive system:

Adrenogenital syndrome (five different enzyme defects)
Cystic fibrosis
Smith-Lemli-Opitz syndrome
Male pseudohermaphroditism due to defects in androgen synthesis (four different enzyme defects)
Female pseudohermaphroditism
Rokitansky-Kuster-Hauser syndrome
Pseudovaginal perineal scrotal hypospadias

Knowledge of the genetic nature of these disorders is essential both for ascertainment of the "at-risk" relatives and for genetic counseling directed to the affected individual, his parents, and his siblings.

For some autosomal recessive disorders that affect the genitourinary tract, prenatal diagnosis by amniocentesis is available at 14 to 16 weeks of gestation. A currently experimental technique of chorionic biopsy will make fetal tissues available for prenatal diagnosis at 8 to 10 weeks of gestation. When the enzyme defect is known and the deficit is expressed in amniocytes, prenatal diagnosis can be made by biochemical assay. Even when the enzyme defect cannot be directly determined by examination of the amniocytes, prenatal diagnosis may be possible with the use of restriction enzymes (restriction endonucleases). Another technique that can be used in prenatal diagnosis relates to genetic linkage. For example, the enzyme 21-hydroxylase (congenital adrenal hyperplasia) is in close linkage to the HLA locus. Although 21-hydroxylase is not expressed in amniocytes, HLA is expressed. Therefore, prenatal diagnosis is possible in families at risk by determination of the HLA haplotypes on the parents, a previously affected sibling, and the fetus.

X-Linked Recessive Inheritance

Genes that are located on the sex chromosomes are unequally distributed to males and females. The inequality results in characteristic, easily recognizable patterns of inheritance. Technically, sex-linked genes may be X-linked or Y-linked. By common usage, however, sex-linked and X-linked have come to be used interchangeably. Genes for male sex determination appear to be in the short arm and/or the very proximal part of the long arm of the Y chromosome. With the exception of "hairy pinnae" and the H-Y antigen (Wachtel et al.,

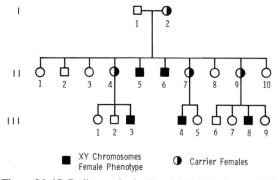

■ XY Chromosomes
Female Phenotype

◐ Carrier Females

Figure 36–15. Pedigree of a family with X-linked recessively inherited testicular feminization syndrome.

Pure gonadal dysgenesis of the XY type
Male pseudohermaphroditism due to a defect in androgen synthesis (17,20-desmolase deficiency)
Male pseudohermaphroditism due to defects in androgen action
   a. Testicular feminization syndrome
   b. Partial testicular feminization syndrome
   c. Incomplete male pseudohermaphroditism (four forms)

1975), no Y-linked genes are known. Since a male can have only one representative of any X-linked gene, he is said to be "hemizygous," rather than homozygous or heterozygous. Since a female has two X chromosomes, she is either homozygous or heterozygous for each X-linked gene.

The pedigree of a family in which the X-linked gene for testicular feminization syndrome (Prader, 1974) is segregating is diagrammed in Figure 36–15. In this disorder, a chromosomal and gonadal male has the external genitalia of a female and is usually assigned a female sex of rearing. The abnormal phenotype is due to any one of several inborn errors of metabolism that result in a defect of androgen action at the cellular level. The intracellular action of testosterone is necessary for the labioscrotal folds to fuse and for the phallus to enlarge to the size of a normal penis. These inborn errors of metabolism therefore result in a male pseudohermaphrodite with apparently normal female external genitalia and vaginal introitus.

The characteristics of X-linked recessive inheritance include the following:

1. The trait is much more frequent in males than in females.

2. The trait cannot be transmitted from a father to a son.

3. A carrier female transmits the trait to half of her sons. The trait may be transmitted through a series of carrier females.

4. Half of the daughters of an affected female are carriers.

Among the X-linked recessive conditions that involve the genitourinary tract are the following (McKusick, 1983).

Renal tubular acidosis (one form)
Fabry's disease
Familial anorchia

X-Linked Dominant Inheritance

Hypophosphatemia (vitamin D–resistant rickets) is an X-linked dominant condition of interest to the urologist (Winters et al., 1957). Affected individuals have low serum phosphorus and skeletal changes resembling those in rickets. The renal phosphate maximum tubular transport capacity (Tm) is reduced to about 50 per cent of normal. Treatment includes high doses of vitamin D, but the high vitamin D dosage can cause hypercalcemia, polyuria, and renal disease.

In X-linked dominant inheritance, affected males transmit the trait to all their daughters but never to a son. Affected heterozygous females transmit the trait to half their offspring, regardless of sex.

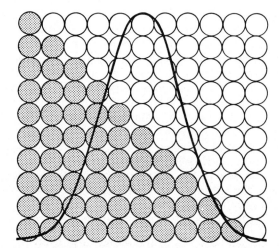

Figure 36–16. The gaussian distribution of a population in which 10 pairs of genes (gray and white) influencing a morphologic phenotype are segregating. Most of the population has four to six of each allele (gray and white). These persons are represented by the large central area under the curve. The few individuals who have mostly "gray" or mostly "white" genes are represented by the areas under the extreme right or left ends of the curve.

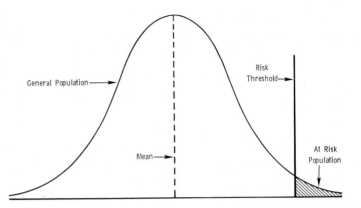

Figure 36–17. A normal distribution curve of a population demonstrating the individuals at risk for a multifactorial disorder and the concept of threshold effects.

Polygenic Inheritance and Environmental Factors

Figures 36–16 to 36–18 illustrate the concepts of multifactorial inheritance and the threshold effect. Figure 36–16 illustrates the normal distribution within a population of ten different genes that influence a hypothetical trait. The mutant and normal alleles are represented by gray and white circles. It can be seen that by random distribution of these genes in the population, rare individuals will have nine or ten of the genes represented by the white circles. Most of this hypothetical population will have approximately equal numbers of these alleles, with the median being five and five.

The concept of threshold effect is illustrated in Figure 36–17. Only those individuals who have at least eight of the genes represented by the white circles can manifest the abnormal trait. It is also possible for environmental factors to come into play. There are developmental abnormalities in which an environmental factor must act upon a predisposing genetic matrix

before the defect is manifested. The development of meningomyelocele is probably an example of a disorder that results from the interaction of an environmental agent and a fetus having the appropriate genetic constitution.

Different populations have very different incidences of meningomyelocele. In the United States, approximately 1 in every 1000 live-born infants has a major defect of central nervous system closure, whereas in some areas of Wales, the incidence approaches 1 in 100 (Elwood and Nevin, 1973). Furthermore, the offspring of affected individuals have an even higher risk for the defect. This suggests a genetic component to the etiologic basis. The seasonal variation in occurrence suggests an environmental component.

Once parents have produced a child with a defect that is due to polygenic inheritance, the risk to subsequent offspring increases greatly over that of the population at large. For example, in one study the risk for the population at large of having a male child with hypospadias was found to be 1 in 500 (Pettersson, 1964).

Figure 36–18. The superimposed distribution curve represents the change in distribution of the population of first-degree relatives of affected individuals. The increased number of individuals at risk is illustrated by the right-hand end of the curve.

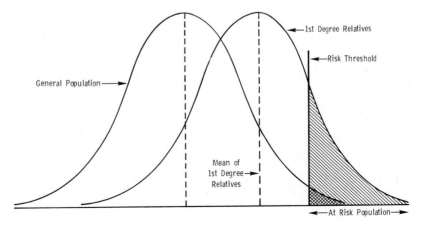

After parents had had one child with hypospadias, the risk of having another similarly affected child increased dramatically. If we assume that in order to be predisposed to hypospadias an affected child must have at least eight of the genes represented by the white circles, then his parents cannot belong to the population represented by the extreme left-hand side of Figure 36–16. The distribution of genes in first-degree relatives of affected individuals is shifted to the right. As the result of this shift, the number of individuals at risk increases markedly (Fig. 36–18).

Genetic counseling regarding recurrence risks for parents who have had one child with a defect thought to be multifactorial in origin must be on the basis of empirical risk data. Empirical risk is the risk as determined by observation and not on the basis of genetic theory. The risk varies with each anomaly. For example, the recurrence risk of midline central nervous system defect after the birth of a child with meningomyelocele is approximately 5 per cent, while the risk of hypospadias to a subsequent male offspring after the birth of an affected sibling is 10 per cent (Sorensen, 1953).

Understanding of underlying genetic principles as they apply to disorders of the genitourinary tract is essential for genetic counseling and is also of value in case finding.

References

Barr, M. L., and Bertram, E. G.: A morphological distinction between neurones of the male and female and the behavior of the nucleolar satellite during accelerated nucleoprotein synthesis. Nature (Lond.), *163*:676, 1949.

Carter, C. O.: Multifactorial genetic disease. Hosp. Pract., *5*:45, 1970.

Caspersson, T., Zech, L., Johansson, C., and Modest, E. J.: Identification of human chromosomes by DNA-banding fluorescent agents. Chromosoma, *30*:215, 1970.

Cassidy, S. B., McGee, van Eys, J., Nance, W. E., and Engel, E.: Trisomy 8 syndrome. Pediatrics, *56*:826, 1975.

Cohen, M. M., Cassady, G., and Hanna, B. L.: A genetic study of hereditary renal dysfunction with associated nerve deafness. Am. J. Hum. Genet., *13*:379, 1961.

Edwards, J. H., Harnden, D. G., Cameron, A. H., Crosse, V. M., and Wolff, O. H.: A new trisomic syndrome. Lancet, *1*:787, 1960.

Egli, F., and Stalder, G.: Malformations of kidney and urinary tract in common chromosomal aberrations. Humangenetik, *18*:1, 1973.

Elwood, J. H., and Nevin, N. C.: Factors associated with an encephalus and spina bifida in Belfast. Br. J. Prev. Soc. Med., *27*:73, 1973.

Ferguson-Smith, M. A.: Karyotype-phenotype correlations in gonadal dysgenesis and their bearing on the pathogenesis of malformations. J. Med. Genet., *2*:142, 1965.

Freedom, R. M., and Gerald, P. S.: Congenital cardiac disease and the "cat eye" syndrome. Am. J. Dis. Child., *126*:16, 1973.

Hamerton, J. L.: Human Cytogenetics. Vols. I and II. New York, Academic Press, 1971.

Hortling, H.: Congenital kidney anomalies in Turner's syndrome. Acta Endocrinol., *18*:548, 1955.

Lejune, J., Gautier, M., and Turpin, R.: Etude des chromosomes somatiques de neuf enfants mongoliens. C. R. Acad. Sci. (Paris), *248*:1721, 1959.

Lewy, P. R., and Belman, A. B.: Familial occurrence of nonobstructive noninfectious vesicoureteral reflux with renal scarring. J. Pediatr., *86*:851, 1975.

Macri, J. N., Haddow, J. E., and Weiss, R. R.: Screening for neural tube defects in the United States. Am. J. Obstet. Gynecol., *133*:119, 1979.

Magenis, R. E., Webb, M. J., McKeon, R. S., Brown, M. J., Allen, L. J., Tomer, D., Kammer, H., Van Dyke, D. L., and Lovien, E.: Translocation (X:Y) (p. 22, 33; p. 11.2) in XX males: etiology of male phenotype. Hum. Genet., *62*:271, 1982.

McKusick, V. A.: Mendelian Inheritance in Man. 6th ed. Baltimore, Johns Hopkins University Press, 1983.

Miller, R. W., Fraimeni, J. F., and Manning, M. D.: Association of Wilms' tumor with aniridia, hemihypertrophy and other congenital malformations. N. Engl. J. Med., *270*:922, 1964.

Milunsky, A., Macri, J. N., Weiss, R. R., Alpert, E., McIsaac, D. G., and Joshi, M. D.: Prenatal detection of neural tube deficits. Am. J. Obstet. Gynecol., *122*:313, 1975.

Ohno, S. T., and Makino, S.: The single-X nature of sex chromatin in man. Lancet, *1*:78, 1961.

Paris Conference (1971): Standardization in human cytogenetics. Birth Defects: Original Article Series, VIII:7. New York, The National Foundation, 1972.

Pettersson, F.: Meclozine and congenital malformations. Lancet, *1*:675, 1964.

Prader, A.: Male pseudohermaphroditisms. Pediatr. Annu., *3*:57, 1974.

Robinson, A., and Puck, T. T.: Studies on chromosomal nondisjunction in man. II. Am. J. Hum. Genet., *19*:112, 1967.

Sahney, S., Weiss, L., and Levin, N. W.: Genetic counseling in adult polycystic kidney disease. Am. J. Med. Genet., *11*:461, 1982.

Schinzel, A.: Catalogue of Unbalanced Chromosome Aberrations in Man. New York, Walter De Grugter, 1984.

Smith, D. W.: Personal communication, 1975.

Sorensen, H. R.: Hypospadias with Special Reference to Etiology. Copenhagen, Munksguard, 1953.

Stanbury, J. B., Wyngaarden, J. B., Fredrickson, D. S., Goldstein, J. L., and Brown, M. S.: The Metabolic Basis of Inherited Disease. 5th ed. New York, McGraw Hill Book Co., 1983.

Taylor, H., Barter, R. H., and Jacobson, C. B.: Neoplasms of dysgenetic gonads. Am. J. Obstet. Gynecol., *96*:816, 1966.

Thompson, J. S., and Thompson, M. W.: Genetics in Medicine. 3rd ed. Philadelphia, W. B. Saunders Co., 1980.

Van Dyke, D. L., Weiss, L., and Robertson, J. R.: The frequency of balanced autosomal rearrangements in man estimated from prenatal genetic studies for advanced maternal age. Am. J. Med Genet., *35*:301, 1983.

Wachtel, S. S., Koo, G. C., Breg, W. R., Ellis, S., Boyse, W. A., and Miller, O. J.: Expression of H-Y antigen in human cells with two Y chromosomes. N. Engl. J. Med., *293*:1070, 1975.

Warkany, J., Passarge, E., and Smith, L. B.: Congenital malformations in autosomal trisomy syndromes. Am. J. Dis. Child., *112*:502, 1966.

Weiss, L., Reynolds, W. A., Saeed, S. M., and Cabal, L.: Congenital hepatic fibrosis and polycystic disease of kidneys with the roentgen appearance of medullary sponge kidney. Birth Defects: Original Article Series, X:22. New York, The National Foundation, 1974.

Winters, R. W., Graham, J. B., Williams, T. F., et al.: A genetic study of familial hypophosphatemia and vitamin D resistant rickets. Trans. Assoc. Am. Physicians, *70*:234, 1957.

CHAPTER 37

Normal Development of the Urinary Tract

MAX MAIZELS, M.D.

Understanding the normal development of the human urinary tract helps the clinical urologist better treat his patients. Grasping this understanding can be difficult because the urologist is expected to use schematic drawings in order to reconstruct visually the actual appearances of embryonic tissues. This chapter attempts to provide a "realistic" view of normal development of the urinary tract by including many "real" pictures of urinary development, even if they represent nonhuman tissues.

Understanding abnormal urinary tract development is probably more useful to the clinical urologist than understanding normal development. It is surprising that few embryos with urinary malformations have been available for study. Although it is logical to project that common urinary malformations arise from aberrations of normal development, such projections may not always be accurate. Unscientific speculation, inaccurate description, and logical mistakes have led to notions about abnormal development that may or may not be accurate (Hamilton and Mossman, 1976a). To reduce such misconceptions, recent experimental observations of urinary development are described in this chapter.

MORPHOGENESIS OF THE GERM LAYERS

Period of the Zygote (Conception–1st Week)

Development begins after a sperm fertilizes an ovum. The combined cell, a zygote, begins its development by division, cleavage, into about 30 smaller cells, blastomeres. The blastomeres arrange themselves as a hollow sphere, the blastula, which is about the same size as the parent zygote (Fig. 37–1A). Darkly colored cells form an inner cell mass that will give rise to the tissues of the embryo.

Period of the Laminar Embryo (2nd–3rd Weeks)

During the second week, the inner cell mass flattens. A separate sheet of cells, the endoderm, appears on the undersurface of the inner cell mass. The cells that appose the endoderm compose the ectoderm. The lamination of the inner cell mass into an endoderm and an ectoderm marks the blastoderm. A cleft appears above the ectoderm and enlarges as the amnion cavity (Fig. 37–1B). During the third week, cells migrate between the ectoderm and endoderm to streak the smooth surface of the blastoderm (Fig. 37–1C and D). These cells develop into mesoderm. At the caudal end of the primitive streak, the endoderm remains apposed to the ectoderm without intervening mesoderm. This area of apposition persists during later stages of development as the cloacal membrane (see Development of the Cloaca). These three tissue types are the germs for organogenesis of the embryo to 8 weeks of development and for maturation of the fetus to term.

OVERVIEW OF NORMAL DEVELOPMENT OF THE URINARY SYSTEM

The definitive urinary system results from complex and poorly understood interactions of

TABLE 37–1. Timetable of the Development of the Human Urinary System

Days After Ovulation	Events During Development
18	Cloacal membrane at caudal end of primitive streak (Fig. 37–1)
20	Para-axial mesoderm and lateral plate mesoderm (Figs. 37–2 and 37–3); tail end of embryo folds to create cloaca
22	Intermediate mesoderm; pronephric duct present (Fig. 37–3)
24	Nephrotomes of the pronephros disappear; mesonephric ducts and tubules appear (Fig. 37–3)
26	Caudal portions of the wolffian ducts end blindly short of the cloaca
28	Wolffian duct has fused to the cloaca; ureteral buds appear (Figs. 37–4 and 37–5); septation of cloaca begins (Fig. 37–15)
32	Common excretory ducts dilate and extend into the cloaca (Fig. 37–17); metanephric mesenchyma caps the ureteral buds (Figs. 37–4 to 37–6 and 37–8)
33	Ureteral buds have extended and appear as primitive pelves (Fig. 37–5)
37	Metanephroi are reniform; ureteral bud ampullae divide into cranial and caudal poles (Fig. 37–5)
41	Müllerian ducts appear (Figs. 37–22 and 37–24); cloaca partitioning (Fig. 37–15); genital tubercle prominent (Figs. 37–14 and 37–16); lumen of ureter is discrete
44	Urogenital sinus separate from rectum (Fig. 37–15); wolffian ducts and ureters drain separately into the urogenital sinus (Fig. 37–17)
48	First nephrons apppear (Fig. 37–6); collecting tubules appear; urogenital membrane ruptures
51	Kidneys in lumbar region (Fig. 37–9); orifices of ureters cranial to those of the wolffian ducts; Müllerian ducts descend adjacent to the mesonephric ducts (Fig. 37–22)
52	Glomeruli appear in the kidney
54	Müllerian ducts are fused behind the urogenital sinus; Müller's tubercle distinct (Fig. 37–18); testis distinguishable
8 weeks	*Period of the fetus begins* Primary and secondary urethral grooves (Fig. 37–16C)
9 weeks	First likelihood of renal function
10 weeks	Genital ducts of opposite sex degenerate
12 weeks	External genitalia become distinctive for sex; male penile urethra forming; urogenital union (Fig. 37–23); apex of bladder separates from allantoic diverticulum; prostate appears (Fig. 37–20); Cowper's glands (Fig. 37–21) and Skene's glands appear
13 weeks	Bladder becomes muscularized
14 weeks	Ureter begins to attain submucosal course in bladder
16 weeks	Mesonephros involuted; glandar urethra forms (Fig. 37–19)
18 weeks	Ureteropelvic junction apparent (Fig. 37–13)
20–40 weeks	Further growth and development complete the urogenital organs

embryonic mesoderm with itself and with endoderm. This development is commonly viewed to repeat phases of development of lower vertebrates: the pronephros persists in adult cyclostomes (i.e., lamprey); the mesonephros is the functional kidney of most anamniotes (i.e., fish); and although the mesonephros functions temporarily, the metanephros is the definitive kidney of most amniotes (i.e., birds and mammals). These phases are repeated in man: the pronephros is the first urinary tissue to appear, next the mesonephros, and finally the metanephros.

PRONEPHROS

During the fourth week of development, condensed mesoderm adjacent to the midline segments into blocklike units, somites (Fig. 37–2). The pronephros appears in the cervical region of the 10-somite embryo between the second and sixth somites (Potter, 1972). Cells presumably derive from the intermediate mesoderm, cluster, and differentiate into pronephric tubules. The tubules do not function. It is believed that the duct of the pronephric tubules continues caudally as the mesonephric duct (Fig. 37–3A). The pronephros is not apparent by 30 days.

MESONEPHROS

The mesonephric duct descends from the cervical somites to the caudal region of the embryo. This descent is mediated by caudal growth of the terminus of the duct. The duct is

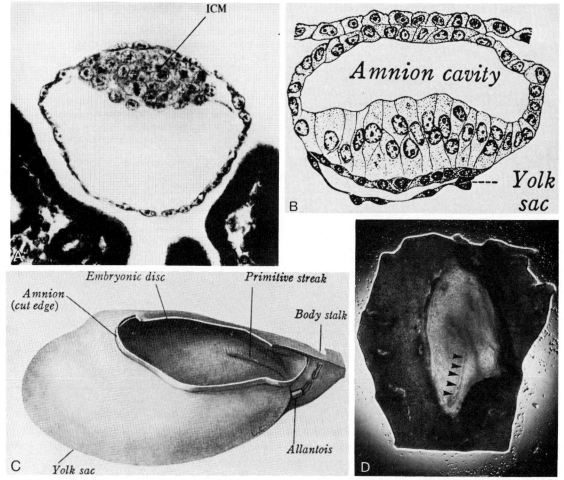

Figure 37–1. Morphogenesis of the germ layers. *A,* Blastocyst consists of cells arranged as a sphere. Some cells aggregate as the inner cell mass (ICM) (blastocyst of bat). *B,* The inner cell mass laminates into endoderm and ectoderm. Clefts above and below the cell layers develop into the amnion cavity and the yolk sac, respectively (monkey). Cell migration between the endoderm and ectoderm streaks the smooth blastoderm. These migrating cells develop into mesoderm. *C,* Primitive streak of the human. *D,* Primitive streak (arrowheads) is located in the center of the clear blastoderm (wet mount of the chick embryo viewed by transillumination). (*A* from Austin, C. R., and Shart, R. V.: Reproduction in Mammals. Cambridge, Cambridge University Press, 1973. *B* and *C* from Arey, L. B.: Developmental Anatomy. Philadelphia, W. B. Saunders Co., 1974. Used by permission.)

adjacent to mesoderm intermediate between the somites and the coelom (primitive peritoneum) (Fig. 37–3B). After the duct and mesoderm appose, mesonephric tubules appear. The nephrons of the mesonephros are induced by the advancing ampulla of the mesonephric duct analogous to the induction of nephrons of the kidney during Period 3 of ureteral bud development (see Development of the Ureteral Bud). During its descent, the mesonephric duct induces about 40 pairs of tubules (Potter, 1972). By 28 days the mesonephric duct has descended to contact the urogenital sinus, and it later drains into the sinus. By 37 days the mesonephroi are fully developed, and they appear as paired retroperitoneal organs close to the midline that bulge into the peritoneum (Fig. 37–4). After 10 weeks of development, many mesonephric nephrons degenerate (Stephens, 1983), but some tubules become incorporated into the genital duct system (see Development of the Ducts of the Genitalia).

We infer that the human mesonephros functions based upon morphologic and physiologic observations. Dilatation of the allantois and bulging followed by rupture of the cloacal membrane are interpreted to result from the hydrostatic pressure generated from mesonephric secretion (Muecke, 1979). Convolution of the tubules and appearance of glomeruli are also interpreted as evidence of function. As the mesonephroi of several mammals can excrete

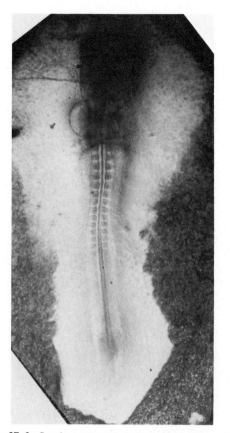

Figure 37–2. Somite stage of development. Mesenchyme condenses as blocklike structures, the somites. A row of somites flanks each side of the midline (wet mount of chick embryo).

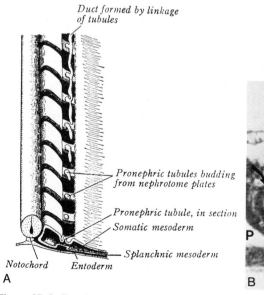

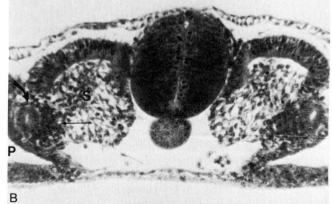

A

B

Figure 37–3. Development of the pronephros and mesonephros. *A,* The pronephric duct of lower vertebrates forms by linkage of pronephric tubules. In man the pronephric duct probably continues caudally as the mesonephric duct. *B,* The mesonephric duct (curved arrow) apposes mesoderm (straight arrow) intermediate between the somite (S) and the coelom (P). Mesonephric tubules appear after the inductive interaction between the duct and mesoderm (chick embryo). (*A* from Arey, L. B.: Developmental Anatomy. Philadelphia, W. B. Saunders Co., 1974. *B* from Maizels, M., and Stephens, F. D.: Invest. Urol., *17:*209, 1979. Used by permission.)

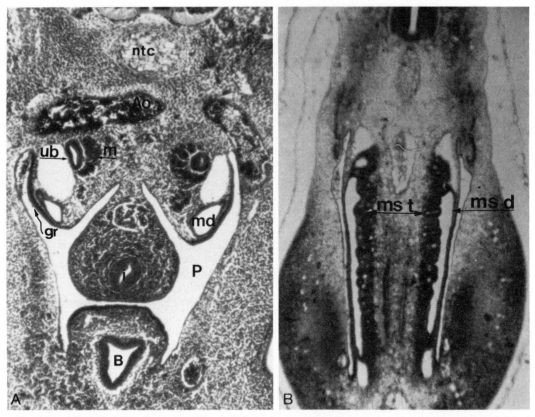

Figure 37–4. Spatial relationship of retro- and intraperitoneal organs. *A,* Kidney blastema consists of ureteral bud (ub) and its apposed mesenchyme (m). The mesonephric duct (md) is between the renal blastema and gonadal ridge (gr) (note thickened epithelium). Bladder (B) is an epithelial tube (intestine, i; aorta, Ao; notochord, ntc; peritoneum, P). (Transverse section of chick embryo.) *B,* Mesonephric tubules (Ms) extend longitudinally along retroperitoneum and drain into mesonephric duct (Msd). (Coronal section of chick embryo.)

marker dyes such as ferrocyanide or phenol red (Hamilton and Mossman, 1976b), it is believed the human mesonephros can clear the plasma of unwanted metabolites.

KIDNEY

Development of the Ureteral Bud

After the mesonephric duct reaches and drains into the urogenital sinus, the ureteral bud appears. The bud originates as a diverticulum from the posteromedial aspect of the mesonephric duct at the point where the terminus of the duct bends to enter the cloaca (Fig. 37–5*A*). Potter (1972) has offered the most cohesive view of the later development of the ureteral bud. The ureteral bud is viewed to develop further during four periods based upon tedious microdissections of human embryonic kidney specimens at various stages of development.

Period 1 (5th–14th Week)

The initial four to six dichotomous branchings of the ampullae contribute to the renal pelvis. The metanephrogenic blastema proliferates so as to remain apposed to all of the new ampullae of the new ureteral bud branches. The initial branch establishes the inferior and superior poles of the future kidney. Branching near the poles of the kidney occurs faster than does branching near the midsection. Because of this asynchrony, by 7 weeks there are about six generations of ampullae at the poles of the kidney and only four generations of ampullae at the midsection of the kidney. The asynchronous branching helps maintain the reniform shape of the kidney (Hamilton and Mossman, 1976b).

This primitive network of ureteral bud branches dilates and creates the appearance of the pelvis and calyces (Fig. 37–5*B* and *C*). Because the dilatation is not uniform, the appearance of the pelvis and calyces in the new-born may be varied.

The subsequent three to five generations of branchings contribute to the calyces. The branchings occur so rapidly that the many branches appear to arise from a common stem. This common stem initially resembles a bulbous chamber (Fig. 37–5D and E). With later growth, the renal parenchyma projects into this chamber as a conical papilla. This projection converts the bulbous chamber into the cup shape of the definitive calyx (Fig. 37–5F). These branchings begin to occur after 7 weeks and are the first to induce nephrons (Fig. 37–6).

The next five to seven generations of branchings of the ampulla of the ureteral bud create the collecting tubules. During this interval the bud branches progressively more slowly. Therefore, as the ampullae extend toward the periphery of the kidney, the collecting tubules laid down close to the calyces are short and wide, whereas the collecting tubules laid down close to the periphery are long and slender.

Period 2 (15th–22nd Week)

During this period the ampullae divide infrequently and a family of nephrons is induced by a single ampulla. Interstitial growth of the collecting tubules causes the ampullae to extend centrifugally toward the surface of the kidney. As each ampulla extends, a family of about four (range of two to eight) nephrons is laid down seriatim as "arcades" or tiers of nephrons (Fig. 37–7). The site where the collecting tubules begin centrifugal growth is the corticomedullary junction. The central zone, the medulla, contains the mass of collecting tubules; the peripheral zone, the cortex, contains the nephrons, which are attached to collecting tubules. The collecting tubules in the cortex are straight, since they do not branch.

Period 3 (22nd–36th Week)

As the ampulla grows, it extends farther toward the cortex of the kidney. As the ampulla migrates, it induces about four to six nephrons in series (Fig. 37–7). This period of development creates nephrons whose glomeruli lie in the outer half of the cortex. About 75 per cent of the complement of glomeruli are induced during Periods 2 and 3 of development

Period 4 (32nd–36th Week to Adulthood)

The ureteral bud ampullae cease to induce new nephrons and are no longer apparent. During this period the collecting ducts elongate, the proximal tubules convolute, and the loops of Henle penetrate deeper into the medulla. A typical collecting duct drains about nine to 11 nephrons. Nephron induction by a branching ureteral bud causes the surface of the kidney to appear lobular at birth.

Induction of the Nephron

Nephrons are always induced by the interaction between an ampulla of the ureteral bud and its adjacent metanephrogenic mesenchyme. They interact during Period 1 when the ampullae branch dichotomously, during Period 2 when the ampullae establish tiers of nephrons, and during Period 3 when the ampullae advance centrifugally.

The specific mechanisms that lead the undifferentiated metanephrogenic blastema to convert into a nephron are becoming better understood. Grobstein (1956) demonstrated the metanephrogenic blastema will not differentiate into tubules if it does not closely contact the ureteral bud or another inductor tissue. Cell processes from the ureteral bud will reach out to the metanephrogenic blastema to initiate induction (Lehtonen et al., 1975). If the tissues are separated and are not permitted close contact, the ureteral bud does not branch and the metanephrogenic blastema does not differentiate. This pattern of biologic behavior is an example of an inductive tissue interaction whereby one cell population significantly alters the behavior of an adjacent cell population (see development of prostate and regression of müllerian duct). This inductive interaction differs from other organs, since the renal mesenchyme converts into an epithelium and attains a basement membrane. Tissues other than the ureteral bud, especially thoracic spinal cord, can induce the metanephrogenic blastema to differentiate into tubules (Unsworth and Grobstein, 1970). However, the only tissue known capable of differentiating into renal tubules is the metanephrogenic blastema.

Our knowledge of the biology of nephron development was expanded when it became appreciated that the extracellular matrix may participate to initiate nephrogenesis. With the

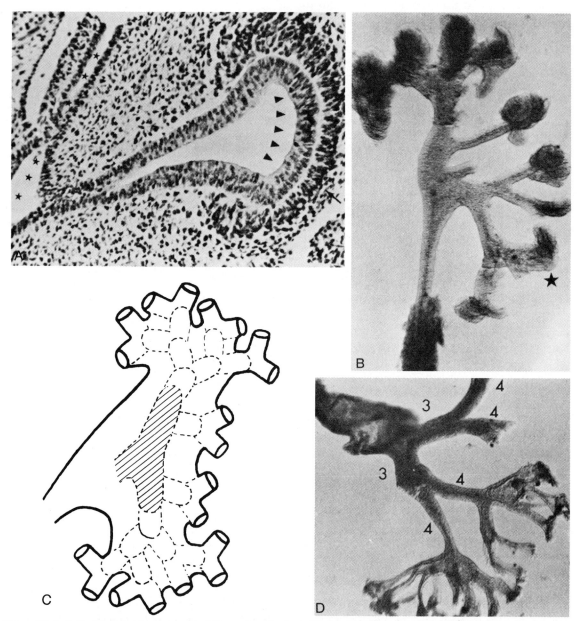

Figure 37–5. Period 1 of the development of the ureteral bud. *A,* Ureteral bud (arrowheads) arises as a diverticulum from the mesonephric duct (asterisks). Metanephric mesenchyme (black arrow) surrounds the ampulla of the ureteral bud (28-day embryo) (see also Fig. 37–4*A*). *B,* The ampullae branch dichotomously; the branches then dilate to establish the primitive pelvis and calyces (asterisk, see *D*) (8-week human embryo). *C,* Schematic of *B* to show how dichotomous branchings (dashed lines) of the primitive ureteral bud (hatches) dilate to create the renal pelvis (solid outline). *D,* Rapid branchings of the ampullae (see asterisk in *B*) create a bushlike appearance. The base of the bush becomes a bulbous chamber, a calyx (10-week human fetus). Numbers refer to generations of ampullary divisions. *E,* Schematic of *D* to show development of a calyx. Rapid division of an ampulla (solid black) produces multiple short branches of the ureteral bud (hatches and stippling). The resultant bulbous chamber is the primitive calyx. *F,* Development of a papilla. With secretion of urine and growth of nephrons, the renal tissue flattens the contour of the calyx (left) and then intrudes into the lumen of the calyx as the renal papilla (right). (From Potter, E. L.: Normal and Abnormal Development of the Kidney. Chicago, Year Book Medical Publishers, 1972. Used by permission.)

Illustration continued on opposite page

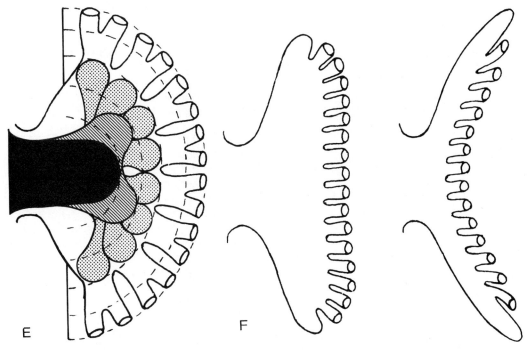

E   F

Figure 37–5 *(Continued).*

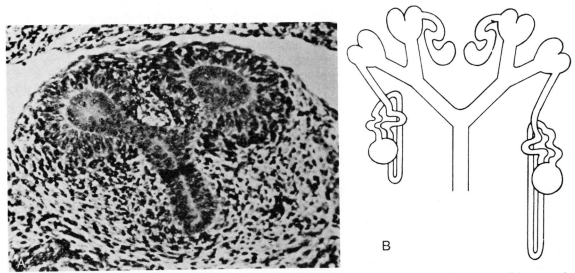

B

Figure 37–6. Induction of nephrons during Period 1 of development of the ureteral bud. *A,* Ampullae branch dichotomously; each branch remains capped by condensed mesenchyme. *B,* Each branch induces a nephron from its cap of undifferentiated metanephric mesenchyme (schematic). (From Potter, E. L.: Normal and Abnormal Development of the Kidney. Chicago, Year Book Medical Publishers, 1972. Used by permission.)

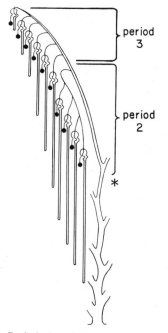

Figure 37–7. Periods 2 and 3 of the development of the ureteral bud. During Period 2 as the ampullae migrate towards the cortex, a family of about four nephrons is induced seriatim as "arcades" or tiers by each ampulla. During Period 3 a series of about five nephrons are induced, which attach directly to the collecting duct. (Asterisk marks site of corticomedullary junction.) (After Potter.)

use of immunohistologic techniques, it was shown that connective tissue antigens are lost during induction (Ekblom, 1981). It was noted the metanephrogenic blastema elaborates interstitial collagens and fibronectin. After induction the collagens are lost at the ampullae, and fibronectin is lost from the mesenchyme. Then, the nephric vesicle emerges from the metanephrogenic blastema. At this stage, a discontinuous basement membrane is detectable.

The two phases of induction, change in the extracellular matrix and overt tubulogenesis, appear to differ metabolically. Inhibitors of DNA, RNA, or protein synthesis impair the morphogenesis of tubules when the inhibitors are applied to the metanephrogenic blastema during induction but not when they are applied later (Ekblom, 1981).

Morphogenesis of the Nephron

The condensed cells of the metanephrogenic blastema first laminate into a comma-shaped, double-layered structure, then swell as a vesicle, and finally connect with the collecting tubule. The cells that participate in creating the visceral layer of Bowman's capsule flatten and angiogenic cells proliferate to create vascular tufts. Potter (1972) counted the kidney of a 40-week-old fetus, which contained 822,300 glomeruli.

In summary, it appears the nephron may develop in phases:

1. Mesenchyme is determined to become the metanephrogenic blastema, which will form renal tubules. The factors responsible for this determination are unknown.

2. Metanephrogenic mesenchyme is induced by the ampulla of the ureteral bud. This induction requires close cell contacts between the two cell types and is associated with a loss of components of the extracellular matrix. The appearance of the nephric vesicle, the earliest morphologic structure resembling a renal tubule, is associated with the appearance of components of the basement membrane of the renal tubule.

3. The nephric vesicle segregates into the glomerulus, proximal and distal tubule, and loop of Henle. The factors leading to this further differentiation are also unknown.

MORPHOGENESIS OF RENAL DYSPLASIA

Understanding normal development of the kidney can be reinforced by viewing its dysplastic development. Metanephrogenic cells are required for normal nephrogenesis, and it appears absence of the cells can lead to dysplasia experimentally (Maizels and Simpson, 1983). Chick renal blastemas can be depleted of condensed metanephrogenic mesenchyme by tissue culture. Such renal blastemas develop further as "primitive ducts" consistent with those seen in human renal dysplasia (Fig. 37–8).

Clinical observations led to inferences that obstruction of urine drainage may cause renal dysplasia (Bernstein, 1971), but the accuracy of these inferences has been challenged by experimental observations. Simple ligation of renal blastemas of the chick embryo (Berman and Maizels, 1982) or of mammalian fetuses (Tanagho, 1972; Fetterman et al., 1974; Javadpour et al., 1974) is associated only with the future development of hydronephrosis, not dysplasia. Although obstruction alone does not cause dysplasia, ureteral buds that are denuded of condensed metanephrogenic mesenchyme and are also ligated show dysplasia more often than such ureteral buds without ligation of the ureter (Maizels et al., 1983).

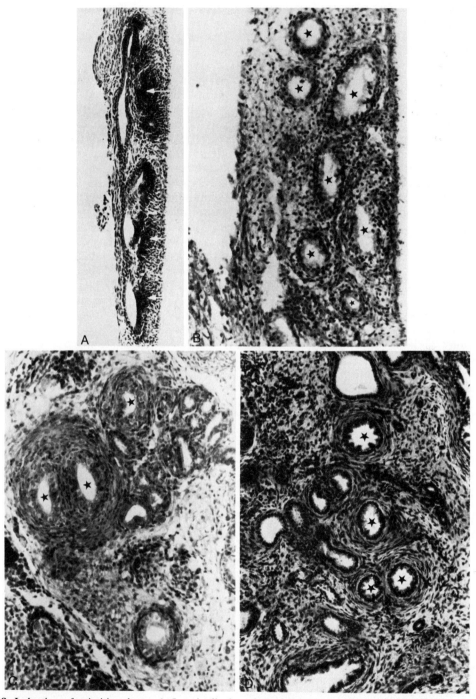

Figure 37–8. Induction of primitive ducts. *A,* Longitudinal section of renal blastema microdissected from chick embryo after 8 days of incubation. Visible are segmental branches of the ureteral bud and condensed metanephrogenic mesenchyme (arrows). *B,* Renal blastema microdissected from chick embryo and then cultured in vitro. Ureteral bud branches (asterisks) area numerous, but the metanephrogenic mesenchyme is no longer condensed or apparent. Renal tubules do not develop in vitro. *C,* Renal blastema microdissected from chick embryo, then cultured in vitro to provide branched ureteral buds without condensed metanephrogenic mesenchyme, and finally further cultured in ovo as a graft develops into tissue composed primarily of primitive ducts (asterisks). The ducts are lined by tall epithelium and are surrounded by whorled mesenchymal cells. *D,* Nephrectomy specimen in newborn with prune belly syndrome. Primitive ducts (asterisks) typical of renal dysplasia are surrounded by whorled fibromuscular cells and resemble those induced in the chick embryos. (From Maizels, M., and Simpson, S. B., Jr.: Science, *219*:509, 1983. Used by permission.)

Clinical observations are consistent with the view that renal dysplasia may follow an abnormal interaction between the ureteral bud and metanephrogenic mesenchyme. When the ureters of duplex kidneys drain onto the trigone, their associated renal units are normally formed; on the other hand, when the ureters of duplex kidneys drain outside the trigone (e.g., urethra or bladder diverticulum), the associated renal units are poorly formed (hypoplasia or dysplasia). Ureters that drain outside the trigone are presumed to have originated from ureteral buds that were abnormally positioned on the wolffian duct. Such malpositioned buds may meet only a deficient complement of metanephrogenic mesenchyme; hypoplasia or dysplasia may follow (Stephens, 1983).

ASCENT OF THE KIDNEY

The renal blastema originates at the level of the upper sacral segments. The final position of the kidney at the level of the upper lumbar vertebrae is attributed to ascent of the renal blastema. Elucidating the mechanisms that lead to normal renal ascent has been approached in the past by studying the microscopic anatomy of human and animal embryos and recently experimentally.

By anatomic studies, normal ascent of the renal primordium from the level of the sacral segments of the human embryo to the level of the lumbar segments of the newborn seems to occur by four mechanisms:

1. 30 days. Caudal growth of the spine causes the ureteral bud to appear to "ascend" the pelvis from the level of the cloaca (Gruenwald, 1943; Friedland and De Vries, 1975).

2. 32 days. Active elongate growth of the ureter into the metanephrogenic blastema causes further ascent in the pelvis. The bud migrates cranially and dorsally, and the kidney reaches the umbilical artery (Friedland and De Vries, 1975).

3. 38 days. When the kidney reaches the umbilical artery, intrinsic growth and moulding of the renal parenchyma hurdles the kidney over the umbilical arteries: first, the umbilical artery tilts the upper pole of the kidney ventrally and the lower pole dorsally; the lower pole abuts on the sacrum; next, the kidney parenchyma elongates and causes further cranial ascent; and finally, the renal parenchyma increases in its transverse diameter and rounds itself to elevate the lower pole of the kidney above the umbilical artery (Boyden, 1932; Gruenwald, 1943).

4. 56 days. The kidney fixes to the tissues of the retroperitoneum, which permits axial growth of the spine to elevate the kidney to its final position (Fig. 37–9) (Gruenwald, 1943).

The belief that elongate growth of the spine participates in renal ascent was examined experimentally (Maizels and Stephens, 1979). The caudal spine of the developing chick embryo was deformed mechanically. In the surviving chick, induced scoliosis was statistically associated with incomplete ascent of the kidneys up the retroperitoneum, namely renal ectopia. This observation supports the belief that normal development of the spine is important to renal ascent above the umbilical arteries.

The dependence of renal ascent upon elongate growth of the spine may be similar to the passive ascent of the spinal cord. For example, the caudal portion of the spinal cord, the conus medullaris, ascends from the level of the coccygeal vertebrae in the adult because the spine grows faster longitudinally than the spinal cord (Langman, 1969).

In addition to scaling the retroperitoneum, the kidney also rotates around its longitudinal

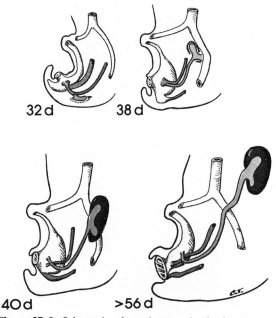

Figure 37–9. Schematic of renal ascent in the human embryo. The ureteral bud has originated from the mesonephric duct and actively elongates to reach the umbilical arteries. By 38 days the umbilical artery tilts the upper pole of the kidney ventrally. At 40 days the renal parenchyma elongates, and by 44 days the kidney rounds itself to elevate the lower pole of the kidney above the umbilical artery. After 56 days the kidney fixes to the tissues of the retroperitoneum; axial growth of the spine then elevates the kidney to its final position.

axis to cause the pelvis to face the spine. Kidneys ectopic within the pelvis are often shaped abnormally. This abnormal shape may reflect an arrest of the moulding of the renal parenchyma during its attempt to hurdle the umbilical artery;

DEVELOPMENT OF THE RENAL ARTERIES

Three groups of branches of the dorsal aorta appear early in development. They course ventrally to the intestine, laterally to the intermediate mesoderm, and dorsolaterally to the body wall and spine. The lateral branches are well developed only in the areas of the developing mesonephroi. Endothelial branchings continue to originate from the aorta until the aorta has developed a mesodermal coat (tunica media). The branchings create two to three arteries at each segmental level between the mesonephric arteries and the dorsolateral segmental arteries. The arterial branches anastomose as a plexus (Fig. 37–10A and B). This plexus anastomoses with renal vessels at more cranial segmental levels as the kidneys ascend the retroperitoneum. Portions of the plexus contribute to the adult pattern of the renal arteries. Local mechanical forces may determine which portions of the plexus will involute. In species having large mesonephroi, the segmental

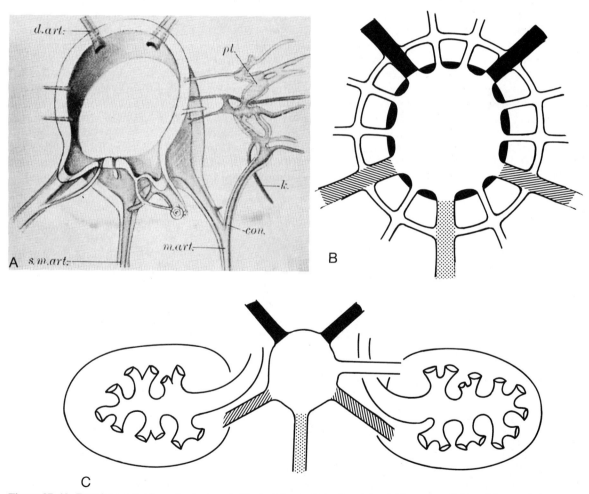

Figure 37–10. Development of renal arteries. *A,* Ventral (s.m. art.), dorsolateral (d. art.), and lateral (m. art.) groups of branches appear at each segmental level of the aorta. A capillary vascular plexus (pl.) exists laterally and supplies the kidney. The lateral plexus connects to the mesonephric artery (m. art.) by a thick-walled vessel (con.) and to the aorta by three slender vessels of endothelium only (reconstruction of cat embryo at second lumbar segment). The left side of the drawing is incomplete (after Bremer). *B,* Schematic of *A. C,* The lateral vascular plexus may be the framework for variability of the renal arteries. If the plexus involutes, there will be a single renal artery (left). If the plexus persists, there may be double or multiple renal arteries (right).

vessels may be pulled ventrally to obliterate the periaortic plexus; in species having an acute curvature of the caudal trunk, the segmental vessels may be pulled dorsally to obliterate the periaortic plexus. Because human embryos do not have large mesonephroi or an acute curvature of the caudal trunk, the portions of the periaortic plexus that persist may be variable, and thereby the renal vasculature may also be variable (Fig. 37–10*C*) (Bremer, 1915).

FUNCTION OF THE FETAL KIDNEY

The first renal tubules are induced after 7 weeks. Correlations of morphologic features with renal function of animal embryos have led to projections that the tubules of the human fetus probably function after about 9 weeks of development (Gersh, 1937). The tubules secrete dyes in vitro by 14 weeks (Cameron and Chambers, 1983). In the laboratory, the exteriorized fetus model (Alexander and Nixon, 1961) permits one to measure normal rates of glomerular and tubular clearance, blood flow, and tubular resorption of electrolytes, water, and solutes. Such measurements have not yet been applied to aid our understanding or treatment of the fetus with a renal malformation.

DEVELOPMENT OF THE URETER

The ureteral bud originates from the mesonephric duct after 28 days of development. The ureteral bud then simply elongates as a hollow tube to ascend the pelvis. However, Ruano-Gil et al. (1975) presented a new view of the early development of the ureter. They studied human embryos and showed the patency of the ureter changes during development. Between 28 and 35 days of development, the ureter is patent in its entire length. This patency may relate to the hydrostatic pressure generated by mesonephric urine, which fills the ureter since the cloaca is still imperforate at this stage. Between 37 and 40 days of development, the lumen of the ureter is not apparent histologically except perhaps at the midportion. Intense elongate growth of the ureter may obliterate the lumen. At the end of this time interval, the lumen extends cranially and caudally from the midportion of the ureter. After 40 days, the lumen is again apparent along the entire length of the ureter (Fig. 37–11). These observations may handily help understand the genesis of congenital strictures at the ureteropelvic or ureterovesical junctions. The lumen at these sites would become patent last. Failure to become patent would cause a stricture. A similar mech-

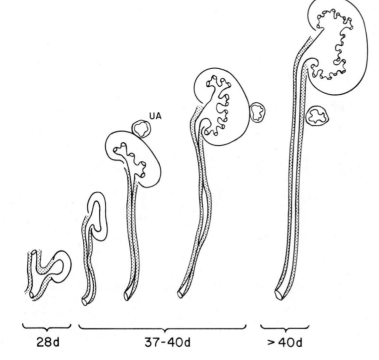

Figure 37–11. Early development of the ureter. At 28 days the ureteral bud appears from the mesonephric duct. Between 37 and 40 days the lumen of the ureter is first progressively lost beginning at its midportion; then the lumen of the ureter becomes apparent again beginning at its midportion. After 40 days the lumen of the ureter is apparent throughout its length (UA, umbilical artery).

28d   37-40d   >40d

anism may account for instances of subglottic stenosis of the larynx (O'Rahilly and Tucker, 1973).

Thereby, by 8 weeks of development the ureter is a patent tube without muscle that has elongated pari passu with ascent of the kidney. After 10 weeks the epithelium of the ureter becomes two-layered, and by 14 weeks a transitional epithelium has appeared. By 18 weeks the ureter demonstrates relative intrinsic narrowings at the ureteropelvic junction, pelvic brim, and ureterovesical junction, and complementary intrinsic dilatations of the upper, middle, and lower spindles of the ureter. However, the ureter may elongate in excess of that needed to accompany ascent of the kidney. To absorb the excess length, the ureter may become tortuous or invaginate its wall as pleats, the "fetal folds" of Ostling (1942) (Fig. 37–12). Smooth muscle of the ureter first appears at the extravesical ureter after about 14 weeks (Felix, 1912a); muscularization gradually extends toward the kidney and is completed by about 18 weeks. By 36 weeks the muscle coat of the intravesical ureter is complete (Stephens, 1983).

Postnatally, the infant's growth rate exceeds that of the ureter. The ureter may lose its tortuosity and unfolds its pleats (Ostling, 1942). The pleats are not ordinarily obstructive. However, a pleat that intrudes into the lumen of the ureter and that is fixed by adventitia of the ureter may obstruct urine drainage as a valve (Fig. 37–13) (Maizels and Stephens, 1980).

DEVELOPMENT OF THE CLOACA

During the period of the laminar embryo, the cloacal membrane is in the caudal region of the embryo where ectoderm apposes endoderm without any intervening mesoderm. Growth of mesenchyme near the cloacal membrane lifts the tail end of the embryo off of the blastoderm. This lifting folds the tail end and creates a chamber, the cloaca, the dilated terminal portion of the hindgut. The cloaca is lined with endoderm. Further growth of the tail fold flexes the tail end of the embryo and the cloacal membrane lies on the ventrum of the embryo. Growth of mesenchyme lateral to the cloacal membrane elevates the tissue as labioscrotal swellings; growth of mesenchyme cranial to the cloacal membrane becomes confluent as the genital tubercle, the primordium of the phallus (Fig. 37–14). The mesoderm extends cranially and the infraumbilical body wall becomes prominent.

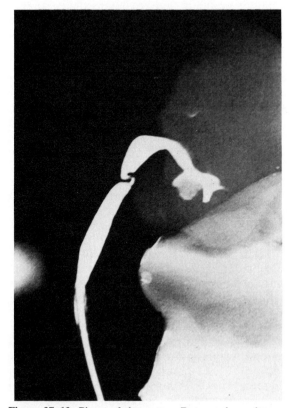

Figure 37–12. Pleats of the ureter. Retrograde pyelogram of a newborn kidney and ureter specimen shows the wall of the ureter folds and pleats the lumen of the ureter. These pleats probably do not usually obstruct urine drainage.

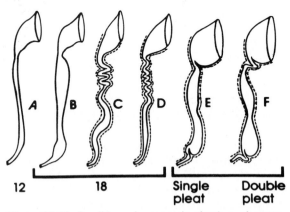

Figure 37–13. Possible embryogenesis of valves of ureter. *A,* By 12 weeks of gestation the caliber of the lumen of the ureter is uniform. *B,* At 18 weeks, pelvic and abdominal spindles of ureter appear. If elongate growth of the ureter occurs faster than that of the trunk, the ureter may become tortuous *(C)* or acquire pleats *(D)*. *E* and *F,* Pleats are normally not obstructive but may persist as valves. (From Maizels, M., and Stephens, F. D.: J. Urol., *123*:742, 1980. Used by permission.)

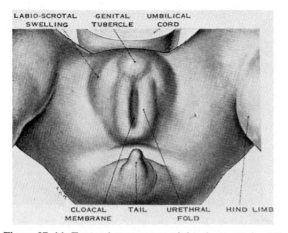

Figure 37–14. External appearance of the cloaca at about 7 weeks of gestation. Growth of the mesenchyme at the caudal end of the embryo lifts the embryo off of the blastoderm and creates the tail fold. Further growth and migration of the mesenchyme around the cloacal membrane create the genital tubercle and the labioscrotal swellings. (From Hamilton, W. J., and Mossman, H. W.: *In* Human Embryology. New York, Macmillan, 1976. Used by permission.)

Septation of the cloaca begins at about 28 days (Stephens, 1983). The urorectal septum, Tourneux's fold, extends in the coronal plane toward the cloacal membrane. At the same time, Rathke's plicae appear as two tissue folds from the lateral aspects of the hindgut. These plicae meet each other in the midline to complete the septation of the cloaca. A separate rectum and primitive urogenital sinus appear by 44 days of development (Fig. 37–15). The portion of the primitive urogenital sinus cranial to the mesonephric ducts is the vesicourethral canal; that caudal to the mesonephric ducts is the definitive urogenital sinus (Fig. 37–16) (Hamilton and Mossman, 1976b).

DEVELOPMENT OF THE TRIGONE AND BLADDER

Understanding the development of the trigone is based predominantly upon reconstructions of embryos that are examined histologically and upon studies of the bladders of children that are examined clinically.

By 28 days of development, the mesonephric ducts have already reached and fused with the urogenital sinus. This fusion involves the coalescence of the epithelium of the urogenital sinus (endoderm derivative) with that of the mesonephric duct (mesoderm derivative). At this time the ureter originates from the meso-nephric duct (see earlier). The segment of the mesonephric duct distal to the site of origin of the ureteral bud dilates as the common excretory duct, the precursor of the trigone. The common excretory duct is absorbed into the urogenital sinus either directly or after the terminus of the duct loops (Hamilton and Mossman, 1976b). After the right and left common excretory ducts have been absorbed into the urogenital sinus, the epithelia of the ducts fuse toward the midline as a triangular area, the primitive trigone. The terminus of the ureter enters the bladder directly.

Our view of the detailed pattern of absorption of the primitive ureter into the trigone is based upon inferences derived from clinical observations of duplex kidneys (Fig. 37–17). As the common excretory duct is absorbed into the urogenital sinus, the orifice of the duct migrates caudally and the orifice of the ureteral bud migrates cranially. Continued growth of the epithelium and mesoderm of the absorbed common excretory duct separates the orifices of the ureters laterally and establishes the framework of the primitive trigone. The ureteral orifice, which drains the upper pole of the kidney, migrates cranially and rotates medially so that it lies caudal to the orifice of the ureter of the lower pole. Weigert and later Meyer recognized the regularity of this disposition, which has come to be known as the Weigert-Meyer rule. Similarly, when the orifices of the ureters of duplex kidneys are adjacent to each other on the trigone, they are situated next to each other such that the orifice of the upper pole ureter is medial to the orifice of the lower pole ureter (Stephens, 1958). Ureteral buds that originate high on the wolffian duct may become abnormally situated on the trigone (Mackie and Stephens, 1979) or retain a direct connection with the wolffian duct (Stephens, 1983). Triplicate ureters do not appear to conform regularly to the Weigert-Meyer rule (Stephens, 1983).

The separate development of the trigone and bladder may account for the fact that the muscle laminae of the trigone are contiguous with the muscle of the ureter and not with the bladder detrusor. This separate development may also account for pharmacologic responses of the musculature of the bladder neck and trigone, which differ from those of the bladder detrusor. The mesenchyme of both common excretory ducts is believed to migrate toward each other, since the endodermal mucosa of the bladder does not persist in the midsection of the trigone (Hamilton and Mossman, 1976b). The mesonephric ducts also migrate caudally and

Text continued on page 1657

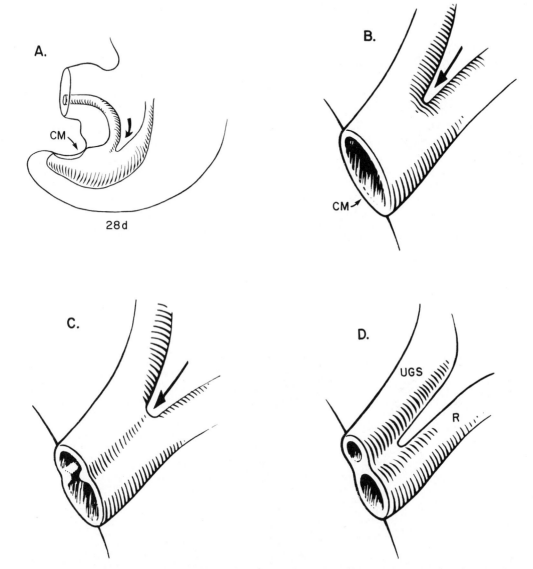

Figure 37–15. Septation of the cloaca. *A,* Lateral view of caudal embryo. (CM, cloacal membrane). Septation of the cloaca occurs in a coronal plane as Tourneux's fold *(B)* extends to the cloacal membrane from above, and *(C)* as Rathke's plicae extend toward each other from the sides. *D,* Septation establishes the primitive urogenital sinus (UGS) and rectum (R). (From Stephens, F. D., and Smith, E. D.: Anorectal Malformations in Children. Chicago, Year Book Medical Publishers, 1971. Used by permission.)

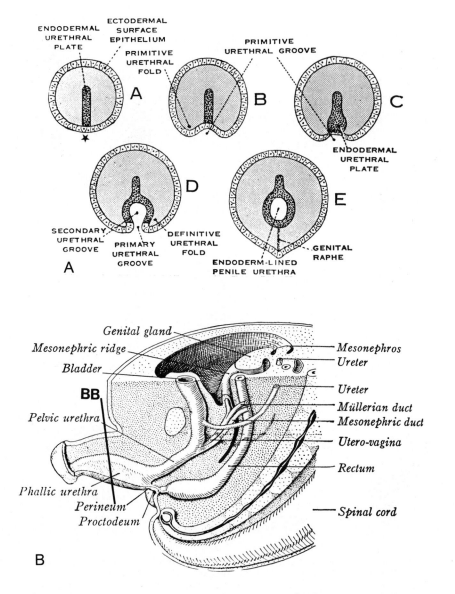

See legend on opposite page

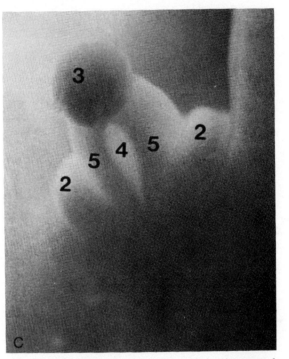

Figure 37–16. Development of the urogenital sinus. *A,* By 9 weeks of development the urogenital sinus consists of a narrow pelvic part near the bladder and an expanded phallic part near the urogenital membrane (anterior portion of cloacal membrane). *B,* Transverse section through phallic part of urogenital sinus (plane BB seen in *A*). The endodermal cells lining the phallic portion of the cloacal membrane (urogenital membrane [asterisk]) thicken and then degenerate to create the secondary urethral groove. The secondary urethral groove remains as the vestibule in the female and closes as the penile urethra in the male. *C,* Transillumination of phallus of 9-week human fetus viewed from below (2, labioscrotal fold; 3, phallus; 4, urethral groove continuous with urogenital sinus; 5, urethral fold). (*A* from Arey, L. B.: Developmental Anatomy. Philadelphia, W. B. Saunders Co., 1974; *B* from Hamilton, W. J., and Mossman, H. W.: *In* Human Embryology. New York, Macmillan, 1976; *C* from England, M. A.: Color Atlas of Life Before Birth. Chicago, Year Book Medical Publishers, 1983. Used by permission.)

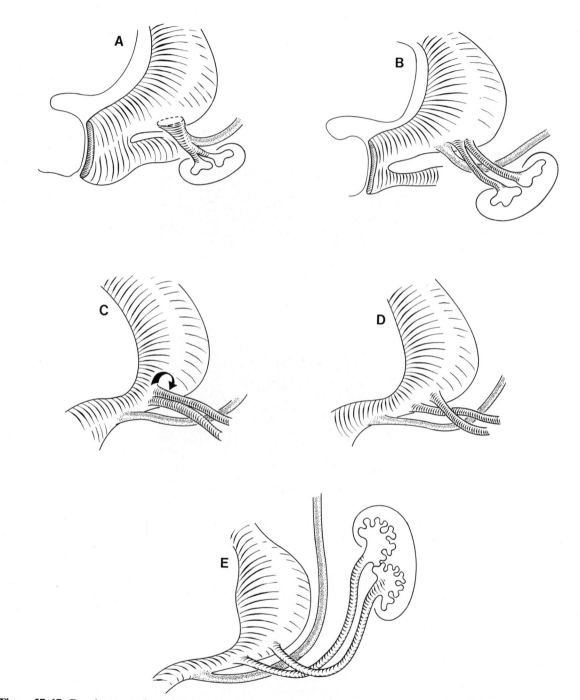

Figure 37–17. Development of a hemitrigone is schematized for a duplex kidney. *A,* The ureteral buds drain into the common excretory duct (shaded). *B,* The buds and duct are absorbed into the urogenital sinus such that the orifice of the mesonephric duct is caudal and medial to that of the ureteral orifices. Continued absorption of the ureters into the trigone is associated with medial rotation of the ureter draining the upper pole around the ureter draining the lower pole (*C* to *E*).

flank the paramesonephric ducts at the level of the urogenital sinus. This is the site of the future verumontanum (Fig. 37–18). The period when the ureter attains the oblique submucosal course of the newborn bladder is uncertain, but occurs after 14 weeks (Felix, 1912b).

By 10 weeks, the bladder is a cylindrical tube lined by connective tissue (Fig. 37–4) (Lowsley, 1912). The wall of the bladder over the trigone is twice as thick as elsewhere. The apex of the vesicourethral canal tapers as the urachus. The urachus is contiguous with the allantoic duct, but the allantois probably does not contribute to the formation of the urachus or bladder (Felix, 1912c; Arey 1974). By 12 weeks, the segment of the bladder contiguous with the allantoic diverticulum involutes. This segment is between the apex of the bladder and the umbilicus. It becomes a thick tube and then a fibrous cord, the median umbilical ligament (Moore, 1977).

By 13 weeks, mesenchyme surrounding the bladder develops into circular, interlacing, and longitudinal strands of smooth muscle. The muscle fibers of the ureters are contiguous with those of the trigone. Muscularization is more abundant at the bladder base, especially at the upper limit of the trigone, than elsewhere. Rapid muscularization causes the wall of the trigone to become 5 times as thick as elsewhere. The bladder lumen narrows at the internal ves-

ical sphincter. By 16 weeks, the entire bladder has discrete inner and outer longitudinal layers and a middle circular layer. Fascicles from the longitudinal layer interlace with the circular layer (Stephens, 1983). The internal sphincter forms from a mass of circular fibers that surrounds the neck of the bladder. The sphincteric muscle is even thicker at 20 weeks. Development to term results in further increase in the size of the muscles of the detrusor, trigone, and sphincter. As imaged by ultrasonography, the fetal bladder varies in size, emptying about 16 ml every 90 minutes near term (Abramovich et al., 1979).

DEVELOPMENT OF THE UROGENITAL SINUS

By 6 weeks of development the urogenital sinus is apparent. The portion of the sinus near the bladder is narrow (pelvic urethra), and the portion near the urogenital membrane is expanded (phallic urethra) (Fig. 37–16A). Between 5 and 10 weeks, the phallic portion of the definitive urogenital sinus is sexually indifferent. During the fifth week, the endodermal portion of the urogenital membrane thickens as a plate of cells. This plate extends distally toward the genital tubercle. Mesenchyme along the lateral margins of the phallic portion of the urogenital sinus raises the overlying ectoderm to create the primitive urethral groove. In the seventh week, the urogenital membrane disintegrates (Fitz-Gerald, 1978). The phallic part of the urogenital sinus becomes exposed and appears as an endoderm-lined trough. By 8 weeks the thickened plate of endodermal cells disintegrates. This cell death establishes the superficial primary and deep secondary urethral grooves (Fig. 37–16*B* and *C*). By this sequence of events, the secondary urethral groove is lined by endoderm and the primary urethral groove is lined by ectoderm. After 10 weeks of development, the external genitalia of the male and female appear different.

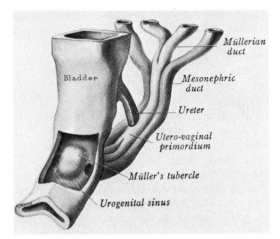

Figure 37–18. Development of the ducts of the genitalia. The paramesonephric ducts descend toward the pelvis medial to the mesonephric ducts. After the mesonephric ducts are absorbed into the trigone, they migrate medially and caudally, flanking the paramesonephric ducts. The termini of these four ducts are at the site of the verumontanum in the male and the cervix in the female. (From Arey after Broman.)

The Urogenital Sinus in the Male

The phallic portion of the urogenital sinus develops into the bulbar and penile urethra. The genital tubercle grows and elongates into a cylindrical phallus. The endodermal edges of the secondary urethral groove fuse to tubularize the penile urethra. The ectodermal edges of the

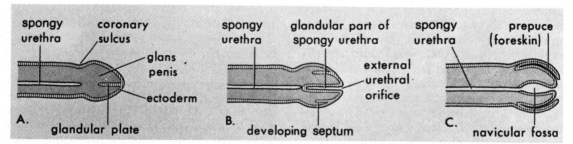

Figure 37–19. Development of the glandar urethra. *A,* The ectoderm of the glans proliferates into the substance of the glans as a plug of cells (11 weeks). *B,* The plug cavitates (12 weeks). *C,* The lumina of the penile and glandar urethra become contiguous (14 weeks). (From Moore, K. L.: The Developing Human. 3rd ed. Philadelphia, W. B. Saunders Co., 1982. Used by permission.)

groove fuse as the median raphe. The scrotal swellings round, migrate caudally, and fuse to form the scrotum at the base of the penis. During the fourth month, the glandar urethra appears. First, the glandar ectoderm proliferates to create a plug of tissue; next, the plug burrows into the glans to meet the penile urethra; and finally, the ectodermal plug cavitates as the glandar urethra (Fig. 37–19). The glandar ectoderm disintegrates similarly to the urethral plate ectoderm.

The pelvic part of the urogenital sinus develops into the lower portion of the prostatic urethra and the membranous urethra (Hamilton and Mossman, 1976b). By 12 weeks, prostate gland rudiments begin to appear as five separate groups of tubules: (1) the middle lobe is made up of about 10 branching tubules, which originate on the floor of the urethra between the bladder and the orifices of the ejaculatory ducts; the middle lobe is rarely absent; (2) and (3) the lateral lobes originate from about 35 tubules on the lateral walls of the urethra; (4) the posterior lobe originates from the floor of the urethra distal to the openings of the ejaculatory ducts; the tubules of the posterior lobe grow back behind the lateral lobes, from which they are separated by a fibrotic capsule; and (5) the anterior lobe is prominent until the 16th week of development and then involutes to become an insignificant structure by 22 weeks (Fig. 37–20) (Lowsley, 1912).

After 16 weeks, the subcervical glands of Albarráns originate from the floor of the urethra below and within the internal sphincter and grow back to lie directly within the bladder mucosa; after 20 weeks, the subtrigonal glands appear (Fig. 37–20*B*) (Lowsley, 1912).

Cowper's glands are present by 12 weeks of development. They originate as endodermal buds of the urogenital sinus. The buds penetrate the surrounding compact mesenchyme of the corpus spongiosum. The buds enlarge as racemose glands at the level of the membranous urethra and remain as small glands at the level of the bulbar urethra. After 18 weeks a glandular epithelium appears (Fig. 37–21).

Dihydrotestosterone mediates the differentiation of the derivatives of the urogenital sinus: the prostate (Cunha, 1972) from the pelvic portion of the urogenital sinus, and the external genitalia from the phallic portion of the urogenital sinus (Siiteri and Wilson, 1974).

The Urogenital Sinus in the Female

The pelvic part of the urogenital sinus develops into the lower portion of the definitive urethra and vagina (Hamilton and Mossman, 1976b). Epithelial tubules originate from the primitive urethra after about 11 weeks (Stephens, 1983). The tubules become the paraurethral glands of Skene (Hamilton and Mossman, 1976b). These glands are the female homologues of the prostate.

The phallic portion of the urogenital sinus remains as a vestibule because the urethral plate does not extend as far to the genital tubercle as in the male (Fig. 37–16*B*). The urethra and vagina open into the vestibule. The labial swellings grow posterior to the vestibule and meet to form the posterior commissure. The swellings also grow lateral to the vestibule to form the labia majora. Urethral folds that flank the urogenital sinus develop into the labia minora (Hamilton and Mossman, 1976b). After the ninth week of development, Bartholin's glands begin as evaginations of the vestibule endoderm, which grow into the labia majora (Stephens, 1983). These glands are the homologues of Cowper's glands.

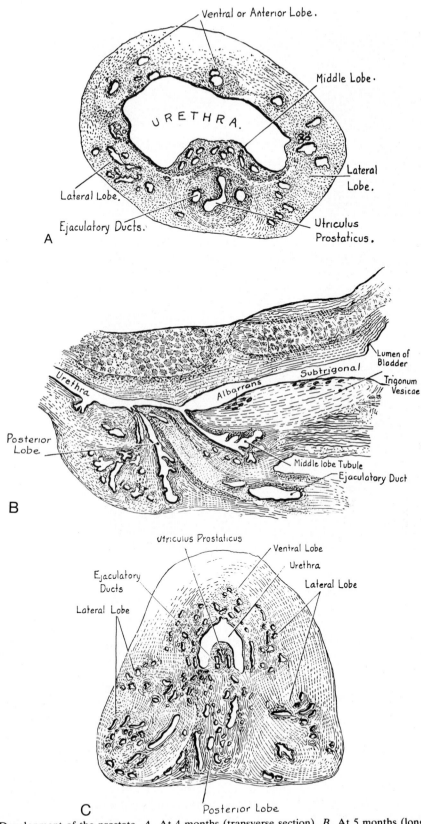

Figure 37–20. Development of the prostate. *A*, At 4 months (transverse section). *B*, At 5 months (longitudinal section). *C*, At 7½ months (transverse section).

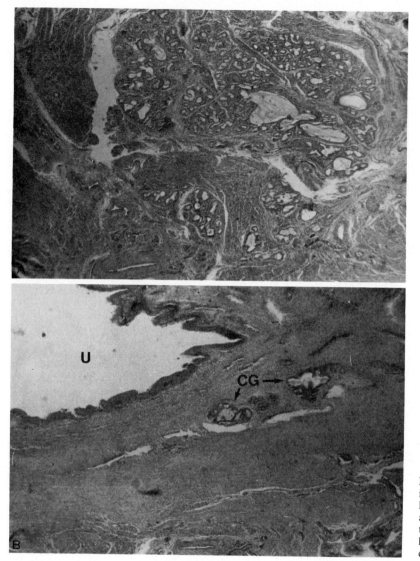

Figure 37–21. Cowper's glands exist as *(A)* racemose glands at the level of the membranous urethra and *(B)* as small glands (CG) near the bulbar urethra (U). (Histologic section of stillborn fetus courtesy of F. D. Stephens.)

DEVELOPMENT OF THE DUCTS OF THE GENITALIA

The genital system appears during the fifth to sixth weeks. Between 5 and 10 weeks of development, genital ducts and gonads of genetically male and female embryos are similar, and this is the sexually indifferent stage. During this stage the mesonephroi begin to degenerate. Between 4 and 8 weeks, the thoracic portions of the mesonephroi degenerate, but formation of new tubules caudally maintains the bulk of the gland in the lumbar region (Felix, 1912d). Of the remaining tubules, the upper five to 12 tubules compose the epigenitalis, and a similar number of tubules at the lower portion compose the paragenitalis.

The paramesonephric (müllerian) ducts originate as a tubular invagination of the coelomic epithelium (peritoneum) near the developing diaphragm (Fig. 37–22). The paramesonephric ducts descend to the pelvis alongside the basement membrane of the lateral portion of the mesonephric ducts (Gruenwald, 1941). The segments of the paramesonephric ducts behind the bladder fuse anterior to the mesonephric ducts to form the uterovaginal primordium (Fig. 37–18). The primordium later penetrates the urogenital sinus (Figs. 37–16 and 37–18). This primordium elevates the dorsal wall of the pelvic portion of the urogenital sinus to create the müllerian tubercle. This tubercle lies between and caudal to the orifices of the mesonephric ducts. The glomeruli of the epigenitalis

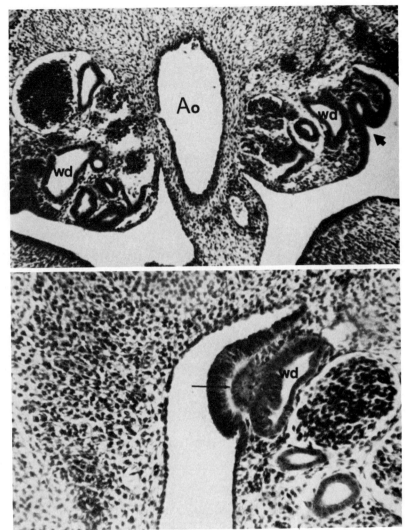

Figure 37–22. Early formation of the müllerian ducts. *Upper panel,* The ducts begin as an invagination of the "peritoneum" (arrow) near the developing diaphragm (aorta, Ao). *Lower panel,* They descend as a solid core (arrow) toward the pelvis alongside the mesonephric duct (wd) (chick embryo). (From Maizels, M. and Stephens, F. D.: Invest. Urol., *17*:209, 1979. Used by permission.)

degenerate, but their connections to the collecting ducts of the mesonephric duct remain. The ends of the collecting ducts become surrounded by the indifferent gonad. After the seventh week, the first morphologic sign of the sex of the fetus appears. The male gonad differentiates into a testis. The female gonad differentiates into an ovary later, during midgestation.

In the male after 12 weeks, rete tubules in the testis connect to the collecting ducts of the mesonephros. The collecting ducts are now referred to as the efferent ducts (Felix, 1912e, f), and the mesonephric duct as the vas deferens. During the fourth month, the portion of the efferent ducts adjacent to the testis remains straight, whereas the portion of the efferent ducts adjacent to the vas deferens becomes coiled. The upper portion of the vas deferens also coils and becomes the epididymis, whereas the lower portion near the müllerian tubercle dilates to almost 4 times its original size as an ampulla (Felix, 1912g). Epigenital tubules that do not participate in urogenital union remain as the appendix of the epididymis. The lower portion of the vas deferens develops concentric layers of mesenchyme by about 12 weeks, but muscle fibers are not seen until 28 weeks (Felix, 1912g). The ejaculatory duct and seminal vesicles appear after 12 weeks by septation of the ampulla of the distal portion of the vas deferens (Fig. 37–23) (Felix, 1912g).

The paradidymis comprises the lower group of the lumbar mesonephric tubules (paragenitalis). The paragenitalis degenerates, but tubules between the head of the epididymis and the testis may remain as the organ of Giraldés.

After the tenth week, the müllerian ducts begin to degenerate in a craniocaudal direction.

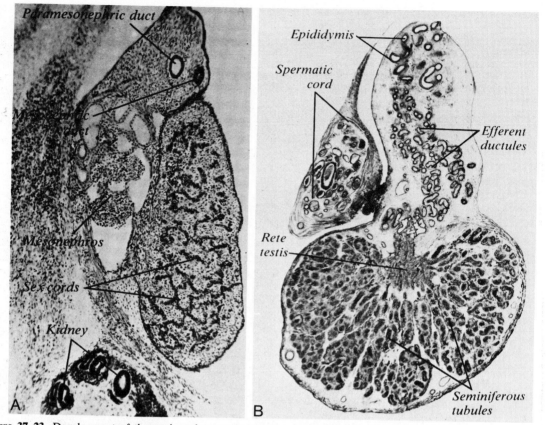

Figure 37–23. Development of the testis and urogenital union. *A*, By 8 weeks the medullary sex cords have begun to differentiate. The glomeruli of the epigenitalis degenerate, and the collecting tubules will later drain the tubules of the testis. *B*, By 20 weeks the rete tubules of the testis drain into the coiled efferent ducts. (From FitzGerald, M. J. T.: Human Embryology. New York, Harper & Row; 1978. Used by permission.)

The cranial end of the degenerating paramesonephric duct may persist as the appendix of the testis (Fig. 37–24). By 16 weeks, the müllerian ducts are obliterated to the level of the ejaculatory ducts (Lowsley, 1912). At this level the müllerian ducts are fused as the uterovaginal primordium. This primordium persists as the prostatic utricle (Fig. 37–20). The utricle becomes quite large and surrounded by a dense layer of stroma. The utricle opens into the urogenital sinus in the midline just below the orifices of the ejaculatory ducts (Lowsley, 1912). By 22 weeks, the utricle and ejaculatory ducts expand under the floor of the urethra and elevate the wall of the urethra to create the verumontanum (Lowsley, 1912). The verumontanum causes the lumen of the prostatic urethra to appear semilunar (Fig. 37–20C). Later the utricle contracts to become only a small structure on the tip of the verumontanum. By 30 weeks, the seminal vesicles have grown back behind the base of the bladder and the ejaculatory ducts are surrounded by thick musculature. Testosterone mediates the differentiation of the derivatives of the wolffian duct: epididymis, vas deferens, and seminal vesicles.

The biologic mechanisms involved in the regression of the müllerian ducts are becoming better understood. Regression of the ducts is mediated largely by a polypeptide, müllerian-inhibiting substance (MIS) (Josso, 1973; Donahoe et al., 1977). MIS is probably produced by the fetal Sertoli cells. The steroids testosterone, medroxyprogesterone, and progesterone augment the effect of MIS in an in vitro assay (Ikawa et al., 1982). This augmentation is believed to be mediated by binding of the steroids to receptors of the mesenchyme that surrounds the müllerian duct. The mesenchyme may then alter the extracellular matrix by increased hyaluronidase activity or fibronectin lysis. These alterations may facilitate breakdown of the müllerian duct basement membrane (Ikawa et al., 1982; Trelstad et al., 1982). MIS can act as a hormone (Donahoe et al., 1976). In the rat, only 24 hours of exposure of the müllerian duct

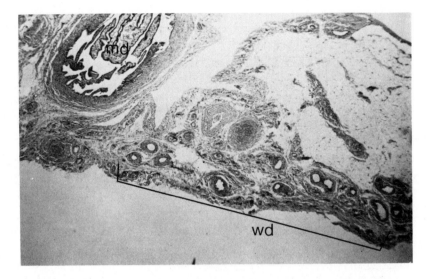

Figure 37–24. Development of müllerian and wolffian ducts. Excisional biopsy of ducts draining a streak gonad in a child with intersex. Müllerian duct (md) elaborates to resemble an oviduct, and wolffian duct (wd) has coiled as a rudimentary epididymis.

to MIS is needed to cause the duct to degenerate (Donahoe et al., 1977). It appears the cranial portion of the duct is more sensitive to the effects of MIS than the caudal portion of the duct (Donahoe et al., 1977).

In the female, the uterovaginal primordium remains Y-shaped until the twelfth week (FitzGerald, 1978). The cranial unfused portion of the paramesonephric ducts becomes the oviducts; the caudal fused portion becomes the uterus and cervix. The bicornuate uterus becomes a single chamber by upward expansion as the fundus (FitzGerald, 1978). The müllerian ducts develop in a feminine manner spontaneously unless they are inhibited by MIS. The mesonephric duct degenerates, but remnants may remain as the duct of Gartner. The duct lies along the margin of the oviduct and uterus and opens adjacent to the cervix.

References

Abramovich, D. R., Garden, A., Jandial, L., and Page, K. R.: Fetal swallowing and voiding in relation to hydramnios. Obstet. Gynecol., *54*:15, 1979.

Alexander, D. P., and Nixon, D. A.: The fetal kidney. Br. Med. Bull., *17*:112, 1961.

Arey, L. B.: Developmental Anatomy. 7th ed. Philadelphia, W. B. Saunders Co., 1974.

Berman, D. J., and Maizels, M.: The role of urinary obstruction in the genesis of renal dysplasia: A model in the chick embryo. J. Urol., *128*:1091, 1982.

Bernstein, J.: The morphogenesis of renal parenchymal maldevelopment (renal dysplasia). Pediatr. Clin. North Am., *18*:395, 1971.

Boyden, E. A.: Congenital absence of the kidney. An interpretation based on a 10 mm human embryo exhibiting unilateral renal agenesis. Anat. Rec., *52*:325, 1932.

Bremer, J. L.: The origin of the renal artery in mammals and its anomalies. Am. J. Anat., *18*:179, 1915.

Cameron, G., and Chambers, R.: Direct evidence of function in kidney of an early human fetus. Am. J. Physiol., *123*:482, 1983.

Cunha, G.: Epithelio-mesenchymal interactions in primordial gland structures which become responsive to androgen stimulation. Anat. Rec., *172*:179, 1972.

Donahoe, P. K., Ito, Y., Marfatia, S., and Hendren, W. H., III: The production of Mullerian inhibiting substance by the fetal, neonatal and adult rat. Biol. Reprod., *15*:329, 1976.

Donahoe, P. K., Ito, Y., and Hendren, W. H., III: A graded organ culture assay for detecting of Mullerian inhibiting substance. J. Surg. Res., *23*:141, 1977.

Ekblom, P.: Determination and differentiation of the nephron. Med. Biol., *59*:139, 1981.

Felix, W.: The development of the urinogenital organs. *In* Keibel, F., and Mall, F. P. (Eds.): Manual of Human Embryology. Vol. II. Philadelphia, J. B. Lippincott Co., 1912: a, p. 866; b, p. 880; c, p. 752; d, p. 815; e, p. 829; f, p. 830; g, p. 938.

Fetterman, G. H., Ravitch, M. M., and Sherman, F. F.: Cystic changes in fetal kidneys following ureteral ligation. Kidney Int., *5*:111, 1974.

FitzGerald, M. J. T.: Abdominal and pelvic organs. *In* FitzGerald, M. J. T. (Ed.): Human Embryology. New York, Harper & Row, 1978, p. 106.

Friedland, G. W., and De Vries, P.: Renal ectopia and fusion—embryologic basis. Urology, *5*:698, 1975.

Gersh, I.: The correlation of structure and function in the developing mesonephros and metanephros. Contrib. Embryol., *26*:35, 1937.

Grobstein, C.: Trans-filter induction of tubules in mouse metanephrogenic mesenchyme. Exp. Cell Res., *10*:424, 1956.

Gruenwald, P.: The relation of the growing Mullerian duct to the Wolffian duct and its importance for the genesis of malformations. Anat. Rec., *81*:1, 1941.

Gruenwald, P.: The normal changes in the position of the embryonic kidney. Anat. Rec., *85*:163, 1943.

Hamilton, W. J., and Mossman, H. W.: Determination, differentiation, the organizer mechanism, abnormal development, and twinning. *In* Human Embryology: Prenatal Development of Form and Function. 4th ed. New York, The Macmillan Press, 1976a, p. 201.

Hamilton, W. J., and Mossman, H. W.: The urogenital system. *In* Human Embryology: Prenatal Development of Form and Function. 4th ed. New York, The Macmillan Press, 1976b.

Ikawa, H., Hutson, J. M., Budzik, G. P., MacLaughlin, D. T., and Donahoe, P. K.: Steroid enhancement of Mullerian duct regression. J. Pediatr. Surg., *17*:453, 1982.

Javadpour, N., Graziano, A. B., and Terril, R.: Experimental induction of patent allantoic duct by intrauterine bladder outlet obstruction. J. Surg. Res., *17*:341, 1974.

Josso, N.: In vitro synthesis of Mullerian inhibiting hormone by seminiferous tubules isolated from the calf fetal testis. Endocrinology, *93*:829, 1973.

Langman, J.: Medical Embryology. 2nd ed. Baltimore, The Williams & Wilkins Co., 1969, p. 301.

Lehtonen, E., Wartiovaara, J., Nordling, S., and Saxen, L.: Demonstration of cytoplasmic processes in millipore filters permitting kidney tubule induction. J. Embryol. Exp. Morphol., *33*:187, 1975.

Lowsley, O. S.: The development of the human prostate gland with reference to the development of other structures at the neck of the urinary bladder. Am. J. Anat., *13*:299, 1912.

Mackie, G. G., and Stephens, F. D.: Duplex kidneys: A correlation of renal dysplasia with position of the ureteral orifice. J. Urol., *114*:274, 1979.

Maizels, M., and Simpson, S. B., Jr.: Primitive ducts of renal dysplasia induced by culturing ureteral buds denuded of condensed renal mesenchyme. Science, *219*:509, 1983.

Maizels, M., and Stephens, F. D.: The induction of urologic malformations: Understanding the relationship of renal ectopia and congenital scoliosis. Invest. Urol., *17*:209, 1979.

Maizels, M., and Stephens, F. D.: Valves of the ureter as a cause of primary obstruction of the ureter: Anatomic, embryologic and clinical aspects. J. Urol., *123*:742, 1980.

Maizels, M., Simpson, S. B., Jr., and Firlit, C. F.: Simulation of human renal dysplasia in a chick embryo model.

Abstract #765. Las Vegas, American Urological Association, Inc., 1983.

Moore, K. L.: The Developing Human. 2nd ed. Philadelphia, W. B. Saunders Co., 1977.

Muecke, E. C.: The embryology of the urinary system. *In* Campbell's Urology. 4th ed. Philadelphia, W. B. Saunders Co., 1979, p. 1286.

O'Rahilly, R., and Tucker, J. A.: The early development of the larynx in staged human embryos. Part 1. Embryos of the first five weeks. Ann. Otol. Rhinol. Laryngol., *82*:[Suppl. 7]1, 1973.

Ostling, K.: The genesis of hydronephrosis: Particularly with regard to the changes at the ureteropelvic junction. Acta Chir. Scand. [Suppl.], *86*:72, 1942.

Potter, E. L.: Normal and Abnormal Development of the Kidney. Chicago, Year Book Medical Publishers, Inc., 1972.

Ruano-Gil, D., Coca-Payeras, A., and Tejedo-Mateu, A.: Obstruction and normal recanalization of the ureter in the human embryo: Its relation to congenital ureteric obstruction. Eur. Urol., *1*:293, 1975.

Siiteri, P. K., and Wilson, J. D.: Testosterone formation and metabolism during male sexual differentiation in the human embryo. J. Clin. Endocrinol. Metab., *38*:113, 1974.

Stephens, F. D.: Anatomical vagaries of double ureters. Aust. N. Z. J. Surg., *28*:27, 1958.

Stephens, F. D.: Congenital Malformations of the Urinary Tract. New York, Praeger Publishers, 1983.

Tanagho, E. A.: Surgically induced partial ureteral obstruction in the fetal lamb. III. Ureteral obstruction. Invest. Urol., *10*:35, 1972.

Trelstad, R. L., Hayashi, K., et al.: The epithelial-mesenchymal interface of the male Mullerian duct: Basement membrane integrity and ductal regression. Dev. Biol., *92*:27, 1982.

Unsworth, B., and Grobstein, C.: Induction of kidney tubules in mouse metanephrogenic mesenchyme by various embryonic mesenchymal tissues. Dev. Biol., *21*:547, 1970.

CHAPTER 38

Anomalies of the Upper Urinary Tract

ALAN D. PERLMUTTER, M.D.
ALAN B. RETIK, M.D.
STUART B. BAUER, M.D.

Congenital anomalies of the upper urinary tract comprise a diversity of abnormalities, ranging from complete absence to aberrant location, orientation, and shape of the kidney as well as aberrations of the collecting system and blood supply. This wide range of anomalies results from a multiplicity of factors that interact to influence renal development in a sequential and orderly manner. Abnormal maturation or inappropriate timing of these processes at critical points in development can produce any number of deviations in the development of the kidney and ureter.

The embryology of the urinary tract is described in Chapter 37. The reader is encouraged to review this material in order to appreciate the complexity of renal and ureteral development and the factors involved in the formation of an abnormality.

The classification of renal and ureteral anomalies used in this chapter is based on structure rather than function. The chapter is divided into four sections, including anomalies of the kidney, the collecting system, the ureteropelvic junction, and the ureter.

ANOMALIES OF THE KIDNEY

Anomalies of the kidney may be classified as follows:

I. Anomalies of number
    A. Agenesis
        1. Bilateral
        2. Unilateral
    B. Supernumerary kidney
II. Anomalies of volume and structure
    A. Hypoplasia
    B. Multicystic kidney
    C. Polycystic kidney
        1. Infantile
        2. Adult
    D. Other cystic disease
    E. Medullary sponge kidney
    F. Medullary cystic disease

III. Anomalies of ascent
    A. Simple ectopia
    B. Cephalad ectopia
    C. Thoracic kidney
IV. Anomalies of form and fusion
    A. Crossed ectopia with and without fusion
        1. Unilateral fused kidney (inferior ectopia)
        2. Sigmoid or S-shaped kidney
        3. Lump kidney
        4. L-shaped kidney
        5. Disc kidney
        6. Unilateral fused kidney (superior ectopia)
    B. Horseshoe kidney
V. Anomalies of rotation

   A. Incomplete
   B. Excessive
   C. Reverse
VI. Anomalies of renal vasculature
   A. Aberrant, accessory, or multiple vessels
   B. Renal artery aneurysms
   C. Arteriovenous fistula

ANOMALIES OF NUMBER

Agenesis

BILATERAL RENAL AGENESIS

Of all the anomalies of the upper urinary tract, bilateral renal agenesis has the most profound effect on the individual. Fortunately, it occurs infrequently when compared with other renal abnormalities. Although bilateral agenesis was first recognized in 1671 by Wolfstrigel, it was not until Potter's eloquent and extensive description of the constellation of associated defects that the full extent of the syndrome could be appreciated and easily recognized (Potter, 1946a and b, 1952). Subsequently, many investigators have attempted to understand all facts of this syndrome and explain them by one common etiology (Fitch and Lachance, 1972).

Incidence. The anomaly is quite rare, only slightly more than 400 cases having been cited in the literature. Potter (1965) estimated that bilateral agenesis occurs once in 4800 births, and Davidson and Ross (1954) noted a 0.28 per cent incidence in autopsies of infants and children. As with most anomalies, there is significant male predominance (nearly 75 per cent). Neither maternal age, nor a specific complication of pregnancy, nor any maternal disease appears to influence its development (Davidson and Ross, 1954). The anomaly has been observed in siblings (Rizza and Downing, 1971) and even in monozygotic twins (Thomas and Smith, 1974). Interestingly, in two pairs of monozygotic twins, one sibling was anephric while the other had normal kidneys (Kohler, 1972; Mauer et al., 1974). If there is a genetic predisposition to this syndrome, it must have a low level of penetrance.

Embryology. Complete differentiation of the metanephric blastema into adult renal parenchyma requires the presence and orderly branching of a ureteral bud. This occurs normally between the fifth and seventh weeks of gestation after the ureteral bud arises from the mesonephric or wolffian duct. It is theorized that induction of ureteral branching into major

and minor calyces depends on the presence of normal metanephric blastema (Davidson and Ross, 1954). The absence of a nephrogenic ridge on the dorsolateral aspect of the celomic cavity or the failure of a ureteral bud to develop from the wolffian duct will lead to agenesis of the kidney. The absence of both kidneys, therefore, requires a common factor causing renal or ureteral maldevelopment on both sides of the midline.

It is impossible to say which of these two factors is paramount. Certainly no kidney can form in the absence of a metanephric blastema, but the presence of a ureteral bud and orderly branching are also necessary for the renal anlage to reach its normal potential. In an extensive autopsy analysis, Ashley and Mostofi (1960) found many clues to the multifactorial nature of this developmental process and shed some light on the causes of renal agenesis. Most anephric children in their series had at least a blindending ureteral bud of variable length. Thus the embryologic insult in some cases was thought to affect the ureteral bud just as or soon after it arose from the mesonephric duct. Even with complete ureteral atresia, structures of wolffian duct origin (vas deferens, seminal vesicle, and epididymis) were usually present and normally formed, suggesting that the injury occurred at about the time the ureteral bud originated (the fifth or sixth week of gestation). When the ureter was absent, Ashley and Mostofi (1960) discovered a rudimentary kidney in only a few instances, supporting the concept of the interdependency of the two processes. Conversely, in some instances the ureter was normal in appearance up to the level of the ureteropelvic junction, where it ended abruptly. In those cases, no recognizable renal parenchyma could be identified. In a small number of autopsies the gonads were absent as well, indicating an abnormality or insult to the entire urogenital ridge (Carpentier and Potter, 1959). Although the nephric and genital portions of the urogenital ridge are closely approximated on the dorsal aspect of the celomic cavity, an extensive lesion affecting this area of the developing fetus is necessary to produce this condition. Thus, several etiologies have been implicated in absence of the kidney(s).

Description. The kidneys are generally completely absent on gross inspection. Occasionally, there might be a small mass of mesenchymal tissue, poorly organized and containing primitive glomerular elements. Tiny vascular branches from the aorta may be seen penetrating into this structure, but no identifiable main

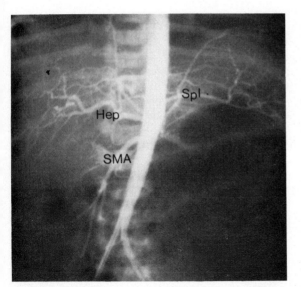

Figure 38–1. Aortogram via an umbilical artery catheter in a newborn with Potter's facies outlines major branches of the aorta but fails to demonstrate either renal artery or kidney.

renal artery is present (Ashley and Mostofi, 1960) (Fig. 38–1).

Besides the absence of functioning kidneys, each ureter is either wholly or partially absent. Complete ureteral atresia is observed in slightly more than 50 per cent of affected individuals (Ashley and Mostofi, 1960). The trigone, if developed, is poorly formed owing to failure of mesonephric duct structures to be incorporated into the base of the bladder. The bladder, when present (about 50 per cent of cases), is usually hypoplastic from the lack of stimulation by fetal urine production. Alternatively, it has been postulated that ureteral bud and wolffian duct structures migrating into the ventral cloacal region are needed to stimulate bladder development (Katz and Chatten, 1974; Levin, 1952).

Associated Anomalies. The other findings in this syndrome have been extensively described by Dr. Potter following an exhaustive investigation of these unfortunate babies. The infants have low birth weights, ranging from 1000 to 2500 gm. At birth, oligohydramnios (absent or minimal amniotic fluid) is present. In addition, a characteristic appearance of the face and extremities sets these children apart. The infants generally look prematurely senile and have "a prominent fold of skin that begins over each eye, swings down in a semi-circle over the inner canthus and extends onto the cheek" (Potter, 1946a and b). Dr. Potter feels that this is the most prominent facial feature and even suggests that its absence confirms the presence

of kidneys (Fig. 38–2A). The nose is blunted, and a prominent depression between the lower lip and chin is evident. The ears appear to be somewhat low-set and drawn forward and are often pressed against the side of the head, making the lobes seem unusually broad and exceedingly large (Fig. 38–2B). The ear canals are not displaced downward, but the appearance of the ear lobes gives this impression. The legs are often bowed and clubbed, with excessive flexion at the hip and knee joints. Occasionally, the lower extremities are completely fused as well (sirenomelia) (Bain et al., 1960).

The skin is excessively dry and appears too loose for the body. This may be secondary to severe dehydration or loss of subcutaneous fat. The hands are relatively large and clawlike.

It is thought that these characteristic facial abnormalities and limb features are caused by the effects of oligohydramnios rather than by multiple organ system defects (Fitch and Lachance, 1972; Thomas and Smith, 1974). Compression of the fetus against the internal uterine walls without a cushioning effect from the amniotic fluid could explain all the findings of this syndrome. Normally, urine produced by the developing kidneys is the major source of amniotic fluid (Thomas and Smith, 1974), but the skin, gastrointestinal tract, and central nervous system also contribute small amounts. Thus, the absence of kidneys reduces severely the amount of amniotic fluid produced.

Pulmonary hypoplasia and a bell-shaped chest are common. Originally, these findings were thought to be secondary to uterine wall compression of the thoracic cage due to the oligohydramniotic state (Bain and Scott, 1960). Subsequently, it was felt that the amniotic fluid itself is responsible for pulmonary development (Fitch and Lachance, 1972). However, this theory was discounted when it was discovered there is a significant reduction in the number of airway generations as well as a decrease in acini formation (Hislop et al., 1979). Pulmonary airway divisioning occurs between the twelfth and sixteenth weeks of gestation (Reid, 1977). A reduction in the number of divisions implies an interference with this process before the sixteenth week. The contribution of the kidney to the amniotic fluid at that time is small, if any. Therefore, the oligohydramnios seen in cases of bilateral renal agenesis is a late finding in pregnancy, occurring long after the structural groundwork of the lung has been laid out. Hislop et al. (1979) suggest that the anephric fetus fails to produce proline, which is needed for collagen formation in the bronchiolar tree.

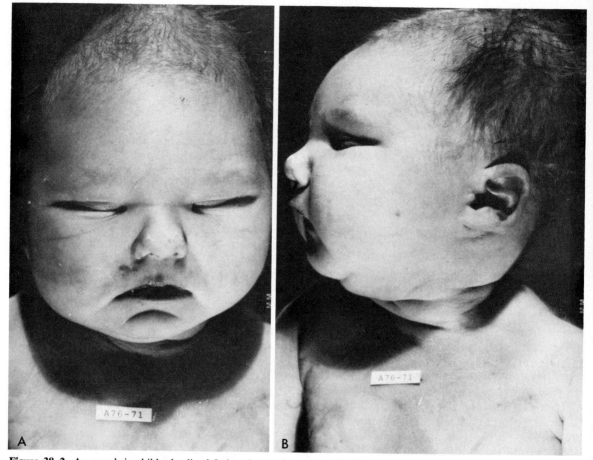

Figure 38–2. An anephric child who lived 2 days has typical Potter facial appearance. *A,* Note the prominent fold and skin crease beneath each eye, blunted nose, and depression between lower lip and chin. *B,* The ears give an impression of being low-set because lobes are broad and drawn forward, but actually the ear canals are located normally.

The kidney is the primary source of proline (Clemmons, 1977), and thus pulmonary hypoplasia results from absence of renal parenchyma and not from diminished amniotic fluid. In support of this hypothesis is the finding of normal lungs in two babies with prolonged leakage of amniotic fluid beginning at a time when one would have expected pulmonary hypoplasia if the amniotic fluid alone were responsible for the defect (Perlman et al., 1976).

In the male, penile development is usually normal. Hypospadias is rare, but its occurrence is not related to the presence or absence of testes. In 33 per cent of cases, however, the testes are undescended (Carpentier and Potter, 1959). They did not find any infants without testes, but Ashley and Mostofi (1960) noted testicular agenesis in 10 per cent. The vas deferens is normal in most cases. The presence of vasa implies that whatever caused the agenesis influenced the ureteral bud only after it was

formed or the insult affected only the nephrogenic ridge.

Although this syndrome occurs uncommonly in females, they have a relatively high incidence of genitourinary anomalies (Carpentier and Potter, 1959). The ovaries are frequently hypoplastic or absent. The uterus is usually either rudimentary or bicornuate; occasionally, it is absent entirely, as in sirenomelia. In addition, the vagina either is a short blind pouch or is completely absent.

The adrenal glands are rarely malpositioned or absent (Davidson and Ross, 1954), but anomalies of other organ systems are seen. The legs are frequently abnormal, with clubbed or even fused feet producing sirenomelia. A lumbar meningocele with or without the Arnold-Chiari malformation is not infrequently observed (Ashley and Mostofi, 1960; Davidson and Ross, 1954). Other malformations include abnormalities of the cardiovascular and gastrointestinal systems, which are present in up to 50 per cent of the infants.

Diagnosis. The characteristic Potter facies and the presence of oligohydramnios are pathognomonic and should alert one to this severe urinary malformation. Amnion nodosum—small white keratinized nodules found on the surface of the amniotic sac—may also suggest this defect (Bain et al., 1960; Thompson, 1960). In addition, 90 per cent of newborns void within the first day of life (Clark, 1977; Sherry and Kramer, 1955). Anuria after the first 24 hours of life without bladder distention should suggest renal agenesis (Williams, 1974). However, most of the infants who are born alive suffer from severe respiratory distress within the first 24 hours of life. This becomes the focus of attention, and the renal anomaly may be thought of only secondarily.

When the association is made, excretory urography may be attempted but is generally fruitless. Renal ultrasound is probably the easiest way to identify the kidneys and the bladder to confirm the presence or absence of urine. If abdominal ultrasonography is inconclusive, a renal scan should be performed. The absence of uptake of the radioisotope in the renal fossa above background activity will confirm the diagnosis of bilateral agenesis. Umbilical artery catheterization and an aortogram will most certainly define the absence of renal arteries and kidneys (Fig. 38–1).

Prognosis. Nearly 40 per cent of the affected infants are stillborn. Most of the infants born alive do not survive beyond the first 24 to 48 hours because of respiratory distress associated with pulmonary hypoplasia. Those infants who do not succumb at this time generally remain alive for variable periods, depending on the rate at which renal failure develops. The longest surviving child lived 39 days (Davidson and Ross, 1954).

UNILATERAL RENAL AGENESIS

Complete absence of one kidney occurs more frequently than does bilateral renal agenesis. In general, there are no telltale signs (as with bilateral agenesis) that suggest an absent kidney (Campbell, 1928). The diagnosis is usually not suspected and remains undetected unless careful examination of the external and internal genitalia uncovers an abnormality that is associated with renal agenesis.

Incidence. The clinically silent nature of this anomaly precludes a completely accurate account of its incidence. Most autopsy series, however, suggest that unilateral agenesis occurs once in 1100 births (Doroshow and Abeshouse, 1961). In a survey of excretory urograms performed at the Mayo Clinic, the clinical incidence approached 1 in 1500 (Longo and Thompson, 1962).

The higher incidence of bilateral renal agenesis noted in males is not nearly as striking in the unilateral condition, but males still dominate in a ratio of 1.8:1 (Doroshow and Abeshouse, 1961). This is not surprising considering the timing of embryologic events. Wolffian duct differentiation occurs earlier in the male than does müllerian duct development in the female, taking place closer to the time of ureteral bud formation. Thus, it is postulated that the ureteral bud is influenced more by abnormalities of the wolffian duct than by those of the müllerian duct.

Absence of one kidney occurs somewhat more frequently on the left side. A familial tendency has been noted. Siblings within a single family and even monozygotic twins have been affected (Kohn and Borns, 1973).

Embryology. The embryologic basis for unilateral renal agenesis does not differ significantly from that described for the bilateral type. The fault lies most probably with the ureteral bud. Complete absence of a bud or aborted ureteral development prevents maturation of metanephric blastema into adult kidney tissue.

It is unlikely that the metanephros is responsible because the ipsilateral gonad (derived from adjacent mesenchymal tissue) is rarely absent, malpositioned, or nonfunctioning (Ashley and Mostofi, 1960). The high incidence of absent or malformed proximal mesonephric duct structures in the male and müllerian duct structures in the female strengthens the argument that the embryologic insult affects the ureteral bud early in its development or even influences its precursor, the mesonephric duct. The abnormality probably occurs no later than the fourth or fifth week of gestation, when the ureteral bud forms and the mesonephric or wolffian duct in the male begins to develop into the seminal vesicle, prostate, and vas deferens. The müllerian duct in the female at this time starts its medial migration, crossing over the degenerating wolffian duct (sixth week) on its way to differentiating into the fallopian tube, uterine horn and body, and proximal vagina (Woolf and Allen, 1953; Yoder and Pfister, 1976).

Magee et al. (1979) proposed an embryologic classification based on the timing of the faulty differentiation (Fig. 38–3). If the insult occurs before the fourth week (Type I), nondifferentiation of the nephrogenic ridge with retar-

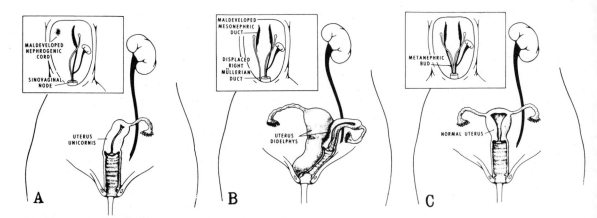

Figure 38–3. A proposed categorization of genital and renal anomalies in females. (From Magee, M.: J. Urol., *121*:265, 1979. Used by permission.)

dation of the mesonephric and müllerian components results, leading to complete unilateral agenesis of genitourinary organs. The individual has a solitary kidney and a unicornuate uterus. In Type II anomalies, the defect occurs early in the fourth week of gestation, affecting mesonephric and ureteral buds. The maldeveloped mesonephric duct prevents crossover of the müllerian duct and subsequent fusion. A didelphys uterus, with ipsilateral obstruction of one horn and the vagina, is produced. If the insult occurs after the fourth week (Type III lesions), the mesonephric and müllerian ducts develop normally and only the ureteral bud and metanephric blastema are affected. Normal genital architecture is present despite the absence of one kidney.

Associated Anomalies. The ipsilateral ureter is completely absent in slightly more than half the patients (Ashley and Mostofi, 1960; Collins, 1932; Fortune, 1927). In many of the remaining individuals, the ureter is only partially developed. In no instance is the ureter totally normal. Partial ureteral development is associated with either complete luminal atresia or variable patency. A hemitrigone (in association with complete ureteral agenesis) or an asymmetric trigone (in the presence of a partially developed ureter) is recognizable at cystoscopy. Segmental ureteral atresia on one side has been associated with contralateral ureteral or renal ectopia (Limkakeng and Retik, 1972). Except for renal ectopia and malrotation, anomalies of the contralateral kidney are very infrequently encountered (Longo and Thompson, 1952).

Ipsilateral adrenal agenesis is rare with renal agenesis, occurring in less than 10 per cent of autopsy reports (Ashley and Mostofi, 1960; Collins, 1932; Fortune, 1927). This is not surprising in view of the different embryologic

derivations of the adrenal cortex and medulla, which arise separately from the metanephros.

Genital anomalies, on the other hand, are much more frequently observed. Despite the predominance of males with unilateral renal agenesis, a greater number of reproductive organ abnormalities seem to appear in females, occurring in 25 to 50 per cent compared with 10 to 15 per cent of males. It may be that a specific genital anomaly is easier to detect in a female, and this may account for the difference in incidence between the two sexes. The incidence of a genital organ malformation for both sexes varies from 20 to 40 per cent (Doroshow and Abeshouse, 1961; Smith and Orkin, 1945; Thompson and Lynn, 1966).

In either sex the gonad is usually normal, but structures derived from the müllerian or wolffian duct are most often anomalous. In the male, the testis and globus major, which contains the efferent ductules and arises from mesonephric tubules, are invariably present; all structures proximal to that which develop from the mesonephric duct (the globus minor, vas deferens, seminal vesicle, ampulla, and ejaculatory duct) are frequently absent, with an incidence approaching 50 per cent (Charny and Gillenwater, 1965; Collins, 1932; Ochsner et al., 1972; Radasch, 1908). Occasionally, the mesonephric duct structures may be rudimentary or ectopic rather than absent (Holt and Peterson, 1974); seminal vesicle cyst is but one example of this (Beeby, 1974; Furtado, 1973). Rarely, ipsilateral cryptorchidism has been noted.

In the female, a variety of anomalies may result from incomplete or altered müllerian development caused by mesonephric duct maldevelopment. Approximately one third of women with renal agenesis have an abnormality of the internal genitalia (Thompson and Lynn,

1966). Conversely, 43 per cent of women with genital anomalies have unilateral renal agenesis (Semmens, 1962). Most frequent of these is a true unicornuate uterus with complete absence of the ipsilateral horn and fallopian tube or a bicornuate uterus with rudimentary development of one horn. The fimbriated end of the fallopian tube, however, is usually fully formed and corresponds in its development to the globus major in the male (Shumacker, 1938).

Complete or incomplete midline fusion of the müllerian ducts may result in a double or septate uterus with either a single or a duplicated cervix (Fortune, 1927; Radasch, 1908). Duplication of the vagina, septate vagina, proximal vaginal atresia associated with a small vaginal dimple, and even complete absence of the vagina have been reported (D'Alberton et al., 1981; Woolf and Allen, 1953). Obstruction of one system is not uncommon, and unilateral hematocolpos or hydrocolpos associated with a pelvic mass or pain, or both, has been reported in the pubertal girl (Gilliland and Dick, 1976; Vinstein and Franken, 1972; Weiss and Dykhuizen, 1967; Wiersma et al., 1976; Yoder and Pfister, 1976) (Fig. 38–4). In rare instances, this

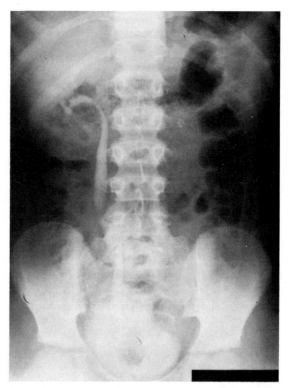

Figure 38–5. A 4-year-old girl had an excretory urogram because of imperforate anus and duplicate vagina. Note absence of left kidney and medial placement of the splenic flexure. At cystoscopy, a hemitrigone was noted.

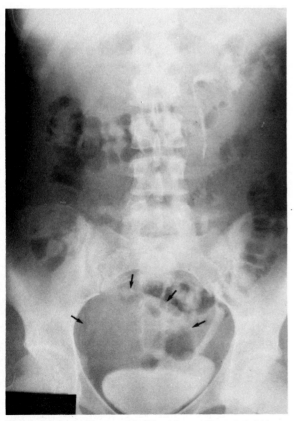

Figure 38–4. A 16-year-old girl with a solitary left kidney had abdominal pain and a pelvic mass that proved to be an obstructed duplicate vagina with hematocolpos.

has been mistaken for a large or infected Gartner's duct cyst. Sometimes a true Gartner's duct cyst has been found in a prepubertal girl in association with an ectopic ureter that is blind-ending at its proximal end or that is connected to a rudimentary kidney (Currarino, 1982).

Investigation of the urinary tract in patients with anomalies of the internal genitalia often will lead to the discovery of an absent kidney on the affected side (Bryan et al., 1949; Phelan et al., 1953). In fact, because unilateral renal agenesis is so frequently associated with anomalies of the internal female genitalia, the physician should evaluate the entire genitourinary system in any girl with one of these anomalies.

Anomalies of other organ systems are found more frequently in these individuals. The more common ones involve the cardiovascular (30 per cent), gastrointestinal (25 per cent), and musculoskeletal (14 per cent) systems (Emanuel et al., 1974) (Fig. 38–5). These include septal and valvular cardiac defects; imperforate anus and anal or esophageal strictures or atresia; and vertebral or phalangeal abnormalities (Jancu et al., 1976). Several syndromes are associated with unilateral agenesis—Turner's syndrome, Poland's syndrome (Mace et al., 1972), and dysmorphogenesis (Say and Gerald, 1968). Thus, a comprehensive review of all organ systems should be undertaken when one or more anomalies are discovered. In a small number of children the composition of defects is incompatible with life, and gestational or neonatal death ensues.

Diagnosis. Generally there are no specific symptoms heralding an absent kidney. Most reports are surveys from autopsy series. In addition, the contralateral kidney does not appear to be more prone to disease because it is solitary.

The diagnosis, however, may be suspected during a physical examination when the vas deferens or body and tail of the epididymis is missing, or when an absent, septate, or hypoplastic vagina is associated with a unicornuate or bicornuate uterus (Bryan et al., 1949). Radiologically, an absent left kidney can be surmised when a plain film of the abdomen demonstrates a medial position of the gas pattern of the splenic flexure of the colon in the area normally occupied by the left kidney (Mascatello and Lebowitz, 1976) (Fig. 38–5). A similar finding showing the hepatic flexure positioned in the right renal fossa suggests congenital absence of the right kidney (Curtis et al., 1977). The diagnosis can be confirmed by renal ultrasonography or excretory urography, which will reveal an absent kidney or nephrogram on that side and compensatory hypertrophy of the contralateral kidney (Cope and Trickey, 1982; Hynes and Watkin, 1970).

Failure of one kidney to "light up" during the total body image phase of a radionuclide technetium scan may be compatible with the diagnosis of an absent kidney but is not infallible. Radionuclide imaging of the kidney using an isotope that characterizes the renal blood flow will clearly differentiate renal agenesis from other conditions in which the kidney may be functioning minimally or not at all. Isotope scanning and ultrasonography have largely replaced arteriography in defining this condition. Fluoroscopic monitoring of the renal fossa at the end of a cardiac catheterization has demonstrated an absent kidney on occasion.

Cystoscopy, if performed, usually reveals an asymmetric trigone or hemitrigone, suggesting either partial or complete ureteral atresia. Cystoscopy has not been needed to confirm the diagnosis since the development of other, more sophisticated noninvasive radiographic studies.

Prognosis. There is no clear-cut evidence of increased susceptibility to disease in patients with a solitary kidney. Most reviews were conducted in the preantibiotic era, and they report a high incidence of "pyelitis," nephro- and ureterolithiasis, tuberculosis, and glomerulonephritis. The increased ability to prevent infection and its sequelae certainly has reduced the incidence of death among patients with a solitary kidney. In Ashley and Mostofi's series (1960), only 15 per cent of the patients died as a result of renal disease, the nature of which in almost every case would have been bilateral had two kidneys been present initially. Trauma resulted in death in 5 per cent; some patients in this group might have lived had there been two kidneys (because the source of the autopsy material included many military personnel, the potential risk of injury was accentuated, however). In other words, unilateral renal agenesis with an otherwise normal contralateral kidney is not incompatible with normal longevity and does not predispose the remaining contralateral kidney to greater than normal risks (Dees, 1960; Gutierrez, 1933).

Supernumerary Kidney

Total renal parenchymal development is controlled, in part, by an unidentified substance that acts to limit the amount of functioning renal tissue. It is, therefore, interesting to find that nature has created, albeit rarely, a condition in which the individual has three separate kidneys and an excessive amount of functioning renal parenchyma (the two main kidneys are usually normal in size and the third is small). The supernumerary kidney is truly an accessory organ with its own collecting system, blood supply, and distinct encapsulated tissue. It may be either totally separate from the normal kidney on that side or connected to it by loose areolar tissue (Geisinger, 1937). The ureters may be bifid or completely separate. This condition is different from the single kidney associated with ureteral duplication, in which each collecting system drains portions of one parenchymatous mass surrounded by a single capsule.

Incidence. The true incidence of this anomaly cannot be calculated because of its very infrequent occurrence. Approximately 66 cases have been reported since it was first described in 1656; it represents a very rare anomaly of the urinary system (Sasidharan et al., 1976). It appears to affect males and females equally but has a higher predilection for the left side (N'Guessan and Stephens, 1983). Campbell (1970) recorded one case involving bilateral supernumerary kidneys, an anomaly that has even been observed in other animal species, i.e., cow and pig.

Embryology. The sequence of interdependent events involved in ureteral bud formation and metanephric blastema development, which are required for the maturation of the normal kidney, probably also allows for the occurrence of a supernumerary kidney. It is postulated that a deviation in both these processes must have taken place to create the anomaly. A second ureteral outpouching off the wolffian duct or a branching from the initial ureteral bud appears necessary as a first step. Next, the nephrogenic cord may divide into two metanephric tails, which separate entirely when induced to differentiate by the separate or bifid ureteral buds (N'Guessan and Stephens, 1983). The twin metanephroi develop only when the bifid or separate ureteral buds enter them. These investigators, however, do not believe that this condition is the result of widely divergent bifid or separate ureteral buds. Geisinger (1937) proposed that the separate kidneys may have been caused either by fragmentation of a single metanephros or by linear infarction producing separate viable fragments that develop only when a second ureteral bud is present.

Description. The supernumerary kidney is a distinct parenchymatous mass that may be either completely or loosely attached to the major kidney on the ipsilateral side. In general, it is located somewhat caudad to the dominant kidney, which is normally situated in the renal fossa. Occasionally, it lies either posterior or craniad to the main kidney, or it may even be a midline structure anterior to the great vessels and loosely attached to each of the other two kidneys (Fig. 38–6).

The kidney is usually normal in shape but smaller than the ipsilateral organ. In about one third of cases, the kidney or its collecting system is abnormal. The collecting system may appear normal, but in almost half the reported cases it is severely dilated and the parenchyma is thinned, indicating an obstructed ureter.

The ureteral interrelationships on the side of the supernumerary kidney are quite variable (Kretschmer, 1929). Convergence of the ipsilateral distal ureters to form a common stem and a single ureteral orifice occurs in 50 per cent of the cases (Exley and Hotchkiss, 1944; N'Guessan and Stephens, 1983). Two completely independent ureters, each with its own entrance into the bladder, were seen in the other 50 per cent of cases. The Weigert-Meyer principle usually is obeyed, but in 10 per cent the caudal kidney has a ureter that does not follow the rule and enters on the trigone below the ipsilateral ureter (Tada et al., 1981) (Fig. 38–7). Rarely, the supernumerary kidney has a completely

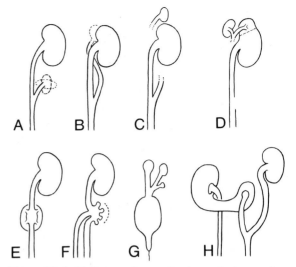

Figure 38–6. Various patterns of urinary drainage when ureters form a common stem. All kidney positions are relative only and are depicted on the left side for ease of interpretation. Dashed lines indicate that detail was not defined. (From N'Guessan, G., and Stephens, F. D.: J. Urol., *130*:649, 1983. Used by permission.)

ectopic ureter opening into the vagina or introitus (Carlson, 1959; Rubin, 1948). Individual case reports have described calyceal communications between the supernumerary and domi-

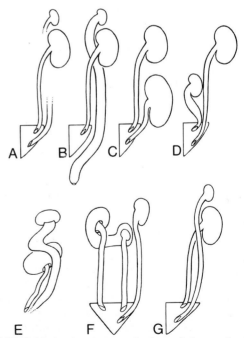

Figure 38–7. Various patterns of urinary drainage of supernumerary and ipsilateral kidneys when ureters are completely separated. All kidney positions are relative only and are depicted on the left side for ease of interpretation. Dashed lines indicate that detail was not defined. (From N'Guessan, G., and Stephens, F. D.: J. Urol., *130*:649, 1983. Used by permission.)

nant kidney or fusion of the dominant kidney's ureter with the pelvis of the supernumerary kidney (Kretschmer, 1929) to create a single distal ureter, which then enters the bladder (Fig. 38–6). The vascular supply to the supernumerary kidney is, as one might expect, very anomalous, depending on its position in relation to the major ipsilateral kidney.

Associated Anomalies. Most often, the ipsilateral and contralateral kidneys are normal. Except for an occasional ectopic orifice from the ureter draining the supernumerary kidney, no genitourinary abnormalities are present in any consistent pattern. Few of the case reports describe anomalies of other organ systems.

Symptoms. Although this anomaly is obviously present at birth, it may not produce symptoms until early adulthood. The average age at diagnosis in all reported cases was 36 years. It is rarely discovered in childhood. Pain, fever, and a palpable abdominal mass are the usual presenting complaints. Urinary infection or obstruction, or both, are the major pathologic conditions leading to urologic evaluation. Ureteral ectopia from the supernumerary kidney may produce urinary incontinence, but this is rarely seen because of the hypoplastic nature of the involved renal element (Hoffman and McMillan, 1948; Shane, 1942).

A palpable abdominal mass secondary to development of a carcinoma in the supernumerary kidney has been noted in two patients. In 25 per cent of all reported cases, however, the supernumerary kidney remains completely asymptomatic and is discovered only at autopsy (Carlson, 1950).

Diagnosis. When the supernumerary kidney is normal and not symptomatic, it is usually diagnosed when excretory urography is performed for other reasons. The kidney may be inferior and distant enough from the ipsilateral kidney so that it does not disturb the latter's architecture. If it is nearby, its mere presence may displace the major kidney or its ureter slightly.

Many times, however, the supernumerary organ is hydronephrotic, and it distorts the normal kidney and ureter on that side. When the collecting system is bifid, the dominant kidney is usually involved in the same disease process. When the ureters are separate, the ipsilateral kidney is pathologic. Voiding cystourethrography, ultrasonography, and even retrograde pyelography may be needed to help delineate the disease process. Cystoscopy will reveal one or two ureteral orifices on the ipsilateral side, depending on whether or not the

ureters are completely duplicated and, if so, to what extent ureteral ectopia exists in or outside the bladder. Occasionally a supernumerary kidney may not be accurately diagnosed until the time of surgery or at autopsy.

ANOMALIES OF VOLUME AND STRUCTURE

These anomalies, as outlined at the beginning of this section, are discussed in Chapter 39.

ANOMALIES OF ASCENT

Simple Renal Ectopia

When the mature kidney fails to reach its normal location in the "renal" fossa, the condition is known as renal ectopia. The term is derived from the Greek *ek* (out) and *topos* (place) and literally means out of place. It is to be differentiated from renal ptosis, in which the kidney initially is located in its proper place (and has normal vascularity) but moves downward in relation to body position. The ectopic kidney, on the other hand, has never resided in the appropriate location.

An ectopic kidney can be found in one of the following positions: pelvic, iliac, abdominal, thoracic, and contralateral or crossed. Only the ipsilateral retroperitoneal location of the ectopic kidney will be discussed here. Thoracic kidney and crossed renal ectopia (with and without fusion) will be dealt with subsequently.

Incidence. Renal ectopia has been known to exist ever since it was described by sixteenth century anatomists, but it did not achieve clinical interest until the mid-nineteenth century. In recent times, with greater emphasis on diagnostic acumen and uroradiographic visualization, this condition has been noted with increasing frequency.

The actual incidence among autopsy series varies from 1 in 500 (Campbell, 1930) to 1 in 1200 (Anson and Riba, 1939; Bell, 1946; Stevens, 1937; Thompson and Pace, 1937), but the average occurrence is about 1 in 900 (Abeshouse and Bhisitkul, 1959). With increasing clinical detection, the incidence among hospitalized patients is now approaching the autopsy rate (Abeshouse and Bhisitkul, 1959). In autopsy studies there is no significant difference in incidence between the sexes. Clinically, renal ectopia is more readily recognized in females because they undergo uroradiologic evaluation more frequently than males as a result of the higher rate of urinary infection or associated genital anomalies (Thompson and Pace, 1937).

The left side is favored slightly over the right. Pelvic ectopia has been estimated to occur once in 2100 to once in 3000 autopsies (Stevens, 1937). Solitary ectopic kidneys occur once in 22,000 autopsies (Delson, 1975; Hawes, 1950; Stevens, 1937). At last count in 1973, 165 cases of a solitary pelvic kidney have been recorded (Downs et al., 1973). Bilateral ectopic kidneys have been observed even more rarely and are reported in only 10 per cent of patients with renal ectopia (Malek et al., 1971).

Embryology. The ureteral bud first arises from the wolffian duct at the end of the fourth week of gestation. It then grows craniad toward the urogenital ridge and acquires a cap of metanephric blastema by the end of the fifth week. At this point, the nephrogenic tissue is opposite the upper sacral somites.

As elongation and straightening of the caudal end of the embryo commence, the developing reniform mass migrates on its own, is forcibly extruded from the true pelvis, or appears to move as the tail uncurls and differential growth between the body and tail of the embryo occurs. Whatever the mechanism or driving force for renal ascent, it is during this migration that the upper ureteral bud matures into a normal collecting system and medial rotation of the renal pelvis takes place. This process of migration and rotation is completed by the end of the eighth week of gestation. Factors that may prevent the orderly movement of kidneys include the following: ureteral bud maldevelopment (Campbell, 1930); defective metanephric tissue that by itself fails to induce ascent (Ward et al., 1965); genetic abnormalities; and maternal illnesses or teratogenic causes (because there is an increased association of genital anomalies) (Malek et al., 1971). A vascular barrier that prevents upward migration secondary to persistence of the fetal blood supply has also been postulated (Baggenstoss, 1951), but the existence of this "early" renal blood supply does not appear to influence position. More probably it is the end result, not the cause, of renal ectopia.

Description. The classification of ectopia is based on the position of the kidney within the retroperitoneum: The *pelvic* kidney is opposite the sacrum and below the aortic bifurcation; the *lumbar* kidney rests opposite the sacral promontory in the iliac fossa and anterior to the iliac vessels; and the *abdominal* kidney is so named

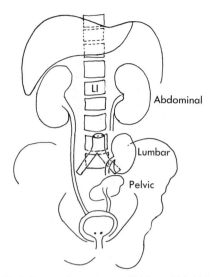

Figure 38–8. Incomplete ascent of kidney: The kidney may halt at any level of the ascent from the pelvis. (From Gray, S. W., and Skandalakis, J. E.: Embryology for Surgeons. Philadelphia, W. B. Saunders Co., 1972.)

when it is above the iliac crest and adjacent to the second lumbar vertebra (Fig. 38–8). The ectopic kidney may be found in any one of these locations with equal frequency (Dretler et al., 1971).

The kidney is generally smaller and may not conform to the usual reniform shape owing to the presence of fetal lobulations. The renal pelvis is usually anterior to the parenchyma because there is an aborted attempt at rotation of the kidney. The axis of the renal pelvis is vertical, but it may be tilted as much as 90 degrees and may lie in a true horizontal plane (Fig. 38–9).

The ureter is usually short and only slightly tortuous. It is not redundant, unlike a ptotic kidney (Fig. 38–10). The ureter usually enters the bladder on the ipsilateral side, and the orifice is not ectopic. Cystoscopy will not distinguish renal ectopia from a normal kidney.

The vascular supply, both arterial and venous, is predictable only by the fact that it is anomalous and dependent on the ultimate resting place of the kidney (Anson and Riba, 1939). There may be one or two main renal arteries arising from the distal aorta or the aortic bifurcation, with one or more aberrant arteries coming off the common or external iliac artery or even from the inferior mesenteric artery. The kidney may be supplied entirely by multiple branches, none of which arises from the aorta. In no instance does the main arterial supply arise from that level of the aorta which would

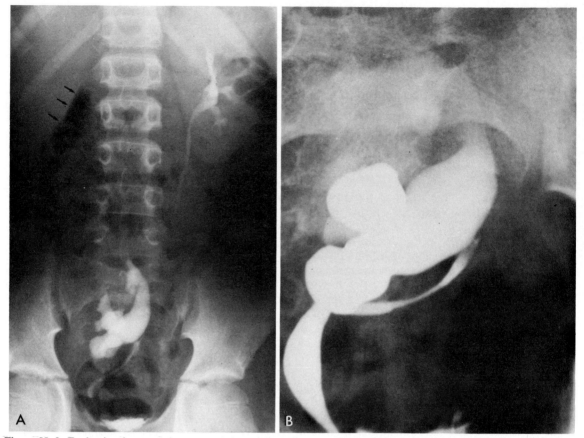

Figure 38–9. Evaluation for one urinary tract infection in a 13-year-old boy reveals: *A,* A right pelvic kidney. Position of the hepatic flexure suggests failure of renal ascent. *B,* Voiding cystourethrography reveals vesicoureteral reflux.

be the proper origin for a normally positioned kidney.

Associated Anomalies. Although the contralateral kidney is frequently normal, there may be an increased number of congenital defects associated with it (Malek et al., 1971; Thompson and Pace, 1937). In this group, the incidence of contralateral agenesis is rather high, suggesting that a teratogenic factor affecting both ureteral buds and/or metanephric blastemas may be responsible for the anomaly (Fig. 38–11). Bilateral ectopia is seen in a very small number of patients (Fig. 38–12).

The most striking feature is the association of genital anomalies in the patient with ectopia. The incidence varies from 15 per cent (Thompson and Pace, 1937) to 45 per cent (Downs et al., 1973), depending on how carefully the patient is evaluated. Twenty to 66 per cent of females have one or more of the following abnormalities of the reproductive organs: bicornuate or unicornuate uterus with atresia of one horn (McCrea, 1942); rudimentry or absent uterus and proximal or distal vagina (D'Alberton et al., 1981; Tabisky and Bhisitkul, 1965);

and duplication of the vagina. In males, 10 to 20 per cent have an associated genital defect; undescended testes, duplication of the urethra, and hypospadias are the most common (Thompson and Pace, 1937).

Rarely, the adrenal gland is absent or abnormally positioned. A small number of patients (21 per cent) have anomalies of other organ systems (Downs et al., 1973); most of these are skeletal or cardiac deformities.

Diagnosis. With the increasing use of radiography, ultrasonography, and radionuclide scanning, the incidence of fortuitous discovery of an asymptomatic ectopic kidney is also increasing. The steady rise in reported cases in recent years attests to this fact.

Most ectopic kidneys are clinically asymptomatic. Vague abdominal complaints of frank ureteral colic secondary to an obstructing stone are still the most frequent symptoms leading to discovery of the misplaced kidney. The abnormal position of the kidney results in patterns of direct and referred pain that are generally atypical for colic and may be misdiagnosed as acute appendicitis or as pelvic organ disease in the

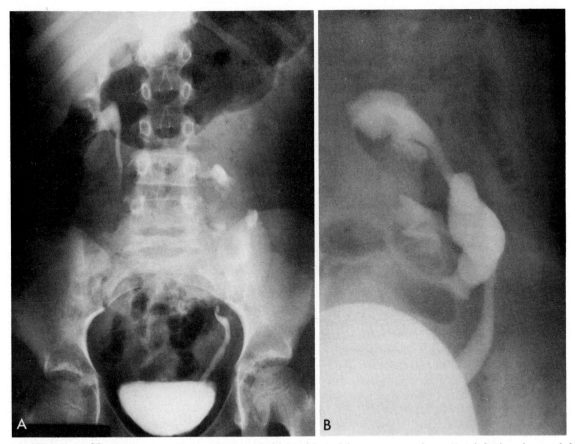

Figure 38–10. *A,* Excretory urography in a 9-year-old girl investigated for recurrent urinary tract infection shows a left lumbar kidney. *B,* Voiding cystourethrography demonstrates reflux to the ectopic kidney. At cystoscopy, the ureteral orifice was located at the bladder neck.

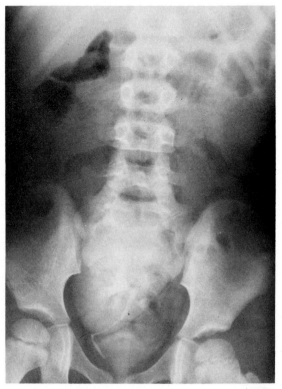

Figure 38–11. A 6-year-old boy with mild infundibular pulmonic stenosis underwent cardiac catheterization; a late abdominal film reveals a solitary pelvic kidney. At cystoscopy, a hemitrigone with an absent left ureteral orifice was discovered.

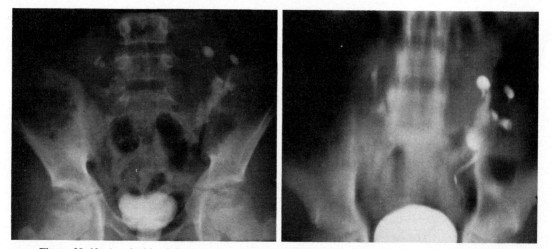

Figure 38–12. A palpable abdominal mass in an 8-year-old girl proved to be bilateral pelvic kidneys.

female. It is rare to find symptoms of compression from organs adjacent to the ectopic kidney. Renal ectopia may also present initially with urinary infection or a palpable abdominal mass.

Malposition of the colon (as discussed in the section on renal agenesis) may be a clue to the ectopic position of a lumbar or pelvic kidney. The diagnosis is easily made when the excretory urogram fails to show the kidney in its proper location. The fact that many of these kidneys overlie the bony pelvis can obscure the collecting system, leading to a misdiagnosis.

Nephrotomography during an excretory urogram examination (if the diagnosis is suspected early enough), radionuclide scanning, or retrograde pyelography will usually satisfy the diagnostician. Cystoscopy alone is rarely useful because the trigone and ureteral orifices are invariably normal unless the ureteral orifice is also ectopic (a rare event). Arteriography may be helpful in delineating the renal vascular supply in anticipation of surgery on the ectopic kidney. This is especially important in cases of solitary ectopia.

Prognosis. The ectopic kidney is no more susceptible to disease than the normally positioned kidney except for the development of hydronephrosis or urinary calculus formation. This is due, in part, to the anteriorly placed pelvis and malrotated kidney, which may lead to impaired drainage of urine from a high ureteropelvic junction or an anomalous vasculature that partially blocks one of the major calyces or the upper ureter.

Renovascular hypertension secondary to an anomalous blood supply has been reported, but a higher than normal incidence is yet unproved. Anderson and Harrison (1965), in a review of pregnant women with renal ectopia, could find no increased occurrence of difficult deliveries or maternal or fetal complications related to the ectopic kidney (Anderson and Harrison, 1965; Delson, 1975). Dystocia from a pelvic kidney is a very rare finding, but when it does occur, early recognition is mandatory and cesarean section is indicated. Although two cases of cancer within an ectopic kidney have been reported, there does not appear to be any increased risk of malignant change.

No deaths have been directly attributable to the ectopic kidney, but in at least five instances a solitary ectopic kidney has been mistakenly removed, with disastrous results, because the kidney was thought to represent a pelvic malignancy (Downs et al., 1973).

Cephalad Ectopia

The mature kidney may be positioned more craniad than normal in patients who have had a history of omphalocele (Pinckney et al., 1978). When the liver herniates into the omphalocele sac with the intestines, the kidneys continue to ascend until they are stopped by the diaphragm. In all reported cases, both kidneys were affected and lay immediately beneath the diaphragm at the level of the tenth thoracic vertebra (Fig. 38–13). The ureters are excessively long but otherwise normal. An angiogram in these patients demonstrates that the origin of the renal artery is more cephalad than normal, but no other abnormality of the vascular pattern is present. Patients with this anomaly usually have no symptoms referable to the malposition, and urinary drainage is not impaired.

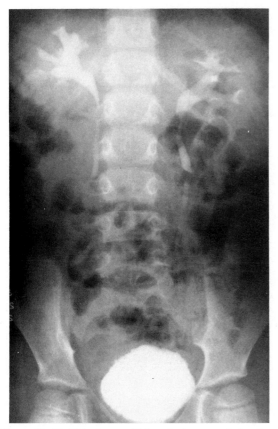

Figure 38–13. This 6-year-old boy had an omphalocele at birth; at the time the liver was noted to be in the sac. An excretory urogram following a urinary tract infection revealed the kidneys more cephalad than usual and opposite T10.

Thoracic Kidney

A very rare form of renal ectopia exists when the kidney is positioned very much higher than normal. Intrathoracic ectopia denotes either a partial or a complete protrusion of the kidney above the diaphragm into the posterior mediastinum. Less than 5 per cent of all patients with renal ectopia have an intrathoracic kidney (Campbell, 1930). This condition is to be differentiated from a congenital or traumatic diaphragmatic hernia, in which other abdominal organs as well as the kidney have protruded into the chest cavity.

Incidence. Prior to 1940, all reports of this entity involved only autopsy findings (DeCastro and Shumacher, 1969). Since 1940, however, at least 83 per cent have been collected in the literature, and three of these have involved bilateral kidneys (Berlin et al., 1957; Hertz and Shakin, 1969; Lundius, 1975; N'Guessan and Stephens, 1984). There appears to be a slight left-sided predominance of 1.5:1, and the sex ratio favors males 3:1 (Lozano and Rodriguez, 1975). This condition has been discovered in all age groups, from a neonate (Shapira et al., 1965) to a 75-year-old man evaluated for prostatic hypertrophy (Burke et al., 1967).

Embryology. The kidney reaches its adult location by the end of the eighth week of gestation. At this time, the diaphragmatic leaflets are formed as the pleuroperitoneal membrane separates the pleural cavity from the peritoneal cavity. Mesenchymal tissue associated with this membrane eventually forms the muscular component of the diaphragm. It is uncertain whether delayed closure of the diaphragmatic anlage allows for accentuated renal ascent above the level of the future diaphragm, or whether the kidney overshoots its usual position because of accelerated ascent prior to normal diaphragmatic closure (Burke et al., 1967; N'Guessan and Stephens, 1984; Spillane and Prather, 1952). Renal angiography has demonstrated a normal site of origin for the renal artery from the aorta supplying the thoracic kidney (Lundius, 1975); however, a more cranial origin than normal has also been encountered (Franciskovic and Martincic, 1959).

Description. The kidney is situated in the posterior mediastinum and generally has completed the normal rotation process (Fig. 38–14). Except for location, the renal contour and collecting system are normal. The kidney usually lies in the posterolateral aspect of the diaphragm in the foramen of Bochdalek. The diaphragm at this point thins out, and a fine membrane surrounds the protruding portion of kidney. Thus, the kidney is not within the pleural space, and there is no pneumothorax (N'Guessan and Stephens, 1984). The lower lobe of the adjacent lung may be hypoplastic. The renal vasculature and the ureter exit from the pleural cavity through the foramen of Bochdalek.

Associated Anomalies. The ureter is elongated to accommodate the excessive distance to the bladder, but it does not enter ectopically into the bladder or other pelvic sites. The adrenal gland has been mentioned in only two reports; in one it accompanied the kidney into the chest (Barloon and Goodwin, 1957), and in the other it did not (Paul et al., 1960). However, N'Guessan and Stephens (1984) analyzed ten cases and found that the adrenal gland is below the kidney in its normal location in the majority of patients. The contralateral kidney is normal, and no other consistent anomalies have been described. However, one child did have trisomy-18 (Shapira et al., 1965), and another patient

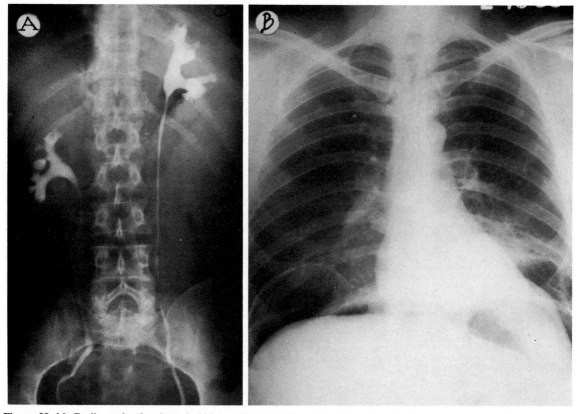

Figure 38–14. Radiograph of a thoracic kidney. The left kidney lies above the diaphragm. *A,* Diagnostic urogram. *B,* Diagnostic pneumoperitoneum. (From Hill, J. E., and Bunts, R. C.: J. Urol., *5*:98, 1960.)

had multiple pulmonary and cardiac anomalies in addition to the thoracic kidney (Fusonie and Molnar, 1966).

Symptoms. The vast majority of patients with this anomaly have remained asymptomatic. Pulmonary symptoms are exceedingly rare, and even more infrequent are urinary ones. Most cases are discovered on routine chest radiographs or at the time of thoracotomy for a suspected mediastinal tumor (DeNoronha et al., 1974).

Diagnosis. The diagnosis is most commonly made following a routine chest x-ray in which the affected hemidiaphragm is elevated slightly. On the lateral chest film a smooth, rounded mass is seen extending into the chest from the posterior aspect of the diaphragmatic leaflet, and in the anteroposterior view this mass is positioned medially. Excretory urography usually suffices to clarify the diagnosis. In some instances, retrograde pyelography is needed. Rarely, when arteriography has been employed to delineate a cardiac or pulmonary anomaly, it has revaled the presence of a thoracic kidney at the same time (Fusonie and Molnar, 1966).

Prognosis. Neither autopsy series nor clinical reports suggest that a thoracic kidney results in serious urinary or pulmonary complications. Because the majority of these patients are discovered fortuitously and have no specific symptoms referable to the misplaced kidney, no treatment is necessary once the diagnosis has been confirmed.

ANOMALIES OF FORM AND FUSION

Crossed Ectopia With and Without Fusion

When an ectopic kidney is located on the opposite side of the midline from its ureteral insertion into the bladder, the condition is known as crossed ectopia. Ninety per cent of crossed ectopic kidneys are fused to the ipsilateral kidney and, except for the horseshoe anomaly, account for the majority of fusion defects. Thus, the various renal fusion abnormalities associated with ectopia will be included in this

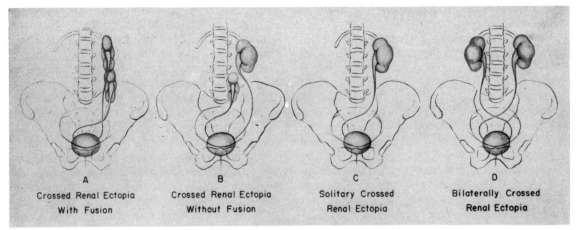

A	B	C	D
Crossed Renal Ectopia With Fusion	Crossed Renal Ectopia Without Fusion	Solitary Crossed Renal Ectopia	Bilaterally Crossed Renal Ectopia

Figure 38–15. Four types of crossed renal ectopia.

discussion. Horseshoe kidney, the most common form of renal fusion, will be presented separately in the next section.

McDonald and McClellan (1957) classified crossed ectopia as follows: crossed ectopia with fusion, crossed ectopia without fusion, solitary crossed ectopia, and bilaterally crossed ectopia (Fig. 38–15).

Fusion anomalies of the kidney were first logically categorized by Wilmer (1938), but McDonald and McClellan (1957) again refined and expanded this classification (Fig. 38–16). These anomalies have been designated as (1) unilateral fused kidney with inferior ectopia; (2) sigmoid or S-shaped; (3) lump or cake; (4) L-shaped or tandem; (5) disc, shield, or doughnut,

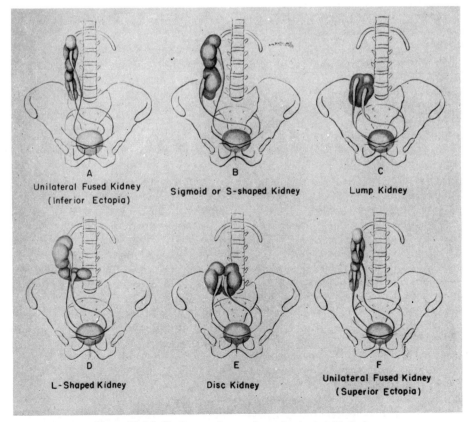

A	B	C
Unilateral Fused Kidney (Inferior Ectopia)	Sigmoid or S-shaped Kidney	Lump Kidney
D	E	F
L-Shaped Kidney	Disc Kidney	Unilateral Fused Kidney (Superior Ectopia)

Figure 38–16. Six forms of crossed renal ectopia with fusion.

and (6) unilateral fused kidney with superior ectopia.

Although this classification has little clinical significance, it does lend some order to understanding the embryology of renal ascent and rotation.

INCIDENCE

The first reported case of crossed ectopia was described by Pamarolus in 1654. Abeshouse and Bhisitkul, in 1959, conducted the last significant review of the subject and collected exactly 500 cases of crossed ectopia with and without fusion. Subsequently, numerous case reports have been published.

Sixty-two patients with crossed ectopia without fusion have been reported (Diaz, 1953; Winram and Ward-McQuaid, 1959). This represents approximately 10 per cent of all crossed ectopic kidneys (Lee, 1949). The anomaly occurs more commonly in males in a ratio of 2:1, and left-to-right ectopia is seen three times more frequently than right-to-left (Lee, 1949).

Solitary crossed ectopia has been reported in 24 patients. Males predominate in a ratio of 2:1. Generally, the crossed ectopia involves migration of the left kidney to the right side with absence of the right kidney, rather than the reverse (Kakei et al., 1976). Bilateral crossed renal ectopia has been described in five patients (Abeshouse and Bhisitkul, 1959; McDonald and McClellan, 1957) and is considered the rarest form.

Abeshouse and Bhisitkul (1959) compiled 433 reports of crossed ectopia with fusion and estimated its occurrence at 1 in 1000. This figure varies with the type of fusion anomaly; the unilaterally fused kidney with inferior ectopia is the most common, while unilateral fusion with superior ectopia is the least common. The autopsy incidence has been calculated at 1 in 2000 (Baggenstoss, 1951). Crossed ectopia with fusion has been discovered in a newborn (Bauer, 1977) but also has been reported in a 70-year-old man undergoing urologic evaluation for benign prostatic hypertrophy. There is a slight male predominance (3:2), and the left-to-right crossover occurs somewhat more frequently than its counterpart.

EMBRYOLOGY

The ureteral bud enters the metanephric blastema while the latter is situated adjacent to the anlage of the lumbosacral spine. During the next 4 weeks the developing kidney comes to lie at the level of L1–L3. Since the factor(s) responsible for the change in kidney position during gestation is still undetermined, the reasons for crossed ectopia are similarly uncertain. Wilmer (1938) suggested that crossover occurs as a result of pressure from abnormally placed umbilical arteries that prevent cephalad migration of the renal unit, which then follows the path of least resistance to the opposite side.

Potter (1952) and Alexander et al. (1950) theorized that crossed ectopia is strictly a ureteral phenomenon, with the developing ureteral bud wandering to the opposite side and inducing differentiation of the contralateral, nephrogenic anlage. Ashley and Mostofi (1960) deduced that strong but undetermined forces are responsible for renal ascent and that these forces attract one or both kidneys to their final place on the opposite side of the midline

Cook and Stephens (1977) postulated that crossover is the result of malalignment and abnormal rotation of the caudal end of the developing fetus, with the distal curled end of the vertebral column being displaced to one side. This results either in the cloaca and wolffian duct structures lying on one side of the vertebral column, allowing one ureter to cross the midline and enter the opposite nephrogenic blastema; or in the kidney or ureter being transplanted to the opposite side of the midline during "normal" renal ascent (Hertz et al., 1977).

In addition, teratogenic factors have been implicated (Kelalis et al., 1973) because there is an increased incidence of associated genitourinary and other organ system anomalies. Finally, genetic influences may play a role because similar anomalies have occurred within a single family (Greenberg and Nelsen, 1971; Hildreth and Cass, 1978).

Fusion of the metanephric masses may occur when they are still in the true pelvis prior to or at the start of cephalad migration, or it may occur during the latter stages of ascent. An abnormally positioned umbilical artery has been questioned as a cause, for it may lead to compression of the two metanephric masses as they migrate from the true pelvis. The extent of fusion is determined by the proximity of the renal anlage to one another. Following fusion, further advancement of the kidneys toward their normal location is impeded by midline retroperitoneal structures—the aortic bifurcation, the inferior mesenteric artery, and the base of the small bowel mesentery (Joly, 1940).

Fusion of a crossed ectopic kidney is related to the time at which it comes in contact with its mate. The crossed kidney usually lies caudad to its normal counterpart on that side. Migration

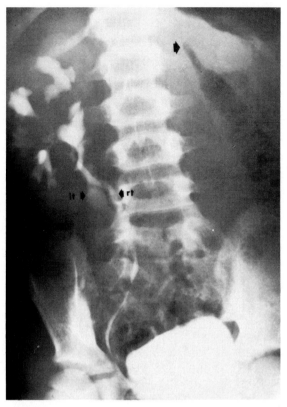

Figure 38–17. An 8-year-old boy with a left to right crossed, fused ectopia, in which the two kidneys lie abreast of one another. Splenic flexure lies in empty right renal fossa.

and proper orientation, while the ectopic kidney is inferior and in a diagonal or horizontal position with an anteriorly placed renal pelvis. The two kidneys in this situation are usually separated by a variable but definite distance, and each is surrounded by its own fascia (Gerota's capsule). In all cases of crossed ectopia without fusion, the ureter from the normal kidney enters the bladder on the ipsilateral side, while that of the ectopic kidney crosses the midline at the pelvic brim and enters the bladder on the contralateral side.

In cases of solitary crossed ectopia, the kidney is usually located in the opposite renal fossa at the level of L1–L3 and is oriented normally, having completed rotation on its vertical axis (Alexander et al., 1950; Purpon, 1963). When the kidney remains in the pelvis or ascends only to the lower lumbar region, it may assume a horizontal line with an anteriorly placed pelvis (Tabrisky and Bhisitkul, 1965) (Fig. 38–18). In either case, the ureter crosses the midline and enters the bladder on the opposite side. The contralateral ureter, if present, is usually rudimentary (Caine, 1956). The pa-

of each kidney begins simultaneously, but ascent of the ectopic unit probably lags behind because of crossover time. Thus, it is the superior pole of the ectopic kidney that generally joins with the inferior aspect of the normal kidney. Ascent continues until either the normal kidney reaches its proper location or one of the retroperitoneal structures impedes further migration of the fused mass. The final shape of the fused kidneys depends on the time and extent of fusion and the degree of renal rotation that has occurred. No further rotation is likely once the two kidneys have joined (Fig. 38–17).

The position of each renal pelvis may provide a clue to the chronology of the congenital defect. An anteriorly placed pelvis suggests early fusion, whereas a medially positioned renal pelvis indicates that fusion probably occured after rotation was completed.

DESCRIPTION

Most cases of crossed ectopia involve fusion of the ectopic kidney with its mate (90 per cent). When they are not fused, the uncrossed kidney generally is in its normal dorsolumbar location

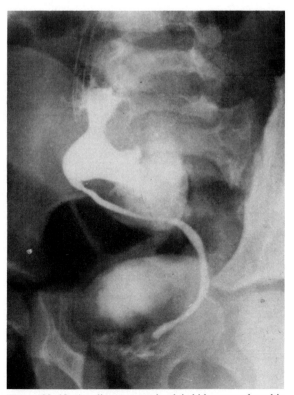

Figure 38–18. A solitary crossed pelvic kidney was found in a 7-year-old girl with recurrent urinary infection and abdominal pain. Voiding cystogram reveals vesicoureteral reflux with pyelotubular backflow.

tient with bilateral crossed ectopia may have perfectly normal-appearing kidneys and renal pelves; however, the ureters cross the midline at the level of the lower lumbar vertebrae (Abeshouse and Bhisitkul, 1959).

Inferior Ectopia. Two thirds of all unilaterally fused kidneys involve inferior ectopia. The upper pole of the crossed kidney is attached to the inferior aspect of the normally positioned kidney (Fig. 38–19). Both renal pelves are anterior; thus, fusion probably occurs relatively early.

Sigmoid or S-shaped Kidney. The sigmoid or S-shaped kidney is the second most common anomaly of fusion. The crossed kidney is again inferior, and the two kidneys are fused only at their adjacent poles. Each kidney, however, has rotated on its respective vertical axis. Thus, each renal pelvis is oriented correctly (except that the ectopic kidney has crossed the midline) and faces in the opposite direction to that of its mate. The lower convex border of one kidney is directly opposed to the outer border of its counterpart, and there is an S-shaped appearance to the entire renal outline. The ureter from the normal kidney courses downward anterior to the outer border of the inferior kidney, and the ectopic kidney's ureter crosses the midline before entering the bladder. Fusion of the two kidneys occurs relatively late after complete renal rotation has taken place.

Lump Kidney. The lump or cake kidney is

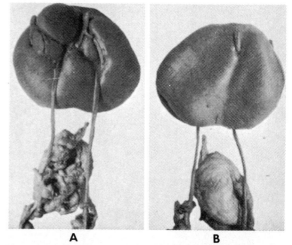

Figure 38–20. *A,* Lump kidney showing the unusual anatomy with the anterior blood supply coming from above and the ureters leaving from below. *B,* Posterior view of *A,* with the blood supply entering from above and a deep grooving of the parenchyma indicating where the kidney pressed against the spine. (Courtesy of Dr. H. S. Altman.)

a relatively rare form of fusion (Fig. 38–20). Extensive joining has taken place over a wide margin of maturing renal anlage. The total kidney mass is irregular and lobulated. Generally, ascent progresses only as far as the sacral promontory, but in many instances the kidney remains within the true pelvis. Both renal pelves are anterior and drain separate areas of parenchyma. The ureters do not cross.

L-shaped Kidney. The L-shaped or tandem kidney occurs when the crossed kidney assumes

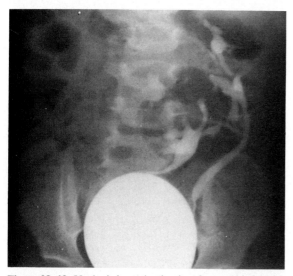

Figure 38–19. Urologic investigation in a 3-year-old girl with facial clefting syndrome and hypertelorism revealed a unilateral fused kidney with inferior ectopia. Voiding cystourethrography reveals bilateral reflux into each collecting system. At cystoscopy, both ureteral orifices were lateral, and the trigone was poorly formed.

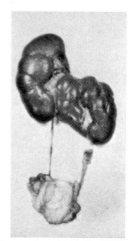

Figure 38–21. Renal fusion. L-kidney in a 1-year-old child in whom a considerable portion of the left renal segment lies across the lower lumbar spine. On each side the pelvic outlet faces anteriorly. (From Campbell, M. F.: *In* Campbell, M. F., and Harrison, J. H. (Eds.): Urology, Vol. 2, 3rd ed. Philadelphia, W. B. Saunders Co., 1970.)

a transverse position at the time of its attachment to the inferior pole of the normal kidney (Fig. 38–21). The crossed kidney lies in the midline or in the contralateral paramedian space anterior to the L4 vertebra (Fig. 38–22). Rotation about the long axis of the kidney may produce either an inverted or a reversed pelvic position. The ureter from each kidney enters the bladder on its respective side.

Disc Kidney. Disc, shield, doughnut, or pancake kidneys, as labeled by various authors, are kidneys that join at the medial borders of each pole to produce a doughnut or ring-shaped mass; when there is more extensive fusion along the entire medial aspect of each kidney, a disc or shield shape is created. The lateral aspect of each kidney retains its normal contour. Thus, this type of fusion differs from the lump or cake kidney in that the reniform shape is better preserved and more normal, and there is a less extensive degree of fusion. The pelves are anteriorly placed, and the ureters remain uncrossed. Each collecting system drains its respective half of the kidney and does not communicate with the opposite side (Fig. 38–23).

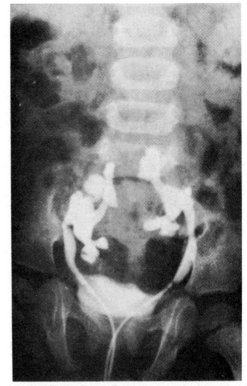

Figure 38–23. Pelvic fused kidney in a 2-year-old girl examined because of the low abdominal mass thought by some to be an ovarian cyst. (From Campbell, M. F.: *In* Campbell, M. F., and Harrison, J. H. (Eds.): Urology, Vol. 2, 3rd ed. Philadelphia, W. B. Saunders Co., 1970.)

Superior Ectopic Kidney. The least common variety of renal fusion is the crossed ectopic kidney that lies superior to the normal kidney. The lower pole of the crossed kidney is fused to the upper pole of the normal kidney. Each kidney retains its fetal orientation with both pelves lying anteriorly.

The vascular supply to each kidney is variable. The crossed ectopic kidney is supplied by one or more branches from the aorta or common iliac artery (Rubinstein et al., 1976). The normal kidney frequently has an anomalous blood supply, with multiple renal arteries arising from various levels along the aorta. In one rare instance, Rubinstein discovered that one renal artery had crossed the midline to supply the tandem ectopic kidney. The solitary crossed ectopic kidney has been found to receive its blood supply generally from that side of the aorta or iliac artery on which it is positioned (Tanenbaum et al., 1970).

ASSOCIATED ANOMALIES

In all the fusion anomalies the ureter from each kidney is usually not ectopic. Except for

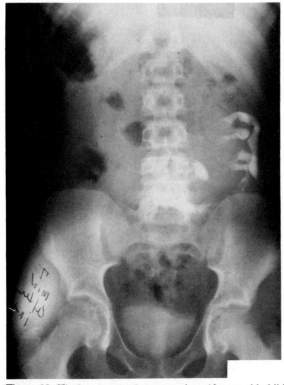

Figure 38–22. An excretory urogram in a 13-year-old child with abdominal pain reveals a tandem or L-shaped crossed ectopia.

solitary crossed ectopia, in which there may be a hemitrigone or a poorly developed trigone with a rudimentary or absent ureter on the side of the ectopic kidney, most patients with crossed ectopia have a normal trigone with no indication that an anomaly of the upper urinary tract is present (Magri, 1961; Tanenbaum et al., 1970; Yates-Bell and Packham, 1972). An ectopic ureteral orifice from the crossed renal unit has been observed about 3 per cent of the time (Abeshouse and Bhisitkul, 1959; Hendren et al., 1976; Magri, 1961). Occasionally, the ureter from the uncrossed renal segment of a fusion anomaly may have an ectopic orifice (Hendren et al., 1976). In one instance Malek and Utz (1970) discovered an ectopic ureterocele associated with the uncrossed kidney. Vesicoureteral reflux was noted frequently in the ectopic kidney (Kelalis et al., 1973) (Figs. 38–18 ·and 38–19). Most orthotopic units are normal. If an abnormality is present, it usually involves the ectopic kidney and consists of cystic dysplasia, ureteropelvic junction obstruction, and carcinoma (Abeshouse and Bhisitkul, 1959; Caldamone and Rabinowitz, 1981; Gerber et al., 1980; Macksood and James, 1983).

The highest incidence of associated anomalies involving both the genital organs and other symptoms occurs in children with solitary crossed renal ectopia. This seems to be related more to renal agenesis than to the ectopic anomaly per se. Fifty per cent of patients with solitary crossed renal ectopia have a genital abnormality consisting of either cryptorchidism or absent vas deferens in the male or vaginal atresia or a unilateral uterine abnormality in the female (Kakei et al., 1976; Yates-Bell and Packham, 1972). Skeletal anomalies and imperforate anus are also observed in 25 and 20 per cent of these patients, respectively.

In general, the occurrence of an associated anomaly in crossed renal ectopia, excluding solitary crossed ectopia, is low; the most frequent are imperforate anus (4 per cent), orthopedic anomalies (4 per cent), skeletal abnormalities, and septal cardiovascular defects.

SYMPTOMS

Most people with crossed ectopic anomalies have no symptoms. The defects are often discovered incidentally at autopsy. If they do occur, common signs and symptoms usually develop in the third or fourth decades of life and include vague low abdominal pain, pyuria, hematuria, and urinary tract infection. Hydronephrosis and renal calculi have been discovered in conjunction with some of these symptoms. It

is believed that the abnormal kidney position and anomalous blood flow may impede urinary drainage from the renal collecting system and thus create a predisposition to urinary tract infection and calculus formation.

In one third of the patients, an asymptomatic abdominal mass may be the presenting sign (Abeshouse and Bhisitkul, 1959). In a smaller number of individuals, hypertension has led to the discovery of an ectopic fusion anomaly (Abeshouse and Bhisitkul, 1959), and in one case, this was attributable to a vascular lesion in one of the anomalous vessels (Mininberg et al., 1971).

DIAGNOSIS

This abnormality has been detected usually by excretory urography, but ultrasonography and radionuclide scanning (for other reasons) have been discovering more asymptomatic cases recently. Nephrotomography can be used when necessary to define further the renal outlines (Dretler et al., 1971). Renal angiography may be a requirement prior to extensive surgery on the ectopic or normal kidney because the blood supply to the kidneys is usually very anomalous.

PROGNOSIS

Most patients with crossed renal ectopia have a good prognosis and normal longevity. However, some patients are at a risk for developing urinary tract infection or a renal calculus, or both (Kron and Meranze, 1949). Boatman et al. (1972) noted that one third of their symptomatic patients required a pyelolithotomy for an obstructing stone. Stubbs and Resnick (1977) reported a struvite staghorn calculus in a patient with crossed renal ectopia. Urinary infection in association with either vesicoureteral reflux or hydronephrosis has been implicated in the formation of these calculi.

Horseshoe Kidney

The horseshoe kidney is probably the most common of all renal fusion anomalies. It is not to be confused with asymmetric or off-center fused kidneys, which may give the impression of being horseshoe-shaped. The anomaly consists of two distinct renal masses that lie vertically on either side of the midline and are connected at their respective lower poles by a parenchymatous or fibrous isthmus that crosses the midplane of the body. It was first recognized during an autopsy by DeCarpi in 1521, but Botallo in 1564 presented the first extensive description and illustration of a horseshoe kidney (Benjamin and Schullian, 1950). In 1820 Morgagni described the first diseased horseshoe kidney, and since then more has been written about this condition than about any other renal anomaly. Almost every renal disease has also been described in the horseshoe kidney.

Incidence. Horseshoe kidney occurs in 0.25 per cent of the population, or about 1 in 400 (Bell, 1946; Campbell, 1970; Dees, 1941; Glenn, 1959; Nation, 1945). As in other fusion anomalies, it is found more commonly in males by a 2 to 1 margin. The abnormality has been discovered clinically in all age groups ranging from 2 days to 80 years, but in autopsy series it is more prevalent in children (Segura et al., 1972). This age incidence is related to the high incidence of multiple congenital anomalies associated with the horseshoe kidney, some of which are incompatible with long-term survival.

Horseshoe kidneys have been reported in identical twins (Bridge, 1960) and among several siblings within the same family (David, 1974). From the rarity of these reports and the relative frequency of the anomaly, it is doubtful that this represents a genetic predisposition. However, it might be the result of a genetic expression with a low penetrance (Leiter, 1972).

Embryology. The abnormality occurs between the fourth and sixth weeks of gestation, after the ureteral bud has entered the renal blastema but, in view of the ultimate spatial configuration of the horseshoe kidney, prior to rotation and considerable renal ascent. Boyden (1931) described a 6-week-old embryo with a horseshoe kidney, the youngest fetus ever discovered with this anomaly. He postulated that at the 14-mm (4½ week) stage, the developing metanephric masses lie close to one another; any disturbance in this relationship might result in their joining at one pole. A slight change in the position of the umbilical or common iliac artery could change the orientation of the migrating kidneys, thus leading to contact and fusion (Fig. 38–24). It is also theorized that an abnormality in the formation of the tail of the embryo or another pelvic organ could account for the fusion process.

Whatever the actual mechanism responsible for horseshoe kidney formation, the fusion process occurs before the kidneys have rotated on their long axis. In its mature form, the pelves and ureters of the horseshoe kidney are usually anteriorly placed, and the later cross ventral to the isthmus (Fig. 38–25). Very rarely, the pelves are anteromedial, suggesting that fusion occurred later, after some rotation had taken place. In addition, migration is usually incomplete, with the kidneys lying somewhat lower than normal. It is presumed that the inferior mesenteric artery obstructs the isthmus and prevents further ascent.

Description. There are many variations in the basic shape of the horseshoe kidney (Fig. 38–26). In 95 per cent of patients, the kidneys join at the lower pole; in a small number, the isthmus connects both upper poles instead (Love and Wasserman, 1975).

Generally, the isthmus is bulky and consists of parenchymatous tissue with its own blood supply (Glenn, 1959; Love and Wasserman, 1975). Occasionally it is just a midline structure of fibrous tissue that tends to draw the renal masses close together. It is located adjacent to

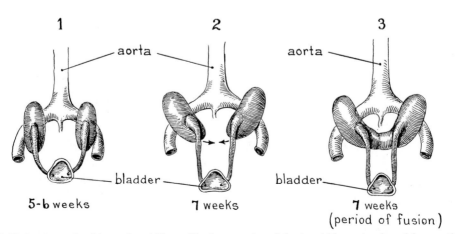

Figure 38–24. Embryogenesis of horseshoe kidney. The lower poles of the two kidneys touch and fuse as they cross the iliac arteries. Ascent is stopped when the fused kidneys reach the junction of the aorta and inferior mesenteric artery. (From Benjamin, J. A., and Schullian, D. M.: J. Hist. Med., 5:315, 1950, after Gutierrez, 1931.)

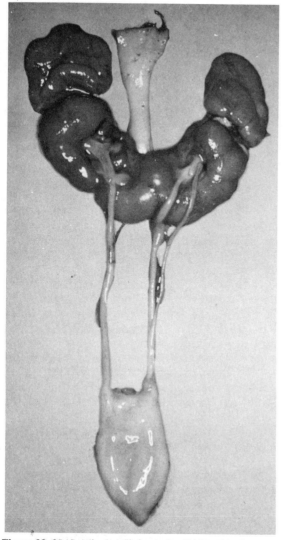

Figure 38–25. Specimen of a horseshoe kidney in a neonate who had multiple anomalies, including congenital heart disease. Note thick parenchymatous isthmus.

the L3 or L4 vertebra just below the junction of the inferior mesenteric artery and the aorta. As a result, the paired kidneys tend to be somewhat lower than normal in the retroperitoneum. In some instances, the anomalous kidneys are very low, anterior to the sacral promontory or even in the true pelvis behind the bladder (Campbell, 1970). The isthmus usually lies anterior to the aorta and vena cava, but it is not unusual for it to pass between the inferior vena cava and the aorta or even behind both vessels (Dajani, 1966; Jarmin, 1938; Meek and Wadsworth, 1940).

The calyces, normal in number, are atypical in orientation. Because the kidney fails to rotate, the calyces point posteriorly, and the axis of each pelvis remains in the vertical or obliquely lateral plane (on a line drawn from lower to upper poles). The lowermost calyces extend caudally or even medially to drain the isthmus and may overlie the vertebral column.

The ureter may insert high on the renal pelvis and lie laterally, probably as the result of incomplete renal rotation. It courses downward and has a characteristic bend as it crosses over and anterior to the isthmus, a deviation that is proportionate to the thickness of the midline structure. Despite upper ureteral angulation, the lower ureter usually enters the bladder normally and rarely is ectopic.

The blood supply to the horseshoe kidney can be quite variable (Fig. 38–27). In 30 per cent of cases, it consists of one renal artery to each kidney (Glenn, 1959), but it may be asymmetric, with duplicate or even triplicate renal arteries supplying one or both kidneys. The blood supply to the isthmus and lower poles is also very variable. The isthmus and adjacent parenchyma may receive a branch from each main renal artery, or they may have their own arterial supply from the aorta originating either above or below the level of the isthmus. Not infrequently this area may be supplied by branches from the inferior mesenteric, common or external iliac, or sacral arteries (Boatman et al., 1971; Kolln et al., 1972). Three cases of retrocaval ureter and isthmus have been reported (Eidelman et al., 1978; Heffernan et al., 1978).

Associated Anomalies. The horseshoe kidney, even though it may produce no symptoms, is frequently associated with other congenital anomalies. Boatman et al. (1972) discovered that nearly one third of the 96 patients they studied had at least one other abnormality. Many newborns and young infants with multiple congenital anomalies have a horseshoe kidney. Judging from autopsy reports, the incidence of other anomalies is certainly greater in patients who die at birth or in early infancy than in those who reach adulthood (Zondek and Zondek, 1964). This implies that horseshoe kidney may occur more often in patients with another serious congenital anomaly. The organ systems most commonly involved include the skeletal, cardiovascular, and central nervous systems. Anorectal malformations are frequently encountered in these patients. Horseshoe kidney may also be seen in 20 per cent of patients with trisomy 18 and in 60 per cent of patients with Turner's syndrome (Smith, 1970).

Boatman and his colleagues (1972) also discovered an increased occurrence of other

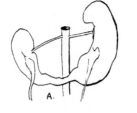
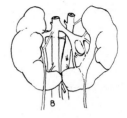

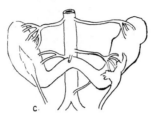
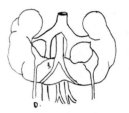

Figure 38–26. Variations in the horse-shoe kidney and the number of their ureters. (From Benjamin, J. A., and Schullian, D. M.: J. Hist. Med., 5:315, 1950, after Gutierrez, 1931.)

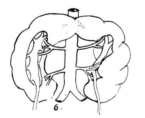
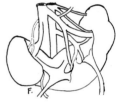

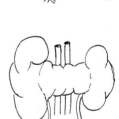

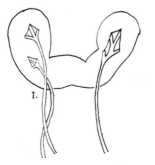
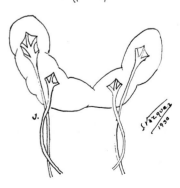

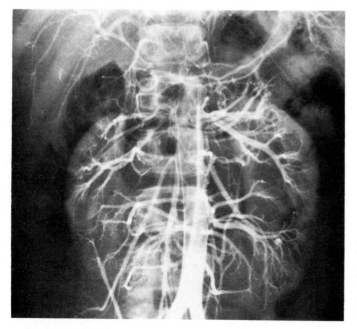

Figure 38–27. Arteriogram in a patient with a horseshoe kidney, showing multiplicity of arteries supplying kidney arising from aorta and common iliac arteries. (From Kelalis, P. P.: *In* Kelalis, P. P., and King, L. R. (Eds.): Clinical Pediatric Urology. Philadelphia, W. B. Saunders Co., 1976.)

genitourinary anomalies in patients with a horseshoe kidney. Hypospadias and undescended testes each occurred in 4 per cent of the males, and bicornuate uterus or septate vagina (or both) were noted in 7 per cent of the females.

Ureteral duplication occurs in 10 per cent of patients (Boatman et al., 1972; Zondek and Zondek, 1964), and in some cases there has been an associated ectopic ureterocele. Vesicoureteral reflux has been noted in more than half the patients (Pitts and Muecke, 1975; Segura et al., 1972). Cystic disease, including multicystic dysplasia (Novak et al., 1977) and adult polycystic kidney disease, has been reported in the horseshoe kidney (Campbell, 1970; Correa and Paton, 1976; Gutierrez, 1934; Pitts and Muecke, 1975).

Symptoms. Nearly one third of all patients with horseshoe kidney remain asymptomatic (Glenn, 1959; Kolln et al., 1972). In most instances, it is an incidental finding at autopsy (Pitts and Muecke, 1975). When symptoms are present, however, they are related to hydronephrosis, infection, or calculus formation. The most common symptom that reflects these conditions is vague abdominal pain that may radiate to the lower lumbar region. Gastrointestinal complaints may be present also. The so-called Rovsing sign—abdominal pain, nausea, and vomiting on hyperextension of the spine—has been infrequently observed. Signs and symptoms of urinary tract infection occur in 30 per cent of patients, and calculi have been noted in

one fifth of patients (Evans and Resnick, 1981; Glenn, 1959; Kolln et al., 1972; Pitts and Muecke, 1975). Five to 10 per cent of horseshoe kidneys present initially as an abdominal mass (Glenn, 1959; Kolln et al., 1972).

Ureteropelvic junction obstruction causing significant hydronephrosis occurs in as many as one third of the patients (Whitehouse, 1975) (Fig. 38–28). The high insertion of the ureter into the renal pelvis, its abnormal course anterior to the isthmus, and the anomalous blood supply to the kidney may individually or collectively contribute to this obstruction.

Diagnosis. Except for the possibility of a palpable midline abdominal mass, the horseshoe kidney does not itself produce symptoms. The complex of clinical findings from a diseased kidney, however, is often vague and nonspecific. The anomaly, therefore, may not be suspected until an excretory urogram is obtained, but then the classic radiologic features are easily recognizable and lead readily to the diagnosis (Fig. 38–29). Findings that suggest a horseshoe kidney singly or collectively include the following: kidneys that are somewhat low-lying and close to the vertebral column; a vertical or outward axis, so that a line drawn through the midplane of each kidney bisects the midline inferiorly; a continuation of the outer border of the lower pole of each kidney toward and across the midline; the characteristic orientation of the collecting system, which is directly posterior to each renal pelvis, with the lowermost calyx pointing caudally or even medially; and the high

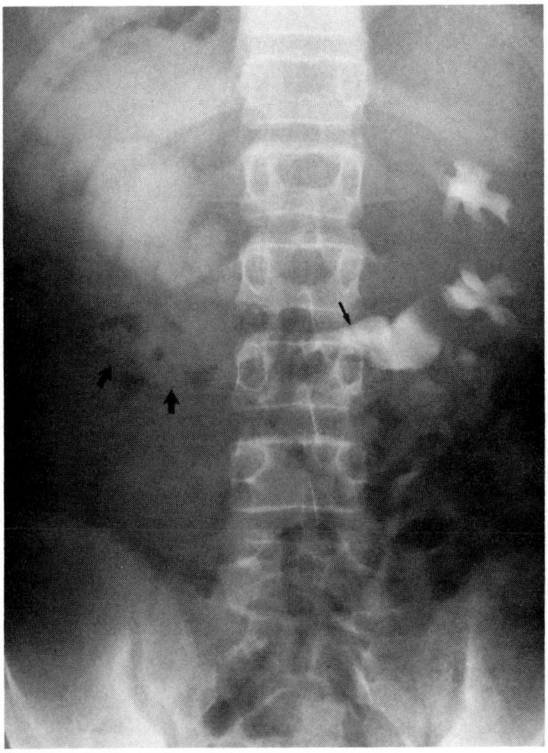

Figure 38–28. An excretory urogram in a 14-year-old boy with gross, painless hematuria following minor trauma revealed a horseshoe kidney with a right-sided ureteropelvic junction obstruction. Arrows identify the lower pole of each kidney. The left ureter can be seen crossing over the isthmus.

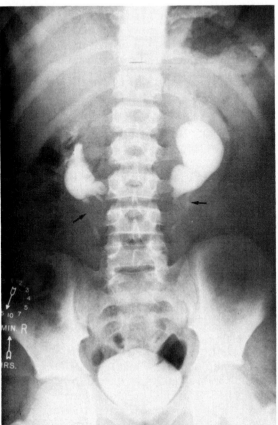

Figure 38–29. Excretory urogram in an 11-year-old boy evaluated for nocturnal incontinence reveals a horseshoe kidney. Note vertical renal axis and medial orientation of the collecting system. The ureters (arrows) are laterally displaced and bow over the isthmus.

ureteral insertion and the laterally and anteriorly displaced upper ureter that appears to cross a midline mass. However, obstruction from either a calculus or a ureteropelvic junction stricture may obscure the radiologic picture (Christoffersen and Iversen, 1976; Love and Wasserman, 1975). Other confirmatory studies, such as retrograde pyelography, ultrasonography, or computed tomography, may be necessary to make the diagnosis.

Prognosis. Although Smith and Orkin (1945) felt that horseshoe kidneys are almost always associated with disease, subsequent investigators have not found this to be so. Glenn (1959) followed patients with horseshoe kidney for an average of 10 years after discovery and found that nearly 60 per cent remained symptom-free. Only 13 per cent had persistent urinary infection or pain, and 17 per cent developed recurrent calculi. Operations to remove these stones or relieve obstruction were necessary in only 25 per cent. In his series, no patients benefited from division of the isthmus for relief of pain, and this indication for surgery has now been largely repudiated (Glenn, 1959; Pitts and Muecke, 1975).

Many patients with a horseshoe kidney have other congenital anomalies, some of which contribute to neonatal or infant death. Excluding that group, survival is not reduced merely by the presence of this anomaly. Often a horseshoe kidney is found incidentally, and it rarely contributes to the cause of death (Boatman et al., 1972; Dajani, 1966).

Many disease processes have been associated with horseshoe kidney, but again this reflects the relative frequency of the congenital defect. One hundred and eleven cases of renal cancer within a horseshoe kidney have been reported (Buntley, 1976); more than half of these were hypernephromas. However, renal pelvic tumors and Wilms' tumor each account for 25 per cent of the total. Except for renal pelvic tumors, a surprisingly high number of these cancers appear to have arisen in the isthmus (Blackard and Mellinger, 1968).

It has been suggested that the increased occurrence of chronic infection, obstruction, and stone formation may be instrumental in producing a higher than expected incidence of renal pelvic tumors in this group (Castro and Green, 1975; Shoup et al., 1962). Wilms' tumor, which is also commonly seen, frequently originates in the isthmus (Beck and Hlivko, 1960), creating a very bizarre radiologic picture (Walker, 1977). The incidence of tumors within horseshoe kidneys seems to be increased when

compared with the general population (Dische and Johnston, 1979). Survival from these tumors is related to the pathology and stage of the tumor at diagnosis and not to the renal anomaly (Murphy and Zincke, 1982).

Because it is located above the pelvic inlet, a horseshoe kidney does not adversely affect pregnancy or delivery (Bell, 1946). The development of renal failure associated with adult polycystic kidney disease is not enhanced by the presence of a horseshoe kidney (Correa and Paton, 1976). Finally, the last Transplantation Registry report failed to reveal any patient with a horseshoe kidney receiving a renal transplant (Advisory Committee to the Human Transplant Registry, 1975).

ANOMALIES OF ROTATION

The adult kidney as it assumes its final location in the "renal" fossa orients itself so that the calyces point laterally and the pelvis faces medially. When this alignment is not exact, the condition is known as malrotation. Most often, this inappropriate orientation is found in conjunction with another renal anomaly, such as ectopia with or without fusion or horseshoe kidney. This discussion centers on malrotation as an isolated renal entity. It must be differentiated from other conditions that mimic it as the result of extraneous forces such as an abnormal retroperitoneal mass.

INCIDENCE

The true incidence of this developmental anomaly cannot be accurately calculated because minor degrees of malrotation are never reported and generally do not cause much concern. Campbell (1963) found renal malrotation once in 939 autopsies, and Smith and Orkin (1945) noted 1 case per 390 admissions. It is frequently observed in patients with Turner's syndrome (Gray and Skandalakis, 1972). Males are affected twice as often as females, but there does not appear to be any predilection for one side. In other animals, e.g., reptiles and birds, the "malrotated kidney" is actually properly oriented for these individual species.

EMBRYOLOGY

Medial rotation of the collecting system occurs simultaneously with renal migration. Thus the kidney starts to turn during the sixth week when it is leaving the true pelvis and completes this process, having rotated 90 degrees toward the midline, by the time that ascent is completed at the end of the ninth week of gestation.

It has been postulated (Felix, 1912) that rotation is actually the result of unequal branching of successive orders of the ureteral tree, with two branches extending ventrally and one dorsally during each generation of division. Each branch then induces metanephrogenic tissue to differentiate and encase it as a cap. More parenchyma develops ventrally than dorsally, and the pelvis rotates medially. Weyrauch (1939) accepted this theory of renal rotation as the result of excessive ventral versus dorsal branching of the ureteral tree and concluded that the fault of malrotation lies entirely with the ureter. A late-appearing ureteral bud may insert into an atypical portion of the renal blastema and may lead to a lessened propensity for the developing nephric tissue to shift. Late appearance of the ureteral bud is almost always associated with an abnormal origin from the wolffian duct; this translates into ureteral ectopia at the bladder or lower urinary tract level. Mackie et al. (1975) did not describe any malrotation anomalies in their study of ureteral ectopia, however. The renal blood supply does not appear to be the cause or the limiting factor in malrotation but rather follows the course of renal hyporotation, hyper-rotation, or reverse rotation.

DESCRIPTION

The kidney and renal pelvis normally rotate 90 degrees ventromedially during ascent. Weyrauch (1939), in an exhaustive and detailed study, outlined the various abnormal phases of medial and reverse rotation and labeled each according to the position of the renal pelvis (Fig. 38–30).

Ventral Position. The pelvis is ventral and in the same anteroposterior plane as the calyces, which point dorsally, since they have undergone no rotation at all. This is the most common form of malrotation. Very rarely, this position may represent excessive medial rotation, in which a complete 360 degree turn has occurred. In one such presumed case reported by Weyrauch (1939), the vasculature had rotated with the kidney and passed around dorsally and laterally to it before entering the anteriorly placed hilus.

Ventromedial Position. The pelvis faces ventromedially because of an incompletely rotated kidney. Excursion probably stops during the seventh week of gestation, when the kidney and pelvis normally reach this position. The calyces thus point dorsolaterally.

Dorsal Position. Renal excursion of 180 degrees occurs to produce this position. The pelvis is dorsal to the parenchyma, and the vessels pass behind the kidney to reach the hilum. This is the rarest form of malrotation.

Lateral Position. When the kidney and pelvis rotate more than 180 degrees but less than 360 degrees, or when reverse rotation of up to 180 degrees takes place, the pelvis faces laterally and the kidney parenchyma resides medially. The renal vascular supply provides the only clue to the actual direction of excursion. Vessels that course ventral to the kidney to

Figure 38–30. Rotation of the kidney during its ascent from the pelvis. The left kidney with its renal artery and the aorta are viewed in transverse section to show normal and abnormal rotation during its ascent to the adult site. *A,* Primitive embryonic position, hilus faces ventrad (anterior). *B,* Normal adult position, hilus faces mediad. *C,* Incomplete rotation. *D,* Hyperrotation, hilus faces dorsad (posterior). *E,* Hyperrotation, hilus faces laterad. *F,* Reverse rotation, hilus faces laterad. (From Gray, S. W., and Skandalakis, J. E.: Embryology for Surgeons. Philadelphia, W. B. Saunders Co., 1972.)

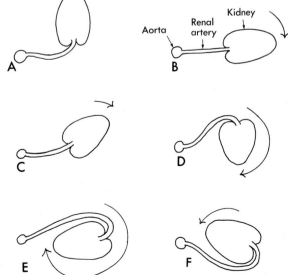

enter a laterally or dorsolaterally placed hilum suggest reverse rotation, whereas a patch dorsal to the kidney implies excessive ventral rotation. Both types of anomalous turning have been cited in Weyrauch's series (1939).

In cases of isolated malrotation, certain other characteristic features may be present. The kidney itself is discoid, elongated, oval, or triangular, with flattened anterior and posterior surfaces. Fetal lobulations are invariably present and accentuated beyond normal limits. A dense amount of fibrous tissue encases the hilar area, possibly even distorting and fixing the pelvis. The ureteropelvic junction may be distorted as well. The upper ureter initially courses laterally, and it too may be encased in this fibrous tissue. The pelvis is elongated and narrow, and the calyces, especially the superior calyx, may be stretched. The blood supply, as previously described, may vary widely, depending on the direction and degree of rotation. The vasculature may consist of a single vessel with or without multiple additional branches entering the parenchyma along the course of the renal artery. In addition, there may be a polar vessel in conjunction with the main renal artery. The manner of the vascular orientation around the kidney provides the only clue to the type and extent of renal rotation, i.e., whether medial or lateral rotation has occurred.

SYMPTOMS

Rotation anomalies per se do not produce specific symptoms. The excessive amount of fibrous tissue encasing the pelvis, ureteropelvic junction, and upper ureter, however, may lead to a relative or actual obstruction. Vascular compression from an accessory artery may contribute to diminished drainage. Symptoms of hydronephrosis, namely, dull aching flank pain, may be experienced during periods of increased urine production. This is the most frequent cause of symptoms. Hematuria, which occurs occasionally with a hydronephrotic collecting system, may be noted as well. Infection and calculus formation, each with its attendant symptoms, may also occur secondary to poor urinary drainage.

DIAGNOSIS

The diagnosis may be surmised by the presence of a renal calculus in an abnormal location, but confirmation should be obtained only from an excretory urogram or retrograde pyelogram (Fig. 38–31). This reveals the abnormal orientation of the renal pelvis and calyces, a flattened and elongated pelvis, a stretched superior calyx

with blunting of the remaining calyces, and a laterally displaced upper third of the ureter. Bilaterality is not uncommon and may lead to the diagnosis of a horseshoe kidney. However, careful inspection for an isthmus and observation of the lower pole renal outline should help to distinguish the two entities.

PROGNOSIS

No abnormality of function of the kidney has been detected secondary to the malrotation, and this anomaly is therefore compatible with normal longevity. Hydronephrosis resulting from impaired urinary drainage may lead to infection and calculus formation with their sequelae.

ANOMALIES OF RENAL VASCULATURE

Aberrant, Accessory, or Multiple Vessels

Knowledge of the anatomy of the renal blood supply is important to every urologic surgeon, and fortunately this subject lends itself to easy investigation. Anatomists were keenly interested in renal vascular patterns before the turn of the century, but the advent of aortography in the 1940's and 1950's spearheaded a systematic clinical approach to this topic. Most of the classic work was performed by investigators in the middle to late 1950's and early 1960's (Anson and Kurth, 1955; Anson and Daseler, 1961; Geyer and Poutasse, 1962; Graves, 1954, 1956; Merklin and Michels, 1958).

The kidney is divided into various segments, each supplied by a single "end" arterial branch that generally courses from one main renal artery. "Multiple renal arteries" is the correct term to describe any kidney supplied by more than one vessel. The term "anomalous vessels" or "aberrant vessels" should be reserved for those arteries that originate from vessels other than the aorta or main renal artery. The term "accessory vessels" denotes two or more arterial branches supplying the same renal segment.

Incidence. Seventy-one (Merklin and Michels, 1958) to 85 per cent (Geyer and Poutasse, 1962) of kidneys have one artery that supplies the entire renal parenchyma. A slightly higher percentage of right-sided kidneys (87 per cent) have a single renal artery (Geyer and Poutasse, 1962). This figure is not influenced significantly by either sex or race. True aberrant

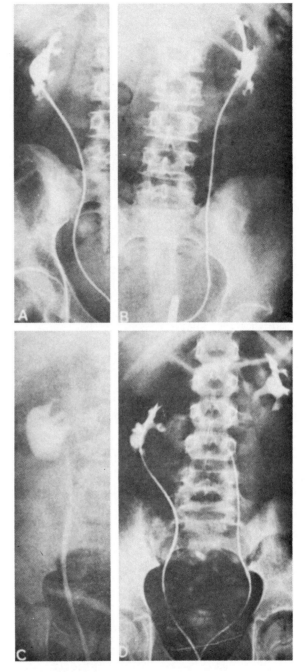

Figure 38–31. Congenital renal malrotation. *A,* Complete; the pelvis faces median. *B,* Pelvis faces posteriorly. *C,* Complete renal rotation in a 20-month-old girl with abnormally high insertion of the ureter into the pelvis. *D,* Diminutive malrotated pelvis in a 5-year-old girl. Urinary infection was the indication for urologic examination in cases *A* to *D.* (From Campbell, M. F.: *In* Campbell, M. F., and Harrison, J. H.: Urology, Vol. 2, 3rd ed. Philadelphia, W. B. Saunders Co., 1970.)

vessels are rare except in patients with renal ectopia with and without fusion and in patients with horseshoe kidney.

Embryology. The renal arterial tree is derived from three groups of primitive vascular channels that coalesce to form the mature vascular pattern for all retroperitoneal structures. The cranial group consists of two pairs of arteries dorsal to the suprarenal gland that shift dorsally to form the phrenic artery. The middle group is made up of three pairs of vessels that pass through the suprarenal area. They retain the same lateral position and become the adrenal artery. Finally, the caudal group has four pairs of arteries that cross ventral to the suprarenal area and become the main renal artery, but sometimes they are joined by the most inferior pair from the middle group (Guggemos, 1962). It is believed that during renal migration this network of vessels selectively degenerates, and the remaining adjacent arteries assume a progressively more important function. By a process of elimination, one primitive renal arterial pair eventually becomes the dominant vessel, the completed process being dependent on the final position of the kidney (Graves, 1956). Polar arteries or multiple renal arteries to the normally positioned kidney represent a failure of complete degeneration of all primitive vascular channels. The multiple vessel pattern that has been described for renal ectopia should be considered an arrested embryonic state for that particular renal position (Gray and Skandalakis, 1972).

Description. On the basis of vascular supply, the renal parenchyma is divided into five segments—apical, upper, middle, lower, and posterior (Fig. 38–32). The main renal artery divides initially into anterior and posterior branches. The anterior branch almost always supplies the upper, middle, and lower segments of the kidney. The posterior branch invariably nourishes the posterior segment. The vessel to the apical segment has the greatest variation in origin; it arises from (1) the anterior division (43 per cent); (2) the junction of the anterior and posterior divisions (23 per cent); (3) the main stem renal artery or aorta (23 per cent); or (4) the posterior division of the main renal artery (10 per cent) (Graves, 1954). Rarely, the upper segment is supplied from a branch totally separate from the main renal artery (Merklin and Michels, 1958).

The lower renal segment, however, is often fed by an accessory vessel. This vessel is usually the most proximal branch when it arises from the main renal artery or its anterior division (Graves, 1954). However, it may originate directly from the aorta near the main renal artery, or it may be aberrant, arising from the gonadal vessel. A summary of findings by Merklin and Michels (1958), who analyzed reports of almost 11,000 kidneys, is depicted in Table 38–1. The relationship of the main renal artery and its proximal branches to the renal vein can be seen in Figure 38–33.

Symptoms. The symptoms attributable to renal vascular anomalies are those that result from inadequate urinary drainage. Multiple, aberrant, or accessory vessels may constrict an infundibulum, a major calyx, or the ureteropelvic junction (Fig. 38–34). Pain or hematuria secondary to hydronephrosis or signs and symptoms of urinary tract infection or calculus formation may result.

Diagnosis. Excretory urography may suggest multiple renal vessels or an aberrant artery when (1) a filling defect in the pelvis is consistent with an anomalous vascular pattern; (2) hydronephrosis is noted with a sharp cutoff in the superior infundibulum (Fraley, 1966, 1969); (3) ureteropelvic junction obstruction is present; or (4) differences are noted in the timing and concentration of one renal segment or the entire kidney (especially when hypertension is present).

Prognosis. The various patterns of renal blood supply do not increase the kidney's susceptibility to disease. Hydronephrosis secondary to a vascular anomaly is indeed a very rare finding, especially when one considers the relative frequency of all renal vascular variations. Hypertension is no more frequent in the patient with multiple renal arteries than in the patient with a single renal vessel (Geyer and Poutasse, 1962). Nathan (1958) did report the development of orthostatic proteinuria in seven patients with a lower pole renal artery that wrapped around and compressed the main renal vein.

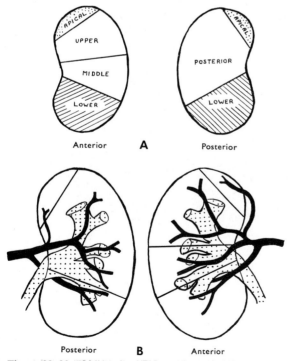

Figure 38–32. Usual pattern of arteries to the kidney. *A*, The five vascular lobes of Graves. *B*, Relationships of renal artery branch and renal pelvis to the five lobes. (From Graves, F. T.: Br. J. Surg., *42*:132, 1954.)

Renal Artery Aneurysm

Aneurysm was the first disease of the renal artery to be recognized (Poutassse, 1957), and until selective renal angiography came into vogue, it was considered a rare occurrence. The

TABLE 38–1. VARIATIONS IN THE ARTERIAL SUPPLY TO THE KIDNEY*

	Condition	Per Cent
	1 Hilar artery	71.1
	1 Hilar artery and 1 upper pole branch	12.6
	2 Hilar arteries	10.8
	1 Hilar artery and 1 upper pole aortic artery	6.2
	1 Hilar artery and 1 lower pole aortic artery	6.9
	1 Hilar artery and 1 lower pole branch	3.1
	3 Hilar arteries	1.7
	2 Hilar arteries, one with upper pole branch	2.7
	Other variations	—

*From Gray, S. W., and Skandalakis, J. E. (Eds.): Embryology for Surgeons. Philadelphia, W. B. Saunders Co., 1972.

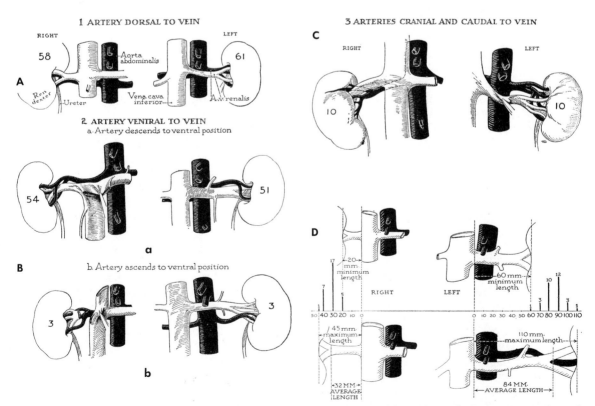

Figure 38–33. Relationships of renal arteries and veins. *A,* Artery dorsal to vein (47.6 per cent). *B,* Artery ventral to vein (*B a,* 42 per cent; *B b,* 2.4 per cent). *C,* Artery cranial and caudal to vein (8.0 per cent). *D,* Maximum, minimum, and average lengths of the renal pedicle in 30 successive specimens. (From Anson, B. J., and Daseler, E. H.: Surg. Gynecol. Obstet., *112*:439, 1961. By permission of Surgery, Gynecology & Obstetrics.)

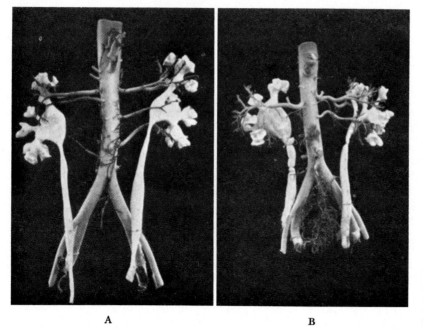

A

B

Figure 38–34. Accessory renal vessels demonstrated by celluloid corrosion preparation. *A,* In a full-term fetus. The renal pelves and ureters are shown in relationship to the main arterial distribution. On each side there are two accessory renal vessels above and one below, the lower one on the left being in proximity to the uretero-vesical junction. *B,* In an 8-month-old fetus in which the kidney on the right had one renal artery but the organ on the left had an accessory branch to the lower renal pole. Yet the location of the lower accessory vessel on the left does not suggest that it might cause ureteral obstruction. On the right there are early hydronephrosis, secondary kinking, and narrowing at the ureterovesical junction. (Courtesy of Dr. Duncan Morison.)

overall incidence has been calculated to be between 0.1 and 0.3 per cent. Abeshouse (1951), in a comprehensive review, classified renal artery aneurysms as follows: saccular, fusiform, dissecting, and arteriovenous. The saccular aneurysm, a localized outpouching that communicates with the arterial lumen by a narrow or wide opening, is the most common type, accounting for 93 per cent of all aneurysms (Hageman et al., 1978; McKeil et al., 1966; Stanley et al., 1975; Zinman and Libertino, 1982). When it is located where the main artery bifurcates into anterior and posterior divisions or at one of the more distal branchings, it is considered to be congenital in origin and is called a fusiform type (Poutasse, 1957). The presence of similar aneurysms at branching points in the vasculature of other organ systems attests to this possible origin. Acquired aneurysms may be located anywhere and result from inflammatory, traumatic, or degenerative factors. A localized defect in the internal elastic tissue and the media allows the vessel to dilate at that point. It is a true aneurysm because its walls are composed of one or more layers of the renal artery (Poutasse, 1957). The outpouchings may vary in size from 1 to 2 cm up to 10 cm (Garritano, 1957).

Most renal artery aneurysms are silent, especially in children. Some produce symptoms at a later age in relation to their size. Pain, hematuria (microscopic and macroscopic), and hypertension secondary to compression of adjacent parenchyma or to altered blood flow

within the vascular tree can occur (Glass and Uson, 1967). This latter sign is renin-mediated, secondary to relative parenchymal ischemia.

The diagnosis may be suspected when a pulsatile mass is palpated in the region of the renal hilus or when a bruit is heard on abdominal auscultation. A wreathlike calcification in the area of the renal artery or its branches (30 per cent) is highly suggestive (Silvis et al., 1956). Selective renal angiography (Cerny et al., 1968) or digital subtraction angiography is needed to confirm the diagnosis.

Many asymptomatic renal artery aneurysms come to light following discovery of hypertension. Fifty per cent are diagnosed when a renal arteriogram is performed for other reasons (Zinman and Libertino, 1982). Generally, excision is recommended if (1) the hypertension cannot be easily controlled; (2) incomplete ringlike calcification is present; (3) the aneurysm is larger than 2.5 cm (Poutasse, 1975); (4) the patient is likely to become pregnant; or (5) the aneurysm increases in size on serial angiograms or an arteriovenous fistula is present. The likelihood of spontaneous rupture (about 10 per cent) with its dire consequences dictates attentive treatment in the foregoing situations.

Renal Arteriovenous Fistula

Although rare, renal arteriovenous fistulas have been discovered with increasing frequency since they were first described by Varela in

1928. Two types exist, congenital and acquired (Maldonado et al., 1964), with the latter (secondary to trauma, inflammation, renal surgery, or postpercutaneous needle biopsy) accounting for the recent increased incidence. Only the congenital variant will be discussed here.

Less than 25 per cent of all arteriovenous fistulas are of the congenital type, which is identifiable by its cirsoid configuration and multiple communications between the main or segmental renal arteries and veins (Crummy et al., 1965; Cho and Stanley, 1978). Although it is considered congenital (because of similar arteriovenous malformations elsewhere in the body), it rarely presents clinically before the third or fourth decade. Females are affected three times as often as males, and the right kidney is involved slightly more than the left (Cho and Stanley, 1978). The lesion is generally located in the upper pole (45 per cent of cases), but not infrequently it may be found in the midportion (30 per cent) or lower pole (25 per cent) of the kidney (Yazaki et al., 1976). A total of 91 cases have been reported (Takaha et al., 1980).

The exact cause remains an enigma, but the condition is thought to be either present at birth or the result of a congenital aneurysm that erodes ino an adjacent vein and slowly enlarges (Thomason et al., 1972). The pathophysiology involved in the shunting of blood, which bypasses the renal parenchyma and rapidly joins the venous circulation and returns to the heart, results in a varied clinical picture. The myriad symptoms are based on the size of the arteriovenous malformation and the length of time it has existed (Messing et al., 1976).

The hemodynamic derangement often produces a loud bruit (in 75 per cent of cases). Diminished perfusion of renal parenchyma distal to the fistulous site leads to relative ischemia and renin-mediated hypertension (40 to 50 per cent) (McAlhany et al., 1971). The increased venous return and high cardiac output with concomitant diminution in peripheral resistance may result in left ventricular hypertrophy and eventually in high-output cardiac failure (50 per cent) (Maldonado et al., 1964). In addition, the arteriovenous fistula usually is located close to the collecting system, and macroscopic and microscopic hematuria may occur in more than 75 per cent of affected individuals (Messing et al., 1976; Cho and Stanley, 1978). Although flank or abdominal pain may be present, a mass is rarely felt (10 per cent).

Excretory urography may reveal diminished or absent function in either one segment of the involved kidney or the entire renal unit (DeSai and DeSautels, 1973), an irregular filling defect in the renal pelvis or calyces (secondary to either clot or encroachment by the fistula), and calyceal distortion or obstruction distal to the site of the lesion (Gunterberg, 1968). Despite these specific radiographic features, an abnormality may be noted in only 50 per cent of excretory urograms. Selective renal arteriography is the most definitive method for diagnosing the lesion. A cirsoid appearance with multiple small tortuous channels, prompt venous filling, and an enlarged renal and possibly gonadal vein are pathognomonic for a renal arteriovenous fistula (DeSai and DeSautels, 1973).

The symptomatic nature of this lesion, which causes a progressive derangement in the cardiovascular system, often dictates surgical intervention. The congenital variant rarely behaves like its acquired counterpart, which may disappear spontaneously after several months. Nephrectomy, partial nephrectomy, vascular ligation (Boijsen and Kohler, 1962), selective embolization (Bookstein and Goldstein, 1973), and balloon catheter occlusion (Bentson and Crandalls, 1972) have been employed to obliterate the fistula.

ANOMALIES OF THE COLLECTING SYSTEM

Anomalies of the collecting system may be classified as follows:

I. Calyx and infundibulum
  A. Calyceal diverticulum
  B. Hydrocalycosis
  C. Megacalycosis
  D. Unipapillary kidney
  E. Extrarenal calyces
  F. Anomalous calyx (pseudotumor of kidny)
  G. Infundibulopelvic dysgenesis
II. Pelvis
  A. Extrarenal pelvis
  B. Bifid pelvis

CALYX AND INFUNDIBULUM

Calyceal Diverticulum

A calyceal diverticulum is a cystic cavity, lined by transitional epithelium, lying in the renal substance and situated peripheral to a minor calyx to which it is connected by a narrow channel. This abnormality, first described by Rayer in 1841, may be multiple, with the upper calyx being most frequently affected.

An incidence of 4.5 per 1000 excretory urograms has been reported (Timmons et al., 1975). A similar incidence has been noted in both children and adults, with no predilection for either side or sex.

Congenital and acquired factors have been suggested to explain the formation of calyceal diverticula. The similarity of incidence in children and adults is consistent with an embryologic etiology (Abeshouse, 1950; Devine et al., 1969; Mathieson, 1953; Middleton and Pfister, 1974). At the 5-mm stage (of the embryo), some of the ureteral branches of the third and fourth order, which ordinarily degenerate, may persist as isolated branches, resulting in the formation of a calyceal diverticulum.

A localized cortical abscess draining into a calyx has also been postulated as an etiologic factor. Other proposed causes include obstruction secondary to stone formation or infection, renal injury, achalasia, and spasm or dysfunction of one of the sphincters surrounding a minor calyx. Small diverticula are usually asymptomatic and are found incidentally at excretory urography. Calyceal distention with urine sometimes causes pain. Infection and stone formation are complications of stasis or obstruction that can produce symptoms (Siegel and McAlister, 1979). Hematuria may be seen in the presence of stones. In the Mayo Clinic series (Timmons et al., 1975), 39 per cent of patients with calyceal diverticula had calculi.

The diagnosis is made by excretory urography; delayed films are helpful in demonstrating pooling of contrast material in the diverticulum. Retrograde pyelography (Fig. 38–35) and, more recently, computerized tomography are sometimes useful in making the diagnosis and in defining the precise anatomy.

Asymptomatic patients in general do not require treatment. Persistent pain, resistant urinary infections, hematuria, and calculi are indications for surgery (Siegel and McAlister, 1979); if feasible, partial nephrectomy is the treatment of choice.

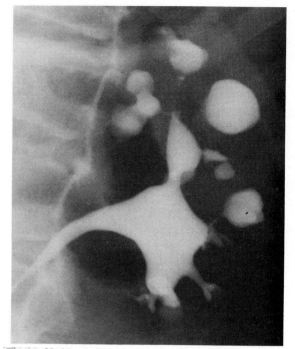

Figure 38–35. A 13-year-old girl with hematuria had a retrograde pyelogram demonstrating multiple calyceal diverticula.

Hydrocalycosis

Hydrocalycosis is a cystic dilatation of a major calyx with a demonstrable connection to the renal pelvis; it is lined by transitional epithelium. It may be caused by a congenital or acquired intrinsic obstruction (Fig. 38–36). This abnormality is rare.

Dilatation of the upper calyx due to obstruction of the upper infundibulum by vessels or stenosis has been described (Fraley, 1966; Johnston and Sandomirsky, 1972). Cicatrization of an infundibulum may result from infection or trauma. Conversely, hydrocalycosis has been reported to occur without an obvious cause (Williams and Mininberg, 1968). It has been postulated (Moore, 1950; Williams and Mininberg, 1968) that achalasia of a ring of muscle at the entrance of the infundibulum into the renal pelvis causes a functional obstruction.

Mild upper calyceal dilatation due to partial infundibular obstruction is relatively common but usually asymptomatic. The most frequent presenting symptom is upper abdominal or flank pain. A mass may be palpated on occasion. Stasis can lead to hematuria or urinary infection, or both.

Hydrocalycosis must be differentiated from

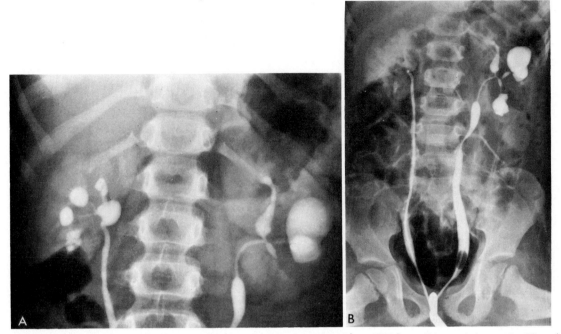

Figure 38–36. Hydrocalycosis of infundibulopelvic stenosis in 3-year-old boy with bilaterally ectopic ureteral orifices (at vesical neck) and other congenital anomalies, who presented with urinary infection. Reflux was not demonstrable, and patient has remained uninfected on chronic suppressive treatment. There has been no urographic change for 5 years. *A,* Excretory urogram. Right infundibular and left infundibulopelvic stenosis. *B,* Retrograde ureteropyelogram (bilateral). Mildly dilated left ureter. Note diffuse tubular backflow on right. (From Malek, R. S.: *In* Kelalis, P. P., and King, L. R. (Eds.): Clinical Pediatric Urology. Philadelphia, W. B. Saunders Co., 1976.)

multiple dilated calyces secondary to ureteral obstruction, calyceal clubbing as a result of recurrent pyelonephritis or medullary necrosis, renal tuberculosis, a large calyceal diverticulum, and megacalycosis. These entities can be differentiated by a combination of excretory urography, findings at surgery, histopathology of removed tissue, and bacteriology.

Hydrocalycosis due to vascular obstruction is usually treated by dismembered infundibulopyelostomy, thus changing the relationship of the infundibulum to the vessel. When the cystic dilatation is due to an intrinsic stenosis of the infundibulum, an intubated infundibulotomy or partial nephrectomy is performed. Although clinical improvement is apparent in most instances, the radiologic appearance often is not altered significantly.

Megacalycosis

Megacalycosis is best defined as nonobstructive enlargement of calyces due to a malformation of the renal papillae (Fig. 38–37). It was first described by Puigvert in 1963. The calyces are generally dilated and malformed and may be increased in number. The renal pelvis is not dilated nor is its wall thickened, and the ureteropelvic junction is normally funneled without evidence of obstruction. The cortical tissue around the abnormal calyx is normal in thickness and shows no signs of scarring or chronic inflammation. The medulla, however, is underdeveloped, assuming a falciform crescent appearance instead of its normal pyramidal shape. The collecting tubules are not dilated but are definitely shorter than normal, and they are oriented transversely rather than vertically from the corticomedullary junction (Puigvert, 1963). A mild disorder of maximum concentrating ability has been reported (Gittes and Talner, 1972), but acid excretion is normal after an acid load (Vela-Navarrete and Garcia Robledo, 1983). Other functions of the kidney—glomerular filtration, renal plasma flow, and iostope uptake—are not altered (Gittes, 1984).

Megacalycosis is most likely to be congenital. It occurs predominantly in males in a ratio of 6:1 and has been found only in Caucasians. Bilateral disease has been seen mostly in males, whereas segmental unilateral involvement oc-

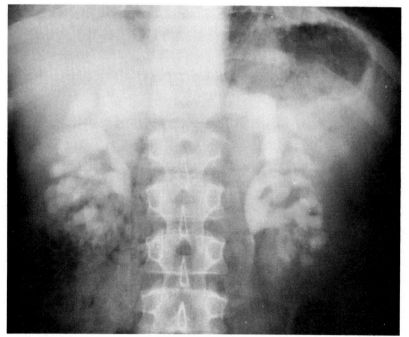

Figure 38–37. Bilateral megacalyces discovered in an 11-year-old boy with abdominal pain and hematuria. He had no history of urinary infection, and voiding cystography did not demonstrate vesicoureteral reflux.

curs only in females. This suggests an X-linked partially recessive gene with reduced penetrance in females (Gittes, 1984).

It has been theorized by Puigvert (1964) and endorsed by Johnston and Sandomirsky, 1972) that there is transient delay in the recanalization of the upper ureter after the branches of the ureteral bud hook up with the metanephric blastema. This produces a short-lived episode of obstruction when the embryonic glomeruli start producing urine. The fetal calyces may dilate and then retain their obstructed appearance despite the lack of evidence of obstruction in postnatal life (Gittes and Talner, 1972). The increased number of calyces frequently seen in this condition may be an aborted response to the obstruction.

Primary hypoplasia of juxtamedullary glomeruli has been suggested as an etiology by Galian et al. (1970), which explains nicely the reason for the lack of concentrating ability; this theory has not been corroborated by others, however.

The abnormality is noticed in children, usually when x-rays are obtained following a urinary tract infection or as part of an evaluation when other congenital anomalies are present. Adults frequently present with hematuria secondary to renal calculi, which leads to excretory urographic investigation.

The calyces are dilated and usually increased in number, but the infundibuli and pelvis may not be enlarged. Although the ureteropelvic junction does not appear obstructed, there may be segmental dilatation of the distal third of the ureter (Kozakewich and Lebowitz, 1974). This anatomic picture not infrequently has been mistaken for congenital ureteropelvic or ureterovesical junction obstruction, with surgery being performed to correct the suspected defect. Postoperatively, the calyceal pattern remains unchanged.

Diuretic renography reveals a normal pattern for the uptake and washout of the isotope, while the Whitaker test does not generate high pressures in the collecting system. Thus, an obstructive picture cannot be delineated. Long-term follow-up of patients with this anomaly does not reveal any progression of the anatomic derangement or functional impairment of the kidney (Gittes, 1984).

Unipapillary Kidney

The unipapillary kidney is an exceptionally rare anomaly in humans. Only six cases have been reported (Harrison et al., 1976; Morimoto et al., 1979; Neal and Murphy, 1960; Sakatoku and Kitayama, 1964; Toppercer, 1980). This anomaly is present not uncommonly in monkeys, rabbits, dogs, marsupials, insectivores, and monotremes. The etiology is thought to be due to a failure of progressive branching after the first three to five generations (which create the pelvis) of the ureteral bud (Potter, cited by Harrison et al., 1976). The solitary calyx drains a ridgelike papilla. Nephrons attach to fewer collecting tubules, which then drain directly into the pelvis.

The kidney is smaller than normal but usually is in its correct location. The arterial tree, although sparse, has a normal configuration. The opposite kidney is frequently absent. Genital anomalies are often present. The condition is frequently asymptomatic, being discovered fortuitously in most instances.

Extrarenal Calyces

Extrarenal calyces is an uncommon congenital anomaly in which the major calyces as well as the renal pelvis are outside the mass of the kidney (Fig. 38–38). This entity was originally reviewed by Eisendrath in 1925 and then more extensively by Malament et al. in 1961. The kidney is usually discoid, with the pelvis and the major and minor calyces located outside the renal parenchyma. The renal vessels have an anomalous distribution and enter the kidneys usually at the circumferential edge of the flat, widened hilus. Malament considered this condition embryologically to be the result of an abnormal nephrogenic anlage or an early and rapidly developing ureteral bud.

Extrarenal calyces usually do not produce symptoms, although failure to drain normally may lead to stasis, infection, and calculi. The dilated, blunted calyces may mimic the radiographic changes usually seen with pyelonephritis or obstruction and should be distinguished from these entities. Surgery is reserved for cases in which infection or obstruction is demonstrated.

Anomalous Calyx (Pseudotumor of the Kidney)

A number of normal variants of the pyelocalyceal system in the kidney have been described. One such entity presents as a localized mass, usually situated between the infundibula of the upper and middle calyceal groups, and is called a hypertrophied column of Bertin (Fig. 38–39). The column may be sufficiently large to compress and deform the adjacent pelvis and calyces, suggesting a mass on the excretory urogram; this is the so-called pseudotumor. The individual calyces, however, are normally shaped and developed.

It is important to differentiate this calyceal anomaly from true disease of the calyx or from a parenchymal tumor. A renal scan will show normal uptake of the isotope in this area (Parker et al., 1976).

Infundibulopelvic Dysgenesis

Infundibulopelvic stenosis most likely forms a link between the cystic dysplastic kidney and

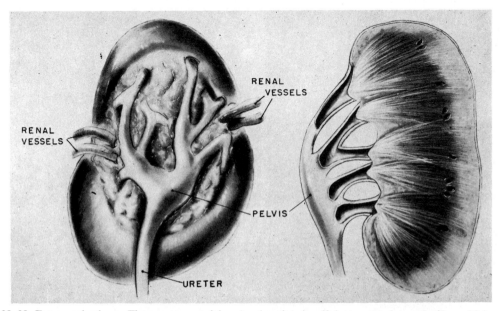

Figure 38–38. Extrarenal calyces. These represent delayed rather than insufficient ureteral growth. (From Malament, M., et al., Am. J. Roentgenol., *86*:823, 1961.)

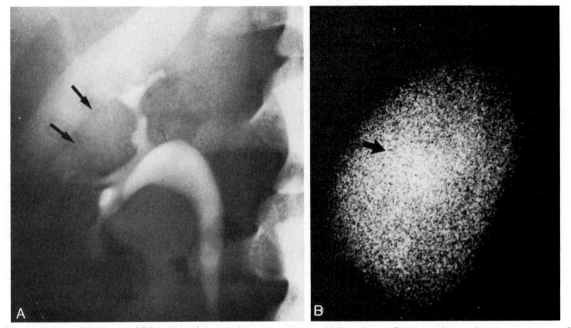

Figure 38–39. *A,* This child has a mass effect with splaying of the middle calyces. *B,* A renal scan demonstrates normal uptake in the area (arrow) suggesting the "pseudotumor" is really a hypertrophied column of Bertin.

the grossly hydronephrotic one (Kelalis and Malek, 1981). This condition includes a variety of roentgenographically dysmorphic kidneys with varying degrees of infundibular or infundibulopelvic stenosis that may be associated with renal dysplasia (Fig. 38–40).

Infundibulopelvic stenosis is usually bilateral and is commonly associated with lower urinary tract abnormalities, such as posterior urethral valves or vesicoureteral reflux. It must be differentiated from renal malignancies and the usual forms of hydronephrosis.

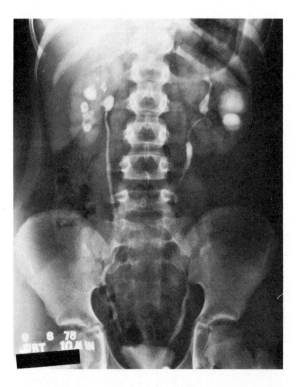

Figure 38–40. Excretory urogram in an 18-year-old boy with one urinary tract infection shows severe stenosis of the infundibula and left ureteropelvic junction and a milder form of infundibulopelvic dysgenesis in the right kidney. Vesicoureteral reflux was absent on voiding cystourethrography. (Courtesy of Dr. Panos Kelalis.)

PELVIS

Extrarenal Pelvis

An extrarenal pelvis is of clinical importance only when drainage is impaired. This is sometimes associated with a variety of kidney abnormalities, including malposition and malrotation, that predispose to urinary stasis, infection, and calculous disease.

Bifid Pelvis

Approximately 10 per cent of normal renal pelves are bifid, the pelvis dividing first at or just within its entrance to the kidney to form two major calyces. Bifid pelvis should be considered a variant of normal. No increased incidence of disease has been reported in patients with this entity. When further division of the renal pelvis occurs, triplication of the pelvis may result, but this is extremely rare.

ANOMALIES OF THE URETEROPELVIC JUNCTION

Anomalies of the ureteropelvic junction may be classified as follows:
I. Ureteropelvic junction obstruction
  A. Intrinsic
  B. Extrinsic
  C. Secondary

URETEROPELVIC JUNCTION OBSTRUCTION

Hydronephrosis due to congenital ureteropelvic junction obstruction is one of the more common anomalies seen in childhood. It is defined as an impediment to urinary flow from the renal pelvis into the ureter. Inefficient drainage of urine at this point leads to progressive dilatation of the collecting system and a further diminution in the efficiency of pelvic emptying (Whitaker, 1975). Initially, the muscle of the renal pelvis hypertrophies, and glomerular filtration diminishes to accommodate the obstruction process. Eventually, when the limit of kidney compromise is reached, destruction of renal parenchyma and impairment of function ensue.

Only primary congenital ureteropelvic junction obstruction is considered in this chapter. Other conditions that delay proximal urinary drainage and secondarily affect the ureteropelvic junction will be discussed in Chapter 65.

INCIDENCE

Ureteropelvic junction obstruction is seen in all pediatric age groups. Nearly 25 per cent of cases, however, are discovered within the first year of life (Fig. 38–41) (Williams and Kenawi, 1976). With the increased use of pre-natal ultrasound studies, it is being discovered routinely in utero. In fact, it is *the* most common cause of dilatation of the collecting system in the fetal kidney, far exceeding the incidence of multicystic dysplastic kidneys (Colodny et al., 1980). Relatively few cases are noted beyond puberty and into adulthood. It occurs more commonly in males (Johnston et al., 1977; Kelalis et al., 1971; Williams and Karlaftis, 1966),

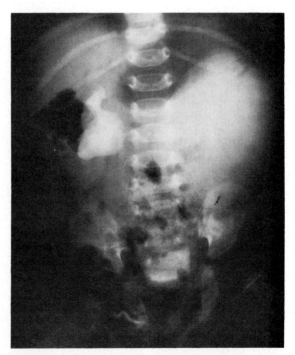

Figure 38–41. Palpation of a smooth, soft abdominal mass that transilluminated in a 3-year-old boy led to this excretory urogram, which at 6 hours reveals a ureteropelvic junction obstruction with severe hydronephrosis. An intrinsic narrowing at the ureteropelvic junction was found at surgery.

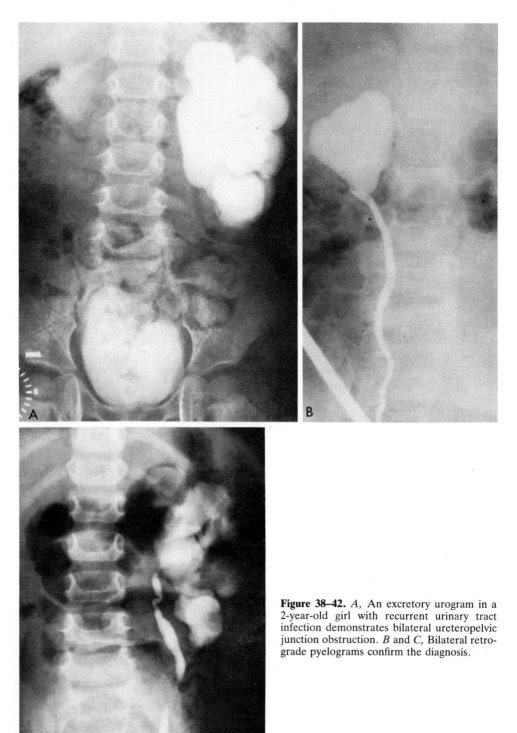

Figure 38–42. *A*, An excretory urogram in a 2-year-old girl with recurrent urinary tract infection demonstrates bilateral ureteropelvic junction obstruction. *B* and *C*, Bilateral retrograde pyelograms confirm the diagnosis.

especially in the newborn period, when the ratio exceeds 2:1 (Johnston et al., 1977; Robson et al., 1976; Williams and Kenawi, 1976). Left-sided lesions predominate, and in the neonate more than two thirds occur on this side. Bilateral ureteropelvic obstruction is present in 10 to 40 per cent of cases (Fig. 38–42) (Johnston et al., 1977; Lebowitz and Griscom, 1977; Nixon, 1953; Robson et al., 1976; Uson et al., 1968; Williams and Kenawi, 1976), and again this occurs most frequently in the newborn or the infant less than 6 months of age (Perlmutter et al., 1980; Snyder et al., 1980). Unilateral and bilateral ureteropelvic junction obstruction affecting members of more than one generation has been reported in several families (Cohen et al., 1978). A dominant autosomal pattern of inheritance with variable penetrance has been suggested.

ETIOLOGY

The exact etiology of ureteropelvic junction obstruction sometimes remains an enigma despite investigations along embryologic (Allen, 1973; Osathanondh and Potter, 1963; Ruano-Gil et al., 1975), anatomic (Johnston, 1969, Nixon, 1953), functional (Whitaker, 1975), and histologic (Hanna et al., 1976; Murnaghan, 1958; Notley, 1968) lines. Hydronephrosis is most often due to a narrowing at the ureteropelvic junction (Allen, 1973; Lebowitz and Griscom, 1977). A localized area of developmental arrest, produced by fetal vessels compressing the ureter, has been suggested by Allen (1973) and Osathanondh and Potter (1963). Ruano-Gil et al. (1975) showed that the embryonic ureter goes through a solid phase with subsequent recanalization. Failure of complete canalization of the upper end of the ureter may be the cause of ureteropelvic junction obstruction.

Intrinsic. An intrinsic lesion within the ureteropelvic wall may sometimes be the basis for obstruction even in the absence of a gross anatomic cause. Murnaghan (1958) demonstrated an interruption in the development of the circular musculature of the ureteropelvic junction. Whitaker (1975) incorporated these findings and theorized that the renal pelvis cannot effectively create a bolus of fluid at its junction with the ureter when it is not funnel-shaped. During an episode of diuresis, the pelvis distends more and loses its already poorly funneled appearance, so that emptying is further impeded (Whitaker, 1975). Notley (1968) and Hanna and associates (1976) learned from electron microscopic studies of the ureteropelvic junction that the muscle cell orientation is normal but that there is an excessive amount of collagen fibers and ground substance between and around the muscle cells. As a result, muscle fibers are widely separated, and their points of connection, or nexuses, are attenuated. Many cells are actually atrophic. These findings are thought to be responsible for a functional discontinuity of ureteropelvic muscular contractions that result in inefficient emptying and apparent ureteropelvic junction obstruction.

Less common causes of intrinsic ureteropelvic junction obstruction include valvular mucosal folds (Maizels and Stephens, 1980), persistent fetal convolutions (Leiter, 1979), and upper ureteral polyps (Colgan et al., 1973; Gup, 1975; Thorup et al., 1981; Williams and Kenawi, 1976; Williams et al., 1980).

Congenital folds are a variant of ureteral valves and are a common finding in the upper ureter of fetuses after the fourth month of development, a finding that may persist until the newborn period (Fig. 38–43). They are mucosal infoldings with an axial offshoot of

Figure 38–43. Congenital mucosal folds are outlined on a retrograde injection of this specimen taken from an 8-month-old gestational age stillborn fetus. The convolutions do not distend during the injection.

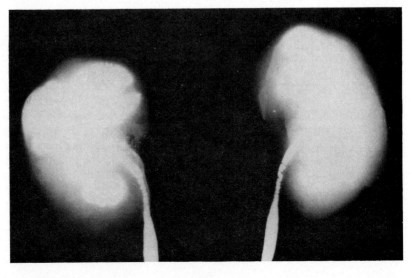

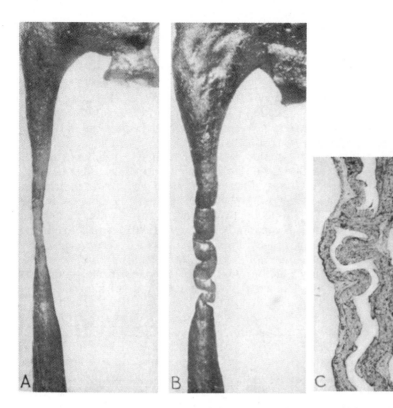

Figure 38–44. Embryologic considerations in the genesis of ureteral fold, kinks, and strictures. *A,* Cast of the ureter and the renal pelvis in a newborn. There is physiologic narrowing of the upper ureter below, which is the normal main spindle of the ureter. No ureteral folds are present. *B,* Cast of the ureter and the renal pelvis in the newborn. The ureteral folds proceed alternately from the opposite sides. *C,* Ureteral kinks that appear as muscular folds with axial offshoots of the loose adventitia. (Courtesy of Dr. Karl Östling.) (From Campbell, M. F.: *In* Campbell, M. F., and Harrison, J. H. (Eds.): Urology, Vol. 2, 3rd ed. Philadelphia, W. B. Saunders Co., 1970.)

adventitia that does not flatten out when the ureter is distended or stretched (Fig. 38–44). The exterior surface has a smooth appearance owing to adventitial bridges (Johnston, 1969). The epithelial folds are secondary to different growth rates of the ureter and the body of the child, with excessive ureteral length occurring early in gestation. This provides a "length reserve" for the ureter, which traverses a shorter distance in the newborn than in the adult (Östling, 1942). Others have felt that congenital folds may represent a phenomenon similar to persistence of Chwalla's membrane in the lower ureter, which produces a ureteral valve (Mering et al., 1972). Östling thought that folds were a precursor of actual ureteropelvic junction obstruction because they are frequently discovered in babies who have contralateral ureteropelvic obstruction. Ordinarily, folds are not obstructive and disappear with growth (Leiter, 1979). They are rarely seen in the older child or the adult. Exaggerated or persistent fetal infoldings containing muscle, or high insertion of a valvular leaflet at the ureteropelvic junction, however, might indeed become obstructive (Maizels and Stephens, 1980). This type of obstruction sometimes can be relieved by dissecting the folds and eliminating the kinking (Johnston, 1969), but more commonly the ureteral portion containing the valve must be excised. Severe vesicoureteral reflux can produce kinking and angulation of the upper ureter that resembles this picture of fetal folds and may well represent a return to the fetal state. Obstruction at the ureteropelvic junction secondary to severe reflux can be a consequence of this condition.

Extrinsic. The most common cause of extrinsic ureteropelvic obstruction is an aberrant, accessory, or early branching vessel to the lower pole of the kidney. These vessels pass anterior to the ureteropelvic junction or upper ureter and have been suggested as a cause of obstruction. Nixon (1953) reported that 25 of 78 cases of ureteropelvic obstruction were secondary to vascular compression (Fig. 38–45). The incidence in other series has varied from 15 to 38 per cent (Ericsson et al., 1961; Johnston et al., 1977; Stephens, 1982; Williams and Kenawi, 1976). Recently, this association has been questioned. It is felt by a number of observers that the vessel may well exacerbate a pre-existing intrinsic lesion, since freeing the involved vessel does not always appear to relieve the obstruction. However, there is no doubt that a certain number of ureteropelvic obstructions are vascular in origin. Stephens (1982) has theorized that when an aberrant or accessory renal artery to the lower pole of the kidney is present and the ureter courses behind it, the ureter may angulate at two places—the ureteropelvic junction and the point at which it drapes over the vessel as the pelvis fills and bulges anteriorly.

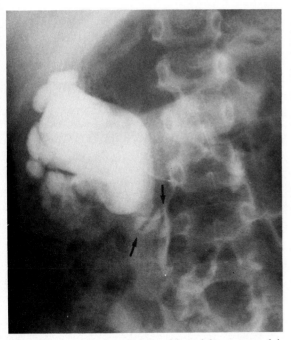

Figure 38–45. A 7-year-old boy with a right ureteropelvic junction obstruction. A retrograde study demonstrates a double kink at the upper end of the ureter. At surgery the ureter was draped over a vessel to the lower pole.

The angulated ureter at the ureteropelvic junction becomes fixed to the pelvis by an array of fascial adhesions. Second, as the ureter arches over the vessel its lumen is compromised by kinking (Fig. 38–46). Thus, a two-point obstruction is created (Johnston, 1969; Nixon, 1953). Freeing the ureter of its adhesions and lifting it off the vessel allow the free flow of urine in most cases. Stephens (1982) found no evidence of fibrosis or stricture at these points when this was done in his series of patients. In addition, he noted that the lumen had a generous caliber in these patients; however, he suggested that with time these areas may become ischemic, fibrotic, and finally stenotic.

Secondary. Ureteropelvic obstruction may also be due to severe vesicoureteral reflux (Lebowitz and Blickman, 1983) or to lower urinary tract obstruction that may cause kinking or tortuosity at the ureteropelvic junction (Hutch et al., 1962; Shopfner, 1966) (Fig. 38–47).

ASSOCIATED ANOMALIES

The incidence of associated congenital anomalies, especially contralateral renal malformations, is high. Another urologic abnormality

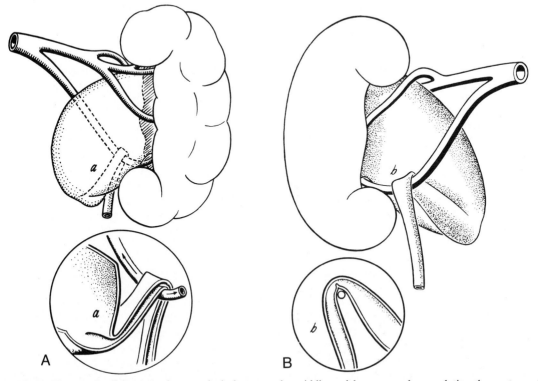

A   B

Figure 38–46. The renal pelvis protrudes anteriorly between the middle and lower vessels, angulating the ureteropelvic junction and hooking the ureter over the vessel. *A* and *B* are anterior and posterior views, respectively, with insets showing flattening and obstructive mechanisms at the ureteropelvic junction and upper ureter. (From Stephens, F. D.: J. Urol., *128*:984, 1982. Used by permission.)

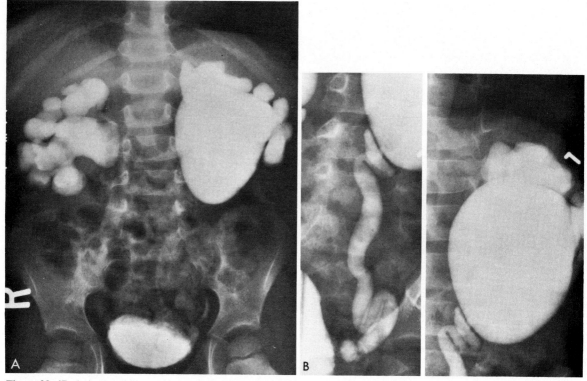

Figure 38–47. A 4-year-old boy with recurrent abdominal pain and episodic low-grade fever had *(A)* an excretory urogram that reveals bilateral ureteropelvic junction obstruction. *B,* A preoperative voiding cystogram demonstrates severe bilateral vesicoureteral reflux with a markedly redundant and kinked left upper ureter producing a secondary ureteropelvic junction obstruction. The milder right-sided obstruction was relieved following correction of the reflux.

may be found in almost 50 per cent of affected babies (Lebowitz and Griscom, 1977; Robson et al., 1976; Uson et al., 1968). Ureteropelvic junction obstruction is the most common anomaly encountered in the opposite kidney; it occurs in 10 to 40 per cent of cases (Fig. 38–48). Renal dysplasia and multicystic kidney disease are the next most frequently observed contralateral lesions (Williams and Karlaftis, 1966). In addition, unilateral renal agenesis has been noted in almost 5 per cent of children (Johnston et al., 1977; Robson et al., 1976; Williams and Kenawi, 1976). Ureteropelvic junction obstruction may also occur in either the upper or the lower half (usually the latter) of a duplicated collecting system (Amar, 1976) (Fig. 38–49) or of a horse-shoe or ectopic kidney.

Minor degrees of vesicoureteral reflux have been noted in as many as 40 per cent of affected children (Lebowitz and Blickman, 1983; Williams and Kenawi, 1976). Generally, this degree of reflux does not contribute to the upper urinary tract obstruction, subsides spontaneously, and is thought to result possibly from the presence of urinary tract infection. Anomalies of other organ systems are infrequently observed and have no consistent pattern of association.

SYMPTOMS

Ureteropelvic junction obstruction usually presents in the neonate or infant as an asymptomatic mass that is palpated on routine examination (Johnston et al., 1977; Robson et al., 1976; Williams and Karlaftis, 1966). Nearly 50 per cent of cases are discovered in this manner. However, it is being diagnosed with increasing frequency prenatally as the use of maternal ultrasonography has gained wide popularity (Fourcroy et al., 1983). Occasionally, failure to thrive, feeding difficulties, or sepsis secondary to urinary tract infection lead the pediatrician to suspect the diagnosis and obtain an excretory urogram. Urinary tract infection is the presenting sign in 30 per cent (Snyder et al., 1980). In the older child, intermittent flank or upper abdominal pain, sometimes associated with vomiting, is a prominent symptom (Kelalis et al., 1971; Williams and Kenawi, 1976). Hematuria, which is seen in 25 per cent of the children (Fig. 38–50), may occur following minor abdom-

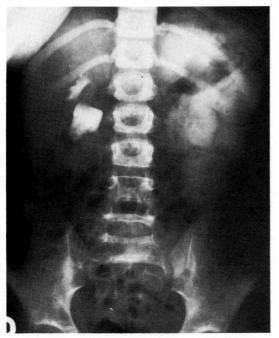

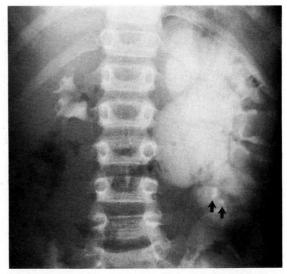

Figure 38–50. A 7-year-old boy with flank pain and hematuria has an obvious ureteropelvic junction obstruction on the left and several stones (arrows) in the lowermost calyx, the result of stasis of urine.

Figure 38–48. An excretory urogram in a 5-year-old girl demonstrates a high-grade obstruction on the left (presumably at the ureteropelvic junction) with a suggestion of a minor ureteropelvic junction obstruction on the right.

inal trauma (Kelalis et al., 1971; Williams and Kenawi, 1976). The hematuria is most probably due to rupture of mucosal vessels in the dilated collecting system (Kelalis et al., 1971).

In the young adult, episodic flank pain, especially during a diuresis, is a common manifestation. Hypertension has also been noted as a presenting sign of ureteropelvic junction obstruction in both adults and children (Grossman et al., 1981; Johnston et al., 1977; Munoz et al., 1977; Squitieri et al., 1974). The pathophysiology is thought to be due to a functional ischemia with reduced renal blood flow (as a result of the enlarged collecting system), producing a renin-mediated hypertension (Belman et al., 1968).

DIAGNOSIS

Whenever the diagnosis of hydronephrosis is suspected prenatally it must be confirmed by a postnatal examination. The fetal and neonatal kidney may show a picture suggesting hydronephrosis on ultrasonography because the pyramids and medullary areas are sometimes sonolucent in the immature kidney. The diagnosis may be confirmed by radioisotopic scanning in the newborn period and by excretory urography in the somewhat older child. Often, children with gastrointestinal complaints have a complete gastrointestinal work-up that is normal, after which the urinary tract is evaluated.

The excretory urogram reveals a distended renal pelvis and calyces, with an abrupt cutoff at the ureteropelvic junction. It is important to obtain delayed films to determine that hydroureter is not present as well (Lebowitz and Griscom, 1977; Snyder et al., 1980). Severe partial obstruction may be present even when the ureter can be visualized beyond the ureter-

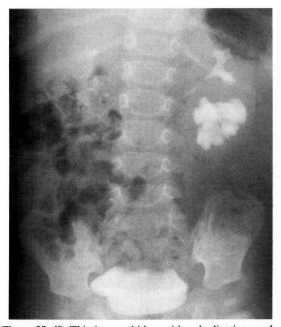

Figure 38–49. This 1-year-old boy with a duplication on the left has an obstruction at the ureteropelvic junction of the lower pole collecting system.

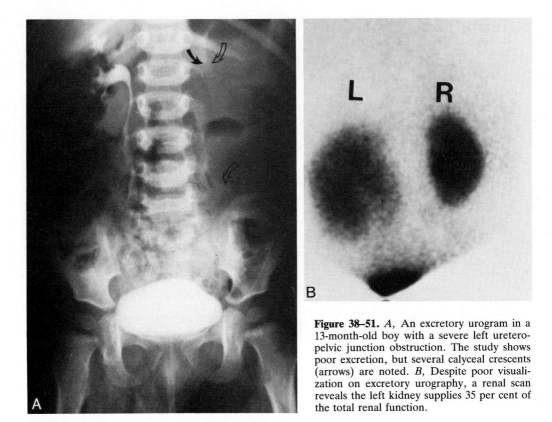

Figure 38–51. *A,* An excretory urogram in a 13-month-old boy with a severe left ureteropelvic junction obstruction. The study shows poor excretion, but several calyceal crescents (arrows) are noted. *B,* Despite poor visualization on excretory urography, a renal scan reveals the left kidney supplies 35 per cent of the total renal function.

opelvic junction. The appearance of calyceal crescents is the result of dilated collecting ducts that have become oriented transversely; it is a reliable sign of upper urinary tract obstruction with recoverable renal function (Fig. 38–51). A retrograde pyelogram performed at the time of surgical correction often helps to delineate the limits of the stricture and the anatomy of the entire ureter.

If the obstruction is equivocal, it is sometimes worthwhile to obtain a diuretic renogram. The rate of uptake of the isotope will delineate the degree of function, and the washout curve following the administration of furosemide will determine the severity of the obstruction (Krueger et al., 1980; O'Reilly et al., 1979). Some patients have intermittent obstruction, which is precipitated only by a diuresis. They may have a normal excretory urogram when asymptomatic but an obstructed picture during an episode of pain (Malek, 1983) (Fig. 38–52). To help define these less clear-cut conditions, a fluoroscopic pressure-flow study can be performed by injecting contrast medium through a percutaneously placed nephrostomy tube and recording intrapelvic pressures during the constant infusion (Krueger et al., 1980; Whitaker, 1973). Alter-

natively, a furosemide-induced diuresis during an excretory urogram or renal scan (Koff, 1982) can be done to determine the efficiency of pelvic emptying (Segura et al., 1974). The diuresis created during the test may also reproduce flank pain if the patient has given a history of it (Nesbit, 1956). The intermittent nature of the signs and symptoms in these patients is usually associated with a vessel crossing the ureteropelvic junction, causing the obstruction.

It is imperative to obtain a voiding cystourethrogram on every patient with ureteropelvic junction obstruction to rule out the possibility of obstruction secondary to vesicoureteral reflux (Lebowitz and Blickman, 1983: Whitaker, 1976).

PROGNOSIS

Severe chronic obstruction may lead to progressive loss of renal function. With severe stasis and infection, stone formation sometimes occurs. Renin-mediated hypertension secondary to obstruction may also develop.

Most obstructed kidneys, however, can be salvaged by pyeloplasty. A quantitative renal scan, using technetium 99–labeled DMSA, that determines individual renal function is some-

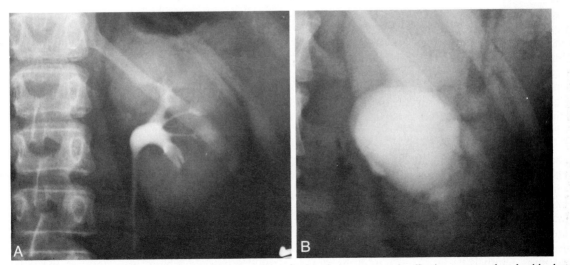

Figure 38–52. *A* and *B,* A 16-year-old boy with intermittent flank pain has a normal collecting system when healthy but severe obstruction when symptomatic.

times helpful in deciding whether to do nephrectomy or pyeloplasty, especially when the excretory urogram reveals a kidney with poor concentrating ability. Most affected kidneys provide at least one third of overall renal function; these can be salvaged. Even poorly functioning kidneys will show some improvement after surgery (Belis et al., 1982; Parker et al., 1981). Only rarely will such kidneys have less than 10 per cent of overall renal function at presentation, and these should probably be removed. The techniques of surgical correction will be discussed in Chapter 65.

ANOMALIES OF THE URETER

Anomalies of the ureter may be classified as follows:

I. Anomalies of number
  A. Agenesis
  B. Duplication
    1. Blind-ending duplication
    2. Inverted Y duplication
  C. Triplication and supernumerary ureters
II. Anomalies of structure
  A. Atresia and hypoplasia
    1. Distal ureteral atresia
  B. Megaureter
    1. Reflux
    2. Obstructed
    3. Nonreflux-nonobstructed
    4. Megaureter in prune belly syndrome
    5. Dysplastic
  C. Ureteral stenosis and stricture
  D. Ureteral valves
  E. Spiral twists and folds of the ureter
  F. Ureteral diverticula
  G. Congenital high insertion of the ureter

III. Anomalies of termination
  A. Vesicoureteral reflux
  B. Ectopic ureter
  C. Ureterocele
    1. Simple
    2. Ectopic
IV. Anomalies of position
  A. Vascular anomalies
    1. Accessory renal vessels
    2. Preureteral vena cava
    3. Preureteral iliac artery (retroiliac ureter)
    4. Ovarian vein syndrome
    5. Distal ureteral vascular obstructions
  B. Herniation of the ureter

Embryology

Before the individual conditions are considered in detail, the disordered embryogenesis common to many ureteral anomalies will be reviewed. Normal embryology of the kidney and ureter is presented in Chapter 37. The stages of normal embryogenesis are well documented, and there are widely accepted explanations and theories for some of the more common primary ureteral anomalies as well. In a review article, Tanagho (1976) correlated and synthesized these into a unified hypothesis for the development of lower ureteral anomalies. These concepts are used as the basis of the following summary.

Briefly, the ureteral bud normally develops from the mesonephric duct at its "elbow," where the duct swings ventrally and medially to join the cloaca. The segment of mesonephric duct between the ureteral bud and the future urogenital sinus is termed the *combined nephric duct* or the *common excretory duct*. Tanagho also calls it the *trigone precursor*, as it will become absorbed progressively into the developing sinus (vesicourethral canal) and contributes mesenchyme to the muscularization of the trigone and underlying detrusor of that area. As the common excretory duct is absorbed into the urogenital sinus, the ureteral bud and meso-

nephric duct acquire separate openings, with the ureteral bud initially located medial and distal to the mesonephric duct. The two orifices migrate in opposing directions, rotating as they do so. The ureteral orifice migrates cephalad and laterally with the developing vesicourethral canal, and the mesonephric duct crosses over the ureter as it moves medially and caudally. Muscularization of the bladder begins after the orifices are well separated, resulting in a separate hiatus for each duct.

Variations in the site of origin of the ureteral bud on the mesonephric duct and supernumerary budding explain a variety of ureterorenal anomalies. The anomalous budding, cephalic or caudal, is associated with varying hypoplasia or dysplasia, or both, of the affected renal segment, related in general to the degree of dislocation (Mackie and Stephens, 1975, Schwarz et al., 1981). This hypothesis of embryogenesis will now be applied to vesicoureteral reflux, ureteral duplication, and ectopic ureter.

Vesicoureteral Reflux (Fig. 38–53). In pri-

PRIMARY REFLUX

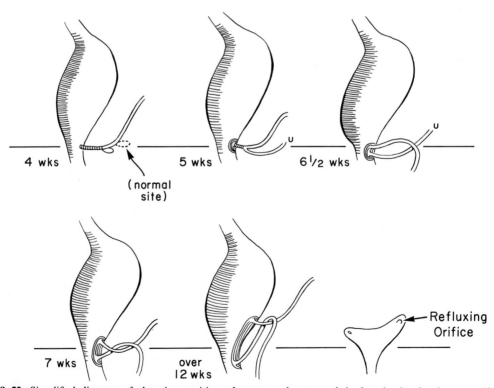

Figure 38–53. Simplified diagram of changing position of ureter and mesonephric duct in the development of primary reflux. (In Figures 38–53 through 38–56, the caudomedial looping of the distal mesonephric duct against the urogenital sinus, which contributes to its absorption, is omitted to simplify the structural relationships. Close position of the ureteral bud to the urogenital sinus results in early absorption into the sinus and more time for cranial and lateral migration of the orifice. See text.) (Modified and redrawn from Tanagho, 1977.)

mary reflux the ureteral bud arises more caudally than normally from the mesonephric duct, resulting in a short common excretory duct. Absorption of the short duct is completely early, giving the now separated ureteral duct a longer period to migrate cranially and laterally before completing its movement. As a result, the separation between the ureter and the mesonephric duct is greater than normal, and there is a large trigone with superior and lateral ureteral orifices. Because the common duct was short, its mesenchymal contribution to the muscular development of the trigone is decreased. Thus, the trigone is not only large but also poorly muscularized. Because there has been less time for the common mesenchyme to accumulate around the developing ureteral bud, the intramural ureter will also be deficient in musculature.

The ultimate result is a large, poorly muscularized trigone with a poorly fixated, laterally positioned ureteral orifice and decreased musculature of the terminal ureter. Owing to the poor attachments of the ureter, the orifice is patulous or gaping and has a deficient submucosal tunnel. The variations encountered clinically in severe vesicoureteral reflux and in altered ureterotrigonal anatomy can be related directly to the degree of dislocation of the ureteral bud toward the urogenital sinus. Additional considerations regarding developmental anatomy in vesicoureteral reflux are found in Chapter 49.

Complete Ureteral Duplication (double ureters) (Fig. 38–54). The commonly accepted explanation of duplication is that an additional ureteral bud arises from the mesonephric duct. The bud closest to the urogenital sinus becomes the lower pole ureter. This bud is absorbed first. The second, higher bud migrates with the mesonephric duct, rotating with it medially and then caudally, before it is attached adjacent but distal to the lower pole orifice at the otherwise normal trigonal location (the Weigert-Meyer law). For additional discussion of the relationship of the ureteral orifices in duplication, see

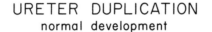

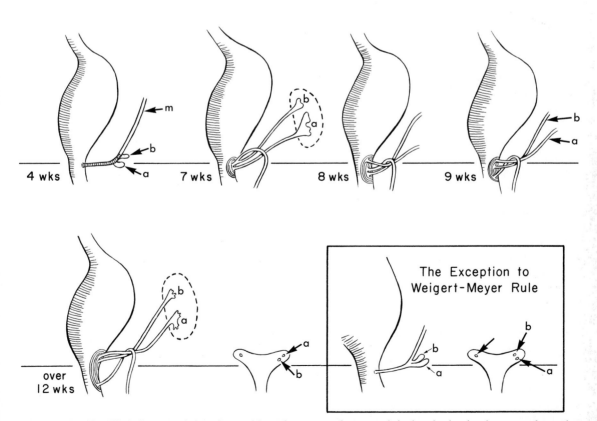

Figure 38–54. Simplified diagram of changing position of ureters and mesonephric duct in the development of complete duplication. (Modified and redrawn from Tanagho, 1977.)

the later section in this chapter, Duplication of the Ureter.

An alternative theory of the genesis of complete duplication is that of immediate fission of a single bud (junctional bud). Just as a bud dividing during its early growth results in a bifid ureter, a junctional bud dividing immediately could result in complete duplication, for the common base would ultimately be absorbed into the urogenital sinus after absorption of the common excretory duct is completed. Stephens (1958, 1963) suggests that this explanation accounts for rarely encountered exceptions to the Weigert-Meyer law (Fig. 38–40). The attachment of the two orifices to the urogenital sinus occurs somewhat later in this circumstance, providing less time for full rotation of the two ureters. (See the later section on duplications of the ureter.)

The terms *orthotopic*, referring to the lower pole ureteral orifice, and *ectopic* or *accessory*, referring to the upper pole ureteral orifice, have been in common use despite the fact that at times either or both orifices may occupy a dislocated position. For this reason and to avoid ambiguity, The Committee on Terminology, Nomenclature and Classification of the Section on Urology, American Academy of Pediatrics, has proposed an alternative terminology (Glassberg et al., 1984). The following terms will be used throughout this chapter: The kidney with two pyelocalyceal systems is a *duplex kidney*. A *bifid system* relates to two pelves joining at the ureteropelvic junction *(bifid pelvis)* or two ureters joining above the bladder *(bifid ureter)*. Two ureters associated with complete duplication are *double ureters*. The ureter draining the upper pole of a duplex kidney is the *upper pole ureter*, and its orifice is the *upper pole orifice*; similarly, the lower pole pelvis is drained by the *lower pole ureter*, and its orifice is the *lower pole orifice*.

An *ectopic ureter* is one draining to a site on the proximal lip of the bladder neck or beyond, whether associated with a duplex or a single system. *Lateral ectopia* of a ureteral orifice is one lateral to the normal position; caudal or medial ectopia of an orifice is one situated at the proximal lip of the bladder neck or beyond. The terminology for ureterocele is also simplified. *Intravesical ureterocele* is located entirely within the bladder. It is usually associated with a single system, uncommonly with an upper pole of a completely duplicated system, and rarely with a lower pole ureter. *Ectopic ureterocele* has some portion of its structure situated at the bladder neck or in the urethra. Its orifice,

however, may be within the bladder, bladder neck, or urethra. Most ectopic ureteroceles are associated with complete duplication, rarely with a single system.

It should be apparent that a number of anomalies of ureteral termination associated with double ureters can result from various alterations in the sites of origin of the two ureteral buds. Clinically, reflux via the lower pole orifice into the lower pelvis is the most common anomaly. Here the first ureteral bud originates too close to the urogenital sinus, and the second or upper pole bud arises from a normal location at the elbow of the mesonephric duct. As a result, the lower pole orifice will be high and lateral, allowing reflux to occur, and the upper pole orifice will terminate more normally on the trigone.

Other combinations can be explained by the same hypothesis. As an example, Figure 38–55 shows the origin of the refluxing lower pole orifice in combination with an ectopic orifice to the bladder neck. In this instance the two ureteral ducts originated well apart on the mesonephric duct, one caudally and one cranially, and they became widely separated by rotation and migration before muscularization began, with the result that separate hiatuses formed in the bladder musculature.

It is not uncommon to encounter symmetric parenchymal thinning of the lower pole segment of a duplicated ureter in the presence of severe reflux to that unit, and diffuse narrowing is more consistent with segmental primary hypoplasia than scarring. Mackie and associates (1975) and Mackie and Stephens (1975) have related this finding to an abnormality of segmental renal development, specifically to the portion of the nephrogenic ridge encountered by the ureteral bud. The normally positioned bud will strike the normal central portion of the ridge, and a normal kidney will result. A bud caudally or cranially misplaced may strike the poorer lower or upper end zones of nephrogenic ridge, resulting in variable degrees of hypoplasia and dysplasia of the affected renal segment. Schwarz and colleagues (1981) graded hypodysplasia and compared this with degrees of lateral or caudal ectopy of the associated ureteric orifice; despite considerable overlap, the degree of hypodysplasia generally correlated with the degree of orifice ectopia.

Ectopic Ureter (Fig. 38–56). Ectopic termination of a single system or of the accessory ureter in a duplex system can be explained by a high (cranial) origin of the involved ureteral bud from the mesonephric duct. As a result, the

URETER DUPLICATION
reflux and ectopy

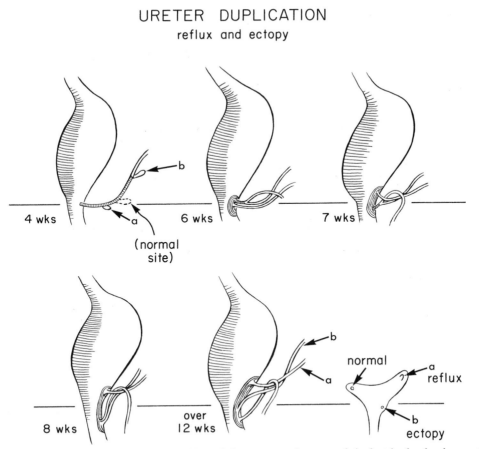

Figure 38–55. Simplified diagram of changing position of the ureters and mesonephric duct in the development of reflux and ectopia in complete duplication. High origin of the second ureteral bud results in migration with the mesonephric duct before delayed absorption in the ectopic position into the urogenital sinus. See text. (Modified and redrawn from Tanagho, 1977.)

ureter migrates for a longer time and for a greater distance attached to the mesonephric duct before the long common segment is completely absorbed and the ureter separates from it. There is little or no time for migration and ascent of the ureter. In the most extreme cases, there is no separation, and in the male the ureter remains attached to the mesonephric duct—i.e., to the ejaculatory duct or to the seminal vesicle, which develops at 13 weeks as a diverticulum from the mesonephric duct (Arey, 1965).

In both sexes, the ectopic ureter can insert along an ectopic pathway (Stephens, 1963) onto the trigone, bladder neck, or urethra. In both sexes, failure of the ureter to separate from the mesonephric duct results in drainage via the genital tract. In the male, urine drains into mesonephric duct–derived structures and never beyond the normal opening of the future ejaculatory duct proximal to the external urinary sphincter. In the female, however, urine drains through the genital tract into paramesonephric (müllerian duct)-derived structures—uterus, cervix, and vagina—causing incontinence (Fig. 38–57).

In the female the mesonephric duct degenerates except for a vestigial remnant, the duct of the epoophoron, which to a varying degree remains in the medial and distal portion as Gartner's duct. In its full extent Gartner's duct lies within the muscular wall of the genital tract, extending from the level of the internal cervical os along the lateral or anterolateral vaginal wall to the hymen. Distention of Gartner's duct with urine causes it to rupture through the thin tissue plane between the duct and the developing genital tract, establishing an extraurinary tract for drainage (Ellerker, 1958; Gray and Skandalakis, 1972; Meyer, 1946). The terminal portion of an incontinent ectopic ureter, therefore, might actually include a segment of the common excretory duct, although this is unproved (Ellerker, 1958).

SINGLE ECTOPIC URETER

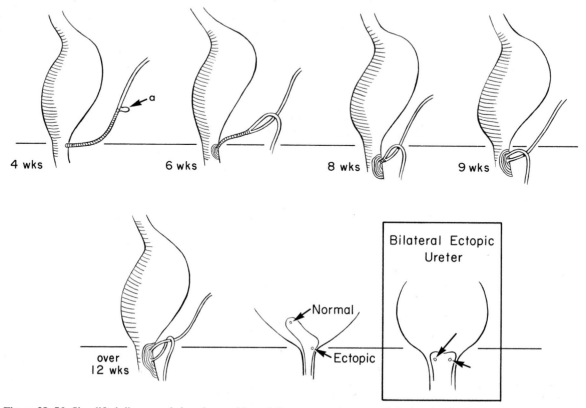

Figure 38–56. Simplified diagram of changing position of the ureter and mesonephric duct in the development of a single ectopic ureter. High origin of the ureteral bud results in migration with the mesonephric duct before delayed absorption in the ectopic position into the urogenital sinus. In bilateral single ectopy, the bladder is small and the bladder neck poorly developed or nonexistent. See text. (Modified and redrawn from Tanagho, 1977.)

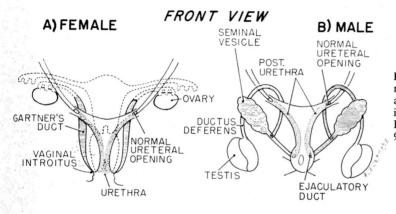

Figure 38–57. Ectopic ureteral orifices in male and female. Stippled and shaded areas indicate sites at which such openings may occur. (From Uson, A. C., and Donovan, J. T.: Am. J. Dis. Child., *98*:152, 1959.)

In patients with bilateral single-system ectopia into the urethra (a rare lesion), the bladder is small and poorly formed, and the bladder neck is ill defined or nonexistent. Since the mesenchyme from the common excretory duct intended for the muscularization of the trigone and bladder neck region is displaced bilaterally along with the ectopic ureter, these normal structures fail to develop. Embryologic development specific to ureterocele is considered in a later section of this chapter.

ANOMALIES OF NUMBER

Ureteral Agenesis

Bilateral ureteral agenesis can occur, along with bilateral renal agenesis, in monsters with multiple anomalies. Because it is incompatible with life, the condition is a medical curiosity.

Unilateral ureteral agenesis should in theory indicate complete failure of ureteral bud development and be accompanied by ipsilateral renal agenesis. The hemitrigone will be totally absent because no mesonephric duct or ureteral bud anlage has been absorbed into the urogenital sinus. If some degree of ipsilateral trigonal development is evident, ureteral hypoplasia or atresia may be present (see later section on ureteral atresia and hypoplasia).

Clinically apparent unilateral ureteral agenesis when the hemitrigone is totally absent is not incompatible but actually consistent with the probability of a single-system ectopic ureter on the affected side. The subject of ureteral ectopia is presented in a subsequent section.

Duplications of the Ureter

A duplicated ureter usually drains a duplex kidney (double collecting system), or rarely a normal supernumerary kidney. Ureteral duplications may be classified as *bifid ureter* (partial duplication) or *double ureters* (complete duplication); in the latter a second orifice enters the bladder, urethra, or other structure. Table 38–2 summarizes the gradations in ureteral and renal duplications, excluding ectopia and ureterocele. Duplication is the most common ureteral anomaly, and in many situations it is an incidental finding causing no functional disturbance. However, there is a higher than expected incidence of duplication in cases of urinary infection, and

it may be associated with upper urinary tract stasis, obstruction, or reflux. Among the manifestations of double ureters are ectopic insertion of the upper pole ureter and ectopic ureterocele.

Incidence. The reported incidence of ureteral duplication varies widely among different series, depending in part on whether the survey was based on autopsy or clinical data, on the composition of patient material in the latter, and on whether or not bifid pelves were separately recorded. As it is generally recognized that clinical series usually contain a disproportionate number of duplication anomalies, unselected autopsy data are more accurate in predicting the true incidence. At least two large autopsy series have provided data not too dissimilar regarding partial and complete ureteral duplication (Campbell, 1970; Nation, 1944) (Table 38–3). Nation (1944) reviewed 230 cases of duplication; 121 of these were clinical. He identified 109 cases in approximately 16,000 autopsies, an incidence of 1 in 147, or 0.68 per cent. Campbell's personal series of 51,880 autopsies in adults, infants, and children included 342 ureteral duplications, an incidence of 1 in 152, or 0.65 per cent. There were 281 duplications in the 32,834 adults, an incidence of 1 in 117, or 0.85 per cent, but only 61 of the 19,046 children had this abnormality, 1 in 312, or 0.32 per cent. Since the anomaly should be found with equal frequency in unselected autopsies on adults or children, he concluded that some of the duplications in children had been overlooked. Combining Nation's autopsy series and Campbell's adult series, the projected incidence of duplication is 1 in 125, or 0.8 per cent.

Despite a wealth of information about sex differences in the incidence of duplication in clinical series (the anomaly is identified in females at least two times more frequently), there are no reliable data on sex differences in unselected series. Campbell's autopsy data do not document such a difference. Of Nation's 109 autopsy cases, 56 were female and 53 male. However, only 40 per cent of the 16,000 autopsies were done in women. Calculating a correction for this difference, one could project a female to male ratio of 1.6 to 1, or 62 per cent. These statistics, however, may not be reliable in view of the small number of cases recorded.

Clinical and autopsy data are in substantial agreement about other aspects of duplication, however (Table 38–3). Unilateral duplication occurs about six times more often than bilateral, with the right and left sides being involved about

TABLE 38–2. GRADATIONS IN URETERAL AND KIDNEY DUPLICATIONS*

Temporal Relationships	Spatial Relationships

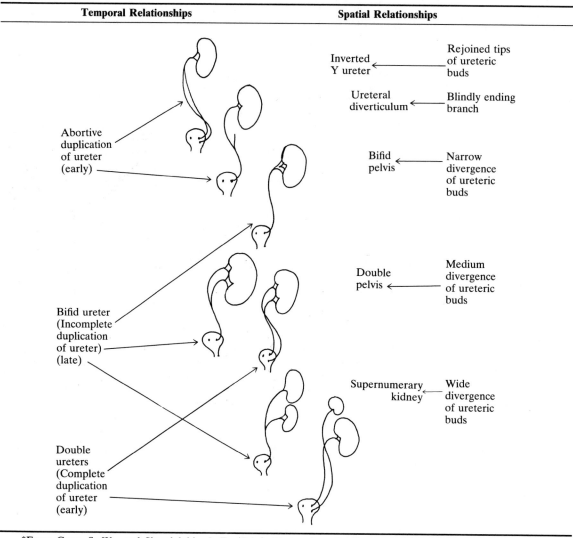

*From Gray, S. W., and Skandalakis, J. E. (Eds.): Embryology for Surgeons. Philadelphia, W. B. Saunders Co., 1972.

equally. Excluding bifid pelvis, there does not appear to be a difference in the literature in the incidence of bifid ureter versus double ureters. A small percentage of individuals with bilateral duplication have a mixed condition, i.e., bifid ureter on one side and double ureters on the other.

Genetics. There is evidence that duplication may be genetically determined by an autosomal dominant trait with incomplete penetrance (Cohen and Berant, 1976). In parents and siblings of probands with duplication, the incidence of duplication increases from the predicted 1 in 125 to 1 in 8 (Whitaker and Danks, 1966) or 1 in 9 (Atwell et al., 1974).

Position of Orifices. In *double ureters* the two orifices are characteristically inverted in relation to the collecting systems they drain, i.e., the orifice to the lower pole ureter occupies the more cranial and lateral position and that of the upper pole ureter has a caudal and medial position. This relationship is so consistent that it has been termed the *Weigert-Meyer law*, which is based on the original description of Weigert (1877) as modified by Meyer (1946). When the two orifices are not immediately adjacent, the orifice from the upper pole can be found anywhere along a predictable pathway, which Stephens (1958, 1963) has called the ectopic pathway (Fig. 38–58).

TABLE 38-3. URETERAL DUPLICATION: CLINICAL, RADIOGRAPHIC, AND AUTOPSY STUDIES

Author, Year	Data Base	No. Duplications	Female	Male	Unilateral	Bilateral	Complete	Partial	Unilateral Complete/Partial	Bilateral Complete/Partial	Bilateral Mixed
Archangelski, 1926	110	R 619 A 3 (2.7%)			502 (80%)	117 (20%)					
Colosimo, 1938	1500	X 50 (3.3%)	(68%)								
Nation, 1944	16000	A 109 (0.68%) C 121 230 total	* (63%) 88 (73%)	* 33	177 (77%)	53 (23%)	102 (44%)	118 (51%)	78 (44%)/99 (56%)	35 (45%)/19 (36%)	10 (4.3%)
Nordmark, 1948	4744	X 138 (2.8%)			119 (86%)	19 (14%)	70 (51%)	65 (47%)	59/60	11/5	3 (2.1%)
Payne, 1959	5000	C 141 X 83	87 (62%)	54	120 (85%)	21 (15%)	45	78 +18 bifid pelvis			
Johnston, 1961		C 73 A 9 82	57 (70%)	25			63 (77%)	19 (33%)			
Kaplan and Elkin, 1968	(partial dupls. only)	X 51	33 (65%)	18	43 (84%)	8 (16%)					
Campbell, 1970	51880 (19046 child) (32834 adult)	A 342 (0.65%) 61 (0.32%) 281 (0.85%)			293 (85%)	53 (15%)	101 (30%)			4	"one in five cases"
Timothy et al., 1971		C 46	39 (85%)	7			24 (52%)	16 (35%)	13/15	11/1	6 (13%)
Privett et al., 1976	5196 (1716 child) (3480 adult) (2896 male) (2300 female)	X 91 (1.8%)	63 (66%)	32	79 (85%)	16 (15%)	33 (29%) (but 21 not known)	57 (52%)			

A = Autopsy.
C = Clinical.
R = Review.
X = X-ray.
* = See text.

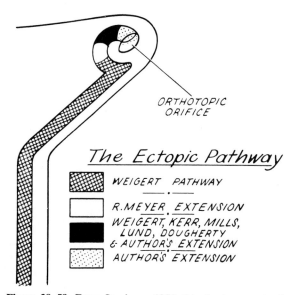

Figure 38–58. From Stephens, 1958. "Author's extension" refers to Stephens' observations. (Stephens, F. D.: Aust. N.Z. J. Surg., *28*:28, 1958.)

Rare exceptions to the Weigert-Meyer law have been observed, in which the upper pole orifice is cranial, although still medial, to the orthotopic orifice. Stephens collected four examples from the literature and added seven more. The pattern of rotation of the ectopic orifice around the orthotopic orifice in this situation is also shown in Figure 38–58. Stevens studied the positional relationship between the lower portions of the ureters and noted that it too varies according to the terminal position of the upper pole orifice. With the rare cranially placed upper pole orifice, the ureter lies anterior to the lower pole ureter, the ureters being uncrossed; with a medial orifice, the upper pole ureter lies medially; and with a caudally placed orifice, it spirals in an anterior to medial direction around the lower pole ureter as it descends, terminating posterior to the lower pole orifice.

An embryologic hypothesis to explain the exception to the Weigert-Meyer law was proposed by Stephens (1958) and is based on the premise that an upper pole orifice located craniomedially arises from a junctional ureteral bud—one that bifurcated immediately—rather than from a second bud. This hypothesis is presented in detail on page 1716, and the embryology is diagrammed in Figure 38–54.

Associated Findings. The distribution of the renal mass drained by each ureter in duplication varies somewhat; about one third of the renal parenchyma is served by the upper collecting system, on the average. In a detailed

radiographic review, Privett and associates (1976) reported a number of observations about duplication. The mean total number of calyces for single-system kidneys was 9.4, and for duplex units it was 11.3, with a mean of 3.7 calyces in the upper and 7.6 in the lower collecting systems. These investigators also observed that 97 per cent of the single-system kidneys in their series were radiographically normal, whereas 29 per cent of the duplex units had scarring or dilatation, or both. Reflux also was more common in the duplex units in patients who had voiding cystograms. Two out of 17 nonduplex units refluxed (12 per cent) compared with 13 of 31 duplex units (42 per cent).

Hydronephrosis of the lower pole segment is not infrequent and is generally associated with severe reflux into that unit. However, primary ureteropelvic junction obstruction can involve the lower pelvis (Cristoffersen and Iversen, 1976; Dahl, 1975; Johnston, 1961; Privett et al., 1976).

Other anomalies are encountered with increased frequency. Twenty-seven (12 per cent) of Nation's (1944) series had other urinary tract anomalies, with just over half of these being on the same side; they included renal hypoplasia and aplasia (today probably termed dysplasia) and various ureteral anomalies, among them ectopic insertion of the upper pole ureter in four cases (3 per cent of the complete duplications). Coexisting urologic anomalies were encountered in 129 of Campbell's (1970) series of 342 duplications, and nonurologic anomalies were found in 63 cases. These were not recorded in detail, but most of the urologic anomalies were, as in Nation's series, a variety of ipsilateral renal and ureteral lesions; 22 were anomalies of the contralateral kidney. The nonurologic lesions mainly involved the gastrointestinal tract plus a few cardiopulmonary lesions. Both these series, however, were autopsy series. Rarely, the pelvocalyceal systems communicate, presumably from late fusion of the ureteral buds during pelvocalyceal expansion (Beer and Mencher, 1938; Braasch, 1912).

The increased incidence of duplications in investigations of childhood urinary infection is well established. Campbell (1970) reported a personal series of 1102 children with pyuria, 307 of whom proved to have ureteropelvic anomalies. Eighty-two (27 per cent) of these were duplications, or 7.5 per cent of the total group. Kretschmer (1937) reviewed 101 cases of hydronephrosis in infancy and childhood and noted 24 renoureteral anomalies, over half of which were duplications.

Based on three cases of duplication with some form of ureteral ectopy, coexistent renal dysplasia and nodular renal blastema, Cromie and colleagues (1980) raised the possibility that this pattern of findings might be more than a coincidental association, accounting for an increased risk of neoplasm (Pendergrass, 1976). This concept deserves further investigation.

Bifid ureter is often clinically unimportant, but stasis and pyelonephritis do occur. When the Y junction is extravesical, free to-and-fro peristalsis of urine from one collecting system to the other may be present, with preferential retrograde waves passing into slightly dilated limbs instead of down the common stem. This results in stasis that is more marked when the Y junction is more distal, when the bifid limbs are wide, or when the Y junction is large. Increased urinary reprocessing from vesicoureteral reflux may enhance this phenomenon. Treatment by ureteroneocystostomy is effective when the junction is sufficiently close to the vesical wall that resection of the common sheath or common stem will permit placement of both orifices within the bladder. Reimplantation of the common stem may be effective when vesicoureteral reflux is severe and the Y junction is higher up. In the absence of reflux, ureteropyelostomy or pyelopyelostomy with resection of one ureteral limb, preferably the upper limb, down to the Y junction is effective in eliminating regurgitation of urine (Kaplan and Elkin, 1968; Lenaghan, 1962).

BLIND-ENDING DUPLICATION OF THE URETER

Rarely, a ureteral duplication does not drain a renal segment; hence the term *blind-ending*. Less than 70 of these have been reported, although they occur considerably less infrequently than the published data indicate. Most blind-ending ureteral duplications involve one limb of a bifid system; even more unusual is one involving a complete duplication (Szokoly et al., 1974; Jablonski et al., 1978). Although the Y junction in the bifid type may be at any level, most are found in the mid- or distal ureter. Blind-ending segments are diagnosed three times more frequently in women than in men and twice as often on the right side (Albers et al., 1971; Schultze, 1967). The condition has been reported in twins (Bergman et al., 1977).

Many of these blind segments cause no problems; symptomatic patients mostly complain of vague abdominal or chronic flank pain, sometimes complicated by infection or calculi, or both (Marshall and McLoughlin, 1978). The

majority of cases are not diagnosed until the third or fourth decade of life.

As the blind segment does not always fill on excretory urography, retrograde pyelography may be required for diagnosis (Fig. 38–59). At times, however, urinary stasis from disordered peristalsis (ureteroureteral reflux) (Lenaghan, 1962) may be demonstrated, with secondary dilatation of the branch, and this is felt to be the cause of the pain (van Helsdingen, 1975). As the lesion is more common in women and

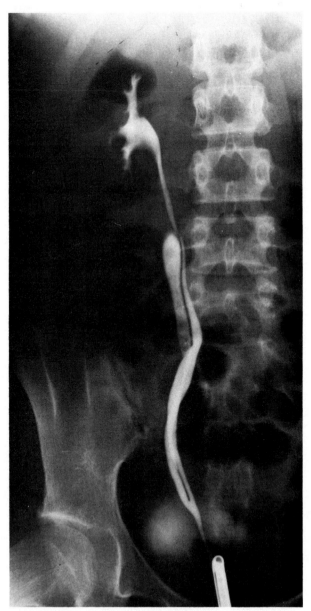

Figure 38–59. Retrograde pyelogram. Blind-ending duplication in an 18-year-old girl noted in evaluation of transitory hematuria. Only the distal portion of this blind-ending duplication has visualized on IVP.

on the right side, the propensity for dilation of the right urinary tract with pregnancy might explain the relatively late age at onset of symptoms.

Embryology. The embryogenesis of blind-ending ureteral duplication is similar to that for duplications in general. It is postulated that the affected ureteral bud is abortive and fails to make contact with the metanephros. Histologically, the blind segment contains all normal ureteral layers. Anatomically, the blind end tends to have a bulbous dilatation. Most of these blind segments are not surrounded by any abortive renal tissue, but in a few there is a fibrous stalk (ureteral atresia) extending into a dysplastic renal segment. The blind limb may vary from a short stump of a few centimeters to one extending all the way into the renal fossa.

The area of union between the two limbs is invested in a common sheath that may be attenuated proximally. The blind segment of the adjacent normal ureter share a common blood supply (Albers et al., 1968; Peterson et al., 1975). When surgery is necessary, excision of the blind segment is indicated. Because the ensheathment is less dense at the upper or proximal end, the dissection should start there, and care should be taken to denude only the blind segment and not to enter the normal ureter. Some investigators suggest leaving a short stump at the junction with the common stem (Peterson et al., 1975; Rao, 1975).

Diverticula of the ureter have also been described. There is confusion in the literature about the distinction between some diverticula and blind-ending duplications, however; in some cases it may simply be a matter of terminology. For example, Campbell (1936) described a case of a finger-like extension from the lower ureter that he called a ureteral diverticulum, but he ascribed it developmentally to an abortive duplication. Similarly, Youngen and Persky (1965) labeled as a diverticulum a tubular, finger-like appendage from the pelvis, but they too ascribed its origin to an abortive budding. Rank et al. (1960) and Gray and Skandalakis (1972) agree that congenital ureteral diverticula have the same embryogenesis as blind duplications. Gray and Skandalakis specifically note that a diverticulum from the mid- or distal ureter originates as a blind ureteral duplication, whereas a diverticulum arising from the ureteropelvic area represents a primitive calyx that has failed to meet nephrogenic mesenchyme.

The distinction between a diverticulum and a blind-ending ureter is one of morphology, the typical blind-ending ureteral segment of a Y-ureter joining the normal ureter at an acute angle and extending upward parallel to the normal ureter; it is at least twice as long as it is wide (Culp, 1947). A congenital diverticulum, on the other hand, has a ballooned appearance. Histologically, both are similar, and both arise from disordered ureteral budding.

Additional description of ureteral diverticula is presented in a subsequent section.

INVERTED Y URETERAL DUPLICATION

This is the rarest of the anomalies of ureteral branching. It consists of two ureteral limbs distally that fuse proximally to become a single channel draining the kidney. Klauber and Reid (1972) reported a female with an ectopic limb to an ectopic ureterocele. In one woman (Britt et al., 1972) the ectopic limb ended blindly behind the trigone and had a further fibrous extension caudally to an unidentified termination. Suzuki and colleagues (1977) similarly reported a 12-year-old girl with bilateral inverted Y duplication and an atretic distal limb on each side, one of which contained a calculus. They found 27 cases in the literature. In reviewing 18 of these, they noted that only 4 were male; 4 had an ectopic ureteral opening. Four cases, including theirs, had ureteral atresia of one limb.

The embryology of inverted Y ureteral duplication is ascribed to two separate ureteral buds whose tips coalesce and fuse into a single duct before joining the metanephros. The frequently ectopic position of one limb is caused by widely separated buds on the mesonephric duct, with the second bud relatively cephalad. To explain the distal atresia of the ectopic limb in their case, Britt and associates offered two possibilities. One is failure of Chwalle's membrane to rupture. The second, postulated by Hawthorne (1936), is atresia of the wolffian duct—a normal regression in the female—prior to absorption of the too cephalad second ureteral bud into the urogenital sinus distally.

Treatment is directed toward any problems resulting from the ectopic limb, generally resection of the accessory channel.

Ureteral Triplication and Supernumerary Ureters

Just as two buds from the mesonephric duct or premature fission of a single bud can explain double and bifid ureters, so the presence of three buds from the mesonephric duct or two with early fission of one of them can account for complete and partial triplications. In the most recent literature review, Marc and colleagues (1977) collected 70 cases, and a few have been reported subsequently. In an earlier review, Smith (1946) classified four varieties of triplicate ureter: (1) complete triplication—three ureters from the kidney with three draining orifices to the bladder, urethra, or elsewhere; (2) incomplete triplication—a bifid ureter plus a single ureter, with three ureters from the kidney and two orifices draining below; (3) trifid ureter—all three ureters unite and drain through a single orifice (this appears to be the most common form encountered); and (4) two ureters from the kidney, one becoming an inverse Y bifurcation, resulting in three draining orifices below. In one apparently unique case, Fairchild et al. (1979) reported a typical bifid system with a third, lateral ureter that appeared to communicate with the lower pole calyx.

Triplication may, of course, present with symptoms and signs of reflux or obstruction, ureterocele (Arap et al., 1982), or ectopia, as for duplication anomalies. Treatment is based on the same principles (see Chapter 50).

ANOMALIES OF STRUCTURE

Atresia and Hypoplasia

Atresia and hypoplasia of the ureter are both caused by varying degrees of failure of ureteral bud development. The trigone on the same side may appear normal or hypoplastic and have a tiny dimple for an orifice (total atresia). A fibrous stalk may represent the ureter, or there may be a hypoplastic or normal ureteral segment of varying length that terminates blindly or in an atretic segment (fibrous stalk) capped by some form of an anomalous dysplastic renal remnant. In ureteropelvic atresia with a multicystic kidney the fibrous segment may contain a minute lumen (Mackie, 1977).

In a study of the morphology of intrinsic ureteral lesions in infants and children derived from both autopsy and clinical sources, Cussen (1971) noted 5 of 147 dilated ureters that had an atretic segment below the dilated area. The lumen and its epithelium were absent for a distance of from 0.5 to 5 cm, and the ureter was replaced by a fibrous strand, sometimes surrounded by a peripheral band of smooth muscle. Distal to the lesion, the morphology of the ureter was normal in every case.

When the atresia involves the ureteropelvic area only, a multicystic dysplastic kidney will cap the atretic segment (see Chapter 39). Ureteral atresia of longer lengths or lower positions will alter the prognosis. In 29 cases of congenital multicystic dysplastic kidney, DeKlerk and colleagues (1977) noted that 13 of 14 infants with isolated ureteropelvic atresia had no contralateral renal anomaly, the one exception being a simple cyst. On the other hand, 6 of 15 infants with a lower level or long segment ureteral atresia with or without associated pelvic atresia had contralateral renal anomalies, generally multicystic dysplasia or hydronephrosis. Only 7 of 15 survived 1 year.

Segmental atretic lesions involving the ureter, regardless of the associated renal anomaly, are apparently related to defective development of the ureteral bud.

Blind-ending single ureters per se that are associated with segmental ureteral atresia should cause no symptoms and generally require no treatment. Treatment should be directed toward any contralateral disease. In some institutions, including those of the authors', there is currently a question as to whether a palpable but otherwise asymptomatic multicystic kidney with a ureteropelvic atresia justifies excision in the newborn. A number of such patients are being followed nonoperatively without any difficulty, at least for short-term follow-up.

DISTAL URETERAL ATRESIA

The term "distal ureteral atresia" is preferred to "blind-ending ureter," which has been used as a synonym for atresia of the proximal ureter (Campbell, 1970) but also can describe atresia at the distal end. Here the ureter has developed proximally and can end blindly distally, at an orthotopic or ectopic position relative to the bladder base. The maldevelopment occurs early in the formation of the ureter; if it occurs after the onset of urinary secretion, a greatly dilated cystic or tubular segment of ureter and nonfunctioning kidney may be present. The surgical importance lies in the differential diagnosis, often during the neonatal period, of a palpable, cystic abdominal mass, which may be of spectacular size and may displace other viscera. Cystography, excretory urography, and ultrasonography are aids to diagnosis. At times gastrointestinal contrast studies will be helpful. Surgical exploration may be the ultimate diagnostic test as well as definitive therapy. With ectopic termination, a duplicated segment may be involved, and ipsilateral lower pole may be obstructed from the mass (Gordon and Reed, 1962; Kornblum and Ritter, 1939; Slater, 1957; Uson et al., 1972).

Megaureter

The term "megaureter" simply means a large ureter. Caulk (1923) first described a condition he called megaloureter in a young woman with a disproportionately dilated ureter almost to the ureterovesical junction and a near-normal pyelocalyceal system. Most typically, megaureter of this type has minimal or no tortuosity and is not associated with a demonstrable anatomic obstruction, although because the ureter appears to be obstructed at its lower end, it has given rise to terms such as ureteral achalasia (Creevy, 1970), primary obstructive megaureter (Williams and Hulme-Moir, 1970), aperistaltic distal ureteral segment, and the functionally obstructed megaureter. Disagreements about terminology and differences in interpretation of morphologic observations have caused confusion in the literature. However, recent studies of ureteral structure and ultrastructure may eventually bring about a better understanding of the pathophysiology and a consensus of opinion on the subject.

Gradually the term *megaureter* has acquired a wider usage so that it now includes a variety of secondary as well as primary lesions, despite the feeling of some that it should be limited to the functionally obstructed condition. It is not likely that the issue of terminology and classification will be resolved here, but a review of the subject of megaureter, including a classification proposed at the International Pediatric Urologic Seminar in 1976 (Smith, 1977), may provide the practicing urologist with a better perspective and, possibly, a workable classification.

In trying to develop a working classification of megaureter, a group at this meeting first devised a flow chart showing the method by which a large (wide) ureter is usually evaluated (Table 38–4, Scheme 1). The classification (Table 38–4, Scheme 2) was not accepted by all members of the working committee but is published here as the current thinking of many pediatric urologists (Table 38–4, Scheme 2). Examples of the various kinds of megaureter as listed are not intended to be complete. The remainder of this section will describe mainly the various forms of primary megaureter outlined in Table 38–4, Scheme 2.

Table 38–5 summarizes a review by Stephens (1974) of the changes of muscular hyperplasia and hypertrophy in various forms of megaureter, compared with the normal. His data are derived from studies by Cussen (1967, 1971), who used a graph and grid technique to quantitate numbers of muscle cells and their size per unit area.

REFLUX MEGAURETER

Reflux megaureter can be a manifestation of primary reflux or of secondary elevated intravesical pressure. There is no site of obstruction in primary reflux megaureter in contrast to primary obstructed megaureter, although its cystographic appearance resembles the intravenous pyelogram (IVP) of the latter. The degree of muscular hypertrophy and hyperplasia is less (Table 38–5). Additional descriptions of reflux megaureter can be found in Chapter 49.

OBSTRUCTED MEGAURETER

The primary form of obstructed megaureter is associated most commonly with a distal adynamic segment (the functionally obstructed megaureter), but infrequently it is linked with a demonstrable anatomic obstruction (stenosis). The typical radiographic appearance is that of a dilated upper ureter without appreciable tortuosity that becomes progressively widened distally. The most distal portion has a marked fusiform or bulbous dilatation, which abruptly changes into a short, undilated ureteral segment, 0.5 to 4 cm in length, which enters the bladder (Pfister et al., 1971; Williams and Hulme-Moir, 1970). Despite the ureteral dilatation, the calyces are generally normally cupped, and the pelvis is normal or somewhat plump. Renal function usually remains near-normal, and radiographic visualization is good.

Fluoroscopic study shows disturbed peristalsis, with failure of at least the more distal portion of the dilated segment to coapt, during contraction, behind the bolus of contrast material. This causes much of the bolus to be regurgitated into the upper ureter after reaching the bottom of the dilated segment, simulating reverse peristalsis, and only a small portion passes through the undilated segment into the bladder. The result is a churning or "yo-yo" effect (Pfister et al., 1971). However, retrograde catheterization of the undilated segment generally is unimpeded and fails to confirm any anatomic obstruction, although in a small minority of cases some narrowing is present (Williams and Hulme-Moir, 1970). If untreated, the condition can at times progress, with development of advancing hydronephrosis and increasing ureteral dilatation and tortuosity (Williams and Hulme-Moir, 1970). An occasional primary obstructed megaureter will reflux to a limited degree into the lower ureter. In this situation, the orifice is somewhat underdeveloped.

Primary obstructed megaureter occurs 3.5 to 5 times more often in males, 2 to 3 times more commonly on the left side, and bilaterally in 15 to 25 per cent of patients. In a few cases, there is contralateral agenesis or dysplasia (Johnston, 1967; Pfister et al., 1971; Williams and Hulme-Moir, 1970). Familial megaureter was recently described in a mother and her adult daughter and is exceedingly rare (Tatu and Brennan, 1981).

Pathology. A number of histologic findings in the undilated segment and the adjacent portion of dilated ureter have been described by different investigators. Some specimens appear normal by light microscopy, while in others the musculature of the proximal end of the undilated segment may be disorganized, abnormal, or absent. An excessive amount of circular fibers has been described (Murnaghan, 1957; Tanagho et al., 1970). The ureteral musculature is normally organized in a feltwork of opposing helixes except for the mainly longitudinal pattern of the intramural segment. In some megaureters, the undilated distal segment has an excessively tight helix, which results in a predominantly circular orientation (Hanna et al., 1976b; McLaughlin et al., 1973).

In many cases, the area of abrupt transition between the dilated and normal-sized ureter shows faulty muscular development, with a segment partially or completely deficient in muscle; the muscle that is found is maloriented. There tends to be an excessive amount of collagen within the undilated segment of ureter and in its adventitia as well (Gregoir and Debled, 1969; MacKinnon et al., 1970).

Regardless of whether or not light microscopic studies show obvious pathology, ultrastructure studies have consistently revealed an increase in collagen between the muscle bundles of the obstructing segment and between the individual muscle cells (Hanna et al., 1976b; Notley, 1972). The adjacent muscle cells in the most distal portion of the dilated segment are abnormal ("sick") as well (Hanna et al., 1976b). Hanna and his associates noted a progressive improvement in muscle cell morphology extending more proximally up the dilated portion of the megaureter; muscular hypertrophy and hyperplasia are quite marked (Table 38–5) (Cussen, 1971; Hanna et al., 1976b). In the absence of an anatomic stenosis, obstruction may be due to failure of peristaltic transmission through the distal ureteral segment. Although various authors have blamed this on a preponderance of circular fibers, increased collagen, or focal absence of muscle, the common mechanism appears to be attenuation or frank disruption of muscular continuity, either grossly or at the cellular level; this separates nexus and thus prevents spread of the action potential (Hanna et al., 1976b).

Tokunaka and Koyanagi, with various other associates, have published a series of recent articles involving light and electron microscopic studies in nonrefluxing megaureter, further defining the pathogenesis of the condition (Tokunaka et al., 1980, 1982, 1984; Tokunaka and Koyanagi, 1982). They identified two groups of nonrefluxing megaureters: a larger group (Group 1), with relatively normal histopathology of the dilated segment and abnormalities limited to the intravesical segment; and a smaller group (Group 2), in which the abnormalities involved the dilated portion of the ureter. In Group 1, the abnormal findings of the intravesical ureter included deranged muscle bundle orientation and increased connective tissue. A generously developed ("bulky") periureteral sheath appeared to contribute to obstruction, especially with bladder filling. The kidneys of these megaureters were normal or showed hydronephrosis without dysmorphism. In Group 2, the length of the distal narrowed segment was variable, in some cases extending extravesically; histology was normal. The dilated portion of the ureter, on the other hand, was abnormal with a marked reduction of muscle cells, which were small and widely separated in a collagen matrix. Muscle bundles were absent, nexus were attenuated, and no thick myofilaments were present. The renal units were dysmorphic with varying hypodysplasia.

In the secondarily obstructed megaureter from posterior urethral valves, muscular hypertrophy and hyperplasia tend to be more marked than in intrinsic obstruction (Table 38–5). In either case, the hypertrophy and hyperplasia are a response to an increased work load and appear in utero. The favorable results often achieved with corrective surgery in infancy may be related to the increased numbers of mesenchymal cells still present at that age that can continue to differentiate into muscle postoperatively. Chronic or recurrent infection may damage the muscle cells of the megaureter, altering the expected histologic findings and interfering with muscle cell function (Hanna et al., 1977).

NONREFLUX-NONOBSTRUCTED MEGAURETER (IDIOPATHIC MEGAURETER)

The primary form is quite uncommon and appears to be a developmental variant wherein the ureteral bud widens excessively during its

TABLE 38–4.*

SCHEME 1. Megaureter—Investigative Flow Chart

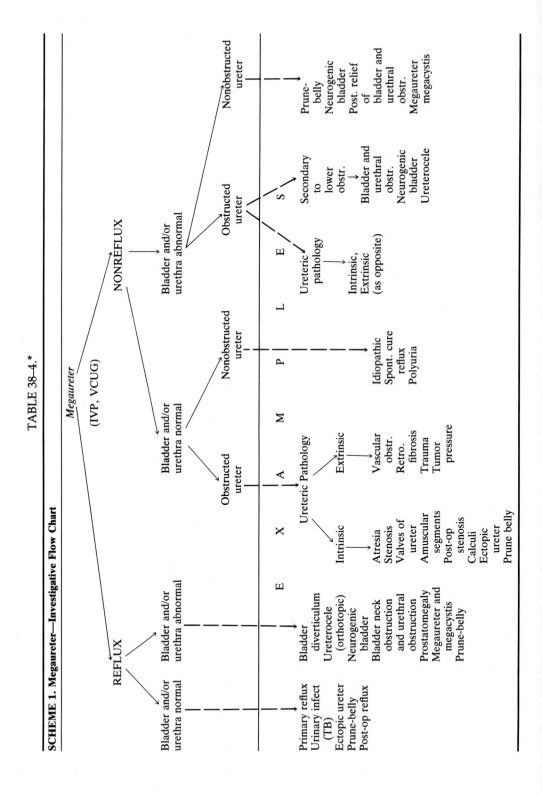

SCHEME 2. Megaureter—A Proposed Classification

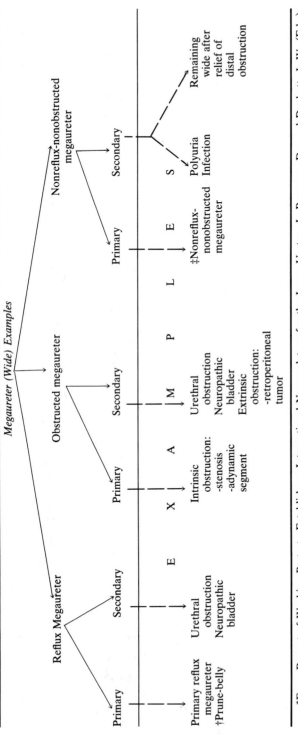

Megaureter (Wide) Examples

*From Report of Working Party to Establish an International Nomenclature for the Large Ureter. *In* Bergsma, D., and Duckett, J. W. (Eds.): Urinary system malformations in children. Birth Defects: Original Article Series, *13*, No. 5. New York, Alan R. Liss for The National Foundation-March of Dimes, 1977.

†Some conditions (e.g., prune-belly, ureteroceles, ectopic ureters, etc.) may appear under several other columns.

‡As proved not to be obstructed.

Note: An occasional megaureter may show reflux and apparent obstruction.

TABLE 38–5. Muscle Hypertrophy and Hyperplasia in Large Ureters*

Disorder	No. Ureters	Hypertrophy (Cell Size)	Hyperplasia (Cell Density)
Obstruction			
intrinsic ureteral	129	2 to 3 times normal	3 to 5 times normal
urethral	72	3 to 5 times normal	5 to 50 times normal
Reflux		slight; normal range	slight; 1 to 3 times normal
Idiopathic megaureter	18	slight; normal range	none

*After Stephens (1974).

differentiation, resulting in a large-caliber ureter. Characteristically, there is a normal-appearing pyelocalyceal system that drains into a wide ureter without evidence of anatomic or functional obstruction. Intraluminal pressures remain in the normal range during measurement of physiologic flow rates and during perfusion study (Hanna and Edwards, 1972; Whitaker, 1973). Muscular hypertrophy is negligible, and there is no hyperplasia (Table 38–5) (Cussen, 1971).

MEGAURETER IN PRUNE BELLY SYNDROME

The dilated ureter in this condition has features that make it relatively unique. It is most often nonobstructed. Reflux is usually but not invariably present. There is a diffuse abnormality of the ureteral musculature consisting of a marked decrease in muscle bundles, and there may be patchy areas in which fibrous tissue has replaced muscle. The individual muscle bundles are surrounded by increased amounts of collagen. The individual muscle cells are also abnormal—there is a developmental myopathy, with ultrastructure studies showing attenuation of myofilaments (Hanna et al., 1977; Palmar and Tesluk, 1974; Williams and Burkholder, 1967) (see also Chapter 53).

DYSPLASTIC MEGAURETER

This condition possibly belongs in a category of miscellaneous primary or acquired lesions. Hanna and associates (1977) studied two such ureters associated with dysplastic renal segments by light and electron microscopy. In addition to a marked unit reduction in muscle cells, there was an increase in inflammatory cells and collagen. The individual muscle cells were severely abnormal, with marked atrophy and various degenerative changes. The authors could not determine whether the findings were related to underdevelopment or to deterioration from repeated infections. Tokunaka and colleagues (1984) studied muscle dysplasia using light and electron microscopy in nonreflux and reflux megaureters, ureteroceles, and ectopic ureters from single and double systems. They defined ureteral muscle dysplasia as small, smooth muscle cells widely separated with connective tissue (collagen), attenuated nexus, and a lack of thick myosin filaments. They found muscle dysplasia in each category of megaureter studied, although the incidence varied by category. Like Hanna, they noted that extensive dysplasia involving the length of the ureter was associated with a high incidence of renal dysmorphism.

The management of megaureter and additional details of evaluation are presented in Chapter 49.

Ureteral Stenosis and Stricture

Congenital anatomic narrowing or narrowing of the ureteral lumen as detected by calibration is referred to as congenital ureteral stenosis and has also been termed congenital ureteral stricture, but developmentally the term "stricture" should refer only to obstructions involving a histologic lesion in the ureter. Cussen (1971), in his series of 147 ureteral lesions, noted 81 (55 per cent) with ureteral stenosis. His histologic studies of the stenotic zone revealed normal transitional epithelium, a diminished population of otherwise normal-appearing smooth muscle cells, and no increase in fibrous tissue in the wall of the stenotic zone. Ultrastructure studies were not done.

The cause of congenital ureteral stenosis is not certain, but ultrastructure studies such as those of Notley (1972) and Hanna and associates (1976a and b, 1977) may provide the answer. Developmentally, simple narrowing probably results from a disturbance in embryogenesis around the eleventh to twelfth week, with disturbed development of the mesenchyme contributing to the ureteral musculature (Allen,

1977). A spectrum of histologic abnormalities, with or without demonstrable anatomic narrowing, may occur at the zone of obstruction (Hanna et al., 1976b). The reader is referred to the previous discussion of megaureter for a description of the reported ultrastructure abnormalities and additional discussion.

Three areas of the ureter are particularly liable to ureteral stenosis. They are, in order of decreasing frequency, the distal ureter just above the ureterovesical junction, the ureteropelvic junction, and rarely, the midureter at the pelvic brim (Allen, 1970; Campbell, 1952). More than one area of segmental stenosis may be present in the same ureter with a widened length of ureter between the segments, suggesting a developmental defect that affects the entire ureteral bud.

The clinical manifestations and treatment of ureteral stenoses and strictures involving the ureteropelvic junction are included in the previous section in this chapter on ureteropelvic junction obstruction and in Chapter 65; for the distal ureter see Chapter 49.

Ureteral Valves

Ureteral valves are uncommon causes of ureteral obstruction consisting of transverse folds of redundant mucosa that contain smooth muscle (Wall and Wachter, 1952). As described and depicted in the earlier literature, these are single annular or diaphragmatic lesions with a pinpoint opening (Figs. 38–60 and 38–61). The ureter is dilated above the obstruction and normal below it. As determined in a review of 40 congenital ureteral valves, ureteral valves are distributed throughout the length of the ureter, though least commonly in the middle third or at the pelviureteral junction (Dajani et al., 1982).

Transverse, nonobstructing mucosal folds are present in 5 per cent of ureters in newborns and gradually disappear with growth (Wall and Wachter, 1952); they may be one of the normal findings described by Östling (1942) and Kirks et al. (1978). Cussen (1971, 1977) has identified what he terms ureteral valves in 46 of 328 abnormal ureters from infants and children at

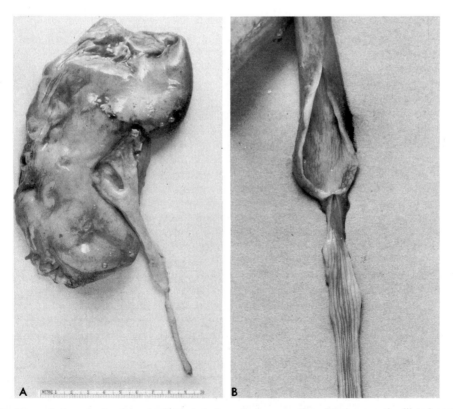

Figure 38–60. Congenital ureteral valve: *A*, Extended view. *B*, Long section showing greatly dilated ureter above the valve and normal size below. (From Simon, H. B., et al.: J. Urol., *74*:336, 1955.)

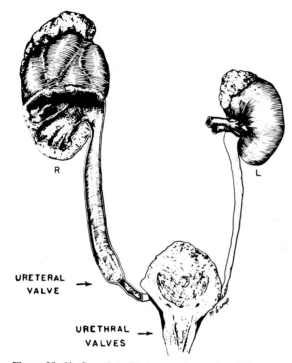

URETERAL
VALVE

URETHRAL
VALVES

Figure 38–61. Complete diaphragm obstructing right ureter, with hydroureter and hydronephrosis above. (From Roberts, R. R.: J. Urol., 76:62, 1956.)

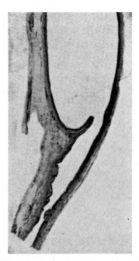

Figure 38–62. Twelve-year-old girl with obstructing distal congenital ureteral valve in ectopic, duplicated ureter. (Specimen courtesy of Dr. Laurence R. Wharton.)

autopsy or surgery. Unlike the diaphragmatic valves described previously, these are cusps demonstrated by perfusing the upper ureter with fixative, dilating the lumen, flattening the mucosa, and accentuating the valves. In patients with valvular obstruction, Cussen noted that the long axis of the distal ureter was eccentric relative to the long axis of the dilated proximal segment, with the fold being an eccentric cusp (Fig. 38–62). He also noted that these flaps could be found in the presence of a normal or stenotic distal ureter. In his series of 328 intrinsic ureteral lesions, he reported 24 primary valves with no distal obstruction—i.e., the valves were considered the cause of the obstruction—and 19 valves in association with a more distal obstruction, these valves being, he felt, either primary or secondary. Others have observed ureteral obstruction from eccentric cusps, believed to be distinct from secondary folds and kinks associated with ureteral dilation and elongation (Gosalbez et al., 1983; Maizels and Stephens, 1980). However, Williams (1977) felt that eccentric obstructing valves may be more infrequent than Cussen believed; many of the apparent valves may be artifacts of distention as the dilated ureter at its junction with the undilated segment assumes a kinked and eccen-

tric position from elongation and from the pull of the surrounding adventitia.

In summary, diaphragmatic annular valves are a rare, though definite, form of ureteral obstruction. Eccentric, cusplike flaps or folds can be obstructing but can also be secondary to the elongation and tortuosity that occurs with ureteral distention at the site of an underlying anatomic or functional obstruction.

Spiral Twists and Folds of the Ureter

Campbell (1970) observed this anomaly only twice in 12,080 autopsies in children (Fig. 38–63). He ascribed it to failure of the ureter to rotate with the kidney. This explanation may be simplistic, as the sketch shows more than one twist. Obstruction and hydronephrosis may result from spiral twists. The condition may arise from one of a number of possible persistent manifestations of normal fetal upper ureteral development, as described by Östling (1942) (Figs. 38–44 and 38–63). These manifestations include ureteral mucosal redundancy (see previous discussion of ureteral valves) and apparent folds and convolutions that may have a spiral appearance. Radiographic evidence of such findings is often present in otherwise normal newborn excretory urograms. However, most of these will gradually disappear with normal growth of the infant. Occasionally, ureteral convolutions that are enclosed by investing fascia persist as a form of ureteropelvic obstruction

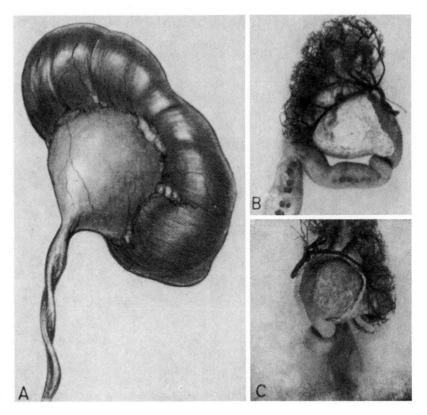

Figure 38–63. Torsion (spiral twists) of the ureter. *A,* As observed in an infant at autopsy at Bellevue Hospital; there is secondary hydronephrosis. Ureteral twists of the ureter of late fetal life; corrosion specimens. *B,* Anterior view. *C,* Lateral view from pelvic aspect. (Courtesy of Dr. Karl Östling.)

(Gross, 1953) (see earlier section in ureteropelvic junction obstruction and Chapter 65).

Persistent fetal folds are described in the previous paragraph. An isolated single fold or "kink" demonstrated radiographically with otherwise normal upper tracts may be acquired, nonobstructing, and reversible, and represents acute or intermittent elongation of the ureter with distal obstruction or reflux. Campbell (1970) felt that isolated primary obstructing congenital kinks could occur as an uncommon disorder, but the example he presented did not demonstrate convincing obstruction. Nevertheless, this sort of deformity is often one manifestation of ureteropelvic junction obstruction in association with ensheathment by dense fibrous bands (Gross, 1953).

Ureteral Diverticula

Diverticula of the ureter have been classified by Gray and Skandalakis (1972) into three categories: (1) abortive ureteral duplications (blind-ending bifid ureters) (see earlier section on blind-ending ureteral duplications); (2) true congenital diverticula, containing all tissue layers of the normal ureter; and (3) acquired diverticula, representing mucosal herniations. Congenital diverticula are very uncommon and have been reported as arising from the distal ureter above the ureterovesical junction, midureter, and ureteropelvic junction (Culp, 1947; McGraw and Culp, 1952; Rathbun, 1927; Richardson, 1942; Williams and Goodman, 1965). These can become very large, and secondary hydronephrosis can ensue. The patient may present with abdominal pain or renal colic and a palpable cystic mass. McGraw and Culp's patient, a 64-year-old woman, had a cystic lesion at surgery extending from under the right costal margin to the pelvic brim. A typical congenital diverticulum in a 20-year-old man is shown in Figure 38–64. Even small diverticula may be symptomatic; Sharma et al. (1980) reported two cases—a man with repeated infections and a girl with intermittent colic. Fluoroscopy in the latter patient demonstrated stasis and peristaltic dysfunction with to-and-fro (yo-yo) ureter to diverticulum reflux. She was cured by diverticulectomy.

As discussed in the previous section on blind-ending duplications, congenital diverticula below the level of the ureteropelvic junction arise from premature cleavage of the ureteral bud with abortive development of the accessory

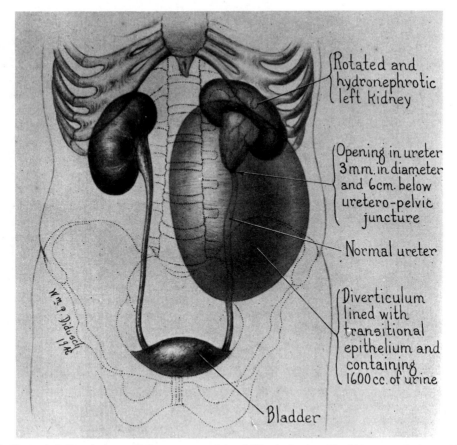

Figure 38–64. Congenital diverticulum of left ureter containing 1600 ml of urine. The kidney was hydronephrotic. (From Culp, O. S.: J. Urol., *58:*309, 1947.)

limb. Those from the ureteropelvic junction region arise from primitive calyceal formation that similarly failed to encounter metanephric tissue (Gray and Skandalakis, 1972).

Single acquired diverticula may be associated with strictures or calculi or may follow trauma (Culp, 1947). There are also reports of multiple diverticula, small in size (under 5 mm), that are ascribed to the effect of chronic infection alone (Holly and Sumcad, 1957; Rank et al., 1960). However, Norman and Dubowy (1966) reported two cases of multiple diverticula that were demonstrable on retrograde pyelography but not on high-dose pyelography even with compression, and Hansen and Frost (1978) reported a third case demonstrated by retrograde ureteropyelography. Such lesions, demonstrable only by unphysiologic pressures, may be congenital variants with weaknesses of the ureteral wall rather than acquired conditions (Hansen and Frost, 1978). However, the published reports do not contain histologic observations to support either hypothesis.

Large diverticula can generally be removed without sacrificing the kidney unless it is irreversibly involved in a dense inflammatory process.

Congenital High Insertion of the Ureter

This rare malformation may drain on otherwise normal and unobstructed kidney (Fig. 38–65). Most high insertions, however, are encountered with ureteropelvic junction obstruction, as discussed earlier.

ANOMALIES OF TERMINATION

Vesicoureteral Reflux

Primary congenital vesicoureteral reflux is classified as a disorder of ureteral termination in which the orifice is too high and lateral and

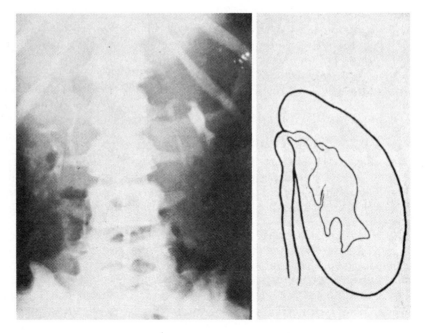

Figure 38–65. Four-year-old girl with high ureteropelvic insertion and no obstruction.

is loosely attached to the angle of a poorly developed trigone. The embryologic origin is described in the introduction to this section of the chapter (p. 1714). In summary, the ureteral bud is felt to originate more caudally than normal from the mesonephric duct, placing it too close to the future bladder. Thus, it separates prematurely from the mesonephric duct as the normally short common segment is absorbed into the developing bladder. Because it has more time to migrate, the orifice finally comes to rest in a high and lateral position, resulting in a large and poorly developed trigone. The mesenchymal precursors of the trigonal and ureteral musculature are deficient as well, thereby contributing to the defect (Ambrose and Nicolson, 1962; Stephens and Lenaghan, 1962; Tanagho, 1976). The degree of caudal displacement of the ureteral bud varies, and the range of severity of ureterovesical incompetence varies with it.

Vesicoureteral reflux is relatively common in total ureteral duplication (Privett et al., 1976) and most frequently involves the lower pole ureter, the so-called orthotopic orifice. The upper pole ureter is less likely to reflux. Even when it inserts close to the orthotopic lower pole orifice, its migratory pathway (Fig. 38–54) almost always places it more distally, so that its intravesical segment is longer. However, it too can reflux, generally to a lesser degree, when both buds have originated more caudally than normal so that the two orifices both terminate too high and lateral. Primary reflux into the

upper pole segment may also occur, often alone, when its orifice into the distal trigone or bladder neck is ectopic, entering through a separate muscular hiatus (Ambrose and Nicolson, 1964; Tanagho, 1976).

The reader is referred to Chapter 49 for a full presentation of vesicoureteral reflux and an extensive bibliography.

Ectopic Ureter

An ectopic ureter is one that does not open at the normal location at the angle of the trigone. Although a refluxing ureteral orifice might be considered to belong in this category because of its tendency to have a more cranial and lateral position (called by some "lateral ectopia"), the term *ectopic ureter* by convention refers to any ureter in which the ultimate termination is determined by a delay in, or lack of, separation from the mesonephric duct. This is the converse of reflux, which results from early separation of the ureteral bud from the mesonephric duct. Eighty per cent of all ectopic ureters are associated with a duplicated system, and most of these occur in females (Schulman, 1976). The embryology of ectopic ureter is detailed on page 1716.

ANATOMY

The ectopic ureteral orifice may open into the urinary or genital tract (Fig. 38–57), following an ectopic pathway (Fig. 38–58) (Stephens,

1958, 1963). When located anywhere along the trigone to the level of the vesical neck, it is unlikely to cause symptoms and is rarely of clinical concern; openings from the vesical neck distally can cause clinical symptoms from obstruction, reflux, and, in the female, incontinence.

Stephens (1963) divided the female urethra into an upper urethral internal sphincter zone and a lower urethral external sphincter zone. An orifice in the internal sphincter region is apt to be obstructed, but the patient will be continent. An orifice in the distal urethra will have a lesser obstruction, but the patient will be incontinent.

Openings also occur in the vestibule and vagina, and rarely, in the cervix or uterus. These openings result from rupture of Gartner's duct into the developing ureterovaginal canal at some point along their common wall (see page 1717). The vestibular opening is the most common form and represents the terminal extent of Gartner's duct. It is likely that the terminal portion of the mesonephric duct (commonly excretory duct) fails to regress totally in some cases, although proof of this is not conclusive (Ellerker, 1958). Abeshouse (1943) found several reports of a ureter opening into a dilated Gartner's duct and, in one case, into a dilated vaginal (Gartner's) cyst. Termination of an ectopic ureter into a Gartner's cyst is the least common manifestation of ureteral ectopy and has been described with a single-system vaginal ectopic ureter. The associated kidney is small and dysplastic or absent (Currarino, 1982). The cyst may be closed or may communicate with the vagina, bladder, bladder neck, or urethra (Kjaeldgaard and Fianau, 1982). In one patient with a bifid system, there was sufficient renal function that treatment included ureteroneocystostomy (Kjaeldgaard et al., 1981).

Three cases of an ectopic ureter entering an apparent urethral diverticulum have been reported, the latter probably representing the terminal mesonephric duct. Two of these were in infant girls (Vanhouette, 1970) who had a small outpouching below the bladder neck. In his search, the author was unable to find any true congenital urethral diverticula in little girls and emphasized that this radiographic finding should indicate an ectopic ureter. The third case was a 26-year-old woman with lifelong incontinence (Wilmarth, 1948). Here the "diverticulum" was large but eccentric, opening at the side of the ectopic ureter, which suggests its congenital origin.

Rarely,. hydrocolpos (urocolpos) and a single vaginal ectopic ureter occur in combination with a vaginal atresia (transverse vaginal septum), the latter representing arrested development of the vaginal plate (Feldman and Ross, 1980). Another rare variant is a vesicoureterovaginal communication in which the ureter has a connection with both bladder and vagina (Kondo et al., 1982). In one girl treated by nephrectomy at age 3 years for a single ectopic system, recurrent incontinence occurred 5 years later from spontaneous vesicovaginal fistula through the stump of the ectopic ureter, suggesting rupture of a thin, hypoplastic membrane (Koyanagi et al., 1977).

Cases of ectopic ureter opening at the vestibule or distal urethra without incontinence have been described. In some, incontinence never developed, and the lesion was discovered during investigation of urinary infection or flank pain. In others, incontinence did not appear until adolescence or after pregnancy. In all these cases, the ectopic ureter presumably passed through some portion of the external urethral sphincter musculature, allowing ureteral drainage only during voiding. It is likely that the changes of puberty or of childbirth cause attenuation of this muscular support in some patients, allowing late-onset incontinence (Childlow and Utz, 1970; Davis, 1930; DeWeerd and Litin, 1958; Honke, 1946; Koyanagi et al., 1980; Moore, 1952; Ogawa et al., 1976; Wesson, 1934; Verbaeys et al., 1980).

In the male, ectopic ureters are found at any level of the ectopic pathway into the prostatic urethra at the level of the verumontanum proximal to the external urinary sphincter. Incontinence is not a symptom. The ectopic ureter can also drain into the genital tract through the seminal vesicle, vas deferens, or ejaculatory duct. The ipsilateral mesonephric derivatives may also be maldeveloped; seminal vesical cysts have been reported as well as one case of agenesis of the corresponding testis (Das and Amar, 1980; Deilmann and Moormann, 1978). Two cases are described of a single-system ectopic ureter terminating in the epididymis (Jona et al., 1979; Ostermayer and Frei, 1981). In a few instances, the ectopic ureter has drained into the utriculus, which is of paramesonephric (müllerian) duct origin. As the mesonephric and paramesonephric ducts lie closely applied in a common mesenchyme at their early attachment to the cloaca, it is likely that a communication develops between them in this situation (Ellerker, 1958) from shifting or fusion of the bud with the paramesonephric duct (Abeshouse, 1943). Based on the termination of the ectopic ureter described earlier, Das and Amar (1981) have classified it as: Type I—urogenital sinus ectopia, in which the ureter terminates in the posterior urethra; and Type II—mesonephric duct ectopia, in which ureter terminates in a mesonephric derivative.

An unusual variant of a persistent common excretory duct involves an ectopic vas deferens opening into the ureter, with a common duct terminating on the trigone in a relatively normal location. This common duct has been termed a persisting mesonephric duct, the terminal portion of which resembles the ureter rather than the vas (Schwarz and Stephens, 1978). In one 7-year-old boy, the orifice was entirely normal and there was no reflux (Alfert and Gillenwater, 1972), and in two infants, vesicoureteral reflux was present (Borger and Belman, 1975). All three patients had other anomalies. In another example, a 13-year-old boy with bilateral ectopic vasa had a large, poorly emptying, hypotonic bladder with a megatrigone and bilateral reflux but no other anomalies (Redman and Sulieman, 1976). Gibbons et al. (1978) reviewed 11 cases with 13 ectopic vasal insertions; ureteral ectopia was encountered in one third of the cases, and vesicoureteral reflux was present in 9 of the 13 renal units. In five instances the vas terminated in the bladder. Although strictly speaking these cases of ectopic vasa do not involve ectopic ureters, the embryologic features, which are similar to those for ectopic insertion of the ureter into the seminal tract, justify inclusion here. Although the embryology of the ectopic vas is not fully understood, the common excretory duct appears to have failed to absorb completely but did not migrate distally, apparently behaving instead like a ureteral duct in its migration and development.

Ureteral openings into the rectum are extremely rare. Leef and Leader (1962) noted three instances in the literature and described an adult with a single-system ectopic ureter into the rectum plus a 2-cm blind-ending ureteral stump into the ipsilateral trigone. Uson and Schulman (1972) provided long-term follow-up data on an infant reported earlier with bilateral duplication–ectopic orifice into the rectum on one side and an ectopic ureterocele on the other.

Occasionally, ureters terminate blindly in a site ectopic from the trigonal region; these present clinically as tubular or rounded cystic masses draining a dysplastic, nonfunctioning kidney. Conversely, the upper end of an ectopic ureter may end blindly, representing an abortive ectopic ureteral bud (Gray and Skandalakis, 1972; Varney and Ford, 1954.)

INCIDENCE

The true incidence of ectopic ureter is uncertain, as many cause no symptoms. Campbell (1970) noted ten examples in 19,046 autopsies in children (1 in 1900) but felt that some had been overlooked. Eighty per cent of ectopic orifices are associated with a duplicated collecting system; in females, more than 80 per cent are duplicated, whereas in males the majority of ectopic ureters drain single systems (Schulman, 1976); this is particularly true if ectopic ureteroceles are excluded from consideration.

Ectopic ureter appears more commonly in females—clinically, from 2 to 12 times more frequently—with the lesser frequency probably reflecting the incidence more accurately (Burford et al., 1949; Eisendrath, 1938; Lowsley and Kerwin, 1956; Mills, 1939). Ellerker (1958) noted 366 females and 128 males in his review of 494 ectopic ureters, including autopsies, for a female-to-male ratio of 2.9:1. Between 7.5 and 17 per cent of ectopic ureters appear bilaterally (Eisendrath, 1938; Ellerker, 1958). A small percentage involve a solitary kidney. With unilateral ectopic ureter, a contralateral ureteral duplication is not uncommon.

The distribution of ectopic ureters by location is itemized in Table 38–6. In the male, the posterior urethra is the most common site of ectopic ureter. Drainage into the genital tract involves the seminal vesicle three times more often than the ejaculatory duct and vas deferens combined (Ellerker, 1958; Lucius, 1963; Riba et al., 1946). In the female, the urethra and vestibule are the most common sites.

TABLE 38–6. LOCATION OF 494 ECTOPIC URETERS (INCLUDING AUTOPSIES)*

	Number	Per Cent
128 Males		
Posterior urethra	60	47
Prostatic utricle	13	10
Seminal vesicle	42	33
Ejaculatory duct	7	5
Vas deferens	6	5
366 Females		35
Urethra	129	34
Vestibule	124	25
Vagina	90	5
Cervix or uterus	18	<1
Gartner's duct	3	<1
Urethral diverticulum	2	

*From Ellerker, A. G.: Br. J. Surg., 45:344, 1958.

The age at diagnosis ranges widely, with many examples not detected during life (Ellerker, 1958).

ASSOCIATED ANOMALIES

The earlier literature fails to provide adequate descriptions of the upper tracts, but more recent reports emphasize that the degree of ectopia is related directly to the degree of renal maldevelopment—i.e., the more remote the ureteral opening, the greater the degree of renal maldevelopment (Schulman, 1976). With duplicated systems this means hypoplasia or dysplasia of the upper pole segment. In ten cases of ectopic ureter that drained a single system and opened into the male seminal tracts, the kidney was nonvisualized radiographically in all (Rognon et al., 1973). Of 16 single renal ducts drained by an ectopic ureter, renal dysplasia was present in 7 (Prewitt and Lebowitz, 1976). The anomalous single kidney may be ectopic in position as well. The ectopic ureter itself is also abnormal, usually to a greater degree in the single than in the duplicated system. Usually the ureter is variably dilated and drainage is impaired (Williams and Royle, 1969). Muscle cells may show severe alterations on ultrastructure studies; whether these changes are developmental or acquired is not yet known (Hanna et al., 1977).

SYMPTOMS

In males an ectopic ureter may remain undiagnosed unless symptoms of ureteral obstruction or infection appear. Although urinary incontinence should not be a complaint, urgency and frequency can be a response to the continuous trickle of urine into the posterior urethra (Ellerker, 1958; Williams, 1954). Incontinence in males, in fact, may be a feature of the uncommon circumstance of bilateral single ectopic ureters, for reasons to be discussed later in this section.

When the ectopic ureter drains into the seminal tract, it often does not become symptomatic until the inset of sexual activity. In addition to dysuria and frequency, symptoms and signs may include prostatitis, seminal vesiculitis and epididymitis, painful defecation, constipation, pelvic pain, epididymal swelling, bloody or painful ejaculation, and a palpable painful cystic mass on rectal palpation (Brannan and Henry, 1973; Schnitzer, 1965). At cystoscopic evaluation, a hemitrigone will be present with a single system, and the posterolateral floor of the bladder may be displaced or elevated by a cystic mass behind it. The intravesical bulge of the dilated ureter can resemble an ectopic ureterocele (Cumes et al., 1981).

In females, about half present with urinary incontinence. The diagnosis may be suspected after toilet training, if not before. Typically, normal cyclic bladder function will be evident despite constant dampness or wetness.

When the offending renal unit is small and poorly functioning, identification may be difficult even with ultrasonography. At times, angiography has defined a tiny, dysplastic, duplicated segment (Kittredge and Levin, 1973). Diagnostic approaches and treatment are detailed in Chapter 50.

TREATMENT AND PROGNOSIS

Progress is generally good for the ectopic ureter in a duplicated system. Partial nephrectomy and ureterectomy, ureteroneocystostomy, or pyelopyelostomy with distal ureterectomy is the usual choice of therapy.

SINGLE ECTOPIC URETER—ADDITIONAL FEATURES

In reports from Caucasian countries, single-system ectopic ureters constitute 20 per cent of all ectopic ureters and most occur in males. In Japan, by contrast, 70 per cent of all ectopic ureters are single systems, mostly in females with vaginal drainage (Gotoh et al., 1983). Single-system ectopic ureters present some differences from those involving double ureters, and, when bilateral, they present more problems. Prewitt and Lebowitz (1976) reported that of 16 patients, 7 had other anomalies—congenital heart disease in 3 and high imperforate anus in 4. The high incidence of ipsilateral renal hypoplasia and dysplasia has been described earlier. Poor function or nonfunction of these anomalous and often ectopically located kidneys and a tiny blood supply make their detection difficult at times (Gibbons and Duckett, 1978; Schulman, 1976, 1978; Scott, 1981).

With *unilateral single ectopic ureter,* the ipsilateral hemitrigone fails to develop, and one side of the bladder neck is incompletely developed. Nevertheless, with unilateral ectopia, the hemitrigone is generally adequate for urinary control provided that, in the female, the ectopic ureter is above the continence zone of the urethra (Mogg, 1974).

With *bilateral single ectopic ureter* into the urethra, the bladder fails to develop properly (Fig. 38–56). The trigone is absent. The bladder is generally small, since it never contains more urine than is regurgitated from the urethra. Continuous incontinence is usual, although not inevitable; even males tend to dribble, although they are generally able to retain enough volume to void as well. Boys appear to have a lesser degree of bladder underdevelopment. The bladder neck region is not clearly defined; the vesical outflow is widely funneled and shortened, resembling the condition seen in epispadias. In extreme cases, the bladder fails to develop at all, and the ureters enter the vestibule, a condition often incompatible with life because of severe renal insufficiency or other anomalies. Most of these patients are females (Koyanagi et al., 1977; Mogg, 1974; Noseworthy and Persky, 1982; Sorenson and Middleton, 1983; Williams and Lightwood, 1972). Survival is possible, however, and rehabilitation is accomplished by intestinal diversion (Glenn, 1959).

In their review of bilateral single ectopic ureters, Williams and Lightwood (1972) added 10 cases, 7 girls and 3 boys, to the 23 previously reported. The girls generally had more severe renal deformities and a lesser degree of bladder development. The results of surgical reconstruction, namely, ureteral reimplantation and construction of a vesical neck, were disappointing, especially for the girls. Only three of the seven gained adequate control; one of these underwent diversion later for upper tract dilatation, and three of the other four failures also underwent diversion. The authors pointed out that success or failure of the reconstruction was related to the severity of the underlying condition.

Ureterocele

Ureterocele is a cystic dilation of the intravesical submucosal ureter. The size may vary from a small bulge of 1 or 2 cm in diameter to a lesion that almost fills the bladder. The appearance is that of a thin walled often translucent mass. The outer surface is vesical epithelium and the inner is ureteral epithelium; between them is a thin layer of patchy muscle and collagen. Ureterocele may involve either a single collecting system or the ureter to the upper pole of a duplicated system; the opening for either may be intravesical in location or ectopic, at the bladder neck or more distal.

CLASSIFICATION AND ANATOMY

A number of classifications of varying complexity have appeared through the years, but a simple one in common use is that of Ericsson (1954). He divided ureterocele into two groups: simple and ectopic. Henceforth, simple ureter-

ocele will be described as intravesical ureterocele. *Intravesical ureterocele* is entirely contained within the urinary bladder. It may arise from a single or occasionally supernumerary ureter that always ends in a normal or near normal bladder location. Intravesical ureteroceles when associated with a single system, tend to be small in size. *Ectopic ureterocele* extends into the bladder neck or urethra. The orifice terminates ectopically. As with ectopic ureters generally, most involve the upper pole of a double ureter; a single system is uncommon. Three recent reports describe the rare finding of a ureterocele involving the lower pole ureter of a double system. In two cases, the upper segment ureter was ectopic and its renal unit was dysplastic and nonfunctioning; in the third case, the upper segment was normal (Ahmed, 1981; Arap et al., 1983; Lima and Cavalcanti, 1981). Ectopic ureteroceles tend to be much larger than intravesical ureteroceles. Intravesical ureteroceles have also been termed *adult ureteroceles* because they resemble the small lesions of the adult that typically involve a single system. The ureter proximal to the ureterocele is variably dilated, to a lesser degree than the ureterocele itself. However, with the largest ectopic ureteroceles, immense dilatation and tortuosity of the ureter may occur.

Although Ericsson's classification of ureterocele has wide clinical applicability, Stephens' (1963) classification is useful for a more detailed understanding of the pathologic anatomy. He defined three major types—stenotic, sphincteric, and sphincterostenotic. The *stenotic ureterocele* has a narrowed orifice location on the dome of a rounded intravesical mass and is usually located in a normal or near-normal intravesical location—i.e., the equivalent of Ericsson's "simple" ureterocele. The degree of stenosis may vary; when slight, the size of the ureterocele varies with peristalsis, and when extreme the ureterocele remains tense and urine dribbles from the orifice between periodic, needle-like jets. Histologically, the wall of a stenotic ureterocele contains a surprising amount of muscle, although it is less dense than that in the ureteral wall above. Its orientation tends to be longitudinal.

The *sphincteric ureterocele* is a form of ectopic ureterocele in which the orifice is within the internal sphincter (bladder neck or proximal urethra). The orifice may be normal or even generous in size, the ureterocele being obstructed by the sphincter-like action of the vesical outlet, emptying only during voiding when the bladder neck opens. At times there is reflux during voiding through this large proximal urethral orifice. Histologically, the sphincteric and the sphincterostenotic ureterocele contain variable muscle bundles, which are considerably less dense than those in the normal distal ureter but are oriented in a more random or helical pattern than the mainly longitudinal bundles of the normal intravesical ureter (Stephens, 1963; Tanagho, 1976). At times the ureterocele is apparently not obstructed; five children have been described with a small, dysplastic renal unit and undilated ureter in association with the ectopic ureterocele (Bauer and Retick, 1978).

The *sphincterostenotic ureterocele* is another variant of ectopic ureterocele in which the orifice is tiny as well as ectopic. This form of ureterocele achieves a larger size, often almost filling the bladder. It is continuously distended and may extend into the vesical outlet, obstructing it to a varying degree. Prolapse of a large ureterocele through the urethra onto the perineum may occasionally occur (Diard et al., 1981; Eklöf et al., 1978; Fenelon and Alton, 1981; Klauber and Crawford, 1980; Orr and Glanton, 1953).

In addition to these three forms of ureterocele, there is an uncommon variant of ectopic ureterocele, the so-called *cecoureterocele*. Here, upward migration of the developing ectopic ureteral orifice leaves a tongue of more distal ureter underneath the urethral mucosa. The orifice in a cecoureterocele is proximal to the bladder neck (Stephens, 1968). Rarely, a ureterocele may end blindly if regression of the mesonephric duct has involved the termination of the ectopic ureter as well (Ericsson, 1954; Stephens, 1968).

Ureteroceles are not inevitably obstructed (Bauer and Retik, 1978), and some intact ureteroceles also reflux (Borden and Martinez, 1977; Leong et al., 1980). Large ectopic ureteroceles can obstruct the lower pole ipsilateral ureter or even the contralateral side as well as the bladder neck. The lower pole ipsilateral ureter at times refluxes. On occasion, dilation of the lower pole segment is due to an intrinsic rather than an extrinsic obstruction (Androulakakis et al., 1981). As is true for ectopic ureters generally, the renal segment associated with an ectopic ureterocele tends to be abnormal and is often poorly functioning or nonfunctioning. Hypoplasia, dysplasia, and hydronephrotic atrophy are frequently present, as is superimposed pyelonephritis (Perrin et al., 1974; Williams and Woodard, 1964). The generally smaller sized intravesical ureterocele associated with a single system often causes a relatively mild degree of obstruction when encountered in adults. When diagnosed in children, however, it can be associated with a severe degree of hydronephrosis and hydroureter; Snyder and Johnston (1978) noted nonfunction of the involved kidney in 5 of 20 intravesical ureteroceles.

All of these forms of ureterocele and their clinical import are illustrated and described in detail in Chapter 50.

INCIDENCE

Incidence has varied in the reports of different authors. Campbell (1951) noted an autopsy incidence in children of 1 in 4000. Uson and associates (1961) observed 6 in 3200 pediatric autopsies, or 1 in 500. Undoubtedly, some small ureteroceles at autopsy are not recognized because they have collapsed. The clinical incidence varies also. In one series, ureterocele occurred in 1 in 100 pediatric urologic admissions (Uson et al., 1961) and in from 1 in 5000 to 1 in 12,000 general pediatric admissions (Malek et al., 1972). Ureterocele is three to four times more frequent in girls. It is more common on the left side. Between 10 and 15 per cent are bilateral (Bruézière et al., 1979; Campbell, 1951; Gross, 1953; Malek et al., 1972; Mandell et al., 1980). Familial occurrence of ureterocele has been described. Two siblings had simple ureteroceles (Abrams et al., 1980); nonidentical twins had ectopic ureteroceles (Ayalon et al., 1979); a mother and daughter had ectopic ureteroceles, and all their first-degree relatives had some degree of ureteral duplication (Babcock et al., 1977).

In most pediatric series, ectopic ureteroceles are more common than intravesical ureteroceles; they composed 14 of 20 in Ericsson's (1954) series and 21 of 30 in Stephens' (1963) series, most of these being duplicated systems. In a series of 93 ureteroceles, 34 were intravesical, 24 of these being single systems. Fifty-nine were ectopic, with double ureters (Bruézière et al., 1979). Ectopic single systems are uncommon; none of Ericsson's series had this anomaly, but in his review of the literature he found two single systems in 14 ectopic ureteroceles. Similarly, Williams and Royle (1969) found 3 single systems in 15 ectopic ureteroceles, and Malek and associates (1972) had 2 in 14; there are other sporadic reports (Prewitt and Lebowitz, 1976). Single-system ectopic ureterocele is more common in males and appears to have a high likelihood of other anomalies. There are two reports of crossed renal ectopia involving the ureterocele (Farkas et al., 1978; Fishman and Borden, 1982). Johnson and Perlmutter (1980) reported seven children with single-system ectopic ureteroceles; six were boys. Five children had a nonfunctioning hypodysplastic kidney; four had major cardiac anomalies and three boys had abdominal testes—two with bilateral nonunion to the vas.

EMBRYOLOGY

The details of the embryology of ureterocele are incompletely understood. Most authors ascribe the formation of intravesical ureterocele to delayed rupture of Chwalle's membrane (Chwalle, 1927)—an occluding, two-layered epithelial membrane normally present in the 15-mm embryo and located between the developing ureter and the urogenital sinus—when the ureter has established its separate attachment to the sinus. This membrane then bulges and the adjacent primitive ureter expands, presumably from early metanephric secretion, before the membrane disappears by the 35-mm stage (Gyllensten, 1949). Delayed opening of the membrane results in further dilatation of the terminal ureteral segment and stenosis of the orifice.

The explanation of ectopic ureterocele includes delayed separation of the ureteral bud from the mesonephric duct because of its too cranial origin. This allows more time for the occurrence of ampullary terminal ureteral dilatation (Tanagho, 1976). When the ectopic orifice is in the proximal urethral or bladder neck region, there may be no intrinsic stenosis. Developmental expansion of the vesicourethral canal may also involve the developing ectopic orifice, causing it to enlarge. Obstruction of the ureterocele in this instance occurs because of sphincteric action from the vesical neck region; this explains the tendency for these ureteroceles to empty somewhat during voiding or, alternatively, for vesicoureteral reflux to occur during voiding (Stephens, 1963, 1968).

These explanations do not account for the fact that not all ectopic ureters are associated with ureterocele formation. An intrinsic alteration in ureteral bud development with excessive expansion of the developing terminal ureter and altered development of the musculature of the developing intravesical ureter in the ectopic ureterocele segment may explain the difference (Stephens, 1963). Stephens compared the intravesical ureteral musculature of ectopic ureteroceles with ectopic ureters that had a long intravesical course and orifices terminating in the internal sphincter zone. The intravesical portion of the ectopic ureter was well muscularized, and the fibers were not limited to the longitudinal orientation typical of a normal ure-

ter. The ectopic ureterocele, on the other hand, had a variable deficiency of musculature; the muscle fibers that were present included bundles oriented in both circular and longitudinal axis. The relatively muscular-deficient distal ureter expanded more than the better muscularized, more proximal ureter. Tokunaka and associates (1981) studied muscle structure, by light and electron microscopy, of several ureteroceles, both intravesical and ectopic. They noted a paucity of muscle bundles in the dome of the ureterocele in contrast to well-developed bundles in the proximal ureter. Muscle cells were smaller in the ureterocele than in the proximal ureter; thick myofibrils were absent in the muscle of the ureterocele. They concluded that these findings indicated a segmental embryonic arrest of the most distal ureter, which plays a role in ureterocele formation.

Stephens did note that some ectopic ureters were deficient in musculature. However, these ureters terminated more distally, below the internal sphincter zone. He felt that when the ureteral orifice was in this location the ultimate size of the ectopic ureter was less predictable, as it was related more to alterations of ureteral bud development than to muscular endowment (Stephens, 1963). In contrast to ectopic ureteroceles, ectopic ureters may enter the lower urinary tract through a hiatus separate from that for the orthotopic ureter, as the mesenchyme of the developing trigone accumulates between the widely separated ureteral buds (Tanagho, 1976). This would tend to keep the terminal ectopic ureter from expanding excessively, even if it is poorly muscularized.

In summary, embryonic obstruction, delayed absorption of the developing ureter into the urogenital sinus, and altered ureteral bud differentiation consisting of arrested muscular development of the most caudal ureter associated with excessive caudal widening have all been proposed as factors in ureterocele formation.

ANOMALIES OF POSITION

Vascular Anomalies Involving the Ureter

A variety of vascular lesions can cause ureteral obstruction; in these, the vascular system rather than the collecting system is generally anomalous. With the exception of accessory renal blood vessels, all of these lesions are relatively uncommon, though all have clinical relevance.

ACCESSORY RENAL BLOOD VESSELS

Accessory or aberrant vessels to the lower pole of the kidney can cross ventral to the ureteropelvic junction, causing obstruction. These are presented earlier in this chapter under Anomalies of the Kidney—Anomalies of Renal Vasculature and in Chapter 65.

PREURETERAL VENA CAVA

Anatomy. This anomaly is commonly known to the urologist as *circumcaval ureter* or *retrocaval ureter,* terms that are anatomically descriptive but developmentally misleading. Of the two terms, circumcaval ureter is preferred, because rarely a ureter may lie behind (dorsal to) the vena cava for some portion of its lumbar course without encircling the cava, and this form of retrocaval ureter appears to be developmentally different (Dreyfuss, 1959; Lerman et al., 1956; Peisojovich and Lutz, 1969). In the case of Dreyfuss (1959) there was also a small branch vein between the vena cava and right iliopsoas muscle, over which (cephalad to it) the ureter coursed to enter the retrocaval area. The term "preureteral vena cava" emphasizes that

the circumcaval ureter arises from altered vascular, rather than ureteral, development.

This disorder involves the right ureter, which typically deviates medially behind (dorsal to) the inferior vena cava, winding about it and crossing in front of it from a medial direction to a lateral one, to resume a normal course distal to the bladder. The renal pelvis and upper ureter are typically elongated and dilated in a J or "fishhook" shape before passing behind the vena cava (Fig. 38–66). However, the collecting system is not inevitably obstructed. Bateson and Atkinson (1969), Crosse and associates (1975), and Kenawi and Williams (1976) have classified circumcaval ureters into two clinical types: The more common Type I has hydronephrosis and a typically obstructed pattern demonstrating some degree of "fishhook" deformity of the ureter to the level of the obstruction, and Type II has a lesser degree of or absent hydronephrosis. Here the upper ureter is not kinked but passes behind the vena cava at a higher level, the renal pelvis and upper ureter lying nearly horizontal before encircling the vena cava in a smooth curve. In Type I the obstruction appears to occur at the edge of the iliopsoas muscle, at which point the ureter deviates cephalad before passing behind the vena cava; in Type II the obstruction, when present, appears to be at the

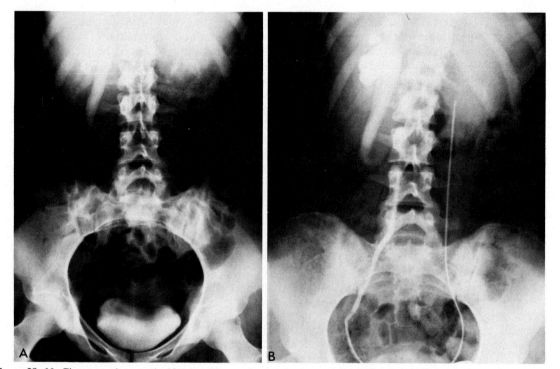

Figure 38–66. Circumcaval ureter in 20-year-old woman with intermittent flank pain. *A,* IVP. *B,* Retrograde ureteropyelogram.

lateral wall of the vena cava as the ureter is compressed against the perivertebral tissues.

Embryology. The definitive inferior vena cava develops on the right side from a plexus of fetal veins (Fig. 38–67). Initially, the venous retroperitoneal pathways consist of symmetrically placed vessels, both ventral and dorsal. The posterior cardinal and supracardinal veins lie dorsally, and the subcardinals lie ventrally. These channels, with their anastomoses, form a collar on each side through which the ascending kidneys pass. Normally, the left supracardinal vein and the lumbar portion of the right posterior cardinal vein atrophy. The subcardinals become the internal spermatic veins. The definitive right-sided inferior vena cava forms from the right supracardinal vein. If the subcardinal vein in the lumbar portion fails to atrophy and becomes the primary right-sided vein, the ureter is trapped dorsal to it.

When the definitive vena cava forms normally and the ventral portion of the primitive ring also persists, a double right vena cava is formed because of the persistence of both the right subcardinal vein dorsally and the right subcardinal vein ventrally; this double vena cava traps the right ureter between its limbs (Fig. 38–68) (Gruenwald and Surks, 1943).

Although bilateral and left-sided venae cavae can occur (Clements et al., 1978), a bilateral circumcaval ureter has been reported only once, in an acardiac monster (Gladstone, 1905), and a left circumcaval ureter has been described in a case of situs inversus (Brooks, 1962). In cases of bilateral venae cavae associated with a circumcaval ureter, the circumcaval ureter has been reported only on the right side, denoting that the right vena cava developed abnormally from a persistent subcardinal vein, whereas the left vena cava developed from the left supracardinal vein but otherwise normally (Pick and Anson, 1940).

Incidence. The incidence of preureteral vena cava is about 1 in 1500 cadavers (Heslin and Mamonas, 1951) and is three to four times more common in male than in female cadavers. Gray and Skandalakis (1972) consider this frequency too high because of the preponderance of male autopsies performed. Clinically, preureteral vena cava occurs 2.8 times more frequently in males; Kenawi and Williams (1976), in reviewing the literature, recorded 114 males

Figure 38–67. Diagrammatic representation depicting: *A,* fetal venous ring, *B,* normal vena cava and *C,* preureteric vena cava. (Redrawn from Hollinshead, W. H.: Anatomy for Surgeons, Vol. 2, New York, Hoeber Medical Division of Harper and Row, 1956.)

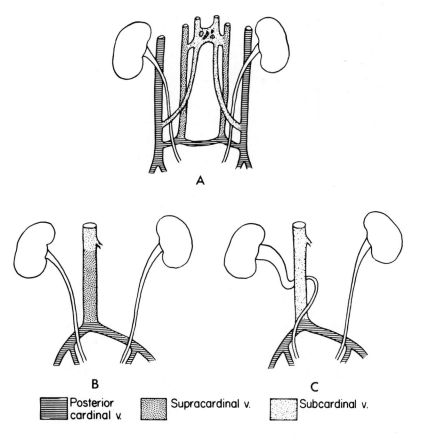

A

B

C

▤ Posterior cardinal v.   ▦ Supracardinal v.   ▧ Subcardinal v.

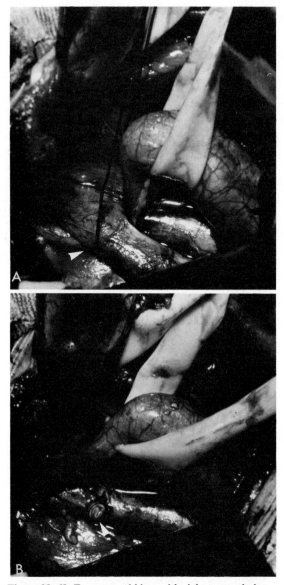

Figure 38–68. Four-year-old boy with right ureteral obstruction from double right vena cava. Site of obstruction is apparent distally, as ureter lies between ventral and dorsal limbs of double cava. Arrow points to ventral limb. Before *(A)* and after *(B)* division.

and 41 females, with 7 not known. The symptoms of preureteral vena cava are those of obstruction. Although the lesion is congenital, most patients do not present until the third or fourth decade of life (Kenawi and Williams, 1976).

Other Anomalies. Several instances of horseshoe kidney have been reported (Cendron and Reis, 1972; Cukier et al., 1969; Eidelman et al., 1978; Hefferman et al., 1978; Kumeda et al., 1982). Contralateral anomalies include a variety of left renal anomalies, such as agenesis, hydronephrosis, malrotation, and hypoplasia (Kenawi and Williams, 1976). There has been one case of left hydronephrosis with ensheathing of both ureters by a single fibrous membrane below the level of the venous anomaly (Salem and Luck, 1976).

Diagnosis. Excretory urography often fails to visualize the portion of the ureter beyond the J hook (i.e., extending behind the vena cava), but retrograde ureteropyelography will demonstrate an S curve to the point of obstruction (Fig. 38–66), with the retrocaval segment lying at the level of L3 or L4 (Kenawi and Williams, 1976). Treatment of the obstruction is detailed in Chapter 68. Briefly, surgical correction involves ureteral division, with relocation and ureteroureteral or ureteropelvic reanastomosis, generally with excision or bypass of the retrocaval segment, which can be aperistaltic.

PREURETERAL ILIAC ARTERY (RETROILIAC URETER)

An extremely rare lesion, the ureter lying behind the iliac artery, has been described six times (Corbus et al., 1960; Dees, 1940; Hanna, 1972; Iuchtman et al., 1980; Seitzman and Patton, 1960; Radhkrishnan et al., 1980). Either side can be involved; in two cases it was bilateral (Hanna, 1972; Radhkrishnan et al., 1980). Obstruction occurs at the level of L5 or S1 as the ureter is compressed behind the artery. Gray and Skandalakis (1972) feel that the anomaly is vascular in origin. Normally the primitive ventral root of the umbilical artery is replaced by development of a more dorsal branch between the aorta and the distal umbilical artery. Persistence of the ventral root as the dorsal root fails to form will trap the ureter dorsally (Fig. 38–69). Dees (1940) also considered the possibility that aberrant upward migration of the kidney in his case might have placed it dorsal to the iliac artery, which was redundant. Ureteral or mesonephric duct ectopia is often present. In Dees' case there was evidence, although not definite proof, that the ureteral orifice was ectopic in the vesical neck, supporting the concept of anomalous renoureteral development. The case of Seitzman and Patton (1960) involved an ectopic ureter emptying, along with the ipsilateral vas deferens, via a persistent common mesonephric duct into the proximal posterior urethra. The case of Radhkrishnan and colleagues (1980) with bilateral retroiliac ureters also involved bilateral ectopic termination of the vas deferentia into the ureters. Iuchtman and associates (1980) described ectopic vaginal

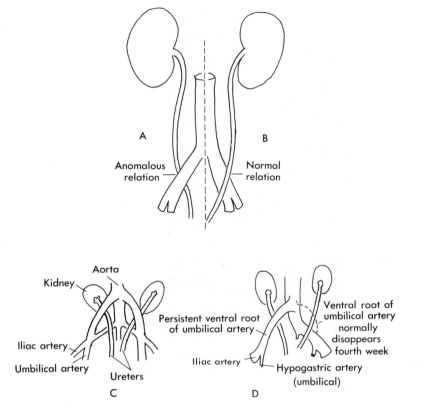

Figure 38–69. Preureteral iliac artery (postarterial ureter). *A,* Anomalous relationship of ureter and artery. *B,* Normal relationship of ureter and artery. *C,* Relationships of ureter and iliac and umbilical arteries in the embryo. *D,* Development of normal iliac channel on the right, anomalous iliac channel (persistence of proximal umbilical artery) on the left. (From Gray, S. W., and Skandalakis, J. E.: Embryology for Surgeons. Philadelphia, W. B. Saunders Co., 1972.)

termination of the involved ureter with urometrocolpos from an imperforate hymen.

VASCULAR OBSTRUCTION OF THE DISTAL URETER

Obstruction of the distal ureter from uterine, umbilical, obturator, and hypogastric vessels close to the bladder has been described (Campbell, 1933, 1936, 1970; Greene et al., 1954; Hyams, 1929; Scultety and Varga, 1975; Young and Kiser, 1965). However, it is not always clear that vascular impressions upon a dilated ureter are the cause of the obstruction. At times these findings may be an artifact, as when a dilated ureter from an intrinsic obstruction is secondarily compressed against the adjacent vessel (Campbell, 1970). Judging from the paucity of contemporary reports describing this lesion, it is likely that primary terminal ureteral obstruction by vascular lesions is a rare occurrence.

Herniation of the Ureter

This is an extremely rare condition. Dourmashkin (1937) searched the literature and tabulated a series of inguinal, scrotal, and femoral herniations of the ureter. Most of these were *paraperitoneal*—i.e., a loop of herniated ureter extended alongside a peritoneal hernial sac; only a minority were *extraperitoneal*—i.e., no hernial sac was present. In the paraperitoneal ureteral hernias, the ureteral loop always lay medial to the peritoneal sac. Of six scrotal hernias, four did not have peritoneal sacs. When the ureter extended into the scrotum it was more likely to be dilated, causing upper tract obstruction.

Watson (1948) collected 102 cases of inguinal or femoral hernia involving the ureter. Jewett and Harris (1953) described a case of left ureteral hernia into the scrotum in a 9-year-old boy with left hydronephrosis (Fig. 38–70). This hernia was of the extraperitoneal type: a mesentery-like blood supply supplied two loops of ureter within the scrotum that were adherent to the cord structures.

Dourmashkin (1937) felt that herniation of the ureter could be acquired or congenital, the acquired form being a "sliding hernia" and the congenital form being present since birth. In the latter form, he proposed that the loop of ureter had been drawn down with the descent of the testis, and the developing ureter had adhered

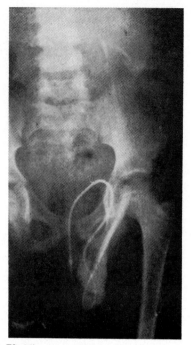

Figure 38–70. Nine-year-old boy with herniation of the left ureter into scrotum. No hernial sac is present. Obstructed system was treated by ureteral resection and reanastomosis. (Courtesy of Dr. Hugh J. Jewett and Journal of Urology.)

to migrating vas. Internal hernias of the ureter are even more exceptional. There have been two reports of sciatic hernia containing ureter (Beck et al., 1952; Lindblom, 1947) and one of herniation between the psoas muscle and iliac vessels (Page, 1955).

References

A note to the reader regarding the bibliography:

The authors intend that these references be comprehensive but not exhaustive. Because the urologic literature has been growing, some early historical reports and articles of an anecdotal nature have been excluded, as a number of the more recent articles cited contain reviews with extensive bibliographies as well as contemporary approaches to diagnosis.

Anomalies of the Kidney

Bilateral Renal Agenesis

Ashley, D. J. B., and Mostofi, F. K.: Renal agenesis and dysgenesis. J. Urol., 83:211, 1960.

Bain, A. D., and Scott, J. S.: Renal agenesis and severe urinary tract dysplasia: A review of 50 cases, with particular reference to associated anomalies. Br. Med. J., 1:841, 1960.

Bain, A. D., Beath, M. M., and Flint, W. F.: Sirenomelia and monomelia with renal agenesis in amnion nodosom. Arch. Dis. Child., 35:250, 1960.

Carpentier, P. J., and Potter, E. L.: Nuclear sex and genital malformation in 48 cases of renal agenesis with special reference to nonspecific female pseudohermaphroditism. Am. J. Obstet. Gynecol., 78:235, 1959.

Clark, D. A.: Times of first void and first stool in 500 newborns. Pediatrics, 60:457, 1977.

Clemmons, J. J. W.: Embryonic renal injury: a possible factor in fetal malnutrition. Pediatr. Res., 11:404, 1977.

Davidson, W. M., and Ross, G. I. M.: Bilateral absence of the kidneys and related congenital anomalies. J. Pathol. Bacteriol, 68:459, 1954.

Fitch, N., and Lachance, R. C.: The pathogenesis of Potter's syndrome of renal agenesis. Can. Med. Assoc. J., 107:653, 1972.

Hislop, A., Hey, E., and Reid, L.: The lungs in congenital bilateral renal agenesis and dysplasia. Arch. Dis. Child., 54:32, 1979.

Katz, S. H., and Chatten, J.: The urethra in bilateral renal agenesis. Arch. Pathol., 97:269, 1974.

Kohler, H. G.: An unusual case of sirenomelia. Teratology, 6:659, 1972.

Levin, H.: Bilateral renal agenesia. J. Urol., 67:86, 1952.

Mauer, S. M., Dobrin, R. S., and Vernier, R. L.: Unilateral and bilateral renal agenesis in monoamniotic twins. J. Pediatr., 84:236, 1974.

Perlman, M., Williams, J., and Hirsh, M.: Neonatal pulmonary hypoplasia after prolonged leakage of amniotic fluid. Arch. Dis. Child., 51:349, 1976.

Potter, E. L.: Bilateral renal agenesis. J. Pediatr., 29:68, 1946a.

Potter, E. L.: Facial characteristics in infants with bilateral renal agenesis. Am. J. Obstet. Gynecol., 51:885, 1946b.

Potter, E. L.: Pathology of the Fetus and the Newborn. Chicago, Year Book Medical Publishers, 1952.

Potter, E. L.: Bilateral absence of ureters and kidneys. A report of 50 cases. Obstet. Gynecol., 25:3, 1965.

Reid, L.: The lung: its growth and remodeling in health and disease. Am. J. Roentgenol., 129:777, 1977.

Rizza, J. M., and Downing, S. E.: Bilateral renal agenesis in two female siblings. Am. J. Dis. Child., 121:60, 1971.

Selby, G. W., and Parmelee, A. H., Jr.: Bilateral renal agenesis and oligohydramnios. J. Pediatr., 48:70, 1976.

Sherry, S. N., and Kramer I.: The time of passage of first stool and first urine by the newborn infant. J. Pediatr., 46:158, 1955.

Thomas, I. T., and Smith, D. W.: Oligohydramnios, cause of the nonrenal features of Potter's syndrome, including pulmonary hypoplasia. J. Pediatr., 84:811, 1974.

Thompson, V. M.: Amnion nodosum. J. Obstet. Gynaecol. Br. Commonw., 67:611, 1960.

Williams, D. I.: Personal communication, 1974.

Wolf, E. L., Berdon, W. E., Baker, D. H., Wigger, H. J., and Blanc, W. A.: Diagnosis of oligohydramnios-related pulmonary hypoplasia (Potter syndrome): Value of portable voiding cystourethrography in newborns with respiratory distress. Radiology, 125:769, 1977.

Unilateral Renal Agenesis

Anders, J. M.: Congenital single kidney with report of a case. The practical significance of the condition with statistics. Am. J. Med. Sci., 139:313, 1910.

Anderson, E. E., and Harrison, J. H.: Surgical importance of the solitary kidney. N. Engl. J. Med., 273:683, 1965.

Beeby, D. I.: Seminal vesicle cysts associated with ipsilateral renal agenesis: Case report and review of literature. J. Urol., 112:120, 1974.

Bryan, A. L., Nigro, J. A., and Counseller, V. S.: One hundred cases of congenital absence of the vagina. Surg. Gynecol. Obstet., 88:79, 1949.

Campbell, M. F.: Congenital absence of one kidney: Unilateral renal agenesis. Ann. Surg., 88:1039, 1928.

Charny, C. W., and Gillenwater, J. Y.: Congenital absence of the vas deferens. J. Urol., 93:399, 1965.

Collins, D. C.: Congenital unilateral renal agenesia. Ann. Surg., 95:715, 1932.

Cope, J. R., and Trickey, S. E.: Congenital absence of the kidney: problems in diagnosis and management. J. Urol., 127:10, 1982.

Currarino, G.: Single vaginal ectopic ureter and Gartner's duct cyst with ipsilateral renal hypoplasia and dysplasia (or agenesis). J. Urol., 128:988, 1982.

Curtis, J. A., Sadhu, V., and Steiner, R. M.: Malposition of the colon in right renal agenesis, ectopia and anterior nephrectomy. Am. J. Roentgenol., 129:845, 1977.

D'Alberton, A., Reschini, E., Ferrari, N., and Candiani, P.: Prevalence of urinary tract abnormalities in a large series of patients with uterovaginal atresia. J. Urol., 126:623, 1981.

Dees, J. E.: Prognosis of the solitary kidney. J. Urol., 83:550, 1960.

Doroshow, L. W., and Abeshouse, B. S.: Congenital unilateral solitary kidney: Report of 37 cases and a review of the literature. Urol. Surv., 11:219, 1961.

Emanuel, B., Nachman, R., Aronson, N., and Weiss, H.: Congenital solitary kidney: A review of 74 cases. Am. J. Dis. Child., 127:17, 1974.

Fortune, C. H.: The pathological and clinical significance of congenital one-sided kidney defect with the presentation of three new cases of agenesia and one of aplasia. Ann. Intern. Med., 1:377, 1927.

Furtado, A. J. L.: The three cases of cystic seminal vesicle associated with unilateral renal agenesis. Br. J. Urol., 45:536, 1973.

Gilliland, B., and Dick, F.: Uterus didelphys associated with unilateral imperforate vagina. Obstet. Gynecol., 48:Suppl. 1, 5s, 1976.

Gutierrez, R.: Surgical aspects of renal agenesis: With special reference to hypoplastic kidney, renal aplasia and congenital absence of one kidney. Arch. Surg., 27:686, 1933.

Holt, S. A., and Peterson, N. E.: Ectopia of seminal vesicle: Associated with agenesis of ipsilateral kidney. Urology, 4:322, 1974.

Hynes, D. M., and Watkin, E. M.: Renal agenesis—roentgenologic problem. Am. J. Roentgenol., 110:772, 1970.

Jancu, J., Zuckerman, H., and Sudarsky, M.: Unilateral renal agenesis associated with multiple abnormalities. South. Med. J., 69:94, 1976.

Kohn, G., and Borns, P. F.: The association of bilateral and unilateral renal aplasia in the same family. J. Pediatr., 83:95, 1973.

Limkakeng, A. D., and Retik, A. B.: Unilateral renal agenesis with hypoplastic ureter: Observations on the contralateral urinary tract and report of four cases. J. Urol., 108:149, 1972.

Longo, V. J., and Thompson, G. J.: Congenital solitary kidney. J. Urol., 68:63, 1952.

Mace, J. W., Kaplan, J. M., Schanberger, J.E., and Gotlin, R. W.: Poland's syndrome: Report of seven cases and review of the literature. Clin. Pediatr., 11:98, 1972.

Magee, M. C., Lucey, D. T., and Fried, F. A.: A new embryologic classification for uro-gynecologic malformations: the syndromes of mesonephric duct induced mullerian deformities. J. Urol., 121:265, 1979.

Mascatello, V., and Lebowitz, R. L.: Malposition of the colon in left renal agenesis and ectopia. Radiology, 120:371, 1976.

Ochsner, M. G., Brannan, W., and Goodier, E. H.: Absent vas deferens associated with renal agenesis. JAMA, 222:1055, 1972.

Phelan, J. T., Counseller, V. S., and Greene, L. F.: Deformities of the urinary tract with congenital absence of the vagina. Surg. Gynecol. Obstet., 97:1, 1953.

Radasch, H. E.: Congenital unilateral absence of the urogenital system and its relation to the development of the Wolffian and Muellerian ducts. Am. J. Med. Sci., 136:111, 1908.

Say, B., and Gerald, P. S.: A new polydactyly/imperforate-anus/vertebral anomalies syndrome? Lancet, 1:688, 1968.

Semmens, J. P.: Congenital anomalies of the female genital tract: functional classification based on review of 56 personal cases and 500 reported cases. Obstet. Gynecol., 19:328, 1962.

Shumacker, H. B.: Congenital anomalies of the genitalia associated with unilateral renal agenesis. Arch. Surg., 37:586, 1938.

Smith, E. C., and Orkin, L. A.: A clinical and statistical study of 471 congenital anomalies of the kidney and ureter. J. Urol., 53:11, 1945.

Thompson, D. P., and Lynn, H. B.: Genital anomalies associated with solitary kidney. Mayo Clin. Proc., 41:538, 1966.

Vinstein, A. L., and Franken, E. A., Jr.: Unilateral hematocolpos associated with agenesis of the kidney. Radiology, 102:625, 1972.

Weiss, J. M., and Dykhuizen, R. F.: An anomalous vaginal insertion into the bladder: A case report. J. Urol., 98:60, 1967.

Wiersma, A. F., Peterson, L. F., and Justema, E. J.: Uterine anomalies associated with unilateral renal agenesis. Obstet. Gynecol., 47:654, 1976.

Woolf, R. B., and Allen, W. M.: Concomitant malformations: The frequent simultaneous occurrence of congenital malformations of the reproductive and urinary tracts. Obstet. Gynecol., 2:236, 1953.

Yoder, I. C., and Pfister, R. C.: Unilateral hematocolpos and ipsilateral renal agenesis: Report of two cases and review of the literature. Am. J. Roentgenol., 127:303, 1976.

Supernumerary Kidney

Campbell, M. F.: Anomalies of the Kidney. In Campbell, M. F., and Harrison, J. H. (Eds.): Urology. Vol. 2, 3rd ed., p. 1422. Philadelphia, W. B. Saunders Co., 1970.

Carlson, H. E.: Supernumerary kidney: A summary of fifty-one reported cases. J. Urol., 64:221, 1950.

Exley, M., and Hotchkiss, W. S.: Supernumerary kidney with clear cell carcinoma. J. Urol., 51:569, 1944.

Geisinger, J. F.: Supernumerary kidney. J. Urol., 38:331, 1937.

Hoffman, R. L., and McMillan, T. E.: Discussion. Trans. South Central Sec., American Urology Assoc., 82, 1948.

Kretschmer, H. L.: Supernumerary kidney. Report of a case with review of the literature. Surg. Gynecol. Obstet., 49:818, 1929.

N'Guessan, G., and Stephens, F. O.: Supernumerary kidney. J. Urol., 130:649, 1983.

Rubin, J. S.: Supernumerary kidney with aberrant ureter terminating externally. J. Urol., 61:405, 1948.

Sasidharan, K. Babu, A. S., Rao, M. M., and Bhat, H. S.: Free supernumerary kidney. Br. J. Urol., 48:388, 1976.

Shan, J. H.: Supernumerary kidney with vaginal ureteral orifice. J. Urol., *47*:344, 1942.

Tada, Y., Kokado, Y., Hashinaka, Y., et al.: Free supernumerary kidney: a case report and review. J. Urol., *126*:231, 1981.

Simple Renal Ectopia

Abeshouse, B. S., and Bhisitkul, I.: Crossed renal ectopia with and without fusion. Urol. Int., *9*:63, 1959.

Anderson, E. E., and Harrison, J. H.: Surgical importance of the solitary kidney. N. Engl. J. Med., *273*:683, 1965.

Anderson, G. W., Rice, G. G., and Harris, B. A., Jr.: Pregnancy and labor complicated by pelvic ectopic kidney. J. Urol., *65*:760, 1951.

Anderson, G. W., Rice, G. G., and Harris, B. A., Jr.: Pregnancy and labor complicated by pelvic ectopic kidney anomalies. A review of the literature. Obstet. Gynecol. Surv., *4*:737, 1949.

Anson, B. J., and Riba, L. W.: The anatomical and surgical features of ectopic kidney. Surg. Gynecol. Obstet., *68*:37, 1939.

Baggenstoss, A. H.: Congenital anomalies of the kidney. Med. Clin. North Am., *35*:987, 1951.

Bell, E. T.: Renal Diseases. Philadelphia, Lea & Febiger, 1946.

Campbell, M. F.: Renal ectopy. J. Urol., *24*:187, 1930.

D'Alberton, A., Reschini, E., Ferrari, N., and Candiani, P.: Prevalence of urinary tract abnormalities in a large series of patients with uterovaginal atresia. J. Urol., *126*:623, 1981.

Delson, B.: Ectopic kidney in obstetrics and gynecology. N.Y. State J. Med., *75*:2522, 1975.

Downs, R. A., Lane, J. W., and Burns, E.: Solitary pelvic kidney: Its clinical implications. Urology, *1*:51, 1973.

Dretler, S. P., Olsson, C. A., and Pfister, R. C.: The anatomic, radiologic and clinical characteristics of the pelvic kidney, an analysis of 86 cases. J. Urol., *105*:623, 1971.

Fowler, H. A.: Bilateral renal ectopia. A report of four additional cases. J. Urol., *45*:795, 1941.

Hawes, C. J.: Congenital unilateral ectopic kidney: A report of two cases. J. Urol., *64*:453, 1950.

Malek, R. S., Kelalis, P. P., and Burke, E. C.: Ectopic kidney in children and frequency of association of other malformations. Mayo Clin. Proc., *46*:461, 1971.

McCrea, L. E.: Congenital solitary pelvic kidney, J. Urol., *48*:58, 1942.

Stevens, A. R.: Pelvic single kidneys. J. Urol., *37*:610, 1937.

Tabisky, J., and Bhisitkul, I.: Solitary crossed ectopic kidney with vaginal aplasia: A case report. J. Urol., *94*:33, 1965.

Thompson, G. J., and Pace, J. M.: Ectopic kidney: A review of 97 cases. Surg. Gynecol. Obstet., *64*:935, 1937.

Ward, J. N., Nathanson, B., and Draper, J. W.: The pelvic kidney. J. Urol, *94*:36, 1965.

Cephalad Ectopia

Pinckney, L. E., Moskowitz, P. S., Lebowitz, R. L., and Fritzsche, P.: Renal malposition associated with omphalocele. Radiology, *129*:677, 1978.

Thoracic Kidney

Ang, A. H., and Chan, W. F.: Ectopic thoracic kidney. J. Urol., *108*:211, 1972.

Barloon, J. W., and Goodwin, W. E.: Thoracic kidney: Case reports. J. Urol., *78*:356, 1957.

Berlin, H. S., Stein, J., and Poppel, M. H.: Congenital superior ectopia of the kidney. Am. J. Roentgenol., *78*:508, 1957.

Burke, E. C., Wenzl, J. E., and Utz, D. C.: The intrathoracic kidney. Report of a case. Am. J. Dis. Child., *113*:487, 1967.

Campbell, M. F.: Renal ectopy. J. Urol., *24*:187, 1930.

DeCastro, F. J., and Shumacher, H.: Asymptomatic thoracic kidney. Clin. Pediatr., *8*:279, 1969.

DeNoronha, L. L., Costa, M. F. E., and Godinho, M. T. M.: Ectopic thoracic kidney. Am. Rev. Respir. Dis., *109*:678, 1974.

Franciskovic, V., and Martincic, N.: Intrathoracic kidney. Br. J. Urol., *31*:156, 1959.

Fusonie, D., and Molnar, W.: Anomalous pulmonary venous return, pulmonary sequestration, bronchial atresia, aplastic right upper lobe, pericardial defect and intrathoracic kidney. An unusual complex of congenital anomalies in one patient. Am. J. Roentgenol., *97*:350, 1966.

Gray, S. W., and Skandalakis, J. E.: The diaphragm. In Embryology for Surgeons, pp. 359–366, Philadelphia, W. B. Saunders Co., 1972.

Hertz, M., Shahin, N.: Ectopic thoracic kidney. Isr. J. Med. Sci., *5*:98, 1969.

Hill, J. E., and Bunts, R. C.: Thoracic kidney: Case reports. J. Urol., *84*:460, 1960.

Lozano, R. H., and Rodriguez, C.: Intrathoracic ectopic kidney: Report of a case. J. Urol., *114*:601, 1975.

Lundius, B.: Intrathoracic kidney. Am. J. Roentgenol., *125*:678, 1975.

N'Guessan, G., and Stephens, F. D.: Congenital superior ectopic (thoracic) kidney. Urology, *24*:219, 1984.

Paul, A. T. S., Uragoda, C. G., and Jayewardene, F. L. W.: Thoracic kidney with report of a case. Br. J. Surg., *47*:395, 1960.

Robbins, J. J., and Lich, R., Jr.: Thoracic kidney. J. Urol., *72*:133, 1954.

Shapira, E., Fishel, E., and Levin, S.: Intrathoracic kidney in a premature infant. Arch. Dis. Child., *40*:86, 1965.

Spillane, R. J., and Prather, G. C.: Right diaphragmatic eventration with renal displacement. Case report. J. Urol., *68*:804, 1952.

Crossed Renal Ectopia With and Without Fusion

Abeshouse, B. S.: Crossed ectopia with fusion: Review of literature and a report of four cases. Am. J. Surg., *73*:658, 1947.

Abeshouse, B. S., and Bhisitkul, I.: Crossed renal ectopia with and without fusion. Urol. Int., *9*:63, 1959.

Alexander, J. C., King, K. B., and Fromm, C. S.: Congenital solitary kidney with crossed ureter. J. Urol., *64*:230, 1950.

Ashley, D. J. B., and Mostofi, F. K.: Renal agenesis and dysgenesis. J. Urol., *83*:211, 1960.

Bagenstoss, A. H.: Congenital anomalies of the kidney. Med. Clin. North Am., *35*:987, 1951.

Bauer, S. B.: Personal communication, 1977.

Bissada, N. K., Fried, F. A., and Redman, J. F.: Crossed-fused renal ectopia with a solitary ureter. J. Urol., *114*:304, 1975.

Boatman, D. L., Culp, D. A., Jr., Culp, D. A., and Flocks, R. H.: Crossed renal ectopia. J. Urol., *108*:30, 1972.

Caine, M.: Crossed renal ectopia without fusion. Br. J. Urol., *28*:257, 1956.

Caldamone, A. A., and Rabinowitz, R.: Crossed fused renal ectopia, orthotopic multicystic dysplasia and vaginal agenesis. J. Urol., *126*:105, 1981.

Campbell, M. F.: Renal ectopy, J. Urol., *24*:187, 1930.

Cass, A. S., and Vitko, R. J.: Unusual variety of crossed renal ectopy with only one ureter. J. Urol., *107*:1056, 1972.

Cook, W. A., and Stephens, F. D.: Fused kidneys: Morphologic study and theory of embryogenesis. In Bergsma, D., and Duckett, J. W. (Eds.): Urinary System Malformations in Children. New York, Allen R. Liss, Inc., 1977.

Diaz, G.: Renal ectopy: Report of a case with crossed ectopy without fusion, with fixation of kidney in normal position by the extraperitoneal route. J. Int. Coll. Surg., *19*:158, 1953.

Dretler, S. P., Olsson, C. A., and Pfister, R. C.: The anatomic, radiologic and clinical characteristics of the pelvic kidney: An analysis of eighty-six cases. J. Urol., *105*:623, 1971.

Gerber, W. L., Culp, D. A., Brown, R. C., Chow, R. C., and Platz, C. E.: Renal mass in crossed-fused ectopia, J. Urol., *123*:239, 1980.

Glenn, J. F.: Fused pelvic kidney. J. Urol., *80*:7, 1958.

Greenberg, L. W., and Nelsen, C. E.: Crossed fused ectopia of the kidneys in twins. Am. J. Dis. Child., *122*;175, 1971.

Hendren, W. H., Donahoe, P. K., and Pfister, R. C.: Crossed renal ectopia in children. Urology, *7*:135, 1976.

Hertz, M., Rabenstein, Z. J., Shalrin, N., and Melzer, M.: Crossed renal ectopia: clinical and radiologic findings in 22 cases. Clin. Radiol., *28*:339, 1977.

Hildreth, T. A., and Cass, A. S.: Cross renal ectopia with familial occurrence. Urology, *12*:59, 1978.

Joly, J. S.: Fusion of the kidneys. Proc. R. Soc. Med., *33*:697, 1940.

Kakei, H., Kondo, A., Ogisu, B. I., and Mitsuya, H.: Crossed ectopia of solitary kidney: A report of two cases and a review of the literature. Urol. Int., *31*:40, 1976.

Kelalia, P. P., Malek, R. S., and Segura, J. W.: Observations on renal ectopia and fusion in children. J. Urol., *110*:588, 1973.

Kretschmer, H. L.: Unilateral fused kidney. Surg. Gynecol. Obstet., *40*:360, 1925.

Kron, S. D., and Meranze, D. R.: Completely fused pelvic kidney. J. Rol., *62*:278, 1949.

Lee, H. P.: Crossed unfused renal ectopia with tumor. J. Urol., *61*:333, 1949.

Looney, W. W., and Dodd, D. L.: An ectopic (pelvic) completely fused (cake) kidney associated with various anomalies of the abdominal viscera. Ann. Surg., *84*:522, 1956.

Macksood, M. J., and James, R. E., Jr.: Giant hydronephrosis in ectopic kidney in a child. Urology, *22*:532, 1983.

Magri, J.: Solitary crossed ectopic kidney. Br. J. Urol., *33*:152, 1961.

Malek, R. S., and Utz, D. C.: Crossed, fused, renal ectopia with an ectopic ureterocele. J. Urol., *104*:665, 1970.

McDonald, J. H., and McClellan, D. S.: Crossed renal ectopia. Am. J. Surg., *93*:995, 1957.

Mininberg, D. T., Roze, S., Yoon, H. J., and Pearl, M.: Hypertension associated with crossed renal ectopia in an infant. Pediatrics. *48*:454, 1971.

Pathak, I. C.: Crossed renal ectopia without fusion associated with giant hydronephrosis. J. Urol., *94*:323, 1965.

Potter, E. L.: Pathology of the Fetus and the Newborn. Chicago, Year Book Medical Publishers, 1952.

Purpon, I.: Crossed renal ectopy with solitary kidney: A review of the literature. J. Urol., *90*:13, 1963.

Rubinstein, Z. J., Hertz, M., Shahin, N., and Deutsch, V.: Crossed renal ectopia: Angiographic findings in six cases. Am. J. Roentgenol., *126*:1035, 1976.

Shah, M. H.: Solitary crossed renal ectopia. Br. J. Urol., *47*:512, 1975.

Srivastava, R. N., Singh, M., Ghai, O. P., and Sethi, U.: Complete renal fusion ("cake"/"lump" kidney). Br. J. Urol., *43*:391, 1971.

Stubbs, A. J., and Resnick, M. I.: Struvite staghorn calculi in crossed renal ectopia. J. Urol., *118*:369, 1977.

Tabrisky, J., and Bhisitkul, I.: Solitary crossed ectopic kidney with vaginal aplasia: A case report. J. Urol., *94*:33, 1965.

Tanenbaum, B., Silverman, N., and Weinberg, S. R.: Solitary crossed renal ectopia. Arch. Surg., *101*:616, 1970.

Thompson, G. J., and Allen, R. B.: Unilateral fused kidney. Surg. Clin. North Am., *14*:729, 1934.

Wilmer, H. A.: Unilateral fused kidney: A report of five cases and a review of the literature. J. Urol., *40*:551, 1938.

Winram, R. G., and Ward-McQuaid, J. N.: Crossed renal ectopia without fusion. Can. Med. Assoc. J., *81*:481, 1959.

Yates-Bell, A. J., and Packham, D. A.: Giant hydronephrosis in a solitary crossed ectopic kidney. Br. J. Surg., *59*:104, 1972.

Horseshoe Kidney

Advisory Committee to the Renal Transplant Registry: The twelfth report of Human Renal Transplant Registry. JAMA, *233*:787, 1975.

Beck, W. C., and Hlivko, A. E.: Wilms' tumor in the isthmus of a horseshoe kidney. Arch. Surg., *81*:803, 1960.

Bell, R.: Horseshoe kidney in pregnancy. J. Urol., *56*:159, 1946.

Benjamin, J. A., and Schullian, D. M.: Observation on fused kidneys with horseshoe configuration: The contribution of Leonardo Botallo (1564). J. Hist. Med., *5*:315, 1950.

Blackard, C. E., and Mellinger, G. T.: Cancer in a horseshoe kidney. Arch. Surg., *97*:616, 1968.

Boatman, D. L., Cornell, S. H., and Kolln, C. P.: The arterial supply of horseshoe kidney. Am. J. Roentgenol., *113*:447, 1971.

Boatman, D. L., Kolln, C. P., and Flocks, R. H.: Congenital anomalies associated with horseshoe kidney. J. Urol., *107*:205, 1972.

Boyden, E. A.: Description of a horseshoe kidney associated with left inferior vena cava and disc-shaped suprarenal glands, together with a note on the occurrence of horseshoe kidneys in human embryos. Anat. Rec., *51*:187, 1931.

Bridge, R. A. C.: Horseshoe kidneys in identical twins. Br. J. Urol., *32*:32, 1960.

Buntley, D.: Malignancy associated with horseshoe kidney. Urology, *8*:146, 1976.

Campbell, M. F.: Anomalies of the kidney. *In* Campbell, M. F., and Harrison, J. H. (Eds.): Urology, pp. 1447–1452,. Philadelphia, W. B. Saunders Co., 1970.

Castor, J. E., and Green, N. A.: Complications of horseshoe kidney. Urology, *6*:344, 1975.

Christoffersen, J., and Iversen, H. G.: Partial hydronephrosis in a patient with horseshoe kidney and bilateral duplication of the pelvis and ureter. Scand. J. Urol. Nephrol., *10*:91, 1976.

Correa, R. J., Jr., and Paton, R. R.: Polycystic horseshoe kidney. J. Urol., *116*:802, 1976.

Dajani, A. M.: Horseshoe kidney: A review of twenty-nine cases. Br. J. Urol., *38*:388, 1966.

David, R. S.: Horseshoe kidney: A report of one family. Br. Med. J., *4*:571, 1974.

Dees, J.: Clinical importance of congenital anomalies of upper urinary tract. J. Urol., *46*:659, 1941.

Dische, M. R., and Johnston, R.: Teratoma in horseshoe kidneys. Urology, *13*:435, 1979.

Eidelman, A., Yuval, E., Simon, D., and Sibi, Y.: Retrocaval ureter. Eur. Urol., *4*:279, 1978.

Evans, W. P., and Resnick, M. I.: Horseshoe kidney and urolithiasis. J. Urol., *125*:620, 1981.

Glenn, J. F.: Analysis of 51 patients with horseshoe kidney. N. Engl. J. Med., *261*:684, 1959.

Gutierrez, R.: The clinical management of horseshoe kidney: A study of horseshoe kidney disease, its etiology, pathology, symptomatology, diagnosis and treatment. New York, Paul B. Hoeber, Inc., 1934.

Hefferman, J. C., Lightwood, R. G., and Snell, M. E.: Horseshoe kidney with retrocaval ureter: second reported case. J. Urol., *120*:358, 1978.

Jarmin, W. D.: Surgery of the horseshoe kidney with a postaortic isthmus: Report of two cases of horseshoe kidney. J. Urol., *40*:1, 1938.

Kolln, C. P., Boatman, D. L., Schmidt, J. D., and Flocks, R. H.: Horseshoe kidney: A review of 105 patients. J. Urol., *107*:203, 1972.

Leiter, E.: Horseshoe kidney: Discordance in monozygotic twins. J. Urol., *108*:683, 1972.

Love, L., and Wasserman, D.: Massive unilateral nonfunctioning hydronephrosis in horseshoe kidney. Clin. Radiol., *26*:409, 1975.

Meek, J. R., and Wadsworth, G. H.: A case of horseshoe kidney lying between the great vessels. J. Urol., *43*:448, 1940.

Murphy, D. M., and Zincke, H.: Transitional cell carcinoma in the horseshoe kidney: report of 3 cases and review of the literature. Br. J. Urol., *54*:484, 1982.

Nation, E. F.: Horseshoe kidney, a study of thirty-two autopsy and nine surgical cases. J. Urol., *53*:762, 1945.

Novak, M. E., Baum, N. H., and Gonzales, E. T.: Horseshoe kidney with multicystic dysplasia associated ureterocele. Urology, *10*:456, 1977.

Pitts, W. R., and Muecke, E. C.: Horseshoe kidneys: A 40 year experience. J. Urol., *113*:743, 1975.

Roy, J. B., and Stevens, R. K.: Polycystic horseshoe kidney. Urology, *6*:222, 1975.

Segura, J. W., Kelalis, P. P., and Burke, E. C.: Horseshoe kidney in children. J. Urol., *108*:333, 1972.

Shoup, G. D., Pollack, H. M., and Dou, J. H.: Adenocarcinoma occurring in a horseshoe kidney. Arch. Surg., *84*:413, 1962.

Silagy, J. M.: The horseshoe kidney and its disease. J. Mt. Sinai Hosp., *18*:297, 1952.

Smith, D. W.: Recognizable patterns of human malformation; genetic embryologic and clinical aspects. Major Problems in Clinical Pediatrics, *7*, p. 50. Philadelphia, W. B. Saunders Co., 1970.

Smith, E. C., and Orkin, L. A.: A clinical and statistical study of 471 congenital anomalies of the kidney and ureter. J. Urol., *53*:11, 1945.

Walker, D.: Personal communication, 1977.

Whitehouse, G. H.: Some urographic aspects of the horseshoe kidney anomaly—a review of 59 cases. Clin. Radiol., *26*:107, 1975.

Zondek, L. H., and Zondek, T.: Horseshoe kidney in associated congenital malformations. Urol. Int., *18*:347, 1964.

Anomalies of Rotation

Campbell, M. F.: Anomalies of the kidney. *In* Campbell M. F. (Ed.): Urology. Vol. 2, 2nd ed., p. 1589. Philadelphia, W. B. Saunders Co., 1963.

Felix, W.: The development of the urogenital organs. *In* Keibel, F., and Mall, F. P. (Eds.): Manual of Human Embryology. Vol. 2, p. 752. Philadelphia, J. B. Lippincott Co., 1912.

Gray, S. W., and Skandalakis, J. E.: The kidney and ureter. *In* Embryology for Surgeons, p. 480. Philadelphia, W. B. Saunders Co., 1972.

Mackie, G. G., Awang, H., and Stephens, F. D.: The ureteric orifice: The embryologic key to radiologic status of duplex kidneys. J. Pediatr. Surg., *10*:473, 1975.

Smith, E. C., and Orkin, L. A.: A clinical and statistical study of 471 congenital anomalies of the kidney and ureter. J. Urol., *53*:11, 1945.

Weyrauch, H. M., Jr.: Anomalies of renal rotation. Surg. Gynecol. Obstet., *69*:183, 1939.

Anomalies of the Renal Vasculature
Aberrant, Accessory, or Multiple Vessels

Anson, B. J., and Daseler, E. H.: Common variations in renal anatomy, affecting the blood supply, form and topography. Surg. Gynecol. Obstet., *112*:439, 1961.

Anson, B. J., and Kurth, L. E.: Common variations in the renal blood supply. Surg. Gynecol. Obstet., *100*:157, 1955.

Fraley, E. E.: Dismembered infundibulopyelostomy: Improved technique for correcting vascular obstruction of the superior infundibulum. J. Urol., *101*:144, 1969.

Fraley, E. E.: Vascular obstruction of superior infundibulum causing nephralgia. A new syndrome. N. Engl. J. Med., *275*:1403, 1966.

Geyer, J. R., and Poutasse, E. F.: Incidence of multiple renal arteries on aortography. JAMA, *182*:118, 1962.

Graves, F. T.: The aberrant renal artery. J. Anat., *90*:553, 1956.

Graves, F. T.: The anatomy of the intrarenal arteries and its application to segmental resection of the kidney. Br. J. Surg., *42*:132, 1954.

Gray, S. W., and Skandalakis, J. E.: Anomalies of the kidney and ureter. *In* Embryology for Surgeons, P. 485. Philadelphia, W. B. Saunders Co., 1972.

Guggemos, E.: A rare case of an arterial connection between the left and right kidneys. Ann. Surg., *156*:940, 1962.

Merklin, R. J., and Michele, N. A.: The variant renal and suprarenal blood supply with data on the inferior phrenic, ureteral and gonadal arteries. A statistical analysis based on 185 dissections and review of the literature. J. Int. Coll. Surg., *29*:41, 1958.

Nathan, H.: Observation on aberrant renal arteries curving around and compressing the renal vein: Possible relationship to orthostatic proteinuria and to orthostatic hypertension. Circulation, *18*:1131, 1958.

Pick, J. W., and Anson, B. J.: The renal vascular pedicle. J. Urol., *44*:411, 1940.

White, R. R., and Wyatt, G. M.: Surgical importance of aberrant renal vessels in infants and children. Am. J. Surg., *58*:48, 1942.

Renal Artery Aneurysms

Abeshouse, B. S.: Renal aneurysm: Report of two cases and review of the literature. Urol. Cutan. Rev., *55*:451, 1951.

Cerny, J. C., Chang, C. Y., and Fry, W. J.: Renal artery aneurysms. Arch. Surg., *96*:653, 1968.

Garritano, A. P.: Aneurysm of the renal artery. Am. J. Surg., *94*:638, 1957.

Glass, P. M., and Uson, A. C.: Aneurysms of the renal artery: A study of 20 cases. J. Urol., *98*:285, 1967.

Hageman, J. H., Smith, R. F., Szilagyi, D. E., and Elliot, J. P.: Aneurysms of the renal artery: problems of prognosis and surgical management. Surgery, *84*:563, 1978.

McKeil, C. F., Jr., Graf, E. C., and Callahan, D. H.: Renal artery aneurysms: A report of 16 cases. J. Urol., *96*:593, 1966.

Poutasse, E. F.: Renal artery aneurysms. J. Urol., *113*:443, 1975.

Poutasse, E. F.: Renal artery aneurysm: Report of 12 cases, two treated by excision of the renal aneurysm and repair of renal artery. J. Urol., *77*:697, 1957.

Rhodes, J. F., and Johnson, G., Jr.: Renal artery aneurysm. J. Urol., *105*:155, 1971.

Silvis, R. S., Hughes, W. F., and Holmes, F. H.: Aneurysm of the renal artery. Am. J. Surg., *91*:339, 1956.

Stanley, J. C., Rhodes, E. L., Gewertz, G. L., Chang, C. Y., Walter, J. F., and Fry, W. J.: Renal artery aneurysms: significance of macroaneurysms exclusive of dissections and fibrodysplastic mural dilations. Arch. Surg., *110*:1327, 1975.

Zinman, L., and Libertino, J. A.: Uncommon disorders of the renal circulation: renal artery aneurysm. *In* Breslin, D. J., Swinton, N. W., Libertino, J. A., and Zinman, L. (Eds.): Renovascular Hypertension. Baltimore, Williams & Wilkins, 1982, pp. 110–114.

Arteriovenous Fistula

Bentson, J. R., and Crandall, P. H.: Use of the Fogarty catheter in arteriovenous malformations of the spinal cord. Radiology, *105*:65, 1972.

Boijsen, E., and Kohler, R.: Renal arteriovenous fistulae. Acta Radiol., *57*:433, 1962.

Bookstein, J. J., and Goldstein, H. M.: Successful management of post biopsy arteriovenous fistula with selective arterial embolization. Radiology, *109*:535, 1973.

Cho, K. J., and Stanley, J. C.: Non-neoplastic congenital and acquired renal arteriovenous malformations and fistula. Radiology, *129*:333, 1978.

Crummy, A. B. Jr., Atkinson, R. J., and Caruthers, S. B.: Congenital renal arteriovenous fistulas. J. Urol., *93*:24, 1965.

DeSai, S. G., and DeSautels, R. E.: Congenital arteriovenous malformation of the kidney. J. Urol., *110*:17, 1973.

Gunterberg, B.: Renal arteriovenous malformation. Acta Radiol., *7*:425, 1968.

Maldonado, J. E., Sheps, S. G., Bernatz, P. E., DeWeerd, J. H., and Harrison, E. G., Jr.: Renal arteriovenous fistula. Am. J. Med., *37*:499, 1964.

McAlhany, J. C., Jr., Black, H. C., Hanback, L. D., Jr., and Yarbrough, D. R., III: Renal arteriovenous fistula as a cause of hypertension. Am. J. Surg., *122*:117, 1971.

Messing, E., Kessler, R., and Kavaney, P. B.: Renal arteriovenous fistula. Urology, *8*:101, 1976.

Takaha, M., Matsumoto, A., Ochi, K., Takeuchi, M., Takemoto, M., and Sonoda, T.: Intrarenal arteriovenous malformation. J. Urol., *124*:315, 1980.

Thomason, W. B., Gross, M., Radwin, H. M., Hulse, C. M., and Dobbs, R. M.: Intrarenal arteriovenous fistulas. J. Urol., *108*:526, 1972.

Yazaki, T., Tomita, M., Akimoto, M., Konjiki, T., Kawai, H., and Kumazaki, T.: Congenital renal arteriovenous fistula: Case report, review of Japanese literature and description of nonradical treatment. J. Urol., *116*:415, 1976.

Anomalies of the Collecting System

Abeshouse, B. S.: Serous cysts of the kidney and their differentiation from other cystic diseases of the kidney. Urol. Cutan. Rev., *54*:582, 1950.

Dacie, J. E.: The "central lucency" sign of low bar dysmorphism (pseudotumour of the kidney). Br. J. Radiol., *49*:39, 1976.

Devine, C. J., Jr., Guzman, J. A., Devine, P. C., and Poutasse, E. F.: Calyceal diverticulum. J. Urol., *101*:8, 1969.

Eisendrath, D. N.: Report of case of hydronephrosis in kidney with extrarenal calyces. J. Urol., *13*:51, 1925.

Fraley, E. E.: Vascular obstruction of superior infundibulum causing nephralgia—new syndrome. N. Engl. J. Med., *275*:1403, 1966.

Galian, P., Forest, M., and Aboulker, P.: La megacaliose. Nouv. Presse Med., *78*:1663, 1970.

Gittes, R. F.: Congenital magacalices. Monogr. Urol., *5*:(1):1, 1984.

Gittes, R. F., and Talner, L. B.: Congenital megacalyces vs. obstructive hydronephrosis. J. Urol., *108*:833, 1972.

Harrison, R. B., Wood, J. L., and Gillenwater, J. Y.: A solitary calyx in a human kidney. Radiology, *121*:310, 1976.

Johnston, J. H., and Sandomirsky, S. K.: Intrarenal vascular obstruction of the superior infundibulum in children. J. Pediatr. Surg., 7:318, 1972.

Kelalis, P. P., and Malek, R. S.: Infundibulopelvic stenosis. J. Urol., *125*:568, 1981.

Kleeman, F. J.: Unilateral megacalicosis. J. Urol., *110*:387, 1973.

Kozakewich, H. P. W., and Lebowitz, R. L.: Congenital megacalices. Pediatr. Radiol., *2*:251, 1974.

Malament, M., Schwartz, B., and Nagamatsu, G. R.: Extrarenal calyces: their relationship to renal disease. Am. J. Roentgenol., *86*:823, 1961.

Mathieson, A. J. M.: Calyceal diverticulum: A case with a discussion and a review of the condition. Br. J. Urol., *25*:147, 1953.

Middleton, A. W., Jr., and Pfister, R. C.: Stone-containing pyelocaliceal diverticulum: Embryogenic, anatomic, radiologic and clinical characteristics. J. Urol., *111*:1, 1974.

Moore, T.: Hydrocalycosis. Br. J. Urol., *22*:304, 1950.

Morimoto, S., Sangen, H., Takamatsu, M., et al.: Solitary calix in siblings. J. Urol., *122*:690, 1979.

Neal, A., and Murphy, L.: Unipapillary kidney: an unusual developmental abnormality of the kidney. J. Coll. Radiol. Aust., *4*:81, 1960.

Parker, J. A., Lebowitz, R., Mascatello, V., and Treves, S.: Magnification renal scintigraphy in differential diagnosis of septa of Bertin. Pediatr. Radiol., *4*:157, 1976.

Puigvert, A.: Megacaliosis: diagnostico diferencial con la hidrocaliectasia. Med. Clin., *41*:294, 1963.

Puigvert, A.: Megacalicose—Diagnostic differentiel avec l'hydrocaliectasie. Helv. Chir. Acta, *31*:414, 1964.

Rao, D. V. N., Sharma, S. K., Rao, N. S., and Bapna, B. C.: Extrarenal calyces with complications: A case report. Aust. N.Z. J. Surg., *42*:178, 1972.

Sakatoku, J., and Kitayama, T.: Solitary unipapillary kidney: presentation of a case. Acta Urol. Jpn., *10*:349, 1964.

Siegel, M. J., and McAlister, W. H.: Calyceal diverticula in children: unusual features and complications. Radiology, *131*:79, 1979.

Timmons, J. W., Jr., Malek, R. S., Hattery, R. R., and DeWeerd, J.: Caliceal diverticulum. J. Urol., *114*:6, 1975.

Toppercer, A.: Unipapillary human kidney associated with urinary and genital abnormalities. Urology, *16*:194, 1980.

Vela Navarrete, R., and Garcia Robledo, J.: Polycystic disease of the renal sinus: structural characteristics. J. Urol., *129*:700, 1983.

Webb, J. A. W., Fry, I. K., and Charlton, C. A. C.: An anomalous calyx in the mid-kidney: An anatomical variant. Br. J. Radiol., *48*:674, 1975.

Williams, D. I., and Mininberg, D. T.: Hydrocalycosis: Report of three cases in children. Br. J. Urol., *40*:541, 1968.

Anomalies of the Ureteropelvic Junction

Allen, T. D.: Congenital ureteral stricture. J. Urol., *104*:196, 1970.

Allen, T. D.: Congenital ureteral strictures. *In* Lutzeyer, W., and Melchior, H. (Eds.): Urodynamic. Upper and

Lower Urinary Tract. Berlin, Springer-Verlag, 1973, pp. 137–147.

Amar, A. D.: Congenital hydronephrosis of lower segment in duplex kidney. Urology, 7:480, 1976.

Belis, J. A., Belis, T. E., Lai, J. C. W., Goodwin, C. A., and Gabrielle, O. F.: Radionuclide determination of individual kidney function in the treatment of chronic renal obstruction. J. Urol., 127:898, 1982.

Belman, A. B., Kropp, K. F., and Simon, N. M.: Renal pressor hypertension secondary to unilateral hydronephrosis. N. Engl. J. Med., 278:1133, 1968.

Cohen, B., Goldman, S. M., Kopilnick, M., Khurana, A. V., and Salik, J. O.: Ureteropelvic junction obstruction: its occurrence in 3 members of a single family. J. Urol., 120:361, 1978.

Colgan, J. R., III, Skaist, L., and Morrow, J. W.: Benign ureteral tumors in childhood: A case report and a plea for conservative management. J. Urol., 109:308, 1973.

Colodny, A. H., Retik, A. B., and Bauer, S. B.: Antenatal diagnosis of fetal urologic abnormalities by intrauterine ultrasonography; therapeutic implications. Presented at Annual Meeting of the American Urological Association, San Francisco, May 18, 1980.

Ericsson, N. O., Rudhe, U., and Livaditis, A.: Hydronephrosis associated with aberrant renal vessels in infants and children. Surgery, 50:687, 1961.

Foote, J. W., Blennerhassett, J. B., Wiglesworth, F. W., and MacKinnon, K. J.: Observations on the ureteropelvic junction. J. Urol., 104:252, 1970.

Fourcroy, J. L., Blei, C. L., Glassman, L. M., and White, R.: Prenatal diagnosis by ultrasonography of genitourinary abnormalities. Urology, 22:223, 1983.

Grossman, I. C., Cromie, W. J., Wein, A. J., and Duckett, J. W.: Renal hypertension secondary to ureteropelvic junction obstruction. Urology, 17:69, 1981.

Gup, A.: Benign mesodermal polyp in childhood. J. Urol., 114:610, 1975.

Hanna, M. K., Jeffs, R. D., Sturgess, J. M., and Barkin, M.: Ureteral structure and ultrastructure. Part II. Congenital ureteropelvic junction obstruction and primary obstructive megaureter. J. Urol., 116:725, 1976.

Hutch, J. A., Hinman, F., Jr., and Miller, E. R.: Reflux as a cause of hydronephrosis and chronic pyelonephritis. J. Urol., 88:169, 1962.

Johnston, J. H.: The pathogenesis of hydronephrosis in children. Br. J. Urol., 41:724, 1969.

Johnston, J. H., Evans, J. P., Glassberg, K. I., and Shapiro, S. R.: Pelvic hydronephrosis in children: A review of 219 personal cases. J. Urol., 117:97, 1977.

Kelalis, P. P., Culp, O. S., Stickler, G. B., and Burke, E. C.: Ureteropelvic obstruction in children: Experiences with 109 cases. J. Urol., 106:418, 1971.

Koff, S. A.: Ureteropelvic junction obstruction: role of newer diagnostic methods. J. Urol., 127:898, 1982.

Krueger, R. P., Ash, J. M., Silver, M. M., Kass, E. J., et al.: Primary hydronephrosis: assessment of diuretic renography, pelvis perfusion pressure, operative findings and renal and ureteral histology. Urol. Clin. North Am., 7:231, 1980.

Lebowitz, R. L., and Blickman, J. G.: The coexistence of ureteropelvic junction obstruction and reflux. Am. J. Roentgenol., 140:231, 1983.

Lebowitz, R. l., and Griscom, N. T.: Neonatal hydronephrosis: 146 cases. Radiol. Clin. North Am., 15:49, 1977.

Leiter, E.: Persistent fetal ureter. J. Urol., 122:251, 1979.

Maizels, M., and Stephens, F. D.: Valves of the ureter as a cause of primary obstruction of the ureter: anatomic, embryologic and clinical aspects. J. Urol., 123:742, 1980.

Malek, R. S.: Intermittent hydronephrosis. The occult ureteropelvic junction obstruction. J. Urol., 130:863, 1983.

Mering, J. H., Steel, J. F., and Gittes, R. F.: Congenital ureteral valves. J. Urol., 107:737, 1972.

Munoz, A. I., Pascual y Baralt, J. F., and Melendez, M. T.: Arterial hypertension in infants with hydronephrosis. Am. J. Dis. Child, 131:38, 1977.

Murnaghan, G. F.: The dynamics of the renal pelvis and ureter with reference to congenital hydronephrosis. Br. J. Urol., 30:321, 1958.

Nesbit, R. M.: Diagnosis of intermittent hydronephrosis: Importance of pyelography during episodes of pain. J. Urol., 75:767, 1956.

Nixon, H. H.: Hydronephrosis in children: A clinical study of seventy-eight cases with special reference to the role of aberrant renal vessels and the results of conservative operations. Br. J. Surg., 40:601, 1953.

Notley, R. G.: Electron microscopy of the upper ureter and the pelviureteric junction. Br. J. Urol., 40:37, 1968.

O'Reilly, P. H., Lawson, R. S., Shields, R. A., and Testa, H. J.: Idiopathic hydronephrosis—the diuresis renogram: a new non-invasive method of assessing equivocal pelvioureteral junction obstruction. J. Urol., 121:153, 1979.

Osathanondh, V., and Potter, E. L.: Development of the kidney as shown by microdissection. Arch. Pathol., 76:271, 1963.

Östling, K.: The genesis of hydronephrosis. Acta Chir. Scand., 86:Suppl. 72, 1942.

Parker, R. M., Rudd, T. G., Wonderly, R. K., and Ansell, J. S.: Ureteropelvic junction obstruction in infants and children: functional evaluation of the obstructed kidney preoperatively and postoperatively. J. Urol., 126:509, 1981.

Perlmutter, A. D., Kroovand, R. L., and Lai, Y. W.: Management of ureteropelvic obstruction in the first year of life. J. Urol., 123:535, 1980.

Robson, W. J., Rudy, S. M., and Johnston, J. H.: Pelviureteric obstruction in infancy. J. Pediatr. Surg., 11:57, 1976.

Ruano-Gil, D., Coca-Payeras, A., and Tejedo-Maten, A.: Obstruction and normal re-canalization of the ureter in the human embryo: its relation to congenital ureteric obstruction. Eur. Urol., 1:287, 1975.

Segura, J. W., Hattery, R. R., and Hartman, G. W.: Fluoroscopic evaluation of intermittent ureteropelvic junction obstruction after furosemide stimulation. J. Urol., 112:449, 1974.

Shopfner, C. E.: Ureteropelvic junction obstruction. Am. J. Roentgenol., 98:148, 1966.

Snyder, H. M., III, Lebowitz, R. L., Colodny, A. H., Bauer, S. B., and Retik, A. B.: Ureteropelvic junction obstruction in children. Urol. Clin. North Am., 7:273, 1980.

Squitieri, A. P., Ceccarelli, F. E., and Wurster, J. C.: Hypertension with elevated renal vein renins secondary to ureteropelvic junction obstruction. J. Urol., 111:284, 1974.

Stephens, F. D.: Ureterovascular hydronephrosis and the "aberrant" renal vessels. J. Urol., 128:984, 1982.

Thorup, J., Pederson, P. V., and Clausen, N.: Benign ureteral polyps as a cause of hydronephrosis in a child. J. Urol., 126:796, 1981.

Ulmsten, U., and Diehl, J.: Investigation of ureteric function with simultaneous intraureteric pressure recordings and ureteropyelography. Radiology, 117:283, 1975.

Uson, A. C., Cox, L. A., and Lattimer, J. K.: Hydronephrosis in infants and children. I. Some clinical and pathological aspects. JAMA, 205:323, 1968.

Whitaker, R. H.: Methods of assessing obstruction in dilated ureters. Br. J. Urol., *45*:15, 1973.

Whitaker, R. H.: Some observations and theories on the wide ureter and hydronephrosis. Br. J. Urol., *47*:377, 1975.

Whitaker, R. H.: Reflux induced pelviureteric obstruction. Br. J. Urol., *48*:555, 1976.

Williams, D. I., and Karlaftis, C. M.: Hydronephrosis due to pelviureteric obstruction in the newborn. Br. J. Urol., *38*:138, 1966.

Williams, D. I., and Kenawi, M. M.: The prognosis of pelviureteric obstruction in childhood: A review of 190 cases. Europ. Urol., *2*:57, 1976.

Williams, P. R., Fegetter, J., Miller, R. A., and Wickham, J. E. A.: The diagnosis and management of benign fibrous ureteric polyps. Br. J. Urol., *52*:253, 1980.

Anomalies of the Ureter

General

Arey, L. B.: Developmental Anatomy: A Textbook and Laboratory Manual of Embryology. 7th ed. Philadelphia, W. B. Saunders Co., 1965.

Frazer, J. E.: The terminal part of the Wolffian duct. J. Anat., *69*:455, 1935.

Glassberg, K. I., Braren, V., Duckett, J. W., Jacobs, E. C., King, L. R., Lebowitz, R. L., Perlmutter, A. D., and Stephens, F. D.: Suggested terminology for duplex systems, ectopic ureters and ureteroceles: Report of the Committee on Terminology, Nomenclature and Classification, Section on Urology, American Academy of Pediatrics. J. Urol., *132*:1153, 1984.

Gray, S. W., and Skandalakis, J. E.: Embryology for Surgeons. The Embryological Basis for the Treatment of Congenital Defects. Philadelphia, W. B. Saunders Co., 1972.

Koyanagi, T., and Tsuji, I.: Experience of complete duplication of the collecting system. Int. Urol. Nephrol., *11*:27, 1979.

Mackie, G. G., and Stephens, F. D.: Duplex kidneys: A correlation of renal dysplasia with position of the ureteral orifice. J. Urol., *114*:274, 1975.

Mackie, G. G., Awang, H., and Stephens, F. D.: The ureteric orifice: The embryologic key to radiologic status of duplex kidneys. J. Pediatr. Surg., *10*:473, 1975.

Ruano-Gil, D., Coca-Payeras, A., and Tejedo-Mateu, A.: Obstruction and normal recanalization of the ureter in the human embryo. Its relation to congenital ureteric obstruction. Eur. Urol., *1*:287, 1975.

Schwartz, R. D., Stephens, F. D., and Cussen, L. J.: The pathogenesis of renal dysplasia. II. The significance of lateral and medial ectopy of the ureteric orifice. Invest. Urol., *19*:97, 1981.

Smith, E. C., and Orkin, L. A.: A clinical and statistical study of 471 congenital anomalies of the kidney and ureter. J. Urol., *53*:11, 1945.

Stephens, F. D.: Congenital Malformations of the Rectum, Anus and Genito-urinary Tracts. London, E & S Livingstone Ltd., 1963.

Tanagho, E. A.: Embryologic basis for lower ureteral anomalies: A hypothesis. Urology, *7*:451, 1976.

Wharton, L. R., Jr.: Double ureters and associated renal anomalies in early human embryos. Contrib. Embryol. Carnegie Inst. Wash., *33*:103, 1949.

Anomalies of Number
Ureteral Duplication

Archangelskj, S.: Verdoppelung Der Ureteren Und Ihre Chirurgische Bedeutung, Zentralorgan Fuer Die Gesamte Chirurgie Und Ihre Grenzebiete, *37*:137, 1927.

Atwell, J. D., Cook, P. L., Howell, C. J., et al.: Familial incidence of bifid and double ureters. Arch. Dis. Child., *49*:390, 1974.

Beer, E., and Mencher, W. H.: Heminephrectomy in disease of the double kidney. report of fourteen cases. Ann. Surg., *108*:705, 1938.

Braasch, W. F.: The clinical diagnosis of congenital anomaly in the kidney and ureter. Ann. Surg., *56*:756, 1912.

Campbell, M. F.: Anomalies of the ureter. *In* Campbell, M. F., and Harrison, J. H. (Eds.): Urology. 3rd ed., Philadelphia, W. B. Saunders Co., 1970.

Christofferson, J., and Iversen, H. G.: Partial hydronephrosis in a patient with horseshoe kidney and bilateral duplication of the pelvis and ureter. Scand. J. Urol. Nephrol., *10*:91, 1976.

Cohen, N., and Berant, M.: Duplications of the renal collecting system in the hereditary osteo-onychodysplasia syndrome. J. Pediatr., *89*:261, 1976.

Colosimo, C.: Double and bifid ureters. Urologia, *5*:239, 1938.

Cromie, W. J., Engelstein, M. S., and Duckett, J. W., Jr.: Nodular renal blastema, renal dysplasia and duplicated collecting systems. J. Urol., *123*:100, 1980.

Dahl, D. S.: Bilateral complete renal duplication with total obstruction of both lower pole collecting systems. Urology, *6*:727, 1975.

Hawthorne, A. B.: Embryologic and clinical aspect of double ureter. JAMA, *106*:189, 1936.

Johnston, J. H.: Urinary tract duplication in childhood. Arch. Dis. Child., *36*:180, 1961.

Kaplan, N., and Elkin, M.: Bifid renal pelves and ureters. Radiographic and cinefluorographic observations. Br. J. Urol., *40*:235, 1968.

Kretschmer, H. L.: Hydronephrosis in infancy and childhood: Clinical data and a report of 101 cases. Surg. Gynecol. Obstet., *64*:634, 1937.

Lenaghan, D.: Bifid ureters in children: An anatomical, physiological and clinical study. J. Urol., *87*:808, 1962.

Meyer, R.: Normal and abnormal development of the ureter in the human embryo—a mechanistic consideration. Anat. Rec., *96*:355, 1946.

Nation, E. F.: Duplication of the kidney and ureter: A statistical study of 230 new cases. J. Urol., *51*:456, 1944.

Nordmark, B.: Double formations of the pelves of the kidneys and the ureters. Embryology, occurrence and clinical significance. Acta Radiol., *30*:267, 1948.

Payne, R. A.: Clinical significance of reduplicated kidneys. Br. J. Urol., *31*:141, 1959.

Pendergrass, T. W.: Congenital anomalies in children with Wilms' tumor: a new survey. Cancer, *37*:403, 1976.

Privett, J. T. J., Jeans, W. D., and Roylance, J.: The incidence and importance of renal duplication. Clin. Radiol., *27*:521, 1976.

Stephens, F. D.: Anatomical vagaries of double ureters. Aust. N.Z. J. Surg., *28*:27, 1958.

Timothy, R. P., Decter, A., and Perlmutter, A. D.: Ureteral duplication: Clinical findings and therapy in 46 children. J. Urol., *105*:445, 1971.

Weigert, C.: Ueber einige Bildunsfehler der Ureteren. Virchows Arch. (Pathol. Anat.), *70*:490, 1877.

Wharton, L. R., Jr.: Double ureters and associated renal anomalies in early human embryos. Contrib. Embryol. Carnegie Inst. Wash., *33*:103, 1949.

Whitaker, J., and Danks, D. M.: A study of the inheritance of duplication of the kidney and ureters. J. Urol., *95*:176, 1966.

Blind-ending Ureteral Duplications and Ureteral Diverticula

Albers, D. D., Geyer, J. R., and Barnes, S. D.: Clinical significance of blind-ending branch of bifid ureter: Report of 3 additional cases. J. Urol., *105*:634, 1971.

Albers, D. D., Geyer, J. R., and Barnes, S. D.: Blind-ending branch of bifid ureter: Report of 3 cases. J. Urol., 99:160, 1968.

Barbalias, G. A., and DiGioacchino, R.: Rudimentary branched ureter. A report of four cases. Del. Med. J., 46:511, 1974.

Bergman, B., Hansson, G., and Nilson, A. E. V.: Duplication of the renal pelvis and blind-ending bifid ureter in twins. Urol. Int., 32:49, 1977.

Caller, C., Cendron, J., and Trotot, P.: Uretere double à branche borgne. J. Urol. Nephrol. (Paris), 85:473, 1979.

Campbell, M. F.: Diverticulum of the ureter. Am. J. Surg., 34:385, 1936.

Culp, O. S.: Ureteral diverticulum: Classification of the literature and report of an authentic case. J. Urol., 58:309, 1947.

de Filippi, G., dal Forno, S., and Bianchi, M.: Blind ureteric buds. Pediatr. Radiol., 5:160, 1977.

Dublin, A. B., Stadalnik, R. C., DeNardo, G. L., et al.: Scintigraphic imaging of a blind-ending ureteral duplication. J. Nucl. Med., 16:208, 1975.

Hanley, H. G.: Blind-ending duplication of the ureter. Br. J. Urol., 17:50, 1945.

Hansen, E. I., and Frost, B.: Multiple diverticula of the ureter. Scand. J. Urol. Nephrol., 12:93, 1978.

Harris, A.: Ureteral anomalies with special reference to partial duplication with one branch ending blindly. J. Urol., 38:442, 1937.

Holly, L. E., and Sumcad, B.: Diverticular ureteral changes: a report of four cases. Am. J. Roentgenol., 78:1053, 1957.

Jablonski, J. P., Voldman, C., and Bruéziere, J.: Duplication totale de la voie excrétrice dont un uretere est borgne. J. Urol. Nephrol. (Paris), 84:837, 1978.

Kontturi, M., and Kaski, P.: Blind-ending bifid ureter with uretero-ureteral reflux. Scand. J. Urol. Nephrol., 6:91, 1972.

Kretschmer, H. L.: Duplication of the ureters at their distal ends, one pair ending blindly. So-called diverticula of the ureters. J. Urol., 30:61, 1933.

Lenaghan, D.: Bifid ureters in children: An anatomical and clinical study. J. Urol., 87:808, 1962.

Marshall, F. F., and McLoughlin, M. G.: Long blind-ending ureteral duplications. J. Urol., 120:626, 1978.

McGraw, A. B., and Culp, O. S.: Diverticulum of the ureter: Report of another authentic case. J. Urol., 67:262, 1952.

Miller, E. V., and Tremblay, R. E.: Symptomatic blindly ending bifid ureter. J. Urol., 92:109, 1964.

Norman, C. H., Jr., and Dubowy, J.: Multiple ureteral diverticula. J. Urol., 96:152, 1966.

Peterson, L. J., Grimes, J. H., Weinerth, J. L., et al.: Blind-ending branches of bifid ureters. Urology, 5:191, 1975.

Ponthieu, A., Anfossi, G., Guidicelli, C., and Boutboul, R.: Dedoublement segmentaire congenital de l'uretere lombaire. J. Urol. Nephrol. (Paris), 83:211, 1977.

Rank, W. B., Mellinger, G. T., and Spiro, E.: Ureteral diverticula: Etiologic considerations. J. Urol., 83:566, 1960.

Rao, K. G.: Blind-ending bifid ureter. Urology, 6:81, 1975.

Richardson, E. H.: Diverticulum of the ureter: A collective review with report of a unique example. J. Urol., 47:535, 1942.

Schultze, R.: Der blind endende Doppelureter. Z. Urol., 4:27, 1967.

Sharma, S. K., Malik, N., Kumar, S., and Bapna, B. C.: Bilateral incomplete ureteric duplication with a ureteric diverticulum. Aust. N. Z. J. Surg., 51:204, 1981.

Sharma, S. K., Subudhi, C. L., Kumar, S., Bapna, B. C., and Suri, S.: Ureteric diverticula: ureterodiverticular reflux and yo-yo effect. Br. J. Urol., 52:345, 1980.

Szokoly, V., Veradi, E., and Szporny, G.: Blind ending bifid and double ureters. Int. Urol. Nephrol., 6:174, 1974.

van Helsdingen, P. J. R. O.: A case of bifid ureter with blind-ending segment as the cause of chronic pain in the flank. Arch. Chir. Nederl., 27:277, 1975.

Youngen, R., and Persky, L.: Diverticulum of the renal pelvis. J. Urol., 94:40, 1965.

Inverted Y Ureteral Duplication

Britt, D. B., Borden, T. A., and Woodhead, D. M.: Inverted Y ureteral duplication with a blind-ending branch. J. Urol., 108:387, 1972.

Hawthorne, A. B.: Embryologic and clinical aspect of double ureter. JAMA, 106:189, 1936.

Klauber, G. T., and Reid, E. C.: Inverted Y reduplication of the ureter. J. Urol., 107:362, 1972.

Suzuki, S., Tsujimura, S., and Sugiura, H.: Inverted Y ureteral duplication with a ureteral stone in atretic segment. J. Urol., 117:248, 1977.

Ureteral Triplication

Arap, S., Lopes, R. N., Mitre, A. I., Menezes De Goes, G.: Triplicité urétérale complète associée à une urétérocèle ectopique. J. Urol. (Paris), 88:167, 1982.

Begg, R. C.: Sextuplicitas renum: A case of six functioning kidneys and ureters in an adult female. J. Urol., 70:686, 1953.

Blumberg, N.: Ureteral triplication. J. Pediatr. Surg., 11:579, 1976.

Delaere, K., and Debruyne, F.: Triplication and contralateral duplication of ureter. Urology, 19:302, 1982.

Fairchild, W. V., Solomon, H. D., Spence, C. R., and Gangai, M. P.: Case profile: unusual ureteral triplication. Urology, 14:95, 1979.

Gill, R. D.: Triplication of the ureter and renal pelvis. J. Urol., 68:140, 1952.

Gilmore, O. J. A.: Unilateral triplication of the ureter. Br. J. Urol., 46:585, 1974.

MacKelvie, A. A.: Triplicate ureter: Case report. Br. J. Urol., 27:124, 1955.

Marc, J., Drouillard, J., Bruneton, J. N., and Tavernier, J.: La triplication urétérale. J. Radiol. Electrol. Med. Nucl., 58:427, 1977.

Parker, R. M., Pohl, D. R., and Robison, J. R.: Ureteral triplication with ectopia. J. Urol., 103:727, 1970.

Parvinen, T.: Complete ureteral triplication. J. Pediatr. Surg., 11:1039, 1976.

Patel, N. P., and Lavengood, R. W.: Triplicate duplicate ureters. Br. J. Urol., 54:436, 1982.

Patel, N. P., and Lavengood, R. W.: Triplicate ureter. Urology, 5:242, 1975.

Perkins, P. J., Kroovand, R. L., and Evans, A. T.: Triplication of ureter: A case report. Radiology, 108:533, 1973.

Redman, J. F.: Triplicate ureter with contralateral ureteral duplication. J. Urol., 116:805, 1976.

Ringer, M. G., and MacFarlan, S. M.: Complete triplication of the ureter: A case report. J. Urol., 92:429, 1964.

Smith, I.: Triplicate ureter. Br. J. Surg., 34:182, 1946.

Soderdahl, D. W., Shiraki, I. W., and Schamber, D. T.: Bilateral ureteral quadruplication. J. Urol., 116:255, 1976.

Spangler, E. B.: Complete triplication of the ureter. Radiology, 80:795, 1963.

Wolpowitz, A., Evan, P., and Botha, P. A. G.: Triplication of ureter on one side and duplication on the other. Br. J. Urol., *47*:622, 1975.

Anomalies of Structure
Ureteral Atresia and Hypoplasia

Campbell, M. F.: Anomalies of the ureter. *In* Campbell, M. F., and Harrison, J. H. (Eds.): Urology. 3rd ed., p. 1512. Philadelphia, W. B. Saunders Co., 1970.

Cussen, L. J.: The morphology of congenital dilatation of the ureter: Intrinsic ureteral lesions. Aust. N.Z. J. Surg., *41*:185, 1971.

DeKlerk, D. P., Marshall, F. F., and Jeffs, R. D.: Multicystic dysplastic kidney. J. Urol., *118*:306, 1977.

Dewolf, W. C., Fraley, E. E., and Markland, C.: Congenital hypoplasia of the proximal ureter. J. Urol., *113*:236, 1975.

Gordon, M., and Reed, J. O.: Distal ureteral atresia. Am. J. Roentgenol., *88*:579, 1962.

Griscom, N. T., Vawter, G. F., and Fellers, F. X.: Pelvo-infundibular atrèsia: The usual form of multicystic kidney: 44 unilateral and two bilateral cases. Semin. Roentgenol., *10*:125, 1975.

Kornblum, K., and Ritter, J. A.: Retroperitoneal cyst with agenesia of the kidney. Radiology, *32*:416, 1939.

Mackie, G. G.: Personal communication, 1977.

Slater, G. S.: Ureteral atresia producing giant hydroureter. J. Urol., *78*:135, 1957.

Uson, A. C., Womack, C. E., and Berdon, W. E.: Giant ectopic ureter presenting as an abdominal mass in a newborn infant. J. Pediatr., *80*:473, 1972.

Megaureter, Ureteral Stenosis, and Stricture

Allen, T. D.: Discussion. *In* Bergsma, D., and Duckett, J. W., Jr. (Eds.): Urinary System Malformation in Children. Birth Defects: Original Article Series, Vol. 13, No. 5, p. 39. New York, Alan R. Liss, 1977.

Allen, T. D.: Congenital ureteral strictures. J. Urol., *104*:196, 1970.

Bellman, A. B.: Megaureter—Classification, etiology, and management. Urol. Clin. North Am., *1*:497, 1974.

Bischoff, P.: Observations on genesis of megaureter. Urol. Int., *11*:257, 1961.

Campbell, M.: Primary megalo-ureter. J. Urol., *68*:584, 1952.

Caulk, J. R.: Megaloureter—The importance of the uretero-vesical valve. J. Urol., *9*:315, 1923.

Chwalle, R.: The process of formation of cystic dilations of the vesical end of the ureter and of diverticula at the ureteral ostium. Urol. Cutan. Rev., *31*:499, 1927.

Creevy, C. D.: The atonic distal ureteral segment (ureteral achalasia). J. Urol., *97*:457, 1970.

Cussen, L. J.: The morphology of congenital dilatation of the ureter: Intrinsic ureteral lesions. Aust. N.Z. J. Surg., *41*:185, 1971.

Cussen, L. J.: The structure of the normal human ureter in infancy and childhood. J. Invest. Urol., *5*:179, 1967a.

Cussen, L. J.: Dimensions of the normal ureter in infancy and childhood. J. Invest. Urol., *5*:167, 1967b.

Gregoir, W., and Debled, G.: L'etiologie du reflux congénital et du méga-uretère primaire. Urol. Int., *24*:119, 1969.

Hanna, M. K., and Edwards, L.: Pressure perfusion studies of the abnormal uretero-vesical junction. Br. J. Urol., *44*:331, 1972.

Hanna, M. K., and Wyatt, J. K.: Primary obstructive megaureter in adults. J. Urol., *113*:328, 1975.

Hanna, M. K., Jeffs, R. D., Sturgess, J. M., et al.: Ureteral structure and ultrastructure. Part III. The congenitally dilated ureter (megaureter). J. Urol., *117*:24, 1977.

Hanna, M. K., Jeffs, R. D., Sturgess, J. M., et al.: Ureteral structure and ultrastructure. Part 1. The normal human ureter. J. Urol., *116*:718, 1976a.

Hanna, M. K., Jeffs, R. D., Sturgess, J. M., et al.: Ureteral structure and ultrastructure. Part II. Congenital ureteropelvic junction obstruction and primary obstructive megaureter. J. Urol., *116*:725, 1976b.

Hutch, J. A., and Tanagho, E. A.: Etiology of non-occlusive ureteral dilatation. J. Urol., *93*:177, 1965.

Johnston, J. H.: Reconstructive surgery of mega-ureter in childhood. Br. J. Urol., *39*:17, 1967.

Lewis, E. L., and Kimbrough, J. C.: Megalo-ureter. New concept in treatment. South. Med. J., *45*:171, 1952.

McLaughlin, P., Pfister, R. C., III, Leadbetter, W. F., et al.: The pathophysiology of primary megaloureter. J. Urol., *109*:805, 1973.

MacKinnon, K. J., Foote, J. W., Wiglesworth, F. W., et al.: The pathology of the adynamic distal ureteral segment. J. Urol., *103*:134, 1970.

Mark, L. K., and Moel, M.: Primary megaloureter. Radiology, *93*:345, 1969.

Murnaghan, G. F.: Experimental investigation of the dynamics of the normal and dilated ureter. Br. J. Urol., *29*:403, 1957.

Notley, R. G.: The structural basis for normal and abnormal ureteric motility. The innervation and musculature of the human ureter. Ann. R. Coll. Surg. Engl., *49*:250, 1971.

Notley, R. G.: Electron microscopy of the primary obstructive megaureter. Br. J. Urol., *44*:229, 1972.

Nunn, I. N., and Stephens, F. D.: The triad syndrome: A composite anomaly of the abdominal wall, urinary system and testes. J. Urol., *86*:782, 1961.

Palmer, J. M., and Tesluk, H.: Ureteral pathology in the prune belly syndrome. J. Urol., *111*:701, 1974.

Pfister, R. C., McLaughlin, A. P., III, and Leadbetter, W. F.: Radiological evaluation of primary megaloureter. Radiology, *99*:503, 1971.

Smith, D. E.: Report of Working Party to Establish an International Nomenclature for the Large Ureter. *In* Bergsma, D., and Duckett, J. W., Jr. (eds.): Urinary System Malformations in Children. Birth Defects: Original Article Series, Vol. 13, No. 5, p. 3. New York, Alan R. Liss, 1977.

Stephens, F. D.: Idiopathic dilations of the urinary tract. J. Urol., *112*:819, 1974.

Swenson, O., MacMahon, H. E., Jaques, W. E., et al.: A new concept of the etiology of megaloureters. N. Engl. J. Med., *246*:41, 1952.

Tanagho, E. A., Smith, D. R., Guthrie, T. H.: Pathophysiology of functional obstruction. J. Urol., *104*:73, 1970.

Tatu, W., and Brennan, R. E.: Primary megaureter in a mother and daughter. Urol. Radiol., *3*:185, 1981.

Tokunaka, S., and Koyanagi, T.: Morphologic study of primary nonreflux megaureters with particular emphasis on the role of ureteral sheath and ureteral dysplasia. J. Urol., *128*:399, 1982.

Tokunaka, S., Gotoh, T., Koyanagi, T., and Miyabe, N.: Muscle dysplasia in megaureters. J. Urol., *131*:383, 1984.

Tokunaka, S., Koyanagi, T., and Tsuji, I.: Two infantile cases of primary megaloureter with uncommon pathological findings: ultrastructural study and its clinical implication. J. Urol., *123*:214, 1980.

Tokunaka, S., Koyanagi, T., Tsuji, I., and Yamada, T.: Histopathology of the nonrefluxing megaloureter: a clue to its pathogenesis. J. Urol., *127*:238, 1982.

Whitaker, R. H.: Some observations and theories on the

wide ureter and hydronephrosis. Br. J. Urol., *47*:377, 1975.

Whitaker, R. H.: Methods of assessing obstruction in dilated ureters. Br. J. Urol., *45*:15, 1973.

Whitaker, R. H., and Johnston, J. H.: A simple classification of wide ureters. Br. J. Urol., *47*:781, 1975.

Williams, D. I.: The chronically dilated ureter. Ann. R. Coll. Surg. Engl., *14*:107, 1954.

Williams, D. I., and Burkholder, G. V.: The prune belly syndrome. J. Urol., *98*:244, 1967.

Williams, D. I., and Hulme-Moir, I.: Primary obstructive megaureter. Br. J. Urol., *42*:140, 1970.

Ureteral Valves

Cussen, L. J.: Valves of the ureter. *In* Bergsma, D., and Duckett, J. W., Jr. (Eds.): Urinary System Malformations in Children. Birth Defects: Original Article Series. Vol. 13, No. 5, p. 19. New York, Alan R. Liss, 1977.

Cussen, L. J.: The morphology of congenital dilatation of the ureter: Intrinsic ureteral lesions. Aust. N.Z. J. Surg., *41*:185, 1971.

Dajani, A. M., Dajani, Y. F., and Dahabrah, S.: Congenital ureteric valves—a cause of urinary obstruction. Br. J. Urol., *54*:98, 1982.

Fitzer, P. M.: Congenital ureteral valve. Pediatr. Radiol., *8*:54, 1979.

Foroughi, E., and Turner, J. A.: Congenital ureteral valve. J. Urol., *81*:272, 1959.

Fried, A. M., Mulcahy, J. J., Bhathena, D. B., and Oliff, M.: Hydronephrosis with ureteral valve: diagnosis by ultrasonography and antegrade pyelography. J. Urol., *120*:754, 1978.

Gosalbez, R., Garat, J. M., Piro, C., Martin, J. A., and Cortes, F.: Congenital ureteral valves in children. Urology, *21*:237, 1983.

Kirks, D. R., Currarino, G., and Weinberg, A. G.: Transverse folds in the proximal ureter: a normal variant in infants. Am. J. Roentgenol., *130*:463, 1978.

Maizels, M., and Stephens, F. D.: Valves of the ureter as a cause of primary obstruction of the ureter: anatomic, embryologic and clinical aspects. J. Urol., *123*:742, 1980.

Noe, H. N., and Scaljon, W.: Case profile: ureteral valves. Urology, *14*:411, 1979.

Passaro, E., Jr., and Smith, J. P.: Congenital ureteral valve in children: A case report. J. Urol., *84*:290, 1960.

Roberts, R. R.: Complete valve of the ureter: Congenital urethral valves. J. Urol., *76*:62, 1956.

Simon, H. B., Culp, O. S., and Parkhill, E. M.: Congenital ureteral valves: Report of two cases. J. Urol., *74*:336, 1955.

Wall, B., and Wachter, H. E.: Congenital ureteral valve: Its role as a primary obstructive lesion: classification of the literature and report of an authentic case. J. Urol., *68*:684, 1952.

Whiting, J. C., Stanisic, T. H., and Drach, G. W.: Congenital ureteral valves: report of 2 patients, including one with a solitary kidney and associated hypertension. J. Urol., *129*:1222, 1983.

Williams, D. I.: Discussion. *In* Bergsma, D., and Duckett, J. W., Jr. (Eds.): Urinary System Malformations in Children. Birth Defects: Original Article Series. Vol. 13, No. 5, p. 39. New York, Alan R. Liss, 1977.

Spiral Twists of the Ureter, Folds, and Kinks

Campbell, M. F.: Anomalies of the ureter. *In* Campbell, M. F., and Harrison, J. H. (Eds.): Urology. 3rd ed. Philadelphia, W. B. Saunders Co., 1970.

Gross, R. E.: Uretero-Pelvic Obstruction. *In* The Surgery of Infancy and Childhood. Philadelphia, W. B. Saunders Co., 1953.

Östling, K.: The genesis of hydronephrosis. Acta Chir. Scand., *86*:Suppl. 72, 1942.

Diverticulum

See *Anomalies of Number:*
Blind-ending duplication and diverticula.

Anomalies of Termination

Reflux

Ambrose, S. S., and Nicolson, W. P.: Ureteral reflux in duplicated ureters. J. Urol., *92*:439, 1964.

Ambrose, S. S., and Nicolson, W. P., III: The causes of vesicoureteral reflux in children. J. Urol., *87*:688, 1962.

Privett, J. T. J., Jeans, W. D., and Roylance, J.: The incidence and importance of renal duplication. Clin. Radiol., *27*:521, 1976.

Stephens, F. D., and Lenaghan, D.: The anatomical basis and dynamics of vesicoureteral reflux. J. Urol., *87*:669, 1962.

Tanagho, E. A., Hutch, J. A., Meyers, F. H., et al.: Primary vesicoureteral reflux: Experimental studies of its etiology. J. Urol., *93*:165, 1965.

Ectopic Ureter

Abeshouse, B. S.: Ureteral ectopia: Report of a rare case of ectopic ureter opening in the uterus and a review of the literature. Urol. Cutan. Rev., *47*:447, 1943.

Alfert, H. J., and Gillenwater, J. Y.: Ectopic vas deferens communicating with lower ureter: Embryological considerations. J. Urol., *108*:172, 1972.

Ayyat, F., Palmer, M. D., and Tingley, J. O.: Ectopic vas deferens communicating with lower ureter. Urology, *19*:423, 1982.

Bard, R. H., and Welles, H.: Nonduplication of upper urinary tract associated with horseshoe kidney and bilateral ureteral ectopia. Urology, *5*:784, 1975.

Brannan, W., and Henry, H. H., II: Ureteral ectopia: Report of 39 cases. J. Urol., *109*:192, 1973.

Borger, J. A., and Belman, A. B.: Uretero–vas deferens anastomosis associated with imperforate anus: An embryologically predictable occurrence. J. Pediatr. Surg., *10*:255, 1975.

Burford, C. E., Glenn, J. E., and Burford, E. H.: Ureteral ectopia: A review of the literature and 2 case reports. J. Urol., *62*:211, 1949.

Cendron, J., and Bonhomme, C.: 31 cas d'uretere à abouchement ectopique sous-sphincterien chez l'enfant du sexe feminin. J. Urol. Nephrol. (Paris), *74*:1, 1968a.

Cendron, J., and Bonhomme, C.: Uretere à terminaison ectopique extra-vesicale chez des sujets de sexe masculin (à propos de 10 cas). J. Urol. Nephrol. (Paris), *74*:31, 1968b.

Childlow, J. H., and Utz, D. C.: Ureteral ectopia in vestibule of vagina with urinary continence. South. Med. J., *63*:423, 1970.

Cox, C. E., and Hutch, J. A.: Bilateral single ectopic ureter: A report of 2 cases and review of the literature. J. Urol., *95*:493, 1966.

Cumes, D. M., Sanfelippo, C. J., and Stamey, T. A.: Single ectopic ureter masquerading as ureterocele in incontinent male. Urology, *17*:60, 1981.

Currarino, G.: Single vaginal ectopic ureter and Gartner's duct cyst with ipsilateral renal hypoplasia and dysplasia (or agenesis). J. Urol., *128*:988, 1982.

Das, S., and Amar, A. D.: Extravesical ureteral ectopia in male patients, J. Urol., *125*:842, 1981.

Das, S., and Amar, A. D.: Ureteral ectopia into cystic seminal vesicle with ipsilateral renal dysgenesis and monorchia. J. Urol., *124*:574, 1980.

Deilmann, W., and Moormann, J. G.: Komplexe urogenital-missbildung im bereich der wolffschen gänge. Urologe A, *17*:313, 1978.

Davis, D. M.: Urethral ectopic ureter in the female without incontinence. J. Urol., 23:463, 1930.

DeWeerd, J. H., and Litin, R. B.: Ectopia of ureteral orifice (vestibular) without incontinence: Report of case. Proc. Staff Meet. Mayo Clin., 33:81, 1958.

Eisendrath, D. N.: Ectopic opening of the ureter. Urol. Cutan. Rev., 42:401, 1938.

Ellerker, A. G.: The extravesical ectopic ureter. Br. J. Surg., 45:344, 1958.

Feldman, S., and Ross, L.: Hydrocolpos with vaginal ureteral ectopia: a case report. J. Urol., 123:573, 1980.

Fuselier, H. A., and Peters, D. H.: Cyst of seminal vesicle with ipsilateral renal agenesis and ectopic ureter: Case report. J. Urol., 115:833, 1976.

Gibbons, M. D., and Duckett, J. W., Jr.: Single vaginal ectopic ureter: a case report. J. Urol., 120:493, 1978.

Gibbons, M. D., Cromie, W. J., and Duckett, J. W., Jr.: Ectopic vas deferens. J. Urol., 120:597, 1978.

Glenn, J. F.: Agenesis of the bladder. JAMA, 169:2016, 1959.

Gordon, H. L., and Kessler, R.: Ectopic ureter entering the seminal vesicle associated with renal dysplasia. J. Urol., 108:389, 1972.

Gotoh, T., Morita, H., Tokunaka, S., Koyanagi, T., and Tsuji, I.: Single ectopic ureter. J. Urol., 129:271, 1983.

Gravgaard, E., Garsdal, L., and Moller, S. H.: Double vas deferens and epididymis associated with ipsilateral renal agenesis simulating ectopic ureter opening into the seminal vesicle. Scand. J. Urol. Nephrol., 12:85, 1978.

Grossman, H., Winchester, P. H., and Muecke, E. C.: Solitary ectopic ureter. Radiology, 89:1069, 1967.

Honke, E. M.: Ectopic ureter. J. Urol., 55:460, 1946.

Johnston, J. H., and Davenport, T. J.: The single ectopic ureter. Br. J. Urol., 41:428, 1969.

Jona, J. Z., Glicklich, and Cohen, R. D.: Ectopic single ureter and severe renal dysplasia: an unusual presentation. J. Urol., 121:369, 1979.

Kittredge, R. D., and Levin, D. C.: Unusual aspect of renal angiography in ureteric duplication. Am. J. Roentgenol., 119:805, 1973.

Kjaeldgaard, and Fianau, S.: Classification and embryological aspects of ectopic ureters communicating with Gartner's cysts. Diagn. Gynecol. Obstet., 4:269, 1982.

Kjaeldgaard, A., Fianau, S., Thorgeirsson, T., and Ekman, P.: Single bifid ectopic left ureter presenting clinically as a vaginal cyst. Diagn. Gynecol. Obstet., 3:321, 1981.

Kondo, A., Sahashi, M., and Mitsuya, H.: A rare variant of ureteric ectopia: opening in vagina and vesico-uretero-vaginal communication. Br. J. Urol., 54:486, 1982.

Koyanagi, T., Hisajima, S., Sakashita, S., Goto, T., and Tsuji, I.: Ureteral ectopia in vestibule without urinary incontinence. Urology, 16:508, 1980.

Koyanagi, T., Takamatsu, T., Kaneta, T., Terashima, M., and Tsuji, I.: A spontaneous vesico-ectopic ureterovaginal fistula in a girl. J. Urol., 118:871, 1977.

Koyanagi, T., Tsuji, I., Orikasa, S., and Hirano, T.: Bilateral single ectopic ureter: report of a case. Int. Urol. Nephrol., 9:123, 1977.

Leef, G. S., and Leader, S. A.: Ectopic ureter opening into the rectum: A case report. J. Urol., 87:338, 1962.

Levisay, G. L., Holder, J., and Weigel, J. W.: Ureteral ectopia associated with seminal vesicle cyst and ipsilateral renal agenesis. Radiology, 114:575, 1975.

Lowsley, O. S., and Kerwin, T. J.: Clinical Urology. Vol. 1, 3rd ed. Baltimore, The Williams & Wilkins Co., 1956.

Lucius, G. F.: Klinik und Therapie der dystopen Hernleitermundungen in die Samenwege. Urologe, 2:360, 1963.

Malek, R. S., Kelalis, P. P., Stickler, G. B., et al.: Observations on ureteral ectopy in children. J. Urol., 107:308, 1972.

Mellin, H. E., Kjaer, T. B., and Madsen, P. O.: Crossed ectopia of seminal vesicles, renal aplasia and ectopic ureter. J. Urol., 115:765, 1976.

Mills, J. C.: Complete unilateral duplication of ureter with analysis of the literature. Urol. Cutan. Rev., 43:444, 1939.

Mogg, R. A.: The single ectopic ureter. Br. J. Urol., 46:3, 1974.

Moore, T.: Ectopic openings of the ureter. Br. J. Urol., 24:3, 1952.

Moore, T.: Ectopic openings of the ureter. Br. J. Urol., 24:3, 1952.

Noseworthy, J., and Persky, L.: Spectrum of bilateral ureteral ectopia. Urology, 19:489, 1982.

Ogawa, A., Kakizawa, Y., and Akaza, H.: Ectopic ureter passing through the external urethral sphincter: Report of a case. J. Urol., 116:109, 1976.

Ostermayer, H., and Frei, A.: Nebenhoden und samenblase als mundungsort ektoper harnleiter. Urologe A, 20:389, 1981.

Prewitt, L. H., and Lebowitz, R. L.: The single ectopic ureter. Am. J. Roentgenol., 127:941, 1976.

Redman, J. F., and Sulieman, J. S.: Bilateral vasal-ureteral communications. J. Urol., 116:808, 1976.

Riba, L. W., Schmidlapp, C. J., and Bosworth, N. L.: Ectopic ureter draining into the seminal vesicle. J. Urol., 56:332, 1946.

Rognon, L., Brueziere, J., Soret, J. Y., et al.: Abouchement ectopique de l'ureter dans le tractus seminal: A propos de 10 cas. Chirurgie (Paris), 99:741, 1973.

Schnitzer, B.: Ectopic ureteral opening into seminal vesicle: A report of four cases. J. Urol., 93:576, 1965.

Schulman, C. C.: Fehlbildung des ureters und nierendysplasia—eine embryologische hypothese. Urologe A, 17:273, 1978.

Schulman, C. C.: The single ectopic ureter. Eur. Urol., 2:64, 1976.

Schulman, C. C.: Les implantations ectopiques de l'uretere. Acta Urol. Belg., 40:201, 1972.

Schwarz, R., and Stephens, F. D.: The persisting mesonephric duct: high junction of vas deferens and ureter. J. Urol., 120:597, 1978.

Scott, J. E. S.: The single ectopic ureter and the dysplastic kidney. Br. J. Urol., 53:300, 1981.

Seitzman, D. M., and Patton, J. F.: Ureteral ectopia: Combined ureteral and vas deferens anomaly. J. Urol., 84:604, 1960.

Sorenson, C. W., Jr., and Middleton, A. W., Jr.: The single ectopic ureter: 3 case reports. J. Urol., 129:132, 1983.

Uson, A. C., and Schulman, C. C.: Ectopic ureter emptying into the rectum: Report of a case. J. Urol., 108:156, 1972.

Uson, A. C., Womack, C. D., and Berdon, W. E.: Giant ectopic ureter presenting as an abdominal mass in a newborn infant. J. Pediatr., 80:473, 1972.

Vanhoutte, J. J.: Ureteral ectopia into a Wolffian duct remnant (Gartner's ducts or cysts) presenting as a urethral diverticulum in two girls. Am. J. Roentgenol., 110:540, 1970.

Varney, D. C., and Ford, M. D.: Ectopic ureteral remnant persisting as cystic diverticulum of the ejaculatory duct: Case report. J. Urol., 72:802, 1954.

Verbaeys, A., Oosterlinck, W., and Dhont, M.: Ureteric ectopia without incontinence in the female. Acta Urol. Belg., 48:366, 1980.

Wesson, M. B.: Incontinence of vesical and renal origin

(relaxed urethra and a vaginal ectopic ureter): A case report. J. Urol., 32:141, 1934.

Williams, D. I., and Lightwood, R. G.: Bilateral single ectopic ureters. J. Urol., 44:267, 1972.

Williams, D. I.: The ectopic ureter: Diagnosis problems. Br. J. Urol., 26:253, 1954.

Williams, D. I., and Royle, M.: Ectopic ureter in the male child. Br. J. Urol., 41:421, 1969.

Wilmarth, C. L.: Ectopic ureteral orifice within an urethral diverticulum: Report of a case. J. Urol., 59:47, 1948.

Ureterocele

Abrams, H. J., Sutton, A. P., and Buchbinder, M. I.: Ureteroceles in siblings. J. Urol., 124:135, 1980.

Ahmed, S.: Uncrossed complete ureteral duplication with caudal orthotopic orifice and ureterocele. J. Urol., 125:875, 1981.

Ambrose, S. S., and Nicolson, W. P.: Ureteral reflux in duplicated ureters. J. Urol., 92:439, 1964.

Androulakakis, P. A., Ossandon, F., and Ransley, P. G.: Intrinsic pathology of the lower moiety ureter in the duplex kidney with ectopic ureterocele. J. Urol., 125:873, 1981.

Arap, S., Arap-Neto, W., Chedid, E. A., Mitre, A. I., and de Góes, G. M.: Ureterocele of the lower pole ureter and an ectopic upper pole ureter in a duplex system. J. Urol., 129:1227, 1983.

Ayalon, A., Shapiro, A., Rubin, S. Z., and Schiller, M.: Ureterocele—a familial congenital anomaly. Urology, 13:551, 1979.

Babcock, J. R., Belman, A. B., Shkolnik, A., and Ignatoff, J.: Familial ureteral duplication and ureterocele. Urology, 9:345, 1977.

Bauer, S. B., and Retik, A. B.: The non-obstructive ectopic ureterocele. J. Urol., 119:804, 1978.

Bondonny, J. M., Diard, F., Bucco, P., Germaneu, J., and Cadier, L.: Les urétérocèles chez l'enfant: tentative de classification et de schéma thérapeutique à partir de l'etude de vingt-quatre dossiers. Ann. Pediatr. (Paris), 28:763, 1981.

Borden, T. A., and Martinez, A.: Vesicoureteral reflux associated with intact orthotopic ureterocele. Urology, 9:182, 1977.

Bruézière, J., Jablonski, J. P., and Frétin, J.: Les urétérocèles sur duplication pyélo-urétérale à développement intra-vesical chez l'enfant. J. Urol. Nephrol. (Paris), 85:704, 1979.

Campbell, M.: Ureterocele: A study of 94 instances in 80 infants and children. Surg. Gynecol. Obstet., 93:705, 1951.

Chwalle, R.: The process of formation of cystic dilatations of the vesical end of the ureter and of diverticula at the ureteral ostium. Urol. Cutan. Rev., 31:499, 1927.

Diard, F., Eklöf, O., Lebowitz, R., and Maurseth, K.: Urethral obstruction in boys caused by prolapse of simple ureterocele. Pediatr. Radiol., 11:139, 1981.

Eklöf, O., Löhr, G., Ringertz, H., and Thomasson, B.: Ectopic ureterocele in the male infant. Acta Radiol. [Diagn.] (Stockh), 19:145, 1978.

Ericsson, N. O.: Ectopic ureterocele in infants and children. Acta Chir. Scand., Suppl. 197:8, 1954.

Farkas, A., Earon, J., and Firstater, M.: Crossed renal ectopia with crossed single ectopic ureterocele. J. Urol., 119:836, 1978.

Fenelon, M. J., and Alton, D. J.: Prolapsing ectopic ureteroceles in boys. Radiology, 140:373, 1981.

Fishman, M., and Borden, S.: Crossed fused renal ectopia with single crossed ectopic ureterocele. J. Urol., 127:117, 1982.

Friedland, G. W., and Cunningham, J.: The elusive ectopic ureteroceles. Am. J. Roentgenol., 116:792, 1972.

Gyllensten, L.: Contributions to the embryology of the human bladder. Part I. The development of the definitive relations between the openings of the Wolffian ducts and the ureters. Acta Anat., 7:305, 1949.

Gross, R. E.: The Surgery of Infancy and Childhood. Its Principles and Techniques. Philadelphia, W. B. Saunders Co., 1953.

Johnson, D. K., and Perlmutter, A. D.: Single system ectopic ureteroceles with anomalies of the heart, testis and vas deferens. J. Urol., 123:81, 1980.

Kjellberg, S. R., Ericsson, N. O., and Rudhe, U.: The lower urinary tract in childhood; some correlated clinical and roentgenologic observations. Chicago, Year Book Publishers, Inc., 1957.

Klauber, G. I., and Crawford, D. B.: Prolapse of ectopic ureterocele and bladder trigone. Urology, 15:164, 1980.

Leong, J., Mikhael, B., and Schillinger, J. F.: Refluxing ureteroceles. J. Urol., 124:136, 1980.

Lima, S. V. C., and Cavalcanti, A. C. C.: Case profile: ureterocele from lower pole. Urology, 17:286, 1981.

Malek, R. S., Kelalis, P. P., Burke, E. C., et al.: Simple and ectopic ureterocele in infancy and childhood. Surg. Gynecol. Obstet., 134:611, 1972.

Mandell, J., Colodny, A. H., Lebowitz, R., Bauer, S. B., and Retik, A. B.: Ureteroceles in infants and children. J. Urol., 123:921, 1980.

Orr, L. M., and Glanton, J. B.: Prolapsing ureterocele. J. Urol., 70:180, 1953.

Perrin, E. V., Perksy, L., Tucker, A., et al.: Renal duplication and dysplasia. Urology, 4:660, 1974.

Prewitt, L. H., and Lebowitz, R. L.: The single ectopic ureter. Am. J. Roentgenol., 127:941, 1976.

Riba, L. W.: Ureterocele: with case reports of bilateral ureterocele in identical twins. Br. J. Urol., 8:119, 1936.

Snyder, H. M., and Johnston, J. H.: Orthotopic ureteroceles in children. J. Urol., 119:543, 1978.

Stephens, F. D.: Etiology of ureteroceles and effects of ureteroceles on the urethra. Br. J. Urol., 40:483, 1968.

Stephens, F. D.: Congenital Malformations of the Rectum, Anus and Genito-urinary Tracts. London, E & S Livingstone Ltd., 1963.

Tanagho, E. A.: Embryologic basis for lower ureteral anomalies: A hypothesis. Urology, 7:451, 1976.

Tokunaka, S., Gotoh, T., Koyanagi, T., and Tsuji, I.: Morphological study of the ureterocele: a possible clue to its embryogenesis as evidenced by a locally arrested myogenesis. J. Urol., 126:726, 1981.

Uson, A. C., Lattimer, J. K., and Melicow, M. M.: Ureteroceles in infants and children: Report based on 44 cases. Pediatrics, 27:971, 1961.

Weiss, R. M., and Spackman, T. J.: Everting ectopic ureteroceles. J. Urol., 111:538, 1974.

Williams, D. I., and Royle, M.: Ectopic ureter in the male child. Br. Jr. Urol., 41:421, 1969.

Williams, D. I., and Woodard, J. R.: Problems in the management of ectopic ureteroceles. J. Urol., 92:635, 1964.

Williams, D. I., Fay, R., and Lillie, J. G.: The functional radiology of ectopic ureterocele. Br. J. Urol., 44:417, 1972.

Anomalies of Position
Preureteral Vena Cava

Bateson, E. M., and Atkinson, D.: Circumcaval ureter: A new classification. Clin. Radiol., 20:173, 1969.

Brooks, R. J.: Left retrocaval ureter associated with situs invertus. J. Urol., 88:484, 1962.

Cathro, A. J.: Section of the inferior vena cava for retrocaval ureter: A new method of treatment. J. Urol., 67:464, 1952.

Campbell, M. F.: Anomalies of the ureter. *In* Campbell,

M. F., and Harrison, J. H. (Eds.): Urology. 3rd Ed., p. 1493. Philadelphia, W. B. Saunders Co., 1970.

Cendron, J., and Reis, C. F.: L'uretere retro-cave chez l'enfant. A propos de 4 cas. J. Urol. Nephrol., 78:375, 1972.

Clements, J. C., McLeod, D. G., Greene, W. R., and Stutzman, R. E.: A case report: duplicated vena cava with right retrocaval ureter and ureteral tumor. J. Urol., 119:284, 1978.

Crosse, J. E. W., Soderdahl, D. W., Teplick, S. K., et al.: Nonobstructive circumcaval (retrocaval) ureter. Radiology, 116:69, 1975.

Cukier, J., Aubert, J., and Dufour, B.: Uretere retrocave et rein en fer à cheval chez un garçon hypospade de 6 ans. J. Urol. Nephrol., 75:749, 1969.

Derrick, F. C., Jr., Price, R., Jr., and Lynch, K. M., Jr.: Retrocaval ureter. Report of a case and review of literature. J.S.C. Med. Assoc., 72:131, 1966.

Dreyfuss, W.: Anomaly simulating a retrocaval ureter. J. Urol., 82:630, 1959.

Duff, P. A.: Retrocaval ureter: Case report. J. Urol., 63:496, 1950.

Eidelman, A., Yuval, E., Simon, D., and Sibi, Y.: Retrocaval ureter: Eur. Urol., 4:279, 1978.

Gladstone, J.: Acardiac fetus (acephalus omphalositicus). J. Anat. Physiol., 40:71, 1905.

Goodwin, W. E., Burke, D. E., and Muller, W. H.: Retrocaval ureter. Surg. Gynecol. Obstet., 104:337, 1957.

Gruenwald, P., and Surks, S. N.: Pre-ureteric vena cava and its embryological explanation. J. Urol., 49:195, 1943.

Harrill, H. C.: Retrocaval ureter. Report of a case with operative correction of the defect. J. Urol., 44:450, 1940.

Heffernan, J. C., Lightwood, R. G., and Snell, M. E.: Horseshoe kidney with retrocaval ureter: second reported case. J. Urol., 120:358, 1978.

Hellsten, S., Grabe, M., and Nylander, G.: Retrocaval ureter. Acta Chir. Scand., 146:225, 1980.

Heslin, J. E., and Mamonas, C.: Retrocaval ureter: Report of four cases and review of literature. J. Urol., 65:212, 1951.

Hochstetter, F.: Entwicklungsgeschichte des Venen-systems der Amnioten. Morph. Jahrb., 20:543, 1893.

Hollinshead, W. H.: Anatomy for Surgeons. Vol. 2., New York, Hoeber Medical Division, Harper & Row, 1956.

Hradcova, L., and Kafka, V.: Retrocaval ureter in childhood. Urol. Int., 16:103, 1963.

Kenawi, M. M., and Williams, D. I.: Circumcaval ureter: A report of four cases in children with a review of the literature and a new classification. Br. J. Urol., 48:183, 1976.

Kumeda, K., Takamatsu, M., Sone, M., Yasukawa, S., Doi, J., and Ohkawa, T.: Horseshoe kidney with retrocaval ureter: a case report. J. Urol., 128:361, 1982.

Lerman, I., Lerman, S., and Lerman, F.: Retrocaval ureter: Report of a case. J. Med. Soc. N.J., 53:74, 1956.

Lowsley, O. S.: Postcaval ureter, with description of a new operation for its correction. Surg. Gynecol. Obstet., 82:549, 1946.

Marcel, J. E.: Grosse hydronephrose par uretere retrocave. Arch. Franc. Pediat., 10:1, 1953.

Mayer, R. F., and Mathes, G. L.: Retrocaval ureter. South. Med. J., 51:945, 1958.

McClure, C. F. W., and Butler, E. G.: The development of the vena cava inferior in man. Am. J. Anat., 35:331, 1925.

Olson, R. O., and Austen, G., Jr.: Postcaval ureter. Report and discussion of a case with successful surgical repair. N. Engl. J. Med., 242:963, 1950.

Parks, R. E., and Chase, W. E.: Retrocaval ureter. Report of two cases diagnosed preoperatively in childhood. Am. J. Dis. Child., 82:442, 1951.

Peisojovich, M. R., and Lutz, S. J.: Retrocaval ureter: A case report and successful repair with a new surgical technique. Mich. Med., 68:1137, 1969.

Pick, J. W., and Anson, B. J.: Retrocaval ureter: Report of a case, with a discussion of its clinical significance. J. Urol., 43:672, 1940.

Randall, A., and Campbell, E. W.: Anomalous relationship of the right ureter to the vena cava. J. Urol., 34:565, 1935.

Rowland, H. S., Jr., Bunts, R. C., and Iwano, J. H.: Operative correction of retrocaval ureter: A report of four cases and review of the literature. J. Urol., 83:820, 1960.

Salem, R. J., and Luck, R. J.: Midline ensheathed ureters. Br. J. Urol., 48:18, 1976.

Voelkel, V. H. H.: Retrokavaler Verlauf des rechten Ureters. Z. Urol., 56:49, 1963.

Preureteric Iliac Artery

Corbus, B. C., Estrem, R. D., and Hunt, W.: Retro-iliac ureter. J. Urol., 84:67, 1960.

Dees, J. E.: Anomalous relationship between ureter and external iliac artery. J. Urol., 44:207, 1940.

Hanna, M. K.: Bilateral retro-iliac artery ureters. Br. J. Urol., 44:339, 1972.

Iuchtman, M., Assa, J., Blatnoi, I., Ezagui, L., and Simon, J.: Urometrocolpos associated with retroiliac ureter. J. Urol., 124:283, 1980.

Radhrishnan, J., Vermillion, C. D., and Hendren, W. H.: Vasa deferentia inserting into retroiliac ureters. J. Urol., 124:746, 1980.

Seitzman, D. M., and Patton, J. F.: Ureteral ectopia: Combined ureteral and vas deferens anomaly. J. Urol., 84:604, 1960.

Vascular Obstruction of the Distal Ureter

Campbell, M. F.: Anomalies of the ureter. In Campbell, M.F., and Harrison, J. H. (Eds.): Urology. 3rd ed., Philadelphia, W. B. Saunders Co., 1970.

Campbell, M. F.: Vascular obstruction of the ureter in children. J. Urol., 36:366, 1936.

Campbell, M. F.: Vascular obstruction of the ureter in juveniles. Am. J. Surg., 22:527, 1933.

Greene, L. F., Priestley, J. T., Simon, H. B., et al.: Obstruction of the lower third of the ureter by anomalous blood vessels. J. Urol., 71:544, 1954.

Hyams. J. A.: Aberrant blood vessels as factor in lower ureteral obstruction. Surg. Gynecol. Obstet., 48:474, 1929.

Scultety, S., and Varga, B.: Obstructions of the lower ureteral segment caused by vascular anomalies (author's transl.). Urologe (A), 14:144, 1975.

Young, J. D., Jr., and Kiser, W. S.: Obstruction of the lower ureter by aberrant blood vessels. J. Urol., 94:101, 1965.

Herniations of the Ureter

Beck, W. C., Baurys, W., Brochu, J., et al.: Herniation of the ureter into sciatic foramen ("curlicue ureter"). JAMA, 149:441, 1952.

Dourmashkin, R. L.: Herniation of the ureter. J. Urol., 38:455, 1937.

Jewett, H. J., and Harris, A. P.: Scrotal ureter: Report of a case. J. Urol., 69:184, 1953.

Lindblom, A.: Unusual ureteral obstruction by herniation of ureter into sciatic foramen; report of case. Acta Radiol., 28:225, 1947.

Page, B. H.: Obstruction of ureter in internal hernia. Br. J. Urol., 27:254, 1955.

Watson, L. F.: Hernia. 3rd ed. London, Henry Kimpton, 1948.

CHAPTER 39

Renal Cystic Disease and Renal Dysplasia

JAY BERNSTEIN, M.D.
KENNETH D. GARDNER, JR., M.D.

Cystic diseases of the kidney are heterogeneous. Different types of disease have different causes, different clinical manifestations, and different clinical courses. A few are distinctive morphologically, a few are distinctive radiographically, and a few are distinctive clinically, but no single method or discipline offers an adequate basis of classification.

The classification that follows incorporates clinical, radiographic, genetic, and morphologic information. It accommodates developmental, heritable, and acquired disorders; it acknowledges the overwhelming morphologic similarities in genetically diverse conditions; and it provides reasonable clinicopathologic correlations for investigation, prognostication, and genetic counseling.

This classification has evolved over a period of years (Bernstein and Meyer, 1967; Elkin and Bernstein, 1969; Bernstein, 1976). It is similar to the schemes developed by Gleason, McAlister, and Kissane (1967) and by Spence and Singleton (1972b). All are strongly based on morphologic and radiographic observations, modified by clinical findings. All use similar terms with similar meanings.

TERMINOLOGY AND CLASSIFICATION

A suitable classification requires a suitable terminology with widespread acceptance and restricted meanings. The common practice of referring to all renal cysts as "polycystic disease" obviously impedes classification; indeed, the liberal use of that term imposes a considerable disadvantage.

Some cystic lesions are both heritable and developmental, arising during renal morphogenesis. Other heritable abnormalities, however, appear after the cessation of nephrogenesis and are not developmental. This point has important implications for polycystic disease if, for example, it can be shown that those cysts are not themselves inherent but are secondary to a metabolic or structural external defect. Cysts can, of course, be acquired at any time during life, arising from the influence of nephrotoxic, cystogenic agents. Several different cystic conditions have predilections for the loops of Henle and peripheral collecting tubules, but the anatomic localization of cysts does not attest to their etiology.

Polycystic Disease is defined as a heritable disorder with diffuse involvement of both kidneys. Apart from the cysts, there is no evidence of renal parenchymal maldevelopment, such as dysplasia. Polycystic disease comprises at least two separate, genetically different diseases—one typically has an onset in childhood (*infantile polycystic disease*), and the other begins in adulthood (*adult polycystic disease*). Both terms are technically misnomers, since each condition occurs in both children and adults; the two are separated in fact on clinicopathologic and genetic grounds rather than according to age of onset.

Infantile Polycystic Disease (IPCD) may be a heterogeneous group of several clinically overlapping conditions, each with autosomal recessive inheritance, or it may be one disease with age-related differences in clinical and morphologic manifestations. Intrahepatic biliary alterations in IPCD include portal fibrosis, with portal hypertension and its complications. Patients without clinically overt renal manifestations are said to have congenital hepatic fibrosis (CHF), though radiographic studies commonly show renal manifestations of IPCD. It continues to be debated whether IPCD with hepatic involvement and CHF with clinically silent renal involvement are different aspects of the same disease or are genetically different diseases.

Adult Polycystic Disease (APCD) appears to be genetically homogeneous, despite morphologic variation in young infants, who often have a predominance of glomerular cysts. APCD is also associated with intrahepatic biliary alterations, an overlap with IPCD that should no longer cause confusion. The disease is transmitted as an autosomal dominant trait. APCD has been recognized in young infants, in whom the morphologic appearance may be dominated by glomerular cysts.

Renal cysts are encountered in many hereditary syndromes, usually as peripheral cortical microcysts that have no clinical or functional significance. Significant cystic disease, however, has been associated with tuberous sclerosis and the orofaciodigital syndrome in older children and young adults. Renal cysts are encountered in von Hippel-Lindau disease, in which they may be related to the same factors that cause carcinoma in those patients. Severe cystic disease is also found in newborns with the Jeune and Zellweger syndromes, but those conditions are seldom of urologic importance. What has been called *glomerulocystic disease* in children is clearly heterogeneous, since glomerular cysts occur in several forms of cystic disease and cystic dysplasia; a large proportion of cases, perhaps 50 per cent, can be accounted for by autosomal dominant polycystic disease (APCD) of early infantile onset.

Simple Cysts of the Renal Parenchyma are conceptually straightforward, common radiographic and pathologic abnormalities that can, when multiple, be difficult to differentiate from APCD, a distinction that is clearly important to clinical care and genetic counseling. Simple cysts are, almost by definition, nonhereditary and are unassociated with progressive renal failure. Segmental and unilateral cysts may constitute diagnostic problems, and these cysts are also conceptually uncertain; they do not appear to be hereditary or related to other forms of cystic renal disease.

Medullary Cysts are encountered in a complex of genetically unrelated heritable tubulointerstitial nephropathies that have similar clinical and morphologic characteristics. Although the cysts probably have no functional significance, the term *uremic medullary cystic disease* is ingrained in the literature; it comprises

both autosomal dominant *medullary cystic disease* (MCD) and autosomal recessive *familial juvenile nephronophthisis* (FJN). The renal lesion encountered in *renal-retinal dysplasia*—which encompasses tapetoretinal degeneration, familial retinitis pigmentosa, and pigmentary optic atrophy—is functionally and morphologically identical to the renal lesion of FJN. Both MCD and FJN must be differentiated from *medullary sponge kidney* (MSK), which is clinically and genetically a different disease.

Renal Dysplasia has been classified on morphologic grounds into several types that may be correlated with clinical findings. One type that is of urologic interest is the enlarged *multicystic kidney*. Cystic dysplasia of the peripheral cortex is associated with lower urinary tract obstruction. Other forms of cystic dysplasia, either isolated or syndromatic, are occasional causes of chronic renal failure.

These considerations have been incorporated into a classification (Table 39–1) that has been modified to reflect changing concepts and recent developments.

TABLE 39–1. CLASSIFICATION OF RENAL
PARENCHYMAL CYSTS

I. Polycystic Disease
  A. Autosomal recessive polycystic disease (IPCD)
    1. Polycystic disease of newborns and young infants
    2. Polycystic disease of older children and adults
      a. Medullary tubular ectasia
      b. Congenital hepatic fibrosis
      c. Caroli syndrome
  B. Autosomal dominant polycystic disease (APCD)
    1. Glomerulocystic disease of newborn (in part)
    2. Classic polycystic disease of older children and adults

II. Renal Cysts in Hereditary Syndromes
  A. Tuberous sclerosis complex
  B. Orofaciodigital syndrome I
  C. von Hippel-Lindau disease
  D. Zellweger cerebrohepatorenal syndrome and Jeune asphyxiating thoracic dysplasia
  E. Cortical cysts and syndromes of multiple malformations
  F. Glomerulocystic disease of newborn (in part)

III. Simple Cysts, Solitary and Multiple

IV. Segmental and Unilateral Cystic Disease

V. Acquired Cystic Disease

VI. Renal Medullary Cysts
  A. Hereditary tubulointerstitial nephritis
    1. Familial juvenile nephronophthisis
    2. Medullary cystic disease
    3. Renal-retinal dysplasia and congeners
  B. Medullary sponge kidney

VII. Renal Dysplasia
  A. Multicystic and aplastic dysplasia
  B. Diffuse cystic dysplasia, isolated and syndromatic
  C. Cystic dysplasia associated with lower urinary tract obstruction

INFANTILE POLYCYSTIC DISEASE

Autosomal Recessive Type

IPCD, which affects both children and adults, is more accurately designated *autosomal recessive polycystic disease,* which is a term that seems just clumsy enough not to have caught on. IPCD bears no relationship to APCD, a separation supported by clinical, genetic, and morphologic studies. The morphologic and clinical features of IPCD are variable, however, impairing any attempt to define the condition in simple anatomic or clinical terms. We have, therefore, continued to rely on clinicopathologic correlations and on visual recognition, and we have not been able to establish a rigorous definition.

Etiology and Genetics

The cause of IPCD is unknown, except that the basic abnormality is hereditary. The disease has long been recognized as an autosomal recessive trait, a point firmly established by Lundin and Olow (1961) and by Heggö and Natvig (1965) in studies of morphologically homogeneous neonatal cases. Subsequent studies have shown that IPCD is not limited to the neonatal period and that it has a morphologically heterogeneous appearance in older children and adults.

Blyth and Ockenden (1971) thought that the clinical variability was determined genetically, there being four forms of infantile and childhood polycystic disease, each of which was transmitted as an autosomal recessive trait and each of which had different clinical and morphologic characteristics. The four types were characterized according to age at onset, with the same type occurring in all the affected children of a family. In contrast, studies reported by Lieberman and her colleagues (1971) indicated an age-related clinical pattern that they saw as a continuum. The clinical differences seemed to reflect the natural history of IPCD, despite different evolutions in individual cases. Lieberman recognized only two groups, those children with typical IPCD and those older children with portal hypertension and only mild renal involvement. Both Lieberman and co-workers and Chilton and Cremin (1981) recognized that Blyth's and Ockenden's groups did not segregate neatly by families.

Those children with hepatic involvement and portal hypertension can be regarded as having CHF, which is a syndrome of considerable heterogeneity (Murray-Lyon et al., 1973). Most patients, however, have renal involvement in the form of medullary ductal ectasia; in some, the renal involvement remains mild or asymptomatic, whereas in others it progresses to renal failure, even after many years (Dupond et al., 1979). We have regarded CHF with typical renal lesions to be part of the spectrum of IPCD (Bernstein, 1976, 1979). Conversely, Landing and colleagues (1980) have found that the hepatic lesions separate morphometrically into two distinct groups: (1) young patients with typical IPCD—the congenital, perinatal, and infantile groups of Blyth and Ockenden (1971) and (2) older patients, including Blyth's and Ockenden's juvenile group, plus typical cases of CHF. Landing and colleagues suggest a new genetic separation along those lines, despite clinical overlap in the occurrence of renal failure and portal hypertension. All studies (Blyth and Ockenden, 1971; Lathrop, 1959; Lieberman et al., 1971; Weiss et al., 1974) are in agreement that IPCD-CHF is transmitted by recessive inheritance. The validity of separating IPCD into several groups may turn out to be substantiated by additional clinical and genetic evaluations, but considerable uncertainty remains.

Pathogenesis and Morphology

A characteristic of all forms of IPCD, with or without CHF, is medullary ductal ectasia. Gross ductal dilatation within the medullary pyramids is seen in newborns with enlarged spongy kidneys, in older children with scattered cortical cysts, and in young adults with no other apparent involvement. The abnormality is easily confused with MSK, and differentiation of the two conditions rests morphologically on the demonstration of cortical cysts in IPCD; the cysts are usually accompanied by some tubular atrophy and interstitial fibrosis.

The diffuse spongy and enlarged (12 to 16 times normal) kidneys in neonatal IPCD are instantly recognizable (Fig. 39–1). Dilated ducts are grossly visible as rounded medullary cysts and radially arranged elongated cortical cysts. The interstitium usually is severely edematous (a factor that probably contributes to the increased weight of the kidneys), but interstitial fibrosis is only mild. Microdissection has shown the principal sites of dilatation to be in the collecting ducts and the collecting tubules (Heggö and Natvig, 1965; Osathanondh and Potter, 1964c). Osathanondh and Potter (1964c) also observed normal numbers of nephrons with normal attachments to collecting tubules. Both light microscopy and microdissection show var-

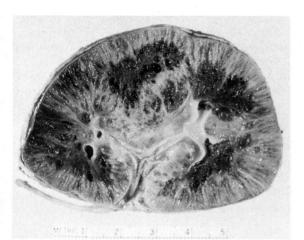

Figure 39–1. IPCD. The kidneys are greatly enlarged, and the cortex is diffusely spongy. The dilated collecting ducts are visible as linear radiations extending from the cortico-medullary junction to the capsule, and the medullary pyramids contain dilated ducts. The kidney typically contains a normal number of lobes, and the pelvis is compressed by the bulky parenchyma.

iable, usually mild nephronic dilatation involving tubules and glomeruli.

Older children have less ductal dilatation, and the cysts, which are irregularly distributed, have rounded rather than saccular configurations. The lesion is bilateral, and is disseminated but not diffuse. The different pattern suggests milder expression of the genetic abnormality (Blyth and Ockenden, 1971), perhaps a regression of cysts (Lieberman et al., 1971). The rounded appearance suggests that the dilatations have become localized, perhaps segmental within the tubule, raising the possibility of secondary and localized ductal obstruction. The implied questions are difficult to answer because the systematic microdissections have not been carried out. Such cases may perhaps be included in Potter's Category 3 (Osathanondh and Potter, 1964b), but the category is heterogeneous, and individual cases are difficult to identify. Glomerular obsolescence, focal tubular atrophy with cast formation, and cortical fibrosis are found in varied mixtures, which are sometimes focal and asymptomatic and other times are diffuse and progress to renal failure. The severe cystic change appears to be the lesion of fetuses and newborns; progression in older individuals seems to take the form of tubular damage without cyst formation. Those patients with the mildest renal involvement are commonly recognized as having CHF.

Despite a large number of theories and considerable speculation, the pathogenesis of

IPCD continues to elude us. Older theories invoking faulty embryogenesis are inapplicable in view of microdissection studies demonstrating normal architectonics. The progressive nature of the lesion and the finding of cortical atrophy in older patients with renal failure strongly indicate that the kidney is subject to continuing injury. The following are possibilities: (1) The genetic abnormality may directly affect epithelial protein in the kidney and liver and (2) the defect may affect the supporting structures and injure tubular and ductal epithelium secondarily. Ultrastructural studies have shown peritubular fibrosis (Thaler et al., 1973), which may contribute to the progression of tubular damage.

The hepatic lesion in IPCD consists of an apparent increase in the number of portal bile ducts, usually with portal enlargement and increased connective tissue. The ducts seem to form an almost continuous system of anastomosing and tortuous channels, which are perhaps flattened cisterns rather than ducts (Jørgensen, 1973; Landing et al., 1973; Bernstein, 1979; Landing et al., 1980). The main interlobular ducts within the portal areas are usually absent, but the intricate biliary network accounts for the lack of functional obstruction. Bile plugs are seen in older children, even though the patients are seldom jaundiced. There is little morphologic evidence of hepatocellular damage. One cause of hepatocellular injury is ascending cholangitis with biliary suppuration, which also leads to increasing portal fibrosis and biliary obstruction. It is not clear whether fibrosis as part of the disease (Albukerk and Duffy, 1971; Thaler et al., 1973) or whether a concurrent maldevelopment of the portal venous system (Odièvre et al., 1977) is responsible for increased vascular resistance, but portal hypertension frequently supervenes. Ductal obstruction does not seem to be present, and communication with the extrahepatic biliary tree can be demonstrated even in those patients with severe intrahepatic ductal ectasia—the so-called Caroli disease, which is a syndrome of multiple etiologies (Murray-Lyon et al., 1972).

Cystic lesions have been described in other organs, but we have observed only minor dilatation of small pancreatic ductules. We have not seen cystic lungs, and the lungs in severely affected newborns are usually hypoplastic. Cerebral berry aneurysms are reported as occasional complications.

Radiography

The radiographic and sonographic findings in IPCD closely reflect the morphologic abnormality. The kidneys are typically enlarged and contain small cysts; larger cysts, 1 to 2 cm in diameter, are sometimes found in older patients.

Excretory urography shows two characteristic patterns: (1) retention and puddling of contrast material within cortical and medullary cysts, producing an irregularly mottled or a streaked nephrogram (Hinkel and Santini, 1956; Gwinn & Landing, 1968; Elkin & Bernstein, 1969) and (2) retention of contrast material in dilated medullary collecting ducts, producing linear medullary opacification (Reilly and Neuhauser, 1960; Bernstein and Meyer, 1967; Six et al., 1975).

The first pattern is seen in the enlarged kidneys of young infants. Contrast material is poorly excreted, and the pelves are barely visualized (Fig. 39–2), though some contrast material often appears in the bladder. The kidneys retain radiopaque material for days, with apparent opacification of cysts and dilated ducts (Figs. 39–2 and 39–3). Older children may have a delayed mottled nephrogram or prompt excretion of contrast material with delineation of the pyelocalyceal system (Lieberman et al., 1971; Vuthibhagdee and Singleton, 1973). Lieberman and colleagues (1971) observed a changing urographic pattern in two cases that were followed

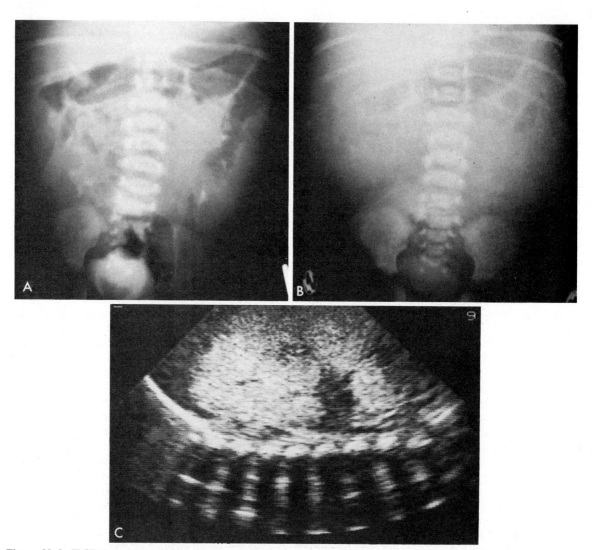

Figure 39–2. IPCD in newborn infant. Excretory urogram at 3 days of age *(A)* shows renal enlargement with a faint pyelogram and some contrast medium in the bladder. Plain film a day later *(B)* shows retention of contrast medium, presumably within renal cysts, producing a mottled nephrogram. A supine parasagittal sonogram of the right kidney *(C)* reveals enlargement and increased echogenicity. (Roentgenograms courtesy of Dr. R. L. Bree, Department of Radiology, William Beaumont Hospital, Royal Oak.)

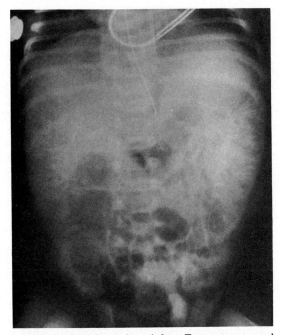

Figure 39–3. IPCD in newborn infant. Excretory urography discloses enlarged kidneys, with retention of contrast medium, presumably in dilated ducts, to produce linear radial opacifications.

over a period of several years; in one case the kidney became smaller and in the other case excretion improved so that a nephrogram performed early in the disease evolved into a mildly abnormal pyelogram. However, alterations in the radiographic pattern have to be interpreted with caution and with regard to the clinical status of the patient, since diminishing renal size

can reflect renal atrophy as well as regression of cysts. Sonographic studies show enlarged kidneys with increased echogeneity and indistinct outlines (Boal and Teele, 1980) (see Fig. 39–2), features that are sufficiently characteristic to allow for prenatal diagnosis (Habif et al., 1982). Whether the pattern is sufficiently characteristic to differentiate fetal IPCD from fetal APCD (Zerres et al., 1982) is not certain.

The second pattern, medullary ductal ectasia (Fig. 39–4), corresponds to "renal tubular ectasia," which was described by Reilly and Neuhauser (1960), and also accounts for at least some of the cases of "familial cystic dysplasia" described by Gwinn and Landing (1968). It may be present both in very young children, in whom the disease progresses to renal failure, and in older individuals with silent renal involvement. Medullary ductal ectasia is also the characteristic renal abnormality that is seen radiographically in patients with CHF (Kerr et al., 1962; Unite et al., 1973; Weiss et al., 1974; Six et al., 1975). We must emphasize that this abnormality is radiographically indistinguishable from MSK, which occurs in a different age group and has a different genetic and clinical background (Bernstein, 1976). The similarity can cause considerable confusion, which has been carried over into the literature (Fairley et al., 1963; Grossman and Seed, 1966; Weiss et al., 1974), but it appears reasonably certain that the patients with a combination of CHF and MSK are indeed victims of IPCD.

The characterization of cases according to radiographic criteria (Chilton and Cremin, 1981) that probably reflect the severity of renal im-

Figure 39–4. Congenital hepatic fibrosis and IPCD. Excretory urography discloses medullary ductal ectasia in an adult with congenital hepatic fibrosis and no clinical evidence of renal disease. The pyramids are opacified, with a brush-like pattern indistinguishable from that seen in medullary sponge kidney. IPCD is, however, a condition that is clinically and genetically different from medullary sponge kidney, despite the identical radiographic pattern. (Roentgenogram courtesy of Dr. J. Farah, Department of Radiology, William Beaumont Hospital, Royal Oak.)

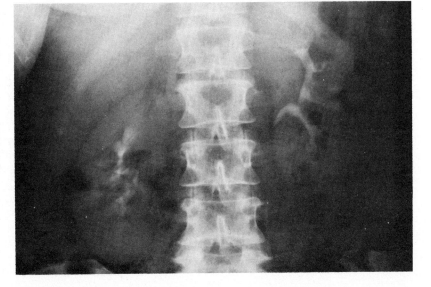

pairment may be helpful in prognostication, though it seems unlikely that the radiographic differences have genetic significance. Similarly, sonographic differences in renal size and severity of cyst formation (Rosenfield et al., 1977; Boal and Teele, 1980) may be very helpful in evaluating individual cases, without providing a basis for further subclassification.

Retrograde pyelography adds little and is seldom performed; it may show mild pyelocalyceal distortion with pyelotubular backflow. Radioisotopic techniques are also of limited value because of the small size of the cysts. Renograms show delayed excretion of radionuclide, confirming excretory impairment.

Radiographic evaluation of the liver has not been helpful as a diagnostic procedure, except in the minority of patients who have hepatic ductal ectasia and Caroli disease.

Renal Function

Children with IPCD have varying degrees of renal insufficiency. Studies by Anand and colleagues (1975) have shown a reduced effective renal plasma flow and a reduced glomerular filtration rate (GFR). Patients with IPCD had an impaired concentrating ability and defective acidification. The GFR was also reduced in several patients with CHF, and the majority had a reduced ability to concentrate urine. The concentrating defect was not dependent on reduced GFR, indicating either a primary tubular abnormality or secondary medullary changes. Cystic abnormalities of the tubules also account for the reduced excretion of acid.

Clinical Features

Newborns with the severe form of the disease die in the first few days of life, usually because of respiratory insufficiency. Many infants have Potter facies and a history of oligohydramnios. The kidneys are massively enlarged, at times causing severe abdominal distention and intrapartum dystocia. Although newborns are usually oliguric after birth, they seldom die of renal failure. Pulmonary hypoplasia is responsible for persistent respiratory distress, and resuscitative measures frequently lead to interstitial emphysema, pneumomediastinum, and pneumothorax. Some infants have hepatomegaly. Congenital malformations of other viscera are uncommon in homogeneous populations of IPCD.

Older children often have smaller kidneys, and Lieberman and colleagues (1971) have observed a progressive reduction in size, beginning between 1 and 2 years of age and stabilizing between 4 and 5 years of age. Some degree of enlargement persists, and the kidneys usually remain palpable. Patients develop renal insufficiency beginning in early childhood, though its progression is variable. Many children die in infancy, but others enjoy prolonged survival (Vuthibhagdee and Singleton, 1973). Almost all patients develop systemic hypertension, and congestive heart failure may be a problem in early infancy. Older children also develop hepatomegaly and splenomegaly. Nonspecific symptoms include abdominal pain, nausea, and vomiting. Growth retardation is common.

Laboratory examinations confirm the presence of renal insufficiency with elevated serum concentrations of urea and creatinine. Patients are acidotic and moderately anemic. Urinalyses show low specific gravity and mild proteinuria. The urine sediment often contains an increased number of pus cells, but bacterial infection is only infrequently demonstrated. The sediment rarely contains a significant number of red blood cells. Hyperphosphatemia and hypocalcemia are late complications. Serum concentrations of albumin are normal or mildly depressed. Liver function tests are usually normal; hepatocellular dysfunction and hepatic insufficiency occur in association with concurrent biliary infection.

Patients who have CHF in addition to IPCD tend to be older and to have milder renal impairment. Renal abnormalities demonstrable on radiography may be limited to medullary ductal ectasia; we have observed several adult patients who had hepatic disease with only radiographic evidence of renal involvement and no apparent renal insufficiency. Late-onset renal insufficiency can occur, however, with progression to renal failure during the third or fourth decade of life (Dupond et al., 1979). Portal hypertension and renal impairment do coexist, and children have been known to suffer from both bleeding esophageal varices and chronic renal failure (Lieberman et al., 1971).

The differential diagnosis in newborns includes other causes of renal enlargement. The most common form of bilateral cystic disease in newborns is multicystic dysplasia; the bilateral malformation is morphologically similar to the more common unilateral condition and is associated with bilateral ureteral atresia. Other forms of diffuse cystic dysplasia are rare. The Meckel syndrome can be recognized by its nonrenal malformations. Renal dysplasia in any of several multiple congenital malformation syndromes may cause renal enlargement, and the diagnosis rests on recognition of the basic syndrome. Bilateral hydronephrosis resulting from urinary tract obstruction produces flank masses; in this regard, the concomitant presence of enlarged kidneys and a suprapubic mass in a male infant should suggest the diagnosis of posterior urethral valves. Hydronephrosis can be recognized by ultrasonography; radionuclide imaging usually shows evidence of delayed excretion and stasis. Bilateral renal tumors also cause renal enlargement. Sonography, excretory urography, and cystography by the direct puncture technique should differentiate these conditions from IPCD, though they might not provide a specific diagnosis. Circulatory disturbances such as renal vein thrombosis cause considerable renal enlargement; significant hematuria is found, even in oliguric patients.

The differential diagnosis in older children should include other causes of progressive renal insufficiency with a concentrating defect. An abnormality that is probably more common than IPCD is FJN, which is one of the hereditary interstitial nephropathies (see page 1783). Children with FJN suffer from severe anemia and growth retardation. Renal function is usually too reduced to allow adequate urographic studies, and the pattern of medullary ductal ectasia is not seen, despite the presence of medullary cysts. The kidneys are very small because of severe cortical atrophy. The development of hepatosplenomegaly is a strong clue to the diagnosis of IPCD, though a few cases with CHF and a renal lesion designated as nephronophthisis have been reported (Boichis et al., 1973).

IPCD in childhood is usually fatal. Progression of the disease, however, is variable, and prolonged survival does occur even with renal impairment (Vuthibhagdee and Singleton, 1973). The presence of similar, though generally milder, renal impairment in patients with predominantly hepatic disease (Anand et al., 1975) makes it difficult to categorize patients for purposes of prognostication. The categories proposed by Blyth and Ockenden (1971) are conceptually important but are of limited clinical applicability. They emphasize that siblings tend to have similar disease, which is an inconstant feature of limited value in prognostication. Other studies (Lieberman et al., 1971; Chilton and Cremin, 1981) indicate greater variability within families, necessitating additional investigation.

Most children with IPCD develop systemic hypertension. Berry aneurysm of the cerebral arteries has been described, but it is much less common in IPCD than in APCD. Many individuals develop portal hypertension with splenomegaly. Bleeding esophageal varices are one of the most important and dangerous complications of IPCD, and hypersplenism is occasionally encountered. Complications of renal failure include growth failure, uremic osteodystrophy, and hyperparathyroidism. Newborns with severe renal involvement also suffer from pulmonary hypoplasia and, as previously noted, they readily develop interstitial emphysema and its sequelae as complications of ventilatory resuscitative measures.

Therapy

Medical treatment of IPCD is supportive. Chronic hemodialysis prolongs survival, and affected children are good candidates for renal allotransplantation. Supportive measures include adequate nutrition to minimize anemia and growth retardation. Children are allowed liberal protein intake, which may be supplemented with amino acid mixtures. It is difficult to maintain normal growth in acidotic children, and supplementation with a base, such as sodium bicarbonate, is often provided. Children run the risk of developing severe dehydration because of their concentrating defects, and generous salt and water intake is encouraged. Secondary hyperparathyroidism may require supplementation with calcium and the administration of vitamin D or one of its newer analogs. Systemic hypertension can be severe enough to require the use of antihypertensive agents, and digitalization for the treatment of congestive heart failure may be necessary in young children.

Hepatic complications rarely cause dysfunction, the major problems being portal hypertension and biliary tract infection. Portacaval shunting is used to treat bleeding esophageal varices (Alvarez et al., 1981; McGonigle et al., 1981), though postoperative hepatocellular dysfunction (Kerr et al., 1978) may vitiate the benefits of venous decompression.

ADULT POLYCYSTIC DISEASE

Autosomal Dominant Type

APCD is the most common form of cystic kidney disease in humans. It ranks third among causes of end-stage renal disease (Advisory Committee to the Renal Transplant Registry, 1973). It is characterized by genetic transmission, diffuse bilateral progressive cystic deformity of both kidneys, hypertension, and death during the sixth decade of life, unless dialysis or transplantation is employed. It may present with hematuria, nephrocalcinosis, progressive renal failure, or acute flank or groin pain. Affected kidneys may harbor infective organisms and thus may repeatedly seed the lower urinary tract or the blood stream.

Genetics and Family Studies

The discovery that heredity plays a role in the transmission of APCD is generally credited to the British urologist H. W. B. Cairns. In 1925, he reported his experience with a single family whose 84 members had spanned four generations and who had transmitted the disease as a dominant trait. Dalgaard (1957) has published the largest study to date: 284 patients and their families.

Adult polycystic disease is inherited as an autosomal dominant trait. Gene penetrance is approximately 100 per cent if the affected individual survives to the age of 80 years (Dalgaard, 1957). Dalgaard also demonstrated that although there was considerable variation among mean ages at onset, there was a remarkably constant adherence to the family mean among the affected members of individual kindreds. The standard deviation (S.D.) for each family's mean age at onset was ± 4 years. Stated differently, Dalgaard's data would indicate that there is a 95 per cent chance (2 S.D.) that the symptoms and signs of APCD will appear during a 16-year span bracketing the mean age at onset in any given family. The observation has more than academic importance; it has practical significance in the selection of related living donors for renal transplantation. It means that a potential donor who has survived without evidence of the disease for 10 years beyond his family's mean age at onset has less than 1 chance in 20 of succumbing to it.

Not all authors have been willing to accept the possibility that APCD is familial. Two groups of workers were unable to document a positive family history in well over 25 per cent of their patients (Hatfield and Pfister, 1972; Rall and Odel, 1949). Such experiences must not be interpreted as indicating that APCD is a nonfamilial condition. They may reflect the frequency with which APCD has been overlooked owing to errors in diagnosis or an absence of symptoms, the number of times that physicians fail to communicate a final diagnosis to bereaved family members, the occurrence of new mutations in the general population, or the effects of environmental influences on genetically susceptible individuals. For diagnosis and for donor selection, therefore, a careful family history is critical.

Etiology and Pathogenesis

The cause and pathogenesis of APCD remain speculative (Bernstein, 1971a). Most available work has come from the study of terminal disease. Only recently have a few studies appeared in which APCD has been observed early in its course or in which laboratory models have been examined. Whatever its cause, APCD appears to affect nephrons that initially possessed normal structure and were capable of normal function.

Virchow (1892) was the first to suggest that APCD was a consequence of tubular obstruction caused by casts or the deposition of "salts." More recent studies provide ample evidence that cystic nephrons are, in fact, not completely occluded. Morphologic studies have identified an admixture of normal and abnormal tubules in the cystic kidney, with the angle of Henle's loop, Bowman's space, and the corticomedullary collecting tubule being the sites most frequently affected by cyst formation (Lambert, 1947; Osathanondh and Potter, 1964b).

Even in the later stages of disease, cystic nephrons communicate with both the glomerulus and the urinary space, and they exhibit functional integrity (Bricker and Patton, 1955; Gardner, 1969; Lambert, 1947). Lambert found inulin in cyst fluid post-mortem following its immediate antemortem injection into the peritoneal cavity. Bricker and Patton extended this study to demonstrate that solute concentrations in cyst fluids sometimes differ dramatically from those in the plasma—for example, cyst fluid:plasma creatinine ratios were as great as 10:1 or 20:1. In general, two populations of nephrons exist in the polycystic kidney (Gardner, 1969; Huseman et al., 1980). They are distinguishable by the characteristics of the fluid within them. One population is composed of cysts that contain fluid with solute concentrations that are similar to those of plasma, suggesting proximal tubular origin. In the second population, cysts contain fluid with solute concentrations that are quite different from those of plasma, including lowered sodium and glucose concentrations and higher creatinine, potassium, and hydrogen ion concentrations, suggesting a distal tubular origin. Recently, Muther and Bennett (1981) demonstrated the appearance of antibiotics in low concentrations in cyst fluid, especially fluid of the distal tubular type.

It is difficult to reconcile with these findings the observation that in vivo hydrostatic pressures are elevated in some, but not all, cysts in APCD (Bjerle et al., 1971). One would expect tubular obstruction in the presence of elevated pressures. It is possible that obstruction in APCD is partial or intermittent, or that it develops late in the evolution of the disease as a consequence of the compression of otherwise normal nephrons by expanding nearby cysts. Quite clearly, further work must be done to determine the role of obstruction, either partial or complete, in the pathogenesis of APCD.

A second hypothesis to account for cyst formation is that growth of the tubular wall is altered, a possibility suggested by studies of rat kidneys exposed to the cystogenetic chemical diphenylamine (Darmady et al., 1970). When fed to rats in low concentrations over a long period of time, diphenylamine produces a renal lesion that is morphologically similar to the one encountered in APCD. Darmady and associates have postulated that the defect underlying APCD is the accumulation of a cystogenetic metabolite that acts on the kidney to cause the tubular deformity.

Work with diphenylthiazole has suggested a third possibility for the pathogenesis of cystic renal disease—that of altered compliance of the tubular wall (Carone et al., 1974). Diphenylthiazole causes diffuse cystic changes throughout the kidneys. Intratubular pressures are normal, a finding that is considered to be supportive of a hypothesis implicating a change in the elasticity of the nephron walls as the primary pathogenetic mechanism of cyst formation.

Apart from obstruction and changes in the growth pattern or character of the tubular wall, other hypotheses of the pathogenesis of cystic renal disease are largely of historical interest (Osathanondh and Potter, 1964b). At the present time, the study of animal models appears to offer the most promising approach to understanding the pathogenesis of cystic renal disease in general and of APCD specifically.

Morphology

The kidney in APCD presents a dramatic appearance. It is enlarged but reniform. Its surface is studded with myriad cysts ranging in size from a few millimeters to several centimeters. Cyst contents are often visible through the semilucent capsule. They range in appearance and color from clear yellow to turbid and from white to opaque dark brown or black (the so-called chocolate cyst). Incision of the capsule is usually attended by a gushing forth of the cyst contents, sometimes several feet into the air.

The cut surface of the end-stage kidney in APCD shows little remaining solid parenchyma. The majority of the renal substance is replaced by cysts of varying sizes (Fig. 39–5). Those cut tangentially often bulge slightly from the surface.

Light microscopy reveals cuboidal epithelium lining cyst walls, the epithelium being a single layer in most areas but hyperplastic and polypoid in some areas (Evan et al., 1979). Between cysts, remnants of what appear to have been normal tubules and glomeruli are evident. Microdissection studies reveal three types of cysts: glomerular, tubular, and excretory (Lambert, 1947). The latter two appear to have anatomic communication with the urinary space.

Untimely deaths of asymptomatic individuals with early APCD have provided an infrequent opportunity to examine kidneys before

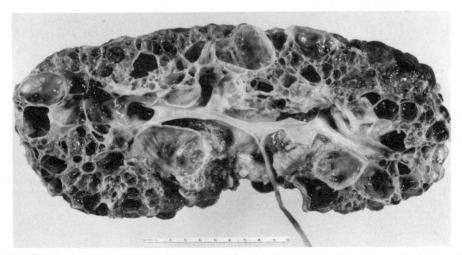

Figure 39–5. APCD. The kidney is enlarged (weight approximately 2500 gm) and, in this terminal stage of disease the parenchyma is almost completely occupied by cysts of varying sizes. Cysts are present in both cortex and medulla, and the pelvis is stretched and compressed by the bulging parenchyma.

they reach the end stage of cyst development. In general, these kidneys are more normal in size, though they are often slightly enlarged, have a substantially greater amount of normal renal parenchyma, and exhibit infrequent cysts in both the cortex and the medulla.

Radiography and Sonography

The radiographic hallmark of APCD is bilateral enlargement of the kidneys. Cysts may be demonstrated with varying degrees of success, depending upon the stage of the lesion and the technique or techniques utilized (Greene and Barrett, 1976; Rosenfield et al., 1977; Milutinovic et al., 1980). Ultrasonography is preferred because it is noninvasive (Greene and Barrett, 1976), but intravenous urography, radionuclide imaging, arteriography, and com-

puterized tomography (CAT scan) also may be used (Figs. 39–6 and 39–7). When a study is negative and reasonable doubt persists, a second technique should be used (Rosenfield et al., 1980).

None of the available radiographic techniques is foolproof. Urography and ultrasonography may fail to detect cysts smaller than 1 to 1.5 cm in diameter, whereas computerized tomography may fail to demonstrate cysts less than 0.5 cm in diameter (Bommer et al., 1980). Occasionally, cyst formation in the two kidneys may be asynchronous. This circumstance has given rise to the impression that APCD may be unilateral, a view often held to be incorrect, perhaps erroneously (Lee et al., 1978).

In addition to aberrant size and shape, the polycystic kidney may exhibit other abnormali-

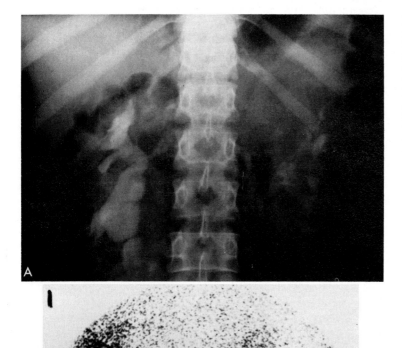

Figure 39–6. APCD. *A,* Excretory urography results in poor visualization of the kidney. The left pelvis and calyces are elongated and distorted; pyelocalyceal dilatation on the right is secondary to ureteropelvic obstruction by a cyst. *B,* Renal scan in same patient demonstrates asymmetric distribution of radioactivity. Surgical intervention to relieve obstruction resulted in improved drainage from the right kidney and improved renal function.

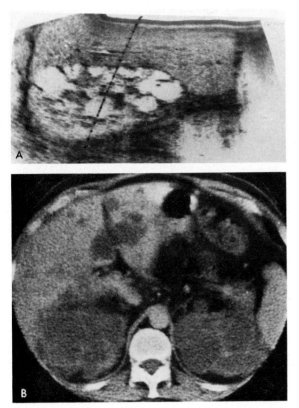

Figure 39–7. APCD. *A,* Ultrasonography demonstrates right polycystic kidney with multiple cysts of variable echogenicity. *B,* Computerized tomography shows bilateral cystic kidneys and a cystic liver.

ties. More than half of 101 cases of APCD in one series exhibited nephrocalcinosis (Greene and Barrett, 1976). Stones may be found in the renal substance and may enter the urinary system to present in the urine, the bladder, or the urethra.

Urinary tract obstruction occurs with unknown frequency, but its incidence may be greater than is usually believed. One series found 17 examples among 100 consecutive cases of APCD (Barbaric et al., 1977). Calculi were the usual cause. In addition to urolithiasis, ureteral obstruction may occur as a consequence of cyst expansion adjacent to the critical ureteropelvic junction. Finally, hepatic cysts may be apparent on the excretory pyelogram, making it worthwhile to examine the liver shadow carefully in suspected cases.

Renal Function

The progressive deterioration that characterizes renal function in APCD has been attributed to two events: the compression of functioning renal tissue by expanding cysts and the

hypertension that appears during the development of renal failure. Inability to concentrate urine maximally may be the first sign of a failing kidney. In an elegant study, Martinez-Maldonado and his associates examined renal function in the members of a family afflicted with APCD (Martinez-Maldonado et al., 1972). Eleven of 13 subjects with demonstrable polycystic kidneys but GFR's of more than 75 ml per minute were unable to concentrate urine to an osmolality greater than 700 mOsm per kg water. Family members with both polycystic disease and renal insufficiency, that is, established disease, had even more marked defects in their urinary concentrating ability.

As APCD progresses, a variety of additional defects in renal function appear. There is a rough correlation between these defects and the degree of renal deformity (Dalgaard, 1957). In any given patient, however, no substantive correlation exists. Proteinuria has been described in 75 to 95 per cent of cases. Casts, usually those of the epithelial series, are relatively uncommon. Pyuria has been described in approximately 50 per cent of cases. Bacteriuria has been documented in one third of patients (Simon and Thompson, 1955).

The GFR may be normal when radiographic evidence of the disease exists. Ultimately, however, it decreases in every affected patient. Uremia, anemia, metabolic acidosis, and azotemia appear concomitantly. Proteinuria rarely achieves 3.5 gm per 24 hours, but the nephrotic syndrome in association with APCD has been described (Ackerman, 1971). Hematuria is such a common complication that a specific discussion of it appears later in this chapter.

Clinical Features

A positive family history, flank masses, hypertension, and azotemia are the cardinal clinical findings of APCD. They are not invariably present, however. The clinical presentation of APCD deserves detailed attention if errors, especially in early diagnosis, are to be avoided.

Signs and Symptoms. A number of authors have attempted to classify the severity of APCD based on clinical presentation. Dalgaard (1957) recognized three stages: Stage 1, no symptoms referable to the disease; Stage 2, a greater or lesser number of symptoms present; Stage 3, the final stage, in which uremia predominates. Overall, the evolution of symptoms in APCD follows a remarkably consistent pattern (Dalgaard, 1957). Among 350 patients with age at onset ranging from less than 10 to more than 90 years of age, pain characteristically preceded the development of flank masses, which, in turn, preceded chemical evidence of renal failure. Thus, the three "D's" of evolving APCD are discomfort, deformity, and then dysfunction.

Pain is generally in the lumbar region but may also appear in the groin or the loin; sometimes it presents as discomfort in the back, the upper abdomen, or the lower chest. Discomfort, generally made worse by activity, characterizes the evolution of APCD in 28 to 60 per cent of patients. It has been attributed to a variety of causes, including tension on the renal capsule, pressure on adjacent organs, hemorrhage into cysts, nephrolithiasis, and infection. Renal colic occurred in 18 per cent of the patients in Dalgaard's series.

Depending upon the limits established for it, hypertension occurs in 50 per cent or more of individuals with APCD (Dalgaard, 1957). Presumably, it arises as a consequence of increased renin production by the involved kidneys. Characteristically, it appears during the middle of the course of the illness. If one accepts a blood pressure of greater than 140 mm Hg systolic to 90 mm Hg diastolic to be indicative of hypertension, more than 70 per cent of individuals with APCD may be classified as hypertensive, and they will show eyeground changes consistent with that diagnosis. Left ventricular hypertrophy is less frequent, and right-sided congestive heart failure has been described only infrequently.

Hematuria, one of the consequences of cyst rupture or of the presence of a renal stone, is common (Dalgaard, 1957). It occurs in approximately half of affected individuals and may be either microscopic or macroscopic. It should be remembered that patients with APCD are also susceptible to hematuria from other causes. Adult polycystic disease should be included in the differential diagnostic evaluation of all patients with bloody urine.

Flank masses, representing bilaterally enlarged kidneys, were present in 64 per cent of Dalgaard's patients. Significantly, only one kidney was palpable in 36 per cent of these patients. Occasionally, the enlarged kidney may be mistaken on physical examination for hepato- or splenomegaly. The careful examiner can often detect a nodular renal surface.

Affected individuals may present for examination because of signs and symptoms arising from involvement of other organs. An aneurysm of the circle of Willis may rupture, bringing an affected individual to a physician's attention because the ensuing picture is that of a cerebrovascular accident. Cysts in other organs may be detected clinically, leading to hospitalization for appropriate surgery. Anuric renal failure, a consequence either of compression of adjacent ureters by cysts or of an obstructing blood clot, also occurs, as does gram-negative sepsis.

The onset in early infancy of APCD has been clearly established in several families with strong histories of autosomal dominant disease (Bengtsson et al., 1975; Kaplan et al., 1977; Shokeir, 1978; Stickler and Kelalis, 1975), and prenatal diagnosis has been accomplished sonographically (Zerres et al., 1982). Morphologic studies have at times shown large numbers or a predominance of glomerular cysts (Bengtsson et al., 1975; Fellows et al., 1976), which is at times an apparent impairment of nephrogenesis (Fellows et al., 1976; Shokeir, 1978). The morphologic variation has made diagnosis uncertain in the absence of a positive family history, and APCD accounts for an uncertain proportion of glomerulocystic kidneys. Although some babies die of renal insufficiency, others survive with stabilization of renal function into later childhood or into adulthood.

Differential Diagnosis

APCD is a relatively common disorder, affecting roughly 1 in every 500 individuals. Although it rarely poses a diagnostic problem in its later stages, APCD can present significant diagnostic challenges to the physician early in its evolution. Differential diagnostic possibilities include the following: renal neoplasm (rarely bilateral, in contrast to APCD), hydronephrosis (bilateral obstruction being rare in conditions other than bladder outlet obstruction), von Hippel-Lindau disease, and pyelonephritis (itself not a cause of nephromegaly). Irregular renal outlines on excretory urography are helpful in distinguishing the polycystic kidney from other conditions in which the kidneys are enlarged, including amyloidosis, acute tubular necrosis, acute glomerulonephritis, and renal vein thrombosis.

There are dangers in utilizing invasive procedures to establish the diagnosis of APCD (Danovitch, 1976). Clinical and laboratory experiences leave little doubt that the polycystic kidney has an increased susceptibility to infection. This fact, coupled with the evidence that instrumentation of the urinary tract carries a significant risk of infection, argues strongly in favor of the tenet that catheterization, cystoscopy, and retrograde pyelography should be avoided when possible in APCD. Owing to technical reasons and the possibility of hemorrhage, most nephrologists avoid the use of percutaneous renal biopsy with this condition.

Course and Prognosis

Among affected individuals, renal failure is relentless, and renal mortality is 100 per cent. The rate at which azotemia progresses is dependent upon the age at onset (Dalgaard, 1957). Generally speaking, onset before the age of 50 years is associated with longer survival (approximately 1 decade), whereas the onset of symptoms after the age of 50 years carries a more ominous prognosis. Once uremia develops, the prognosis for patient survival is poor. Among 17 patients in one series, the average survival was slightly more than 2 years after blood urea concentrations had reached 40 mg per dl (Rall and Odel, 1949).

A number of authors have ascertained the mean age at death for APCD. The figure is remarkably constant: 50 years of age, ranging from 49.3 to 51.5 years, in four series (Dalgaard, 1957). Cardiac disease, uremia, and cerebral hemorrhage accounted for the majority of deaths.

Complications and Associated Anomalies

The complications that characterize APCD may arise as the consequence of renal failure or as the consequence of involvement of other organs.

Hematuria occurs in approximately half the affected individuals, often following a bout of pain. On occasion, it may be sufficiently massive to result in anemia or obstruction of the lower urinary tract by a clot.

Some patients present with anuria or intractable ureteral pain. Excretory urography may reveal ureteropelvic occlusion by a cyst. Signs and symptoms of rapidly progressive renal failure may also appear in the absence of appreciable pain or with a reduction of urine volume. The vicious cycle of vomiting, dehydration, and progressive failure of kidney function that characterizes terminal renal failure from a variety of causes occurs in APCD. Restoration of blood volume may re-establish more tolerable levels of renal function under such conditions.

Infection represents a relatively infrequent but potentially lethal complication of APCD. Less severe infections, evidenced by bacteriuria and pyuria, occur more often. Frequently, treatment, even with appropriate antibiotics, fails to sterilize infected cysts, evidently resulting from the failure of antibiotics to enter the cysts in adequate concentrations (Muther and Bennett, 1981). Ultimately, nephrectomy may be necessary to control recurrent septicemia. Other complications of APCD include stones, malignant changes, and bone and joint disorders. An increased incidence of gouty arthritis has been reported among individuals with APCD. Although the incidence of malignant change in APCD is considered low, it occurs (Sogbein et al., 1981) and is of special interest because of the epithelial hyperplasia that is found along cyst linings in APCD (Evan et al., 1979). Renal angiography is the preferred technique for its demonstration.

Symptoms produced by the developmental anomalies that accompany APCD may occur (Hartnett and Bennett, 1976). Six per cent of patients presenting with cerebrovascular accidents have APCD, whereas as many as 45 per cent of individuals with APCD may have cerebral aneurysms. Roughly one third of patients with APCD have hepatic cysts that present the diagnostic challenge of a mass or filling defect in the liver but are rarely the site of disease. Cysts may occur in other organs, including bladder, epididymis, lungs, ovaries, pancreas, spleen, testes, thyroid gland, and uterus. It has not been established that these lesions are developmentally associated with APCD. They are significant because, on occasion, an individual affected by APCD may present to the physician because of a cystic deformity of an organ other than the kidney.

Therapy

Treatment of APCD is nonspecific. Thus, it must frequently be symptomatic.

Medical Therapy. Medical treatment of APCD includes the use of analgesics for pain, appropriate antibiotics for infection, and the generally recognized therapy for chronic renal failure—attention to protein and sodium intake, avoidance of both over- and underhydration, treatment of metabolic acidosis (sodium bicarbonate, 4 to 6 gm daily), and use of aluminum hydroxide gel in oral doses (generally more than 25 gm per day) sufficient to restore serum phosphate levels to normal. Currently, it is deemed appropriate to start aluminum hydroxide administration early in the evolution of renal failure—that is, when serum creatinine levels reach 2 mg per dl—in an effort to retard the development of renal osteodystrophy. Hypertension can prove recalcitrant, and its management may require the use of several drugs to achieve some level of control. In this regard, care must be taken not to overload the hypertensive patient with sodium (which can worsen any tendency toward elevated blood pressure) while treating metabolic acidosis with sodium bicarbonate.

Surgical Treatment. After almost 50 years, the surgical approach to APCD has run full circle. Currently, there are considered to be few specific indications for surgery in the treatment of APCD (Editorial, 1981). Resolution of anuric renal failure due to ureteral occlusion by an enlarged cyst can be accomplished with drainage of the cyst. A direct surgical approach (cyst drainage and deroofing) is preferable to ureteral catheterization, which carries the risk of infection and often provides only temporary relief from obstruction. If the patient is sufficiently symptomatic from renal failure, hemodialysis may be required in the preparation for surgery. Intractable pain and infection caused by pyonephrosis are also considered indications for surgical intervention. In the former instance, decompression of the painful kidney has been proved to provide only an evanescent cure. The physician may be forced to perform bilateral nephrectomy to remove the source of infection. Ureteral stones or blood clots may be amenable to a transurethral approach, or direct surgery may be required to relieve obstruction.

In its final stages, APCD, like other forms of chronic renal disease, is amenable to treatment with dialysis or renal transplantation. Peritoneal dialysis is usually precluded by the enormous kidneys, which occupy most of the available space in the abdomen. Hemodialysis is effective and may be performed without prior nephrectomy in patients who are not symptomatic from their enlarged kidneys. Renal transplantation appears to be no more or less effective in patients with APCD than in patients with disorders such as chronic glomerulonephritis, which is immunogenic and acquired rather than dysgenic and inherited. The selection of a donor for a patient with APCD obviously must be undertaken with care, since the condition is familial. Preferably, a blood relative from the unaffected side of the family should be found.

The only known form of prevention of APCD is genetic counseling sufficient to motivate potentially affected individuals to go childless. APCD may not appear until after the childbearing years. Since it is a dominant trait, its continuation is assured. Surprisingly, some affected individuals take the attitude that since medical science is helping them, it will help their children, so why not have them? Whether the clinical importance of extrarenal anomalies as causes of morbidity and mortality will increase as we keep individuals with APCD alive

longer than their kidneys remains to be established (Hartnett and Bennett, 1976).

OTHER FORMS OF HERITABLE RENAL CYSTIC DISEASE

Multiple cortical cysts are encountered in several heritable conditions that cannot be regarded as polycystic disease (Bernstein, 1971a). The cysts are most often inconsequential, being inconstant, small, asymptomatic, and of little or no functional significance. Subcapsular cortical "microcysts" are seen, for example, in the trisomy D and trisomy E syndromes, the cerebrohepatorenal syndrome of Zellweger, the asphyxiating thoracic dysplasia of Jeune, and several other syndromes of multiple congenital malformations (Bernstein and Kissane, 1973). There is some question as to whether they are actually inherent components of those syndromes; they could conceivably be secondary developmental abnormalities resulting from renal injury mediated through inherited metabolic nephrotoxic defects. The cysts differ morphologically in both distribution and pattern from those of polycystic disease.

There is no satisfactory terminology to describe these trifling cystic lesions in malformation syndromes. Several designations used in the recent past are "micromulticystic," "microcystic," and "pluricystic." The term *multicystic kidney* is customarily used to signify a form of cystic dysplasia, and the term *microcystic disease* has been used in connection with the congenital nephrotic syndrome. Most authors continue to use the term *polycystic disease* in a descriptive and imprecise fashion, probably because the abnormality lacks sufficient importance to be given a proper designation of its own.

These abnormalities are not, however, minor variants of polycystic disease, and they are not to be confounded with polycystic disease of either the infantile or the adult type. Certainly, there is no advantage to the indiscriminate application of the term; the disadvantage lies in our not having established homogeneous categories with meaningful clinicopathologic correlations.

The kidneys may occasionally be severely cystic. Excluding diffuse cystic dysplasia, for example in the Meckel syndrome, severe cyst formation, with functional and clinical sequelae, has been encountered in several malformation syndromes. Diffuse cystic disease has been observed in some newborns with the Zellweger syndrome and the Jeune syndrome (Bernstein et al., 1974). Severe renal disease leading to chronic renal failure has occurred in several patients with the orofaciodigital syndrome, Type I (Stapleton et al., 1982), and cystic disease has been encountered in the Ehlers-Danlos syndrome (Mauseth et al., 1977), perhaps as part of the syndrome, perhaps as coincidental polycystic disease. The occurrence of significant cystic disease in tuberous sclerosis and in von Hippel-Lindau disease may be of more than passing interest to the urologist, and these conditions are described in greater detail.

Tuberous Sclerosis

Renal failure as a complication of tuberous sclerosis has been attributed to multiple angiomyolipomas (Anderson and Tannen, 1969). The nature and distribution of the tumors have been a source of confusion with polycystic disease (Anderson and Tannen, 1969; Chonko et al., 1974; O'Callaghan et al., 1975), but it must be remembered that diffuse cystic disease occurs in tuberous sclerosis as well, and it is also a cause of chronic renal failure (Dolder, 1975; Rosenberg et al., 1975). The cysts may be more important than the angiomyolipomas in the development of renal failure (Okada et al., 1982).

Renal cysts in children with tuberous sclerosis were described by Arey (1959) as apparently incidental findings. Extensive cortical involvement with large cysts has been found at autopsy (Engström et al., 1962; Kawamura et al., 1969) and on exploratory laparotomy (Bernstein and Meyer, 1967; Elkin and Bernstein, 1969; Wenzl et al., 1970). In one case (Bernstein and Meyer, 1967; Bernstein et al., 1974), a 2-month-old male infant underwent laparotomy because of bilateral renal involvement. He had moderate azotemia and hypertension, and he suffered from mental retardation and recurrent convulsions. Following renal biopsy and decompression of cysts, kidney function improved and hypertension was ameliorated. The diagnosis of tuberous sclerosis became apparent when the patient had reached the age of 5 years, and a skin lesion was diagnosed as adenoma sebaceum. His renal function was still normal. A similar patient (Elkin and Bernstein, 1969) was seen at the age of 4 months because of seizures and renal masses; the diagnosis of tuberous sclerosis was confirmed 7 years later. These cases demonstrate that renal lesions may antedate other stigmas of the syndrome.

The cystic lesion in tuberous sclerosis is a morphologically distinctive, perhaps unique, ab-

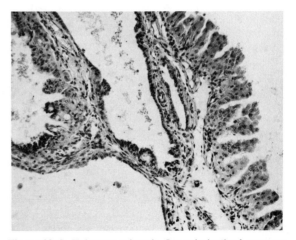

Figure 39–8. Tuberous sclerosis. Irregularly sized cysts are lined with remarkably hyperplastic, eosinophilic epithelium, which is thrown into papillary folds and often forms small intracystic nodules. The intervening parenchyma appears to be compressed, and there is an increase in connective tissue. Hematoxylin and eosin, × 130.

normality (Bernstein et al., 1974). The cysts are usually small, though they can also be large enough to produce radiographic distortion (Elkin and Bernstein, 1969; Engström et al., 1962; Wenzl et al., 1970). The distinctive feature is the microscopic appearance of the epithelium, which typically is extraordinarily hyperplastic (Fig. 39–8). It is tempting to suggest that cellular hyperplasia is the cause of renal tubular enlargement and cyst formation, much as cellular hypertrophy and hyperplasia produce other lesions of the complex. Despite the epithelial hyperplasia, we had seen only one case (unreported) of renal cell carcinoma in a patient with tuberous sclerosis; that complication has now been documented in two recent reports (Honey and Honey, 1977; Suslavich et al., 1979). Microdissection in one newborn revealed thin-walled cysts that were enlargements of Henle's loop and subcapsular cysts, surrounded by connective tissue and arising in collecting tubules (Osathanondh and Potter, 1964b). The renal cysts in patients undergoing chronic hemodialysis may collapse and become sclerotic, leaving a scarred cortex that contains scattered hyalinized masses (Rosenberg et al., 1975). Since renal insufficiency appears to result from both the replacement of renal parenchyma and its compression, it may be assumed that patients with mild degrees of cystic involvement will remain asymptomatic.

The incidence of renal cysts in tuberous sclerosis appears to be low, particularly when compared with a 40 to 50 per cent frequency of

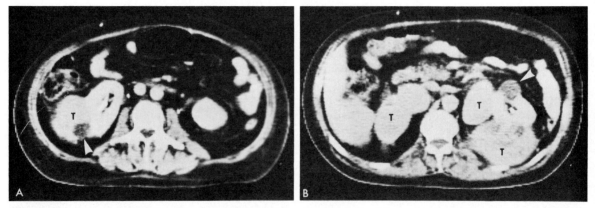

Figure 39–9. Tuberous sclerosis with multiple angiomyolipomas and cysts. Sonograms show bilateral tumors (T), with irregular areas of decreased attenuation. *A,* An area of sharply decreased attenuation (−28 Hounsfield units) in the right kidney (white arrowhead) is identifiable as fat. *B,* The left kidney also contains a cyst (6 Hounsfield units) (white arrowhead), and the combination of findings is strongly suggestive of tuberous sclerosis. (Sonograms courtesy of Dr. M. Bosniak, Department of Radiology, New York University Medical Center, New York, N.Y.)

solid angiomyolipomas. The clinical manifestations have been extremely variable. Severe hypertension often begins early in life (Cree, 1969; Kawamura et al., 1969), and renal cysts have also been associated with hypertension in adults (Gonzalez-Angulo et al., 1964). The disease is transmitted as an autosomal dominant condition with variable expressivity.

Cysts and angiomyolipomas can usually be identified and differentiated by CAT scans (Fig. 39–9). Urographic evaluation may be supplemented by nephrotomography and selective arteriography (Viamonte et al., 1966; Compton et al., 1976) to provide adequate differentiation between the two. In cases not recognized as tuberous sclerosis, the concurrence of cysts and angiomyolipomas provides a strong clue to the diagnosis.

von Hippel-Lindau Disease

Renal involvement in von Hippel-Lindau disease has been known to exist since the first descriptions of the syndrome. Lindau, who in 1926 recognized the connection between von Hippel's retinal angiomatosis and the other manifestations of the syndrome, observed that renal abnormalities were present in two thirds of his cases. The tumors are often multiple and bilateral; they were described originally as benign (Lindau, 1926), but their malignant nature has since been amply demonstrated. The syndrome comprises cerebellar and retinal hemangioblastomas, pancreatic cysts and carcinoma, and renal, epididymal, and other visceral cysts and tumors. The manifestations are variable,

and sporadic cases may go unrecognized. Hemangioblastoma of the cerebellum is usually regarded as the principal cause of death (Horton et al., 1976), and the same tumor may occur elsewhere in the central nervous system. Minimal criteria for diagnosis might include either the cerebellar tumor and one other characteristic manifestation of the syndrome, or a characteristic manifestation together with a suitable family history (Melmon and Rosen, 1964). The disease is transmitted as an autosomal dominant condition with moderate penetrance (Christoferson et al., 1961). Its clinical onset is in early or middle adulthood. Early recognition and genetic counseling are, therefore, of considerable importance to younger members of affected families (Horton et al., 1976; Lee et al., 1977; Frimodt-Møller et al., 1981). Recent papers have emphasized the value of computerized tomography in conjunction with ophthalmologic and neurologic examination of individuals at risk (Fill et al., 1979; Levine et al., 1979; Wesolowski et al., 1981; Levine et al., 1982) (Fig. 39–10).

The initial clinical symptoms are commonly neurologic. Patients often have polycythemia (Richards et al., 1973), a complication associated with both cerebellar henangioblastoma and renal cell carcinoma. The features of urologic interest include renal and epididymal involvement, both of which are important in evaluating members of affected families, and renal tumors, which are of major clinical significance. The discovery of lesions such as epididymal cysts and papillary cystadenomas, renal cysts combined with hypernephroma, and multiple hypernephromas in young patients should prompt a search for other manifestations of the disease. Computerized tomography can be supplemented with angiography and nephrotomography in the evaluation of masses and cysts in individual patients. Early recognition and early surgical intervention are the only means of averting malignant complications of renal involvement, and several authors (Levine et al., 1979; Pearson et al., 1980) have advocated local resection of tumors to conserve renal tissue in a condition that is likely to be bilateral.

The renal cysts are often described as "simple," meaning that they are irregularly distributed and are lined with flattened, nondescript or cuboidal epithelium (Schecterman, 1961). The cysts may be quite numerous, measuring as much as several centimeters in diameter, and they may sufficiently distort the renal parenchyma to be apparent urographically. In several of the few cases that we have reviewed, the cysts were surrounded by dense fibrous collars and appeared to be undergoing involution. In others, the lining epithelium was irregularly hyperplastic and formed mural nodules of clear cells that appeared to be intracystic hypernephromas. We have speculated, therefore, that the hyperplastic epithelium lining the cysts is a direct precursor of malignancy, and that the two abnormalities (cysts and tumors) are more than casually associated (Bernstein and Kissane, 1973).

Glomerulocystic Disease

A form of diffuse cystic disease involving the glomeruli principally or predominantly has been recognized in young infants (McAlister et al., 1979; Taxy and Filmer, 1976). Glomerulocystic disease is not, however, a clinicopathologic entity, since glomerular cysts occur in a large number of renal disorders, including early onset APCD, chromosomal malformation syndromes, orofaciodigital syndrome, renal dysplasia, and urinary tract obstruction, among others. APCD may account for as much as one half of glomerulocystic disease. The clinical presentation has been variable, with varying degrees of renal functional impairment. Some infants die as newborns of respiratory insufficiency, perhaps related to the Potter syndrome, and others succumb to associated malformations. Other

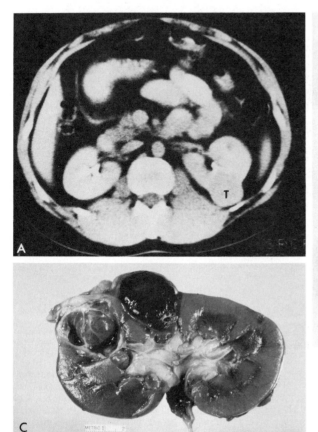

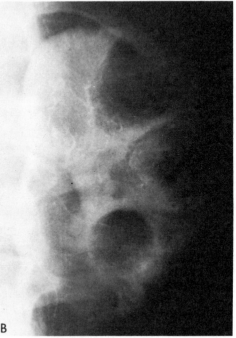

Figure 39–10. Von Hippel-Lindau disease. A sonogram (*A*) shows the left kidney to be severely distorted by tumor (T) of irregular density, and a nephrogram (*B*) shows an irregular pattern, indicating complicated cysts. The nephrectomy specimen (*C*) contains both cysts and tumor.

children seem to have a more favorable course, with stabilization of renal function and stabilization or diminution of renal size. The ultimate prognosis is as yet unclear, except that those patients with APCD can be expected to develop typical signs of that disease in the second or third decade of life.

LOCALIZED CYSTIC DISEASE: SIMPLE CYSTS AND SEGMENTAL CYSTIC DISEASE

The most common cystic abnormality of the kidney is the simple cyst (retention cyst), which may be solitary or multiple, and unilateral or bilateral. Multiple simple cysts are common incidental radiographic and post-mortem findings in elderly patients (Laucks and McLachlan, 1981) (Figs. 39–11 and 39–12). Large cysts occur at any age, though they are uncommon in child-

hood (DeWeerd and Simon, 1956; Siegel and McAlister, 1980). They are to be regarded as acquired abnormalities of undetermined, possibly diverse causes. The origin of the cysts is frequently considered to be vascular nephrosclerosis, a relationship for which there is no direct evidence. There is certainly no compelling reason to regard them as congenital or developmental, despite a common inclination to do so. Even though multiple cysts are conceptually different from and unrelated to heritable cystic disease, their differential diagnosis may be difficult in practice.

Large simple cysts often appear to be solitary, but they are commonly accompanied by a varying number of clinically and radiographically inapparent small cysts (Braasch and Hendrick, 1944; Bernstein, 1976). It is not clear if the cysts arise in ducts or tubules; they contain thin serous fluid variably admixed with altered blood. Hemorrhagic cysts (Jackman and Ste-

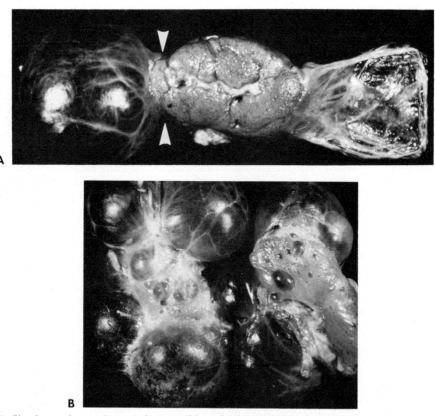

Figure 39–11. *A,* Simple renal cyst. A somewhat atrophic and sclerotic kidney in an elderly patient contains two large, thin-walled cysts, one at each pole. Examination of the other kidney showed only nephrosclerosis, and the patient had not exhibited clinical evidence of renal disease prior to death. Note that cortical tissue is pushed up around the base of the intact cyst (arrowheads), forming a rim that accounts for the radiographic "beak sign." *B,* Multiple simple renal cysts. Multiple cysts involving both kidneys in an elderly patient. Differentiation from APCD is difficult and may be unreliable. The irregular distribution and size of the cysts and the presence of large amounts of intervening solid parenchyma suggest that they are multiple simple cysts rather than polycystic disease.

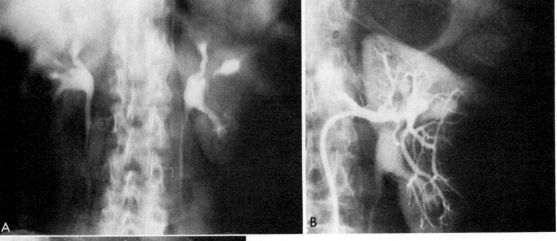

Figure 39–12. Simple renal cysts. Computerized tomography in an elderly patient shows renal enlargement and distortion by multiple cysts (arrows). (Sonogram courtesy of Dr. R. L. Bree, Department of Radiology, William Beaumont Hospital, Royal Oak.)

vens, 1974) arise principally from severe hemorrhage into pre-existing simple cysts and hematoma secondary to trauma enters the differential diagnosis. The cyst walls occasionally undergo calcification, which may be visible radiographically (Becker and Schneider, 1975).

These cysts are often detected as incidental findings during sonography or computerized tomography. The cysts do not opacify on excretory urography, but they do distort the pyelocalyceal system (Fig. 39–13). Selective arteriography, which has become less important in diagnosis

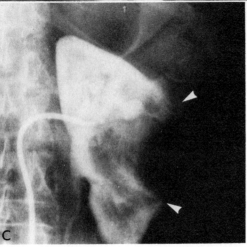

Figure 39–13. Simple renal cyst. *A,* Excretory urography demonstrates distortion of the pyelocalyceal system in the left kidney. *B,* Selective arteriography shows the vessel to be displaced around a lucent nonopacified area, which is also entirely avascular. *C,* The nephrogram demonstrates "beaking" (arrowheads) of the renal parenchyma at the margins of the mass. (Roentgenograms courtesy of Dr. J. Farah, Department of Radiology, William Beaumont Hospital, Royal Oak.)

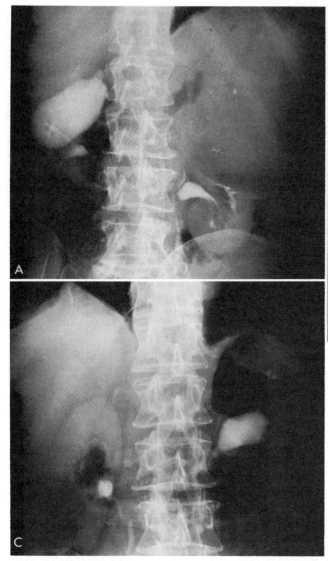

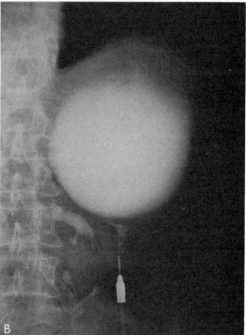

Figure 39–14. Simple renal cyst. *A,* Excretory urography demonstrates an extremely large cyst at upper pole of left kidney. *B,* Tapping the cyst leads to its collapse, as shown by a more normal pyelogram *(C).* (Roentgenograms courtesy of **Dr.** J. Farah, Department of Radiology, William Beaumont Hospital, Royal Oak.)

than other radiographic techniques (Becker and Schneider, 1975), demonstrates avascular masses, and the renal cortex at the margins of large cysts is compressed and displaced outward, the so-called lip or beak sign (Elkin and Bernstein, 1969). Needling or tapping of cysts with the subsequent injection of contrast medium and cytologic evaluation of aspirated fluid has been advocated as a means of differentiating cysts from cystic neoplasms (Lang et al., 1972; Thornbury, 1972), though its value has been challenged (McClennan et al., 1979) (Fig. 39–14). In addition to fine needle aspiration, nephrotomography is helpful in differentiating large cysts from solid tumors. The cysts are characteristically unilocular. They do not communicate with the renal pelvis, except in the event of rupture. The walls are composed of thin fibrous tissue that is lined with flattened or cuboidal epithelium. The adjacent parenchyma, which is usually sharply demarcated, is compressed, and there is secondary glomerular obsolescence and tubular atrophy.

Cysts present clinically as abdominal masses, sometimes as incidental urographic findings. Symptoms are variable and nonspecific. Acute bleeding into a cyst may be responsible for abdominal or lumbar pain, and bleeding into the adjacent parenchyma may lead to hematuria. Secondary infection, which appears to be uncommon, may also be responsible for symptoms. Cysts are occasionally associated with polycythemia. Hypertension as a direct consequence of simple cysts is uncommon; it may be associated with renal and vascular compression. Males are afflicted more often than females, and the left side is involved more often than the right (Sommerkamp, 1970). The cysts may require resection or decompression, either because of their size or because of recurrent pain and bleeding. Percutaneous decompression has had considerable success in some hands (Lang, 1971; Melicow and Becker, 1967). Disorders that are considered in the differential diagnosis include cystic neoplasms, lymphatic cysts (Lindsey, 1970), perirenal effusions, and renal abscesses.

Multiple cysts present a diagnostic dilemma, namely the differentiation of nonprogressive, nonhereditary cysts from polycystic disease (Bernstein, 1976). Many such cases have been labeled "polycystic disease," a diagnosis that places serious clinical and social stigmas on the patient. We believe, on the basis of radiographic and post-mortem observations, that most cases of multiple renal cysts, especially in elderly patients, are not "early" or incipient polycystic disease. In establishing a diagnosis, we rely heavily on the extent of cystic involvement. Multiple cysts are typically irregularly distributed, with a large amount of intervening solid parenchyma (See Fig. 39–11). This criterion, though simply stated, is unfortunately imperfect. Radiographic studies, particularly sonography and computerized tomography early in the course of APCD have shown patterns that

are hardly distinguishable from multiple simple cysts. The cysts are scattered and few in number, and we have come to realize that our concept of APCD as a diffuse disorder stems principally from the study of advanced disease in terminal cases. The dilemma is particularly applicable to the finding of unilateral involvement, and we have observed the subsequent development of bilateral cystic disease in a patient whose initial examination had shown only unilateral involvement by all criteria, including radiography and laparotomy. Simple cysts can also cause parenchymal and pyelocalyceal distortion, the abnormalities that we take to be urographic evidence of severe and diffuse involvement. Cysts large enough and numerous enough to distort the parenchyma also distort the arteriographic pattern. In other words, we know of no sure criteria by which APCD and multiple simple cysts can be differentiated. We must rely strongly on family history, the presence or absence of renal function impairment, and the presence or absence of typical hepatic lesions. There will undoubtedly be times when the diagnosis remains in doubt, and we advocate expressing that doubt in preference to making an unwarranted or unconfirmed diagnosis.

We have also differentiated strictly unilateral lesions (Sellers et al., 1972; Lee et al., 1978; Kossow and Meek, 1982) from polycystic dis-

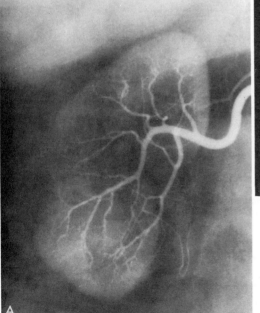
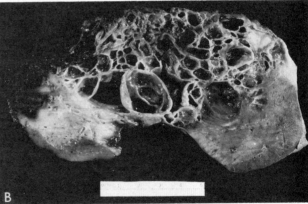

Figure 39–15. Unilateral segmental cystic disease. *A,* An arteriogram taken in the early phase of the disease demonstrates a lucent abnormality within the central portion of the kidney. The arteries are displaced, and the cortical outline is irregular, indicating the presence of a mass or a cystic lesion. *B,* Postmortem examination of the kidney discloses a cystic abnormality involving the central portion only. The cysts are poorly demarcated from adjacent parenchyma, and the trabeculae contain atrophic remnants of renal tissue, differentiating the lesion from multilocular cystadenoma. No other stigmas of polycystic disease were present, and the family history was negative. (Roentgenogram courtesy of Dr. J. Farah, Department of Radiology, William Beaumont Hospital, Royal Oak. Photograph reprinted from Bernstein, J.: A classification of renal cysts. *In* Gardner, K. D., Jr.: Cystic Diseases of the Kidney. Reprinted by permission of John Wiley & Sons, New York, 1976.)

ease, recognizing that APCD may at times be deceptively asymmetric. Like multiple simple cysts, the localized lesion, be it unilateral or segmental, appears not to be familial or progressive (Hutchins et al., 1972; Cho et al., 1979). These segmental lesions must also be differentiated from renal dysplasia, because they lack evidence of abnormal parenchymal differentiation. Arteriography demonstrates parenchymal displacement by a cystic mass (Fig. 39–15) that contained fine blood vessels corresponding to the septa separating the cysts. The segmental lesions do not correspond to multilocular cystic adenomas, because the cystic masses lack demarcation. The cysts are lined with flattened simple epithelium, and the septa among them blend into and incorporate the surrounding parenchyma. Such cases have been so uncommon that clinicopathologic correlations and generalizations cannot yet be made.

ACQUIRED RENAL CYSTIC DISEASE

In 1977, Dunnill, Millard, and Oliver reported the presence of cysts in the kidneys of 14 of 30 patients who had been on long-term hemodialysis. Their initial clinical, pathologic, and radiologic evaluations had failed to disclose the presence of renal cysts. It appeared, therefore, that for reasons unknown these patients had acquired renal cysts during the course of their dialytic therapy (Fig. 39–16).

This observation was quickly confirmed by subsequent studies from several countries. Kidneys with acquired cysts were found in 24 of 80 autopsied patients who had been on dialysis for up to 7 years in the eastern United States (Fayemi and Ali, 1979), in kidneys of 76 of 96 patients dialyzed for more than 3 years in Japan (Ishikawa et al., 1980), and in the kidneys of 21 of 22 patients dialyzed for a mean of 2.8 years in Germany (Krempien and Ritz, 1980).

Cysts that appear in the kidneys of individuals on chronic dialysis are more than a medical curiosity. They have clinical relevance. They can be the site of hemmorhage, infection, rupture, or neoplasia. Consequently, the onset of fever, hematuria, or flank pain is indication for prompt and careful evaluation of renal integrity in the chronic dialysis patient. Currently, computerized tomography appears to be the most reliable means to this end (Ishikawa et al., 1980).

In the setting of chronic dialysis, cyst formation may involve both cortex and medulla. Often, it is accompanied by epithelial hyperplastic and dysplastic changes (McManus and Hughson, 1979), which are reminiscent of those seen in APCD and which have been regarded as premalignant (Hughson, et al., 1980). Heavy deposits of oxalate occur throughout many of these kidneys, but oxalate urolithiasis has not been reported.

Whether renal cysts can be acquired in other settings is debatable. The possibility is suggested by the experience of Hestbech and associates (1977) who reported cysts in the kidneys of two patients following long-term lithium therapy. It was not certain, however, that cysts were absent from their kidneys before therapy was begun. For the moment, cyst formation in the kidneys of chronic hemodialysis patients remains the only convincing example of acquired renal cystic disease in humans.

NEPHRONOPHTHISIS–CYSTIC RENAL MEDULLA COMPLEX

The nephronophthisis-cystic renal medulla complex derives its name from the pathologic appearance of the kidney, which is remarkably consistent in this entity. The renal substance is shrunken, scarred, and punctuated with a variable number of microscopic to pea-sized cysts throughout its corticomedullary and medullary regions. On histologic examination, there are periglomerular fibrosis, tubular atrophy, and interstitial infiltration by round cells, a picture reminiscent of chronic pyelonephritis. Cysts are not considered a necessary component of the disease complex. Some authors have described patients whose kidneys contained no cysts, de-

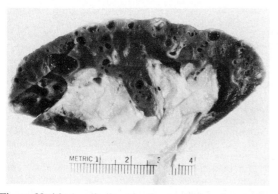

Figure 39–16. Acquired cystic disease. Kidney in a patient with chronic renal failure who was treated with long-term hemodialysis contains multiple small cortical cysts at postmortem examination.

spite the presence of a characteristic clinical course, that is, a family history positive for renal disease, anemia, renal sodium-wasting, and relentless and progressive renal failure (Burke et al., 1982; Richmond et al., 1981).

Credit for recognition of the complex as an entity is generally given to both Fanconi and his associates in Europe and Strauss in the United States. In 1951, Fanconi and coworkers described two families with the condition. Although these workers failed to emphasize that medullary cysts were present, one of the illustrations accompanying their publication shows them clearly. In contrast, Strauss in 1962 found only 2 of 18 families with a positive history for renal disease. Thus, although he emphasized that cysts were present, he considered the complex not to be a heritable disorder. More than 230 cases of the condition have now been described, and undoubtedly more have gone unreported (Gardner, 1976). This complex has been cited as one of the more common causes of renal failure among children.

Genetics and Family Studies

In spite of many similarities in clinical progression and renal lesions that appear virtually identical in all affected cases, several variants of the nephronophthisis-medullary cystic disease complex can be distinguished by genetic criteria. These variants include isolated cases in which the family history is clearly negative for renal disease, recessively inherited illness that may or may not be associated with degenerative changes of the retina, and dominantly transmitted disease.

A relatively small number of sporadic cases of the nephronophthisis-medullary cystic disease complex have been described (Gardner, 1976). They may represent new dominant mutations, the occurrence of recessive disease in a family with only one child, or perhaps cystic deformity in a kidney affected by some other primary illness, such as chronic glomerulonephritis. Even though sporadic cases do occur, the discovery of medullary cysts in a surgical or autopsy specimen should stimulate an aggressive investigation of members of the patient's family, who may be unaware that they harbor the disease.

The families described by Fanconi and his associates (1951) transmitted nephronophthisis-medullary cystic disease as a recessively inherited trait. This genetic variant of the complex is the most common, accounting for roughly two

thirds of all reported cases. Both sexes are affected equally. The tendency toward a greater than expected ratio of occurrence of one affected sibling: three unaffected siblings has been encountered and is attributed to a self-selective process: The more affected members within one generation, the greater the likelihood of that family's coming to medical attention. Consanguineous mating has been described among several families, strengthening the possibility that recessive inheritance is a likely genetic modality in the complex. Most recessively inherited cases have been reported in the literature under the title *familial juvenile nephronophthisis*. Gardner (1976) has presented evidence that when recessively transmitted, the complex tends to appear at a younger age and to result in terminal renal failure during the second decade of life. Exceptions to this evolutionary pattern have been cited, however (Giangiacomo et al., 1975).

The writings of Senior (1973), Schimke (1969), and others have drawn attention to the finding that in a number of families, recessively inherited disease is accompanied by retinal degeneration. The eye lesion may or may not progress to blindness and cannot be considered a critical determinant in the decision whether to give affected individuals long-term treatment for their renal disease. The number of families reported to have eye and renal lesions is now sufficient to allow the association to be regarded as a special variant of the complex (vide infra).

Approximately ten families have been described in which the complex is transmitted as a dominant trait, probably autosomal but possibly also X-linked. Disease transmitted as a dominant trait tends not to appear until the second or third decade of life. Based on reported experience, it appear to be more fulminant, resulting in terminal renal failure after an average downhill course of only 2 or 3 years (Gardner, 1976). Retinal disease and consanguineous mating have not been encountered in any dominantly transmitted example of the complex.

Associated Syndromes

Renal-retinal dysplasia. This is the name given to that variant of the nephronophthisis-cystic renal medulla complex that is characterized by the typical renal lesion, retinal degeneration, and recessive inheritance. During the 1960's and 1970's it became evident that some families with the nephronophthisis-medullary cystic disease complex were also transmitting ocular defects. These defects primarily affected the retina, usually in the form of retinitis pigmentosa. At least 11 such families have now been identified (Avasthi et al., 1976). In all of them, the mode of inheritance of both eye and renal abnormalities is recessive. Progressive blindness is not invariable. Among these families, 25 affected individuals have had both eyes and kidneys involved, whereas only 8 siblings suffered from either retinal involvement or renal disease. This distribution is strongly suggestive of a gene defect that is pleiotropic rather than multiple. The association of retinitis pigmentosa with the nephronophthisis-cystic renal medulla complex makes it mandatory that individuals with the former be investigated for renal disease, whereas those with the latter should undergo thorough ophthalmologic evaluation.

Alström's syndrome. This condition is a rarely reported, genetically transmitted disorder characterized by obesity, blindness, diabetes mellitus, nerve deafness, and nephropathy (Goldstein and Fialkow, 1973). The renal lesion can be a major clinical component. It is characterized in its early stages by aminoaciduria and a urinary concentrating defect and in its later stages by variably progressive failure of renal function and a pathologic picture similar to that seen in the nephronophthisis–cystic renal medulla complex, with one exception: Several renal biopsies have shown glomerular obsolescence and tubular atrophy, a picture similar to nephronophthisis (Goldstein and Fialkow, 1973). Cysts have not been mentioned in descriptions of post-mortem specimens. Bernstein (1976), nonetheless, has suggested that Alström's syndrome be classified with the renal medullary cystic disorders, based on the clinical and functional similarities to nephronophthisis.

Miscellaneous syndromes. The nephronophthisis-cystic renal medulla complex has also been described in association with the Laurence-Moon-Biedl syndrome (Hurley et al., 1975), horseshoe kidney (Whelton et al., 1974), and hepatic fibrosis (Boichis et al., 1973). (There is some question in the last instance whether the renal lesion is typical, inasmuch as glomerular but not medullary cysts are described.) It has been emphasized that individuals with the complex may have blond or red hair (Rayfield and McDonald, 1972). Although such has not been true in our experience, the existence of blond or red hair in a patient with kidney disease should suggest the possibility that the patient is suffering from a variant of the nephronophthisis-cystic renal medulla complex.

Etiology and Pathogenesis

Virtually nothing concerning the cause and pathogenesis of the complex is known. Comments made earlier in this chapter concerning studies of experimental models are applicable to the nephronophthisis-cystic renal medulla complex, as well as to APCD. At present, it can be said only that genetic factors participate in the transmission of this condition and that at least three genotypes are responsible for the phenotypic expression of the renal lesion. Because recurrence of the typical pathologic picture has not been described in a transplanted kidney, a circulating nephrotoxic cystogenetic metabolite is considered an unlikely pathogenetic mechanism.

Morphology

No differences in renal morphology have been detected in these kidneys; the disease may be recessively or dominantly transmitted, renal-retinal dysplasia may or may not be present, or the nephronophthisis-medullary cystic disease may be familial or nonfamilial.

On gross examination, the kidney with nephronophthisis-medullary cystic disease is typically shrunken, firm, and pale. The subcapsular surface is granular. An occasional typical retention cyst may be visible.

On sectioning, the lesions from which the complex derives its name become visible. The cortex is thin. Cysts ranging in size from microscopic to as much as a centimeter in diameter are characteristically seen in the corticomedullary and medullary regions (Fig. 39–17). The loss of renal substance is seen to extend from capsule to papillae. Microscopic examination reveals further changes. Periglomerular fibrosis is widespread. Occasional glomeruli may be hyalinized; some appear normal. Tubular atrophy is pronounced, especially in regions of glomerular hyalinization, but elsewhere dilation and tortuosity are evident. Foci of lymphocytes and plasma cells scattered throughout the interstitium complete the picture. Few studies of these kidneys with scanning electron microscopy have been performed. Many medullary cysts, however, exhibit a progressive flattening of their cells, from the point at which the tubule enters or leaves the cyst to out over the cyst wall. The most dramatic finding with the transmission electron microscope is basement membrane thickening (Pascal, 1973).

It must be emphasized that aside from the

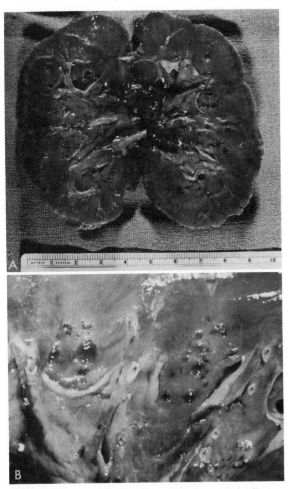

Figure 39–17. Nephronophthisis–medullary cystic disease. *A,* The kidney is small, and the cut surface reveals an atrophic scarred cortex. The medulla is punctuated with scattered cysts that measure 1 to 4 mm in diameter. *B,* Closeup view of the medulla in another case discloses variation in the number and size of cysts.

corticomedullary and medullary cysts, none of the renal changes seen in the complex are specific. All have been described in other forms of renal disease. For the moment, the importance to the diagnosis of finding cysts remains questionable. More than three quarters of the cases described in the literature do have cysts, but a substantial number do not (Gardner, 1976). In some of these latter cases, complete examination of the kidney has not been performed. Ample evidence exists in the literature to indicate that cysts can frequently be overlooked until the involved kidney is directly examined by the pathologist. There are instances, however, in which careful examinations of kidneys have been made and cysts, even though looked for, were not seen.

Microdissection studies have shown that though nephrons may be strikingly heterogeneous in size with diverticula scattered along their entire lengths, cysts tend to be restricted in location to the distal convoluted and collecting tubular segments (Sherman et al., 1971).

The cysts in this lesion are nonspecific in appearance. Usually, they are lined with cuboidal epithelium and often contain proteinaceous material. Calcification is rare, if it occurs at all, as opposed to its frequency in MSK. No analyses of the composition of cyst fluid are available, though Gardner (1969) has mentioned that sodium concentrations may be dramatically low (7 mEq per L).

Radiography and Sonography

Generally, the radiographic diagnosis of the nephronophthisis-cystic renal medulla complex has been disappointing. Excretory urography cannot be counted on to disclose the presence of medullary cysts, especially late in the course of the disease. Similar experience has also been described with renal arteriography (Gardner, 1976). In contrast, Mena and his associates (1974), are among those who believe that the angiographic features of the complex are usually fairly characteristic. In four of five patients, they procured angiograms that demonstrated small kidneys, diminished renal blood flow as judged by the backflow technique, reduction in size of the main renal artery, identifiable cysts during the nephrogram phase, sparing of the outer cortex by cysts, and distortion of the interlobar arcuate arteries (Fig. 39–18). Their study is particularly helpful because they correlated angiographic findings with nephrectomy specimens from three cases. Reported experience with sonography and computerized tomography is too sparse to permit generalizations concerning their usefulness. They should be utilized in suspected cases because of their ability to detect cysts in the 3- to 5-mm range.

Renal Function Evaluation

Affected individuals generally come to medical attention in one of two ways: They present with well-established renal failure or they are identified early in the course of their renal disease because another member of their family has the condition. Although an inability to concentrate urine maximally is a functional hallmark of all forms of progressive renal dis-

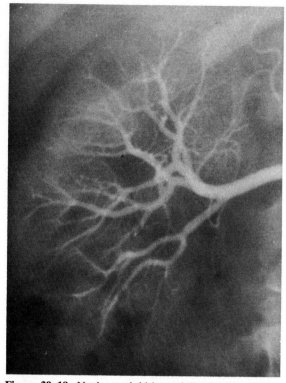

Figure 39–18. Nephronophthisis–medullary cystic disease. Arteriography reveals a general reduction in renal size and a thinning of the cortex. Bowing of the intrarenal arteries reflects the presence of cysts within the deeper renal tissue.

tions of renal sodium handling (Gardner, 1976). Of these, frank salt-wasting was found in 24 cases. It may reach prodigious proportions and may necessitate a compensatory salt intake in excess of 200 mEq daily to maintain adequate extracellular volume. With one exception, aminoaciduria has not been detected among cases reported to date.

Clinical Features

Signs and Symptoms. Among those patients coming to medical attention, polydipsia and polyuria are reported to be the most frequent primary presenting complaints. Especially among children, these disorders have often been present for years, sometimes dating to infancy. Less frequent presenting complaints include failure to thrive, pallor, weakness, and the characteristic symptoms of advanced azotemia (Gardner, 1976). In contrast to both polycystic kidney disease and MSK, pain is absent from the history. The sexes are affected equally. Cases of this disorder may be more common among individuals with red or blond hair. Anemia, which has been highly publicized as a feature of the syndrome, is probably the consequence of renal failure per se.

ease, a urinary concentrating defect may well be the earliest sign of renal involvement in the nephronophthisis-cystic renal medulla complex. The literature contains references to at least six instances in which a concentrating defect was the presenting abnormality in renal function, occurring in the presence of relatively normal glomerular filtration (Gardner, 1976).

Significantly, urinalysis is relatively unhelpful. Proteinuria rarely exceeds 2+ qualitatively, and formed elements are found infrequently on examination of the sediment. Hematuria, red blood cell casts, and hemoglobin casts are not characteristic. The presence of significant proteinuria (in excess of 4 gm), gross hematuria, or blood casts in the urinary sediment should suggest other diagnostic possibilities. Urinary acidifying ability is intact in most affected subjects (Gardner, 1976).

Renal sodium-wasting is considered a clinical characteristic of the disease, yet relatively few cases have been studied adequately. It has been described in both the presence and the absence of cysts. A recent review of published experience revealed that only 35 of 110 well-studied cases included the results of observa-

Differential Diagnosis

The nephronophthisis-cystic renal medulla complex poses a definite diagnostic challenge to the clinician. Inasmuch as the kidneys are small, the urinalysis is not remarkable, and the roentgenographic findings are often nonspecific, the clinician is faced with distinguishing the complex from all diseases characterized by small kidneys and progressive renal failure. A family history that is positive for renal disease provides a significant clue. Frequently, such a history is uncovered only by careful questioning. It is advantageous to record the age at death of family members; the occurrence of multiple premature deaths among relatives of an individual with undiagnosed renal disease can be a valuable clue to the presence of familial nephropathy. Also helpful is a search for any renal tissue from other family members that might be available from nephrectomy or autopsy specimens.

The nephronophthisis-cystic renal medulla complex is distinguished from MSK by virtue of its familial occurrence, the absence of hematuria and nephrocalcinosis, and the lack of specific diagnostic changes on excretory urography. The Alport syndrome and hereditary nephritis have several features similar to this complex, but they can be distinguished from it by the presence of nephritic elements in the urine and by the frequent association of deafness with renal disease in the Alport syndrome. Bilateral oligonephronic hypoplasia is a relatively rare form of congenital renal dysplasia that affects children, who present with vomiting, polyuria, and dehydration. It may pose a problem in the differential diagnosis. In contrast to the nephronophthisis-cystic renal medulla complex, however, the GFR tends to remain relatively stable, and the family history is negative for renal disease. In questionable cases, renal arteriography or biopsy can be a useful diagnostic aid.

Course, Prognosis, and Complications

Renal failure is progressive and relatively rapid, once diagnosed. The interval between diagnosis and death or terminal renal failure averages less than 5 years. Hypertension is relatively uncommon, even in the later stages, if renal salt-wasting is present. Anemia tends to become more pronounced as renal failure progresses. Among children, renal osteodystrophy due to secondary hyperparathyroidism appears often and can become a major problem in clinical management. In contrast to the polycystic kidney, the kidney with nephronophthisis–medullary cystic disease appears not to exhibit any special propensity for infection. Urinary tract infection has been documented in fewer than 10 reported cases (Gardner, 1976), a somewhat surprising fact in view of the histologic picture of the renal lesion, which is reminiscent of chronic interstitial nephritis.

Therapy

In general terms, treatment is nonspecific and is directed toward the nutritional and chemical abnormalities that arise as a result of renal failure. Metabolic acidosis does occur but is less severe among these patients. The loss of increased amounts of sodium through the kidneys provides the physician with the opportunity to treat both salt loss and any tendency toward metabolic acidosis, with sodium bicarbonate, usually without worsening arterial hypertension. Both hemodialysis and renal transplantation have been performed on affected individuals with success. No reports have appeared documenting recurrence of the lesion in a transplanted kidney, an experience suggesting that circulating factors do not play a role in pathogenesis.

MEDULLARY SPONGE KIDNEY

MSK is a relatively common, calcinotic, cystic, and possibly congenital lesion of the innermost regions of the kidney that is diagnosed on radiologic examination. Lenarduzzi (1939) and Cacchi and Ricci (1948) are generally given credit for establishing the lesion as a specific entity. A recent review indicates that more than 600 case descriptions have appeared in the literature, most of them in the past 25 years (Kuiper, 1976). The lesion is of special interest to urologists because it predisposes to nephrolithiasis and its associated complications. In its most flagrant forms, MSK is diagnosed with relative ease with excretory urography. Estimates of its frequency in the general population range from 1 in 5000 to 1 in 20,000, and it occurs in approximately 1 of 200 patients with urologic disease.

Genetics and Pathogenesis

Most workers regard MSK as a congenital deformity of the renal medulla (Ekström et al., 1959; Pyrah, 1966). It has been found in children, but most patients are diagnosed during their adult years. Nothing is known of its pathogenesis. At least three etiologic hypotheses have been advanced (Kuiper, 1976): infection, obstruction, and heredity. None has gained acceptance. Although many histologic features of MSK suggest chronic pyelonephritis, chronic papillary infection is considered an unlikely cause by most authorities; infection is generally considered a secondary, not a primary, feature. In utero obstruction of the distal nephron by salts of calcium or uric acid is considered a remote possibility, but in stillborns distal nephron deformity is unusual, whereas deposits of uric acid are commonplace (Potter and Osathanondh, 1963). Finally, two bits of evidence suggest that hereditary factors play a role (Kuiper, 1976). Nine families have been described in which MSK affected two or more members; in one, three consecutive generations were affected. Also, instances of the association of MSK with other hereditary diseases (e.g., the

Ehlers-Danlos syndrome) have been reported (Kuiper, 1976; Levine and Michael, 1967). Any argument that MSK is genetically transmitted, however, is weakened by the fact that in the vast majority of cases, neither a positive family history nor associated congenital or hereditary abnormalities can be documented.

The question of why MSK is more susceptible to stone formation is under current study (Yendt, 1982). Prolonged transit times through ectatic ducts, and differences in the biochemical composition of urine are cited but no clear-cut answer is available yet.

Morphology

In the absence of a complication such as chronic infection or obstruction, the characteristic pathologic features of MSK are restricted to the innermost regions of the kidney. Grossly, the kidney is normal in size but may be slightly enlarged (30 per cent of cases) if cystic changes are striking. The cut surface exhibits "cysts" that contain calcareous deposits in 40 to 60 per cent of cases. The "cysts," which represent dilated collecting tubules, are variable in size (as large as 8 to 10 mm) and may be localized to one or two renal pyramids or, as in the majority of cases, may involve all of them. Microdissection of affected nephrons confirms diffuse enlargement of the intrapapillary collecting tubules.

With the light microscope, it can be seen that cysts are lined with a variety of types of epithelium. Most lumens appear to communicate with the urinary space. Even in kidneys from patients in whom no urinary tract infection can be demonstrated, changes highly suggestive of pyelonephritis can be seen, with round cell infiltration and foci of tubular atrophy. Evidence may be found of erosion of stones through cyst walls. The most constantly demonstrated microscopic feature is a more or less severe inflammatory cell infiltration, which is usually most pronounced nearest the renal pelvis (Ekström et al., 1959).

Radiography and Sonography

The radiographic criteria for MSK are diagnostic. During excretory urography, the contrast medium can be seen to concentrate in the ectatic or cystic tubules at the pyramidal apices. Calculi are located in the same region. In films taken after the nephrographic phase and before complete pelvocalyceal filling, contrast medium often can be seen to fill ectatic pyramidal tubules. Subsequently, after the calyces have emptied, contrast medium persists in the pyramidal tubules.

There is considerable debate in the literature regarding the significance of less dramatic changes in renal pyramids during urography. Whether these lesions are earlier stages of true MSK and whether they progress with time are also controversial questions. The roentgenographic appearance of the intrapyramidal cavities in MSK (Fig. 39–19) has been categorized as follows: (1) fan-shaped, (2) resembling a bunch of flowers, (3) resembling a cluster of grapes, or (4) presenting a mosaic pattern (DiSieno and Guareschi, 1956). Ekström and his associates (1959) also described four general types of urographically visible cavities: generally dilated collecting tubules and oval, rounded, or triangular or irregular cavities. Of these lesions, they considered the first to have a similar appearance on urography to the normal pyramidal blush that is frequently seen in otherwise normal urograms. Although *pyramidal blush* without identifiable tubular streaking is regarded as insignificant or nondiagnostic by some radiologists, others consider it the earliest sign of MSK. They argue that it occurs frequently in some pyramids of kidneys that exhibit more dramatic involvement of adjacent pyramids. Those opposed to the idea point out that there is no evidence of progression, that is, a pyramid initially shown to demonstrate *pyramidal blush* has not later been shown to contain the frank cyst formation and calcification typical of advanced MSK. The issue remains unsettled.

Sonography, retrograde urography, and arteriography are generally considered unnecessary diagnostic efforts, in view of the ease with which pyramidal deformities are demonstrated with excretory urography.

Renal Function

One might anticipate that the pattern of renal dysfunction in MSK would be characterized by loss of those activities that are most dependent on intact medullary structures, namely urinary concentrating ability and acidification. Maximal urinary concentrating ability has been shown to be impaired in more than two thirds of affected individuals in two relatively large series (Ekström et al., 1959; Granberg et al., 1971). Most patients with MSK, however, have intact urinary acidifying mecha-

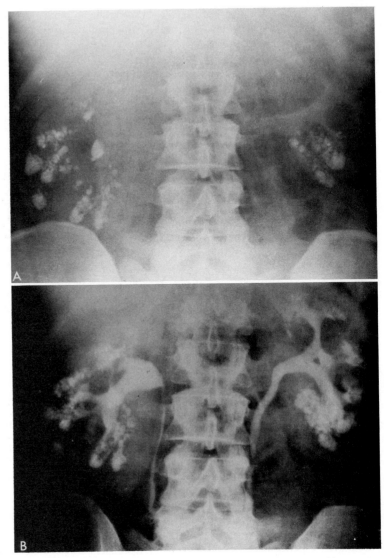

Figure 39–19. MSK. *A*, Plain film of the abdomen showing bilateral calcinosis in an advanced stage of the disease. *B*, Excretory urography in the same patient discloses increased opacification due to the accumulation of contrast medium within medullary cysts.

nisms. Five instances of distal renal tubular acidosis have been reported (Hamburger et al., 1968; Kuiper, 1976).

Hypercalciuria occurred in 40 per cent of the patients described by Ekström et al. (1959). Its causes are the same as the metabolic abnormalities found among stone formers in general (O'Neill, et al., 1981). Women with MSK tend to form stones more frequently than do men, and they are at higher risks for infection, cystoscopy, and hospitalization (Parks et al., 1982). In general, glomerular filtration remains normal in MSK, unless the lesion is complicated by chronic infection or obstruction. Levels of serum calcium, phosphorus, bicarbonate, and chloride are also within normal limits in the uncomplicated case.

Clinical Features

When uncomplicated, MSK is asymptomatic and only comes to light as an incidental finding. When there are complications, MSK may present in several ways. In the series of Ekström and coworkers (1959), renal colic was the most frequent presenting complaint, occurring in 25 of their 44 patients, and was associated with the verified passage of a stone in 19 cases. Silent and macroscopic hematuria in six of eight additional patients, and acute cystopyelitis in a further seven patients were the next most frequent initial symptoms.

Hypertension and azotemia are decidedly unusual in this disease complex.

The age and sex of the patient are of little

diagnostic help. Hamburger et al. (1968), in more than 100 cases, noted the first symptoms to occur at ages varying from 3 weeks to 71 years. Males and females appear to be involved with equal frequency. Proteinuria and hyperuricemia have been described in approximately 50 per cent of cases in at least one series (Hamburger et al., 1968).

Differential Diagnosis

The roentgenographic appearance of MSK, even though relatively specific, shares many of the features of a number of pathologic conditions. The issue of whether *papillary blush* alone represents an early stage of MSK has already been discussed. In the absence of more advanced lesions elsewhere in the kidney, of nephrocalcinosis, or of symptoms referable to the urinary tract, a papillary blush may be regarded as clinically benign or even normal.

A number of conditions are associated with nephrocalcinosis, all of which should be considered in the differential diagnosis of MSK. They include the hypercalcemic conditions associated with hyperparathyroidism, sarcoidosis, vitamin D intoxication, multiple myeloma, tuberculosis, and the milk-alkali syndrome. Of these, Ekström (1959) regards the commonest cause of renal pyramidal calcification to be hyperparathyroidism, which can now be diagnosed with direct measurement of serum parathormone levels. Renal tuberculosis must be considered in all cases; skin testing, chest x-rays, and urine cultures should also be performed.

The appearance of renal papillary necrosis on excretory urography may, on occasion, be confused with that of MSK. The clinical course of papillary necrosis, however, is generally acute and often fulminant. It tends to predominate in patients with diabetes mellitus, sickle cell anemia, obstruction, or recurrent urinary tract infections. During its acute phase, a "ring sign" can often be seen on the excretory urogram. A history of analgesic abuse can sometimes be obtained. IPCD (vide supra) may be confused on pyelography with MSK, but there are distinctive differences.

Calyceal diverticula and cysts may contain calculi; though they usually occur as single lesions, they may be multiple within the same kidney. Their cavities are generally larger than those seen in MSK. Generally, they pose no problem for the experienced radiologist.

Course and Prognosis

The course of uncomplicated MSK is benign. Radiographic evidence of progression of the disease can be obtained in fewer than 10 to 15 per cent of patients, and it almost always consists of only minimal change in the size or the distribution of dilated collecting tubules (Kuiper, 1976). Once symptomatic, however, MSK generally does not follow a silent clinical course. At some time during their lives, 60 per cent of affected individuals experience ureteral colic from the extrusion of stones, and an additional 30 per cent suffer with gross hematuria. The disease runs a variable course among these patients. One individual may enjoy a long period free of symptoms, whereas another may require repeated hospitalization for recurrent infection or colic (Ekström et al., 1959). Kuiper (1976) has estimated that 10 per cent of symptomatic patients, however, must be regarded as having a poor prognosis, with ureterolithiasis, septicemia, or renal failure being the major causes of morbidity. Surgical intervention, especially in cases with unilateral involvement, may be rewarding. Ekström and his associates (1959) considered five patients to be cured with radical surgery (three nephrectomies and two partial nephrectomies). Considerable care is required to avoid performing nephrectomy when there is bilateral renal involvement, inasmuch as complications of the disease can progress asynchronously in the two kidneys.

Complications

Lithiasis. Nephrolithiasis, as discussed, will complicate the course of 50 per cent of patients with MSK. It occurs more frequently in women than in men (Parks et al., 1982; Yendt, 1982). On chemical analysis, stones are usually found to contain calcium phosphates, with oxalate being present less frequently. Although there is little evidence to suggest that stone formation is retarded or prevented with the use of phosphate binders in MSK, there is ample evidence to indicate that stone formation can be progressive if not treated. Consequently, efforts to prevent stone formation seem warranted. They include ensurance of an ample fluid intake, attention to limitation of dietary calcium and sodium intake, and the use of cellulose phosphates—5 gm orally two or three times daily. In addition to retrieval with partial or complete nephrectomy, an occasional stone may be accessible through a direct surgical approach. Ekström and his colleagues (1959) succeeded in extracting ureteral stones transurethrally in four patients. In addition, they performed eight ureterolithotomies and five pyelolithotomies or pyelonephrolithotomies in 11 of their 44 patients.

As in polycystic kidney disease, it is unwise to use instruments in the lower urinary tract in patients with MSK. The susceptibility of these kidneys to infection is undoubtedly increased. The risk of introducing unwanted pathogenic bacteria during instrumentation of the lower urinary tract is great. Therefore, procedures such as cystoscopy must be undertaken only after careful consideration of the consequences.

Infection. After nephrolithiasis, urinary tract infection represents the greatest threat to the health and life of patients with MSK. In most instances, infection is associated with nephrocalcinosis. The series of Ekström et al. (1959) contains 12 patients in whom infection more or less dominated the clinical picture. Only two of the seven operated on for stones became free from infection, and in those cases palliative surgery was supplemented with radical resection. Four patients in the series suffered recurrent attacks of acute pyelonephritis. They were treated successfully with appropriate antibiotic therapy. In general, there are no secrets about the treatment of infection in patients with MSK. Work-up includes urine and blood cultures, laboratory determination of antibiotic sensitivities, and, ultimately, treatment with the appropriate agent. There is no evidence in these patients that long-term antibiotic therapy suppresses episodes of infection or reduces the incidence of stone formation.

Associated Conditions

MSK has been reported to accompany a variety of other pathologic states which include mongolism, ectopic kidney, horseshoe kidney, and the Ehlers-Danlos syndrome (Kuiper, 1976). MSK has also been reported to accompany congenital total hemihypertrophy in at least 17 instances (Sprayregen et al., 1973). (By definition, hemihypertrophy is one-sided.) Among these patients, four instances of unilateral MSK occurred, three on the side ipsilateral to the hemihypertrophy and one on the contralateral side. Hemihypertrophy itself shows no preference for laterality.

Cases of MSK have been reported to be associated with hyperparathyroidism. This probably represents a coincidental coexistence of the two conditions, but it does illustrate the importance of a careful and complete work-up in those tending to form renal stones (Stella et al., 1973).

MSK has also been reported to develop in association with congenital hepatic fibrosis (Spence and Singleton, 1972a), a lesion that is known to occur in association with IPCD. In our opinion, these reports are based on a misinterpretation of radiographic evidence. In IPCD, as in MSK, the typical renal medullary lesion is a dilation of the intrapyramidal collecting ducts, sometimes to the point that small cysts are formed. IPCD, however, also involves the cortex, with atrophy, interstitial fibrosis, and even cyst formation. Also, in contrast to MSK, IPCD and CHF are found most frequently in infants and adolescents. Thus, the age group and pathologic picture found in IPCD associated with CHF are clearly different from those found in MSK.

RENAL DYSPLASIA

The term *dysplasia* is used to designate abnormalities in renal morphogenesis, differentiation, and structural organization (Baggenstoss, 1951; Marshall, 1953; Ericsson and Ivemark, 1958; Bernstein, 1968; Risdon, 1971). Dysplasia is distinguished from hypoplasia, though the two abnormalities often coexist; dysplasia refers to altered morphogenesis and hypoplasia refers to reduced renal mass. Dysplasia may result from an arrest of development, with failure of cytodifferentiation and persistence of incompletely developed structures, but the abnormalities that constitute dysplasia do not correspond to normal stages of fetal development. Dysplasia is not simply a retention of fetal renal structures.

Renal dysplasia should not be regarded as a specific malformation, but rather as a group of heterogeneous malformations that are characterized by abnormal parenchymal development (Bernstein, 1971b). Dysplastic kidneys may be large or small, functioning or nonfunctioning, reniform or misshapen, and solid or cystic. The defects involve the cortex or the medulla, or both, and they may be diffuse or segmental. The gross features of renal dysplasia include cysts and abnormal lobar configuration, though cysts can be acquired, and apparent lobar disorganization can result from scarring.

The usual histopathologic criteria include (1) primitive ducts, which are lined with undifferentiated columnar epithelium, are surrounded by fibromuscular collars, and derive from the metanephric duct (Ericsson and Ivemark, 1958) and (2) nests of metaplastic cartilage, which are usually cortical and derive from the metanephric blastema (Voth, 1961). More subtle abnormalities, which are often difficult to evaluate, include altered architectonics. The metanephric kidney—by virtue of specialized anatomic relationships between nephrons and ducts and among nephrons, ducts, and blood vessels—operates as more than simply the sum of filtering glomeruli and resorbing tubules. Recognizable forms of abnormal architecture include the so-called delta-like medulla (Marshall, 1953), in which the medullary pyramids contain primitive ducts with excessive connective tissue and a paucity of tubules and blood vessels. Another example of developmentally altered anatomic relationships is incomplete demarcation of the medullary pyramids with rudimentary calyceal and fornical development.

Dysplastic kidneys also contain primitive glomeruli and tubules (Pasternack, 1960), but they are not reliable signs of dysplasia, since they can result from circulatory disturbances and inflammatory scarring in fully formed kidneys (Bernstein, 1968, 1971b). Glomeruli and tubules may, as a consequence of ischemic injury, acquire a fetal appearance that is suggestive of abnormal differentiation, but regarding such lesions as dysplastic introduces an unacceptable degree of heterogeneity. The interpretation of cartilaginous metaplasia as evidence of dysplasia has also been challenged (Taxy and Filmer, 1975), though most investigators continue to regard it as evidence of altered metanephric differentiation. Dysplasia is neither the result nor the cause of chronic pyelonephritis; inflammation is found only in association with urinary stasis or reflux and is lacking in dysplastic kidneys with atretic ureters (Risdon, 1971).

Renal dysplasia is commonly associated with urinary tract obstruction. The association is neither necessary nor universal, but the incidence of anatomic abnormalities of the ureters, bladder, and urethra is approximately 90 per cent (Rubenstein et al., 1961). Unilateral dysplasia is associated with ipsilateral ureteral obstruction, and bilateral dysplasia is associated with lower tract obstruction. Segmental dysplasia is associated with segmental obstruction, as in ureteral duplication with ectopic ureterocele (Newman et al., 1974; Perrin et al., 1974). The renal dysplasia that accompanies meningomyelocele has been attributed to neurogenic vesical dysfunction and obstruction (Forbes, 1972).

The patterns of dysplasia bear a relationship to the type of urinary tract obstruction (Bernstein, 1971b). First, it may be said that all dysplastic kidneys contain some evidence of metanephric corticomedullary differentiation. The nephronic derivatives (glomeruli and tubules) may be very rudimentary, but they are present and have the same relationship to primitive ducts as normal cortex has to medulla. Second, all forms of dysplasia contain an admixture of primitive, atrophic, and cystic ductular and nephronic elements. The lack of sharp distinctions among them has been interpreted to indicate that nephrogenesis continues despite the pathologic processes and that the agents responsible for the maldevelopment must have continued to act on the developing kidney over a period of time. Third, morphologic examination shows that cortical dysplasia is usually most marked in the outer cortex, suggesting that the responsible agent is operative after the formation of the inner cortex and presumably after the early secretion of urine. Fourth, in general, the more severe the obstruction, the more severe the dysplasia. Ureteropelvic occlusion is associated with a severely deformed multicystic kidney; severe infravesical obstruction due to posterior urethral valves is associated with peripheral cortical dysplasia. These observations have also been used to support the argument that urinary tract obstruction bears a causal relationship to renal dysplasia.

Clearly, however, renal dysplasia is not always associated with urinary tract obstruction. Renal dysplasia occurs in heritable syndromes of multiple malformations without obstruction (Bernstein, 1975). Moreover, renal dysplasia in association with posterior urethral valves is often asymmetric, without a constant relationship to either concurrent reflux or the severity of obstruction (Cussen, 1971), except that urethral atresia seems always to be associated with renal dysplasia. Another hypothesis that has gained recent attention relates dysplasia, which is in a sense a poor quality of metanephric induction, to concomitant ureteral ectopy because of abnormal positioning of the ureteric bud (Mackie and Stephens, 1975; Schulman, 1978; Henneberry and Stephens, 1980; Schwarz et al., 1981).

The classification of renal dysplasia is, to a large degree, descriptive. Dysplastic kidneys are often cystic, but they must be differentiated from polycystic kidneys (Bernstein, 1973). Although they may be divided into several broad clinicopathologic categories (Bernstein, 1971*b*; Risdon, 1975; Risdon et al., 1975), many specimens remain unclassified.

Multicystic and Aplastic Dysplasia

The multicystic kidney (Schwartz, 1936) is large, cystic, and disorganized, and the aplastic kidney (Gutierrez, 1933; Nation, 1944) is small, noncystic, and less severely disorganized. They differ principally in the severity of cyst formation, which also influences the severity of disorganization; intermediate degrees make a clear separation difficult. The two prototypes can be regarded as the opposite ends of a spectrum and are conveniently considered together. Multicystic kidneys are more common and more easily recognized, clinically and radiographically.

In our experience, the multicystic kidney has always been associated with either ureteropelvic occlusion or ureteral atresia (or agenesis). The aplastic kidney is also associated with ureteral atresia and agenesis, but its differentiation from less severe degrees of dysplasia has been uncertain, and numerous patients have been said to have patent and even dilated ureters. Failure to visualize the ureteric orifice in cystoscopic examination does not, therefore, differentiate between the two conditions. Nevertheless, the severity of the malformation and the customary absence of a patent urinary tract are responsible for excretory nonfunction, and bilateral involvement is lethal in newborns (Johannessen et al., 1973). Bilateral involvement is one cause of the Potter syndrome in the newborn (oligohydramnios, abnormal facies, and amnion nodosum), and bilateral dysplasia is commonly associated with other congenital malformations. Both kidneys may have the same malformation, or one may be aplastic and the other multicystic. Renal aplasia may be transmitted as an autosomal dominant trait in a few families, and it is sometimes associated with other malformations, particularly of the ears and the internal female genitalia (Buchta et al., 1973; Cain et al., 1974; Fitch and Srolovitz, 1976; Schimke and King, 1980). Several families have included offspring with lethal, bilateral renal agenesis or dysplasia. Despite those occurrences, the risk of recurrence of unilateral dysplasia appears to be negligible, approximately 2 per cent (Al Saadi et al., 1984).

Unilateral aplasia occurs as an isolated abnormality, but it is commonly associated with milder contralateral malformations that impair the prognosis and necessitate corrective meas-ures. Isolated unilateral maldevelopment is often asymptomatic and can therefore be encountered in patients of any age. The signs and symptoms of unilateral aplasia are ill-defined, and manifestations in older individuals have included vague intestinal pains, malaise, flank pain, urinary frequency, and dysuria. The clinical manifestations suggest infection, and recurrent pyuria is said to be a problem in older children and adults (Burkland, 1954). The aplastic kidney does not itself appear to be a common site of chronic infection, and the symptoms may be referable to abnormalities of the opposite kidney, including ectopia, hydronephrosis, vesicoureteric reflux, pyelonephritis, and lithiasis (Eisendrath, 1935). Hypertension is regarded as a major complication (Nation, 1944), but its relationship to the aplastic kidney seems tenuous. The literature is clouded by a lack of distinctions among dysplastic, hypoplastic, and atrophic kidneys, and most of the literature antedates the recognition of reflux nephropathy and segmental renal atrophy, which are commonly associated with hypertension. Radiographic studies commonly show lack of both function and visualization, and the extremely small renal arteries supplying aplastic kidneys may be overlooked in arteriographic studies. Small masses can often be demonstrated by sonography and computerized tomography. The differential diagnosis includes other forms of small kidney, and confirmation of the dysplastic nature of the abnormality requires histopathologic examination.

The multicystic kidney is also most often unilateral, though associations with contralateral renal abnormalities (Parkkulainen et al., 1959; Pathak and Williams, 1964; Greene et al., 1971) and other malformations complicate clinical management. It has been suggested (Newman et al., 1972) that patients identified clinically as having unilateral masses have done well on long-term follow-up and have an excellent prognosis; cases recognized at post-mortem examination have shown a much higher frequency of contralateral abnormalities. In a similar sort of way, small multicystic kidneys appear more often to be associated with contralateral abnormalities than do large multicystic kidneys (Bloom and Brosman, 1978). Fewer contralateral abnormalities and good prognoses have also been observed in patients with high ureteropelvic occlusion as opposed to those who have low ureteral atresia (De Klerk et al., 1977). It appears, therefore, that complete clinical evaluation is required in all cases, and careful urographic evaluation of the opposite kidney is

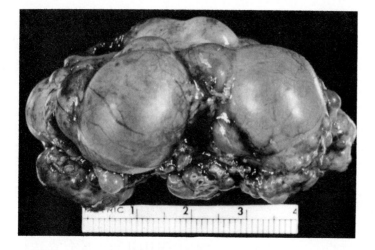

Figure 39–20. Multicystic dysplasia. A unilateral mass was palpable clinically in a 5-day-old male infant, and excretory urography failed to visualize a kidney. Surgical exploration revealed a cystic kidney with ureteral atresia, and pathologic examination demonstrated pyelocalyceal occlusion and parenchymal dysplasia.

mandatory before the patient can be given a good prognosis.

The multicystic kidney, which has often been loosely described as resembling a bunch of irregularly sized grapes, can achieve considerable size, weighing as much as several hundred grams (Fig. 39–20). Actually, the malformation is readily recognized as a cystic kidney, and most specimens have a central, relatively solid area that contains rudimentary renal tissue and dysplastic elements (Bernstein, 1968). The tubules and glomeruli form clusters of cortical tissue in relation to primitive ducts, forming rudimentary lobes (Bernstein, 1968; Vellios and

Garrett, 1961), and metanephric tissue within the septa among the cysts (Elkin and Bernstein, 1969) may account for septal opacification in high-dose excretory urography ("total-body opacification") (Fig. 39–21).

The multicystic kidney is the most common form of renal cystic disease in infancy. The presenting sign is most often a unilateral abdominal mass discovered in newborn or "well-baby" examinations. Male patients predominate, and the lesion is somewhat more common on the left than on the right side. Older patients may complain of pressure symptoms, abdominal or flank pain, or vague intestinal problems that are

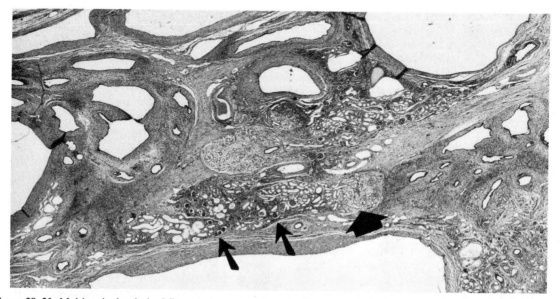

Figure 39–21. Multicystic dysplasia. Microscopic examination of solid tissue within the central portion of the cystic kidney discloses rudimentary lobules of metanephric tissue, in which glomeruli and tubules (arrows) are related to adjacent primitive ducts (broad arrow) in the manner of cortex to medulla. These islands of metanephric tissue may account for opacification of the solid portions and the septa on high-dose excretory urography. Hematoxylin and eosin, × 18.

probably unrelated to the abnormality, which is, in a real sense, an incidental radiographic finding.

Abdominal roentgenograms commonly show a flank mass, and conventional excretory urography shows lack of renal function. The diagnosis can usually be confirmed by sonography, which demonstrates a cystic, septate mass (Bearman et al., 1976; Stuck et al., 1982). Percutaneous cyst puncture and injection with radiopaque material show that the cysts may communicate through tubules (Saxton et al., 1981), confirming our view that the cysts arise in altered metanephric structures (Fig. 39–22). High-dose urography does opacify the walls of cysts (Leonidas et al., 1972; Newman et al., 1972), and roentgenograms delayed as much as 48 hours reveal retention of contrast medium in ill-defined cysts (Young et al., 1973; Cooperman, 1976). Radiographic and endoscopic studies confirm the association of multicystic kidney with ureteral atresia and agenesis (Kyaw, 1973; Newman et al., 1972), though the lower portion of the ureter is sometimes patent, allowing a ureteral catheter to be partially inserted. The upper ureter and pelvis are sometimes dilated in association with lower ureteral atresia, creating confusion between multicystic and hydro-

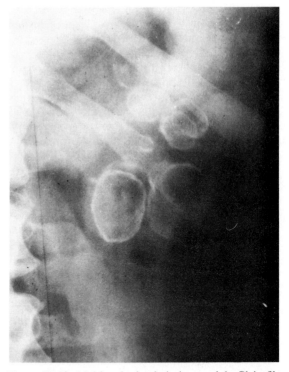

Figure 39–23. Multicystic dysplasia in an adult. Plain film of the abdomen shows that the left kidney contains numerous calcified cysts; the kidney was nonfunctional. (Roentgenogram courtesy of Dr. R. Ellwood, Department of Radiology, William Beaumont Hospital, Royal Oak.)

nephrotic kidneys (Felson and Cussen, 1975). Cyst walls often calcify in older patients, producing the radiographic picture of opaque rings within the mass (Fig. 39–23).

Therapy for both aplastic and multicystic kidneys has traditionally been surgical removal. Under those circumstances, the prognosis clearly depends upon the state of the opposite kidney, which usually undergoes considerable compensatory hypertrophy (Newman et al., 1972). Early reports of good outcome (Spence, 1955; Weinberg et al., 1956) were challenged by studies showing a high incidence—perhaps 30 per cent (Greene et al., 1971)—of contralateral abnormality (Parkkulainen et al., 1959; Pathak and Williams, 1964). Elective nephrectomy as the treatment of choice has itself been challenged now, since the condition is widely regarded as a benign malformation. Hypertension seems to be a rare complication (Javadpour et al., 1970), perhaps because most cases have been identified and treated early in infancy. In a survey of pediatric urologists, however, 15 per cent of respondents offered anecdotal evidence of hypertension (Bloom and Brosman, 1978). The same survey indicated that almost one half

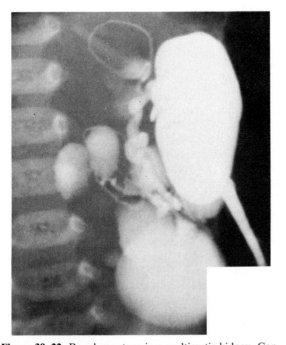

Figure 39–22. Renal puncture in a multicystic kidney. Contrast material injected superiorly into the most lateral cyst flowed through tubules on its medial aspect to enter the other cysts. (From Saxton, H. M., Golding, S. J., Chantler, C., and Haycock, G. D.: Diagnostic puncture in renal cystic dysplasia (multicystic kidney). Br. J. Radiol. *54*:555, 1981.)

of practitioners no longer thought prompt surgical exploration to be mandatory, and a sizable minority thought it not necessary to remove multicystic kidneys. That view would, of course, be modified in the face of signs and symptoms referable to the abnormal organ. Among the complications is an uncertain risk of malignancy (Barrett and Wineland, 1980) that needs to be evaluated critically. Strong sentiments remain in favor of surgical treatment (Ambrose et al., 1982).

Recent developments in sonography have permitted prenatal diagnosis of urinary tract abnormalities, including multicystic kidney (Older et al., 1979; Legarth et al., 1981; Bartley et al., 1977). However, when diagnosable, the condition is probably not correctable through surgical intervention.

Generalized and Segmental Dysplasia

Many dysplastic kidneys retain a reniform configuration, with variable preservation of metanephric architecture (Bernstein, 1968; Risdon, 1975). The lobar architecture and corticomedullary differentiation are readily apparent, and the pelves and ureters are patent. These kidneys also retain a limited ability to excrete urine. They cannot be sharply distinguished from aplastic kidneys, but their functional capacity, despite its limitations, provides the basis for regarding them as a separate group. A suitable terminology for this group has not evolved, perhaps because it is so heterogeneous. Localized or segmental forms of dysplasia are included for convenience (Bernstein, 1971b).

The diagnosis of dysplasia is established on histologic examination. Typical dysplasia with evidence of abnormal differentiation may coexist with hypoplasia, in which there is a reduction in mass and number of renal lobes. The radiographic appearances have been extremely variable, and demonstration of pyelocalyceal deformities does not serve to differentiate this group from secondarily shrunken kidneys, particularly in reflux nephropathy. The ureter may be dilated and is occasionally ectopic. Symptoms have been vague; pain is presumably related to infection and to lithiasis. Hypertension has been said to be common, but many of the patients in question have probably had segmental atrophy—the so-called Ask-Upmark kidney—arising in association with vesicoureteral reflux. Impaired tubular function is commonly present in the form of defective concentration and acidification (Gur et al., 1975).

Bilateral generalized dysplasia is a cause of progressive renal insufficiency in childhood, and in addition to reflux nephropathy, the differential diagnosis includes, familial juvenile nephronophthisis (see page 1783) and oligomeganephronia. All show evidence of tubular dysfunction, especially concentrating defects. Familial juvenile nephronophthisis is distinguished by its autosomal recessive transmission and by the rapid deterioration of renal function. Oligomeganephronia is rarely familial, and affected children go through a long period of stable renal function. Renal dysplasia may be familial, occasionally occurring as an isolated malformation (Cole et al., 1976) but more often in specific syndromes of multiple malformations. One of the most striking examples is found in the Meckel syndrome, a complex that includes microcephaly, posterior encephalocele, polydactyly, cleft palate and lip, genital anomalies, and hepatic dysgenesis. Most infants die shortly after birth. The kidneys vary greatly in size; at times they are huge, and at other times they are hypoplastic. The histologic pattern has, however, been remarkably consistent, with very few exceptions. The cysts are dilated collecting ducts, showing the usual features of dysplasia, and the intervening tissue contains remarkably few nephrons. There is little or no corticomedullary differentiation, and the kidneys are incapable of functioning. Similar renal malformations are encountered in several other syndromes that also involve the brain, and we have suggested that they are closely related abnormalities (Bernstein, 1976). The cerebral malformations include hydrocephalus (Simopoulos syndrome), Dandy-Walker deformity (Goldston syndrome), and cerebral dysgenesis (Miranda syndrome).

Bilateral cystic dysplasia has also been seen in the Jeune syndrome and in the Zellweger syndrome, and the renal findings have been overshadowed by the other abnormalities (Bernstein, 1975). Segmental dysplasia has been observed on occasion in the trisomy D syndrome, but the significance of the lesion to survival, renal function, and hypertension is not known. Medullary dysplasia without clinical and functional correlations has been observed in the Beckwith-Wiedemann syndrome (macroglossia, omphalocele, endocrine abnormalities, and hypoplastic visceromegaly). The kidneys are extremely large, and Wilms tumor is a relatively frequent complication.

The pathogenesis of the renal malformation in each of these syndromes is a matter of conjecture. Urinary tract obstruction is not a factor. The renal lesions in the Zellweger cerebrohepatorenal syndrome run the gamut from scattered small cysts in the peripheral cortex to generalized cystic dysplasia. The renal lesions in the Jeune syndrome of asphyxiating thoracic dysplasia encompass peripheral cortical microcysts, generalized cystic dysplasia, and progressive nephropathy. The renal lesions in the trisomy D syndrome are most often scattered, small, peripheral cortical cysts, at most a trifling abnormality. This much variability may reflect heterogeneity in the syndromes under discussion, but it may also mean that the renal lesion is secondary to another abnormality. If that abnormality is the primary heritable metabolic defect of the syndrome, the morphologic variability may reflect variable developmental timing and severity of expression, rather than genetic heterogeneity.

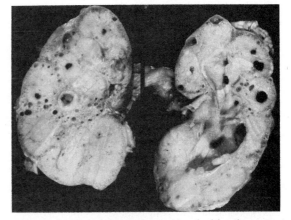

Figure 39–24. Renal dysplasia associated with urinary tract obstruction. Dysplasia typically involves the peripheral cortex, at which point a thin row of cysts is present beneath the capsule and along the columns of Bertin. The inner cortex often is relatively normal in appearance. Hydronephrosis is variable and often asymmetric, with partial obliteration of the medullary pyramids. The specimen is from a male infant with severe infravesical obstruction caused by posterior urethral valves.

Dysplasia Associated with Urinary Tract Obstruction

The association of urinary tract obstruction with dysplasia has been described. The severity and type of dysplasia relate to the severity and type of obstruction. Abnormally increased hydrostatic pressure, whether from stasis or from reflux, affects renal development by producing peripheral cortical dysplasia (usually cystic), and medullary dysplasia.

Renal dysplasia is encountered in any form of congenital urinary tract obstruction and is most common in infants with posterior urethral valves (Bernstein, 1971b; Risdon, 1975). The severity of the cortical abnormality relates to the severity of the obstruction. For example, urethral valvular obstruction that is severe enough to cause difficulty in the newborn is often associated with dysplasia, whereas similar obstruction that is mild enough to be inapparent until later childhood or early adulthood is usually not associated with dysplasia (Rattner et al., 1963). Urethral atresia is regularly associated with severe renal maldevelopment. Renal involvement is frequently asymmetric, perhaps because of asymmetry in the degree of associated reflux, perhaps because of variability in positioning of the ureteric bud. Fetal intervention to relieve lower urinary tract obstruction in the expectation of averting progressive renal maldevelopment may provide the answers to some of our questions about pathogenesis. The typical lesion consists of cysts that are formed of dilated primitive ducts in the subcapsular cortex and along the columns of Bertin (Fig. 39–24). The medullary pyramids may be partially effaced, and they seem to contain a diminished number of ducts in a relatively fibrous stroma that lacks tubules and normal vasculature—the so-called delta-like medulla. Dysplasia of the kidney is a cause of renal nonfunction following relief of the obstructive abnormality, and it vitiates surgical reconstruction (see Chapters 48 and 50).

Renal dysplasia has been found in infants with dilatation and hypertrophy of the bladder that was unaccounted for by anatomic obstruction; it has also been encountered in the "prune-belly" syndrome (see Chapter 53) (Risdon, 1975). Unilateral obstruction has been observed in duplex kidneys with ureteral ectopia. A ureterocele of the upper pole ureter causes severe obstruction and abnormal development of that portion of the kidney (Newman et al., 1974; Perrin et al., 1974). The ectopic ureter may occasionally stem from the lower pole, in which dysplasia may also be encountered. Ectopia of a single ureter may result in obstruction and may be associated with urinary dysplasia (Rattner et al., 1960). The diagnosis and treatment of duplex kidney and ureteral ectopia are discussed elsewhere (see Chapters 38 and 50).

References

Ackerman, G. L.: Nephrotic syndrome in polycystic renal disease. J. Urol., *105*:7, 1971.

Advisory Committee to the Renal Transplant Registry: The eleventh report of the Human Transplant Registry. JAMA, *226*:1197, 1973.

Albukerk, J., and Duffy, J. L.: Fibrogenesis in congenital

hepatic fibrosis. An electron and light microscopic study. Arch. Pathol., *92*:126, 1971.

Al Saadi, A. A., Yoshimoto, M., Bree, R., Farah, J., Chang, C.-H., Sahney, S., Shokeir, M. H. K., and Bernstein, J.: A family study of renal dysplasia. Am. J. Med. Genet. In press.

Alvarez, F., Bernard, O., Brunelle, F., Hadchouel, M., Leblanc, A., Odievre, M., and Alagille, D.: Congenital hepatic fibrosis in children. J. Pediatr., *99*:370, 1981.

Ambrose, S. S., Gould, R. A., Trulock, T. S., and Parrott, T. S.: Unilateral multicystic renal disease in adults. J. Urol., *128*:366, 1982.

Anand, S. K., Chan, J. C., and Lieberman, E.: Polycystic disease and hepatic fibrosis in children. Renal function studies. Am. J. Dis. Child., *129*:810, 1975.

Anderson, D., and Tannen, R. L.: Tuberous sclerosis and chronic renal failure. Potential confusion with polycystic kidney disease. Am. J. Med., *47*:163, 1969.

Arey, J. B.: Cystic lesions of the kidney in infants and children. J. Pediatr., *54*:429, 1959.

Avasthi, P. S., Erickson, D. G., and Gardner, K. D., Jr.: Hereditary renal-retinal dysplasia and the medullary cystic disease-nephronophthisis complex. Ann. Intern. Med., *84*:157, 1976.

Baggenstoss, A. H.: Congenital anomalies of the kidney. Med. Clin. North Am., *35*:987, 1951.

Barbaric, Z. L., Spataro, R. F., and Segal, A. J.: Urinary tract obstruction in polycystic renal disease. Radiology, *125*:627, 1977.

Barrett, D. M., and Wineland, R. E.: Renal cell carcinoma in multicystic dysplastic kidney. Urology, *15*:152, 1980.

Bartley, J. A., Golbus, M. S., Filly, R. A., and Hall, B. D.: Prenatal diagnosis of dysplastic kidney disease. Clin. Genet., *11*:375, 1977.

Bearman, S. B., Hine, P. L., and Sanders, R. C.: Multicystic kidney: A sonographic pattern. Radiology, *118*:685, 1976.

Becker, J. A., and Schneider, M.: Simple cyst of the kidney. Semin. Roentgenol., *10*:103, 1975.

Bengtsson, U., Hedman, L., and Svalander, C.: Adult type of polycystic kidney disease in a new-born child. Acta Med. Scand., *197*:447, 1975.

Bernstein, J.: Developmental abnormalities of the renal parenchyma: Renal hypoplasia and dysplasia. *In* Sommers, S. C. (Ed.): Pathology Annual 1968, New York, Appleton-Century-Crofts, 1968, pp. 213–247.

Bernstein, J.: Heritable cystic disorders of the kidney: The mythology of polycystic disease. Pediatr. Clin. North Am., *18*:435, 1971a.

Bernstein, J.: The morphogenesis of renal parenchymal maldevelopment (renal dysplasia). Pediatr. Clin. North Am., *18*:395, 1971b.

Bernstein, J.: The classification of renal cysts. Nephron, *11*:91, 1973.

Bernstein, J.: Familial renal dysplasia and renal abnormalities associated with malformation syndromes. *In* Rubin, M. I., and Barratt, T. M.: Pediatric Nephrology. Baltimore, The Williams & Wilkins Co., 1975, p. 356.

Bernstein, J.: A classification of renal cysts. *In* Gardner, K. D., Jr.: Cystic Diseases of the Kidney. New York, John Wiley & Sons, 1976, pp. 7–30.

Bernstein, J.: Cystic diseases of the liver in infancy. *In* Javitt, N. B. (Ed.): Neonatal Hepatitis and Biliary Atresia. Bethesda, MD., National Institutes of Health, U.S. Public Health Service, Publication 79-1296, 1979, pp. 331–338.

Bernstein, J., and Kissane, J. M.: Hereditary disorders of

the kidney. *In* Rosenberg, H., and Bolande, R. P.: Perspectives in Pediatric Pathology. Vol. 1. Chicago, Year Book Medical Publishers, 1973, p. 435.

Bernstein, J., and Meyer, R.: Parenchymal maldevelopment of the kidney. Chap. 26. *In* Kelley, V. C.: Brennemann's Practice of Pediatrics. Vol. 3. Hagerstown, Md., Harper & Row, 1967.

Bernstein, J., Brough, A. J., and McAdams, A. J.: The renal lesion in syndromes of multiple congenital malformations: Cerebrohepatorenal syndrome; Jeune asphyxiating thoracic dystrophy; tuberous sclerosis; Meckel syndrome. *In* Bergsma, D. (Ed.): The Fifth Conference on the Clinical Delineation of Birth Defects. Birth Defects: Original Article Series, *10*:35, 1974. Baltimore, Williams & Wilkins Co.

Bjerle, B., Lindqvist, B., and Michaelson, G.: Pressure measurements in renal cysts. Scand. J. Clin. Lab. Invest., *27*:135, 1971.

Bloom, D. A., and Brosman, S.: The multicystic kidney. J. Urol., *120*:211, 1978.

Blyth, H., and Ockenden, B. G.: Polycystic disease of kidneys and liver presenting in childhood. J. Med. Genet., *8*:257, 1971.

Boal, D. K., and Teele, R. L.: Sonography of infantile polycystic kidney disease. AJR, *135*:575, 1980.

Boichis, H., Passwell, J., David, R., and Miller, H.: Congenital hepatic fibrosis and nephronophthisis. A family study. Q.J. Med., *42*:221, 1973.

Bommer, J., Waldherr, R., van Kaick, G., Strauss, L., and Ritz, E.: Acquired renal cysts in uremic patients—in vivo demonstration by computed tomography. Clin. Nephrol., *14*:299, 1980.

Bosniak, M. A.: Angiomyolipoma (hamartoma) of the kidney: A preoperative diagnosis is possible in virtually every case. Urol. Radiol., *3*:135, 1981.

Braasch, W. F., and Hendrick, J. A.: Renal cysts, simple and otherwise. J. Urol., *51*:1, 1944.

Bricker, N. S., and Patton, J. F.: Cystic disease of the kidneys. A study of dynamics and chemical composition of cyst fluid. Am. J. Med., *18*:207, 1955.

Buchta, R. M., Viseskul, C., Gilbert, E. F., Sarto, G. E., and Opitz, J. M.: Familial bilateral renal agenesis and hereditary renal adysplasia. Z. Kinderheilk., *115*:111, 1973.

Burke, J. R., Inglis, J. A., Craswell, P. W., Mitchell, K. R. and Emmerson, B. T.: Juvenile nephronophthisis and medullary cystic disease—the same disease (report of a large family with medullary cystic disease associated with gout and epilepsy). Clin. Nephrol., *18*:1, 1982.

Burkland, C. E.: Clinical considerations in aplasia, hypoplasia, and atrophy of kidney. J. Urol., *71*:1, 1954.

Buttarazzi, P. J., Poutasse, E. F., Devine, C. J., Jr., Fiveash, J. R., Jr., and Devine, P. C.: Aspiration of renal cyst. J. Urol., *100*:591, 1968.

Cacchi, R., and Ricci, V.: Sopra una rara e forse ancora non descritta affezione cistica delle piramidi renali ("rene a spugna"). Atti. Soc. Ital. Urol., *5*:59, 1948.

Cain, D. R., Griggs, D., Lackey, D. A., and Kagan, B. M.: Familial renal agenesis and total dysplasia. Am. J. Dis. Child., *128*:377, 1974.

Cairns, H. W. B.: Heredity in polycystic disease of the kidney. Q.J. Med., *18*:359, 1925.

Carone, F. A., Rowland, R. G., Perlman, S. G., and Ganote, C. E.: The pathogenesis of drug-induced renal cystic disease. Kidney Int., *5*:411, 1974.

Chilton, S. J., and Cremin, B. J.: The spectrum of polycystic disease in children. Pediatr. Radiol., *11*:9, 1981.

Chinn, D. H., and Filly, R. A.: Ultrasound diagnosis of fetal genitourinary tract anomalies. Urol. Radiol., 4:115, 1982.

Cho, K. J., Thornbury, J. R., Bernstein, J., Heidelberger, K. P., and Walter, J. F.: Localized cystic disease of the kidney: Angiographic-pathologic correlation. AJR, 132:891, 1979.

Chonko, A. M., Weiss, S. M., Stein, J. H., and Ferris, T. F.: Renal involvement in tuberous sclerosis. Am. J. Med., 56:124, 1974.

Christoferson, L. A., Gustafson, M. B., and Petersen, A. G.: von Hippel-Lindau's disease. JAMA, 178:280, 1961.

Chynn, K. Y., and Evans, J. A.: Nephrotomography in the differentiation of renal cyst from neoplasm: A review of 500 cases. J. Urol., 83:21, 1960.

Cole, B. R., Kaufman, R. L., McAlister, W. H., and Kissane, J. M.: Bilateral renal dysplasia in three siblings: Report of a survivor. Clin. Nephrol., 5:83, 1976.

Compton, W. R., Lester, P. D., Kyaw, M. M., and Madsen, J. A.: The abdominal angiographic spectrum of tuberous sclerosis. AJR, 126:807, 1976.

Cooperman, L. R.: Delayed opacification in congenital multicystic dysplastic kidney, an important roentgen sign. Radiology, 121:703, 1976.

Cree, J. E.: Tuberous sclerosis with polycystic kidneys. Proc. R. Soc. Med., 62:327, 1969.

Cussen, L. J.: Cystic kidneys in children with congenital urethral obstruction. J. Urol., 106:939, 1971.

Dalgaard, O. Z.: Bilateral polycystic disease of the kidneys: A follow-up study of 284 patients and their families. Acta Med. Scand., 158 (Suppl. 328), 1–255, 1957.

Danovitch, G. M.: Clinical features and pathophysiology of polycystic kidney disease in man. In Gardner, K. D., Jr.: Cystic Diseases of the Kidney. New York, John Wiley & Sons, 1976, pp. 125–150.

Darmady, E. M., Offer, J., and Woodhouse, M. A.: Toxic metabolic defect in polycystic diseases of the kidney. Lancet, 1:547, 1970.

De Klerk, D. P., Marshall, F. F., and Jeffs, R. D.: Multicystic dysplastic kidney. J. Urol., 118:306, 1977.

Devine, C. J., Jr., Buttarazzi, P. J., Devine, P. C., Fiveash, J. G., Jr., and Poutasse, E. F.: Aspiration or exploration to confirm diagnoses of renal masses. JAMA, 204:758, 1968.

DeWeerd, J. H., and Simon, H. B.: Simple renal cysts in children. Review of the literature and report of five cases. J. Urol., 75:912, 1956.

DiSieno, A., and Guareschi, B.: Il quadro radiologico del rene a spugna midollare. Radiol. Clin., 25:80, 1956.

Dolder, E.: Niereninsuffizienz bei tuberose Sklerose (Morbus Bourneville). Schweiz. Med. Wochenschr., 105:406, 1975.

Dunnill, M. S., Millard, P. R., and Oliver, D.: Acquired cystic disease of the kidneys: a hazard of long-term intermittent maintenance haemodialysis. J. Clin. Pathol., 30:868, 1977.

Dupond, J. L., Miguet, J. P., Carbillet, J. P., Saint Hillier, Y., Perol, C., and Leconte des Floris, R.: Polykystose rénale, principale expression de la fibrose hépatique congénitale. 3 observations. Nouv. Presse Méd., 8:2885, 1979.

Editorial: Adult polycystic disease of the kidneys. Br. Med. J., 282:1097, 1981.

Eisendrath, D. N.: Clinical importance of congenital renal hypoplasia. J. Urol., 33:331, 1935.

Ekström, T.: Renal hypoplasia: A clinical study of 179 cases. Acta Chir. Scand., (Suppl. 203), 1–168, 1955.

Ekström, T., Engfeldt, B., Lagergren, C., and Lindvall, N.: Medullary Sponge Kidney. Stockholm, Almqvist and Wiksell, 1959.

Elkin, M., and Bernstein, J.: Cystic diseases of the kidney. Radiological and pathological considerations. Clin. Radiol., 20:65, 1969.

Engström, N., Ljungqvist, A., Persson, B., and Wetterfors, J.: Tuberous sclerosis with a localized angiomatous malformation in the ileum and excessive albumin loss into the lower intestinal tract. Report of a case. Pediatrics, 30:681, 1962.

Ericsson, N. O., and Ivemark, B. I.: Renal dysplasia and pyelonephritis in infants and children. Part I and Part II. Primitive ductules and abnormal glomeruli. Arch. Pathol., 66:255, 264, 1958.

Evan, A. P., Gardner, K. D., Jr., and Bernstein, J.: Polypoid and papillary epithelial hyperplasia: A potential cause of ductal obstruction in adult polycystic disease. Kidney Int., 16:743, 1979.

Fairley, K. F., Leighton, P. W., and Kincaid-Smith, P.: Familial visual defects associated with polycystic kidney and medullary sponge kidney. Br. Med. J., 5337:1060–1063, 1963.

Fanconi, V. G., Hanhart, E., Albertini, A., et al.: Die familiäre juvenile Nephronophthise (die idiopathische parenchymatöse Schrumpfniere). Helv. Paediatr. Acta, 6:1, 1951.

Fayemi, A. O., and Ali, M.: The pathology of end-stage renal disease in hemodialysis patients. Isr. J. Med. Sci., 15:901, 1979.

Fellows, R. A., Leonidas, J. C., and Beatty, E. C., Jr.: Radiologic features of "adult type" polycystic kidney disease in the neonate. Pediatr. Radiol., 4:87, 1976.

Felson, B., and Cussen, L. J.: The hydronephrotic type of unilateral congenital multicystic disease of the kidney. Semin. Roentgenol., 10:113, 1975.

Fill, W. L., Lamiell, J. M., and Polk, N. O.: The radiographic manifestations of von Hippel-Lindau disease. Radiology, 133:289, 1979.

Fitch, N., and Srolovitz, H.: Severe renal dysgenesis produced by a dominant gene. Am. J. Dis. Child., 130:1356, 1976.

Forbes, M.: Renal dysplasia in infants with neurospinal dysraphism. J. Pathol., 107:13, 1972.

Frimodt-Møller, P., Nissen, H. M., and Dyreborg, U.: Polycystic kidneys as the renal lesion in Lindau's disease. J. Urol., 125:868, 1981.

Gardner, K. D., Jr.: Composition of fluid in twelve cysts of a polycystic kidney. N. Engl. J. Med., 281:985, 1969.

Gardner, K. D., Jr.: Evolution of clinical signs in adult-onset cystic disease of the renal medulla. Ann. Intern. Med., 74:47, 1971.

Gardner, K. D., Jr.: Juvenile nephronophthisis and renal medullary cystic disease. In Gardner, K. D., Jr.: Cystic Diseases of the Kidney. New York, John Wiley & Sons, 1976, pp. 173–185.

Giangiacomo, J., Monteleone, P. L., and Witzleben, C. L.: Medullary cystic disease vs. nephronophthisis: A valid distinction. JAMA, 232:629, 1975.

Gleason, D. G., McAlister, W. H., and Kissane, J.: Cystic diseases of the kidney in children. Am. J. Roentegnol. Radium Ther. Nucl. Med., 100:135, 1967.

Goldstein, J. L., and Fialkow, P. J.: The Alström syndrome: Report of three cases with further delineation of the clinical, pathophysiological, and genetic aspects of the disorder. Medicine, 52:53, 1973.

Gonzalez-Angulo, A., Alford, B. R., and Greenberg, S. D.: Tuberous sclerosis. An otolaryngic diagnosis. Arch. Otolaryngol., 80:193, 1964.

Granberg, P. O., Lagergren, C., and Theve, N. O.: Renal

function studies in medullary sponge kidney. Scand. J. Urol. Nephrol., 5:177, 1971.

Greene, L. F., and Barrett, D. M.: Renal cystic disease: Radiologic appearance. *In* Gardner, K. D., Jr.: Cystic Diseases of the Kidney. New York, John Wiley & Sons, 1976, pp. 91–113.

Greene, L. F., Feinzaig, W., and Dahlin, D. C.: Multicystic dysplasia of the kidney: with special reference to the contralateral kidney. J. Urol., 105:482, 1971.

Grossman, H., and Seed, W.: Congenital hepatic fibrosis, bile duct dilatation and renal lesion resembling medullary sponge kidney. Congenital "cystic" disease of the liver and kidneys. Radiology, 87:46, 1966.

Gur, A., Siegel, N. J., Davis, C. A., Kashgarian, M., and Hayslett, J. P.: Clinical aspects of bilateral renal dysplasia in children. Nephron, 15:50, 1975.

Gutierrez, R.: Surgical aspects of renal agenesis: with special reference to hypoplastic kidney, renal aplasia, and congenital absence of one kidney. Arch. Surg., 27:686, 1933.

Gwinn, J. L., and Landing, B. H.: Cystic diseases of the kidneys in infants and children. Radiol. Clin. North Am., 6:191, 1968.

Habif, D. V., Jr., Berdon, W. E., and Yeh, M. -N.: Infantile polycystic kidney disease: *In utero* sonographic diagnosis. Radiology, 142:475, 1982.

Hamburger, J., Richet, G., Crosnier, J., et al. (Eds.): Nephrology. Philadelphia, W. B. Saunders Co., 1968, pp. 1087–1100.

Hartnett, M., and Bennett, W.: Extrarenal manifestations of cystic kidney disease. *In* Gardner, K. D., Jr.: Cystic Diseases of the Kidney. New York, John Wiley & Sons, 1976, pp. 201–219.

Hatfield, J. M., and Pfister, R. C.: Adult polycystic disease of the kidneys (Potter type III). JAMA, 222:1527, 1972.

Heggö, O., and Natvig, J. B.: Cystic disease of the kidneys. Autopsy report and family study. Acta Pathol. Microbiol. Scand., 61:459, 1965.

Henneberry, M. O., and Stephens, F. D.: Renal hypoplasia and dysplasia in infants with posterior urethral valves. J. Urol. 123:912, 1980.

Hestbech, J., Hansen, H. E., Amdisen, A., and Olsen, S.: Chronic renal lesions following long-term treatment with lithium. Kidney Int., 12:205, 1977.

Hinkel, C. L., and Santini, L. C.: Polycystic disease of kidney in infants: Nephrograms following intravenous urography. Am. J. Roentgenol. Radium Ther. Nucl. Med., 76:153, 1956.

Honey, R. J., and Honey, R. M.: Tuberose sclerosis and bilateral renal carcinoma. Br. J. Urol., 49:441, 1977.

Horton, W. A., Wong, V., and Eldridge, R.: von Hippel-Lindau disease. Clinical and pathological manifestations in nine families with 50 affected members. Arch. Intern. Med., 136:769, 1976.

Hughson, M. D., Hennigar, G. R., and McManus, J. F. A.: Atypical cysts, acquired renal cystic disease, and renal cell tumors in end stage dialysis kidneys. Lab. Invest., 42:475, 1980.

Hurley, R. M., Dery, P., Nogrady, M. B., et al.: The renal lesion of the Laurence-Moon-Biedl syndrome. J. Pediatr., 87(z):206, 1975.

Huseman, R., Grady, A., Welling, D., and Grantham, J.: Macropuncture study of polycystic disease in adult human kidneys. Kidney Int., 18:375, 1980.

Hutchins, K. R., Mulholland, S. G., and Edson, M.: Segmental polycystic disease. N.Y. State J. Med., 72:1850, 1972.

Isaac, F., Schoen, I., and Walker, P.: An unusual case of Lindau's disease: Cystic disease of the kidneys and pancreas with renal and cerebellar tumors. Am. J. Roentgenol. Radium Ther. Nucl. Med., 75:912, 1956.

Ishikawa, I., Saito, Y., Onouchi, Z., Kitada, H., Suzuki, S., Kurihara, S., Yuri, T., and Shinoda, A.: Development of acquired cystic disease and adenocarcinoma of the kidney in glomerulonephritic chronic hemodialysis patients. Clin. Nephrol., 14:1, 1980.

Jackman, R. J., and Stevens, G. M.: Benign hemorrhagic renal cysts. Radiology, 110:7, 1974.

Javadpour, N., Chelouhy, E., Moncada, L., Rosenthal, I. M., and Bush, I. M.: Hypertension in a child caused by a multicystic kidney. J. Urol., 104:918, 1970.

Johannessen, J. V., Haneberg, B., and Moe, P. J.: Bilateral multicystic dysplasia of the kidneys. Beitr. Pathol., 148:290, 1973.

Jørgensen, M.: A stereological study of intrahepatic bile ducts. 3. Infantile polycystic disease. Acta Pathol. Microbiol. Scand. (A), 81:670, 1973.

Jørgensen, M.: A stereological study of intrahepatic bile ducts. 4. Congenital hepatic fibrosis. Acta Pathol. Microbiol. Scand (A), 82:21, 1974.

Kaplan, B. S., Rabin, I., Nogrady, M. B., and Drummond, K. N.: Autosomal dominant polycystic renal disease in children. J. Pediatr., 90:782, 1977.

Kawamura, J. Sawanishi, K., Miyake, Y., and Nishio, T.: Bourneville-Pringle phacomatosis with striking renal abnormality: Report of a case of four-year-old boy. Acta Urol. Jap., 15:91, 1969.

Kerr, D. N. S., Okonkwo, S., and Choa, R. G.: Congenital hepatic fibrosis: the long-term prognosis. Gut, 19:514, 1978.

Kerr, D. N. S., Warrick, C. K., and Hart-Mercer, J.: A lesion resembling medullary sponge kidney in patients with congenital hepatic fibrosis. Clin. Radiol., 13:85, 1962.

Kossow, A. S., and Meek, J. M.: Unilateral adult polycystic kidney disease. J. Urol., 127:297, 1982.

Krempien, B., and Ritz, E.: Acquired cystic transformation of the kidneys of haemodialysed patients. Virchows Arch. (Pathol. Anat.), 386:189, 1980.

Kuiper, J. J.: Medullary sponge kidney. *In* Gardner, K. D., Jr.: Cystic Diseases of the Kidney. New York, John Wiley & Sons, 1976, pp. 151–171.

Kyaw, M. M.: Roentgenologic triad of congenital multicystic kidney. Am. J. Roentgenol. Radium Ther. Nucl. Med., 119:710, 1973.

Lalli, A. F.: Percutaneous aspiration of renal masses. Am. J. Roentgenol. Radium Ther. Nucl. Med., 101:700, 1967.

Lambert, P.: Polycystic disease of the kidney: A review. Arch. Pathol., 44:34, 1947.

Landing, B. H., Wells, T. R., and Claireaux, A. E.: Morphometric analysis of liver lesions in cystic diseases of childhood. Hum. Pathol., 11:549, 1980.

Landing, B. H., Wells, T. R., Reed, G. B., and Narayan, M. S.: Diseases of the bile ducts in children. Chap. 22. *In* Gall, E. A., and Mostofi, F. K. (Eds.): The Liver. Baltimore, Williams & Wilkins Co., 1973.

Lang, E. K.: Coexistence of cyst and tumor in the same kidney. Radiology, 101:7, 1971.

Lang, E. K., Johnson, B., Chance, H. L., Enright, J. R., Fontenot, R., Trichel, B. E., Wood, M., Brown, M., and St. Martin, E. C.: Assessment of avascular renal mass lesions: The use of nephrotomography, arteriography, cyst puncture, double contrast study and histochemical and histopathologic examination of the aspirate. South. Med. J., 65:1, 1972.

Lathrop, D. B.: Cystic disease of the liver and kidney. Pediatrics, 24:215, 1959.

Laucks, S. P., Jr., and McLachlan, M. S. F.: Aging and simple cysts of the kidney. Br. J. Radiol., 54:12, 1981.

Lee, J. K. T., McClennan, B. L., and Kissane, J. M.: Unilateral polycystic kidney disease. AJR, 130:1165, 1978.

Lee, K. R., Wulfsberg, E., and Kepes, J. J.: Some important radiological aspects of the kidney in Hippel-Lindau syndrome: The value of prospective study in an affected family. Radiology, *122*:649, 1977.

Legarth J., Verder, H., and Grønvall, S.: Prenatal diagnosis of multicystic kidney by ultrasound. Acta Obstet. Gynecol. Scand., *60*:523, 1981.

Lenarduzzi, G.: Reporto pielografico poco commune dilatazione della vie urinarie intrarenali. Radiol. Med. (Torino), *26*:346, 1939.

Leonidas, J. C., Strauss, L., and Krasna, I. H.: Roentgen diagnosis of multicystic renal dysplasia in infancy by high dose urography. J. Urol., *108*:963, 1972.

Levin, N. W., Rosenberg, B., Zwi, S., et al.: Medullary cystic disease of the kidney with some observations on ammonium excretion. Am. J. Med., *30*:807, 1961.

Levine, A. S., and Michael, A. F.: Ehlers-Danlos syndrome with renal tubular acidosis and medullary sponge kidney. J. Pediatr., *71*:107, 1967.

Levine, E., Collins, D. L., Horton, W. A., and Schimke, R. N.: CT screening of the abdomen in von Hippel-Lindau disease. AJR, *139*:505, 1982.

Levine, E., Lee, K. R., Weigel, J. W., and Farber, B.: Computed tomography in the diagnosis of renal carcinoma complicating Hippel-Lindau syndrome. Radiology, *130*:703, 1979.

Levine, S. R., Witten, D. M., and Greene, L. F.: Nephrotomography in Lindau-von Hippel's disease. J. Urol., *93*:660, 1965.

Lieberman, E., Salinas-Madrigal, L., Gwinn, J. L., Brennan, L. P., Fine, R. N., and Landing, B. H.: Infantile polycystic disease of the kidneys and liver: Clinical, pathological and radiological correlations and comparison with congenital hepatic fibrosis. Medicine, *50*:277, 1971.

Lindau, A.: Studien Über Kleinhirncysten. Bau, Pathogenese und Beziehungen zur Angiomatosis retinae. Acta Pathol. Microbiol. Scand. (Suppl. 1) 1–128, 1926.

Lindsey, J. R.: Lymphangiectasia simulating polycystic disease. J. Urol., *104*:658, 1970.

Ljungqvist, A.: Arterial vasculature of the multicystic dysplastic kidney: A micro-angiographical and histological study. Acta Pathol. Microbiol. Scand., *64*:309, 1965.

Lundin, P., and Olow, I.: Polycystic kidneys in newborns, infants and children. A clinical and pathological study. Acta Paediatr., *50*:185, 1961.

Mackie, G. G., and Stephens, F. D.: Duplex kidneys: A correlation of renal dysplasia with position of the ureteral orifice. J. Urol., *114*:274, 1975.

Malek, R. S., and Greene, L. F.: Urologic aspects of von Hippel-Lindau syndrome. J. Urol., *106*:800, 1974.

Marshall, A. G.: The persistence of foetal structures in pyelonephritic kidneys. Br. J. Surg., *41*:38, 1953.

Martinez-Maldonado, M., Yium, J. J., Eknoyan, G., and Suki, W. N.: Adult polycystic kidney disease: Studies of the defect in urine concentration. Kidney Int., *2*:107, 1972.

Mauseth, R., Lieberman, E., and Heuser, E. T.: Infantile polycystic disease of the kidneys and Ehlers-Danlos syndrome in an 11-year-old patient. J. Pediatr., *90*:81, 1977.

McAlister, W. H., Siegel, M. J., Shackelford, G., Askin, F., and Kissane, J. M.: Glomerulocystic kidney. AJR, *133*:536, 1979.

McClennan, B. L., Stanley, R. J., Melson, G. L., Levitt, R. G., and Sagel, S. S.: CT of the renal cyst: Is cyst aspiration necessary? AJR, *133*:671, 1979.

McGonigle, R. J. S., Mowat, A. P., Bewick, M., Howard, E. R., Snowden, S. A., and Parsons, V.: Congenital hepatic fibrosis and polycystic kidney disease; role of porta-caval shunting and transplantation in three patients. Q. J. Med., *50*:269, 1981.

McManus, J. F. A., and Hughson, M. D.: Studies on end-stage kidneys. V. Unusual epithelial activity or remarkable endothelial metaplasia. Findings in a dialyzed kidney. Am. J. Surg. Pathol., *3*:229, 1979.

Melicow, M. M., and Becker, J. R.: Radiographic simulation of certain solid tumors of the renal corpus to renal cysts. J. Urol., *97*:592, 1967.

Melmon, K. L., and Rosen, S. W.: Lindau's disease. Review of the literature and study of a large kindred. Am. J. Med., *36*:595, 1964.

Mena, E., Bookstein, J. J., McDonald, F. D., et al.: Angiographic findings in renal medullary cystic disease. Radiology, *110*:277, 1974.

Mitnick, J. S., Bosniak, M. A., Hilton, S., Raghavendra, B. N., Subramanyam, B., and Genieser, N. B.: Cystic renal disease in tuberous sclerosis. Radiology. In press.

Milutinovic, J., Fialkow, P. J., Phillips, L. A., et al.: Autosomal dominant polycystic kidney disease: early diagnosis and data for genetic counselling. Lancet, *1*:1203, 1980.

Murray-Lyon, I. M., Ockenden, B. G., and Williams, R.: Congenital hepatic fibrosis—is it a single clinical entity? Gastroenterology, *64*:653, 1973.

Murray-Lyon, I. M., Shilkin, K. B., Laws, J. W., Illing, R. C., and Williams, R.: Non-obstructive dilatation of the intrahepatic biliary tree with cholangitis. Q. J. Med., *41*:477, 1972.

Muther, R. S., and Bennett, W. M.: Cyst fluid antibiotic concentrations in polycystic kidney disease: Differences between proximal and distal cysts. Kidney Int., *20*:519, 1981.

Nation, E. F.: Renal aplasia: A study of sixteen cases. J. Urol., *51*:579, 1944.

Newman, L., McAlister, W. H., and Kissane, J.: Segmental renal dysplasia associated with ectopic ureteroceles in childhood. Urology, *3*:23, 1974.

Newman, L., Simms, K., Kissane, J., and McAlister, W. H.: Unilateral total renal dysplasia in children. Am. J. Roentgenol. Radium Ther. Nucl. Med., *116*:778, 1972.

O'Callaghan, T. J., Edwards, J. A., Tobin, M., and Mookerjee, B. K.: Tuberous sclerosis with striking renal involvement in a family. Arch. Intern. Med., *135*:1082, 1975.

Odièvre, M., Chaumont, P., Montagne, J. P., and Alagille, D.: Anomalies of the intrahepatic portal venous system in congenital hepatic fibrosis. Radiology, *122*:427, 1977.

Okada, R. D., Platt, M. A., and Fleishman, J.: Chronic renal failure in patients with tuberous sclerosis: association with renal cysts. Nephron, *30*:85, 1982.

Older, R. A., Hinman, C. G., Crane, L. M., Cleeve, D. M., and Morgan, C. L.: In utero diagnosis of multicystic kidney by gray scale ultrasonography. AJR, *133*:130, 1979.

O'Neill, M., Breslau, N. A., and Pak, C. Y. C.: Metabolic evaluation of nephrolithiasis in patients with medullary sponge kidney. JAMA, *245*:1233, 1981.

Osathanondh, V., and Potter, E. L.: Pathogenesis of polycystic kidneys. Survey of results of microdissection. Arch. Pathol., *77*:510, 1964a.

Osathanondh, V., and Potter, E. L.: Pathogenesis of polycystic kidneys. Type 3 due to multiple abnormalities of development. Arch. Pathol., *77*:485, 1964b.

Osathanondh, V., and Potter, E. L.: Pathogenesis of polycystic kidneys. Type 1 due to hyperplasia of interstitial portions of collecting tubules. Arch. Pathol., *77*:466, 1964c.

Parkkulainen, , V., Hjelt, L., and Sirola, K.: Congenital multicystic dysplasia of the kidney: Report of 19 cases with discussion on the etiology, nomenclature, and classification of cystic dysplasia of the kidney. Acta Chir. Scand., (Suppl. 244), 1–46, 1959.

Parks, J. H., Coe, F. L., and Strauss, A. L.: Calcium

nephrolithiasis and medullary sponge kidney in women. N. Engl. J. Med., *306*:1088, 1982.

Pascal, R. R.: Medullary cystic disease of the kidney: Study of a case with scanning and transmission electron microscopy and light microscopy. Am. J. Clin. Pathol., *59*:659, 1973.

Pasternack, A.: Microscopic structural changes in macroscopically normal and pyelonephritic kidneys of children. Ann. Paediatr. Fenn., *6* (Suppl. 14), 1–88, 1960.

Pathak, I. G., and Williams, D. I.: Multicystic and cystic dysplastic kidneys. Br. J. Urol., *36*:318, 1964.

Pearson, J. C., Weiss, J., and Tanagho, E. A.: A plea for conservation of kidney in renal adenocarcinoma associated with von Hippel-Lindau disease. J. Urol., *124*:910, 1980.

Perrin, E. V., Persky, L., Tucker, A., and Chrenka, B.: Renal duplication and dysplasia. Urology, *4*:660, 1974.

Potter, E. L., and Osathanondh, V.: Medullary sponge kidney. J. Pediatr., *62*:901, 1963.

Proesmans, W., Van Damme B., Casaer P., and Marchal, G.: Autosomal dominant polycystic kidney disease in the neonatal period: Association with a cerebral arteriovenous malformation. Pediatrics, *70*:971, 1982.

Pyrah, L. N.: Medullary sponge kidney. J. Urol., *95*:274, 1966.

Rall, J. E., and Odel, H. M.: Congenital polycystic disease of the kidney: Review of the literature and data on 207 cases. Am. J. Med. Sci., *218*:399, 1949.

Rattner, W. H., Meyer, R., and Bernstein, J.: Vaginal ureteral ectopy. J. Pediatr., *57*:579, 1960.

Rattner, W. H., Meyer, R., and Bernstein, J.: Congenital abnormalities of the urinary system. IV. Valvular obstruction of posterior urethra. J. Pediatr., *63*:84, 1963.

Rayfield, E. J., and McDonald, F. D.: Red and blond hair in renal medullary cystic disease. Arch. Intern. Med., *130*:72, 1972.

Reilly, B. J., and Neuhauser, E. B. D.: Renal tubular ectasia in cystic disease of the kidneys and liver. Am. J. Roentgenol. Radium Ther. Nucl. Med., *84*:546, 1960.

Richards, R. D., Mebust, W. K., and Schimke, R. N.: A prospective study on von Hippel-Lindau disease. J. Urol., *110*:27, 1973.

Richmond, J. M., Kincaid-Smith, P., Whitworth, J. A., and Becker, G. J.: Familial urate nephropathy. Clin. Nephrol., *16*:163, 1981.

Risdon, R. A.: Renal dysplasia. Part. I. A clinicopathological study of 76 cases. Part II. A necropsy study of 41 cases. J. Clin. Pathol., *24*:57, 1971.

Risdon, R. A.: Renal dysplasia and associated abnormalities of the urinary tract. *In* Rubin, M. I., and Barratt, T. M.: Pediatric Nephrology. Baltimore, Williams & Wilkins Co., 1975, p. 346.

Risdon, R. A., Young, L. W., and Chrispin, A. R.: Renal hypoplasia and dysplasia: A radiological and pathological correlation. Pediatr. Radiol., *3*:213, 1975.

Rosenberg, J. C., Bernstein, J., and Rosenberg, B.: Renal cystic disease associated with tuberous sclerosis complex: Renal failure treated by cadaveric kidney transplantation. Clin. Nephrol., *4*:109, 1975.

Rosenfield, A. T., Siegel, N. J., Kappelman, N. B., Taylor, K. J. W.: Gray scale ultrasonography in medullary cystic disease of the kidney and congenital hepatic fibrosis with tubular ectasia: New observations. AJR, *129*:297, 1977.

Rothermel, F. J., Miller, F. J., Jr., Sanford, E., Drago, J., and Rohner, T. J.: Clinical and radiographic findings of focally infected polycystic kidneys. Urology, *9*:580, 1977.

Rubenstein, M., Meyer, R., and Bernstein, J.: Congenital abnormalities of the urinary system. I. A postmortem survey of developmental anomalies and acquired congenital lesions in a children's hospital. J. Pediatr. *58*:356, 1961.

Saxton, H. M., Golding, S. J., Chantler, C., and Haycock, G. D.: Diagnostic puncture in renal cystic dysplasia (multicystic kidney). Evidence on the aetiology of the cysts. Br. J. Radiol., *54*:555, 1981.

Schechterman, L.: Lindau's disease. Report of an unusual case and two additional cases in a Negro family. Med. Ann. D. C., *30*:64, 1961.

Schimke, R. N.: Hereditary renal-retinal dysplasia. Ann. Intern. Med., *70*:735, 1969.

Schimke, R. N., and King, C. R.: Hereditary urogenital adysplasia. Clin. Genet., *18*:417, 1980.

Schulman, C. C.: Fehlbildung des Ureters und Nierendysplasia—eine embryologische Hypothese. Urologe (A), *17*:273, 1978.

Schwartz, J.: An unusual unilateral multicystic kidney in an infant. J. Urol., *35*:259, 1936.

Schwarz, R. D., Stephens, F. D., and Cussen, L. J.: The pathogenesis of renal dysplasia. II. The significance of lateral and medial ectopy of the ureteric orifice. Invest. Urol., *19*:97, 1981.

Sellers, A. L., Winfield, A., and Rosen, V.: Unilateral polycystic kidney disease. J. Urol., *107*:527, 1972.

Senior, B.: Familial renal-retinal dystrophy. Am. J. Dis. Child. *125*:442, 1973.

Sherman, F. E., Studnicki, F. M., and Fetterman, G. H.: Renal lesions of familial juvenile nephronophthisis examined by microdissection. Am. J. Clin. Pathol., *55*:391, 1971.

Shokeir, M. H. K.: Expression of "adult" polycystic renal disease in the fetus and newborn. Clin. Genet., *14*:61, 1978.

Siegel, M. J., and McAlister, W. H.: Simple cysts of the kidney in children. J. Urol., *123*:75, 1980.

Simon, H. B., and Thompson, G. J.: Congenital renal polycystic disease: A clinical and therapeutic study of three hundred sixty-six cases. JAMA, *159*:657, 1955.

Six, R., Oliphant, M., and Grossman, H.: A spectrum of renal tubular ectasia and hepatic fibrosis. Radiology, *117*:117, 1975.

Sommerkamp, H.: Nierencysten: Diagnostik und Operationsbefunde. Urologe (A), *9*:314, 1970.

Sogbein, S. K., Moors, D. E., and Jindal, S. L.: A case of bilateral renal cell carcinoma in polycystic kidneys. Can. J. Surg., *24*:193, 1981.

Spence, H. M.: Congenital unilateral multicystic kidney: An entity to be distinguished from polycystic kidney disease and other cystic disorders. J. Urol., *74*:693, 1955.

Spence, H. M., and Singleton, R.: Cysts and cystic disorders of the kidney: Types, diagnosis, treatment. Urol. Surv., *22*:131, 1972a.

Spence, H. M., and Singleton, R.: What is sponge kidney and where does it fit in the spectrum of cystic disorders? J. Urol., *107*:176, 1972b.

Sprayregen, S., Strasberg, A., and Naidich, T. P.: Medullary sponge kidney and congenital total hemihypertrophy. N. Y. State J. Med., *73*:2768, 1973.

Stapleton, F. B., Bernstein, J., Koh, G., Roy, S., III, and Wilroy, R. S.: Cystic kidneys in a patient with oral-facial-digital syndrome type I. Am. J. Kidney Dis., *1*(5):288, 1982.

Stapleton, F. B., Johnson, D., Kaplan, G. W., and Griswold, W.: The cystic renal lesion in tuberous sclerosis. J. Pediatr., *97*:574, 1980.

Stella, F. J., Massry, S. G., and Kleeman, C. R.: Medullary sponge kidney associated with parathyroid adenoma. Nephron, *10*:332, 1973.

Stickler, G. B., and Kelalis, P. P.: Polycystic kidney disease. Recognition of the "adult form" (autosomal dominant) in infancy. Mayo Clin. Proc., *50*:547, 1975.

Strauss, M. B.: Clinical and pathological aspects of cystic disease of renal medulla. Ann. Intern. Med., *57*:373, 1962.

Stuck, K. J., Koff, S. A., and Silver, T. M.: Ultrasonic features of multicystic dysplastic kidney: Expanded diagnostic criteria. Radiology, *143*:217, 1982.

Suslavich, F., Older, R. A., and Hinman, C. G.: Calcified renal carcinoma in a patient with tuberous sclerosis. AJR. *133*:524, 1979.

Taxy, J. B., and Filmer, R. B.: Metaplastic cartilage in nondysplastic kidneys. Arch. Pathol., *99*:101, 1975.

Taxy, J. B., and Filmer, R. B.: Glomerulocystic kidney. Report of a case. Arch. Pathol. Lab. Med., *100*:186, 1976.

Thaler, M. M., Ogata, E. S., Goodman, J. R., Piel, C. F., and Korobkin, M. T.: Congenital fibrosis and polycystic disease of liver and kidneys. Am. J. Dis. Child., *126*:374, 1973.

Thornbury, J. R.: Needle aspiration of avascular renal lesions. Correlation of contrast medium injection with cytologic and arteriographic diagnosis. Radiology, *105*:299, 1972.

Unite, I., Maitem, A., Bagnasco, F. M., and Irwin, G. A. L.: Congenital hepatic fibrosis associated with renal tubular ectasia. Radiology, *109*:565, 1973.

Vellios, F., and Garrett, R. A.: Congenital unilateral multicystic disease of the kidney: A clinical and anatomic study of 7 cases. Am. J. Clin. Pathol., *35*:244, 1961.

Viamonte, M., Jr., Ravel, R., Politano, V., and Bridges, B.: Angiographic findings in a patient with tuberous sclerosis. Am. J. Roentgenol Radium Ther. Nucl. Med., *98*:723, 1966.

Virchow, R.: Discussion über den Vortrag des Herrn A. Ewald: Zur totalen cystischen Degeneration der Nieren. Klin. Wochenschr., *29*:104, 1892.

Voth, D.: Zur Genese des hyalinen Knorpelgewebes in hypoplastischen Nieren. Zentralbl. Allg. Pathol., *102*:554, 1961.

Vuthibhagdee, A., and Singleton, E. B.: Infantile polycystic disease of the kidney. Am. J. Dis. Child., *125*:167, 1973.

Weinberg, S. R., O'Connor, W. J., and Senger, F. L.: Unilateral multicystic renal diseases of the newborn. Am. J. Dis. Child., *92*:576, 1956.

Weiss, L., Reynolds, W. A., Saeed, S. M., and Cabal, L.: Congenital hepatic fibrosis and polycystic disease of kidneys with the roentgen appearance of medullary sponge kidney. *In* Bergsma, D. (Ed.): The Fifth Conference on the Clinical Delineation of Birth Defects. Birth Defects: Original Article Series, *10*:22, 1974. Baltimore, Williams & Wilkins Co.

Wenzl, J. E., Lagos, J. C., and Albers, D. D.: Tuberous sclerosis presenting as polycystic kidneys and seizures in an infant. J. Pediatr., *77*:673, 1970.

Wesolowski, D. P., Ellwood, R. A., Schwab, R. E., and Farah, J.: Hippel-Lindau syndrome in identical twins. Br. J. Radiol., *54*:982, 1981.

Whelton, A., Ozer, F. L., Bias, W., et al.: Renal medullary cystic disease: A family study. *In* Bergsma, D. (Ed.): The Fifth Conference on the Clinical Delineation of Birth Defects. Birth Defects: Original Article Series, *10*:154, 1974. Baltimore, Williams & Wilkins Co.

Yendt, E. R.: Medullary sponge kidney and nephrolithiasis. N. Engl. J. Med., *306*:1106, 1982.

Young, L. W., Wood, B. P., Spohr, C. H., et al.: Delayed excretory urographic opacification, a puddling effect in multicystic renal dysplasia. Ann. Radiol. (Paris), *17*:391, 1973.

Zachrisson, L.: Simple renal cysts treated with bismuth phosphate at the diagnostic puncture. Acta Radiol. (Diagn.), *23*:209, 1982.

Zerres, K., Weiss, H., Bulla, M., and Roth, B.: Prenatal diagnosis of an early manifestation of autosomal dominant adult-type polycystic kidney disease. Lancet, *2*:988, 1982.

CHAPTER 40

Embryology of the Genital Tract

FREDRICK W. GEORGE, Ph.D.
JEAN D. WILSON, M.D.

INTRODUCTION

Sexual differentiation is a sequential process beginning with the establishment of chromosomal sex at fertilization, followed by the development of gonadal sex, and culminating with the development of secondary sex characteristics, collectively termed the male and female phenotypes (Fig. 40–1). Each step in this process is dependent on the preceding one, and under normal circumstances the chromosomal sex established at fertilization dictates gonadal development, and hence, the sexual phenotype of the embryo (Jost, 1953, 1972). The process of phenotypic sexual differentiation does not begin immediately following fertilization, however, and the phenotypic development of male and female urogenital tracts in human embryos is identical prior to 6 weeks of gestational age. Only thereafter does anatomic and physiologic development diverge to result in the formation of the male and female phenotypes. Although most aspects of this process are completed by the end of the first trimester, certain functional and structural aspects of sexual development, including maturation of the genital tract and gonads, are not completed until postnatal life.

There is probably no process of embryonic development that is understood as well as sexual differentiation. This is due to the fact that normal sexual development, unlike most other developmental processes, is not essential to the life of the individual. Consequently, a variety of naturally occurring disorders of sexual development are available for systematic study. These aberrations of sexual development occur at many levels and lead to clinical consequences that range from common defects involving the terminal stages of male development (cryptorchidism and microphallus) to more fundamental abnormalities involving hormone formation and action that result in various conditions of intersex.

In this chapter, attention is directed first to the sequence of the anatomic events (Fig. 40–2) and then to the regulatory factors that control sexual differentiation. It should be recognized that complete sexual development involves the maturation of functional, as well as anatomic, processes. The former—which include the development of gender identity, the regulation of gonadotropin secretion by the hypothalamic-pituitary system, and certain aspects of behavior—are not considered here.

SEXUAL DIFFERENTIATION

DEVELOPMENT OF CHROMOSOMAL SEX

Chromosomal sex is established at the moment of fertilization. If the fertilizing sperm contains an X chromosome, the zygote will be 46,XX—the genotype of the female; if the successful sperm carries a Y chromosome, the 46,XY karyotype that is characteristic of the male will result. It is important to note, however, that genes that are essential for normal male development are also located on the X chromosome and that genes that are essential to the development of both the male and female phenotypes are located on the autosomes. Consequently, the process of sexual differentiation is more correctly viewed as the result of interactions between genes on the autosomes and

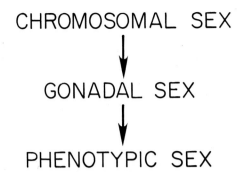

Figure 40–1. Successive events of sexual differentiation.

genetic determinants on the X and Y chromosomes, rather than as the sole consequence of the sex chromosome composition. The complexity of the system is emphasized by the fact that at least 19 genes are involved in sex determination in humans (Wilson and Goldstein, 1975).

DEVELOPMENT OF GONADAL SEX

The genital ridges (the anlage of the gonads) are formed by proliferation of the coe-lomic epithelium and condensation of the underlying mesenchyme on each side of the midline between the primitive kidney (mesonephros) and the dorsal mesentery. These genital ridges are initially devoid of germ cells. During the first 3 weeks of gestation, the germ cells are located in the endoderm of the yolk sac near the allantoic evagination (Witschi, 1948; Peters, 1970) (Fig. 40–3). Shortly thereafter, the germ cells leave the primitive gut and migrate by ameboid movement through the mesentery to the genital ridges. The fact that the germ cells migrate by pseudopodal movement to a specific location in the embryo suggests that the migration is directed by a chemotactic factor (McCarrey and Abbott, 1979). During the migration, the germ cells steadily increase in number by means of mitotic division. Late in the fifth week of gestation, when germ cell migration is completed, the gonads of the male and female embryo are indistinguishable and are composed of three principal cell types: (1) germ cells, (2) supporting cells that are derived from the coelomic epithelium of the genital ridge and that

APPROXIMATE TIME AFTER FERTILIZATION		DEVELOPMENTAL PROCESS		
WEEKS	**TRIMESTER**	**MALE**	**INDIFFERENT**	**FEMALE**
3	First		• GERM CELLS BEGIN MIGRATION	
3.5-4.5			• WOLFFIAN DUCT APPEARS AS PRONEPHRIC DUCT	
5-6			• INDIFFERENT GONADS DEVELOP ON GENITAL RIDGES • MAMMARY LINES PRESENT	
6-7		• APPEARANCE OF TESTICULAR CORDS	• MULLERIAN DUCT DEVELOPMENT BEGINS	
7			• FORMATION OF UROGENITAL SINUS BEGINS	
7.5			• UROGENITAL TUBERCLE AND SWELLINGS COMPLETE • URETHRAL FOLD AND GROOVE COMPLETE	
9		• SERTOLI CELLS APPARENT • MULLERIAN DUCT REGRESSION BEGINS	• UROGENITAL SINUS, MULLERIAN AND WOLFFIAN DUCTS COMPLETE INDIFFERENT DEVELOPMENT	• FORMATION OF VAGINAL PLATE BEGINS • UTERINE DEVELOPMENT COMMENCES
9-10		• LEYDIG CELLS APPEAR IN TESTIS • ONSET OF TESTOSTERONE SYNTHESIS	• MULLERIAN DUCTS ATTACHED TO MULLERIAN TUBERCLE WITHOUT PENETRATING • WOLFFIAN DUCTS OPEN LATERALLY INTO UROGENITAL SINUS	
9-11		• LENGTHENING OF UROGENITAL DISTANCE • FUSION OF LABIO SCROTAL SWELLINGS • GROWTH OF WOLFFIAN DUCTS		
10		• FORMATION OF PROSTATE BEGINS		• CAUDAL FLEXION OF THE GENITAL TUBERCLE BEGINS
11		• MULLERIAN REGRESSION COMPLETE		• REGRESSION OF WOLFFIAN DUCT BEGINS • GERM CELLS ENTER MEIOSIS • CANALIZATION OF VAGINAL PLATE BEGINS
12-13	Second	• FORMATION OF SEMINAL VESICLES		
13-16		• FORMATION OF PROCESSUS VAGINALIS		
15		• PREPUCE FORMATION COMPLETE		• FOLLICLE FORMATION IN OVARY BEGINS
17		• TESTIS COMES TO REST AGAINST ANTERIOR ABDOMINAL WALL		• UTERINE DEVELOPMENT COMPLETE • VAGINAL DEVELOPMENT COMPLETE
28-37	Third	• TRUE TESTICULAR DESCENT BEGINS • GROWTH OF EXTERNAL GENITALIA		

Figure 40–2. Approximate sequence of events in sexual differentiation. (Data compiled from several sources, including Jirasek, J. E.: Development of the Genital System and Male Pseudohermaphroditism, Baltimore, Johns Hopkins Press, 1971; Koff, A. K.: Carnegie Contributions to Embryology No. 140, *24*:59–90, 1933; and Gillman, J.: Carnegie Contributions to Embryology, No. 210, *32*:83–131, 1948.)

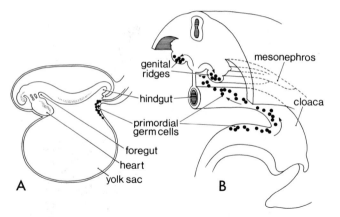

Figure 40–3. *A,* Schematic drawing showing the site of origin of the germ cells in the wall of the yolk sac in a 3-week-old embryo. *B,* Migratory path of the primordial germ cells along the wall of the yolk sac and dorsal mesentery and into the genital ridges. (After Langman, J.: Medical Embryology: Human Development—Normal and Abnormal. 4th ed. Baltimore, Williams & Wilkins Co., 1981.)

differentiate either into the Sertoli cells of the testis or the granulosa cells of the ovary, and (3) stromal (interstitial) cells derived from the mesenchyme of the gonadal ridge. Beginning during the seventh week of gestation, the testis in the human male embryo undergoes rapid development, commencing with the differentiation of the seminiferous tubules, followed by the appearance of interstitial cells and the onset of endocrine function at 8 weeks (see Fig. 40–2) (Gillman, 1948).

During this period, the fetal ovaries grow, but they do not undergo striking histologic changes from the indifferent state. Cells corresponding to those in the testis, which undergo organization into the primordial seminiferous tubules, multiply in the ovary, but characteristic follicular development is not apparent. Later, at approximately 11 weeks of gestation, the germ cells in the ovary become grouped and enter meiosis. The germ cells then become surrounded by follicular cells, and by approximately 15 weeks histologic development of a definitive ovary with follicles and stroma commences, some 8 weeks after the initiation of testicular differentiation in the human male fetus (see Fig. 40–2) (Gillman, 1948; Gondos et al., 1971).

Although the mechanisms that control the differentiation of the indifferent gonad into an ovary or testis are poorly understood, studies of a male-specific cell surface histocompatibility antigen have provided a working model for gonadal differentiation (Silvers and Wachtel, 1977; Ohno, 1979; Wachtel, 1980, 1983). According to this model the expression of a male specific (H-Y) antigen or antigens is dictated by a gene or genes on the Y chromosome. The antigen is expressed by virtually all tissues of the male (Gasser and Silvers, 1972), and in some types of cells the antigen becomes an-

chored in the cell membrane in association with β_2-microglobulin (Beutler et al., 1978). Cells of the developing ovary and testis have receptors for H-Y antigen that are distinct from the membrane anchorage site (Muller et al., 1978), and the presence of H-Y antigen in the male is believed to act via these receptors to organize the cells of the fetal testis into characteristic tubules (Ohno et al., 1978; Zenzes et al., 1978). Despite the powerful explanatory potential of this model for understanding testicular differentiation, it is now clear that several male-specific antigens exist, and there is no invariable relationship between the presence of a given antigen and the development of a testis (Silvers et al., 1982). Furthermore, in humans, the presence of the H-Y antigen does not always correlate with testicular formation (Jones et al., 1979). Consequently, additional work will be required before the validity of the theory can be established.

DEVELOPMENT OF PHENOTYPIC SEX

The internal accessory organs of reproduction in both sexes, as well as the renal collecting ducts, are derived from the mesonephric kidney system (Fig. 40–4). The mesonephric kidney develops from intermediate mesoderm during the fourth week of gestation in the human embryo. Within the substance of the mesonephros, tubules form that connect primitive capillary networks with a longitudinal mesonephric (or wolffian) duct. Caudally, the wolffian duct empties into the primitive urogenital sinus. An outgrowth of the dorsomedial wall of the wolffian duct (the ureteric bud) gives rise to the excretory ducts and collecting tubules of the metanephric (permanent) kidney. At approximately 6 weeks, the development of the paramesonephric, or müllerian, duct commences in embryos of both sexes as an evagination in the

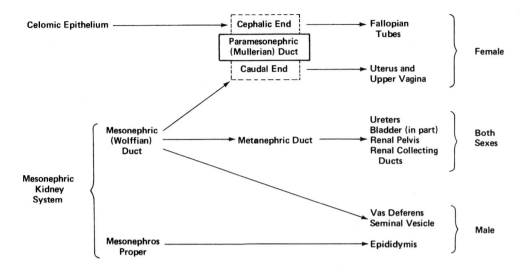

Figure 40–4. Role of the mesonephric kidney system and coelomic epithelium in the development of the urogenital tract. (From Griffin, J. E., Edwards, C., Madden, J. D., Harrod, M. J., and Wilson, J. D.: Ann. Intern. Med., *85*:224–236, 1976. Used by permission.)

coelomic epithelium just lateral to the mesonephros proper. This evagination develops into a tubular structure, the caudal end of which becomes intimately connected with the wolffian duct so that no basement membrane separates their epithelia (Fig. 40–5). Whether the müllerian duct "splits off" from the wolffian duct in its later caudal development to become an in-

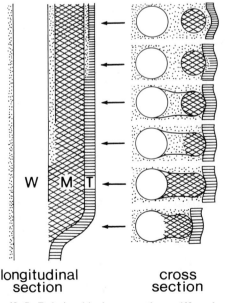

Figure 40–5. Relationship between the wolffian duct and the developing müllerian duct at about 8 weeks of development. The level of each cross section is indicated by an arrow. M, müllerian duct; T, tubal ridge; W, wolffian duct. The mesenchyme is stippled. (After Gruenwald, P.: Anat. Rec., *81*:1–19, 1941.)

dependent duct system that empties into the urogenital sinus or whether the wolffian duct simply acts as a guide for the subsequent evolution of the müllerian duct from the coelomic epithelium is uncertain. However, müllerian duct development cannot take place in the absence of the wolffian duct (Gruenwald, 1941). Thus, at the end of the indifferent phase of phenotypic sexual development (prior to 6 weeks), a dual duct system (wolffian and müllerian) constitutes the anlagen of the internal accessory organs of reproduction (Fig. 40–6).

The termination of the mesonephric ducts in the urogenital sinus divides the sinus into an upper and a lower portion. The upper portion, the vesicourethral canal, is involved in the development of the bladder and the upper urethra. The lower portion contributes to the development of the external genitalia. Prior to 6 weeks of gestation, the anlagen of the external genitalia are indistinguishable in the two sexes. The genital eminence is a rounded mass between the umbilical cord and the tail (Spaulding, 1921). This eminence is composed of a genital tubercle that is flanked by prominent genital swellings. The opening of the urogenital sinus between the genital swellings (the urethral groove) is surrounded by genital folds (Fig. 40–7). At 7 weeks of gestation the genital tubercle begins to elongate, and a shallow circular depression defines the glans of the tubercle. At this stage of development there are no remarkable differences between the external genitalia of male and female embryos.

Male Development. The initial event in

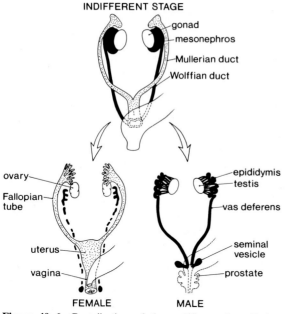

INDIFFERENT STAGE

gonad
mesonephros
Mullerian duct
Wolffian duct

ovary
Fallopian tube
uterus
vagina

FEMALE

epididymis
testis
vas deferens
seminal vesicle
prostate

MALE

Figure 40–6. Contribution of the wolffian and müllerian ducts and the urogenital sinus to the development of the urogenital tract in the male and female.

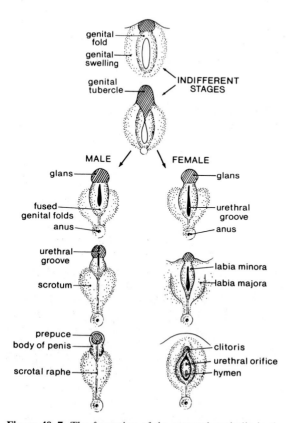

genital fold
genital swelling
genital tubercle

INDIFFERENT STAGES

MALE   FEMALE

glans   glans
fused genital folds   urethral groove
anus   anus

urethral groove
scrotum   labia minora
                               labia majora

prepuce
body of penis   clitoris
                               urethral orifice
scrotal raphe   hymen

Figure 40–7. The formation of the external genitalia in the male and female from common anlagen. (After Langman, J.: Medical Embryology: Human Development—Normal and Abnormal. 4th ed. Baltimore, William & Wilkins Co., 1981.)

the virilization of the male urogenital tract is the onset of müllerian duct regression, which coincides with the development of the spermatogenic cords in the fetal testis between 7 and 8 weeks of gestation (see Fig. 40–2). As a consequence, the müllerian ducts of the male undergo almost complete regression so that only a small cranial portion of the müllerian duct, termed the appendix testis, persists (Fig. 40–8). The remainder of the duct disappears, though the extreme lower end contributes to the prostatic utricle (Glenister, 1962).

The transformation of the wolffian ducts into the male genital tract begins after the onset of müllerian duct regression. Although most of the mesonephric tubules regress, those adjacent to the testis (the epigenital tubules) lose their glomeruli and establish contact with the developing rete and spermatogenic tubules to form the efferent ducts of the testis (see Fig. 40–8). The part of the wolffian duct that is cranial to the gonad becomes the vestigial appendix epididymis. The portion of the duct immediately distal to the efferent ducts becomes elongated and convoluted to form the epididymis, and the central portion of the duct develops thick muscular walls to become the vas deferens. At about the 13th week of gestation the seminal vesicles begin to develop as buds off the lower portions of the wolffian ducts (Watson, 1918). The terminal portions of the ducts between the developing seminal vesicles and the urethra become the ejaculatory ducts and the ampullae of the vas deferens. By the end of the first trimester of gestation, the virilization of the wolffian ducts is largely complete.

The prostatic and membranous portions of the male urethra develop from the pelvic portion of the urogenital sinus. At about 10 weeks of gestation, the endodermal lining of the urethra begins to bud into the surrounding mesenchyme (Lowsley, 1912; Bengmark, 1958; Kellokumpu-Lehtinen et al., 1980). These buds, which are the anlage of the prostatic epithelium, arise from all sides of the urethra but are most extensive in the area surrounding the entry of the wolffian ducts (the ejaculatory ducts) into the male urethra. Differentiation of the prostate occurs early in embryogenesis, and growth and development of the gland continue into postnatal life.

Beginning in the 9th week of gestation, and continuing through the 12th week, development of the external genitalia of the male and female diverge (Spaulding, 1921) (see Fig. 40–7). In the male, the genital swellings enlarge and migrate posteriorly to form the scrotum. Subsequently, the genital folds fuse over the urethral groove to form the penile urethra. The line of

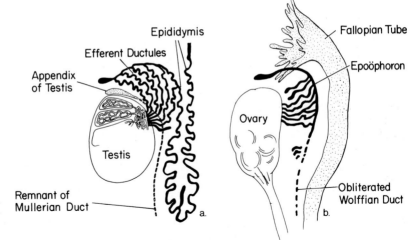

Figure 40–8. The diverse fates of the müllerian and wolffian ducts in the male *(a)* and female *(b)*. The black areas denote wolffian duct–derived structures, and stippled areas denote müllerian duct derivatives. (After Arey, L. B.: Developmental Anatomy. A Textbook and Laboratory Manual of Embryology. 7th ed. Philadelphia, W. B. Saunders Co., 1974.)

closure remains marked by a scar—the penile raphe. Incomplete fusion of the genital folds over the urethral groove results in various degrees of hypospadias. When the formation of the urethra is almost complete, the prepuce starts to develop, and by 15 weeks of gestation it completely covers the glans penis (Hunter, 1933).

Thus, the formation of the male genital tract is accomplished largely between 6 and 13 weeks of gestation. During the latter two thirds of gestation two additional processes occur— the completion of descent of the testes and the growth of the external genitalia.

Testicular descent (Fig. 40–9) is complex and poorly understood. At about the eighth week of development the testis and the mesonephros are attached to the posterior abdominal wall by a broad peritoneal fold. Subsequently as the mesonephros degenerates, the portion of this fold cranial to the testis also degenerates. However, the portion caudal to the testis becomes a narrow ligamentous attachment for the testis—the caudal genital ligament. In the inguinal region, the caudal genital ligament is continuous with a band of mesenchyme extending into the genital swellings. This mesenchymous band, including the caudal genital liga-

Figure 40–9. Descent of the testes. (After Arey, L. B.: Developmental Anatomy. A Textbook and Laboratory Manual of Embryology. 7th ed. Philadelphia, W. B. Saunders Co., 1974.)

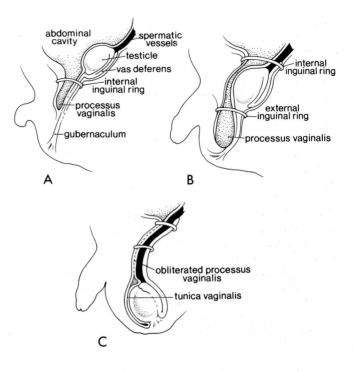

ment, is known as the gubernaculum. The gubernaculum anchors the fetal testis to the inguinal region and probably serves to prevent upward movement (e.g., as happens with the kidney) of the testis during the rapid elongation of the trunk.

During the third month of gestation a herniation of the coelomic cavity (termed the processus vaginalis) forms on each side of the midline through the ventral abdominal wall along the course of the gubernaculum (see Fig. 40–9). Herniation probably results from internal abdominal pressure, which is intensified by rapid organ development after closure of the umbilical cord. Continued pressure results in enlargement of the processus vaginalis around the gubernaculum and in the formation of an inguinal canal. The opening produced by the processus vaginalis in the transversalis fascia is known as the deep inguinal ring, and the opening in the external oblique aponeurosis is the superficial inguinal ring. In human embryogenesis the actual movement of the testis from the abdominal cavity through the inguinal canal and into the scrotum does not take place until after the beginning of the seventh month of gestation. At this time the gubernaculum increases in thickness until the mass in the inguinal canal approaches that of the testis. As a result of abdominal pressure (Frey et al., 1983) and degeneration of the portion of the gubernaculum in contact with the epididymis and testis, the testis descends into the scrotum. The process is androgen-dependent (Rajfer and Walsh, 1977) and may also involve contraction of striated muscle fibers in the gubernaculum (Radhakrishnan et al., 1979; Elder et al., 1982). Continued development of the abdominal musculature causes closure of the deep and superficial inguinal rings and obliteration of the processus vaginalis (see Fig. 40–9).

When formation of the male urethra is largely completed at approximately 11 weeks of gestation, the size of the phallus in the male does not differ substantially from that of the female. However, during the last two trimesters the male external genitalia, prostate, and structures of the wolffian duct grow progressively. At the time of birth the external genitalia of the male are much larger than those of the female.

Female Development. The internal reproductive tract of the female is formed from the müllerian ducts. The wolffian ducts persist only in remnant form; some mesonephric excretory tubules and a portion of the wolffian duct form the epoophoron in the mesovarium (see Fig. 40–8). Remnants of the wolffian duct are occa-

sionally found caudal to the gonad and are termed the Gartner ducts (see Fig. 40–8). The cephalic ends of the müllerian ducts (the portions derived from coelomic epithelium) are the anlagen of the fallopian tubes, whereas the caudal portions fuse to form the uterus (see Fig. 40–6; Fig. 40–10). After fusion of the caudal portions of the ducts at 8 to 9 weeks of development, a septum divides the lumen of the uterus into two cavities. This septum subsequently disappears, and by 10 to 11 weeks of gestation a single cavity lined by cuboidal epithelium is present. The junction of the body and cervix of the uterus can be recognized by 9 weeks of development, but the formation of the muscular walls of the uterus (myometrium) from the mesenchyme that surrounds the müllerian ducts is not completed until approximately 17 weeks of gestation.

Development of the vagina begins at approximately 9 weeks of gestation with the formation of a solid mass of cells (the uterovaginal plate) between the caudal buds of the müllerian ducts and the dorsal wall of the urogenital sinus (see Fig. 40–10) (O'Rahilly, 1977). The relative

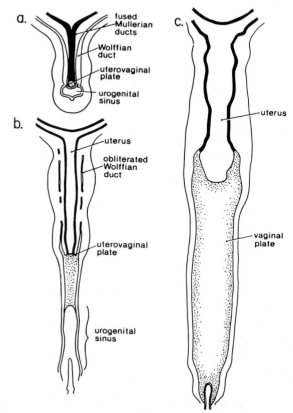

Figure 40–10. Development of the vagina. a, 7 to 8 weeks; b, 10 weeks; c, 20 weeks. (After Koff, A. K.: Carnegie Contributions to Embryology No. 140, 24:59–90, 1933.)

contributions of the müllerian and wolffian ducts and the urogenital sinus to the development of the uterovaginal plate is not known. However, interaction between these tissues is essential for vaginal development (Gruenwald, 1941; Bulmer, 1957; Bok and Drews, 1983). The cells of the uterovaginal plate proliferate, thus increasing the distance between the uterus and urogenital sinus (see Fig. 40–10). At 11 weeks of development a lumen begins to form in the caudal end of the vaginal plate, and by 20 weeks of gestation the vagina is completely canalized (see Fig. 40–10) (Koff, 1933). The lumen of the vagina remains separated from the urogenital sinus by a thin membrane of mesodermal tissue (the hymen).

Because of its ligamentous attachments, the ovary also undergoes an apparent transabdominal descent analogous to that of the testis. The caudal genital ligament forms the suspensory ligament of the ovary and the round ligament of the uterus. Although a processus vaginalis develops in female embryos, no true ovarian descent occurs, and the permanent location of the ovary is just below the rim of the true pelvis.

After 10 weeks of gestation the genital tubercle of the female bends caudally, the lateral portions of the genital swellings enlarge to form the labia majora, and the posterior portions of the genital swellings fuse to form the posterior fourchette. The urethral folds flanking the urogenital orifice do not fuse but persist as the labia minora (see Fig. 40–7). Thus, in contrast to the male in whom the phallic and perineal portions of the urogenital sinus are enclosed by fusion of the urethral folds and genital swellings, most of the urogenital sinus of the female remains exposed on the surface as a cleft into which the vagina and urethra open.

Breast Development. At 5 weeks of development, paired lines of epidermal thickening extend from the forelimb to the hindlimb on the ventral surface of the embryo. Between 6 and 8 weeks of development these "mammary lines" largely disappear except for a small portion on each side of the thoracic region that condenses and penetrates the underlying mesenchyme. This single pair of mammary buds undergoes little change until the fifth month of development when secondary epithelial buds appear and nipples develop. Proliferation of the ductules occurs throughout the remainder of gestation so that by the time of birth 15 to 25 separate glands are present, each of which is connected to the exterior through the nipple. Although in some species sexual dimorphism in breast development is apparent during embry-

ogenesis, such dimorphism has never been documented in humans, and the development of the breast in boys and girls is identical prior to the onset of female puberty (Pfaltz, 1949).

ENDOCRINE CONTROL OF PHENOTYPIC DIFFERENTIATION

Jost (1953, 1972) established that differentiation of the sexual phenotype is ultimately dependent on the type of gonad that develops. The paradigm that chromosomal sex determines gonadal sex and that gonadal sex, in turn, determines phenotypic sex has now become the central dogma of sexual differentiation (see Fig. 40–1). This theory was based on the observation that removing the gonads from embryos of either sex prior to the onset of phenotypic differentiation resulted in the development of a female phenotype. As a consequence of this type of experiment and of studies involving transplantation of embryonic gonads or of hormone administration, or both, it was deduced that the male phenotype is induced by testicular secretions, whereas female development does not require secretions from the embryonic ovary. Jost recognized that two substances from the fetal testis are essential to male development. The first is an androgenic steroid, which is responsible for virilization of the wolffian duct system and urogenital sinus and for formation of the male external genitalia. The second substance (müllerian-inhibiting substance) causes regression of the müllerian ducts in the male.

ONSET OF ENDOCRINE FUNCTION OF THE TESTIS AND THE OVARY

Differentiation of the fetal ovary and testis can first be detected histologically with the development of the spermatogenic tubules in the fetal testis at 7 weeks of gestation (Gillman, 1948). The formation of müllerian-inhibiting substance is associated with the appearance of the spermatogenic tubules in the testis. Thus, müllerian-inhibiting substance is the primordial hormone of the fetal testis, and regression of the müllerian ducts is the first event in male development. Shortly thereafter, at approximately 8 to 9 weeks of gestation, Leydig cells can be recognized in the interstitium of the testis, and the testis begins to synthesize testosterone (Siiteri and Wilson, 1974) (Fig. 40–11). The onset of estrogen formation by the fetal ovary occurs at approximately the same time that the fetal testis begins to synthesize testos-

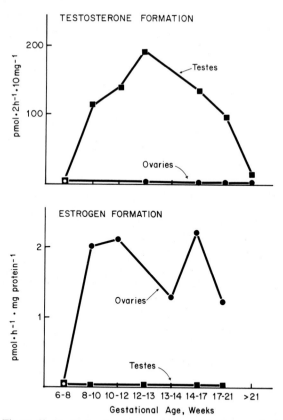

Figure 40–11. Endocrine differentiation of the human fetal ovary and testis. (After Siiteri, P. K. and Wilson, J. D.: J. Clin. Endocrinol. Metab. *38*:113–125, 1974 and George, F. W. and Wilson, J. D.: J. Clin. Endocrinol. Metab., *47*:550–555, 1978.)

terone (George and Wilson, 1978) (Fig. 40–11), despite the fact that development of the ovarian follicle does not commence until the fifth month of gestation. Thus, endocrine differentiation of the ovary and testis occurs at the same time in embryogenesis.

The endocrine differentiation of the fetal ovary and testis has been studied in detail in the rabbit and appears to involve the differential expression of relatively few enzymes in the complex process of synthesizing testosterone and estradiol (George et al., 1979; Wilson et al., 1981). In the 18-day-old rabbit embryo the activity of the rate-limiting enzyme for testosterone synthesis (3β-hydroxysteroid dehydrogenase-$\delta^{4,5}$-isomerase) is greater in the testis than in the ovary, and the conversion of testosterone to estradiol (aromatase activity) is greater in the ovary than in the testis. All other enzyme activities in the steroidogenic pathway are initially equal in the ovary and testis (George et al., 1979). Thus, despite the overall complexity of the mechanisms of gonadal differentiation,

variation in the activity of only a few enzymes have profound effects on the hormones formed, and ultimately on sexual development.

Delineation of the factors that control the initiation of testosterone formation in the fetal testis is of paramount importance in understanding how genetic sex is translated into phenotypic sex. The enzymatic differentiation of the fetal rabbit gonad does not require extragonadal hormones (George et al., 1978; George and Wilson, 1980), and the onset of testosterone secretion also appears to be independent of gonadotropin regulation, despite the fact that luteinizing hormone–human chorionic gonadotropin receptors are detectable in the fetal rabbit testis from the onset of testosterone synthesis (Catt et al., 1975; George et al., 1979). However, control of the onset of testosterone synthesis in the human embryo has not been studied in such detail, and it is possible that gonadotropins from the placenta (chorionic gonadotropin) or fetal pituitary (luteinizing hormone) have a more important role in the human than in the rabbit. Receptors for luteinizing hormone have been detected in the human fetal testis as early as the 12th week of gestation (Huhtaniemi et al., 1977; Molsberry et al., 1982), and the addition of human chorionic gonadotropin in vitro causes increased testosterone synthesis at this time (Abramovich et al., 1974; Huhtaniemi et al., 1977). Furthermore, the possibility that male pseudohermaphroditism can result from a defect in testicular gonadotropin receptors is in keeping with a role for gonadotropin regulation of testocterone synthesis at the time of male phenotypic development (Schwartz et al., 1981). However, until appropriate direct studies are done in the human fetal testis (between 8 and 12 weeks of gestation), the question of whether or not gonadotropin plays a role in the initiation of testosterone synthesis in the human fetal testis will remain open.

ROLE OF HORMONES IN MALE DEVELOPMENT

Müllerian Duct Regression. Regression of the müllerian duct begins in male fetuses at 8 to 9 weeks of gestational age and is mediated by a glycoprotein that has a molecular weight of approximately 124,000 and is synthesized and secreted by the fetal Sertoli cells (Blanchard and Josso, 1974; Picard et al., 1978; Tran and Josso, 1982). Müllerian-inhibiting substance is thought to act locally to suppress müllerian duct development rather than as a circulating hormone (Vigier et al., 1981). The concept that müllerian duct regression is an active process in male development is supported by studies of individuals with the persistent müllerian duct syndrome (Brook, 1980). In this disorder, genetic and phenotypic males who have male wolffian duct–derived structures also have fallopian tubes and a uterus. Family studies suggest that the disorder is due either to an autosomal or X-linked gene defect (Sloan and Walsh, 1976). The exact nature of the defect is uncertain, but it may reside either in a failure of production of müllerian-inhibiting substance by the fetal testis or in a failure of the tissue to respond to the hormone. Little is known about the mechanisms by which regression of the müllerian ducts is accomplished. However, developments in this field, including the formation of monospecific antibodies to müllerian-inhibiting substance (Vigier et al, 1982; Mudgett-Hunter et al., 1982), indicate that substantial progress will be made in unraveling this important embryologic process in the future.

Virilization. This process in the male fetus results from the action of androgen on specific target organs—the wolffian ducts, urogenital sinus, and external genitalia. Although testosterone is the principal androgen secreted by the fetal and adult testis in postnatal life, testosterone is thought to have relatively few actions of its own but instead serves as a prohormone for two other potent hormones that are synthesized in target tissues (Wilson, 1975) (Fig. 40–12). Testosterone can undergo irreversible 5α-reduction to dihydrotestosterone, which mediates many of the differentiating, growth-promoting, and functional actions of the hormone. Alternatively, circulating androgens can be converted to estrogens in the peripheral tissues of both sexes. Estrogens, in some instances, act in con-

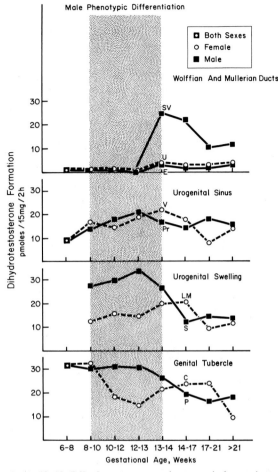

Figure 40–13. Dihydrotestosterone in urogenital tract tissues of the human fetus. SV, seminal vesicle; U, uterus; E, epididymis; V, vagina; Pr, prostate; LM, labia majora; S, scrotum; C, clitoris; P, penis. (After Siiteri, P. K. and Wilson, J. D.: J. Clin. Endocrinol. Metab., *38*:113–125, 1974.)

cert with androgens to influence physiologic processes but may also exert independent effects on cellular function, and on occasion, they have effects that are in opposition to those of androgens. Thus, the physiologic consequences of circulating testosterone in the postnatal state represents the sum of the combined effects of testosterone itself and of the estrogenic and androgenic metabolites of testosterone.

ROLE OF TESTOSTERONE AND DIHYDROTESTOSTERONE. In human development, the 5α-reductase enzyme responsible for the conversion of testosterone to dihydrotestosterone is present in anlagen of the external genitalia (the genital tubercle and urogenital sinus and swellings) prior to the onset of phenotypic differentiation (Siiteri and Wilson, 1974) (Fig. 40–13). The wolffian duct, however, is incapable of convert-

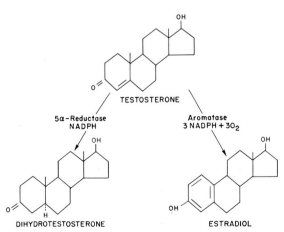

Figure 40–12. Role of testosterone as a circulating prohormone for the formation of other hormones.

ing testosterone to dihydrotestosterone until after male phenotypic differentiation is advanced and the epididymis and seminal vesicle are formed. This difference between the wolffian duct system, on the one hand, and the urogenital sinus and urogenital swellings and tubercle, on the other, is also true for several other mammalian species. Thus, virilization of the external genitalia appears to be mediated by dihydrotestosterone, whereas testosterone itself appears to be responsible for virilization of the wolffian ducts. This view is substantiated by studies of the 5α-reductase deficiency syndrome in humans, in which the external genitalia fail to virilize because of the inability to form dihydrotestosterone in peripheral tissues. However, in affected individuals, the wolffian duct–derived structures—the epididymis, vas deferens, and seminal vesicles—develop normally (Walsh et al., 1974). Thus, to explain the known events in male phenotypic differentiation, at least three hormones must be involved. The regression of the müllerian duct is mediated by müllerian-inhibiting substance, a hormone that is secreted transiently by the fetal testis. The other aspects of male phenotypic development of the embryo are accomplished by two androgens. Testosterone, the androgen secreted by the fetal testis, causes virilization of the wolffian ducts prior to the development of their ability to form dihydrotestosterone, whereas dihydrotestosterone is responsible for virilization of the external genitalia and the male urethra.

ROLE OF THE ANDROGEN RECEPTOR. The current formulation of how androgens act within target cells is depicted in Figure 40–14. Testosterone enters cells passively by diffusion down an activity gradient. Inside the cell, testosterone either binds directly to protein receptors in the cytoplasm or is 5α-reduced to dihydrotestosterone before binding to the androgen receptor. After binding, the receptor-steroid complex undergoes a poorly understood transformation process and is translocated to the nucleus at which point it is presumed to bind to specific acceptor sites on the chromatin. As a consequence, an increase in transcription of messenger RNA occurs, and ultimately new proteins are synthesized in the cell cytoplasm.

The essential role of the androgen receptor in mediating the embryonic action of androgens was established as the result of studies of the testicular feminization (*Tfm*) mutation in the mouse, an X-linked disorder in which affected males have testes and normal testosterone production but differentiate as phenotypic females (Lyon and Hawkes, 1970). Since no müllerian duct derivatives (uterus or fallopian tubes) are present in affected mice, the müllerian-inhibiting function of the fetal testis is unimpaired. However, such animals are profoundly resistant to endogenous and exogenous androgens, and there is total failure of androgen-mediated virilization of the wolffian duct, urogenital sinus, and external genitalia. Dihydrotestosterone formation is normal, but the androgen receptor of the cell cytosol is not detectable (Gehring et al., 1971; Bullock et al., 1971; Goldstein and Wilson, 1972). Consequently, the hormone cannot interact with the chromosomes and fails to elicit a hormone response.

Several disorders of the androgen receptor in humans have provided additional insight into the mechanism of androgen action in embryonic virilization. These abnormalities range from a complete absence of the receptor (or a severe structural abnormality that renders the receptor undetectable by present techniques) to more subtle structural defects in the receptor. In addition, abnormalities in androgen action that occur despite the presence of apparently normal androgen binding have been identified in several patients (Griffin et al., 1982).

It is not clear why testosterone is responsible for one portion of virilization (wolffian duct differentiation) and dihydrotestosterone is responsible for the remainder of the process. However, the observation that dihydrotestosterone binds with greater affinity to the androgen receptor than does testosterone (Wilbert et al.,

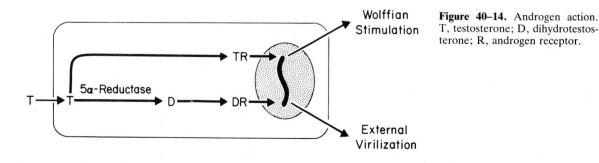

Figure 40–14. Androgen action. T, testosterone; D, dihydrotestosterone; R, androgen receptor.

1983; George and Noble, 1984) suggests that dihydrotestosterone formation probably serves as an amplifying signal for androgen action in peripheral tissues. Since the wolffian ducts are in close proximity to the fetal testes, the concentration of testosterone in the lumen of the wolffian ducts might be sufficiently high to overcome its low affinity for the androgen receptor and thus could mediate the virilization of the ducts. To substantiate this theory, it will be necessary to establish whether the concentration of testosterone in the wolffian ducts is substantially higher than it is in plasma and other androgen target tissues. It is also possible that there is a transient testosterone receptor in the embryonic wolffian duct, but the fact that androgen-dependent tissues of wolffian duct origin fail to develop in animals and people with abnormalities of the androgen receptor suggests that testosterone and dihydrotestosterone act via the same receptor.

Female embryos have the same androgen receptor system and the same ability to respond to androgens as do male embryos. Thus, female embryos virilize when exposed to androgens (Schultz and Wilson, 1974). The most common cause of female virilization in humans is congenital adrenal hyperplasia in which increased secretion of adrenal androgens virilize the external genitalia in affected females (New et al., 1983). Thus, differences in anatomic development between males and females are dependent on differences in the hormonal signals themselves and not on differences in the receptors for hormones.

MESENCHYMAL-EPITHELIAL INTERACTIONS IN SEXUAL DIFFERENTIATION. The androgen-mediated morphologic differentiation of the male genital tract is dependent on the interaction of the epithelium with a hormonally responsive mesenchyme. For example, when tissue recombinants of embryonic urinary bladder epithelium and urogenital sinus mesenchyme are exposed to androgens, the epithelium develops prostatic buds. Recombinants of epithelium from the urogenital sinus and mesenchyme from other embryonic sites are incapable of prostatic development under similar circumstances, however (Cunha et al., 1983). Furthermore, mesenchyme from androgen-insensitive *Tfm* mouse urogenital sinus fails to mediate prostatic growth when recombined with normal urogenital sinus epithelium, whereas epithelium from *Tfm* mouse urogenital sinus undergoes prostate formation in the presence of androgen when recombined with normal mesenchyme (Cunha and Lung, 1978; Lasnitzki and Mizuno, 1980). These results imply that the ability of a tissue to respond to androgenic stimulation resides in the mesenchyme of that tissue.

This is not to say that the epithelium has no role to play in the androgen-mediated cytodifferentiation. For example, it is known that the embryonic mammary bud undergoes androgen-dependent regression in the male mouse and that the target tissue for androgen action in the mammary rudiment is the embryonic mesenchyme (Kratochwil and Schwartz, 1976). However, the ability of the mesenchyme to respond to androgen (the induction of androgen receptors) appears to require the specific interaction of mammary epithelium with mammary mesenchyme (Heuberger et al., 1982). There are also indications that epithelium derived from mesodermal or endodermal germ layers responds differently when recombined with androgen-responsive mesenchyme (Cunha et al., 1983). Understanding the nature of these mesenchymal-epithelial interactions is fundamental to our understanding of the hormonal control of sexual differentiation.

ROLE OF HORMONES IN THE DEVELOPMENT OF THE FEMALE PHENOTYPE AND THE BREAST

Embryogenesis takes place in a sea of hormones (steroid and non-steroid) derived from the placenta, the maternal circulation, the fetal adrenal gland, the fetal testis, and possibly the fetal ovary. Because the embryo develops in the "female environment" of the mother, it has not been possible to devise an experiment analogous to Jost's to determine whether any of these hormones is essential to female development. Even if they are not essential for the differentiation of the female urogenital tract, estrogens and progestins are probably involved in the growth and maturation of the accessory reproductive organs of the female during the latter phases of embryonic life.

Dimorphism in the development of the breast in human males and females has not been documented prior to puberty, and the transient milk secretion in the newborn male and female suggests there is also no functional difference between the two sexes until later in life (Pfaltz, 1949). The endocrinologic control of female breast development and milk formation in postembryonic life is complex. Estrogen plays a key role in the growth and maturation of the normal gland, and the administration of estrogen (or the alteration of the normal male ratio of androgen:estrogen) can result in profound breast development in the male at any phase in life, supporting the concept that embryonic development of the tissue in the male and female embryos is not fundamentally different (Wilson et al., 1980).

SUMMARY

Although genes located on the autosomes as well as on the sex chromosomes contribute to the establishment of genetic sex, determinants on the Y chromosome in the male embryo are paramount in inducing differentiation of the indifferent gonadal primordia into testes. In the absence of the Y chromosome, the indifferent gonad develops into an ovary. The function of the embryonic gonads as endocrine organs determines the development of phenotypic sex; specifically, the secretion by the fetal testis of two hormones—müllerian-inhibiting substance and testosterone—imposes male development on the indifferent fetus. Testosterone and its metabolite dihydrotestosterone act to virilize the male fetus via the same receptor machinery that mediates androgen action in the postnatal state. This receptor machinery is present in both male and female embryos. Consequently, normal phenotypic development is determined solely by the presence (in males) or absence (in females) of the specific hormonal signals at the critical time in embryonic development. The characterization of several single gene defects in humans and animals that result in various forms of abnormal sexual development has aided the elucidation of the genetic, molecular, and endocrine aspects of sexual differentiation.

Nevertheless, many fundamental issues in sexual differentiation are still poorly understood. For example, it is not known how the germ cells find their way to the gonadal ridges from their site of origin in the yolk sac or how histologic differentiation of the gonads controls the endocrine function of the fetal gonads. The process by which embryonic tissues acquire the ability to respond to a hormonal stimulus and consequently initiate anatomic and functional development also remains an enigma. Ultimately, these fundamental problems of embryology must be resolved before we can understand the overall program by which the myriad genetic and regulatory factors interact to cause differentiation of the sexual phenotypes.

References

Abramovich, D. R., Baker, T. G., and Neal, P.: Effect of human chorionic gonadotropin on testosterone secretion by the fetal human testis in organ culture. J. Endocrinol 60:179, 1974.

Arey, L. B.: Developmental Anatomy. A Textbook and Laboratory Manual of Embryology. 7th ed. Philadelphia, W. B. Saunders Co., 1974.

Bengmark, S.: The Prostatic Urethra and Prostatic Glands. Lund, Sweden, Berlingska Boktryckeriet, 1958.

Beutler, B., Nagai, Y., Ohno, S., Klein, G., and Shapiro, I. M.: The HLA-dependent expression of testis-organizing H-Y antigen by human male cells. Cell 13:509, 1978.

Blanchard, M. G., and Josso, N.: Source of the anti-müllerian hormone synthesized by the fetal testis: Müllerian-inhibiting activity of the fetal bovine Sertoli cells in tissue culture. Pediatr. Res. 8(12):968, 1974.

Bok, G., and Drews, U.: The role of the wolffian ducts in the formation of the sinus vagina: an organ culture study. J. Embryol. Exp. Morphol. 73:275, 1983.

Brook, C. G. D.: Persistent müllerian duct syndrome. In Josso, N. (Ed.): The Intersex Child, (Pediatric and Adolescent Endocrinology Ser., Vol. 8 Karger, Basel, pp. 100–104, 1980).

Bullock, L. P., Bardin, C. W., and Ohno, S.: The androgen insensitive mouse: Absence of intranuclear androgen retention in the kidney. Biochem. Biophys. Res. Commun. 44:1537, 1971.

Bulmer, D.: The development of the human vagina. J. Anat. 91:490, 1957.

Catt, K. J., Dufau, M. L., Neaves, W. B., Walsh, P. C., and Wilson, J. D.: LH-hCG receptors and testosterone content during differentiation of the testis in the rabbit embryo. Endocrinology 97:1157, 1975.

Cunha, G. R., and Lung, B.: The possible influence of temporal factors in androgenic responsiveness of urogenital tissue recombinants from wild-type and androgen-insensitive (Tfm) mice. J. Exp. Zool. 205:181, 1978.

Cunha, G. R., Chung, L. W. K., Shannon, J. M., Taguchi, O., and Fujii, H.: Hormone-induced morphogenesis and growth: Role of mesenchymal-epithelial interactions. Recent Prog. Horm. Res., 39:559, 1983.

Elder, J. S., Isaacs, J. T., and Walsh, P. C.: Androgenic sensitivity of the gubernaculum testis: Evidence for hormonal/mechanical interactions in testicular descent. J. Urol. 127:170, 1982.

Frey, H. L., Peng, S., and Rajfer, J.: Synergy of abdominal pressure and androgens in testicular descent. Biol. Reprod. 29:1233, 1983.

Gasser, D. L., and Silvers, W. K.: Genetics and immunology of sex-linked antigens. Adv. Immunol. 15:215, 1972.

Gehring, U., Tomkins, G. M., and Ohno, S.: Effect of the androgen-insensitivity mutation on a cytoplasmic receptor for dihydrotestosterone. Nature New Biol. 232:106, 1971.

George, F. W., and Noble, J. F.: Androgen receptors are similar in fetal and adult rabbits. Endocrinology 115:1451, 1984.

George, F. W., and Wilson, J. D.: Conversion of androgen to estrogen by the human fetal ovary. J. Clin. Endocrinol. Metab. 47:550, 1978.

George, F. W., and Wilson, J. D.: Endocrine differentiation of the fetal rabbit ovary in culture. Nature 283:861, 1980.

George, F. W., Catt, K. J., Neaves, W. B., and Wilson, J. D.: Studies on the regulation of testosterone synthesis in the rabbit fetal testis. Endocrinology 102:665, 1978.

George, F. W., Simpson, E. R., Milewich, L., and Wilson, J. D.: Studies on the regulation of steroid hormone biosynthesis in fetal rabbit gonads. Endocrinology 105:1100, 1979.

Gillman, J.: The development of the gonads in man, with a consideration of the role of fetal endocrines and the histogenesis of ovarian tumors. Carnegie Contributions to Embryology, No. 210, *32*:83, 1948.

Glenister, T. W.: The development of the utricle and of the so-called "middle" or "median" lobe of the human prostate. J. Anat. *96*:443, 1962.

Goldstein, J. L., and Wilson, J. D.: Studies on the pathogenesis of the pseudohermaphroditism in the mouse with testicular feminization. J. Clin. Invest. *51*:1647, 1972.

Gondos, B., Bhinaleus, P., and Habel, C. J.: Ultrastructural observations on germ cells in human fetal ovaries. Am. J. Obstet. Gynecol. *110*:644, 1971.

Griffin, J. E., Edwards, C., Madden, J. D., Harrod, M. J., and Wilson, J. D.: Congenital absence of the vagina. The Mayer-Rokitansky-Kuster-Hauser Syndrome. Ann. Intern. Med. *85*:224, 1976.

Griffin, J. E., Leshin, M., and Wilson, J. D.: Androgen resistance syndromes. Am. J. Physiol. *243*(2):E81, 1982.

Gruenwald, P.: The relation of the growing müllerian duct to the wolffian duct and its importance for the genesis of malformation. Anat. Rec. *81*:1, 1941.

Heuberger, B., Fitzka, I., Wasner, G., and Kratochwil, K.: Induction of androgen receptor formation by epithelium-mesenchyme interaction in embryonic mouse mammary gland. Proc. Natl. Acad. Sci. U.S.A. *79*:2957, 1982.

Huhtaniemi, I. T., Korenbrat, C. C., and Jaffe, R. R.: HCG binding and stimulation of testosterone biosynthesis in the human fetal testis. J. Clin. Endocrinol. Metab. *44*(5):963, 1977.

Hunter, R. H.: Notes on the development of the prepuce. J. Anat. *70*:68, 1933.

Jirasek, J. E.: Development of the Genital System and Male Pseudohermaphroditism. Baltimore, Johns Hopkins Press, 1971.

Jones, H. W., Jr., Rary, J. M., Rock, J. A., and Cummings, D.: The role of the H-Y antigen in human sexual development. Johns Hopkins Med. J. *145*:33, 1979.

Jost, A.: Problems of fetal endocrinology: The gonadal and hypophyseal hormones. Recent Prog. Horm. Res. *8*:379, 1953.

Jost, A.: A new look at the mechanisms controlling sex differentiation in mammals. Johns Hopkins Med. J. *130*:38, 1972.

Kellokumpu-Lehtinen, P., Santti, R., and Pelliniemi, L. J.: Correlation of early cytodifferentiation of the human fetal prostate and Leydig cells. Anat. Rec. *196*:253, 1980.

Koff, A. K.: Development of the vagina in the human fetus. Carnegie Contributions to Embryology, No. 140, *24*:59, 1933.

Kratochwil, K., and Schwartz, P.: Tissue interaction in androgen response of embryonic mammary rudiment of the mouse: Identification of the target tissue for testosterone. Proc. Natl. Acad. Sci. U.S.A. *73*:4041, 1976.

Langman, J.: Medical Embryology: Human Development—Normal and Abnormal. 4th ed. Baltimore, Williams & Wilkins Co., 1981.

Lasnitzki, I., and Mizuno, T.: Prostate induction: Interaction of epithelium and mesenchyme from normal wild-type and androgen insensitive mice with testicular feminization. J. Endocrinol. *85*:423, 1980.

Lowsley, O. S.: The development of the human prostate gland with reference to the development of other structures at the neck of the urinary bladder. Am. J. Anat. *13*:299, 1912.

Lyon, M. F., and Hawkes, S. G.: X-linked gene for testicular feminization in the mouse. Nature *227*:1217, 1970.

McCarrey, J. R., and Abbott, U. K.: Mechanisms of genetic sex determination, gonadal sex differentiation, and germ-cell development in animals. Adv. Genet. *20*:217, 1979.

Molsberry, R. L., Carr, B. R., Mendelson, C. R., and Simpson, E. R.: Human chorionic gonadotropin binding to human fetal testes as a function of gestational age. J. Clin. Endocrinol. Metab. *55*:791, 1982.

Moore, K. L.: The Developing Human. Clinically Oriented Embryology. 2nd ed. Philadelphia, W. B. Saunders Co., 1977.

Mudgett-Hunter, M., Budzik, G. P., Sullivan, M., and Donahoe, P. K.: Monoclonal antibody to Müllerian inhibiting substance. J. Immunol. *128*(3):1327, 1982.

Muller, U., Aschmoneit, I., Zenzes, M. T., and Wolf, U.: Binding studies of H-Y antigen in rat tissues: Indications for a gonad specific receptor. Human Genet. *43*:151, 1978.

New, M. I., Dupont, B., Grunbach, K., and Levine, L. S.: Congenital adrenal hyperplasia and related conditions. *In* Stanbury, J. B., Wyngaarden, J. G., Fredrickson, D. S., Goldstein, J. L., and Brown, M. S. (Eds.): The Metabolic Basis of Inherited Disease. 5th ed. New York, McGraw-Hill, 1983, pp. 973–1000.

Ohno, S.: Major Sex-Determining Genes. New York, Springer-Verlag, 1979.

Ohno, S., Nagai, Y., and Ciccarese, S.: Testicular cells lysostripped of H-Y antigen organize ovarian follicle-like aggregates. Cytogenet. Cell Genet. *20*:351, 1978.

O'Rahilly, R.: The development of the vagina in the human. *In* Blandau, R. J., and Bergsma, D. (Eds.): Morphogenesis and Malformation of the Genital System. Birth Defects Original Article Series. Vol. XIII, 1977, pp. 123-136.

Peters, H.: Migration of gonocytes into the mammalian gonad and their differentiation. Philos. Trans. R. Soc. Lond. (Ser. B) *259*:91, 1970.

Pfaltz, C. R.: Das embryonale and postnatale Verhalten den Männlichen Brustdruse beim Menschern. II Das Mammanorgan in Kurder-, Junglings-Mannes-, und Greisenalten. Acta Anat. *8*:293, 1949.

Picard, J. Y., Tran, D., and Josso, N.: Biosynthesis of labelled anti-müllerian hormone by fetal testes: evidence for the glycoprotein nature of the hormone and for its disulfide-bonded structure. Mol. Cell. Endocrinol. *12*:17, 1978.

Radhakrishnan, J., Morikawa, Y., Donahoe, P. K., and Hendren, W. H.: Observations on the gubernaculum during the descent of the testes. Invest. Urol. *16*:365, 1979.

Rajfer, J., and Walsh, P. C.: Hormonal regulation of testicular descent: Experimental and clinical observations. J. Urol. *118*:985, 1977.

Schultz, F. M., and Wilson, J. D.: Virilization of the wolffian duct in the rat fetus by various androgens. Endocrinology *94*:979, 1974.

Schwartz, M., Imperato-McGinley, J., Petersen, R. E., Cooper, G., Morris, P. L., MacGillivray, M., and Hensle, T.: Male pseudohermaphroditism secondary to an abnormality in Leydig cell differentiation. J. Clin. Endocrinol. Metab. *53*:123, 1981.

Siiteri, P. K., and Wilson, J. D.: Testosterone formation and metabolism during male sexual differentiation in the human embryo. J. Clin. Endocrinol. Metab. *38*:113, 1974.

Silvers, W. K., Gasser, D. L., and Eicher, E. M.: H-Y antigen, serologically detectable male antigen and sex determination. Cell *28*:439, 1982.

Silvers, W. K., and Wachtel, S. S.: H-Y antigen: Behavior and function. Science *195*:956, 1977.

Sloan, W. R., and Walsh, P. C.: Familial persistent müllerian duct syndrome. J. Urol. *115*:459, 1976.

Spaulding, M. H.: The development of the external genitalia in the human embryo. Carnegie Contributions to Embryology, No. 61, *13*:67, 1921.

Tran, D., and Josso, N.: Localization of anti-Müllerian hormone in the rough endoplasmic reticulum of the developing bovine sertoli cell using immunocytochemistry with a monoclonal antibody. Endocrinology *111*(5):1562, 1982.

Vigier, B., Picard, J. Y., Bézard, J., and Josso, N: Anti-Müllerian hormone: A local or long-distance morphogenetic factor? Hum Genet. *58*(1):85, 90, 1981.

Vigier, B., Picard, J. Y., and Josso, N.: A monoclonal antibody against bovine anti-Müllerian hormone. Endocrinology *110*(1):131, 1982.

Wachtel, S. S.: Where is the H-Y structural gene? Cell *22*:3, 1980.

Wachtel, S. S.: H-Y antigen and the Biology of Sex Determination. New York, Grune & Stratton, 1983.

Walsh, P. C., Madden, J. D., Harrod, M. J., Goldstein, J. L., MacDonald, P. C., and Wilson, J. D.: Familial incomplete male pseudohermaphroditism, type 2: decreased dihydrotestosterone formation is pseudovaginal perineoscrotal hypospadias. N. Engl. J. Med. *291*:944, 1974.

Watson, E. M.: The development of the seminal vesicles in man. Am. J. Anat. *24*:395, 1918.

Wilbert, D. M., Griffin, J. E., and Wilson, J. D.: Characterization of the cytosol androgen receptor of the human prostate. J. Clin. Endocrinol. Metab. *56*:113, 1983.

Wilson, J. D.: Metabolism of testicular androgens. *In* Greep, R. O., and Astwood, E. B. (Eds.): Handbook of Physiology. Chap. 25. Section 7: Endocrinology. Vol. V. Male Reproductive System. Washington, D.C., American Physiological Society, pp. 491–508, 1975.

Wilson, J. D., and Goldstein, J. L.: Classification of hereditary disorders of sexual development. *In* Bergsma, D. (Ed.): Genetic Forms of Hypogonadism. Birth Defects Original Article Series. Vol. XI. 1975. pp. 1–16.

Wilson, J. D., Aiman, J., and MacDonald, P. C.: The pathogenesis of gynecomastia. Adv. Int. Med. *25*:1, 1980.

Wilson, J. D., Griffin, J. E., Leshin, M., and George, F. W.: Role of gonadal hormones in development of the sexual phenotypes. Hum. Genet. /2058:78, 1981.

Witschi, E.: Migration of the germ cells of human embryos from the yolk sac to the primitive gonadal folds. Carnegie Contributions to Embryology, No. 209, *32*:69, 1948.

Zenzes, M. T., Wolf, U., Günther, E., and Engel, W.: Studies on the function of H-Y antigen: Dissociation and reorganization experiments on rat gonadal tissue. Cytogenet. Cell. Genet. *20*:365, 1978.

CHAPTER 41

Disorders of Sexual Differentiation

JAMES E. GRIFFIN, M.D.
JEAN D. WILSON, M.D.

Normal sexual differentiation is a sequential and orderly process; chromosomal sex determines gonadal sex, and gonadal sex, in turn, determines phenotypic sex (see Chapter 40). Phenotypic sex encompasses both the normal anatomic development of men and women and the capacity to reproduce. Disorders of sexual differentiation result from disturbances that impair any step in this process during embryonic life.

There are a variety of known mechanisms by which abnormalities in human development can arise: an environmental insult, as in the ingestion of a virilizing drug during pregnancy; nonfamilial aberrations of the sex chromosomes, as in 45,X gonadal dysgenesis; developmental birth defects of multifactorial origin, as in most cases of hypospadias; or hereditary disorders resulting from single-gene mutations, as in the testicular feminization syndrome.

From the standpoint of pathophysiology, abnormalities in sexual development can be categorized as resulting from derangements in any of the three principal processes involved in sexual differentiation, namely disorders of chromosomal sex, disorders of gonadal sex, and disorders of phenotypic sex. Although such a categorization is useful both conceptually and clinically, two problems with such a schematization should be recognized. First, the manifestations of these disorders vary widely from extreme problems of sexual ambiguity in the newborn to inappropriate or impaired pubertal development to infertility in otherwise normal individuals (Table 41–1). This broad spectrum results from the fact that these disorders vary in the severity of their effects (e.g., the 47,XXY karyotype may predominately impair fertility in men, whereas 46,XY/45,X mosaicism commonly results in sexual ambiguity). Second, since the process of sexual differentiation normally is sequential, individual manifestation of abnormal development (such as hypospadias) can result from abnormalities that occur at any stage in the process.

Despite these problems of variability and overlap, the correct diagnosis can usually be ascertained if all relevant clinical information is assembled, including detailed delineation of the chromosomal complement and assessment of the endocrine status.

TABLE 41–1. COMMON MANIFESTATIONS OF ABNORMALITIES OF SEXUAL DIFFERENTIATION

Ambiguous Genitalia in the Newborn
  True hermaphroditism
  Mixed gonadal dysgenesis
  The absent testes syndrome
  Female pseudohermaphroditism
  Male pseudohermaphroditism
Inappropriate pubertal development
  Congenital adrenal hyperplasia due to 21- or 11-
    hydroxylase deficiency
  True hermaphroditism
Impaired pubertal development
  Gonadal dysgenesis
  Klinefelter syndrome
  XX Male syndrome
  Pure gonadal dysgenesis
  The absent testes syndrome
  Congenital adrenal hyperplasia due to 17-hydroxylase
    deficiency in females
  Male pseudohermaphroditism
Infertility
  Klinefelter syndrome
  XX Male syndrome
  Infertile male with androgen resistance

However, diagnosis can be difficult in the prepubertal and neonatal periods, when assessment of ultimate endocrine status is generally not practical. Even in such instances, however, the combination of genetic, phenotypic, and chromosomal assessment usually restricts the diagnostic possibilities to a limited number of conditions so that appropriate gender assignment can be made and appropriate tailoring of phenotype can be carried out.

DISORDERS OF CHROMOSOMAL SEX

Disorders of chromosomal sex (Table 41–2) occur when the number or structure of the X or Y chromosomes is abnormal.

KLINEFELTER SYNDROME

Klinefelter, Reifenstein and Albright (1942) described a disorder in men characterized by small firm testes, varying degrees of impaired sexual maturation, azoospermia, gynecomastia, and elevated levels of urinary gonadotropins. The fundamental defect was shown to be the presence of an extra X chromosome in a male (Jacobs and Strong, 1959). The common karyotype is either a 47,XXY chromosomal pattern (the classic form) or 46,XY/47,XXY (the mosaic form). This disorder is the most common major abnormality of sexual differentiation with an incidence of approximately 1 in 500 males.

Clinical Features. Subjects with the Klinefelter syndrome usually come to medical attention after the time of expected puberty and often are recognized as having the condition only incidentally. Prepubertally, patients have small testes with decreased numbers of spermatogonia, but otherwise they appear normal. After puberty the disorder becomes manifest as infertility, gynecomastia, or occasionally under-androgenization (Fig. 41–1). The frequency of the various clinical features is given in Table 41–3. Damage to the seminiferous tubules and azoospermia are consistent features of the 47,XXY variety. The small firm testes are characteristically less than 2 and are always less than 3.5 cm in length (corresponding to 2 and 12 ml volume, respectively). Typical histologic changes in the testes include hyalinization of the tubules, absence of spermatogenesis, and an apparent increase in Leydig cells.

The increased average body height in the disorder is the result of an increased lower body segment. Gynecomastia ordinarily appears during adolescence, is generally bilateral and painless, and may progress to become disfiguring.

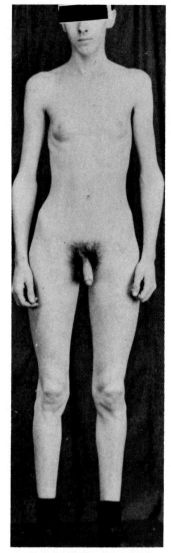

Figure 41–1. A patient with Klinefelter syndrome. (Courtesy of Dr. Harry F. Klinefelter.)

Obesity and varicose veins occur in one third to one half of patients, and mild mental deficiency, social maladjustment, subtle abnormalities of thyroid function, diabetes mellitus, and pulmonary disease may be more common than in the general population. The risk of breast cancer is 20 times that in normal men, though the incidence is only about one-fifth that in women. Most patients have a male psychosexual orientation and are capable of functioning sexually as normal men.

The variant with 46,XY/47,XXY mosaicism composes about 10 per cent of the patients, as estimated by chromosomal karyotypes on peripheral blood leukocytes. The frequency of this

TABLE 41–2. CLINICAL FEATURES OF THE DISORDERS OF CHROMOSOMAL SEX

Disorder	Common Chromosomal Complement	Gonadal Development	External Genitalia	Internal Genitalia	Breast Development	Comment
Klinefelter syndrome	47,XXY or 46,XY/ 47,XXY	Hyalinized testes	Normal male	Normal male	Gynecomastia	Most common disorder of sexual differentiation; tall stature.
XX Male	46,XX	Hyalinized testes	Normal male	Normal male	Gynecomastia	Shorter than normal men; increased incidence of hypospadias. Similar to Klinefelter syndrome. May be familial.
Gonadal dysgenesis (Turner syndrome)	45,X or 46,XX/ 45,X	Streak gonads	Immature female	Hypoplastic female	Immature female	Short stature and multiple somatic abnormalities. May be 46,XX with structurally abnormal X chromosome.
Mixed gonadal dysgenesis	46,XY/45,X or 46,XY	Testis and streak gonad	Variable but almost always ambiguous; 60% reared as female	Uterus, vagina, and one fallopian tube	Usually male	Second most common cause of ambiguous genitalia in the newborn; tumors common.
True hermaphroditism	46,XX or 46,XY or mosaics	Testis and ovary or ovotestis	Variable but usually ambiguous; 75% reared as males	Usually a uterus and urogenital sinus; ducts correspond to gonad	Gynecomastia in 75%	May be familial.

(From Petersdorf, R. G., Adams, R. D., Braunwald, E., et al.: Disorders of sexual differentiation. *In* Harrison's Principles of Internal Medicine. 10th ed. New York, McGraw-Hill Book Co., 1983, pp. 724–739.)

TABLE 41–3. Characteristics of Patients with Classic versus Mosaic Klinefelter Syndrome*

	47,XXY (%)	46,XY/47,XXY (%)
Abnormal testicular histology	100	94†
Decreased length of testis	99	73†
Azoospermia	93	50†
Decreased testosterone	79	33
Decreased facial hair	77	64
Increased gonadotropins	75	33†
Decreased sexual function	68	56
Gynecomastia	55	33†
Decreased axillary hair	49	46
Decreased length of penis	41	21

*Table based on 519 XXY patients and 51 XY/XXY patients.

†Significantly different at p <0.05 or better.

After Gordon, D. L., Krmpotic, E., Thomas, W., Gandy, H. M., and Paulsen, C. A.: Pathologic testicular findings in Klinefelter's syndrome. Arch. Intern. Med., *130*:726, 1972.

variant may be underestimated, since chromosomal mosaicism may be present only in the testes. Thus, the peripheral leukocyte karyotype may be normal, and the patient may still have the Klinefelter syndrome. As summarized in Table 41–3, the mosaic form is usually not as severe as the 47,XXY variety, and the testes may be normal in size (Gordon et al., 1972). The endocrine abnormalities are also less severe, and gynecomastia and azoospermia are less common. Indeed, occasional patients with mosaicism may be fertile. In some individuals the diagnosis may not even be suspected because of the minor degree of the physical abnormalities.

Approximately 30 additional karyotypic varieties of the Klinefelter syndrome have been described, including those with uniform cell lines (such as XXYY, XXXY, and XXXXY) and a variety of mosaicisms of the X chromosome with or without associated structural abnormalities of the X chromosome. In general, the greater the degree of chromosomal abnormality (and in mosaic forms the more cell lines that are abnormal), the more severe the manifestations.

Pathophysiology. The classic form of the Klinefelter syndrome is caused by meiotic nondisjunction of the chromosomes during gametogenesis (Fig. 41–2). About 40 per cent of the responsible meiotic nondisjunctions occur during spermatogenesis, and 60 per cent occur during oogenesis. Advanced maternal age is a predisposing factor in the cases in which the defect occurs during oogenesis. In contrast, the mosaic form of the disorder is thought to result from chromosomal mitotic nondisjunction after fertilization of the zygote and can take place either in a 46,XY zygote (Fig. 41–2) or in a 47,XXY zygote. The latter defect or double nondisjunction (meiotic and mitotic) may be the usual cause of the mosaic form and may thus explain why the mosaic form is less common than the classic disorder.

Endocrine changes in the pituitary-testicular axis are characteristic. Plasma follicle-stimulating hormone (FSH) and luteinizing hormone (LH) levels are usually high; FSH shows the best discrimination, and little overlap occurs with normal individuals, a consequence of the consistent damage to the seminiferous tubules (Leonard et al., 1979). The plasma testosterone level averages half of normal, but the range of values is broad and overlaps the normal range. Mean plasma estradiol levels are elevated, the

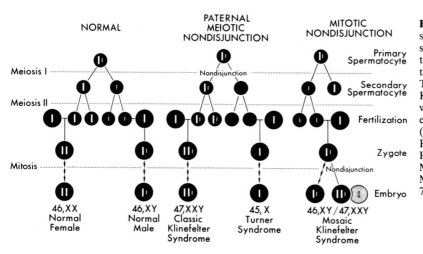

Figure 41–2. Schema for normal spermatogenesis and fertilization showing effects of meiotic and mitotic nondisjunction leading to the classic Klinefilter syndrome, Turner syndrome, and mosaic Klinefelter syndrome. The schema would be similar if the abnormal events took place in oogenesis. (From Petersdorf, R. G., Adams, R. E., Braunwald, E., et al.: *In* Harrison's Principles of Internal Medicine. 10th ed. New York, McGraw-Hill Book Co., 1983, p. 727. Used by permission.)

cause of which is not entirely clear. Early in the course of the disorder, the testes may secrete increased amounts of estradiol in response to the elevated plasma LH, but later in the course the testicular secretion of estradiol (and testosterone) declines. Elevated plasma estradiol levels in this circumstance are probably due to a combination of a decreased metabolic clearance rate and an increased rate of testosterone conversion to estradiol in extraglandular tissues (Wang et al., 1975). The net result both early and late is a variable degree of insufficient androgenization and enhanced feminization. This feminization, including the development of gynecomastia, is thought to depend on the ratio of circulating estrogen:androgen (relative or absolute), and it follows that subjects with the lower plasma testosterone and higher plasma estradiol levels are more likely to develop gynecomastia. The increase in plasma gonadotropins after the administration of luteinizing hormone–releasing hormone (LHRH) is exaggerated after the age of expected puberty, and the normal feedback inhibition of testosterone on pituitary LH secretion is diminished. Older patients with untreated Klinefelter syndrome may have "reactive pituitary abnormalities" in the form of enlarged or abnormal sellae, presumably secondary to the persistent lack of gonadal feedback, and hypertrophy of gonadotropes, in response to stimulation by LHRH (Samaan et al., 1979). It is not known whether there is actual adenoma formation.

Management. No method is available for reversing the infertility, and surgical removal is the only available means for effective treatment of the gynecomastia. Some underandrogenized patients benefit from supplemental androgen, but such treatment may paradoxically worsen the gynecomastia, presumably by providing increased androgen substrate for the conversion to estrogens in the peripheral tissues. Androgen should be administered in the form of injections of testosterone cypionate or testosterone enanthate (Snyder and Lawrence, 1980). Following the administration of testosterone, plasma LH returns to normal, usually only after several months (Caminos-Torres et al., 1977).

XX MALE SYNDROME

The incidence of a 46,XX karyotype in phenotypic males is approximately 1 in 20,000 to 24,000 male births. More than 150 XX males have been reported (de la Chapelle, 1981). Affected individuals lack all female internal genitalia and have male psychosexual identification. The findings resemble those in the Klinefelter syndrome: the testes are small and firm (generally less than 2 cm); gynecomastia is frequent; the penis is normal to small in size; azoospermia and hyalinization of the seminiferous tubules are usual. Mean plasma testosterone levels are low, the plasma estradiol level is elevated, and plasma gonadotropin levels are high (Perez-Palacios et al., 1981; Schweikert et al., 1982). Affected individuals differ from typical Klinefelter patients in that average height is less than in normal men, the incidence of mental deficiency is not increased, and the incidence of hypospadias is increased (Roe and Alfi, 1977).

Four theories have been proposed to explain the pathogenesis of this disorder: (1) mosaicism in some cell lines for a Y-containing cell line or early loss of a Y chromosome; (2) a mendelian gene mutation on an autosome; (3) interchange of a Y-chromosomal gene with the X chromosome; and (4) deletion or inactivation of an X chromosomal gene or genes that normally have a negative regulatory effect on testis development (de la Chapelle, 1981). Although some evidence has been marshaled to support each of these four possibilities in individual instances of XX males, as yet there is no unifying hypothesis that can explain all the facts known about XX males. Although mosaicism appears to be unlikely in most cases, the other listed explanations remain possible. The etiology of the condition may be heterogeneous.

The management of the disorder is similar to that of the Klinefelter syndrome.

GONADAL DYSGENESIS (THE TURNER SYNDROME)

Gonadal dysgenesis is characterized by primary amenorrhea, sexual infantilism, short stature, multiple congenital anomalies, and bilateral streak gonads in phenotypic women with any of several defects of the X chromosome. This condition should be distinguished from three similar disorders: (1) mixed gonadal dysgenesis, in which a unilateral testis and a contralateral streak gonad are present; (2) pure gonadal dysgenesis, in which bilateral streak gonads are associated with a normal 46,XX or 46,XY karyotype, normal stature, and primary amenorrhea; and (3) the Noonan syndrome, which is an autosomal dominant disorder characterized by the presence of webbed neck, short stature, congenital heart disease, cubitus valgus, and other congenital defects in both males and females with normal karyotypes and normal gonads. The eponym associated with gonadal dysgenesis stems from the description by Turner in

1938 of seven patients with sexual infantilism, short stature, congenital webbed neck, and cubitus valgus (Turner, 1938). Subsequently, a 45,X chromosomal complement was found to be present in typical patients (Ford et al., 1959). The term "Turner's syndrome" then came to be applied to such patients. However, not all patients with bilateral streak gonads and some X chromosome abnormality have the characteristic somatic features or a 45,X chromosomal complement. Thus, "gonadal dysgenesis" is the preferred term whether or not the Turner features are present. This disorder is the most common cause of primary amenorrhea, accounting for as many as one third of all such patients (Ross et al., 1981).

Clinical Features. The 45,X complement is the most common chromosomal abnormality in the disorder. It is found in 0.8 per cent of zygotes, but less than 3 per cent of the 45,X embryos survive to term, so the incidence of 45,X in newborns is about 1 in 2700 live phenotypic females. However, this is an underestimate of the incidence of gonadal dysgenesis, since only about half of patients have a 45,X chromosomal complement (see later discussion).

The diagnosis is made either at birth, because of the associated anomalies, or more frequently at puberty, when amenorrhea and failure of sexual development are noted in conjunction with the associated anomalies (Fig. 41–3). The external genitalia are unambiguously female, but they remain immature and there is usually no breast development unless the patient is treated with exogenous estrogen. The internal genitalia consist of small but otherwise normal fallopian tubes and uterus and bilateral streak gonads located in the broad ligaments. Primordial germ cells are present transiently during embryogenesis but disappear as the result of an accelerated rate of atresia (Singh and Carr, 1966). After the age of expected puberty, these streaks contain fibrous tissue that is indistinguishable from normal ovarian stroma but usually lack identifiable follicles and ova.

The associated somatic anomalies primarily affect tissues of mesodermal origin, that is, the skeleton and connective tissue. Lymphedema of the hands and feet, webbing of the neck, a low hair line, redundant skin folds on the back of the neck, a shieldlike chest with widely spaced nipples, and a low birth weight are features that suggest the diagnosis in infancy. In addition, the facies may be distinctively characterized by micrognathia, epicanthal folds, prominent, low set or deformed ears, a fishlike mouth, and ptosis.

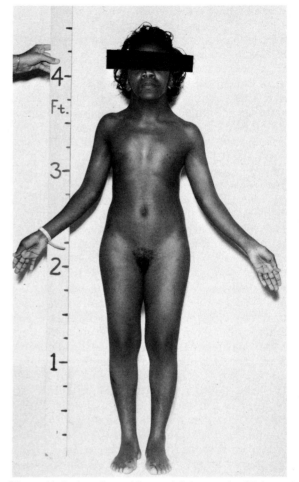

Figure 41–3. A patient with gonadal dysgenesis. (Courtesy of Dr. Peggy Whalley.)

Short fourth metacarpals are present in one half of patients, and 10 to 20 per cent have congenital cardiac abnormalities. Coarctation of the aorta (preductal or postductal) is the most common cardiac abnormality, especially in 45,X patients. Less common cardiac abnormalities include aortic valve disease, ventricular septal defect, atrial septal defect, dextrocardia, and hypoplastic left heart. Pulmonic stenosis (more typical of the Noonan syndrome) is occasionally seen in 45,X patients. Vascular malformations are infrequent but include intestinal telangiectasis, hemangiomas, and lymphangiectasis as potential causes of gastrointestinal bleeding. In adults the average height rarely exceeds 150 cm. The short stature is primarily due to a decrease in the lower segment height. Associated conditions include renal malformations, pigmented nevi, hypoplastic nails, a tendency toward keloid formation, perceptive hearing loss, unexplained hypertension, and certain autoimmune disorders. The renal abnormalities are particularly common, with about 60 per cent of all patients with gonadal dysgenesis having some renal structural abnormality compared with 10 per cent of normal individuals. Horseshoe kidneys, with or without duplication of the collecting ducts and malrotation of the kidney, are the most common abnormality. The associated autoimmune disorders include primary hypothyroidism, inflammatory bowel disease, and diabetes. Frank hypothyroidism is seen in approximately 20 per cent of adult women with gonadal dysgenesis. Both regional enteritis and ulcerative colitis appear to have an increased incidence in these patients as well. The association with diabetes is somewhat less clear, since initial studies were based only on glucose tolerance testing. Impaired insulin release in subjects with gonadal dysgenesis as compared with nonaffected siblings has been reported (AvRuskin et al., 1979).

Pathophysiology. About one half of patients have a 45,X karyotype, and the cytogenetic findings in the remainder are variable. Approximately one fourth have mosaicism with no structural abnormality (46,XX/45,X), and the remainder have a structurally abnormal X chromosome with or without mosaicism (Simpson, 1979). In occasional individuals, the mosaicism may be limited to the streak gonad with a uniform 46,XX karyotype in peripheral blood and skin. The most frequent X chromosome structural abnormality is an isochromosome for the X long arm, or i(Xq), in which there has been abnormal division of the centromere in the transverse rather than the longitudinal plane so that both arms of the chromosome are the same, with duplication of the long arm (Xq) and complete deletion of the short arm (Xp). About two thirds of the time this i(Xq) occurs with mosaicism for 45,X instead of alone. Deletions of the X long arm [del (Xq)] or the X short arm [del (Xp)] are usually incomplete and are less common. The 45,X variety may result from chromosome loss during gametogenesis in either parent or from an error in mitosis during one of the early cleavage divisions of the fertilized zygote (see Fig. 41–2). Short stature and other somatic features result from loss of genetic material on the short arm of the X chromosome. Streak gonads result when genetic material is missing from either the long or short arm of the X chromosome. In individuals with mosaicism or with structural abnormalities of the X chromosome, phenotypes, on average, are intermediate in severity between those seen in the 45,X variety and the normal. In some patients with

hypertrophy of the clitoris, there is an unidentified fragment of a chromosome present in addition to the X chromosome, which is assumed to be an abnormal Y. Rarely, familial transmission of gonadal dysgenesis can be the result of a balanced X-autosome translocation (Leichtman et al., 1978).

Assessment of sex chromatin was previously used as a means of screening for abnormalities of the X chromosome. Normal sex chromatin (the Barr body) is the result of inactivation of one of two X chromosomes, and women with a 45,X chromosome composition, like normal men, are said to be chromatin-negative. However, only about half of the patients with gonadal dysgenesis (those with 45,X and those with the most extreme forms of mosaicism and structural abnormalities) are chromatin-negative, and karyotypic analysis is necessary both to establish the diagnosis and to identify the fraction with Y-chromosomal elements, who have as much as a 15 per cent chance of developing malignancy in the streak gonads.

Although sparse pubic and axillary hair develops at the time of expected puberty, the breasts usually remain infantile, and no menses occur. In contrast to individuals with the Klinefelter syndrome, who have no detectable endocrine abnormality prepubertally, patients with gonadal dysgenesis have elevations of gonadotropins that are detectable from the neonatal period to 4 years of age (Conte et al., 1975). After this period, there is a decline to normal levels of gonadotropins between 4 and 10 years of age, which is followed by a rise to high levels again after 10 years of age. The degree of elevation of FSH is of greater magnitude than that of LH. This pattern of secretion is qualitatively similar to normal children, indicating that the program of secretion is inherent in the hypothalamic-pituitary axis, and only the amounts of gonadotropin secretion are modulated by gonadal function. As in the case of the Klinefelter syndrome, mosaicism with a normal chromosomal complement lessens the severity of the gonadal abnormality. Thus patients with gonadal dysgenesis who are past the age of expected puberty have a greater likelihood of menses and breast development if some of the cells have a normal 46,XX complement. Approximately 3 per cent of 45,X subjects and 12 per cent of mosaic subjects have sufficient residual follicles to allow some menstruation. Moreover, although only 5 per cent of nonmosaic subjects have spontaneous breast development, almost one fifth of mosaic individuals have some

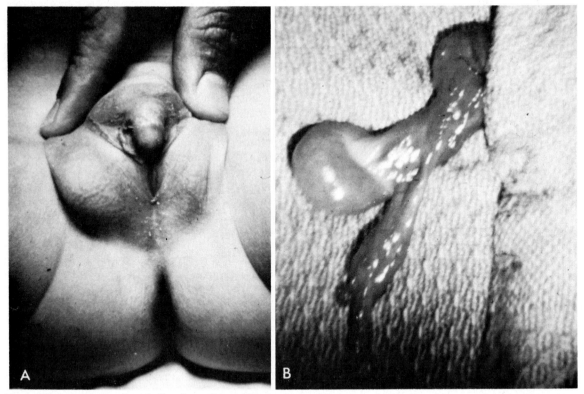

Figure 41–4. *A,* External genitalia of a patient with mixed gonadal dysgenesis. *B,* The right scrotal testis of the same patient, demonstrating the adjacent fallopian tube.

spontaneous feminization (Simpson, 1979). Pregnancy occasionally occurs in the less severely affected individuals with spontaneous menses and secondary sex characteristics. About a dozen pregnancies have been reported in nonmosaic patients, and more than 100 have been noted in mosaic individuals. There is a 50 per cent incidence of fetal wastage and a 33 per cent incidence of chromosomal abnormalities in newborn offspring. The reproductive life of such patients with gonadal dysgenesis is brief and is followed by early menopause.

Management. At the anticipated time of puberty, replacement therapy with estrogen should be instituted in those without spontaneous feminization to induce maturation of the breasts, labia, vagina, uterus, and fallopian tubes. Linear growth and bone maturation rates are approximately doubled during the first year of treatment with estradiol, but the eventual height of patients rarely approaches the predicted height. Ultimate height gain is not affected by the timing of the initiation of hormone therapy. Treatment with growth hormone has not been helpful. Therapy should be initiated with low doses of conjugated estrogens or ethinyl estradiol alone 25 days a month for the first

6 to 12 months with a subsequent increase in the estrogen dose. In many clinics it is customary in addition to add medroxyprogesterone acetate during the last 10 of the 25 days.

Gonadal tumors are rare in 45,X patients. However, gonadal malignancies have occurred in patients with mosaicism involving the Y chromosome. Consequently, streak gonads should be removed in any patient with evidence of virilization or a Y-containing cell line.

MIXED GONADAL DYSGENESIS

Mixed gonadal dysgenesis is an entity in which phenotypic males or females have a testis on one side and a streak gonad on the other (Sohval, 1963). Most have 45,X/46,XY mosaicism, but the clinical entity is by no means confined to that chromosomal pattern. The true incidence is unknown, but in most hospitals it is the second most common cause of ambiguous genitalia in the neonate, after congenital adrenal hyperplasia.

Clinical Features. About two thirds of patients are reared as females, and most phenotypic males are incompletely virilized at birth. The majority exhibit some degree of ambiguous genitalia, including phallic enlargement, a urogenital sinus, and varying degrees of labioscrotal fusion (Fig. 41–4*A*). In most, the testis is located intra-abdominally; individuals with a testis in the inguinal or scrotal position are usually reared as males. A uterus, vagina, and at least one fallopian tube are almost invariably present in phenotypic males as well as in phenotypic females (Fig. 41–4*B* and 41–5).

On histologic examination, the prepubertal testis appears relatively normal. The postpubertal testis contains abundant mature Leydig cells, but the seminiferous tubules contain only Sertoli cells and lack germinal elements. Frequently, the testis is undescended, and when descended it may present in association with a hernia containing the uterus and fallopian tube. The streak gonad—a thin, pale, elongated structure located either in the broad ligament or along the pelvic wall—is composed of fibrous connective tissue that is often arranged in whorls so that it resembles ovarian stroma. At puberty, the testis secretes androgen, and both virilization and phallic enlargement occur. Feminization is rare; when it occurs, estrogen secretion from a gonadal tumor should be suspected.

Approximately one third of patients exhibit the somatic features of 45,X gonadal dysgenesis, that is, low posterior hairline, shield chest, multiple pigmented nevi, cubitus valgus, webbing of the neck, and short stature (height less than 150 cm).

Virtually all are chromatin-negative. About two thirds have the 45,X/46,XY karyotype, and in the remainder a 46,XY karyotype is present, but mosaicism might have been undetected. The origin of 45,X/46,XY mosaicism is best explained by the loss of a Y chromosome during an early mitotic division of an XY zygote similar to the postulated loss of the X chromosome in 46,XY/47,XXY mosaicism, as shown in 41–2.

Pathophysiology. It has been assumed that the 45,XY cell line stimulates testicular differentiation, whereas the 45,X stem leads to the development of the contralateral streak gonad, but actual comparisons between karyotype and phenotypic expression have failed to substantiate such a relationship; furthermore, no clear correlation has been found between the percentage of cells cultured from blood or skin containing 45,X or 46,XY and the degree of gonadal development of somatic anomalies.

Both masculinization and müllerian duct regression in utero are incomplete. Since Leydig cell function is normal at puberty, the inadequate virilization in utero may be the result of delay in the development of a testis that is ultimately capable of normal Leydig cell function. The capacity of the internal duct structures, the urogenital sinus, and the external genitalia to virilize completely in response to androgen is limited to a critical period between 7 and 14 weeks of gestation, and consequently a delayed but otherwise normal onset of endocrine function in the fetal testis might allow incomplete masculinization of the external genitalia and explain persistence of müllerian ducts. Alternatively, the fetal testis may simply be incapable of synthesizing adequate amounts of müllerian-inhibiting substance and androgen.

Management. Several factors must be considered in the management of patients with mixed gonadal dysgenesis. For the older child

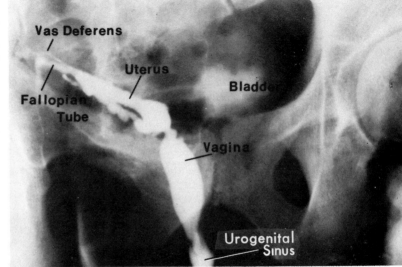

Figure 41–5. Retrograde genitogram, with a blunt-ended syringe placed in the urogenital sinus of a patient with mixed gonadal dysgenesis. The vagina, uterus, fallopian tube, and vas deferens are demonstrated.

or adult in whom gender is fixed prior to diagnosis, the central issue is the possibility of tumor development in the gonads. The overall incidence of gonadal tumors in patients with mixed gonadal dysgenesis is about 25 per cent. Seminomas occur more frequently than gonadoblastomas. The tumors may occur prior to puberty, occur most frequently in patients with a female phenotype who lack the somatic features typical of 45,X gonadal dysgenesis, and are more common in intra-abdominal testes than in the streak gonads. When the diagnosis is established in phenotypic females, early exploratory laparotomy and prophylactic gonadectomy are advisable for two reasons: (1) gonadal tumors may occur in childhood, and (2) the testis secretes androgen at puberty and thus causes virilization. Such subjects, like those with gonadal dysgenesis, are then given estrogen to induce and maintain feminization.

When the diagnosis is established in phenotypic males during late childhood or in adults the management is more complicated. Phenotypic males with mixed gonadal dysgenesis are infertile (no germinal elements are present in the testes) and also have a high risk of developing gonadal tumors. Which testes can be safely conserved? In general the following observations apply: (1) tumors develop in scrotal streak gonads but not in scrotal testes; (2) tumors that develop in intra-abdominal testes are always associated with ipsilateral müllerian duct structures; and (3) tumors in streak gonads are always associated with tumors in the contralateral abdominal testis. Based on these observations, it is recommended that (1) all streak gonads be removed; (2) scrotal testes be preserved; and (3) intra-abdominal testes be excised unless they can be relocated in the scrotum and unless they are not associated with ipsilateral müllerian duct structures. Decisions as to reconstructive surgery of the phallus depends upon the nature of the defect. Gender assignment is usually female in those subjects who are identified because of ambiguous genitalia as a newborn. Resection of the enlarged phallus and gonadectomy in such patients can be accomplished in infancy, usually in one procedure.

TRUE HERMAPHRODITISM

True hermaphroditism is a condition in which both an ovary and a testis or a gonad with histologic features of both (ovotestis) is present. The incidence is unknown, but more than 400 cases have been reported (van Niekerk and Retief, 1981). To justify the diagnosis there must be histologic documentation of both types of gonadal epithelium; the presence of ovarian stroma without oocytes is not sufficient. Three categories are recognized: (1) one fifth are bilateral (testicular and ovarian tissue [ovotestes] on each side); (2) two fifths are unilateral (an ovotestis on one side and an ovary or a testis on the other); and (3) the remainder are lateral (a testis on one side and an ovary on the other). The ovary occurs most commonly on the left side, whereas testicular tissue, occurring either as a testis or an ovotestis, has a greater tendency to occur on the right side of the body.

Clinical Features. The external genitalia display all gradations of the male to female spectrum. Three fourths of patients are sufficiently masculinized to be reared as males. However, less than one tenth have normal male external genitalia; most have hypospadias, and more than half have incomplete labioscrotal fusion. Two thirds of phenotypic females have an enlarged clitoris, and most have a urogenital sinus. Commonly, differentiation of the internal ducts corresponds to the adjacent gonad. Although an epididymis usually develops adjacent to a testis, development of the vas deferens is complete in only one third of patients. Only one duct is usually present next to an ovotestis. On histologic examination about two thirds of the ducts next to an ovotestis have the characteristics of a fallopian tube, and one third have the characteristics of a vas deferens. The more testicular tissue present in an ovotestis, the more likely that the adjacent duct will be a vas deferens (van Niekerk, 1981). A uterus is usually present, though it may be hypoplastic or unicornuate; the latter is characteristic of lateral true hermaphroditism with absence of the horn on the side of the testis. The ovary usually occupies the normal position, but the testis or ovotestis may be found at any level along the route of embryonic testicular descent and is frequently associated with an inguinal hernia. Testicular tissue is present in the scrotum or the labioscrotal fold in one third patients, in the inguinal canal in one third of patients, and in the abdominal area in one third of patients.

At puberty signs of variable feminization and virilization develop; three fourths of patients develop significant gynecomastia, and about half menstruate. In phenotypic men, menstruation presents as cyclic hematuria. Ovulation occurs in approximately a fourth and is more common than spermatogenesis. In phenotypic men ovulation may present as testicular pain. Fertility has been reported in women following removal of an ovotestis and in a man who fathered two children. Congenital malformations of other systems are rare.

Pathophysiology. About two thirds of subjects have a 46,XX karyotype, one tenth have a 46,XY karyotype, and the remainder are chromosomal mosaics. True hermaphroditism associated with chromosomal mosaicism falls into two categories. The first of these, 46,XX/46,XY true hermaphroditism, is about as common as the 46,XY variety and is thought to arise most commonly from chimerism, the presence in a single individual of cells derived from two zygotes, as in the fertilization of an ovum and its polar body. True hermaphroditism has also been described in subjects with a 45,X/46,XY chromosome composition. However, neither ovulation nor spermatogenesis has been described in the latter disorder, and it is likely that it is a form of mixed gonadal dysgenesis, in which, as in other types of gonadal dysgenesis, atresia of the ovarian follicles is incomplete. True hermaphroditism has rarely been reported with other forms of mosaicism such as 46,XY/47,XXY, but these disorders have not been characterized in detail. The mechanism responsible for the gonadal development in true hermaphroditism is unknown. In general, the presence of a Y chromosome increases the likelihood of a testis occurring from about one fifth in the overall population of true hermaphroditism to three-fifths. The most common gonadal distribution pattern in 46,XX patients is an ovary on one side and an ovotestis on the other side. In those individuals without a Y-containing line in the chromosomal complement, it is assumed that testis development occurs as a result of the presence of genetic material derived from the Y chromosome. The rare instances of 46,XX true hermaphroditism associated with a positive family history seem to be most consistent with an autosomal recessive pattern of inheritance.

Because corpora lutea are present in the ovaries of more than one fourth of subjects, it can be deduced that a female neuroendocrine axis is present and that it functions normally in such individuals. Feminization (gynecomastia and menstruation) is the result of the secretion of estradiol by the ovarian tissue that is present (Aiman et al., 1978). It is presumed that secretion of androgen predominates over secretion of estrogen in masculinized patients, and the fact that some patients produce sperm is in keeping with this view. The venous effluent from one ovotestis was shown to contain a concentration of testosterone that was similar to that found in the testicular vein of normal men (Roy et al., 1980).

Management. When the diagnosis is made in a newborn or young infant, gender assignment depends largely upon the anatomical findings. In older children and adults, gonads and internal duct structures that are contradictory to the predominant phenotype (and the gender of rearing) should be removed, and when necessary the external genitalia should be modified appropriately. Although gonadal tumors are rare in true hermaphroditism, gonadoblastoma has been reported in an individual with an XY cell line. Consequently, the possibility of future tumor development in the gonad must be taken into consideration when the decision regarding conservation of gonadal tissue is made.

DISORDERS OF GONADAL SEX

Disorders of gonadal sex result when chromosomal sex is normal, but for one of several reasons differentiation of the gonads is abnormal. Thus, chromosomal sex does not correspond to gonadal and phenotypic sex.

PURE GONADAL DYSGENESIS

The syndrome of "pure gonadal dysgenesis," as the term is used here, is restricted to phenotypic females with gonads and genitalia that are identical to those in patients with gonadal dysgenesis (bilateral streak gonads and usually sexual infantilism), but who have normal height, few if any congenital anomalies, and either a uniform 46,XX or 46,XY chromosomal complement. In one series, this disorder was about one third as common as gonadal dysgenesis (McDonough et al., 1977).

Clinical Features. There is a clear-cut genetic basis for considering this to be a separate disorder from gonadal dysgenesis, but on clinical grounds it cannot be distinguished from those instances of gonadal dysgenesis that are associated with minimal somatic abnormalities. The height is normal or greater than normal, some subjects being more than 170 cm. Estrogen deficiency varies from profound deficiency typical of classic 45,X gonadal dysgenesis to some breast development and appearance of menses that invariably terminate with an early menopause. As many as 40 per cent have some feminization (McDonough et al., 1977). Axillary and pubic hair are scanty, and the internal genitalia consist solely of müllerian derivatives.

Tumors may develop in the streak gonads, particularly dysgerminoma or gonadoblastoma in the 46,XY disorder. Such tumors are frequently heralded by the development of virilizing signs or a pelvic mass.

Pathophysiology. Although a variety of chromosomal mosaicisms have been described under this nosology, the designation as used here is restricted to subjects with uniform 46,XX or 46,XY karyotypes. (Those individuals with mosaicism are actually variants of gonadal dysgenesis or mixed gonadal dysgenesis as already described). The rationale for this restricted definition is based upon the fact that both the XX and XY varieties can result from different single gene mutations. Several sibships have been reported in which more than one individual is affected with the 46,XX type of the disorder, and they are frequently the result of consanguineous matings, suggesting that the disorder is transmitted in an autosomal recessive pattern. Furthermore, several instances of familial occurrence of the 46,XY variety have been described in which the mutation appears to be inherited either as an X-linked recessive mutation or as a male-limited autosomal recessive trait (Simpson et al., 1981). Thus, the familial 46,XY form of pure gonadal dysgenesis is genetically heterogenous. In both the 46,XX and the 46,XY forms the mutation prevents differentiation of the ovary or testis, respectively, by an uncertain mechanism; the development of the female phenotype in both situations is the consequence of the failure of gonadal development.

Management. Management of the estrogen deficiency is identical to that in gonadal dysgenesis; appropriate estrogen replacement therapy is initiated at the time of expected puberty and is maintained in adult life. Because of the high frequency of gonadal tumors in the 46,XY variety, exploratory surgery and removal of the streak gonads should be undertaken once the diagnosis is made. The development of virilizing signs is indication for immediate surgery. The natural history of the gonadal tumors is uncertain, but the prognosis after surgical removal appears to be good.

THE ABSENT TESTES SYNDROME (ANORCHIA, GONADAL AGENESIS, TESTICULAR REGRESSION, AGONADISM)

A spectrum of phenotypes has been described in 46,XY males with absent or rudimentary testes in whom unequivocal evidence exists that endocrine function of the testis (e.g., variable müllerian duct regression and variable testosterone synthesis) was present at some time during embryonic life. This rare disorder can be distinguished from pure gonadal dysgenesis in which no evidence can be inferred for gonadal function during embryonic development. The disorder has been reported under a variety of eponyms and varies in its manifestations from complete failure of virilization through varying degrees of incomplete virilization of the external genitalia to otherwise normal males with bilateral anorchia (Bergada et al., 1962). An analogous disorder may occur in 46,XX phenotypic females in whom gonadal absence is associated with sexual infantilism and müllerian development (Medina et al., 1982).

Clinical Features. The purest form of the syndrome is represented by 46,XY phenotypic females with absent testes, sexual infantilism, and concomitant absence of the müllerian duct derivative and accessory organs of male reproduction. The syndrome in such individuals differs from the 46,XY form of pure gonadal dysgenesis in that no gonadal remnant whatsoever can be identified—there are no streak gonads and no müllerian derivatives. In these women, testicular failure must have occurred during the interval between the onset of formation of müllerian-inhibiting substance and the secretion of testosterone; that is, after development of the seminiferous tubules but before the onset of Leydig cell function. In others, the clinical features indicate that the testicular failure occurred during later phases of gestation, and some of these individuals constitute problems in gender assignment. In some, failure of müllerian regression occurs to a greater extent than the failure of testosterone secretion, but none exhibit complete müllerian development. In individuals with more extensive virilization, the external genitalia are phenotypically male, but rudimentary oviducts and vasa deferentia may coexist internally.

At the final extreme is the syndrome of bilateral anorchia in phenotypic men with absence of müllerian structures and gonads but complete male development of the external genitalia and all of the wolffian system except the epididymis (Aynsley-Green et al., 1976). Microphallus in such subjects implies that failure of androgen-mediated growth occurred during late embryogenesis after anatomic development of the male urethra is complete. Persistent gynecomastia may or may not develop after the time of puberty.

Pathophysiology. The pathogenesis of these disorders is not understood. The karyotype is 46,XY by definition. Whether the testicular regression is the result of mutant genes, teratogen, or trauma is unclear. Multiple instances of agonadism in the same family have been reported, and since unilateral and bilateral agonadism can occur within the same family, it is necessary to obtain a careful family history. There have been five instances of discordance of anorchia in monozygotic twins, suggesting that some nongenetic factor may be involved (Glass, 1982; Aynsley-Green et al., 1976).

The quantitative dynamics of gonadal steroid production have been studied in only a few patients. In two phenotypic females who had primary amenorrhea, sexual infantilism, and no internal genital structures, androgen and estrogen kinetics were similar to those in gonadal dysgenesis. The daily production rates of estrogen were low, and no glandular secretion of testosterone could be documented, confirming the functional as well as anatomic absence of the testes. In one phenotypic male with bilateral anorchia there was no glandular secretion of testosterone; total testosterone and estrogen production was accounted for by peripheral conversion from plasma androstenedione (Edman et al., 1977). However, some subjects in whom no testes can be identified at laparotomy have blood testosterone values that are clearly above the castrate range, presumably derived from remnant testes (Kirschner et al., 1970).

Management. The management of the two extremes in this disorder is clear-cut. Sexually infantile, phenotypic females should be treated like patients with gonadal dysgenesis, namely they should be given adequate estrogen to ensure appropriate breast and female somatic development, and any coexisting vaginal agenesis should be treated by either surgical or medical means. Likewise, phenotypic males with anorchia should be given adequate androgen replacement to allow normal male secondary

sexual development. In one instance of monozygotic twins discordant for anorchia, testicular transplantation was successful (Silber, 1978). Cases with incomplete virilization or ambiguous development of the external genitalia are more complex and require individual assessment as to whether surgical means are appropriate for improving male or female phenotypes. In either case, appropriate hormonal therapy is mandatory at the time of expected puberty.

DISORDERS OF PHENOTYPIC SEX

FEMALE PSEUDOHERMAPHRODITISM

Congenital Adrenal Hyperplasia

The pathways by which glucocorticoids are synthesized in the adrenal gland and androgens are formed in the testis and adrenal gland are schematically summarized in Figure 41–6. A variety of syndromes result from hereditary defects in the enzymes of steroid hormone synthesis. Three enzymes are common to the formation of glucocorticoids and androgens (20,22-desmolase, 3β-hydroxysteroid dehydrogenase, and 17α-hydroxylase); deficiency of any of these enzymes results in deficiency of glucocorticoid and androgen synthesis and consequently results in both congenital adrenal hyperplasia (resulting from enhanced ACTH levels) and defective virilization of the male embryo (male pseudohermaphroditism). Two enzymes are involved exclusively in androgen synthesis (17,20-desmolase and 17β-hydroxysteroid dehydrogenase); deficiency in either results in pure male pseudohermaphroditism with normal glucocorticoid synthesis. A deficiency of either of the terminal two enzymes of glucocorticoid synthesis (21-hydroxylase and 11β-hydroxylase) results

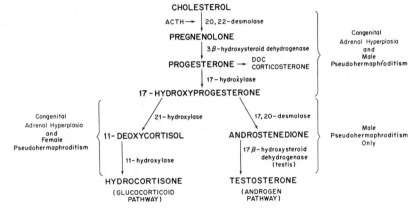

Figure 41–6. The relationship between defects in steroid hormone biosynthesis and the development of male and female pseudohermaphroditism.

in defective formation of hydrocortisone; the compensatory increase in adrenocorticotropic hormone (ACTH) secretion causes enhanced formation of adrenal steroids proximal to the enzymatic defect and a secondary increase in androgen formation. As a consequence, the latter two disorders result in adrenal hyperplasia and either virilization in the female embryo or precocious masculinization in the male. (One disorder, 3 β-hydroxysteroid dehydrogenase deficiency, can cause either male or female pseudohermaphroditism, but because the more common genital defect is incomplete virilization of the male, it will be discussed under male pseudohermaphroditism.)

Clinical Features. The adrenal insufficiency in these disorders may produce equally severe and life-threatening problems in both sexes. The major features of the different forms of congenital adrenal hyperplasia are listed in Table 41–4. From the standpoint of abnormal sexual development it is helpful to consider separately those enzyme defects in steroidogenesis that result in female pseudohermaphroditism and those that cause male pseudohermaphroditism. (One disorder, 3β-hydroxysteroid dehydrogenase deficiency, can cause either male or female pseudohermaphroditism, but since the more common genital defect is incomplete virilization of the male it will be discussed as an abnormality of male phenotypic differentiation.)

Congenital adrenal hyperplasia caused by *21-hydroxylase deficiency* is the most common cause of ambiguous genitalia in the newborn, with an incidence of between 1 in 5000 and 1 in 15,000 in Europe and the United States. Virilization is usually apparent at birth in the female and within the first 2 to 3 years of life in the male. At birth there is hypertrophy of the clitoris associated with ventral binding (chordee), variable fusion of the labioscrotal folds, and differing degrees of virilization of the urethra (Fig. 41–7). The internal female structures and ovaries remain unaltered. The wolffian ducts regress normally, probably because the onset of adrenal function occurs relatively late in embryogenesis. The labioscrotal folds are bulbous and rugated and resemble a scrotum. The external appearance of affected females is similar to that of males with bilateral cryptorchidism and hypospadias. In a small percentage, the virilization is so severe that it results in development of a complete male penile urethra and prostate so that errors in sex assignment may occur at birth (Fig. 41–7). Radiography following the injection of radio-opaque dye into

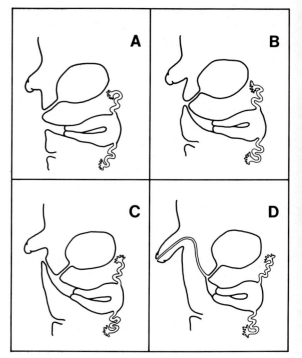

Figure 41–7. The spectrum of external virilization in congenital adrenal hyperplasia. *A,* Clitoromegaly; *B* and *C,* progressive labioscrotal fusion; *D,* complete virilization with penile urethra.

the external genital orifice is helpful in defining the internal structures and, in particular, in demonstrating the presence of vagina, uterus, and sometimes even fallopian tubes. In a few cases, virilization of the female is slight or absent at birth and becomes evident in later infancy, adolescence, or adulthood, presumably as the result of allelic variation of the mutant genes (the so-called late onset or adult form of the disorder).

The untreated female grows rapidly during the first year of life and has progressive virilization. At the time of expected puberty there is a failure of normal female sexual development and absence of menstruation. In both sexes rapid somatic maturation results in premature epiphyseal closure and short adult height. Since male phenotypic differentiation is normal, the condition usually is not recognized in the newborn male in the absence of overt adrenal insufficiency. However, there is early growth and maturation of the external genitalia, and the appearance of secondary sex characteristics, coarsening of the voice, frequent erections, and excessive muscular development are noticeable in the first few years of life. Virilization in the male can follow either of two patterns. Exces-

TABLE 41–4. FORMS OF CONGENITAL ADRENAL HYPERPLASIA

Deficiency	Cortisol	Aldosterone	Degree of Virilization of Females	Failure of Virilization of Males	Dominant Steroid Secreted	Comment
21-Hydroxylase, partial (simple virilizing or compensated)	Normal	↑	++++	0	17-Hydroxyprogesterone	Most common type (~95% of total); from one third to two thirds salt losers
Severe (salt-losing)	↓	↓↓	++++	0	17-Hydroxyprogesterone	
11β-Hydroxylase (hypertension)	↓	↓	++++	0	11-Deoxycortisol and 11-deoxycorticosterone	Hypertension
3β-Hydroxysteroid dehydrogenase	0	0	+	++++	Δ^5-3β-OH compounds (dehydroepiandrosterone)	Probably second most common, usually salt loss
17α-Hydroxylase	↓	↓	0	++++	Corticosterone and 11-deoxycorticosterone	No feminization of female, hypertension
20,22-Desmolase (lipoid adrenal hyperplasia)	0	0	0	++++	Cholesterol (?)	Rare, usually salt loss

(From Petersdorf, R. G., Adams, R. D., Braunwald, E., et al.: Disorders of sexual differentiation. *In* Harrison's Principles of Internal Medicine. 10th ed. New York, McGraw-Hill Book Co., 1983, pp. 724–739.)

sive adrenal androgens can inhibit gonadotropin production so that the testes remain infantile in size despite the acceleration of masculinization. Such untreated adult men are capable of erection and ejaculation but have no spermatogenesis. Alternatively, early adrenal androgen secretion can activate a premature maturation of the hypothalamic-pituitary axis and initiate a true precocious puberty, including early maturation of spermatogenesis. The untreated male is also subject to the development of ACTH-dependent "tumors" of the testis composed of adrenal rest cells.

In 21-hydroxylase deficiency, which accounts for about 95 per cent of congenital adrenal hyperplasia, there is reduced activity of the 21-hydroxylase enzyme, which leads to decreased production of hydrocortisone and consequently to increased release of ACTH, enlargement of the adrenal glands, and partial or complete compensation of the defect in the secretion of hydrocortisone. In about one half the patients, the enzyme defect appears to be partial, and cortisol secretion is normal as the result of the adrenal enlargement. This form is termed "simple virilizing" or "compensated." In the remainder, the enzyme deficiency is more complete; the enlarged adrenal gland fails to produce adequate amounts of cortisol and aldosterone, leading to severe salt wastage with anorexia, vomiting, volume depletion, and collapse within the first few weeks of life, the so called salt-losing form of 21-hydroxylase deficiency. In all untreated patients overproduction of the cortisol precursors prior to the 21-hydroxylase step occurs, leading to an increase in plasma progesterone and 17-hydroxyprogesterone. These act as weak aldosterone antagonists at the receptor level and in the compensated form result in greater than normal aldosterone production to maintain normal sodium balance.

A rare form of congenital adrenal hyperplasia associated with female pseudohermaphroditism is *11β-hydroxylase deficiency*. In this disorder, a block in hydroxylation at the 11-carbon results in the accumulation of 11-deoxycortisol and deoxycorticosterone (DOC), a potent salt-retaining hormone that causes hypertension rather than salt loss. The clinical features that stem from glucocorticoid deficiency and androgen excess are similar to those in 21-hydroxylase deficiency.

Pathophysiology. The reported pedigrees are consistent with an autosomal recessive pattern of inheritance for both disorders. The carrier frequency for 21-hydroxylase deficiency is about 1 in 50. At least three forms of 21-hydroxylase deficiency have been identified, all involving mutations of a gene on the sixth chromosome close to the HLA-B locus: (1) the common type, which acts like an ordinary autosomal recessive enzyme mutation; (2) a cryptic allele, which is clinically silent in homozygous form but causes typical disease when present as a genetic compound with the common variety; and (3) a late-onset variant (New and Levine, 1983). Patients with 21-hydroxylase deficiency and carriers of the disorder within a given family can be identified on the basis of the HLA haplotype. In 11β-hydroxylase deficiency there is no known linkage of the mutation to the HLA system.

Excretion of ketosteroids is elevated, as is the excretion of the major metabolites that accumulate proximal to the enzymatic blocks. In 21-hydroxylase deficiency, 17-hydroxyprogesterone accumulates in blood and is excreted predominantly as pregnanetriol. In 11-hydroxylase deficiency, 11-deoxycortisol accumulates in blood and is excreted predominantly as tetrahydrocortexolone. Plasma ACTH is elevated in untreated patients.

Management. In so far as is possible, gender assignment should correspond to the chromosomal and gonadal sex, and appropriate surgical correction of the external genitalia should be undertaken promptly. This is of particular importance because appropriately treated men and women are capable of fertility. However, if the correct diagnosis is made late (after 2 years of age) gender assignment should be changed only after careful consideration of the psychosexual background.

Medical treatment with appropriate glucocorticoids prevents the consequences of hydrocortisone deficiency, arrests the rapid virilization, and prevents premature somatic advancement and epiphyseal maturation. The suppression of the abnormal steroid secretion results in cure of the hypertension in patients with 11β-hydroxylase deficiency and allows normal onset of menses and development of female secondary sex characteristics in both disorders. In males, glucocorticoid therapy suppresses adrenal androgens and results in normal gonadotropin secretion, testicular development, and spermatogenesis. Measurements of plasma 17-hydroxyprogesterone, androstenedione, ACTH, and renin have all been used to assess the adequacy of replacement therapy. In severe forms of 21-hydroxylase deficiency that are associated with salt loss or elevated plasma renin activity, treatment with mineralocorticoids is also indicated. In such patients, the monitoring of plasma renin activity is useful for determining the adequacy of mineralocorticoid replacement.

Nonadrenal Female Pseudohermaphroditism

At present, nonadrenal causes of female pseudohermaphroditism are rare. In the past, the administration to pregnant women of progestational agents with androgenic side effects (such as 17α-ethinyl-19-nor-testosterone) to prevent abortion resulted in masculinization of female fetuses. Such infants usually virilize less severely than those with congenital adrenal hyperplasia. Female pseudohermaphroditism may also occur in babies born to mothers who have virilizing tumors (e.g., arrhenoblastomas, luteomas of pregnancy) and, rarely, under circumstances in which no etiology can be determined.

Congenital Absence Of The Vagina (Müllerian Agenesis)

Congenital absence of the vagina in combination with some form of abnormal or absent uterus (the Mayer-Rokitansky-Kuster-Hauser syndrome) is second only to gonadal dysgenesis as a cause of primary amenorrhea (Ross et al., 1981).

Clinical Features. In most patients the disorder is ascertained after the time of expected puberty because of a failure to menstruate, and absence or hypoplasia of the vagina is found. Height and intelligence are normal, and the breasts, axillary and pubic hair, and habitus are feminine in character. The uterus may vary from almost normal, lacking only a conduit to the introitus, to the more characteristic rudimentary bicornuate cords with or without a lumen (Fig. 41–8). In some patients, cyclical abdominal pain indicates that sufficient functional endometrium is present to result in retrograde menstruation or hematometra, or both.

Renal, skeletal, and other congenital anomalies are common (Griffin et al., 1976). About one third of patients have abnormal kidneys, most commonly agenesis or ectopy. Fused kidneys of the horseshoe type and solitary ectopic kidneys located in the pelvis also occur. Skeletal abnormalities are present in one tenth of patients; two thirds of them involve the spine, and limb and rib abnormalities account for most of the remainder. Specific bone abnormalities include wedge vertebrae, fusions, rudimentary or asymmetric vertebral bodies, and supernumerary vertebrae. The Klippel-Feil syndrome (congenital fusion of the cervical spine, short neck, low posterior hairline, and painless limitation of cervical movement) is a frequent association.

Pathophysiology. The karyotype is 46,XX. Most cases are believed to be sporadic in nature, but several instances of familial occurrence have been described. The most extensive study of familial occurrence is the report by Shokeir (1978) of ten individuals with a positive family history. In eight of these ten families the pattern of inheritance was most consistent with a sex-limited autosomal dominant mutation. It is not known whether the sporadic cases represent new mutations of the type responsible for the familial disorder or are multifactoral in etiology. In some familial cases variable expressivity of the defect occurs; some affected family members have skeletal or renal abnormalities only, whereas others have abnormalities of müllerian derivation, such as a double uterus (Griffin et al., 1976). Bilateral renal aplasia in stillborn infants is also commonly associated with absence of the

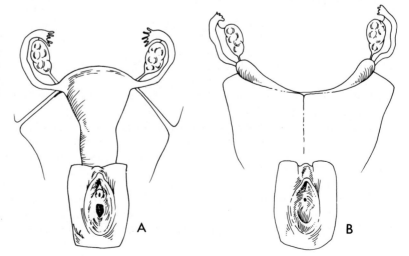

Figure 41–8. *A*, The normal female genital tract. *B*, The genital tract in congenital absence of the vagina. The blind-ending introitus, the replacement of the vagina and most of the uterus with fibrous tissue, and the bicornuate uterine remnants are characteristic findings.

uterus and vagina. Thus, the family histories should be probed for instances of isolated skeletal and renal abnormalities and for stillbirths that might result from the congenital absence of both kidneys.

Documentation of ovulatory peaks of plasma LH and biphasic temperature curves during the cycle suggests that ovarian function is normal, and successful pregnancies have been reported following corrective vaginal surgery in patients who have normal uteri.

Management. Vaginal agenesis can be treated by surgical or nonsurgical means. Surgical repair generally utilizes a split-thickness skin graft around a solid rubber mold for the creation of an artificial vagina. Medical treatment consists of the repeated application of pressure against the vaginal dimple with a simple dilator to cause development of adequate vaginal depth. In view of the overall complication rate of around 5 to 10 per cent in surgical series, medical treatment should be tried in most cases, and surgery should be reserved for patients in whom a well-formed uterus is present and the possibility of fertility exists. Continued coitus or instrumental dilatation is probably essential for maintaining the neovagina formed either by the nonoperative technique or by the surgical method.

MALE PSEUDOHERMAPHRODITISM

Defective virilization of the male embryo (male pseudohermaphroditism) can result from defects in androgen synthesis, defects in androgen action, defects in müllerian duct regression, and uncertain causes. Testosterone synthesis is normal in more than 80 per cent of subjects with male pseudohermaphroditism (Savage et al., 1978; Campo et al., 1979, 1981).

Abnormalities In Androgen Synthesis

Five enzymatic defects have been described that result in defective testosterone synthesis (Fig. 41–6) and incomplete virilization of the male embryo during embryogenesis (Tables 41–4 and 41–5). Each of the enzymes catalyzes a critical biochemical step in the conversion of cholesterol to testosterone (Griffin and Wilson, 1978). Three (20,22-desmolase, 3β-hydroxysteroid dehydrogenase, and 17α-hydroxylase) are common to the synthesis of other adrenal hormones as well; consequently, their deficiency results in congenital adrenal hyperplasia (Table 41–4) as well as male pseudohermaphroditism. The other two (17,20-desmolase and 17β-hydroxysteroid dehydrogenase) are unique to the

pathway of androgen synthesis, and their deficiency results only in male pseudohermaphroditism. Since 19-carbon androgens are obligatory precursors of estrogens, it likewise follows that in all but the terminal defect (17β-hydroxysteroid dehydrogenase deficiency) synthesis of estrogen is also low in affected individuals of both sexes.

Clinical Features. In 46,XY subjects there is usually no trace of uterus or fallopian tubes, indicating that the müllerian inhibiting function of the testis takes place normally during embryogenesis. However, the masculinization of the wolffian ducts, urogenital sinus, and urogenital tubercle and the degree of virilization at puberty vary from almost normal to absent. Therefore, the clinical picture spans the range from phenotypic men with mild hypospadias to phenotypic women who prior to puberty resemble patients with the complete testicular feminization syndrome. This extreme variability is presumed to be the consequence of the varying severity of the enzymatic defects in different patients and of varying effects of the steroids that accumulate proximal to the metabolic blocks in the different disorders. In patients with partial defects and in whom plasma testosterone is normal the diagnosis can only be made by measuring the steroids that accumulate proximal to the metabolic block in question.

20,22-Desmolase deficiency (lipoid adrenal hyperplasia) is a form of congenital adrenal hyperplasia in which virtually no urinary steroids (either 17-ketosteroids or 17-hydroxycorticoids) can be detected and in which the enzyme deficiency occurs prior to the formation of pregnenolone. The abnormality is assumed to involve the enzyme or enzymes of the 20,22-desmolase complex that are responsible for cleavage of the side chain of cholesterol to form pregnenolone. The syndrome is associated with salt wasting and profound adrenal insufficiency, and most affected individuals die during infancy. However, at least one severely affected male was studied at 8 years of age (Kirkland et al., 1973). At autopsy the adrenal glands and the testes were enlarged and infiltrated with lipid.

3β-Hydroxysteroid dehydrogenase deficiency is the second most common cause of congenital adrenal hyperplasia (Bongiovanni, 1978). In male infants it causes a spectrum of defects from varying degrees of hypospadias to complete failure of masculinization associated with the presence of a vagina. Female infants may be modestly virilized at birth resulting from the weak androgenic potency of dehydroepian-

TABLE 41–5. ANATOMIC, GENETIC, AND ENDOCRINE PROFILE OF HEREDITARY MALE PSEUDOHERMAPHRODITISM

Disorder	Inheritance	Phenotype						Endocrine Profile Relative to Normal Male		
		Müllerian Ducts	Wolffian Ducts	Spermato-geneses	Urogenital Sinus	External Genitalia	Breasts	Testosterone Production	Estrogen Production	LH
Defects in Testosterone Synthesis										
Five enzyme deficiencies	Autosomal or X-linked recessive	Absent	Variable development	Normal to decreased	Variable from male to female	Generally female	Usually male	Normal to decreased	Variable	High
Defects in Androgen Action										
5α-Reductase deficiency	Autosomal recessive	Absent	Male	Normal or decreased	Female	Clitoromegaly	Male	Normal	Normal	Normal or increased
Receptor Disorders										
Complete testicular feminization	X-linked recessive	Absent	Absent	Absent	Female	Female	Female	High	High	High
Incomplete testicular feminization	X-linked recessive	Absent	Male	Absent	Female	Clitoromegaly and posterior fusion	Female	High	High	High
Reifenstein syndrome	X-linked recessive	Absent	Variable development	Absent	Variable from male to female	Incomplete male development	Female	High	High	High
Infertile male syndrome	Probably X-linked recessive	Absent	Male	Absent or decreased	Male	Male	Usually male	Normal or High	Normal or High	Normal or High
Receptor-positive resistance	Uncertain	Absent	Variable	Absent or decreased	Variable	Female to male	Variable	Normal or High	Normal or High	Normal or High
Defects in Müllerian Regression										
Persistent müllerian duct syndrome	Autosomal or X-linked	Rudimentary uterus and fallopian tubes	Male	Normal	Male	Male	Male	Normal	Normal	Normal

(From Petersdorf, R. G., Adams, R. D., Braunwald, E., et al.: Disorders of sexual differentiation. *In* Harrison's Principles of Internal Medicine. 10th ed. New York, McGraw-Hill Book Co., 1983, pp. 724–739.)

drosterone, which is the major steroid secreted. In the mild form in women, the disorder may not be recognized until hirsutism develops at the expected time of puberty (Rosenfield et al., 1974). If the enzyme is absent in both the adrenal and the testis, no urinary steroids contain a Δ^4-3-keto configuration, whereas in patients in whom the defect is partial or affects only the testis, the urine may contain normal or even elevated levels of Δ^4-3-keto steroids. Most patients have marked salt wasting and profound adrenal insufficiency, and long-term survival occurs only in states of partial deficiency. There have been reports of several affected males who experienced otherwise normal male puberty except for pathologic gynecomastia (Parks et al., 1971). In these individuals the blood testosterone level is in the low-normal range but is accompanied by elevated Δ^5-precursors (Rosenfield et al., 1974). The enzyme in different tissues must be under complex genetic and regulatory control, since deficiency of the enzyme in the testis may be less severe than that in the adrenal gland and since enzyme activity in the liver may be normal in the face of profound deficiency in the adrenal gland and the testis (Schneider et al., 1975). Individuals with normal liver enzymes can be mistakenly identified as having 21-hydroxylase deficiency if urinary Δ^5-pregnanetriol is not documented to be greater than urinary pregnanetriol (Bongiovanni, 1978).

17α-Hydroxylase deficiency characteristically results in hypogonadism, absence of secondary sex characteristics, hypokalemic alkalosis, hypertension, and virtually undetectable hydrocortisone secretion in phenotypic women (Biglieri et al., 1966). There is elevated secretion of both corticosterone and DOC by the adrenal gland, and urinary 17-ketosteroids are low. Aldosterone secretion is low, presumably as the result of high plasma DOC and depressed angiotensin levels, but it returns to normal after suppressive doses of hydrocortisone are administered. In 46,XX subjects, amenorrhea, lack of pubic hair, and hypertension are common, but since gonadal steroids are not required for female development during embryogenesis, the phenotype is that of a normal prepubertal woman. In males, however, the enzyme deficiency results in defective virilization that varies from complete male pseudohermaphroditism to ambiguous genitalia with perineoscrotal hypospadias (New, 1970). In males with presumed partial enzyme deficiency, pathologic gynecomastia may develop at puberty. Subjects with this disorder do not develop adrenal insufficiency, since the secretion of both corticosterone

(a glucocorticoid and a mineralocorticoid) and DOC (a mineralocorticoid) is elevated. The hypertension and hypokalemia that are prominent features of the disorder (even in the neonatal period) remit after suppression of the DOC secretion by adequate glucocorticoid replacement.

17,20-Desmolase deficiency has been described in 15 subjects from seven families. Affected males have a 46,XY chromosome pattern, normal adrenocortical function, and a variable pattern of male pseudohermaphroditism (Zachmann et al., 1982). The defect leading to male pseudohermaphroditism involves a variable deficiency in the conversion of 17-hydroxyprogesterone to androstenedione. In the majority of patients there is genital ambiguity at birth with some virilization at the time of expected puberty. However, two patients have had a female phenotype with no virilization at the time of expected puberty (Goebelsmann et al., 1976; Zachmann et al., 1982). The disorder has been recognized in one 46,XX woman with sexual infantilism (Larrea et al., 1983).

17β-Hydroxysteroid dehydrogenase deficiency involves the final step in androgen biosynthesis, reduction of the 17-keto group of androstenedione to form testosterone. This disorder is probably the most common enzymatic defect in testosterone synthesis causing male pseudohermaphroditism. Affected 46,XY males usually have a female phenotype with a blind-ending vagina and absence of müllerian derivatives, but inguinal or abdominal testes and virilized wolffian duct structures are present. At the time of expected puberty, both virilization (with phallic enlargement and development of facial and body hair) and a variable degree of female breast development take place. In one patient in the United States and in a large Arab kindred, gender role reversal from female to male occurred at puberty in untreated subjects (Imperato-McGinley et al., 1979; Rösler and Kohn, 1983). Androgen and estrogen dynamics have not been elucidated in detail, but the 17-keto reduction of estrone to estradiol by the gonads is also low. 17β-hydroxysteroid dehydrogenase is normally present in many tissues besides the gonads, but only the gonadal enzyme appears to be defective in this disorder. Plasma testosterone may be in the low-normal range, making it essential to document a significant elevation in plasma androstenedione to make the diagnosis.

Pathophysiology. The available data for the 17α-hydroxylase and 3β-hydroxysteroid dehydrogenase defects are compatible with autosomal recessive inheritance. The limited family data for 17,20-desmolase deficiency and 17β-hydroxysteroid dehydrogenase deficiency are compatible either with autosomal recessive or X-linked recessive mutations. Insufficient data are available for the 20,22-desmolase defect to warrant any conclusions as to the pattern of inheritance.

The pattern of steroid secretion and excretion depends on the site of the various metabolic blocks (see Fig. 41–6). In general, gonadotropin secretion is high, and as a consequence many individuals with incomplete defects are able to compensate so that the steady state concentration of end-products such as testosterone may be normal or almost normal.

Instances of male pseudohermaphroditism have been described in which testosterone formation is deficient for reasons other than a single enzyme defect in androgen synthesis. Included are disorders in which Leydig cell agenesis or unresponsiveness to gonadotropin (Berthezene et al., 1976) or the secretion of a biologically inactive LH molecule (Park et al., 1976) have been thought to be the primary defects. In addition, as already described, a spectrum of defects in testicular development have been characterized, including familial XY gonadal dysgenesis, sporadic dysgenetic testes, and the absent testis syndrome in which deficient testosterone production is secondary to the underlying disorder of gonadal development.

Management. Replacement therapy with glucocorticoids and in some instances mineralocorticoids is indicated in those disorders causing adrenal insufficiency. The decision as to the management of the genital abnormalities depends upon the individual case. Fertility has not been reported, and its consideration does not enter into the decision of sex assignment. In genetic females there is no problem (except in diagnosis) in that affected individuals are raised appropriately as females, and suitable estrogen replacement is indicated at the time of expected puberty to promote development of normal female secondary sex characteristics. The decision as to whether affected newborn males with ambiguous genitalia should be raised as males or females depends upon the anatomic defect; in general, more severely affected individuals should be raised as females, and corrective surgery of the genitalia and removal of the testes should be undertaken as early as possible. In subjects raised as females, estrogen therapy is also indicated at the appropriate age to allow development of normal female secondary sex characteristics. In individuals raised as males,

corrective surgery is indicated for any coexisting hypospadias, and careful monitoring of plasma androgens and estrogens should be undertaken at the time of expected puberty to determine whether long-term supplemental testosterone therapy is appropriate.

Abnormalities In Androgen Action

Several disorders of male phenotypic development result from abnormalities of androgen action. The spectrum of phenotypes is described in Table 41–5. In these disorders, testosterone formation and müllerian regression are normal; however, male development is impaired to a variable degree as a result of resistance to androgen action in the target cells (Wilson et al., 1983).

5α-Reductase deficiency is a form of male pseudohermaphroditism that is inherited in an autosomal recessive fashion and is characterized by (1) severe perineoscrotal hypospadias with a hooded prepuce, a ventral urethral groove, and opening of the urethra at the base of the phallus (Fig. 41–9A); (2) a blind vaginal pouch of variable size opening either into the urogenital sinus or more frequently onto the urethra immediately behind the urethral orifice; (3) well-developed and histologically differentiated testes with normal epididymides, vasa deferentia, and seminal vesicles, and termination of the ejaculatory ducts into the blind-ending vagina (Fig. 41–9B); (4) a female habitus without female breast development but with normal axillary and pubic hair; (5) the absence of female internal genitalia; and (6) normal male plasma testosterone and masculinization to a variable degree at the time of puberty (Walsh et al., 1974; Imperato-McGinley et al., 1974).

The fact that the defective virilization during embryogenesis is limited to the urogenital sinus and the anlage of the external genitalia provided insight into the nature of the fundamental abnormality. Testosterone, the androgen secreted by the fetal testis, is the intracellular mediator for differentiation of the wolffian duct into the epididymis, the vas deferens, and the seminal vesicle, whereas dihydrotestosterone is the functional intracellular hormone responsible for virilization of the urogenital sinus and the anlage of the external genitalia. Consequently, in a male embryo with normal testosterone synthesis and normal androgen receptors, a failure of dihydrotestosterone formation would be expected to result in the phenotype observed in this disorder, namely normal male wolffian duct derivatives with defective masculinization of the structures originating from the urogenital sinus,

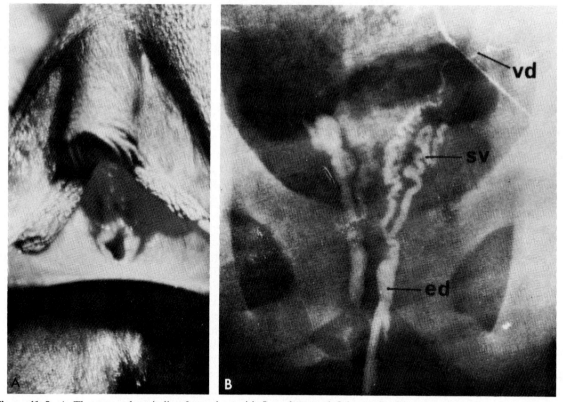

Figure 41–9. *A,* The external genitalia of a patient with 5α-reductase deficiency. *B,* Genitogram of the same patient. vd, vas deferens; sv, seminal vesicle; ed, ejaculatory ducts. (From Walsh, P. C., Madden, J. D., Harrod, M. J., Goldstein, J. L., McDonald, P. C., and Wilson, J. D.: N. Engl. J. Med. *291*:944, 1974. Used by permission.)

genital tubercle, and genital swellings (Fig. 41–10). Since testosterone itself is the hormone that regulates LH secretion, plasma LH is usually only minimally elevated. As a result, testosterone and estrogen production rates are those of normal men, and gynecomastia does not develop.

The fact that the 5α-reductase enzyme is deficient in this disorder was suspected on phenotypic and endocrine grounds and was established by direct enzymatic assay in biopsied tissues and in fibroblasts cultured from affected individuals (Walsh et al.; 1974). There is considerable genetic heterogeneity; in most subjects the 5α-reductase is either profoundly deficient or functionally absent, and in others the enzyme protein is synthesized at a normal rate but is structurally abnormal (Leshin et al., 1978). It is not clear why virilization at puberty appears to be more normal than the virilization that takes place during sexual differentiation.

Androgen receptor disorders may result in several distinct phenotypes (Fig. 41–11). Despite differences in clinical presentation and molecular pathology, these disorders are similar

in regard to endocrinology, genetics, and basic pathophysiology. The major clinical features and issues of management of the disorders will be considered first, followed by a discussion of the similar endocrinology and pathophysiology.

Complete testicular feminization is the most common form of male pseudohermaphroditism, estimates of frequency varying from 1 in 20,000 to 1 in 64,000 male births. It is the third most common cause of primary amenorrhea in phenotypic women after gonadal dygenesis and congenital absence of the vagina (Ross et al., 1981). The clinical features are characteristic, namely a phenotypic female is seen by the physician either because of inguinal hernia (prepubertal) or primary amenorrhea (postpubertal). The development of the breasts after puberty, the general habitus, and the distribution of body fat are female in character, so many patients have a truly feminine appearance (Fig. 41–11*A*). Axillary and pubic hair are absent or scanty, but slight vulval hair is usually present. Scalp hair is that of a normal woman, and facial hair is absent. The external genitalia are unambiguously female (Fig. 41–12*A*), and the cli-

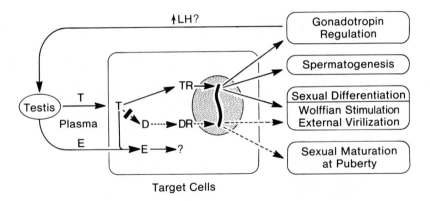

Figure 41–10. Deranged androgen physiology in 5α-reductase deficiency. T, testosterone; D, dihydrotestosterone; E, estradiol.; LH, luteinizing hormone; R, androgen receptor.

toris is normal or small. The vagina is short and blind-ending and may be absent or rudimentary. All internal genitalia are absent except for the gonads, which have histologic features of undescended testes (normal or increased Leydig cells and seminiferous tubules without spermatogenesis).

The testes may be located in the abdomen, along the course of the inguinal canal, or in the labia majora. Occasionally, remnants of müllerian or wolffian duct origin can be identified in the paratesticular fascia or in fibrous bands extending from the testis. Patients tend to be

rather tall, bone age is normal, and intelligence is normal. The psychosexual development is unmistakably female in regard to behavior, outlook, and maternal instincts.

The major complication of undescended testes in this disorder, as in other forms of cryptorchidism, is the development of tumors. Since affected individuals undergo a normal pubertal growth spurt and feminize successfully at the time of expected puberty, and since testicular tumors rarely develop until after puberty in patients with intra-abdominal testes, it is usual to delay castration until after the time

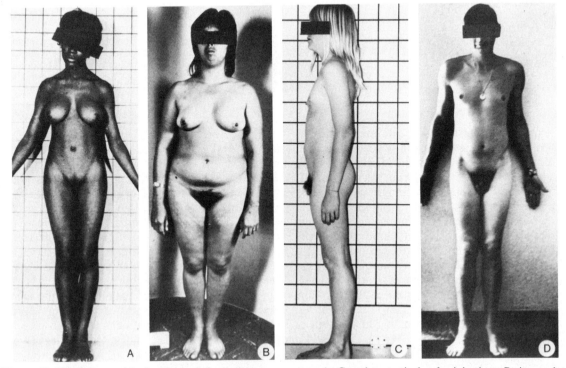

Figure 41–11. Patients with disorders of the androgen receptor. *A,* Complete testicular feminization; *B,* incomplete testicular feminization; *C,* Reifenstein syndrome; *D,* the infertile male syndrome. (*A* courtesy of Dr. Howard Jones, *C* courtesy of Dr. Ronald Swerdloff, and *D* courtesy of Dr. James Aiman.)

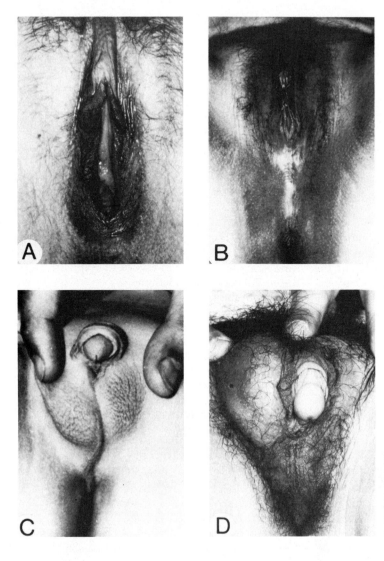

Figure 41-12. External genitalia of four patients with disorders of the androgen receptor. *A,* Complete testicular feminization; *B,* incomplete testicular feminization; *C,* Reifenstein syndrome in a prepubertal subject; *D,* Reifenstein syndrome in a postpubertal subject.

of expected puberty. Surgical intervention is indicated prepubertally if the testes are present in the inguinal region or in the labia majora and result in discomfort or hernia formation. (If hernia repair is indicated prepubertally, most physicians prefer to remove the testes at the same time so as to limit the number of operative procedures.) If the testes are removed prepubertally, estrogen therapy is required at the appropriate age to ensure normal growth and breast development. When castration is performed postpubertally, menopausal symptoms and other evidence of estrogen withdrawal supervene, and suitable estrogen replacement is indicated.

Incomplete testicular feminization is about one tenth as frequent as the complete form. The disorders are similar except that in the incomplete disorder there is a minor virilization

of the external genitalia (partial fusion of the labioscrotal folds and some degree of clitoromegaly, Fig. 41–12*B*), normal pubic hair (Fig. 41–11*B*), and some virilization as well as feminization at the time of expected puberty. The vagina is short and blind-ending. In contrast to the complete form, the wolffian duct derivatives are often partially developed. The family history is usually uninformative, but in several instances multiple family members are affected in a pattern compatible with X-linkage.

The management of patients with the complete and incomplete forms of testicular feminization differs. Since patients with the incomplete disorder virilize at the time of expected puberty, gonadectomy should be performed before the expected time of puberty in prepubertal patients with clitoromegaly or posterior labial fusion.

Reifenstein syndrome is the term now applied to a variety of forms of incomplete male pseudohermaphroditism that were initially described by a number of eponyms (Reifenstein syndrome, Gilbert-Dreyfus syndrome, Lubs syndrome) (Wilson et al., 1974). Each of these phenotypes was originally assumed to be a distinct entity. Since several families have now been described in which affected members exhibit variable manifestations that span the phenotypes described under these terms, these syndromes probably constitute variable manifestations of a single mutation. The most common presentation is a child with perineoscrotal hypospadias (Fig. 41–12C) or a man with perineoscrotal hypospadias and gynecomastia (Figs. 41–11C and 41–12D), but the spectrum of defective virilization in such families ranges from infertile men to men with gynecomastia and azoospermia to phenotypic women with pseudovaginas. Axillary and pubic hair are normal, but chest and facial hair are minimal. Cryptorchidism is common, the testes are usually small, and spermatogenesis is usually incomplete. Some have defects in wolffian duct derivatives such as absence or hypoplasia of the vas deferens.

Since the psychologic development in most is unequivocally male, the hypospadias and cryptorchidism should be corrected surgically. The only successful form of treatment of the gynecomastia is surgical removal.

The *infertile male syndrome* is the most common disorder of the androgen receptor and in contrast to the other disorders is not actually a form of male pseudohermaphroditism (Aiman et al., 1979). Some such individuals are minimally affected subjects in families with Reifenstein syndrome, and azoospermia is the only manifestation of the receptor abnormality. More commonly, the individuals present with male infertility and have negative family histories.

Evaluation of such men with normal external genitalia (Fig. 41-11D), apparently normal wolffian duct structures, and infertility due to azoospermia or severe oligospermia has shown that a disorder of the androgen receptor may be present in one fifth or more of men with idiopathic azoospermia (Aiman and Griffin, 1982). There is no treatment for the infertility in any of these disorders.

The endocrinology and pathophysiology of these four disorders of the androgen receptor are similar (Fig. 41–13). The karyotype is 46,XY and the mutant gene is believed to be located on the X chromosome. The frequency of a positive family history varies from about two thirds of patients with testicular feminization and Reifenstein syndrome to only an occasional patient with the infertile male syndrome. It is assumed the disorder in patients with a negative family history is the result of a new mutation.

Hormone dynamics have been best characterized in complete testicular feminization, but they are similar in all disorders of the androgen receptor. Plasma testosterone levels and rates of testosterone production by the testes are normal or higher than normal. The elevated rate of testosterone production is caused by the high mean plasma level of LH, which, in turn, is due to defective feedback regulation caused by resistance to the action of androgen at the hypothalamic-pituitary level. Elevated LH concentration is probably also responsible for the increased estrogen production by the testes. (In normal men, most estrogen is derived from peripheral formation from circulating androgens, but when plasma LH is elevated, the testes secrete significant amounts of estrogen into the circulation). Thus, resistance to the feedback regulation of LH secretion by circulating androgen results in elevated plasma LH levels, and this, in turn, results in the enhanced secretion of both testosterone and

Figure 41–13. Deranged androgen physiology in receptor disorders. T, testosterone; D, dihydrotestosterone; E, estradiol; LH, luteinizing hormone; R, androgen receptor.

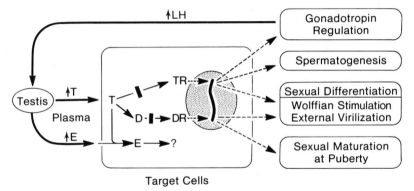

estradiol by the testes. Gonadotropin levels rise even higher (and menopausal symptoms may develop) when the testes are removed, indicating that gonadotropin secretion is under partial regulatory control. Presumably, in the steady state and in the absence of an androgen effect, estrogen alone regulates LH secretion, a control that is achieved at the expense of an elevated plasma estrogen concentration for a male.

Feminization in these disorders is the result of two interlocking phenomena. First, androgens and estrogens have antagonistic effects at the peripheral level, and normal virilization occurs in normal men when the ratio of androgen to estrogen is 100:1 or greater; in the absence of androgen action, the cellular effect of estrogen is unopposed. Second, the production of estradiol in these subjects is greater than that in the normal male (though it is less than that of the normal female) (MacDonald et al., 1979). Variable degrees of androgen resistance, coupled with variably enhanced estradiol production, results in different degrees of defective virilization and enhanced feminization in the four clinical syndromes. The defective virilization is most severe in complete testicular feminization, and the full feminizing effect of the increased estrogen is expressed. Estrogen production in the Reifenstein syndrome is increased to a similar or greater extent as that in testicular feminization, but a less severe androgen resistance results in a predominantly male phenotype with less pronounced feminization (Wilson et al., 1974). Only a few men with the infertile male syndrome have had evaluation of androgen-estrogen dynamics (Aiman et al., 1979). The hormonal changes seem to be similar to those in the other receptor disorders, but are less marked. Some men with this syndrome do not have an elevation of plasma LH or plasma testosterone.

Each of these four syndromes is the result of an abnormality of the androgen receptor.

Initially, fibroblasts cultured from the skin of some subjects with complete testicular feminization were shown to have a near absence of high-affinity dihydrotestosterone binding. Subsequently, other individuals with complete testicular feminization, as well as subjects with incomplete testicular feminization, Reifenstein syndrome, and the infertile male syndrome, have been found to have either a decreased amount of an apparently normal receptor or a qualitatively abnormal androgen receptor. Absent or near-absent binding appears to be associated primarily with complete testicular feminization, and a decreased amount of an apparently qualitatively normal receptor appears to be most common in the two syndromes with predominant male phenotypes. However, a qualitatively abnormal receptor has been detected in families with each of the four clinical phenotypes (Griffin and Durrant, 1982). Except for the lack of binding in complete testicular feminization, there is no consistent correlation between the receptor abnormality as demonstrated in cultured fibroblasts and the clinical severity of the androgen resistance in individual patients.

Receptor-positive resistance is a category of androgen resistance that does not appear to involve either 5α-reductase or the androgen receptor. It was first identified in a family with the syndrome of testicular feminization (Amrhein et al., 1976). Subsequent patients, with a variety of phenotypes ranging from incomplete testicular feminization to findings similar to those in the Reifenstein syndrome, have been described. The hormonal profile is similar to that seen in the receptor disorders. The site of the molecular abnormality in these patients is unclear (Fig. 41–14). It could be due to defects of the androgen receptor that are too subtle to be detected by the usual assay. If the defect is truly distal to the receptor, there could be failure of specific messenger RNA generation or an

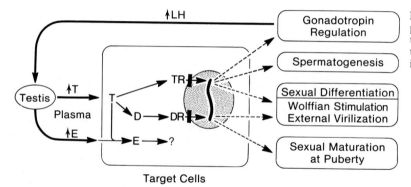

Figure 41–14. Deranged androgen physiology in receptor-positive resistance. T, testosterone; D, dihydrotestosterone; E, estradiol; LH, luteinizing hormone; R, androgen receptor.

Target Cells

abnormality of RNA processing. Indeed, it is not established that a uniform defect is present, and the disorder may represent a heterogeneous group of molecular abnormalities. Studies designed to detect subtle qualitative abnormalities of the receptor are likely to decrease the number of patients in this category. At present they appear to amount to less than one fifth of patients with androgen resistance (Griffin and Durrant, 1982). Management depends on the phenotype.

Persistent müllerian duct syndrome results in normal penile development but, in addition, bilateral fallopian tubes, a uterus, and an upper vagina and variable development of the vas deferens. The subjects commonly present with inguinal hernias that contain the uterus, and cryptorchidism is common. Most have uninformative family histories, but several pairs of siblings have been described in whom the condition must be inherited either as an autosomal recessive or an X-linked recessive mutation. Because the external genitalia are well developed and the patients masculinize normally at puberty, it is assumed that during the critical stage of embryonic sexual differentiation the fetal testes produced a normal amount of androgen. However, müllerian regression does not occur, possibly because of failure of the fetal testis to produce müllerian-inhibiting substance or because of failure of the tissues to respond to this hormone.

The preservation of external male appearance and the maintenance of virilization are essential. A primary or staged orchiopexy should be performed. None of the reported cases has developed a malignancy in the uterus or vagina, and because the vasa deferentia are closely associated with the broad ligaments, the uterus and vagina should be left in place to avoid disruption of the vasa deferentia during removal and consequently to preserve possible fertility.

DIFFERENTIAL DIAGNOSIS AND EVALUATION OF SEXUAL AMBIGUITY

The evaluation of the newborn with ambiguous genitalia is one of the most complicated challenges of medicine. Possibly no other field requires a broader application of both theoretical and practical knowledge, and certainly few decisions have greater social impact on the future of the patient. Indeed, it is no exaggeration to say that the detection of sexual ambiguity in the newborn constitutes a true medical emergency. Untreated sexual ambiguity can lead to confusion about gender identity or role, or both, either because of uncorrected biological abnormalities per se or because of uncertainty as to the correct sex assignment on the part of both the parents and the affected individuals. Therefore, assignment of the sex of rearing should be made as early as possible, preferably in the newborn nursery but not before all necessary diagnostic procedures have been performed.

In this section, the discussion centers on those disorders that most frequently present with ambiguity of the external genitalia, thereby excluding the disorders in which the phenotypic sex of an individual is clear-cut, such as the Klinefelter syndrome, gonadal dysgenesis, testicular feminization, and so on. This limits the differential diagnosis to the four most common causes of ambiguous genitalia: true hermaphroditism, mixed gonadal dysgenesis, female pseudohermaphroditism, and male pseudohermaphroditism.

While the infant with ambigous genitalia is undergoing evaluation, the family should be informed that the development of the external genitalia is incomplete and that additional studies are necessary before the correct gender assignment can be made. The procedures used for the investigation of subjects with ambiguous genitalia includes (1) a detailed history (including a pedigree analysis) and physical examination; (2) evaluation of the chromosomal sex, utilizing nuclear chromatin studies, fluorescent staining of the Y chromosome, and karyotyping; (3) biochemical evaluation of the urinary and plasma steroids with stimulation by human chorionic gonadotropin; (4) evaluation of the urogenital sinus and internal duct structures with roentgenographic and endoscopic procedures; (5) laparotomy and gonadal biopsy; and (6) when available, assessment of androgen action in cultured fibroblasts.

HISTORY AND PHYSICAL EXAMINATION

Because many of the disorders are familial, the family history must be probed not only for cases of identically affected individuals but also for variant forms of abnormal sexual development, unexplained death during infancy, infertility, amenorrhea, and hirsutism. If a similar disorder is present in a maternal aunt, uncle, or cousin, one of the disorders that is inherited as an X-linked recessive trait should be considered. For disorders that are inherited as autosomal recessive traits, the presence of parental consanguinity should be determined. In addition, the mother should be questioned about symptoms of virilization and about the ingestion of androgens, progestational agents, or other drugs during pregnancy.

The most important finding on physical examination is the presence of a gonad in the labioscrotal fold or scrotum. Because ovaries rarely descend, the presence of a palpable gonad excludes the diagnosis of female pseudohermaphroditism. Other findings that are helpful on physical examination include (1) hyperpigmentation of the areola and labioscrotal folds, which is frequently present in patients with congenital adrenal hyperplasia; (2) palpation of the uterus as a midline, thickened structure; (3) evidence of dehydration and failure to thrive; and (4) the existence of other associated congenital anomalies. The size of the phallus and the location of the urethral meatus should be documented, and the contents of any hernias should be examined carefully. Each infant with bilateral cryptorchidism, or unilateral cryptorchidism associated with hypospadias should be considered to have a disorder of sexual differentiation until it is proved otherwise.

CHROMOSOMAL EVALUATION

A quick and often useful laboratory test in the differential diagnosis of intersexuality is the examination of buccal mucosal cells for the presence of chromatin clumps on the nuclear membrane—the Barr body. The Barr body, which represents the second X chromosome, is found in 20 per cent or more of the nuclei of normal females and in less than 2 per cent of the cells of normal males. In the female, counts may be lower during the first few days of life and should therefore be repeated after 1 week to obtain an accurate estimate.

If the buccal mucosal cells are stained with quinacrine or its mustard derivative and are examined with fluorescence microscopy, the Y chromosome (the F body) can be identified. This phenomenon, which was first described by Caspersson and associates (1971), provides a more accurate, rapid means of obtaining insight into the chromosomal composition than other indirect means of estimating sex chromosomes. However, because the fluorescent portion of the Y chromosome is on the long arm of the Y chromosome and the male-determining factors are located on the short arm, the absence of a fluorescent Y body must be interpreted with caution. There are several reports in which absence of the fluorescent portion of the Y chromosome has been associated with normal male sexual differentiation (Meisner and Inhorn, 1972).

The more direct and accurate means of determining the human chromosomal complement involves the culture of peripheral blood leukocytes in medium containing a mitogenic agent (phytohemagglutinin), which induces the lymphocytes to divide after a 3-day period of incubation at 37 degrees C. A mitotic spindle poison such as colchicine, which arrests mitosis at metaphase, is added, and the cells are harvested and stained. The chromosomes of a number of cells in metaphase are assessed to establish their number and histologic characteristics. This technique is valuable in establishing the exact chromosomal complement, the presence of mosaicism, and the presence of structural chromosomal alterations. To determine mosaicism accurately, the study of multiple tissues may be necessary.

BIOCHEMICAL EVALUATION

Biochemical tests are most useful in identifying the presence of congenital adrenal hyperplasia and in determining whether there is a normal capacity to form testosterone. In untreated patients with 21-hydroxylase deficiency, the common variety of congenital adrenal hyperplasia, morning plasma 17-hydroxyprogesterone levels are markedly elevated (usually greater than 2000 ng per dl, whereas the upper limit in control subjects of all ages is rarely greater than 200 ng per dl (Hughes and Winter, 1976). When plasma measurements are not available, the diagnosis can be established by measuring the urinary excretion of 17-ketosteroids and pregnanetriol. Caution must be exercised in interpreting values obtained from infants in the first 3 weeks of life. In normal infants, urinary 17-ketosteroid excretion may be as high as 2.5 mg per day in the first 3 weeks of life and thereafter fall to less than 0.5 mg per day. Pregnanetriol is a metabolic by-product of 17-hydroxyprogesterone, which is a precursor of cortisol, and is normally found in the urine in amounts of less than 0.5 mg per day. It is increased in congenital virilizing adrenal hyperplasia owing to the deficiency of 21-hydroxylase (and to a somewhat lesser extent the deficiency of 11-hydroxylase).

In the rarer forms of defective steroid hormone biosynthesis, it may be necessary to document high levels of plasma pregnenolone and dehydroepiandrosterone (3β-hydroxysteroid dehydrogenase deficiency), profound deficiency of C-21 and C-19 steroids (20,22-desmolase deficiency), high corticosterone and deoxycorticosterone levels (17-hydroxylase deficiency), or deficiency of C-19 steroids and elevation of C-21 precursor steroids (17,20-desmolase deficiency). Again, caution must be exercised in interpreting these values in the newborn.

Although plasma testosterone rises during the neonatal period in normal male infants, the diagnostic implication of the increase has not been documented in pathologic states. Therefore, to evaluate the capacity for testosterone biosynthesis in infants with male pseudohermaphroditism, it is customary to measure plasma androgens before and after the administration of human chorionic gonadotropin (HCG). Indeed, infants with androgen resistance can be separated from those with defective testosterone synthesis (caused either by single enzyme defects or by developmental defects in the testes) by demonstrating that plasma testosterone increases in the former group to levels greater than 2 ng per ml after treatment for 4 days with 2000 IU of HCG per day (Forest, 1979; Walsh et al., 1976). Plasma androstenedione levels should be measured simultaneously in these plasma samples, since HCG causes a greater than normal increase in this hormone in individuals with 17β-hydroxysteroid dehydrogenase deficiency (Levine et al., 1980). Likewise, if the phenotype is suggestive of 5α-reductase

deficiency, measurement of plasma dihydrotestosterone in the post-HCG plasma (and documentation that the ratio of plasma testosterone:plasma dihydrotestosterone is greater than 30) may establish the diagnosis of this condition (Peterson et al., 1977).

As is true for many other inborn errors of metabolism, fibroblasts cultured from skin biopsy have been utilized to diagnosis individuals affected with the syndromes of androgen resistance, and the measurement of steroid 5α-reductase activity or dihydrotestosterone binding in such fibroblasts may be useful in appropriate instances (Wilson et al., 1983).

ENDOSCOPY AND RADIOGRAPHY

Radiographic and endoscopic procedures are useful in evaluating the status of the urogenital sinus and the internal duct structures in patients with ambiguous genitalia. Genitography is easily accomplished with a blunt-ended syringe positioned firmly at the opening of the urogenital sinus. While contrast medium is injected slowly, fluoroscopy is used to select spot films demonstrating the filling of the urogenital sinus and internal duct structures (Cremin, 1974; Peck and Poznanski, 1972) (see Fig. 41–15). This method is superior to voiding cystourethrography. In addition, the location of the

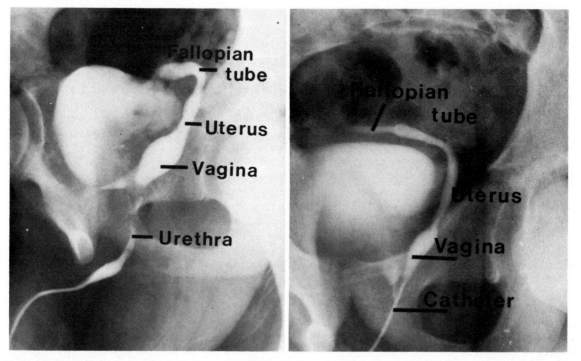

Figure 41–15. Radiograms performed after retrograde instillation of sodium diatrizoate into the prostatic utricles of two patients with familial persistent müllerian duct syndrome. (From Sloan, W. R., and Walsh, P. C.: J. Urol., *115*:459, 1976. © 1976 The Williams & Wilkins Co., Baltimore. Used by permission.)

urogenital sinus and the presence of a cervix can be confirmed on endoscopy.

At endoscopy, the urogenital sinus or the prostatic utricle can be catheterized for retrograde contrast studies (Sloan and Walsh, 1976) (Fig. 41–15). Although the lower vagina may be present in any of the common forms of intersexuality, the presence of a uterus and one fallopian tube excludes the diagnosis of male pseudohermaphroditism caused by a defect in androgen synthesis or androgen action.

When the urogenital sinus cannot be catheterized, or when genitography is unsuccessful, pelvic ultrasonography is a useful ancillary means for documenting the presence and size of the uterus and fallopian tubes (Alzen et al., 1981). At exploratory laparotomy, the differentiation of the distal wolffian duct structures can be determined with anterograde vasography. The technique involves the exposure of the vas deferens and the insertion of a small blunt needle (20 to 25 gauge) through a transverse vasotomy. Following the injection of 1 ml of 50 per cent diatrizoate sodium, appropriate x-ray films are taken to document the presence of the distal vas deferens, seminal vesicle, and ejaculatory duct (Madden et al., 1975; Walsh et al., 1974) (see Fig. 41–9B).

EXPLORATORY LAPAROTOMY AND GONADAL BIOPSY

In the newborn, exploratory laparotomy is very occasionally undertaken for inspection and biopsy (and occasional removal) of gonadal tissue. Laparotomy is indicated only if gonadal biopsy will influence the sex of rearing. The major consideration in establishing the sex of rearing should be the achievement of functional genitalia; fertility is of secondary importance. If the phallus is inadequate, there is no necessity for early exploration; this patient should be reared as a female regardless of gonadal status. In the patient with both a vagina and a well-developed phallus, however, the findings on exploratory laparotomy and gonadal biopsy are occasionally of great importance in assigning the sex of rearing. In a 46,XX patient with normal urinary steroid excretion, a negative family history, and no exposure to exogenous androgens, laparotomy is necessary to distinguish between female pseudohermaphroditism and true hermaphroditism. Similarly, in chromatin-negative patients (either 46,XY or mosaics), exploratory laparotomy is often necessary to distinguish among mixed gonadal dysgenesis, true hermaphroditism, and male pseudohermaphroditism.

Even when all available diagnostic criteria currently available are employed—including pedigree analysis, chromosomal studies, biochemical and molecular assessment, genitography, and exploratory laparotomy—it is not possible to establish the diagnosis in all instances of ambiguous genitalia. In such instances, the gender assignment and the decision regarding appropriate corrective surgery must be made empirically on the basis of the clinical findings and the psychosocial setting. However, it is imperative that a vigorous attempt be made to establish the exact cause in all cases of ambiguous genitalia, since the information may be invaluable in the genetic counseling of the families regarding the risks of involvement in subsequent children.

WORKING SCHEME FOR THE EVALUATION OF PATIENTS

All these procedures do not need to be utilized in the work-up of every patient. In practice, the design of the work-up is influenced by the findings on physical examination. Two scrotal or inguinal gonads suggest that the infant is an incompletely virilized genetic male. A single palpable gonad suggests either mixed gonadal dysgenesis or true hermaphroditism. The failure to find palpable gonads in a child with ambiguous genitalia suggests female pseudohermaphroditism, or, rarely, true hermaphroditism or male pseudohermaphroditism.

The second diagnostic question concerns chromosomal sex. For example, a 46,XX karyotype with palpable gonads is fairly specific for true hermaphroditism. Similarly, a 45,X/46,XY karyotype with or without palpable gonads suggests mixed gonadal dysgenesis. Either combination provides an indication for genitography to define internal duct structures and eventually gonadal biopsy to establish a definitive diagnosis.

If the infant is 46,XY with palpable gonads or 46,XX without palpable gonads, it is necessary to determine whether congenital adrenal hyperplasia is present. (Indeed it may be necessary to perform such tests prior to the availability of information about the karyotype if a suspicion exists as to the presence of a salt-losing form of congenital adrenal hyperplasia). Measurement of serum 17-hydroxyprogesterone or urinary 17-ketosteroid excretion identifies 21-hydroxylase and 11β-hydroxylase deficiencies, and other techniques are employed to identify the less common forms of the disorder.

Different strategies are required for the evaluation of sexual ambiguity in 46,XY and 46,XX infants. In the 46,XY infant, the differential diagnosis is between inadequate production of testosterone and resistance to the action of the hormones. Normal response of plasma testosterone to HCG indicates that the diagnosis is androgen resistance or that the subject has had a temporary interference with androgen production during embryogenesis; most individuals with profound androgen resistance virilize poorly at puberty and are candidates for female sex assignment. The diagnosis can sometimes be substantiated by measuring 5α-reductase and androgen receptor levels in fibroblasts cultured from genital skin. Defects in testosterone synthesis can either be due to hereditary defects in the enzymes required for testosterone biosynthesis or to a variety of developmental defects in testicular development. In either case, virilization is usually satisfactory when androgen replacement is given at puberty.

Infants with 46,XX female pseudohermaphroditism in the absence of congenital adrenal hyperplasia are rare, and the condition usually results either from maternal ingestion of progestational agents during pregnancy or from maternal virilizing syndromes.

SEX ASSIGNMENT

Once the studies are complete, sex assignment should be made after careful consultation with the family. Several general aspects of the problem are clear-cut. As mentioned previously, if the subject has an inadequate phallus, the individual should be reared as a female, regardless of the results of diagnostic tests. In the patient with an adequate phallus, however, as much information as possible should be obtained before a decision is made.

If a diagnosis of female pseudohermaphroditism is made, the patient should be reared as a female. All these patients have ovaries, fallopian tubes, a uterus, and an upper vagina, and all are potentially fertile.

If a diagnosis of mixed gonadal dysgenesis is made, there are many factors that favor rearing these patients as female: (1) Most patients are inadequately masculinized and all have a uterus and vagina; (2) if they are reared as males, the testis in adulthood is infertile, and as many as one fourth of these individuals may develop gonadal tumors; and (3) approximately half the patients will be shorter than 150 cm.

In the true hermaphrodite who has both a vagina and a well-developed phallus, the sex of rearing should be based on the findings at exploratory laparotomy. If there is a normal testis that can be placed in the scrotum, the assignment should be male. If normal müllerian duct

structures and a normal ovary are present on one side and either a testis or an ovotestis is present on the other side, the assignment should be female. These changes will provide the best prospects for future fertility, recognizing that the considerations of fertility are always of secondary importance. The primary decision should be based on the development of the external genitalia, and the question of future fertility should never override this.

Finally, in patients with male pseudohermaphroditism due to abnormalities of androgen synthesis or action, proper gender assignment is complicated because it may be impossible to predict what will occur at puberty: (1) Will there be adequate growth of the phallus? (2) will the patient feminize? and (3) will the patient be fertile? With further refinements in our understanding of male pseudohermaphroditism, it may someday be possible to predict these events accurately. At present, however, in the absence of a definitive diagnosis on genetic, endocrinologic, or biochemical grounds, the major criterion of sex assignment is the degree of masculinization of the external genitalia in utero. Presumably, if this was adequate, there will be sufficient masculinization at puberty, though in many cases the patient will not be fertile.

As summarized by Money and Ehrhardt (1972), gender assignment should be made as early as possible and only after involving the parents in the decision. When feasible, we prefer to complete diagnostic work-ups and perform plastic reconstruction before the infants are discharged. Orchidectomy may be necessary to prevent the neonatal surge of androgen when the decision is made to raise the child as a female. It is our belief the more normal the infant appears, the more favorably the parents usually react. Obviously, many such therapeutic interventions make it necessary to plan lifetime medical follow-ups of patients, with institution of gonadal steroid treatment at the time of expected puberty. After a child has reached the period normally associated with well-differentiated psychosexual identity (1 1/2 to 2 years) reassignment of gender is unwise and should be undertaken only after careful psychiatric, social, and endocrine evaluation.

References

Klinefelter Syndrome

Caminos-Torres, R., Ma, L., and Snyder, P. J.: Testosterone-induced inhibition of the LH and FSH responses to gonadotropin-releasing hormone occurs slowly. J. Clin. Endocrinol. Metab., *44*:1142, 1977.

Ferguson-Smith, M. A., Mack, W. S., Ellis, P. M., Dickson, M., Sanger, R., and Race, R. R.: Parental age and the source of the X chromosomes in XXY Klinefelter's syndrome. Lancet, *1*:46, 1964.

Gordon, D. L., Krompotic, E., Thomas, W., Gandy, H. M., and Paulsen, C. A.: Pathologic testicular findings in Klinefelter's syndrome. 47,XXY vs 46,XY/47,XXY. Arch. Intern. Med., *130*:726, 1972.

Jacobs, P. A., and Strong, J. A.: A case of human intersexuality having a possible XXY sex-determining mechanism. Nature, *183*:302, 1959.

Klinefelter, H. F., Jr., Reifenstein, E. C., Jr., and Albright, F.: Syndrome characterized by gynecomastia, aspermatogenesis without A-leydigism, and increased excretion of follicle-stimulating hormone. J. Clin. Endocrinol., *2*:615, 1942.

Leonard, J. M., Paulsen, C. A., Ospina, L. F., and Burgess, E. C.: The classification of Klinefelter's syndrome. *In* Vallet, H.L., Porter, I. H. (Eds.): Genetic Mechanisms of Sexual Development. New York, Academic Press, 1979, pp. 407–423.

Lubs, H.A., Jr.: Testicular size in Klinefelter's syndrome in men over fifty. Report of a case with XXY/XY mosaicism. N. Engl. J. Med., *267*:326, 1962.

Paulsen, C. A., Gordon, D. L., Carpenter, R. W., Gandy, H. M., and Drucker, W. D.: Klinefelter's syndrome and its variants: A hormonal and chromosomal study. Recent Progr. Horm. Res., *24*:321, 1968.

Ratcliffe, S. G.: The sexual development of boys with the chromosome constitution 47,XXY (Klinefelter's syndrome). Clin. Endocrinol. Metabol., *11*:703, 1982.

Samaan, N. A., Stepanas, A. V., Danziger, J., and Trujillo, J.: Reactive pituitary abnormalities in patients with Klinefelter's and Turner's syndromes. Arch. Intern. Med., *139*:198, 1979.

Snyder, P. R., and Lawrence, D. A.: Treatment of male hypogonadism with testosterone enanthate. J. Clin. Endocrinol. Metab., *51*:1335, 1980.

Wang, C., Baker, H. W. G., Burger, H. G., De Kretser, D. M., and Hudson, B.: Hormonal studies in Klinefelter's syndrome. Clin. Endocrinol., *4*:399, 1975.

XX Male Syndrome

De la Chapelle, A.: Nature and origin of males with XX sex chromosomes. Am. J. Hum. Genet., *24*:71, 1972.

de la Chapelle, A.: The etiology of maleness in XX men. Hum. Genet., *58*:105, 1981.

Kasdan, R., Nankin, H. R., Troen, P., Wald, N., Pan, S., and Yanaihara, T.: Paternal transmission of maleness of XX human beings. N. Engl. J. Med., *288*:539, 1973.

Perez-Palacios, G., Medina, M., Ullao-Aguirre, A., Chavez, B. A., Villareal, G., Dutrem, M. T., Cahill, L. T., and Wachtel, S.: Gonadotropin dynamics in XX males. J. Clin. Endocrinol. Metab., *53*:254, 1981.

Roe, T.F., and Alfi, O. S.: Ambiguous genitalia in XX male children: Report of two infants. Pediatrics, *50*:55, 1977.

Schweikert, H. U., Weissbach, L., Leyendecker, G., Schwinger, E., Wartenberg, H., and Kruck, F.: Clinical, endocrinological, and cytological characterization of two 46,XX males. J. Clin. Endocrinol. Metab., *54*:745, 1982.

Wachtel, S. S., Koo, G. C., Breg, W. R., Thaler, H. T., Dillard, G. M., Rosenthal, I. M., Dosik, H., Gerald, P. S., Saenger, P., New, M., Lieber, E., and Miller, O. J.: Serologic detection of a Y-linked gene in XX males and XX true hermaphrodites. N. Engl. J. Med., *295*:750, 1976.

Gonadal Dysgenesis

AvRuskin, T. W., Crigler, J. F., Jr., Soeldner, J. S.: Turner's syndrome and carbohydrate metabolism. I. Impaired insulin secretion after tolbutamide and glucagon stimulation tests: evidence of insulin deficiency. Am. J. Med. Sci., *277(2)*:145, 1979.

Brook, C. G. D., Murset, G., Zachmann, M., and Prader, A.: Growth in children with 45,XO Turner's syndrome. Arch. Dis. Child., *49*:789, 1974.

Conte, F. A., Grumbach, M. M., and Kaplan, S. L.: A diphasic pattern of gonadotropin secretion in patients with the syndrome of gonadal dysgenesis. J. Clin. Endocrinol. Metab., *40*:670, 1975.

Conte, F. A., Grumbach, M., Kaplan, S. L., and Reiter, E. O.: Correlation of luteinizing hormone-releasing factor-induced luteinizing hormone and follicle-stimulating hormone release from infancy to 19 years with the changing pattern of gonadotropin secretion in agonadal patients: Relation to the restraint of puberty. J. Clin. Endocrinol. Metab., *50*:163, 1980.

Ford, C. E., Jones, K. W., Polani, P. E., De Almedia, J. C., and Briggs, J. H.: A sex-chromosome anomaly in a case of gonadal dysgenesis (Turner's syndrome). Lancet, *1*:711, 1959.

Hall, J. G., Sybert, V. P., Williamson, R. A., Fisher, N. L., and Reed, S. D.: Turner's syndrome. West. J. Med., *137*:32, 1982.

Leichtman, D. A., Schmickel, R. D., Gelehrter, T. D., Judd, W. J., Woodbury, M. C., and Meilinger, K. L.: Familial Turner syndrome. Ann. Intern. Med., *89*:473, 1978.

Lock, J. P., Henry, G., Gotlin, R., and Betz, G.: Spontaneous feminization and menstrual function developing during puberty in Turner's syndrome. Obstet. Gynecol., *54*:496, 1979.

Ross, G. T., Vande Wiele, R. L., and Frantz, A. G.: The ovaries and the breasts. Part 1: The ovaries. *In* Williams, R. H. (Ed.): Textbook of Endocrinology. Philadelphia, W. B. Saunders Co., 1981, p. 355.

Samaan, N. A., Stepanas, A. V., Danziger, J., and Trujillo, J.: Reactive pituitary abnormalities in patients with Klinefelter's and Turner's syndromes. Arch. Intern. Med., *139*:198, 1979.

Simpson, J. L.: Gonadal dysgenesis and sex chromosome abnormalities: Phenotypic-karyotypic correlations. *In* Vallet, H. L., and Porter, I. H. (Eds.): Genetic Mechanisms of Sexual Development. New York, Academic Press, 1979, p. 365.

Singh, R. P., and Carr, D. H.: The anatomy and histology of XO human embryos and fetuses. Anat. Rec., *155*:369, 1966.

Turner, H. H.: A syndrome of infantilism, congenital webbed neck, and cubitus valgus. Endocrinology, *23*:566, 1938.

Mixed Gonadal Dysgenesis

Davidoff, F., and Federman, D. D.: Mixed gonadal dysgenesis. Pediatrics, *52*:727, 1973.

Donahoe, P. K., Crawford, J. D., and Hendren, W. H.: Mixed gonadal dysgenesis, pathogenesis and management. J. Pediatr. Surg. *14*:287, 1979.

Kofman, S., Perez-Palacios, G., Medina, M., Escobar, N., Garcia, M., Ruz, L., Mutchinick, O., and Lisker, R.: Clinical and endocrine spectrum in patients with the 45,X/46,XY karyotype. Hum. Genet., *58*:373, 1981.

Robboy, S. J., Miller, T., Donahoe, P. K., Jahre, C., Welch, W. R., Haseltine, F. P., Miller, W. A., Atkins, L., and Crawford, J. D.: Dysgenesis of testicular and streak gonads in the syndrome of mixed gonadal dysgenesis: Perspective derived from a clinicopathologic analysis of twenty-one cases. Hum. Pathol., *13*:700, 1982.

Schellhas, H. F.: Malignant potential of the dysgenetic gonad. Part I. Obstet. Gynecol., *44*:298, 1974*a*.

Schellhas, H. F.: Malignant potential of the dysgenetic gonad. Part II. Obstet. Gynecol., *44*:455, 1974*b*.

Sohval, A. R.: "Mixed" gonadal dysgenesis: A variety of hermaphroditism. Am. J. Hum. Genet., *15*:155, 1963.

Teter, J., and Boczkowski, K.: Occurrence of tumors in dysgenetic gonads. Cancer, *20*:1301, 1967.

Zah, W., Kalderon, A. E., and Tucci, J. R.: Mixed gonadal dysgenesis. Acta Endocrinol., (Suppl.), *197*:1, 1975.

True Hermaphroditism

Aiman, J., Hemsell, D. L., and MacDonald, P. C.: Production and origin of estrogen in two true hermaphrodites. Am. J. Obstet. Gynecol., *132*:401, 1978.

Gallegos, A. J., Guizar, E., Armendares, S., Cortes-Gallegos, V., Cervantes, C., Bedolla, N., and Parra, A.: Familial true hermaphrodism in three siblings: Plasma hormonal profile and *in vitro* steroid biosynthesis in gonadal structures. J. Clin. Endocrinol. Metab., *42*:653, 1976.

Lee, S.: High incidence of true hermaphroditism in the early human embryos. Biol. Neonate, *18*:418, 1971.

Perez-Palacios, G., Carnevale, A., Escobar, N., Villareal, G., Fernandez, E., and Medina, M.: Induction of ovulation in a true hermaphrodite with male phenotype. J. Clin. Endocrinol. Metab., *52*:1257, 1981.

Roy, C., Roger, M., Boccon-Gibod, L., Fellous, M., Bonno, R., Pasqualini, J., and Harpey, J. P.: Clinical, cytogenetical, histological, immunological and hormonal studies in a case of true hermaphroditism. Clin. Endocrinol., *12*:423, 1980.

Simpson, J. L.: True hermaphroditism: Etiology and phenotypic considerations. Birth Defects, *14(6C)*:9, 1978.

van Niekerk, W. A.: True hermaphroditism. Pediatr. Adolesc. Endocrinol., *8*:80, 1981*a*.

van Niekerk, W. A., and Retief, A. E.:The gonads of human true hermaphrodites. Human. Genet., *58*:117, 1981*b*.

Winters, S. J., Wachtel, S. S., White, B. J., Koo, G. C., Javadpour, N., Loriaux, L., and Sherins, R. J.: H-Y antigen mosaicism in the gonad of a 46,XX true hermaphrodite. N. Engl. J. Med., *300*:745, 1979.

Pure Gonadal Dysgenesis

Aleem, F. A.: Familial 46,XX gonadal dysgenesis. Fertil. Steril., *35*:317, 1981.

Carr, B. R., and Aiman, J.: Steroid production in a woman with gonadal dysgenesis, breast development, and clitoral hypertrophy. Obstet. Gynecol., *56*:492, 1980.

German, J., Simpson, J. L., and Chaganti, R. S. K.: Genetically determined sex-reversal in 46,XY humans. Science *202*:53, 1978.

McDonough, P. G., Byrd, J. R., Tho, P. T., and Mahesh, V. B.: Phenotypic and cytogenetic findings in eighty-two patients with ovarian failure—changing trends. Fertil. Steril., *28*:638, 1977.

Moltz, L., Schwartz, U., Pickartz, H., Hammerstein, J., and Wolf, U.: XY gonadal dysgenesis: Aberrant testicular differentiation in the presence of H-Y antigen. Obstet. Gynecol., *58*:17, 1981.

Passarge, E., and Wolf, U.: Brief clinical report: Genetic heterogeneity of XY gonadal dysgenesis (Swyer syndrome): H-Y antigen–negative XY gonadal dysgenesis

associated with inflammatory bowel disease. Am. J. Med. Genet., *8*:437, 1981.

Phansey, S. A., Satterfield, R., Jorgenson, R. J., Salinas, C. F., Yoder, F. E., Mathur, R. S., and Williamson, H. O.: XY gonadal dysgenesis in three siblings. Am. J. Obstet. Gynecol., *138*:133, 1980.

Simpson, J. L., Blagowidow, N., and Martin, A.O.: XY gonadal dysgenesis: Genetic heterogeneity based upon clinical observations, H-Y antigen status and segregation analysis. Hum. Genet., *58*:91, 1981.

Absent Testes Syndrome

Aynsley-Green, A., Zachmann, M., Illig, R., Rampini, S., and Prader, A.: Congenital bilateral anorchia in childhood: A clinical, endocrine and therapeutic evaluation of twenty-one cases. Clin. Endocrinol., *5*:381, 1976.

Bergada, C., Cleveland, W. W., Jones, H. W., Jr., and Wilkins, L.: Variants of embryonic testicular dysgenesis: Bilateral anorchia and the syndrome of rudimentary testes. Acta Endocrinol., *40*:521, 1962.

Edman, C. D., Winters, A. J., Porter, J. C., Wilson, J., and MacDonald, P. C.: Embryonic testicular regression. A clinical spectrum of XY agonadal individuals. Obstet. Gynecol., *49*:208, 1977.

Glass, A. R.: Identical twins discordant for the "rudimentary testes" syndrome. J. Urol., *127*:140, 1982.

Hall, J. G., Morgan, A., and Blizzard, R. M.: Familial congenital anorchia. *In* Bergsma, D. (Ed.): Genetic Forms of Hypogonadism. Birth Defects: Original Article Series. Vol. XI. No. 4. Baltimore, The Williams & Wilkins Co., 1975, pp. 115–119.

Kirschner, M. A., Jacobs, J. B., and Fraley, E. E.: Bilateral anorchia with persistent testosterone production. N. Engl. J. Med., *282*:240, 1970.

Medina, M., Kofman-Alfaro, S., and Perez-Palacios, G.: 46,XX gonadal absence: a variant of the XX pure gonadal dysgenesis? Acta Endocrinol., *99*:585, 1982.

Silber, S. J.: Transplantation of a human testis for anorchia. Fertil. Steril., *30*:181, 1978.

Congenital Adrenal Hyperplasia

Bongiovanni, A. M.: Acquired adrenal hyperplasia: With special reference to 3β-hydroxysteroid dehydrogenase. Fert. Steril., *35*:599, 1981.

Chrousos, G. P., Loriaux, D. L., Mann, D. L., and Cutler, G. B.: Late-onset 21-hydroxylase deficiency mimicking idiopathic hirsutism or polycystic ovarian disease. Ann. Intern. Med., *96*:143, 1982.

Glenthøj, A., Nielsen, M. D., and Starup, J.: Congenital adrenal hyperplasia due to 11β-hydroxylase deficiency: final diagnosis in adult age in three patients. Acta Endocrinol., *93*:94, 1980.

Hughes, I. A., and Winter, J. S. D.: The application of a serum 170H-progesterone radioimmunoassay to the diagnosis and management of congenital adrenal hyperplasia. J. Pediatr., *88*:766, 1976.

Kuhnle, U., Chow, D., Rapaport, R., Pang, S., Levine, L. S., and New, M.: The 21-hydroxylase activity in the glomerulosa and fasciculata of the adrenal cortex in congenital adrenal hyperplasia. J. Clin. Endocrinol. Metab., *52*:534, 1981.

Lee, P. A., Rosenwaks, Z., Urban, M. D., Migeon, C. J., and Bias, W. D.: Attenuated forms of congenital adrenal hyperplasia due to 21-hydroxylase deficiency. J. Clin. Endocrinol. Metab., *55*:866, 1982.

Levine, L. S., Dupont, B., Lorenzen, F., Pang, S., Pollack, M., Oberfield, S., Kohn, B., Lerner, A., Cacciari, E., Mantero, F., Cassio, A., Scaroni, C., Chiumello, G.,

Rondanini, G. F., Garantini, L., Giovannelli, G., Virdis, R., Bartolotta, E., Migliori, C., Pintor, C., Tato, L., Barboni, F., and New, M. I.: Cryptic 21-hydroxylase deficiency in families of patients with classical congenital adrenal hyperplasia. J. Clin. Endocrinol. Metab., 51:1316, 1980.

Levine, L. S., Zachmann, M., New, M. I., Prader, A., Pollack, M. S., O'Neill, G. J., Yang, S. Y., Oberfield, S. E., and Dupont, B.: Genetic mapping of the 21-hydroxylase-deficiency gene within the HLA linkage group. N. Engl. J. Med., 299:911, 1978.

New, I. M., and Levine, L. S.: Congenital adrenal hyperplasia and related conditions. In Stanbury, J. B., Wyngaarden, J. B., Fredrickson, D. S., Goldstein, J. L., and Brown, M. S. (Eds.): Metabolic Basis of Inherited Disease. 5th ed. New York, McGraw-Hill Book Co., 1983, pp. 973–1000.

Newell, M. E., Lippe, B. M., and Ehrlich, R. M.: Testis tumors associated with congenital adrenal hyperplasia: A continuing diagnostic and therapeutic dilemma. J. Urol., 117:256.

Pang, S., Hotchkiss, J., Drash, A. L., Levine, L. S., and New, M. I.: Microfilter paper method for 17α-hydroxyprogesterone radioimmunoassay: Its application for rapid screening for congenital adrenal hyperplasia. J. Clin. Endocrinol. Metab., 45:1003, 1977.

Rosler, A., Levine, L. S., Schneider, B., Novogroder, M., and New, M. I.: The interrelationship of sodium balance, plasma renin activity and ACTH in congenital adrenal hyperplasia. J. Clin. Endocrinol. Metab., 45:500, 1977.

Weldon, V. V., Blizzard, R. M., and Migeon, C. J.: Newborn girls misdiagnosed as bilaterally cryptorchid males. N. Engl. J. Med., 274:829, 1966.

Nonadrenal Female Pseudohermaphroditism

Grumbach, M. M., and Conte, F. A.: Disorders of sexual differentiation. In Wilson, J. D., and Foster, D. W. (Eds.): Williams' Textbook of Endocrinology. 7th ed. Philadelphia, W. B. Saunders Co., 1985.

Hensleigh, P. A., and Woodruff, J. D.: Differential maternal-fetal response to androgenizing luteoma or hyperreactio luteinalis. Obstet. Gynecol. Surv., 33:262, 1978.

Congenital Absence of the Vagina

Bryans, F. E.: Management of congenital absence of the vagina. Am. J. Obstet. Gynecol., 139:281, 1981.

Evans, T. N., Poland, M. L., and Boving, R. L.: Vaginal malformations. Am. J. Obstet. Gynecol., 141:910, 1981.

Frank, R. T.: The formation of an artificial vagina without operation. Am. J. Obstet. Gynecol., 35:1053, 1938.

Fraser, I. S., Baird, D. T., Hobson, B. M., Michie, E. A., and Hunter, W.: Cyclical ovarian function in women with congenital absence of the uterus and vagina. J. Clin. Endocrinol. Metab., 36:634, 1973.

Griffin, J. E., Edwards, C., Madden, J. D., Harrod, M. J., and Wilson, J. D.: Congenital absence of the vagina. The Mayer-Rokitansky-Kuster-Hauser syndrome. Ann. Intern. Med., 85:224, 1976.

Hauser, G. A., and Schreiner, W. E.: Das Mayer-Rokitansky-Kuster Syndrome. Schweiz. Med. Wochenschr., 91:381, 1961.

Jones, H. W., Jr., and Mermut, S.: Familial occurrence of congenital absence of the vagina. Am. J. Obstet. Gynecol., 114:1100, 1972.

Jones, H. W., Jr., and Wheeless, C. R.: Salvage of the reproductive ducts: 1868-1968-2068. Am. J. Obstet. Gynecol., 104:348, 1969.

Ross, G. T., Vande Wiele, R. L., and Frantz, A. G.: The ovaries and the breasts. In Williams, R.H. (Ed.): Textbook of Endocrinology. 6th ed. Philadelphia, W. B. Saunders, Co., 1981, p. 355.

Shokeir, M. H. K.: Aplasia of the müllerian system: Evidence for probable sex-limited autosomal dominant inheritance. In Summitt, R. L., and Bergsma, D. (Eds.): Sex Differentiation and Chromosomal Abnormalities. Birth Defects: Original Article Series. Vol. XIV. No. 6C. New York, Alan R. Liss, Inc., 1978, pp. 147–165.

Wabrek, A. J., Millard, P. R., Wilson, W. B., Jr., and Pion, R. J.: Creation of a neovagina by the Frank nonoperative method. Obstet. Gynecol., 37:408, 1971.

Male Pseudohermaphroditism (General)

Campo, S., Monteagudo, C., Nicolau, G., Pellizzari, E., Belgorosky, A., Stivel, M., and Rivarola, M.: Testicular function in prepubertal male pseudohermaphroditism. Clin. Endocrinol., 14:11, 1981.

Campo, S., Stivel, M., Nicolau, G., Monteagudo, C., and Rivarola, M.: Testicular function in post pubertal male pseudohermaphroditism. Clin. Endocrinol., 11:481, 1979.

Griffin, J. E., and Wilson, J. D.: Hereditary male pseudohermaphroditism. Clin. Endocrinol., 5:457, 1978.

Savage, M. O., Chaussain, J. L., Evain, D., Roger, M., Canlorbe, O., and Job, J. C.: Endocrine studies in male pseudohermaphroditism in childhood and adolescence. Clin. Endocrinol., 8:219, 1978.

Abnormalities in Androgen Synthesis
20,22-Desmolase

Camacho, A. M., Kowarski, A., Migeon, C. J., and Brough, A. J.: Congenital adrenal hyperplasia due to a deficiency of one of the enzymes involved in the biosynthesis of pregnenolone. J. Clin. Endocrinol., 28:153, 1968.

Kirkland, R. T., Kirkland, J. L., Johnson, C. M., Horning, M. G., Librik, L, and Clayton, G. W.: Congenital lipoid adrenal hyperplasia in an eight-year-old phenotypic female. J. Clin. Endocrinol., 36:488, 1973.

3β-Hydroxysteroid dehydrogenase

Bongiovanni, A. M.: Congenital adrenal hyperplasia and related conditions. In Stanbury, J. B., Wyngaarden, J. B., and Fredericksen, D. S. (Eds.): The Metabolic Basis of Inherited Disease. 4th ed. New York, McGraw-Hill Book Co., 1978, pp. 868–893.

Parks, G. A., Bermudez, J. A., Anast, C. S., Bongiovanni, A. M., and New, M. I.: Pubertal boy with the 3β-hydroxysteroid dehydrogenase defect. J. Clin. Endocrinol., 33:269, 1971.

Rosenfield, R. L., DeNiepomniszsze, A. B., Kenny, F. M., and Genel, M.: The response to human chorionic gonadotropin (HCG) administration in boys with and without Δ⁵-3β-hydroxysteroid dehydrogenase deficiency. J. Clin. Endocrinol. Metab., 39:370, 1974.

Schneider, G., Genel, M., Bongiovanni, A. M., Goldman, A. S., and Rosenfield, R. L.: Persistent testicular Δ⁵-isomerase-3β-hydroxysteroid dehydrogenase (Δ⁵-3β-HSA) deficiency in the Δ⁵-3β-HSD form of congenital adrenal hyperplasia. J. Clin. Invest., 55:681, 1975.

Zachmann, M., Völlmin, J. A., Mürset, G., Curtius, H. C., and Prader, A.: Unusual type of congenital adrenal hyperplasia probably due to deficiency of 3β-hydroxysteroid dehydrogenase. Case report of a surviving girl and steroid studies. J. Clin. Endocrinol. Metab., 30:719, 1970.

17α-Hydroxylase

Biglieri, E. G., Herron, M. A., and Brust, N.: 17-hydroxylation deficiency in man. J. Clin. Invest., *45*:1946, 1966.

Jones, H. W., Lee, P. A., Rock, J. A., Archer, D. F., and Migeon, C. J.: A genetic male patient with 17α-hydroxylase deficiency. Obstet. Gynecol., *59*:245, 1982.

New, M. I.: Male pseudohermaphroditism due to 17α-hydroxylase deficiency. J. Clin. Invest., *49*:1930, 1970.

Sills, I. N., MacGillivray, M. H., Amrhein, J. A., Migeon, C. J., and Peterson, R. E.: 17α-hydroxylase deficiency in a genetic male and female sibling pair. Int. J. Gynaecol. Obstet., *19*:473, 1981.

17,20-Desmolase

Forest, M. G., Lecornu, M., and DePeretti,: Familial male pseudohermaphroditism due to 17-20-desmolase deficiency. I. *In vivo* endocrine studies. J. Clin. Endocrinol. Metab., *50*:826, 1980.

Goebelsmann, U., Zachmann, M., Davajan, V., Israel R., Mestman, J. H., and Mishell, D. R.: Male pseudohermaphroditism consistent with 17,20-desmolase deficiency. Gynecol. Invest., *7*:138, 1976.

Larrea, F., Lisker, R., Banuelos, R., Bermudez, J. A., Herrera, J., Rasilla, V. N., and Perez-Palacios G.: Hypergonadotrophic hypogonadism in an XX female subject due to 17,20 steroid desmolase deficiency. Acta Endocrinol., *103*:400, 1983.

Zachmann, M., Völlmin, J. A., Hamilton, W., and Prader, A.: Steroid 17,20-desmolase deficiency: A new cause of male pseudohermaphroditism. Clin. Endocrinol., *1*:369, 1972.

Zachmann, M., Werder, E. A., Prader, A.: Two types of male pseudohermaphroditism due to 17,20-desmolase deficiency. J. Clin. Endocrinol. Metab., *55*:487, 1982.

17β-Hydroxysteroid dehydrogenase

Akesode, F. A., Meyer, W. J., III, and Migeon, C. J.: Male pseudohermaphroditism with gynecomastia due to testicular 17-ketosteroid reductase deficiency. Clin. Endocrinol., *7*:443, 1977.

Givens, J. R., Wiser, W. L., Summitt, R. L., Kerber, I. J., Andersen, R. N., Pittaway, D. E., and Fish, S. A.: Familial male pseudohermaphroditism without gynecomastia due to deficient testicular 17-ketosteroid reductase activity. N. Engl. J. Med., *291*:938, 1974.

Goebelsmann, U., Horton, R., Mestman, J. H., Arce, J. J., Nagata, Y., Nakamura, R. M., Thorneycroft, I. H., and Mishell, D. R., Jr.: Male pseudohermaphroditism due to testicular 17β-hydroxysteroid dehydrogenase deficiency. J. Clin. Endocrinol. Metab., *36*:867, 1973.

Imperato-McGinley, J., Peterson, R. E., Stoller, R., and Goodwin, W. E.: Male pseudohermaphroditism secondary to 17β-hydroxysteroid dehydrogenase deficiency: Gender role change with puberty. J. Clin. Endocrinol. Metab., *49*:391, 1979.

Rösler, A., and Kohn, G.: Male pseudohermaphroditism due to 17β-hydroxysteroid dehydrogenase deficiency: Studies on the natural history of the defect and effect of androgens on gender role. J. Steroid Biochem., *19*:663, 1983.

Virdis, R., Saenger, P., Seniror, B., and New, M.I.: Endocrine studies in a pubertal male pseudohermaphrodite with 17-ketosteroid reductase deficiency. Acta Endocrinol., *87*:212, 1978.

Leydig Cell Abnormalities

Berthezene, R., Forest, M.G., Grimaud, J. A., Claustrat, B., and Mornex, R.: Leydig-cell agenesis. A cause of male pseudohermaphroditism. N. Engl. J. Med., *295*:969, 1976.

Lee, P. A., Rock, J. A., Brown, T. R., Fichman, K. M., Migeon, C. J., and Jones, H.W., Jr.: Leydig cell hypofunction resulting in male pseudohermaphroditism. Fertil. Steril., *37*:675, 1982.

Park, I. J., Burnett, L. S., Jones, H. W., Jr., Migeon, C. J., and Blizzard, R. M.: A case of male pseudohermaphroditism associated with elevated LH, normal FSH and low testosterone possibly due to the secretion of an abnormal LH molecule. Acta Endocrinol., *83*:173, 1976.

Perez-Palacios, G., Scaglia, H. E., Kofman-Alfaro, S., Saavedra, O. D., Ochoa, S., Larraza, O., and Perez, A. E.: Inherited male pseudohermaphroditism due to gonadotrophin unresponsiveness. Acta Endocrinol., *98*:148, 1981.

Schwartz, M., Imperato-McGinley, J., Peterson, R. E., Cooper, G., Morris, P. L., MacGillivray, M., and Hensle, T.: Male pseudohermaphroditism secondary to an abnormality in Leydig cell differentiation. J. Clin. Endocrinol. Metab., *53*:123, 1981.

Abnormalities in Androgen Action

5α-Reductase Deficiency

Fisher, L. K., Kogut, M. D., Moore, R. J., Goebelsmann, U., Weitzman, J. J., Isaacs, H., Jr., Griffin, J. E., and Wilson, J. D.: Clinical, endocrinological, and enzymatic characterization of two patients with 5α-reductase deficiency: Evidence that a single enzyme is responsible for the 5α-reduction of cortisol and testosterone. J. Clin. Endocrinol. Metab., *47*:653, 1978.

Imperato-McGinley, J., Guerrero, L., Gautier, T., and Peterson, R. E.: Steroid 5α-reductase deficiency in man: An inherited form of male pseudohermaphroditism. Science, *186*:1213, 1974.

Imperato-McGinley, J., Peterson, R. E., Gautier, T., Sturla, E.: Androgens and the evolution of male-gender identity among male pseudohermaphrodites with 5α-reductase deficiency. N. Engl. J. Med., *300*:1233, 1979.

Imperato-McGinley, J., Peterson, R. E., Leshin, M., Griffin, J. E., Cooper, G., Draghi, S., Berenyi, M., and Wilson, J. D.: Steroid 5α-reductase deficiency in a 65-year-old male pseudohermaphrodite: The natural history, ultrastructure of the testes, and evidence for inherited enzyme heterogeneity. J. Clin. Endocrinol. Metab., *50*:15, 1980.

Leshin, M., Griffin, J. E., and Wilson, J. D.: Hereditary male pseudohermaphroditism associated with an unstable form of 5α-reductase. J. Clin. Invest., *62*:685, 1978.

Peterson, R. E., Imperato-McGinley, J., Gautier, T., and Sturla, E.: Male pseudohermaphroditism due to steroid 5α-reductase deficiency. Am. J. Med., *62*:170, 1977.

Price, P., Wass, J. A. H., Griffin, J. E., Leshin, M., Savage, M. O., Large, D. M., Bullock, D. E., Anderson, D. C., Wilson, J. D., and Besser, G. M.: High dose androgen therapy in male pseudohermaphroditism due to 5α-reductase deficiency and disorders of the androgen receptor. J. Clin. Invest., *74*:1496, 1984.

Walsh, P. C., Madden, J. D., Harrod, M. J., Goldstein, J. L., MacDonald, P. C., and Wilson, J. D.: Familial incomplete male pseudohermaphroditism, Type 2. Decreased dihydrotestosterone formation in pseudovaginal perineoscrotal hypospadias. N. Engl. J. Med., *291*:944, 1974.

Wilson, J. D., Griffin, J. E., Leshin, M., and MacDonald, P. C.: The androgen resistance syndromes: 5α-reductase deficiency, testicular feminization, and related disorders. *In* Stanbury, J.B., Wyngaarden, J. B., Fredrickson, D. S., Goldstein, J. L., and Brown, M. S. (Eds.): The Metabolic Basis of Inherited Disease. Chap. 48. New York, McGraw-Hill Book Co., 1983, pp. 1001–1026.

Receptor Disorders—Testicular Feminization, Reifenstein Syndrome, and the Infertile Male Syndrome

Aiman, J., and Griffin, J. E.: The frequency of androgen receptor deficiency in infertile men. J. Clin. Endocrinol. Metab., *54*:725, 1982.

Aiman, J., Griffin, J. E., Gazak, J. M., Wilson, J. D., and MacDonald, P. C.: Androgen insensitivity as a cause of infertility in otherwise normal men. N. Engl. J. Med., *300*:223, 1979.

Amrhein, J. A., Meyer, W. J., III, Jones, H. W., Jr., and Migeon, C. J.: Androgen insensitivity in man: Evidence for genetic heterogeneity. Proc. Natl. Acad. Sci. U.S.A., *73*:891, 1976.

Bowen, P., Lee, C. S. N., Migeon, C. J., Kaplan, N. M., Whalley, P. J., McKusick, V. A., and Reifenstein, E. C., Jr.: Hereditary male pseudohermaphroditism with hypogonadism, hypospadias, and gynecomastia (Reifenstein's syndrome). Ann. Intern. Med., *62*:252, 1965.

Boyar, R. M., Moore, R. J., Rosner, W., Aiman, J., Chipman, J., Madden, J. D., Marks, J. F., and Griffin, J. E.: Studies of gonadotropin-gonadal dynamics in patients with androgen insensitivity. J. Clin. Endocrinol. Metab., *47*:1116, 1978.

Griffin, J. E.: Testicular feminization associated with a thermolabile androgen receptor in cultured human fibroblasts. J. Clin. Invest., *64*:1624, 1979.

Griffin, J. E., and Durrant, J. L.: Qualitative receptor defects in families with androgen resistance: Failure of stabilization of the fibroblast cytosol androgen receptor. J. Clin. Endocrinol. Metab., *55*:465, 1982.

Hauser, G. A.: Testicular feminization. *In* Overzier, C. (Ed.): Intersexuality. London, Academic Press, 1963, pp. 255–276.

Imperato-McGinley, J., Peterson, R. E., Gautier, T., Cooper, G., Danner, R., Arthur, A., Morris, P. L., Sweeney, W. J., and Shackleton, C.: Hormonal evaluation of a large kindred with complete androgen insensitivity: Evidence for secondary 5α-reductase deficiency. J. Clin. Endocrinol. Metab., *54*:931, 1982.

Kaufman, M., Pinsky, L., and Feder-Hollander, R.: Defective up-regulation of the androgen receptor in human androgen insensitivity. Nature, *293*:735, 1981.

Keenan, B. S., Kirkland, J. L., Kirkland, R. T., and Clayton, G. W.: Male pseudohermaphroditism with partial androgen insensitivity. Pediatrics, *59*:224, 1977.

Keenan, B. S., Meyer, W. J., III, Hadjian, A. J., and Migeon, C. J.: Androgen receptor in human skin fibroblasts. Characterization of a specific 17β-hydroxy-5α-androstan-3-one-protein complex in cell sonicates and nuclei. Steroids, *25*:535, 1975.

MacDonald, P. C., Madden, J. D., Brenner, P. F., Wilson, J. D., and Siiteri, P. K.: Origin of estrogen in normal men and in women with testicular feminization. J. Clin. Endocrinol. Metab., *49*:905, 1979.

Madden, J. D., Walsh, P. C., MacDonald, P. C., and Wilson, J. D.: Clinical and endocrinologic characterization of a patient with the syndrome of incomplete testicular feminization. J. Clin. Endocrinol. Metab., *41*:751, 1975.

Meyer, W. J., III, Migeon, B. R., and Migeon, C. J.: Locus on human X chromosome for dihydrotestosterone receptor and androgen insensitivity. Proc. Natl. Acad. Sci. U.S.A., *72*:1469, 1975.

Reifenstein, E. C., Jr.: Hereditary familial hypogonadism. Clin. Res., *3*:86, 1947.

Rosenfield, R. L., Lawrence, A. M., Liao, S., and Landau, R. L.: Androgens and androgen responsiveness in the feminizing testis syndrome. Comparison of complete and "incomplete" forms. J. Clin. Endocrinol. Metab., *32*:625, 1971.

Ross, G. T., Vande Wiele, R. L., and Frantz, A. G.: The ovaries and the breasts. *In* Williams, R.H. (Ed.): Textbook of Endocrinology., Philadelphia, W.B. Saunders Co., 1981, p. 355.

Wilson, J. D., Griffin, J. E., Leshin, M., and MacDonald, P. C.: The androgen resistance syndromes: 5α-reductase deficiency, testicular feminization, and related disorders. *In* Stanbury, J. B., Wyngaarden, J. B., Frederickson, D. S., Goldstein, J. L., and Brown, M. S. (Eds.): The Metabolic Basis of Inherited Disease. Chap. 48. New York, McGraw-Hill Book Co., 1983, pp. 1001–1026.

Wilson, J. D., Harrod, M. J., Goldstein, J. L., Hemsell, D. L., and MacDonald, P. C.: Familial incomplete male pseudohermaphroditism, Type I. Evidence for androgen resistance and variable clinical manifestations in a family with the Reifenstein syndrome. N. Engl. J. Med., *290*:1097, 1974.

Persistent Müllerian Duct Syndrome

Brook, C. G. D., Wagner, H., Zachmann, M., Prader, A., Armendares, S., Frenk, S., Aleman, P., Najjar, S. S., Slim, M. S., Genton, N., and Bozic, C.: Familial occurrence of persistent müllerian structures in otherwise normal males. Br. Med. J., *1*:771, 1973.

Nilson, O.: Hernia uteri inguinalis beim Manne. Acta Chir. Scand., *83*:231, 1939.

Sloan, W. R., and Walsh, P. C.: Familial persistent Müllerian duct syndrome. J. Urol., *115*:459, 1976.

Weiss, E. B., Kiefer, J. H., Rowlatt, U. F., and Rosenthal, I. M.: Persistent müllerian duct syndrome in male identical twins. Pediatrics, *61*:797, 1978.

Chromosomal Evaluation

Caspersson, T., Hulten, M., Jonasson, J., Lindsten, J., Therkelsen, A., and Zech, L.: Translocations causing non-fluorescent Y chromosomes in human XO/XY mosaics. Hereditas, *68*:317, 1971.

Meisner, L.F., and Inhorn, S.L.: Normal male development with Y chromosome long arm deletion (Yq−). J. Med. Genet., *9*:373, 1972.

Simpson, J. L., Jirasek, J. E., Speroff, L., and Kase, N. G.: Disorders of Sexual Differentiation. New York, Academic Press, 1976, p. 466.

Biochemical Evaluation

Forest, M. G.: Pattern of the response of testosterone and its precursors to human chorionic gonadotropin stimulation in relation to age in infants and children. J. Clin. Endocrinol. Metab., *49*:132, 1979.

Hughes, I. A., and Winter, J. S. D.: The application of a serum 17OH-progesterone radioimmunoassay to the diagnosis and management of congenital adrenal hyperplasia. J. Pediatr. *88*:766, 1976.

Levine, L. S., Lieber, E., Pang, S., and New, M. I.: Male pseudohermaphroditism due to 17-ketosteroid reductase deficiency diagnosed in the newborn period. Pediatr. Res., *14*:480, 1980.

Peterson, R. E., Imperato-McGinley, J., Gautier, T., and Sturla, E.: Male pseudohermaphroditism due to steroid 5α-reductase deficiency. Am. J. Med., *62*:170, 1977.

Walsh, P. C., Curry, N., Mills, R. C., and Siiteri, P. K.: Plasma androgen response to hCG stimulation in prepubertal boys with hypospadias and cryptorchidism. J. Clin. Endocrinol. Metab., *42*:52, 1976.

Wilson, J. D., Griffin, J. E., Leshin, M., and MacDonald, P. C.: The androgen resistance syndromes: 5α-reductase deficiency, testicular feminization, and related disorders. *In* Stanbury, J.B., Wyngaarden, J. B., Fredrickson, D. S., Goldstein, J. L., and Brown, M. S. (Eds.): The Metabolic Basis of Inherited Disease. Chap. 48. New York, McGraw-Hill, 1983, pp. 1001–1026.

Endoscopy and Radiography

Alzen, G., Jakobi, R., Dinkel, E., Weitzel, D., and Schönberger, W.: Sonographic contribution to the diagnosis of gynaecological diseases in children. Ultraschall., *2*:135, 1981.

Cremin, B. J.: Intersex states in young children: The importance of radiology in making a correct diagnosis. Clin. Radiol., *25*:63, 1974.

Madden, J. D., Walsh, P. C., MacDonald, P. C., and Wilson, J. D.: Clinical and endocrinologic characterization of a patient with the syndrome of incomplete testicular feminization. J. Clin. Endocrinol. Metab., *40*:751, 1975.

Peck, A. G., and Poznanski, A. K.: A simple device for genitography. Radiology, *193*:212, 1972.

Sloan, W. R., and Walsh, P. C.: Familial persistent Müllerian duct syndrome. J. Urol., *115*:459, 1976.

Walsh, P. C., Madden, J. D., Harrod, M. J., Goldstein, J. L., MacDonald, P. C., and Wilson, J. D.: Familial incomplete male pseudohermaphroditism, Type 2. Decreased dihydrotestosterone formation in pseudovaginal perineoscrotal hypospadias. N. Engl. J. Med., *291*:944, 1974.

Sex Assignment

Money, J.: Psychologic evaluation of the child with intersex problems. Pediatrics, *36*:51, 1965.

Money, J., and Ehrhardt, A. A.: Man and Woman, Boy and Girl. Baltimore, Johns Hopkins University Press, 1972.

Wilson, J. D.: Gonadal hormones and sexual behavior. *In* Besser, G. M., and Martini, L. (Eds.): Clinical Neuroendocrinology. Vol. II. Chap. 1. 1982, pp. 1–29.

CHAPTER 42

Exstrophy, Epispadias, and Other Anomalies of the Bladder

EDWARD C. MUECKE, M.D.

INTRODUCTION

The primary anomalies of the urinary bladder are described in this chapter with emphasis on the exstrophy-epispadias complex. Many bladder anomalies are rare, and only a few cases have been described in the literature. Abnormalities of the distal ureters and ureterovesical junction as well as those of the bladder outlet and urethra other than epispadias are not included in this chapter (see Chapters 38 and 48). In order to understand the complex embryogenesis of vesical exstrophy and its variants, the development of the bladder will be reviewed here as an introduction to congenital anomalies of the bladder.

EMBRYOLOGY OF THE BLADDER

In man the bladder is derived principally from the ventral portion of the cloaca and is not fully separated from the intestinal tract until the embryo is 6 weeks old. The base of the bladder or trigone, on the other hand, is derived from the mesoderm, having incorporated, at least in part, portions of the distal ends of the wolffian ducts (see Chapter 37).

In the early developmental phase of the embryo, the cloaca is a blind, oval pouch with a short extension into the tail portion of the embryo, the tailgut. Superiorly, it receives the midgut and the allantoic duct (Fig. 42–1). Its anterior wall is formed by the cloacal membrane: a two-layered structure composed of an outer ectoderm and an inner entoderm (Fig. 42–2). Seen from outside, this cloacal membrane appears as a rhomboid-shaped area between two lateral mesodermal ridges, and in the 4-mm embryo this membrane may extend superiorly into the body stalk.

In the 4- to 8-mm stage of development, roughly a 2-week span of time, the cloacal membrane is obliterated as mesodermal cells migrate mediad from the primitive node and caudad from the body stalk. In the 6-mm embryo this once prominent membrane now forms only the anterior wall of the lower two thirds of the cloaca; in the 8-mm embryo it begins to rotate away from the body wall to form the floor of the enlarging genital tubercle. Unhindered mesodermal movement is critical at this developmental stage, for any impediment could result in a weak anterior body wall with lateral displacement of its musculoskeletal elements.

As the mesodermal plate wedges itself between the ectodermal and entodermal layers of the cloacal membrane, the original flanking ridges are exaggerated and begin to form paired cloacal or genital folds. These folds fuse superiorly to form the genital tubercle (Fig. 42–3A). As this tubercle enlarges, the cloacal membrane is pushed downward and forward, forming the floor of this primitive phallus. Thus, the once prominent cloacal membrane, which formed almost the entire anterior infraumbilical abdominal wall in the young embryo, has been effectively reduced to a narrow groove in the floor of the now prominent genital tubercle that has

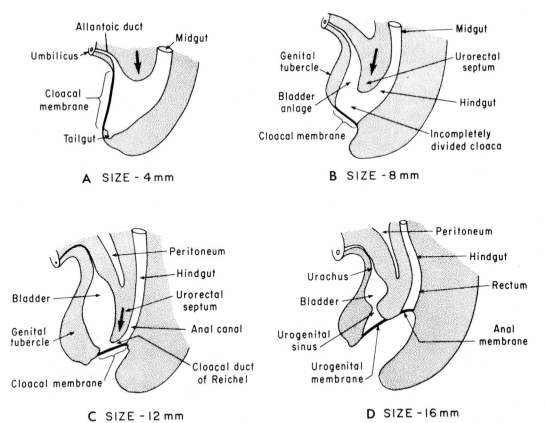

Figure 42–1. Developmental changes of the cloaca and cloacal membrane in the 4-mm to 16-mm embryo. Arrows show direction of growth of the urorectal septum. (Drawings are not to scale.)

taken its place. This occurs in less than 2 weeks and is due to the inflow of mesodermal elements that effectively reinforce the membranous anterior abdominal body wall, which until then has had two layers. Should the mesodermal movement be blocked by an unusually large cloacal membrane or delayed by other factors, the anterior wall of the cloaca would remain a weak bilaminar membrane, and the genital ridges would be forced to fuse inferiorly, carrying the cloacal membrane as a roof rather than as a floor. Sequential developmental steps would then be altered: The musculoskeletal structures would be held apart, the anterior pelvic girdle would be widened, and an open urethral groove would lie on the anterior surface of the phallus. All these anomalies are characteristic of exstrophy of the bladder; thus, this condition is the result of a defect in normal embryogenesis that must have taken place at this early stage.

Concurrent with the normal events just described, the cloaca is divided into hindgut and bladder by the formation of a crescent-shaped partition, the urorectal septum (Fig. 42–1). In

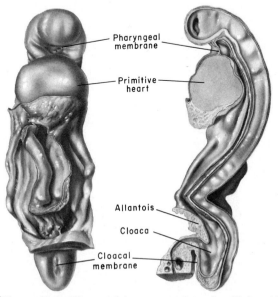

Figure 42–2. Wax model reconstruction of a 30-day-old embryo, Carnegie Collection No. 2053 (Davis, 1923). External (frontal) view on left and midsagittal view on right. The prominent cloacal membrane occupies the central portion of the infraumbilical wall flanked by ridges of mesoderm.

NORMAL

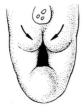
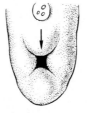
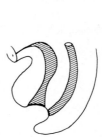

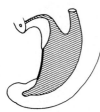
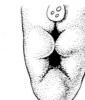

A   4 mm   8 mm   16 mm

EXSTROPHY

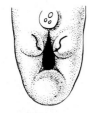
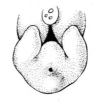
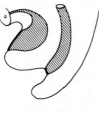

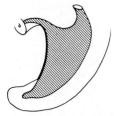

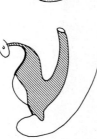

B 4 mm   8 mm   16 mm

Figure 42–3. Schematic view of regression of cloacal membrane and formation of the primitive phallus. *A,* Normal sequential events. *B,* Genesis of the exstrophy group of anomalies by a persistent cloacal membrane impeding mesodermal flow. The paired genital folds fuse inferiorly, carrying the thin cloacal membrane along the anterior surface of the enlarging phallus. A weak, membranous anterior body wall persists, leading to the eventual catastrophic event of exstrophy.

the 6-mm embryo this septum has reached the level of the openings of the wolffian ducts, and in the 12-mm embryo the communication between hindgut and bladder has been restricted to a small connecting passage, the cloacal duct of Reichel. If development is temporarily inhibited at this stage, this cloacal duct may persist; if so, it is recognized as the urethrorectal "fistula" in the newborn male with imperforate anus.

In the 12-mm embryo the urogenital sinus now has a proximal or pelvic component and a distal or phallic portion; on cross section the former is a flattened tube with many folds in its epithelial lining, whereas the latter is trumpet-shaped. Finally, in the 16-mm embryo the urorectal septum meets the cloacal membrane and thereby divides it into the urogenital membrane anteriorly and the anal membrane posteriorly. At about the same time the urogenital membrane dehisces and establishes the urogenital orifice. In the contact of urorectal septum and cloacal membrane, the primitive perineum is formed, and the distal urinary tract is forever separated from the intestinal tract (Fig. 42–1)

The allantoic duct, which originally communicated with the bladder apex (Fig. 42–1) begins to show obliterative changes in its distal lumen in the 10-mm embryo and becomes completely fused in the 16-mm and older embryo. At this stage, the dome of the bladder reaches to the umbilicus; with further growth of the embryo the bladder retains this attachment, but its upper part narrows more and more as it forms the urachus. Thus, the urachus is principally derived from the bladder, and the allantoic duct contributes only to its most proximal or umbilical portion (Chwalla, 1927).

THE EXSTROPHY-EPISPADIAS GROUP OF ANOMALIES

Introduction

Even among deformities in general, exstrophy of the bladder and its variants are exotic conditions. They not only involve the genitourinary tract but also routinely affect the musculoskeletal structures of the lower abdomen and anterior pelvis. In some cases, the lower gastrointestinal tract is also involved, thus presenting a complex anatomic derangement that includes the urinary, genital, musculoskeletal, and intestinal systems. Furthermore, bladder exstrophy rarely if ever appears in animals; when found, it has been recorded as a rare monstros-

ity. It also seems to be unusual when it occurs in a family, for only rarely have two siblings born to the same parents presented with this congenital defect. Although most persons with this anomaly do not reproduce, at least 33 children have been born to 26 mothers with exstrophy, and none had the deformity (Marshall and Muecke, 1962). An anomaly so rare can hardly fail to excite curiosity.

Historical Survey

Reference has been made in the literature to an Assyrian clay tablet of about 2000 B.C. that is believed to describe ectopia vesicae. In more recent times, this condition was first recorded in the English literature in 1735 (Spence et al., 1975). The first truly detailed and exact clinical and anatomic descriptions were given by Mowat in "Medical Essays and Observations," published by the Edinburgh Society in 1747. The typical musculoskeletal separation of the anterior pelvic girdle, the complete epispadias that accompanies exstrophy of the bladder, and the frequently occurring inguinal hernias were well illustrated by Mowat (Fig. 42–4). Perhaps the most famous patient with this anomaly was Matthew Ussem, who exhibited himself more than a century ago in many European medical centers. The first rational treatment appeared near the end of the eighteenth century in the form of a silver bowl fitted to keep the victim dry (Spence et al., 1975). Most patients with untreated exstrophy have lived pitiable, wretched lives and have died young, although at least two have lived for 80 years (Marshall and Muecke, 1962). As a final note of despair, cancer of the exstrophied bladder is no rarity in the hardy few who do survive several decades (Goyanna et al., 1951).

Pathology

Many theories about the faulty embryogenesis have been proposed, but only the wedge effect of an abnormally large or persisting cloacal membrane in the early embryo can readily explain the great variations seen in the exstrophy anomaly. Such a structure would weaken the infraumbilical portion of the anterior abdominal wall; as a wedge it would tend to keep the rectus muscles divergent yet intrinsically normal; the corpora of the penis or clitoris would have an abnormal direction with a definite tendency to be separate; the urethra in the

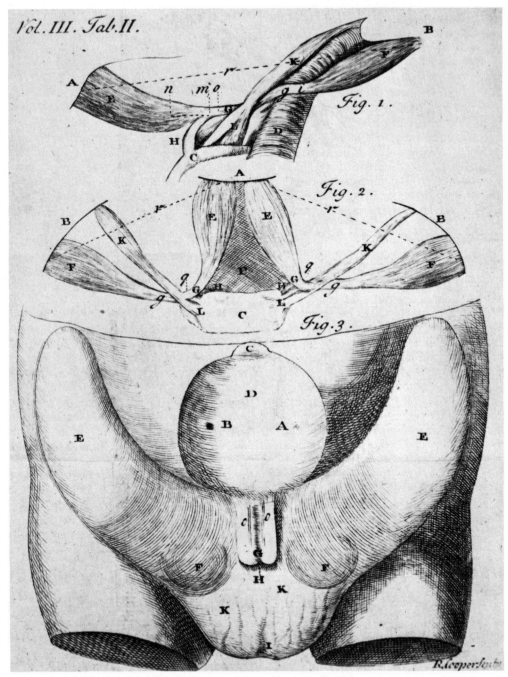

Figure 42–4. Mowat's illustration of exstrophy (1747). Inguinal hernias are dramatized as well as incomplete testicular descent. Note dissection of anterior abdominal wall (compare with Figure 42–2).

male would be located anteriorly rather than posteriorly as in the normal penis. Recognition of an overdeveloped but still unopened cloacal membrane in an early embryo would no doubt be extremely difficult, yet Pohlman in 1911 thought that he had seen this and commented that this embryonic defect could have " . . . a decided bearing on bladder exstrophy and epispadias." Experimental studies in chick embryos (Muecke, 1964) have further supported the concept of a wedgelike effect of a persistent cloacal membrane as theorized by anatomists for almost a century.

The result of a persistent cloacal membrane in the early embryo would be a membranous center in the infraumbilical abdominal wall that would divert mesodermal flow to either side as well as caudal to this structure: Thus, the paired genital tubercles would have to fuse inferiorly, and the pelvis would be widened by this anterior membranous wedge (Fig. 42–3B). This might allow the paired müllerian ducts to remain partially separated, resulting in a bicornuate uterus; in cases of cloacal exstrophy, the paired posterior cardinal veins might survive as a double vena cava (Muecke, 1972). As this membranous

wall eventually dehisces, structures lying immediately behind it will be turned inside out and lie on the surface of the lower anterior abdominal wall. If this dehiscence occurs after the urorectal septum has partitioned the cloaca, classic exstrophy will result (Fig. 42–5); if the rupture occurs earlier, the cloaca itself will protrude (Fig. 42–6), with the still undeveloped hindgut separating the two bladder halves. Should the persistence of the cloacal membrane be only partial and inferior, epispadias will result; if it is superior only, a superior vesical fissure will be the result. These variations in exstrophy are discussed and illustrated later in this chapter.

Classic Exstrophy of the Bladder

GENERAL

Exstrophy of the bladder is the most frequently encountered malformation in this group of anomalies. Uson and coworkers (1958) reported 66 cases of classic exstrophy in their collective series of 72 patients with forms of exstrophy. Of the 158 cases of exstrophy re-

Figure 42–5. Diagram of events leading to classic exstrophy.

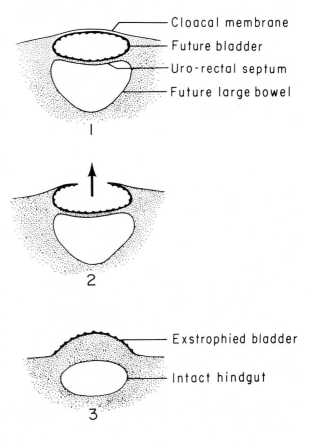

- Cloacal membrane
- Future bladder
- Uro-rectal septum
- Future large bowel

1

2

- Exstrophied bladder
- Intact hindgut

3

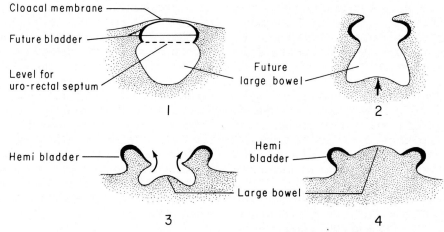

Figure 42–6. Diagram of eventration of cloaca to form cloacal exstrophy.

ported by Higgins (1962), all but 5 were of classic form. Of 52 cases of various forms of exstrophy, reported in 1962 in our series from The New York Hospital, 44 were of the classic variety (Table 42–1).

Exstrophy of the bladder occurs more commonly in males than in females. It is not as rare an anomaly as it was once thought to be, for it has been estimated that more than 100 children with exstrophy are born each year in the United States.

DESCRIPTIVE FEATURES

In the male infant, the bladder lies everted on the lower abdominal wall with the moist mucosal surface exposed (Fig. 42–7). The epispadiac urethra is delineated by the pink smooth epithelium covering the anterior surface of a

TABLE 42–1. VARIATIONS OF EXSTROPHY ANOMALIES REPORTED FROM THE NEW YORK HOSPITAL

Variety	No. Cases
Spade penis only	1
Epispadias with continence	
Balanic	2
Penile	6
Epispadias with incontinence	
Subsymphyseal	1
Penopubic	17
Classic exstrophy	44
Cloacal exstrophy	4
Superior vesical fissure	1
Duplicate exstrophy	1
"Pseudoexstrophy"	2
	79

From Marshall, V. F., and Muecke, E. C.: J. Urol., *88*:766, 1962.

stubby penis that ends in a cleft glans. The ureteral orifices are easily recognized on two mucosal hillocks from which urine flows. The pubic bones are separated, and on palpation a fibrous structure is usually felt just beneath the exposed bladder neck; this is the so-called symphyseal band. The umbilicus is low-set and elongated. A thin, almost triangular sheet of fibrous tissue covered by skin lies in the space between the two divergent rectus muscles; it may bulge outward as a paraumbilical hernia. Bilateral inguinal hernias are frequently present at birth or are recognized shortly thereafter. The testes may not be fully descended. The penis points upward; it is short and stubby, and the glans has a characteristic flattened appearance. The prepuce lies posterior; the midline raphe on the undersurface of the penis is normal, as is the scrotal sac. The shortness of the penis most likely is related to the widened anterior pelvic girdle and to the outward rotation of the puboischial rings. Indeed, the size of the penis seems to reflect the severity of the malformation: In milder cases of epispadias, the penis may be normal or near normal in size, but as the degree of exstrophy worsens, the penis becomes shorter and stubbier until it becomes totally separated and is recognizable only as paired "swell bodies" in the extreme manifestation of this anomaly, cloacal exstrophy. We have measured total penile lengths in our cases of the classic form of male exstrophy (crural attachment plus pendular length) and have not been convinced that such penes are particularly deficient in their entirety. Yet, one cannot deny embryologic observations that the mesodermal build-up that gives rise to the genital tubercles (phallus) must be delayed in those embryos

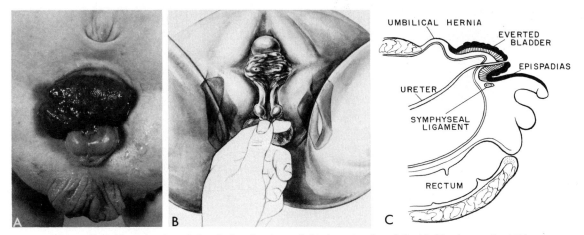

Figure 42–7. Photograph and descriptive drawings of classic exstrophy of the bladder in a male child.

destined to have exstrophy and, therefore, should be deficient in total mass. Thus, the final product may fall short of the expected.

In the female child, the everted bladder occupies the same area as it does in the male with similar associated anomalies of the umbilicus and divergent rectus muscles of the lower anterior abdomen (Fig. 42–8). The labia are separated anteriorly, and the clitoris is bifid. The epispadiac urethra may be difficult to recognize in the usually somewhat edematous and polypoid exstrophic bladder mucosa. The vaginal opening is tilted slightly upward or may be translocated anteriorly; in about two thirds of

female patients with exstrophy the vaginal orifice may be stenotic. Absent or septate vaginas have been reported. The uterus may be bicornuate, or, in more severely afflicted patients, it may be actually duplicated with two cervices (Fig. 42–9)–an example of failure of fusion of the müllerian ducts.

All cases of exstrophy have the characteristic widening of the symphysis pubis (Muecke and Currarino, 1968) caused by the outward rotation of the innominate bones, in relation to the sagittal plane of the body, along both sacroiliac joints. In addition, there is an outward rotation or eversion of the pubic rami at their

Figure 42–8. Female child with exstrophy of the bladder. A patulous anus was also present.

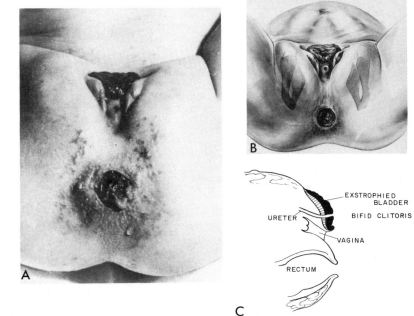

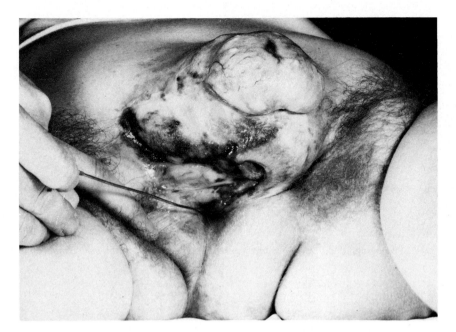

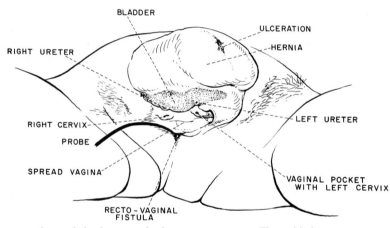

Figure 42–9. An extreme form of classic exstrophy in a young woman. The pubic bones were separated by 17 cm; two cervices and uteri were present, and the vagina communicated with the rectum (marked by probe).

junction with the ischial and iliac bones. A third component is present in more severe cases of exstrophy, namely, a lateral separation of the innominate bones inferiorly, with the fulcrum at the iliosacral joint (Fig. 42–10A-C). It is these rotational deformities of the pelvic skeletal structures that may contribute to a short pendular penis; thus, simple closure of the anterior pelvic girdle by bilateral iliac osteotomies would increase the degree of outward rotation of the puboischial ring, resulting probably in a further shortening of an already stubby penis as its crural attachments separate even more. The outward rotation and lateral displacement of the

innominate bones also account for the increased distance between the hips, the waddling gait, and the outward rotation of lower limbs of these children.

The upper urinary tracts are normal in the neonate. With increase of time and consequent metaplasia of the exposed vesical mucosa, obstructive changes will make their appearance in the older child with uncorrected bladder exstrophy (Fig. 42–11). Maloney et al. (1965) reported that 17 out of 50 patients with exstrophy had bilateral hydronephrosis and hydroureters when first seen; in each case the obstruction appeared to be in the vicinity of the distal

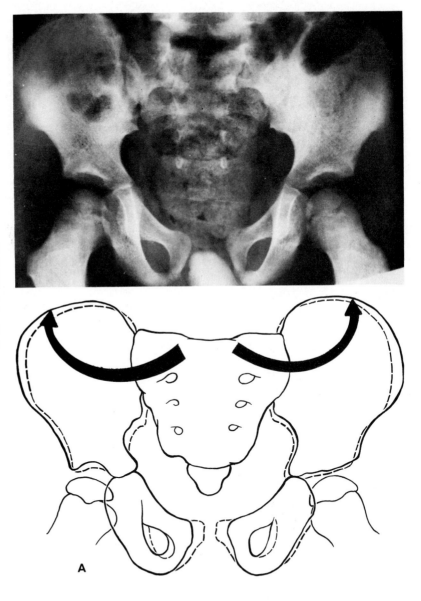

Figure 42–10. Rotational and lateral deformities of the pelvic girdle in cases of exstrophy. *A,* (1) Widening of the symphysis caused by outward rotation of the innominate bones, usually the only skeletal abnormality present in epispadias.

Illustration and legend continued on following page

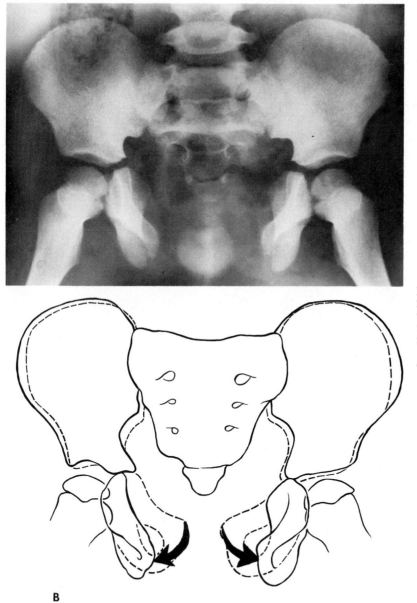

B

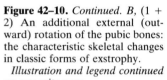

Figure 42–10. *Continued. B,* (1 + 2) An additional external (outward) rotation of the pubic bones: the characteristic skeletal changes in classic forms of exstrophy.

Illustration and legend continued on opposite page

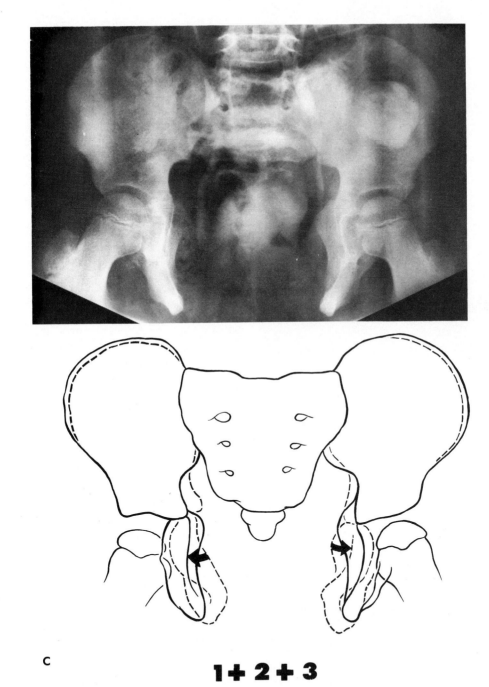

1+ 2+ 3

Figure 42–10. *Continued.* C, (1 + 2 + 3) The final addition of lateral inferior separation of the innominate bones present in the extreme manifestation of the complex, namely, cloacal exstrophy.

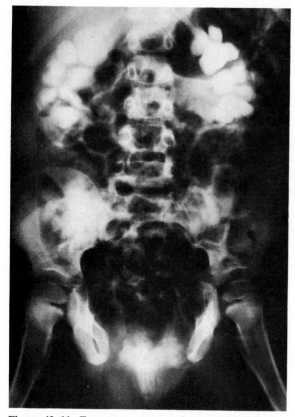

Figure 42–11. Excretory urogram of an untreated 3-year-old boy born with classic form of exstrophy. Points of obstruction were the ureterovesical junctions caused by fibrosis and polypoid metaplasia of the exposed ureteral orifices.

ureters and was caused by fibrosis and metaplasia of the mucosa of the untreated exstrophied bladder.

Although the formation of the anal canal is not directly affected in the malformation leading to the classic presentation of exstrophy of the bladder, the widened pelvic floor does affect endopelvic fascial support of the distal rectum. Thus, a patulous anus (Fig. 42–8) or actual prolapse of the rectum may occur, and this may thereby narrow the choice of surgical management of such an infant (for example, ureterosigmoidostomies as a form of primary urinary diversion would be ill advised). The abnormal bony pelvis, in which there is increased separation of the acetabular fossas, causes the child to walk with a broad-based waddling gait that is self-corrective, for in the older child, the pelvic separation appears to cause little if any handicap to locomotion, and special orthopedic treatment is not required.

Cloacal Exstrophy (Vesicointestinal Fissure)

GENERAL FEATURES

Cloacal exstrophy is a rare and curious anomaly that involves not only the genitourinary system but also the intestinal tract. The first complete description of this anomaly was that of Bartels in 1868. Almost a century later Soper and Kilger (1964) were able to collect 53 cases from the German and English literature and added 5 cases of their own. Although cloacal exstrophy is a more apt term for this complex anomaly, the term "vesicointestinal fissure" (Schwalbe, 1909) is commonly used throughout the literature.

The incidence of this disorder is estimated to be approximately 1 in 200,000 live births. There seems to be no sex preponderance. Many of the afflicted infants are born prematurely, as were our two patients at The New York Hospital.

The causative factor of this anomaly, as in all exstrophy-type abnormalities, is the cloacal membrane–specifically, its large size and early dehiscence. The defect occurs as the abnormally large membrane gives way before the urorectal septum has partitioned the cloacal pouch; thus, the cloaca itself exstrophies. If, as mentioned earlier, the anterior walls of the cloaca are destined to form the bladder and posterior wall, or hindgut (i.e., the colon), then eventration would result in this piece of hindgut lying in the center flanked by a remnant of anterior wall (i.e., bladder) (Fig. 42–6). Hence, bowel mucosa would be present in the middle of the exstrophied tissue with a hemibladder on either side. Because the urorectal septum may have had some slight but significant beginning at the time of the catastrophic dissolution of the cloacal membrane, in the resulting cloacal exstrophy bladder elements would be joined in a somewhat horseshoe shape in its upper portion. As early as 1913 Johnston wrote that if some observer could demonstrate vesical mucosa between the bowel and the umbilicus in any case of cloacal exstrophy, " . . . the case for an abnormally early and excessive rupture of the cloacal membrane will be established beyond doubt." Von Geldern (1924) made this demonstration 10 years later (Fig. 42–12).

EXPERIMENTAL DATA

The wedge effect of a large cloacal membrane in the early embryo was given experimental support by Muecke in 1964. In the early

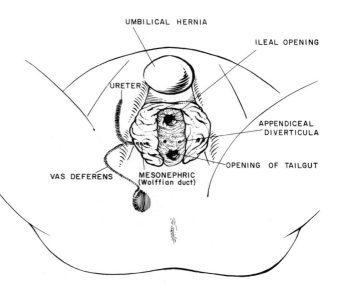

Figure 42–12. Diagram of cloacal exstrophy as described by Von Geldern in 1924. Exstrophied bladder mucosa forms a horseshoe configuration cradling the central intestinal tissue that receives the ileum superiorly and a blind intestinal tube (the tailgut) inferiorly. Ureters terminated in each ipsilateral bladder half. Colon, rectum, and anus are absent.

embryonic stage in the chick the cloacal membrane anlage was surgically altered and made into a nonregressive entity by the insertion of a small bit of plastic material into this region. Theoretically, this small foreign body could be expected to act like a mechanical barrier to mesodermal flow, initiating an abdominal defect and the consequent formation of cloacal exstrophy. Figure 42–13 shows the experimental model of cloacal exstrophy in which the anatomic features are strikingly similar to those seen in the human neonate born with this anomaly.

One interesting comment was made by Muecke (1964) in his experimental studies. In mammals other than man, exstrophy of the bladder has almost never been observed. A plausible explanation for this variation in incidence according to species may be that struc-

tures adjacent to the cloacal membrane, particularly the allantois, are of varying importance to embryonic survival. In domestic animals such as the pig, horse, cow, dog, and sheep, the allantoic vesicle is of vital importance in uterine implantation of the zygote (Mossman, 1937). Thus, an early defect in the allantoic region would make implantation impossible and abortion inevitable. In man, on the other hand, the allantoic has a vestigial role in placentation; thus, abnormalities in the neighboring cloaca might be better tolerated, and a significant number of exstrophied bladders could be expected in any large statistical compilation of live human births.

DESCRIPTIVE FEATURES

The characteristic anatomic features of this congenital abnormality are the presence of two hemibladders, each with its own ureter, separated by an area of intestine (Fig. 42–14). The exposed intestinal structure has a surface of mucosa that is histologically compatible with that of colon; this mucosal surface is readily distinguishable from its neighboring bladder epithelium by its deeper purple hue. This exstrophied intestine most likely represents cecum, as it receives the distal ileum superiorly. Although the midgut development should have been normal, we observed in our surviving patient with cloacal exstrophy that the distal ileum was shorter than normal and its absorptive mucosa was deficient. An attached remnant of tailgut extends as a blind intestinal tube from an opening near the midline toward the posterior or caudal part of the exstrophied colocecum. A

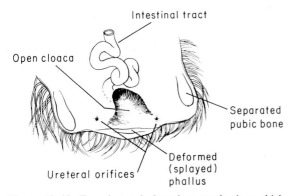

Figure 42–13. Experimental cloacal exstrophy in a chick. The pubic bones are widely separated, and the cloaca lies open to the surface of the abdomen flanked by a hemiurodeum on either side receiving its ipsilateral ureter.

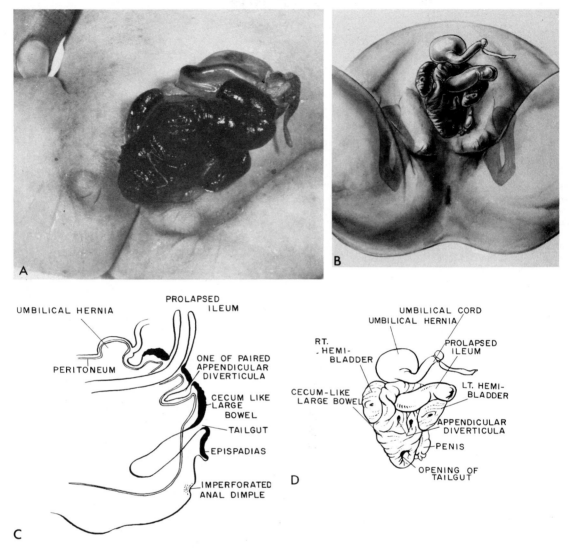

Figure 42–14. *A–D,* Cloacal exstrophy in the newborn. Diagrams emphasize characteristic anatomic features: two hemibladders with their ureteral orifices; cecum-like exstrophied intestine receiving the terminal ileum superiorly and the tailgut inferiorly; paired appendiceal diverticula; two hemipenises or corpora cavernosa.

pair of bowel sacs near the upper or cephalic portion of the exstrophied intestine is frequently found and is thought to be appendiceal diverticula. The appendix-like diverticula have varied greatly in character in reported cases and have been missing in a few, but their tendency to be paired and their large-bowel structure are real. The ureter and wolffian duct normally become completely separated before the embryo is 6 weeks old (see Chapter 37). If eventration occurred well before that event, then ureter and vas may infrequently be found joined in a common, persistent mesonephric duct (Fig. 42–12). Epispadias invariably is present if the penis is intact; however, far more commonly the two

corpora are widely separated, frequently presenting only as two "swell bodies" composed of vascular erectile tissue attached to the widely separated pubic bones. In the series of cloacal exstrophy collected by Soper and Kilger (1964), in 29 infants determined to be male, the penis was absent in 8 and the scrotum in 19. Fifteen of the infants had diphallus, and eight had a bifid scrotum. Of the 24 female neonates reviewed, the clitoris was absent in 14 and bifid in 7. The vagina was absent in 6 and duplicated in 14. Thirty-eight infants had skeletal defects other than the characteristic pelvic deformities, with spina bifida being the most common.

Another interesting feature of cloacal ex-

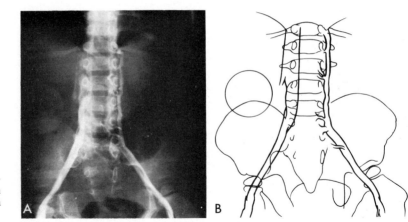

Figure 42–15. Inferior vena cavagram of a year-old child born with cloacal exstrophy. A double vena cava is present.

strophy is the high probability of the occurrence of a double vena cava. The development of a right-sided vena cava appears to be the end result of "tight quarters" in the embryonic pelvis. As the kidneys develop and enlarge, the posterior cardinal veins are compressed laterally and obliterated, and the return flow of blood from the limb buds is channeled through the supracardinal network. Our investigation, based on autopsy material and inferior venograms, has confirmed this surprisingly high incidence of a paired abdominal vena cava (Fig. 42–15) in children born with cloacal exstrophy. The widening of the pelvic girdle by the eventration of

the bladder and hindgut anlagen allowed enough room for persistence of the primitive paired posterior cardinal veins as the metanephroi expanded (Muecke, 1972).

VARIANTS

Since the entire exstrophy group of anomalies represents a spectrum, it is not surprising that transitions between bladder exstrophy and cloacal exstrophy have been reported. The best descriptive series is by Johnston and Penn (1966), and a photograph of one of their cases is shown here (Fig. 42–16). Here the eventration of pelvic structures occurred before the urorec-

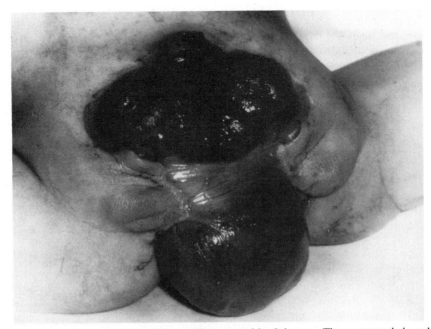

Figure 42–16. Photograph of incomplete cloacal exstrophy reported by Johnston. The eventrated cloacal duct of Reichel bridges the exstrophied bladder to the exstrophied (prolapsed) colon.

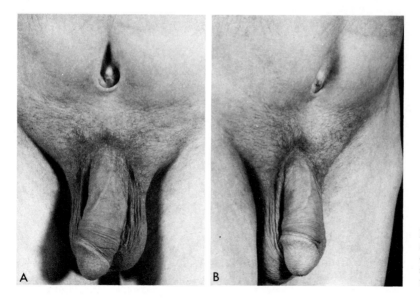

Figure 42–17. Pseudoexstrophy in an adult male patient. Musculoskeletal deformity characteristic of exstrophy is present, but the urinary tract is intact.

tal septum had reached the cloacal membrane (Fig. 42–1). The communicating cloacal duct of Reichel lies exposed, bridging the bladder exstrophy and prolapsed colon. Again, the phallus did not form as such; remnants of erectile tissue are attached to the pubic rami.

Variants of Bladder Exstrophy

PSEUDOEXSTROPHY

The presence of characteristic musculoskeletal defects of the exstrophy anomaly with no major defect in the urinary tract has been reported and named "pseudoexstrophy" (Marshall and Muecke, 1968). About eight cases have been described in the literature; we have seen two such cases. The 58-year-old man shown in the photograph (Fig. 42–17) had transitional cell carcinoma of the bladder, but the urinary tract, which was thoroughly investigated, was otherwise normal. The umbilicus was elongated and low-set; the rectus muscles diverged from just above the umbilicus to attach on the separated pubic bones. When the bladder was full, it would bulge outward between the separated abdominal musculature, mimicking a ventral abdominal hernia. In this rare anomaly, the cloacal membrane persists as a triangular-shaped linea alba. The mesodermal migration had been dammed in its superior aspect only, and perhaps the caudal flow from the umbilical stalk alone was impeded, thus wedging apart the musculoskeletal elements of the lower abdominal wall without displacing the formation of the genital tubercle. All developmental events caudal to this most superior aspect of the cloacal membrane probably continued on sched-

ule; with the opening of the urogenital sinus, pressure within the developing pelvis would be relieved, and the almost membranous abdominal wall could remain intact.

SUPERIOR VESICAL FISSURE

In this group of rare exstrophic manifestations, the musculoskeletal defects characteristic of the whole group are present but the bladder eventration is minimal and is present only below the abnormal umbilicus (Fig. 42–18). This child was seen at The New York Hospital because of a "ruptured bladder." She had indeed an opening into the bladder just below the umbilical bulge that would allow part of the bladder to prolapse; the clitoris was normal, and the patient was continent. Closure of the vesical opening with excision of the exstrophied portion was all that was necessary. The child has no reflux, well-formed upper urinary tracts, and no persistent infection. Uson and Roberts (1958) presented two cases in their series of "pseudoexstrophy" in which the patients had slight urinary leakage from openings just below the umbilicus. Superior vesical fissure is not merely an example of patent urachus, for the musculoskeletal abnormalities of exstrophy are present in the former and never in the latter.

DUPLICATE EXSTROPHY

If a superior vesical fissure should occur and then fuse, bladder elements might remain on the outside. Such an occurrence is even more rare than superior vesical fissure. About six cases have been reported in the literature. Our case seems to be typical of duplicate exstrophy (Fig. 42–19). This boy was referred to us by his pediatrician, who was certain that the youngster

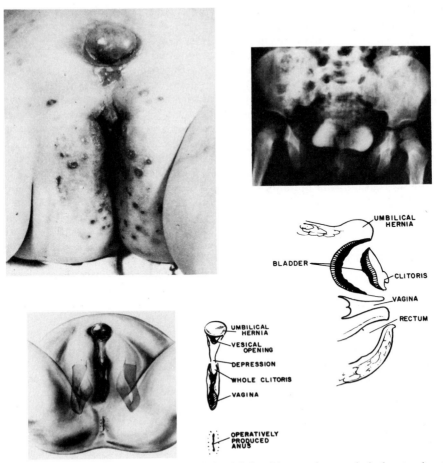

Figure 42–18. Superior vesical fissure in a girl. Musculoskeletal deformities are those typical of exstrophy of the bladder.

Figure 42–19. Duplicate exstrophy in a boy with an intact urinary tract.

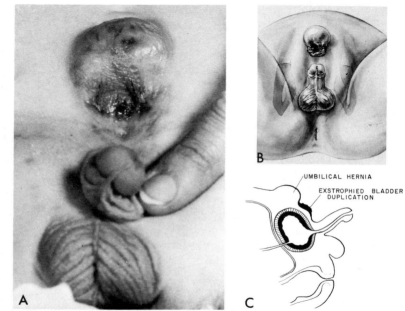

had exstrophy even though he also exhibited normal urinary control. Anatomically, the patient had the characteristic widened symphysis pubis and a somewhat stubby upward-pointing penis. A rudimentary patch of exstrophic bladder mucosa lay immediately below the umbilical bulges; the bladder, trigone, and urethra were normal. A possible transitional case between this one and the one described previously as superior vesical fissure is the case reported by Kittredge and Bradburn (1954). In their patient, a tiny fistula connected the external vesical exstrophy with a normal internal bladder.

Epispadias

GENERAL FEATURES

The epispadiac group of anomalies reflect to a lesser degree abnormal embryogenesis of the entire spectrum of the exstrophy complex. It is easy to speculate that, in this group of lesser exstrophies of the distal urinary tract, the cloacal membrane was successfully reinforced superiorly with mesoderm but persisted as a membrane inferiorly, forming the roof of the somewhat caudally displaced genital tubercle. The urethral groove thus comes to lie on the anterior surface of the developing phallus. The degree of persistence of the cloacal membrane will determine the severity of the epispadiac defect.

The incidence of this anomaly, unlike that of exstrophy, is quite rare: It is the least expressive form of the exstrophy complex. In a collective summary of over 5 million hospital admissions in the United States, Dees (1949) reported only 56 cases, or a statistical incidence of 1 in 100,000 hospital admissions. The sex ratio of incidence favors males 5 to 1. The degree of musculoskeletal derangement, which consists mainly of a widened symphysis, seems to coincide in general with the degree of the urinary defect. Of all patients seen at The New York Hospital with this anomaly (27 patients), roentgenograms showed that the width of the symphysis was increased in 12 and normal in 7; in 8 patients the symphysis pubis had not been measured or commented upon in the hospital records. One may conclude, lacking contrary evidence, that in isolated epispadias the musculoskeletal deformity is less marked than the exstrophy, and indeed is not present in the mildest degree of the anomaly.

DESCRIPTIVE FEATURES

In the male, there are three forms of epispadias–balanic or glandular, penile, and penopubic. The penopubic form, together with the only recognized female form, subsymphyseal epispadias, is always accompanied by urinary incontinence.

Balanic or Glandular Epispadias. Balanic or glandular epispadias is the rarest form as well as the one with the mildest degree of urinary defect (Fig. 42–20). The defect extends anteriorly from the meatus to the corona of the glans penis. The glans is somewhat flattened (spade-shaped) and the penis may show some degree of upward curvature. In The New York Hospital series (Table 42–1) two such cases were recorded. We have observed an even milder case of this defect in a boy with a flattened "spade penis" in whom the most distal urethra was covered by a thin, membrane-like epithelium but the actual meatus was in the tip of the penis. The penis was short and stubby and protruded at right angles to the frontal body plane even in the flaccid condition. A photographic record is not available.

Penile Epispadias. The penile form of epispadias is the next step in the progression toward exstrophy. Here, the urethral meatus terminates somewhere along the anterior shaft of the penis. The penis is short, flattened, and curved anteriorly. Most commonly the urethral opening is near the penopubic angle, and the distal urethra is represented by an open, epithelium-lined groove in the anterior penis (Fig. 42–21). The prepuce may be fully formed, or the penis may have a "tent" shape because of the high ventral insertion of the scrotum and a

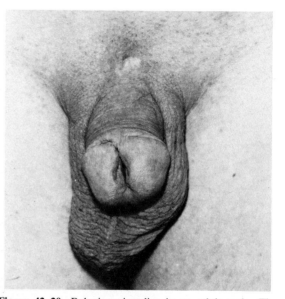

Figure 42–20. Balanic epispadias in an adult male. The ureteral defect, an anterior cleft, extends only to the corona of the glans penis.

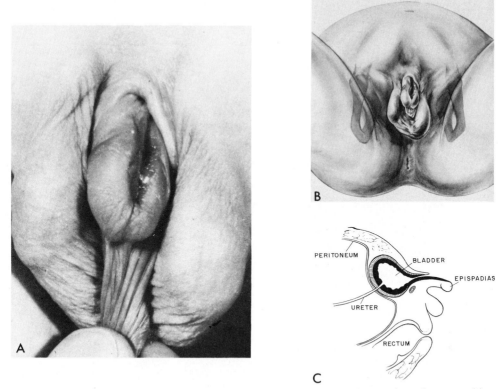

Figure 42–21. Penile epispadias with urinary continence. The open urethral groove extends to the penopubic angle. The sphincter mechanism and proximal urethra are intact.

relative redundancy of penile skin. These boys are continent. The musculoskeletal defect of a widened symphysis was present in one half of our group of six such youngsters.

Penopubic Epispadias (Subsymphyseal Epispadias in the Female). In the male with penopubic epispadias, incontinence is the rule rather than the exception, and a widened anterior pelvis is almost always present (Figs. 42–22 and 42–23). It is the most common form of epispadias in the absence of vesical exstrophy: It represents 17 of our 27 cases of epispadias and 11 of 18 in the series reported by Gross and Cresson (1952), and is the most common form in Dees' collection (1949). In some of these cases, the urethral cleft was so extensive that prolapse of the bladder occurred. Sometimes these cases have been referred to in the literature as "inferior vesical fissure," but they are really only transitions to the more common exstrophy of the bladder.

The clinical features of this most severe type of epispadias anomaly are dramatized in the drawings in Figures 42–22 and 42–23. The anterior urethral cleft extends through the sphincteral mechanism, thereby rendering the patient incontinent. As the shortened, upwardly directed stubby penis is pulled downward, a puddle of urine will flow out, and the open proximal (prostatic) urethra with its exposed verumontanum may be visualized. The urinary opening in the lower abdomen is often large enough to allow portions of the anterior bladder wall to prolapse. The typical musculoskeletal defect of exstrophy is almost always present. The bladder may appear hypoplastic but is otherwise normal. Reflux is not an uncommon finding on cystography.

Complete epispadias also occurs in the female child and is known as subsymphyseal epispadias (Muecke and Marshall, 1968). In these afflicted youngsters the urethra tends to be short and patulous. The labia are not fused anteriorly, and the clitoris is therefore bifid. The mons is flattened, and often its midportion appears to be covered by smooth pink epithelium rather than skin. The symphysis pubis is widened, and the rectus muscles are divergent. This is a rare manifestation of this group of anomalies (Fig. 42–23).

Summary

There is a close relationship among all forms of the exstrophy-epispadias complex, for

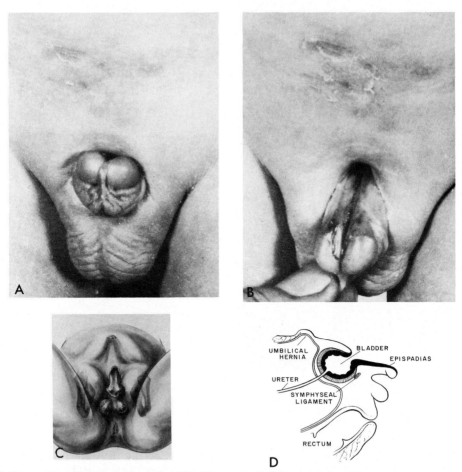

Figure 42–22. Penopubic epispadias in the male child. The urethral cleft extends into the anterior bladder outlet and the verumontanum can be easily visualized as the penis is pulled down. These boys are incontinent.

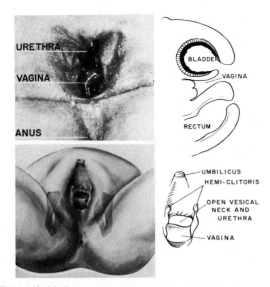

Figure 42–23. Subsymphyseal epispadias in the female child. The clitoris is separated and the anterior labia not fused in the midline. A gaping short urethra leads into the vesical outlet. These youngsters lack urinary control.

the fault in its embryogenesis is common to all; therefore, all clinical manifestations are merely variations on a theme. Figure 42–24 attempts to show this relationship to the classic and most common form of exstrophy. The relative frequency of each form has been suggested by the size of the arrows.

OTHER BLADDER ANOMALIES

Agenesis and Congenital Atresia of the Bladder

Complete absence of a urinary bladder is very rare and is of more interest to students of pathology than to clinicians. When the ureteral orifices are ectopic (as in Glenn's report of congenital hypoplasia of the bladder [1959]), the patient may survive the surgical correction, or urinary diversion may be successfully performed. Marshall and Muecke (1968) collected

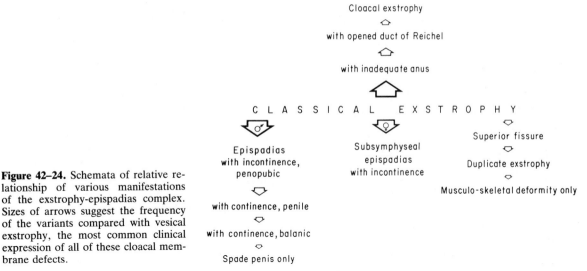

Cloacal exstrophy

⇧

with opened duct of Reichel

⇧

with inadequate anus

⇧

C L A S S I C A L   E X S T R O P H Y

⇩   ⇩   ⇨

Epispadias   Subsymphyseal   Superior fissure
with incontinence,   epispadias
penopubic   with incontinence   ⇨

⇩   Duplicate exstrophy

with continence, penile   ⇨

⇩   Musculo-skeletal deformity only

with continence, balanic

⇨

Spade penis only

Figure 42–24. Schemata of relative relationship of various manifestations of the exstrophy-epispadias complex. Sizes of arrows suggest the frequency of the variants compared with vesical exstrophy, the most common clinical expression of all of these cloacal membrane defects.

25 cases from the world literature in a review of bladder anomalies. It is difficult to arrive at any conclusive figures of incidence, although Campbell (1963) recorded 7 cases among 19,046 autopsies.

Agenesis of the urinary bladder means that the cloaca persists, and thus the urorectal septum fails to fulfill its function of partitioning the cloaca into an anterior bladder and a posterior intestinal tract. Thus a child born with "bladder agenesis" has a persistent cloaca, and the ureters terminate in the rectum. Such a case has been described by Lepoutre (1940). The patient was a 4-month-old boy; his ureters entered the anterior rectal wall, and an excretory urogram was almost normal. Since müllerian duct development is normally unimpeded, the ureters also could conceivably terminate in its end-products, that is, the vagina and uterus. Such cases have been reported by Miller (1948) and Ignatescu et al. (1938). In each case the bladder and urethra remained undeveloped. Finally, an embryonic bladder might persist as a small diverticulum, as described by Glenn (1959) (Fig. 42–25). Here the ureters remained attached to their respective wolffian ducts and terminated in the vaginal introitus—an example of extreme bilateral ureteral ectopia. These last cases are good illustrations of the concept that the embryogenesis of the urinary tract is a dynamic process: organs, tubular structures, sacs, or pouches must not merely be formed but also must function in utero lest they be destined to remain hypoplastic or become atretic.

Duplication of the Bladder

Duplication of the urinary bladder and related anomalies is rare, and only a few cases have been described in the literature. Most of the early cases reported were based on autopsy findings, and many descriptions are vague about the exact nature of the bladder anomaly encountered. As diagnostic roentgenographic and endoscopic methods improved, fewer case reports of bladder septa, multiloculated chambers, and hour-glass deformities have appeared in the urologic literature. Many of the earlier cases undoubtedly represented ureteroceles, dilated

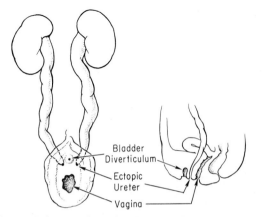

Figure 42–25. Atresia of the bladder with ectopic ureters as reported by Glenn. A small diverticulum persisted in the introitus where the urethra should have been, with both ureters having ectopic openings (probably via Gartner's ducts).

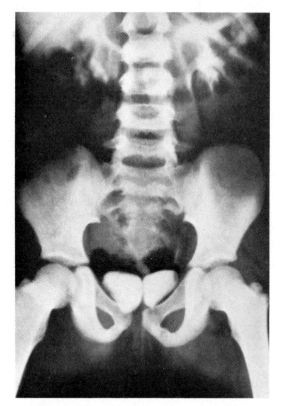

Figure 42–26. Roentgenogram of bladder duplication as reported by Nesbit and Bromme.

If so, why do the skeletal defects in this group of bladder anomalies occur infrequently? In the early German literature concerning the precise origin of the urorectal septum (Keibel, 1896), there are some wax models of early embryos in which this septum arose as lateral and superior folds, which eventually fused to result in a crescent-shaped membrane growing caudad. The occurrence of supernumerary urorectal septa has been proposed by some authors and is supported by Watson's (1920) description of fetal bladders that on cross section showed epithelial folds fused into recognizable septa. Thus it is theoretically possible that a sagittally oriented fold of the primitive urorectal septum could not only halve the embryonic bladder anlage but also quarter the cloaca into the anterior bladders and two hindguts, thus accounting for the complete duplication of the lower intestinal tracts in cases of double bladders. For descriptions of other bladder anomalies, such as partial or multiple bladder septa, hourglass deformities, and other entities, the reader is referred to reviews by Abrahamsom (1961) and Marshall and Muecke (1968).

ABNORMALITIES OF THE URACHUS

The original observation and description of a congenitally patent urachus were made by Bartholomaeus Carbrolius in 1550. The patient was an 18-year-old girl who voided from an umbilical opening as well as through the urethra.

The urachus is formed from the apical portion of the bladder (see earlier under Embryology of the Bladder), and in embryos 10 to 24 mm in size the bladder apex reaches to the umbilicus. As the embryo enlarges, the bladder descends into the pelvis proper, and its apical portion narrows progressively into a fibromuscular strand, the urachus. Even in the adult this fibromuscular strand between the bladder apex and the umbilicus retains a central epithelial canal with frequent cystlike dilatations (Luschka's lacumae). It is this structural formation that allows for variations in urachal abnormalities (Hinman, 1961a, b; Vaughan, 1905) (Fig. 42–27). These variations include (1) congenital patent urachus ("completely patent"): The urachus remains patent or the apex of the bladder fails to narrow into the fibromuscular duct; (2) vesicourachal diverticulum ("blind internal"): The urachus is patent only at its vesical termination; (3) umbilical cyst or sinus ("blind external"): Only the subumbilical portion of the

posterior urethras secondary to valves, and paraureteric diverticula.

The first radiographic diagnosis of true duplication of the bladder and urethra was published by Nesbit and Bromme (1933) (Fig. 42–26). In this anomaly, two bladders are present, each quite distinct and lying side to side; they are separated by a peritoneal fold of varying depth. Each bladder receives a ureter from its ipsilateral kidney, and each bladder empties through a separate urethra. Eighteen cases of this interesting anomaly were reported by Marshall and Muecke (1968). Of these, nine (50 per cent) had duplication of the lower gastrointestinal tract, and of these nine, six had complete duplication from the ileocecal valve caudad! In Ravitch and Scott's review (1953) of 20 cases of hindgut duplication, 12 patients (40 per cent) had a double bladder. Duplication of external genitalia was present in 16 of the 18 cases (90 per cent).

The embryologic defect that results in duplication of the bladder, which is frequently accompanied by hindgut replication, could be partial twinning of the tail portion of the embryo, as suggested by Ravitch and Scott (1953).

Tumors of the urachus are rare; when present, they are as a rule mucus-producing adenocarcinomas. The difference in their histopathology from that of bladder tumors probably reflects the duality of their origin—namely, the allantoic duct and the bladder apex. Surgical treatment of urachal carcinoma is presented elsewhere.

References

Abrahamson, J.: Double bladder and related l anomalies: Clinical and embryological aspects and a case report. Br. J. Urol., *33*:195, 1961.

Bartels, M.: Über die Bauchblasengenitalspalte, einen bestimmten Grad der sogenannten Inversion der Harnblase. Arch. Anat. Physiol., 1868, p. 165.

Campbell, M. F.: Urology. 3rd ed. Philadelphia, W. B. Saunders Co., 1970.

Chwalla, R.: Über die Entwicklung der Harnblase und der primären Harnröhre des Menschen. Z. Anat. Entwickl., *83*:615, 1927.

Connell, F. G.: Exstrophy of the bladder. JAMA, *36*:637, 1901.

Davis, C. L.: Description of a human embryo having twenty paired somites. Contrib. Embryol. Carnegie Institution Wash., *15*:53–54, 1923.

Dees, J. E.: Congenital epispadias with incontinence. J. Urol., *62*:513, 1949.

Duncan, A.: An attempt toward a systematic account of appearances connected with the malformation of the urinary organs. Edinburgh Med. J., *1*:43, 1805.

Glenn, J. F.: Agenesis of the bladder. JAMA, *169*:2016, 1959.

Goyanna, R., Emmett, J. L., and McDonald, J. R.: Exstrophy of the bladder complicated by adenocarcinoma. J. Urol., *65*:391, 1951.

Gross, R. E., and Cresson, S. L.: Treatment of epispadias: A report of 18 cases. J. Urol., *68*:477, 1952.

Higgins, C. C.: Exstrophy of the bladder: Report of 158 cases. Am. Surg., *28*:99, 1962.

Hinman, F.: Urologic aspects of the alternating urachal sinus. Am. J. Surg., *102*:339, 1961*a*.

Hinman, F.: Surgical disorders of the bladder and umbilicus of urachal origin. Surg. Gynecol. Obstet., *113*:605, 1961*b*.

Ignatescu, M., Slobozianu, H., and Athanasiu-Vergu, E.: Absence de la vessie et abouchement des ureteres dans l'uterus chez deux jumelles. J. Urol. Med. Chir., *45*:51, 1938.

Johnston, J. H., and Penn, I. A.: Exstrophy of the cloaca. Br. J. Urol., *38*:302, 1966.

Johnston, T. B.: Extroversion of the bladder, complicated by the presence of intestinal openings on the surface of the extroverted area. J. Anat. Physiol., *48*:89, 1913.

Keibel, F.: Zur Entwicklungsgeschichte des menschlichen Urogenitalapparates. Arch. Anat. Physiol., 55–157, 1896.

Kittredge, W. E., and Bradburn, C.: Incomplete exstrophy of the bladder: Case report. J. Urol., *72*:38, 1954.

Lepoutre, C.: Sur un cas d'absence congenitale de la vessie (persistance du cloague). J. Urol. Med. Chir., *48*:334, 1940.

Maloney, P. K., Gleason, D. M., and Lattimer, J. K.: Ureteral physiology and exstrophy of the bladder. J. Urol., *93*:588, 1965.

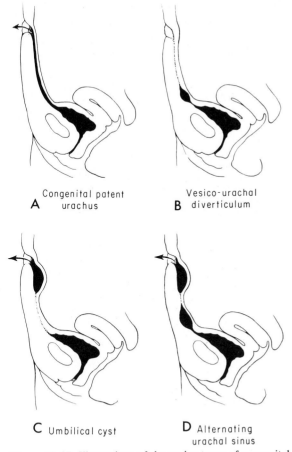

A Congenital patent urachus

B Vesico-urachal diverticulum

C Umbilical cyst

D Alternating urachal sinus

Figure 42–27. Illustrations of the major types of congenital urachal abnormalities.

urachus remains patent; and (4) alternating urachal sinus: Both ends of the urachus are patent, and infection may enter from without.

The symptomatology of urachal abnormalities varies according to the patency of the urachal lumen. In patients with a congenitally patent urachus, distal obstructive uropathy seems to be commonly and causally associated and must be treated prior to any surgical closure of the patent urachal duct. Vesicourachal diverticula are usually asymptomatic unless calculus formation occurs in the diverticula. Umbilical cysts and external urachal sinuses present as inflammations of the umbilicus in the adult. When such a cyst ruptures, it usually drains through the umbilicus and may thereafter remain as an indolent abscess unless it is properly treated by excision. The term "alternating urachal sinus" has been used by Hinman (1961*a*) to describe urachal anomalies that present with clinical findings of both umbilical and urinary infections. Additional discussion of urachal anomalies and details about surgical correction are presented in Chapter 43.

Marshall, V. F., and Muecke, E. C.: Congenital abnormalities of the bladder. *In* Alken, C. E., Dix, V. W., Goodwin, W. E., and Wildbolze, E. (Eds.): Handbuch der Urologie. Berlin, Springer Verlag, 1968.

Marshall, V. F., and Muecke, E. C.: Variations in exstrophy of the bladder. J. Urol., *88*:766, 1962.

Miller, H. L.: Agenesis of the urinary bladder and urethra. J. Urol., *59*:1159, 1948.

Mossman, H. W.: Comparative morphogenesis of the fetal membranes and accessory uterine structures. Contrib. Embryol. Carnegie Institut., *26*:129, 1937.

Mowat, J.: An account of a child born with the urinary and genital organs preternaturally formed. *In* Edinburgh Society: Med. Essays and Observations, 3:220, 1747.

Muecke, E. C.: The role of the cloacal membrane in exstrophy: The first successful experimental study. J. Urol., *92*:659, 1964.

Muecke, E. C., and Currarino, G.: Congenital widening of the pubic symphysis; associated clinical disorders and roentgen anatomy of affected bony pelves. Am. J. Roentgenol. Radium Ther. Nucl. Med., *103*:179, 1968.

Muecke, E. C., and Marshall, V. F.: Subsymphyseal epispadias in the female patient. J. Urol., *99*:622, 1968.

Muecke, E. C., Cook, G. T., and Marshall, V. F.: Duplication of the abdominal vena cava associated with cloacal exstrophy. J. Urol., *107*:490, 1972.

Nesbit, R. M., and Bromme, W.: Double penis and double bladder with report of case. Am. J. Roentgenol., *30*:497, 1933.

Pohlman, A. G.: The development of the cloaca in human embryos. Am. J. Anat., *12*:1, 1911.

Ravitch, M. M., and Scott, W. W.: Duplication of the entire colon, bladder and urethra. Surgery, *34*:843, 1953.

Rickham, P. P.: Vesico-intestinal fissure. Arch. Dis. Child., *35*:97, 1960.

Schwalbe, E.: Die Morphologie der Missbildungen des Menschen und der Tiere: Jena, Gustav Fischer Verlag, 1909.

Soper, R. T., and Kilger, K.: Vesico-intestinal fissure. J. Urol., *92*:490, 1964.

Spence, H. M., Hoffman, W. W., and Pate, V.: Exstrophy of the bladder: II. Historical survey of treatment with personal critique. Urol. Survey, *25*:233, 1975.

Uson, A. C., Lattimer, J. K., and Melicow, M. M.: Types of exstrophy of the bladder and concomitant malformations. Pediatrics, *23*:927, 1958.

Uson, A. C., and Roberts, M. S.: Incomplete exstrophy of the urinary bladder: A report of two cases. J. Urol., *79*:57, 1958.

Vaughan, G. T.: Patent urachus; review of the cases reported: operation on a case complicated with stones in the kidneys; a note on tumors and cysts of the urachus. Trans. Am. Surg. Assoc., *23*:273, 1905.

Von Geldern, C. E.: The etiology of exstrophy of the bladder. Arch. Surg., *8*:61, 1924.

Watson, E. M.: The developmental basis for certain vesical diverticula. JAMA, *75*:1473, 1920.

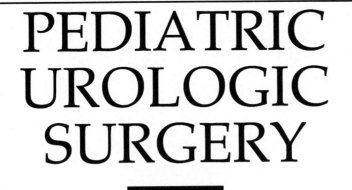

PEDIATRIC UROLOGIC SURGERY

CHAPTER 43

Management of the Exstrophy-Epispadias Complex and Urachal Anomalies

ROBERT D. JEFFS, M.D.
HERBERT LEPOR, M.D.

EXSTROPHY-EPISPADIAS COMPLEX

Bladder exstrophy, cloacal exstrophy, and epispadias are variants of the exstrophy-epispadias complex (Fig. 43–1), the etiology of which is attributed to the failure of the cloacal membrane to be reinforced by an ingrowth of mesoderm (Muecke, 1964). The cloacal membrane, therefore, persists as a bilayered membrane that becomes progressively attenuated. The cloacal membrane is subject to premature rupture; depending upon the extent of the infraumbilical defect and the stage of development when rupture occurs, bladder exstrophy, cloacal exstrophy, or epispadias develops (Ambrose and O'Brien, 1974).

The surgical management of bladder exstrophy, cloacal exstrophy, and epispadias is emphasized in this chapter. The surgical management of bladder exstrophy, however, is exceedingly controversial. Although many reconstructive techniques have been described, a unified approach to the surgical management of this disorder has not evolved, since all modalities are associated with substantial failure and operative morbidity. Until recently, surgical reconstruction of cloacal exstrophy, the most severe deformity of the exstrophy-epispadias variants, was considered futile. Afflicted neonates were left untreated and usually died from sepsis or dehydration. The surgical principles that have evolved for treating bladder exstrophy are being applied to the management of cloacal exstrophy.

The surgical management of epispadias, the least extensive anomaly of the epispadias-exstrophy complex, is straightforward and includes restoration of urinary continence and reconstruction of the genitalia. In this chapter, the techniques for managing the epispadias-exstrophy variants are reviewed, a detailed description of our surgical approach to these anomalies is presented, and the results of surgical intervention are summarized.

BLADDER EXSTROPHY

Incidence and Inheritance

The incidence of bladder exstrophy has been estimated between 1 in 10,000 (Rickham, 1961) to 1 in 50,000 (Lattimer and Smith, 1966a) live births. The male:female ratio of bladder exstrophy, derived from the combined series of Higgins (1962), Gross and Cresson (1952), Jeffs et al., (1982), Bennett (1973), and Harvard and Thomson (1951), is 2.3:1.

The risk of recurrence of bladder exstrophy in a given family is approximately 1 in 100 (Ives et al., 1980). Shapiro et al. (1984) conducted a questionnaire survey of pediatric urologists and surgeons in North America and Europe and identified the recurrence of exstrophy and epispadias in only 9 of approximately 2500 indexed

Types of Syndromes

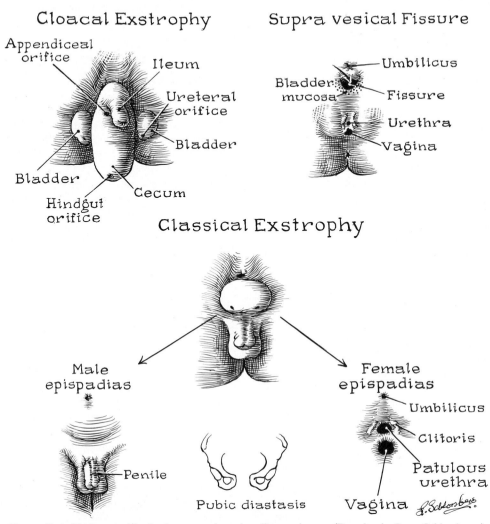

Figure caption labels — Cloacal Exstrophy: Appendiceal orifice, Ileum, Ureteral orifice, Bladder, Bladder, Hindgut orifice, Cecum. Supra vesical Fissure: Umbilicus, Bladder mucosa, Fissure, Urethra, Vagina. Classical Exstrophy: Male epispadias, Penile, Pubic diastasis, Female epispadias, Umbilicus, Clitoris, Patulous urethra, Vagina.

Figure 43–1. Various entities in the exstrophy-epispadias syndrome. (Drawing by Leon Schlossberg.)

cases. Lattimer and Smith (1966*b*) cited a set of identical twins with bladder exstrophy and another set of twins in which only one child had the condition. Higgins (1962) observed two sets of twins and two sets of siblings in the same family with bladder exstrophy. Shapiro's series identified five sets of male and female nonidentical twins in which only one twin was affected with exstrophy; five sets of male identical twins in which both twins were affected; one set of identical male twins in which only one twin was affected; and three sets of female identical twins in which only one twin had the exstrophy anomaly (Shapiro et al., 1984).

The inheritance pattern of bladder exstrophy, in a literature review by Clemetson (1958), identified 45 females with bladder exstrophy who produced 49 offspring; in no instance did any of their offspring demonstrate features of the exstrophy-epispadias complex. Until recently, bladder exstrophy or epispadias had not been reported in offspring of parents with the exstrophy-epispadias complex. Shapiro et al. (1984) reported two females with complete epispadias who each gave birth to a son with bladder exstrophy, and another female with bladder exstrophy who produced a son with bladder exstrophy. The inheritance of these three cases of bladder exstrophy was identified in a total of 225 offspring (75 males and 150 females) produced by individuals with bladder exstrophy and epispadias. Shapiro determined that the risk of bladder exstrophy in offspring of individuals with bladder exstrophy and epispadias is 1 in 70 live births, a 500-fold greater incidence than in the general population.

Anatomic and Pathologic Considerations

Anomalous development of one system in the fetus frequently results in defects in other body systems, apparently because the causal agent interferes with normal development at multiple embryonic sites. In bladder exstrophy, most anomalies are related to defects of the abdominal wall, bladder, genitalia, rectum, and anus (Fig. 43–2). In unpublished data, Charrios observed the following coexisting anomalies in 12 of 43 children with bladder exstrophy: two multiple skin hemangiomas, two corneal opacities, three renal anomalies, one hemihypertrophy, one clubfoot, one pectus excavatum, one epilepsy, and one chylothorax. Gross and Cresson (1952) described seven cases of spina bifida, five omphaloceles, three rectovesical fistulas, two rectoperineal fistulas, and three myelomeningoceles in their series of 80 bladder exstrophy cases. It is difficult to determine whether cases of cloacal exstrophy were included in this series. The relatively high incidence of spinal cord and rectal anomalies has not been observed in our experience. Children presenting with bladder exstrophy are usually robust, full-term babies with the anomalous development confined to structures adjacent to the cloacal membrane.

Williams (1974) organized the pathologic anatomy and clinical problems in bladder exstrophy under the following headings: musculoskeletal, anorectal, male and female genital, and urinary.

MUSCULOSKELETAL DEFECTS

The most obvious skeletal defect is the separation of the pubic symphysis with outward rotation of the innominate bones, which in itself causes little disability. A waddling gait develops secondary to the external rotation of the lower extremities resulting from the posterolateral position of the acetabula (Cracchiolo and Hall, 1970). The wide and waddling gait, noticeable when the child begins to walk, soon corrects itself and leaves no orthopedic problem. Reapproximation of the divergent pubis, therefore, does not provide any functional musculoskeletal advantage.

The triangular defect caused by the premature rupture of the abnormal cloacal membrane is occupied by the open bladder. The fascial defect is limited inferiorly by the intersymphyseal band, which represents the divergent urogenital diaphragm. The tendon and tendon sheath of the rectus muscles, seeking midline attachment, have a fanlike extension behind the urethra and bladder neck that inserts into the intersymphyseal band.

At the upper end of the triangular defect and bladder is the umbilicus. In bladder exstrophy, the distance between the umbilicus and

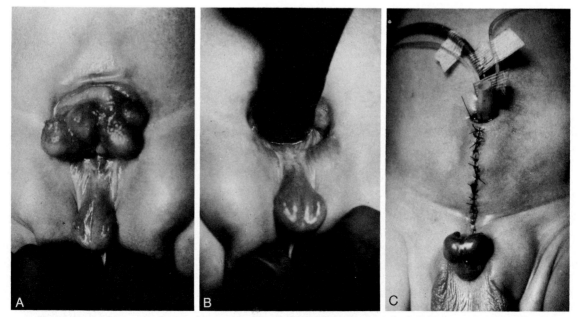

Figure 43–2. Male exstrophy: *A,* At presentation. *B,* With bladder indented. *C,* Following primary closure.

the anus is always foreshortened. Because the umbilicus is situated well below the horizontal line through the iliac crest, there is an unusual expanse of uninterrupted upper abdominal skin. Although an umbilical hernia is always present, it is usually of insignificant size. The umbilical hernia should be repaired at the time of abdominal wall closure. Omphaloceles are rarely seen in bladder exstrophy; however, they are frequently associated with cloacal exstrophy. The omphaloceles associated with the exstrophy-epispadias disorders are usually small and can be closed at the time of bladder closure. Ruptured omphaloceles require immediate surgical attention. A large omphalocele may be treated conservatively by painting it with an antiseptic solution that promotes skin overgrowth, or the omphalocele can be covered using skin flaps (Haller, 1974). We have not encountered large omphaloceles that require these special considerations; however, we recognize that such defects require prompt management at birth.

The frequent occurrence of indirect inguinal hernias is attributed to a persistent processus vaginalis, large internal and external inguinal rings, and lack of obliquity of the inguinal canal. An inguinal hernia should be treated at the time of presentation, and it requires both excision of the hernia sac and repair of the transversalis fascia and muscle defect to prevent recurrence or direct herniation.

ANORECTAL DEFECTS

The perineum is short and broad. The anus, situated directly behind the urogenital diaphragm, is displaced anteriorly and corresponds to the posterior limit of the triangular fascial defect. The anal canal may be stenotic and, rarely, ends ectopically in a rectovaginal or perineal fistula. Anal stenosis is usually treated by dilatation; however, anoplasty is required for the rare rectovaginal fistula. The anal sphincter mechanism is also anteriorly displaced and should be preserved intact in case internal urinary diversion should be required in future patient management.

The divergent levator ani and puborectalis muscles and the distorted anatomy of the external sphincter contribute to varying degrees of anal incontinence and rectal prolapse. Anal continence is usually imperfect at an early age, and in some patients the rectal sphincter mechanism may never be adequate to control liquid content of the bowel. Anorectal control should be assessed prior to ureterosigmoidostomy or other techniques of urinary diversion. Rectal prolapse frequently occurs in untreated patients with widely separated symphyses. It is usually transient and is easily reduced. Rectal prolapse is frequently exacerbated by the child's straining and crying caused by the discomfort of the irritated exposed bladder. Prolapse virtually always disappears after bladder closure or cystectomy and urinary diversion. The appearance of prolapse is an indication to proceed with definitive management of the exstrophied bladder.

MALE GENITAL DEFECT

The male genital defect is severe and may be the most troublesome aspect of the surgical reconstruction, independent of the decision to treat by functional closure or by urinary diversion (Fig. 43–3). The individual corpora cavernosa in bladder exstrophy are usually of normal caliber; however, the penis appears foreshortened because of the wide separation of the crural attachments, the prominent dorsal chordee, and the shortened urethral groove. The urethral groove may be so short and the dorsal chordee so severe that the glans becomes located adjacent to the verumontanum. A functional and cosmetically acceptable penis can be achieved when the dorsal chordee is released, the urethral groove lengthened, and the penis lengthened by mobilizing and reanastomosing the crura in the midline. Duplication of the penis and unilateral hypoplasia of the glans and corpus are rare variants that may further complicate surgical management (Fig. 43–4). Patients with a very small or dystrophic penis should be considered for sex reassignment. The need for sex reassignment in classic exstrophy occurred in only 1 in 50 to 100 cases in our experience.

The vas deferens and ejaculatory ducts are normal providing they are not injured iatrogenically (Hanna and Williams, 1972). Testicular function has not been comprehensively studied in a large series of postpubertal exstrophy males, but it is generally believed that fertility is not impaired. The autonomic innervation of the corpora cavernosa is provided by the cavernous nerves. The cavernous nerves normally course along the posterolateral surfaces of the prostate, traversing the urogenital diaphragm along or within the membranous urethra (Walsh and Donker, 1982). These autonomic nerves must be displaced laterally in patients with exstrophy, since potency is preserved following functional bladder closure, penile lengthening, and dorsal chordee release. Retrograde ejaculation may occur following functional bladder closure, since the internal sphincter remains patent. The testicles frequently appear undescended in their

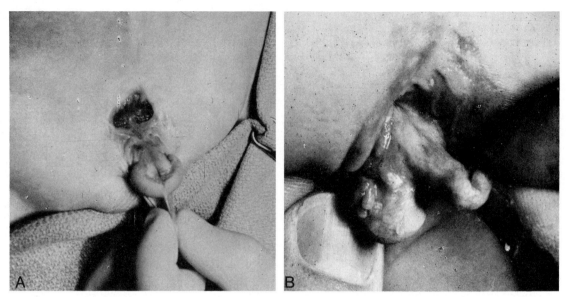

Figure 43–3. Difficult genital reconstruction: *A,* Short penis and very small bladder. *B,* Duplex penis.

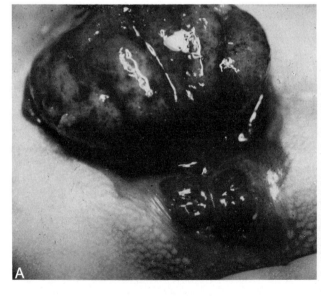

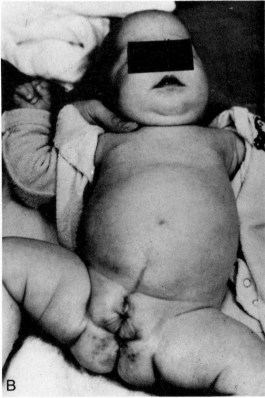

Figure 43–4. *A,* Male exstrophy with rudimentary penis. *B,* Reconstructed and raised as female.

course from the widely separated pubic tubercles to the flat, wide scrotum. Most testicles are retractile and have an adequate length of spermatic cord to reach the scrotum without the need for orchiopexy.

FEMALE GENITAL DEFECT

Reconstruction of the female genitalia presents a less complex problem than reconstruction of the male phallus (Fig. 43–5). The urethra and vagina are short, the vaginal orifice is frequently stenotic and displaced anteriorly, the clitoris is bifid, and the labia, mons pubis, and clitoris are divergent. The uterus, fallopian tubes, and ovaries are normal except for occasional uterine duplication. Approximation of the clitoral halves and the hair-bearing skin of the mons pubic provides satisfactory cosmetic restoration of the external genitalia (Dees, 1949). Vaginal dilatation or episiotomy may be required to allow satisfactory intercourse in the mature female. The defective pelvic floor may predispose mature females to develop uterine prolapse, making uterine suspension necessary. Uterine prolapse does not appear to occur when osteotomy and closure of the anterior defect are performed early in life.

URINARY DEFECT

At birth the bladder mucosa may appear normal; however, ectopic bowel mucosa or an isolated bowel loop may be present on the bladder surface. Abnormal bladder histology was observed in each of 23 bladder specimens

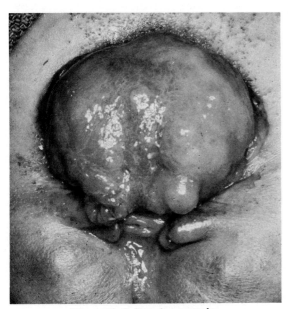

Figure 43–5. Female exstrophy.

obtained from individuals between the ages of 1 month and 52 years with bladder exstrophy. Squamous metaplasia, cystitis cystica, cystitis glandularis, and acute and chronic inflammation were commonly identified in these exstrophied bladder specimens (Culp, 1964). Scanning and transmission electron microscopy of human exstrophied bladders have demonstrated microvilli and the absence of surface ridges on the uroepithelial cells (Clark and O'Connell, 1973). The abnormal histologic features demonstrated by both light and electron microscopy may represent chronic mucosal changes secondary to persistent infection.

The size, distensibility, and neuromuscular function of the exstrophied bladder as well as the size of the triangular fascial defect to which the bladder muscle is attached affect the decision to attempt functional closure. When the bladder is small, fibrosed, and inelastic, functional closure may be impossible. The more normal bladder may be invaginated or may bulge through a small fascial defect, indicating the potential for satisfactory capacity.

It has been suggested that the exstrophied bladder may be incapable of normal detrusor function, since normal bladder function was achieved in only 22 per cent of closed exstrophies (Nisonson and Lattimer, 1972). Persistent reflux and chronic infection may account for the apparent detrusor insufficiency observed in this series. When bladder function was assessed in continent closed exstrophy patients, normal reflexive bladders and normal anal plug electromyograms were demonstrated in 70 per cent and 90 per cent of cases, respectively (Toguri et al., 1978). Muscarinic cholinergic drugs, such as Pro-Banthine and urecholine, clinically and experimentally affect bladder muscle function. Lepor and Kuhar (1984) have characterized the muscarinic cholinergic receptor in the bladder using radioligand receptor binding techniques. Using these techniques, Shapiro et al. (in press) demonstrated that exstrophied and control bladders contain similar levels of muscarinic cholinergic receptors.

The upper urinary tract is usually normal, but anomalous development does occur. We have seen horseshoe kidney, pelvic kidney, hypoplastic kidney, solitary kidney, and dysplastic megaureter. The ureters have an abnormal course and termination. The peritoneal pouch of Douglas between the bladder and rectum is enlarged and unusually deep, forcing the ureter down and laterally in its course across the true pelvis. The distal segment of the ureter approaches the bladder from a point inferior and lateral to the orifice, and it enters the bladder with little or no obliquity. Therefore, reflux in the closed exstrophied bladder occurs in nearly 100 per cent of cases and requires subsequent surgery.

Terminal ureteral dilatation frequently appears on pyelograms and is usually the result of edema, infection, and fibrosis of the terminal ureter acquired after birth. Prenatal ureterovesical obstruction is also encountered and may represent the simultaneous occurrence of an adynamic ureteral segment.

Surgical Management

The primary objectives for surgical management of bladder exstrophy are to obtain the following: secure abdominal wall closure, urinary continence with preservation of renal function, and reconstruction of a functional and cosmetically acceptable penis in the male. These objectives can be achieved following primary bladder closure, bladder neck reconstruction, and epispadias repair; or following urinary diversion, cystectomy, and epispadias repair. Historically, both urinary diversion and functional bladder closure have been fraught with complications and a consensus for the surgical management of bladder exstrophy has not been established. Advocates of urinary diversion concede that functional bladder closure provides the most ideal restoration of the genitourinary tract; however, they argue that the theoretical advantages of primary closure are seldom achieved (Bennett, 1973; Spence et al., 1975). Perez Castro and Martinez-Pineiro (1968) have stated that urinary diversion for bladder exstrophy simply transforms a congenital anomaly into an iatrogenic anomaly; however, urinary continence in their series of functional bladder closures was achieved in only 22 per cent of cases. The ideal surgical management of each bladder exstrophy patient requires detailed study and investigation; knowledge of all possible surgical solutions and their results; and a creative team approach to the overall management of the individual patient.

URINARY DIVERSION

The first ureterosigmoidostomy was performed for bladder exstrophy by Simon (1852), and the patient died 1 year later. Early experiences with ureterosigmoidostomies for bladder exstrophy were fraught with complications that included peritonitis, ureterosigmoid anastomotic strictures, acute and chronic pyelonephri-

tis, stones, intestinal obstruction, anal incontinence, and hyperchloremic, hypokalemic acidosis. The postoperative mortality in a large series of ureterosigmoidostomies performed between 1912 and 1946 was 12.5 per cent (Harvard and Thompson, 1951). The magnitude of early and late complications following ureterosigmoidostomy for bladder exstrophy was reported in Higgins's (1962) personal series of 132 ureterosigmoidostomies. Immediate postoperative complications include acute pyelonephritis, 15; wound infection, 7; evisceration, 5; ureterointestinal leak necessitating nephrostomy drainage, 3; strangulated inguinal hernia, 2; and postoperative mortality, 7. Delayed complications included hyperchloremic acidosis, 49; pyelonephritis, 39; uremia, 7; renal calculus, 5; strangulated inguinal hernia, 3; and intestinal obstruction, 1. Two modifications in operative technique markedly diminished the morbidity of ureterosigmoidostomy. Coffey (1921) described a mucosal-to-mucosal ureterointestinal anastomosis, and Leadbetter (1955) described an antirefluxing ureterointestinal anastomosis that diminished subsequent chronic pyelonephritis and renal failure. The impact of these technical modifications is reflected in the series that compared the surgical results of ureterosigmoidostomies performed prior to 1954 (Group A) with those performed after 1954 (Group B) (Bennett, 1973). The renal units assessed by excretory urography were normal in 59 per cent and 89 per cent of individuals in Groups A and B, respectively. The availability of broad-spectrum antibiotics and regimens for preoperative bowel sterilization are additional factors contributing to the decreased morbidity of ureterosigmoidostomy.

A long-term assessment of 31 ureterosigmoidostomies (Spence et al., 1975) revealed that no immediate postoperative deaths occurred; three subsequent deaths were attributed to ureterosigmoidostomy. Eleven cases (35 per cent) required 13 additional operative procedures for stones, anastomotic strictures, and recurrent pyelonephritis. Of 60 renal units assessed by intravenous pyelography, 41 units (67 per cent) were considered good (no or minimal dilatation of the collecting system, prompt and adequate excretion, and no stones); 5 units were fair; and 15 units were poor. Major infection developed in 14 patients (45 per cent), and 9 individuals (29 per cent) had absolutely no problems with infection. Half the patients developed hyperchloremic acidosis; however, chronic alkalinization was required infrequently. Overall, 50 per cent of patients in this series had no complications as measured by excretory pyelograms, infection, blood chemistries, and clinical assessment.

It is imperative that individuals be followed carefully following ureterosigmoidostomies, since anastomotic strictures, chronic pyelonephritis, urinary calculi, and metabolic abnormalities may develop insidiously. The late occurrence of carcinoma of the bowel adjacent to the ureterocolic anastomosis must also be considered. A recommended follow-up protocol includes IVP and blood chemistries every 6 months for the first 2 years, annual appraisal for the subsequent 5 years, and biannual evaluation thereafter (Spence et al., 1975).

Owing to the many complications associated with ureterosigmoidostomy, several alternative techniques for urinary diversion for bladder exstrophy have been described. Maydl (1894) described the trigonosigmoidostomy. Boyce and Vest (1952) reviewed 23 trigonosigmoidostomies followed for a mean interval of 10 years. Renal function, assessed by excretory urography, was normal in 21 cases (91 per cent); stones formed in two patients (9 per cent); and hyperchloremic acidosis developed in approximately 50 per cent. However, only a few individuals required chronic alkalinization; reoperation was performed in two cases (9 per cent). All the children achieved daytime continence, and, overall, 18 cases (78 per cent) were considered good results.

The Heitz-Boyer and Hovelacque (1912) procedure included diverting the ureters into an isolated rectal segment and pulling the sigmoid colon through the anal sphincter muscle just posterior to the rectum. Taccinoli et al. (1977) reviewed 21 staged Heitz-Boyer and Hovelacque procedures for bladder exstrophy that were followed between 1 and 16 years. They reported 95 per cent fecal and urinary continence; no cases of urinary calculi, electrolyte abnormalities, or postoperative mortality; and 3 patients (14 per cent) who developed ureterorectal strictures requiring surgical revision. Isolated cases treated in North America with this approach have been subject to multiple and severe complications. Boyce (1972) described a technique that also diverted the ureters into a rectal bladder; however, it consisted of construction of a proximal colostomy rather than a pull-through procedure.

The early good results following ileal conduit urinary diversion suggested that this technique might be ideal for urinary drainage in bladder exstrophy patients, since fecal contamination and acidosis due to reabsorption were avoided. Unfortunately, significant long-term complications have developed in children 10 to 15 years following ileal conduit diversion (Jeffs and Schwarz, 1975; Shapiro et al., 1975). Ileal conduit urinary diversion is not acceptable for exstrophy children who may have a normal life expectancy (MacFarlane et al., 1979).

Hendren (1976) described using colon urinary conduits in cases of bladder exstrophy. The nonrefluxing ureterointestinal anastomosis represents the primary advantage of colon conduits. The colon conduit is constructed at 1 year of age. If anal continence is achieved, if the ureterocolonic anastomosis is nonrefluxing, and if there is no upper tract deterioration, the colon conduit is undiverted into the colon at age 4 to 5 years. Sixteen colon conduits and 11 subsequent colocoloplasties have been performed by Hendren, and the only reported postoperative complications were intestinal obstruction in 3 cases (19 per cent) and ureteral obstruction in 1 case (6 per cent). There have been no cases of stomal complications, persistent reflux, pyelonephritis, or upper tract deterioration in Hendren's series. The long-term assessment of renal function and continence following colon conduit diversion and subsequent colocoloplasty requires further investigation. Despite our preference for primary functional bladder closure for bladder exstrophy, colon conduit urinary diversion represents the most attractive alternative, since a nonrefluxing anastomosis is achieved and undiversion can be performed when clinically indicated.

FUNCTIONAL BLADDER CLOSURE (PRIMARY BLADDER CLOSURE AND BLADDER NECK RECONSTRUCTION

Thiersch (1869) raised neighboring skin flaps in order to enclose a narrow space in front of the everted bladder. Urine was retained by an external appliance that occluded the internal sphincter. Trendelenburg (1906) attempted to achieve urinary continence by sacroiliac synchondrosis and bladder closures with narrowing of the patulous urethra. Trendelenburg attributed the lack of success with this procedure to subsequent displacement of the pubis.

Young (1942) reported the first successful functional closure for bladder exstrophy. A narrow strip of posterior urethral mucosa was selected, the mucosa lateral to the posterior urethral strip was excised, the posterior urethral strip was tubularized, and the neourethra was reinforced with the denuded detrusor muscle. The bladder was inverted and closed, and the abdominal wall defect was closed with fascial flaps. The patient eventually developed a 3-hour continent interval; however, preservation of renal function was not mentioned. Marshall and Muecke (1970) reviewed 329 functional bladder closures reported in the literature between 1906 and 1966 and determined that urinary continence with preservation of renal function was achieved in only 16 cases (5 per cent). Dehiscence of the abdominal wall and bladder, urinary fistulas, incontinence, persistent reflux, and pyelonephritis frequently resulted in subsequent urinary diversion. Over the past 20 years, modifications in the management of functional bladder closure have contributed to a dramatic increase in the success of this procedure. The most significant changes in management of bladder exstrophy were (1) reconstructing a competent bladder neck; (2) performing bilateral iliac osteotomies; (3) staging the reconstruction procedures; and (4) defining criteria for the selection of patients suitable for functional closure.

Bladder Neck Reconstruction. Dees (1949) modified the Young technique for reconstructing the bladder neck for complete epispadias. A triangular wedge of tissue was removed from the roof and lateral aspect of the proximal urethra as well as adjacent bladder wall, including a portion of each lateral lobe of the prostate. The remaining posterior urethral mucosal strip was tubularized, and the neourethra was reinforced with the adjacent denuded muscle. Leadbetter (1964) considered that the length and the tone of the muscular reinforcement of the neourethra contributed to the achievement of urinary continence. The Dees procedure was modified by tubularizing a posterior urethral strip, $3\frac{1}{2}$ cm long, that included trigonal mucosa. The neourethra was reinforced with trigonal muscle, and bilateral ureteroneocystotomies were performed. A posterior urethal strip of this length may be excessive, since urethral pressure profilometry in a series of continent bladder exstrophy patients demonstrated that continence can be achieved with a functional closure pressure as low as 20 cm of water pressure and a continence length as low as 0.6 cm (Toguri et al., 1978b). The median functional closure pressure and continence length in this group of continent exstrophies were 40 cm of water pressure and 1.35 cm, respectively.

Osteotomy. Schultz (1964) combined primary bladder closure with bilateral iliac osteotomies. The efficacy of iliac osteotomies is controversial. The primary arguments against osteotomies are that (1) the pubis eventually pulls apart; (2) the penis retracts farther; and

(3) continence can be achieved without osteotomies (Marshall and Muecke, 1970). The advantages of bilateral iliac osteotomies are that (1) reapproximation of the pubic symphysis diminishes the tension of the abdominal closure and eliminates the need for fascial flaps; (2) placement of the urethra within the pelvic ring reduces the excessive urethrovesical angle and permits urethral suspension after bladder neck plasty; and (3) reapproximation of the urogenital diaphragm and approximation of the levator ani may aid in voluntary urinary control (Jeffs et al., 1982). Ezwell and Carlson (1970) observed that urinary diversion was subsequently performed in 20 per cent of functional closures in patients who had undergone osteotomies, whereas 75 per cent of individuals who had not undergone prior osteotomies during bladder closure eventually required urinary diversion. Ninety per cent of patients referred to our institution following partial or complete bladder dehiscence had not undergone a prior osteotomy (Lowe and Jeffs, 1983). Therefore, our recommendation is to perform bilateral iliac osteotomies when primary bladder closure is performed after 72 hours of life.

Staged Surgical Reconstruction. The disadvantage of performing the entire surgical reconstruction of bladder exstrophy as a single-stage procedure is that a single complication jeopardizes the entire repair. Sweetser et al. (1952) first described a staged surgical approach for bladder exstrophy. Bladder closure was performed 4 to 6 days following bilateral iliac osteotomies, and epispadias repair was performed as a separate procedure. The continence procedure was limited to freeing the fibrous intersymphyseal band and wrapping this band around the urethra. A staged approach to functional bladder closure that includes three separate stages (bladder closure, bladder neck reconstruction with an antireflux procedure, and epispadias repair) has been recommended for most cases of exstrophy reconstruction (Jeffs et al., 1972).

Patient Selection. Successful treatment of exstrophy by functional closure demands that the potential for success in each child be considered at birth (Fig. 43–6).

Bladder size and functional capacity of the detrusor muscle are important considerations in the eventual success of functional closure. The correlation between apparent bladder size and the potential bladder capacity must not be confused. In minor grades of exstrophy that approach the condition of complete epispadias with incontinence, the bladder may appear small

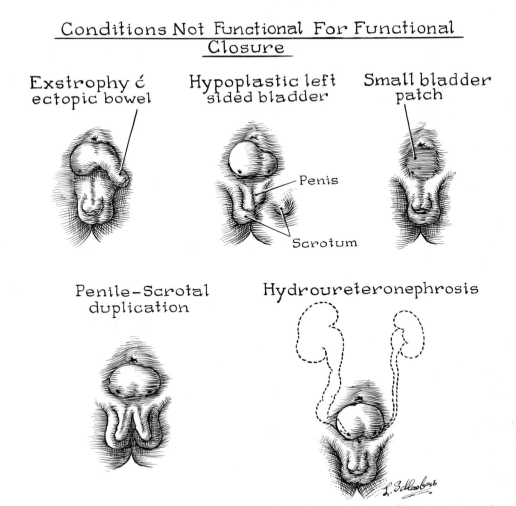

Figure 43–6. Classic exstrophy bladders that may not be suitable for functional closure. (Drawings by Leon Schlossberg.)

yet may demonstrate acceptable capacity either by bulging when the baby cries or by indenting easily when touched by a gloved finger (Chisholm, 1962). Stimulation of the bladder by a stream of cold water will indicate the ability of the detrusor muscle to contract and relax, proving its functional integrity. Once removed from surface irritation and repeated trauma, the small bladder will enlarge and will gradually increase its capacity, even in the absence of continence or outlet resistance. The exstrophied bladder that is estimated at birth to have a capacity of 5 ml or more and that demonstrates elasticity and contractility can be expected to develop useful size and capacity following successful closure. A small fibrotic bladder patch that is stretched between the edges of a small triangular fascial defect without either elasticity or contractility cannot be selected for the usual closure procedure. Bladder augmentation using bowel segments may be required in order to achieve closure (Ransley, 1984), and later bladder augmentation using bowel may be required to achieve adequate capacity (Arap, 1976). Examination under anesthesia may at times be required to adequately assess the bladder, particularly if considerable edema and excoriation have developed between birth and time of assessment. The elasticity of the bladder can be demonstrated in this way, and the size of the triangular abdominal fascial defect can be appreciated by simultaneous abdominal and rectal examination. Neonatal closure of the abdominal defect even when the bladder is small allows for later assessment of bladder potential and provides an initial step in genital reconstruction that is helpful in gaining acceptance by the family.

GENITAL RECONSTRUCTION

The techniques for reconstructing the male genitalia in bladder exstrophy are similar for patients managed by urinary diversion or by functional bladder closure. Since male adolescents consider their odd-looking genitalia a greater psychosocial problem than their incontinence, every effort must be made to restore the penis to a normal appearance (Feinberg et al., 1974). A well-planned program of surgical reconstruction must be designed at the initiation of treatment in order to avoid ineffective use of the limited penile skin.

The reconstruction of the male genitalia includes penile lengthening, release of the dorsal chordee, and urethroplasty. Owing to the extent of the penile deformity and the limited availability of penile skin in patients with bladder exstrophy, a functionally and cosmetically acceptable penis can rarely be achieved in a single operative procedure. Many of the techniques used for reconstructing the male genitalia in bladder exstrophy were described initially for hypospadias and epispadias repair.

Kelly and Eraklis (1971) lengthened the penis by nearly totally mobilizing the crura from their inferior pubic attachments to the level of the ischial tubercles and joining the freed crura in the midline. The dorsal chordee was released by dividing the suspensory ligaments and the attachments of the crura to the skin. Johnston (1974) described a more limited dissection of the corpora that achieved substantial penile length and minimized the potential risk of injuring the neurovascular bundle (Fig. 43–7). The corpora were exposed by elevating a V-flap that extended from the pubic bones to the urethral meatus. The exposed corpora were only partially mobilized from the pubis and were joined in the midline. Skin coverage was provided by preputial flaps and by closing the V incision in a Y fashion. Six months following penile lengthening and release of the chordee, the dorsal penile skin was tubularized into the neourethra.

Hinman (1958) described a three-stage procedure for reconstructing the male genitalia in bladder exstrophy. The penis was lengthened by excising the fibrous attachments of the corpora and dividing the suspensory ligaments. Preputial flaps were used for skin coverage, and a scrotal skin tube was raised for later use. In the second stage the dorsal skin was tubularized into a urethra, and the proximal end of the scrotal tube was transposed adjacent to the prostatic urethra. The mucous membrane of the prostatic urethra was covered with the scrotal tube during the third stage. The number of stages for genital reconstruction can be reduced by performing penile lengthening and release of the dorsal chordee at the time of primary bladder closure (Duckett, 1977).

Construction of the urethra using full-thickness skin grafts obtained from the thigh (Hendren, 1979) and prepuce (Devine et al., 1980) has been described for penile reconstruction in complete epispadias. These techniques can be used for urethral reconstruction in bladder exstrophy when there is insufficient penile skin available for tubularization to form a new urethra.

Staged Functional Reconstruction for Classical Bladder Exstrophy

The primary objective in functional closure of classic bladder exstrophy is to convert the exstrophy to complete epispadias with incontinence while preserving renal function. Secondarily, the best management for the incontinence and epispadias will be determined in a later stage or stages.

THE DELIVERY ROOM AND NURSERY

The disappointment and sense of tragedy that attend the birth of any deformed child affect the obstetric staff, the nursery staff, the pedia-

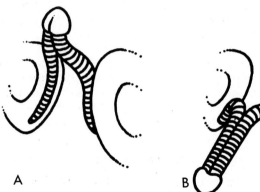

A   B

Figure 43–7. *A,* An important factor in the pathogenesis of the penile shortness is the separation of the pubes. *B,* Lengthening is obtained by partial detachment of the crura from the puboischial rami so that the extra penile parts of the corpora cavernosa can be advanced into the shaft. (From Johnston, J. H.: Epispadias. *In* Harrison, J. H., et al. (Eds.): Campbell's Urology. 4th ed. Philadelphia, W. B. Saunders Co., 1979.)

trician, and most of all, the parents. Usually the child with bladder exstrophy is the first such patient that the obstetrician and obstetric nursing staff have seen. The general practitioner and pediatrician may have seen one or two such patients in training or during lengthy practice but cannot be considered experts. The counseling of the parents and decisions about eventual therapy should be made by surgeons with special interests and experience in managing cases of bladder exstrophy.

At birth the bladder mucosa is usually smooth, thin, and intact; it is sensitive and easily denuded. In the delivery room the umbilical cord should be tied with nylon or Dexon sutures relatively close to the abdominal wall so that the umbilical clamp or long cord does not add to the trauma and excoriation of the bladder surface. The bladder may be covered with a nonadherent film of Saran or Glad wrap to prevent the mucosa from sticking to clothing or diapers. Standard varieties of Vaseline gauze become dry and lift off the delicate epithelium when removed.

The distraught parents, at this stage, need reassurance. An awareness that renal function, locomotion, sexual function, and fertility in bladder exstrophy patients can approach normal will restore hope. The parents should know that a carefully considered decision by an experienced surgeon concerning the management of urinary storage, drainage, and control will be made as soon as possible. The parents can then begin to understand the implications of the problem and help in the medical and social decisions to be made. They will also be relieved to learn that the expectation of bladder exstrophy recurring in their future offspring is low and that patients with exstrophy rarely produce children with the exstrophy-epispadias complex (Shapiro et al., 1984).

The social services offered by the hospital can be of great help to the parents in facing the family problems resulting from prolonged hospitalization and the financial strain of unexpected medical care, family separation, and home-to-hospital travel.

EARLY MANAGEMENT

Cardiopulmonary and general physical assessment can be carried out in the first few hours of life. Immediate intravenous pyelographic assessment of the kidneys in the newborn may lack clarity and detail, but useful information can usually be obtained between 24 and 48 hours of age. Radionuclide scans and ultrasound studies can provide evidence of renal function and drainage even in the first few hours of life. There is an advantage to being able to make a decision about bladder closure within the first 48 hours of life (Ansell, 1983). The ease with which the pelvis can be molded at this time allows approximation of the pubic diastasis and the rectus muscles without the need for osteotomies.

Circumstances may be less than ideal at birth, however, and neonatal assessment may have to be deferred until transportation to a children's medical center can be arranged. In these days of air travel and fast motor transportation, no child should be more than a few hours away from a neonatal center will full diagnostic and consultative services. During travel the bladder should be protected by a plastic membrane (not Vaseline gauze) to prevent contact of dressing or clothing with the delicate bladder mucosa.

THE OPERATIVE PROCEDURE

Osteotomy. When suitable patients are seen within the first 48 hours of life, the bladder and pelvic ring closure can be carried out without osteotomy owing to the malleability of the pelvic ring. However, when the separation is unduly wide or when there is delay in referral and the patient is not seen until he or she is several days of age or older, osteotomy will be required to achieve closure of the pelvic ring. Osteotomy may be carried out at the same time as bladder closure, or it may be done a few days to a week in advance. A well-coordinated surgical and anesthesiologic team can carry out osteotomy and proceed to bladder closure without undue loss of blood or risk to the child from prolonged anesthesia. The osteotomy is performed through bilateral incisions over the sacroiliac region, and iliac osteotomy is performed vertically and close to the midline to allow the two wings of the pelvis to hinge and come together without anterior to posterior flattening of the true pelvic ring (Fig. 43–8). The pelvic ring closure not only allows midline approximation of the abdominal wall structures but also allows the levator ani and puborectalis muscles to lend potential support to the bladder outlet, thereby adding resistance to urinary outflow. Furthermore, the incontinence procedures can be carried out on the bladder neck and urethra within the closed pelvic ring at a distance from the suface and free from independent movement of the two halves of the pubis. When the urethra and bladder neck are set more normally within the true pelvis, they present a normal relationship with the vertical axis of the bladder rather

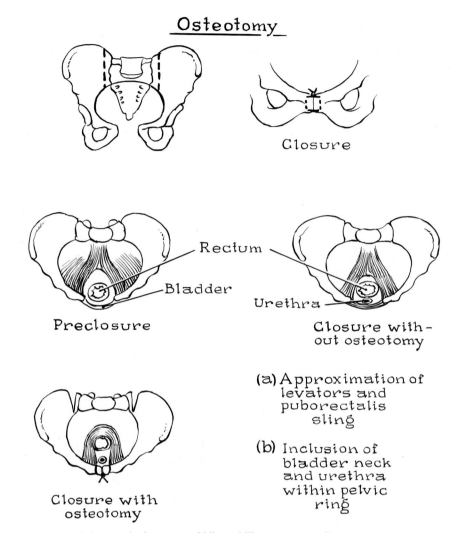

Osteotomy

Closure

Preclosure

Closure without osteotomy

Closure with osteotomy

Rectum

Bladder

Urethra

(a) Approximation of levators and puborectalis sling

(b) Inclusion of bladder neck and urethra within pelvic ring

Figure 43–8. The technique and advantages of bilateral iliac osteotomy. (Drawings by Leon Schlossberg.)

than an acute angulation. Postoperatively, both the bladder exstrophy patients closed without osteotomies in the first 48 hours of life and the patients requiring osteotomies are immobilized by modified Bryant's traction with adhesive skin traction in a position in which the hips have 90 degrees of flexion and the knees are slightly bent to protect the arterial tree (Fig. 43–9). Traction is maintained for a period of 3 to 4 weeks, allowing firm fibrous healing of the pelvic ring anteriorly. The fibrocartilage of the pubic symphysis is united by a horizontal mattress suture tied anterior to the pubic closure using 2-0 nylon. This horizontal mattress suture is placed directly through the calcified portion of the pubis on each side to provide good anchorage and maintain apposition after the suture is tied. Should the suture work loose or cut through the tissues during subsequent healing,

the anterior placement of the knot in the horizontal mattress suture ensures that it will not erode into the urethra and interfere with the bladder or urethral lumen.

Bladder and Prostatic Urethral Closure. The various steps in primary bladder closure are illustrated in Figure 43–10. A strip of mucosa 2 cm wide, extending from the distal trigone to below the verumontanum in the male and to the vaginal orifice in the female, is outlined for prostatic and posterior urethral reconstruction. When the length of the urethral groove that extends from the verumontanum to the glans is so short that it interferes with eventual penile length, the urethral groove is lengthened after the manner of Johnston (1975) and Duckett (1978). The diagrams (Fig. 43–10) indicate that an incision is made outlining the bladder mucosa and the prostatic plate. The urethral groove is

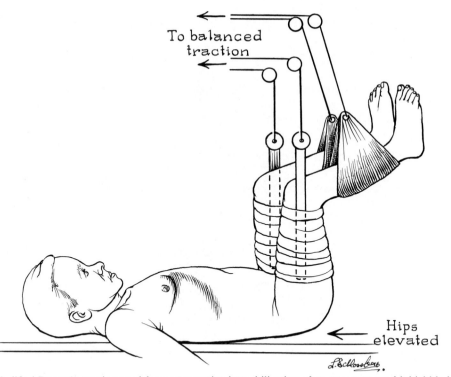

Figure 43–9. Modified Bryant's traction used for postoperative immobilization after osteotomy and initial bladder closure. (Drawing by Leon Schlossberg.)

transected distal to the verumontanum, but continuity is maintained between the thin, mucosa-like, non–hair-bearing skin adjacent to the posterior urethra and bladder neck and the skin and mucosa of the penile shaft and glans. Flaps from the area of thin skin are subsequently moved distally and rotated to reconstitute the urethral groove, which may be lengthened by 2 to 4 cm.

Penile lengthening is achieved by exposing the corpus cavernosum bilaterally and freeing the corpora from their attachments to the suspensory ligaments and anterior part of the inferior pubic rami. The partially freed corpora are joined in the midline and the bare corpora are then covered with flaps of the thin para-exstrophy skin (mentioned previously), which are rotated medially to be attached to the distal mucosa of the posterior plate. These same flaps may also be used to lengthen the urethra in the female by detaching the urethral groove distally and suturing the flap to the urethra in a tubular fashion.

Bladder closure then proceeds by excision of the umbilical area, the redundant skin adjacent to the superior aspect of the bladder mucosa being discarded and the bladder muscle being freed from the fused rectus sheaths on

each side. This dissection is facilitated by exposing the peritoneum above the umbilicus and then carefully dissecting extraperitoneally to enter the retropubic space on each side from above. The wide band of fibrous and muscular tissue representing the urogenital diaphragm is detached subperiostally from the pubis bilaterally. The dissection is extended for 5 to 10 mm in a subperiosteal plane onto the inferior ramus of the pubis, allowing the bladder neck and posterior urethra to fall back and achieve a position within the pelvic ring. The mucosa and muscle of the bladder and posterior urethra are then closed in the midline anteriorly. The posterior urethra and bladder neck are buttressed by the tissues of the urogenital diaphragm, which are closed as a second layer. The bladder is drained by a suprapubic Malecot catheter for a period of 4 weeks. The urethra is not stented in order to avoid pressure necrosis or the accumulation of infected secretions in the urethra. Ureteral stents provide urethral drainage during the first 5 to 7 days when swelling, or the pressure of the bladder closure, may obstruct the ureters and give rise to obstruction and transient hypertension.

When the bladder and urethra have been closed, pressure over the greater trochanters

Text continued on page 1900

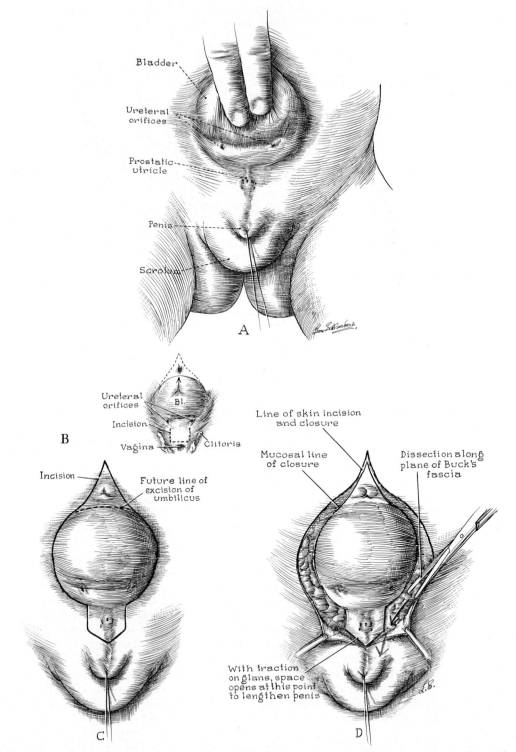

Figure 43–10. *A* to *O*, Steps in primary bladder closure following osteotomy, or without osteotomy, in the newborn less than 72 hours of age.

Illustration continued on opposite page

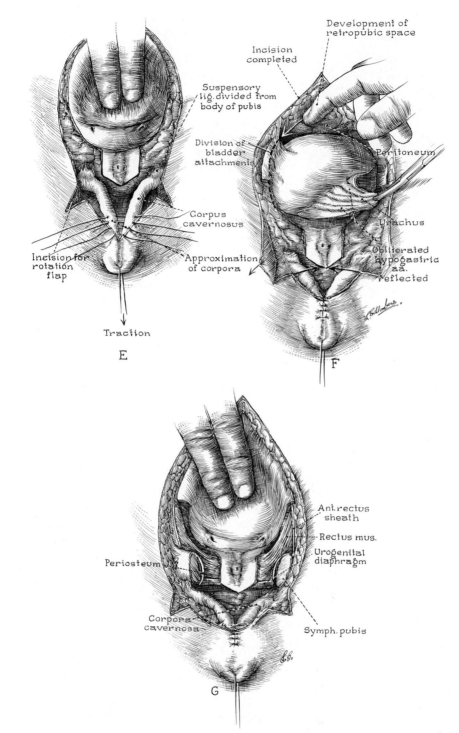

Figure 43–10 *Continued. E,* Lateral skin incision to allow rotation of paraexstrophy skin to cover elongated penis. *F,* Development of retropubic space from area of umbilical dissection to facilitate separation of bladder from the rectus sheath and muscle. *G,* Medial fan of rectus muscle attaching behind prostate to urogenital diaphragm. Diaphragm and anterior corporus freed from pubis in subperiosteal plane.

Illustration continued on following page

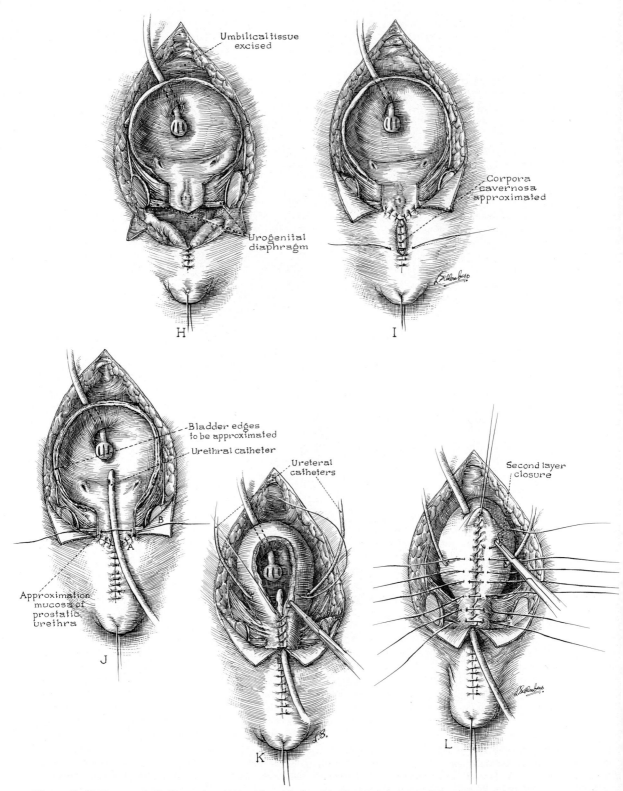

Figure 43–10 *Continued. K,* Ureteral catheters placed before bladder closure to provide renal drainage for 5 to 10 days.

Illustration continued on opposite page

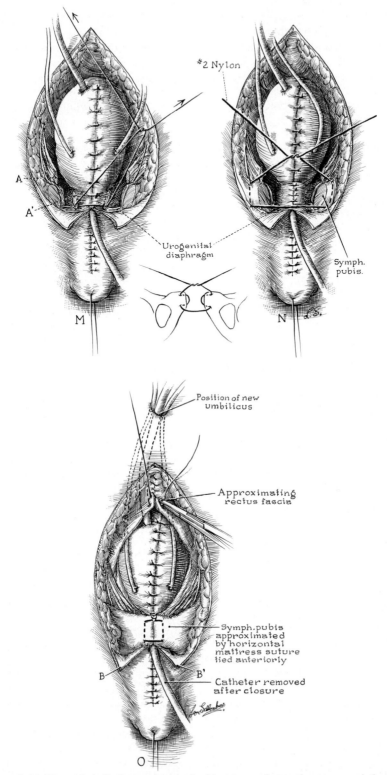

Figure 43–10 *Continued. M,* Urogenital diaphragm is closed with separate layer of sutures, or is brought together when pubic symphysis is united. *N,* Horizontal mattress suture tied on external surface of symphysis. *O,* Catheter removed from closed bladder neck and urethra. Approximation of skin point B to B₁ provides an anterior step from penile closure to abdominal wall closure. (Drawings by Leon Schlossberg.)

allows the pubic bones to be approximated in the midline. The horizontal mattress suture is placed and tied, and the rectus sheath is closed in the midline. The suprapubic tube and ureteral stents emerge from the abdominal skin above the midline skin closure at a point corresponding to the normal position of the umbilicus.

During this procedure, the patient is given broad-spectrum antibiotics in an attempt to convert a contaminated field into a clean surgical wound. Nonreactive sutures of Dexon and nylon are used to avoid undesirable stitch reaction or stitch abscesses.

INTERIM MANAGEMENT AFTER INITIAL CLOSURE

The procedure just described converts a child with exstrophy into one with complete epispadias with incontinence. Prior to removal of the suprapubic tube, 4 weeks postoperatively, the bladder outlet is calibrated by a urethral catheter or by cystoscopy to ensure free outlet drainage. An intravenous pyelogram is obtained to record the status of the pelvis and ureters, and appropriate urinary antibiotics are administered to treat any bladder contamination that may be present after removal of the suprapubic tube. Residual urine is estimated by straight catheterization, and cultures are obtained before the patient leaves the hospital and at subsequent intervals to detect infection and ensure adequate drainage. The intravenous pyelogram is repeated 3 months after discharge from the hospital and will be repeated at intervals of 6 months to 1 year during the next 2 to 3 years to detect any upper tract change caused by reflux or infection. Antibiotics (Septra, Bactrim, or Macrodantin) should be continued at least through the first 6 months, and then as necessary thereafter. Should bladder outlet resistance be such that urine is retained within the bladder, and reflux and ureteral dilatation develop with infected urine, it may be necessary to dilate the urethra or, occasionally, to begin intermittent catheterization. If bladder outlet resistance persists, an antireflux procedure may be required as early as 6 months to 1 year after the initial bladder closure. If a useful continent interval has resulted unexpectedly from the initial closure, no further operation or incontinence may be required.

In the patient converted from exstrophy to complete epispadias with incontinence, the bladder gradually increases in capacity, and inflammatory changes in the mucosa resolve. Cystograms at 2 to 3 years of age will indicate bilateral reflux in nearly 100 per cent of the patients and will provide an estimate of bladder capacity. Even in the completely incontinent patient, bladder capacity gradually increases to the point at which it can be distended at cystography to a capacity of 50 to 60 ml. In some patients with very small bladders, the bladders may require 4 to 5 years to achieve this capacity.

A tight bladder closure, uncontrolled urinary infection, and reflux may cause uncontrollable ureteral dilatation. Judgment is required to know when to abort attempts at functional closure and turn to urinary diversion as a means of preserving renal function. This change of plan is seldom necessary if a wide outlet has been constructed at initial closure and if careful attention has been paid to the details of follow-up.

When the child is 3 to 5 years of age, providing the bladder has achieved a capacity of 50 to 60 ml when distended, treatment of incontinence and reflux is undertaken. Cultures and radiologic studies should indicate sterile urine and good ureteral drainge in the undistended bladder. The rationale for performing bladder neck reconstruction prior to urethral reconstruction is that iatrogenic injury to a reconstructed urethra may result if instrumentation is required for urinary retention immediately following the bladder neck reconstruction. However, if by age 3 years the bladder capacity in boys has not reached 50 ml, we proceed directly to epispadias repair; bladder neck reconstruction is deferred until bladder capacity increases. The formation of the neourethra may produce additional resistance to urine outflow and therefore contribute to increasing bladder capacity.

THE INCONTINENCE AND ANTIREFLUX PROCEDURE

The incontinence and antireflux procedures are illustrated in Figure 43–11. This illustration depicts a Cohen (1975) type of transtrigonal advancement procedure for correcting reflux, in which a new hiatus lateral to the original orifice is selected prior to advancing the ureter across the bladder above the trigone. The bladder is originally opened through a V incision at the bladder neck, but a vertical extension is used. The midline closure of this incision enlarges the vertical dimension of the bladder, which in exstrophy is often short.

The incontinence procedure is begun by selecting a posterior strip of mucosa 18 to 20 mm wide and 30 mm long that extends distally from the midtrigone to the prostate or posterior urethra. The bladder muscle lateral to this mu-

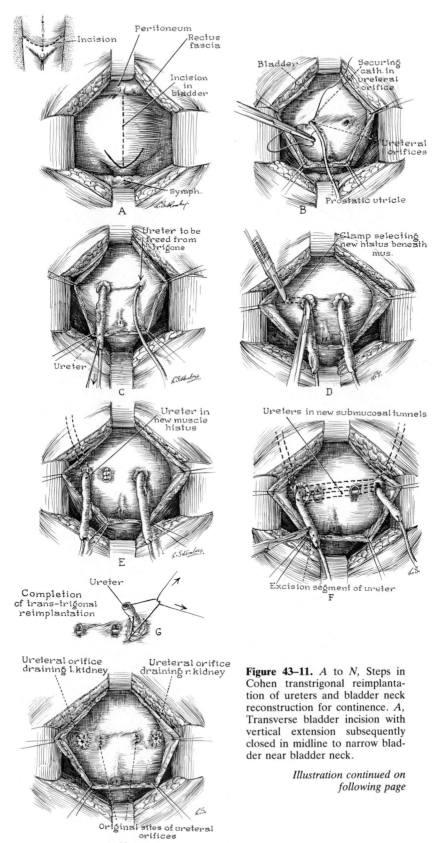

Figure 43–11. *A* to *N*, Steps in Cohen transtrigonal reimplantation of ureters and bladder neck reconstruction for continence. *A*, Transverse bladder incision with vertical extension subsequently closed in midline to narrow bladder near bladder neck.

Illustration continued on following page

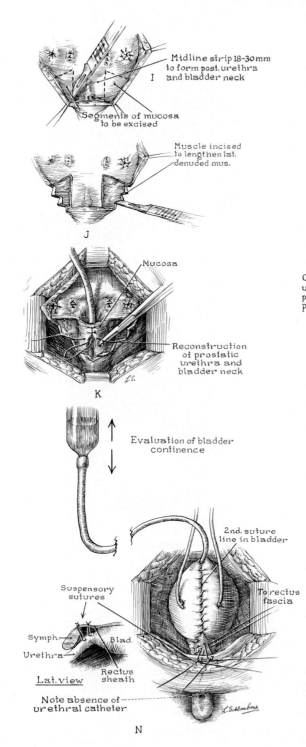

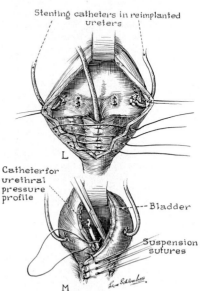

Figure 43–11 *Continued. I* to *L,* Mucosal strip of trigone to form bladder neck and prostatic urethra. Lateral denuded muscle triangles are lengthened by several small incisions to allow easy tailoring of double-breasted muscular closure of bladder neck. *M,* Pressure profile of closed bladder neck and urethra is obtained prior to closure of bladder dome. Suspension sutures are elevated manually to estimate final pressure profile. *N,* Bladder neck and urethra are unstented; drainage is by ureteral catheters and suprapubic tube. Bladder outlet resistance is estimated by water manometer. (Drawings by Leon Schlossberg.)

cosal strip is denuded of mucosa. The edges of the mucosa and the underlying muscle are formed into a tube by interrupted sutures, and the adjacent denuded muscle flaps are overlapped and sutured firmly in place in order to provide reinforcement of the bladder neck and urethral reconstruction. Wide dissection of the bladder, bladder neck, and urethra is required within the pelvis to provide mobility both for this urethral reconstruction and for subsequent anterior suspension of the newly created urethra and bladder neck. Tailoring of the denuded lateral triangles of bladder muscle is aided by multiple small incisions in the free edges bilaterally.

Urethral profiles are obtained intraoperatively to measure continence length and urethral closure pressure. Retrospective comparison of these values with subsequent success or failure in producing continence serves as a guideline for reconstructing the bladder neck. Preliminary results suggest that an intraoperative continence length of 2.5 to 3.5 cm is desirable, and that intraoperative closure pressures ranging between 70 and 100 ml of water are required to prevent leakage when the bladder pressure is raised to 50 cm of water intraoperatively. Undoubtedly, the measurements of continence length and closure pressure will be considerably less in eventual follow-up, when stretching occurs and swelling and edema disappear. At the end of the procedure, the bladder neck reconstruction is further enhanced by suspending the urethra and the bladder neck to the structures of the pubis and anterior rectus sheath in the manner of Marshall, Marchetti, and Krantz (Marshall et al., 1949). Profiles taken after this stage of the procedure indicate that additional continence length and additional closure pressure are achieved (Fig. 43–12).

In the small bladder, ureteral stents are placed in the reimplanted ureters and the bladder is drained once again by suprapubic catheter, which is left indwelling for a 3-week period. Suprapubic catheter drainage prevents stretching or pressure on the reconstructed bladder neck. No urethral stent is used, and catheterization or instrumentation through the urethra is avoided for at least a 3-week period. The adequacy of bladder neck reconstruction is tested by a water manometer at the end of the procedure. The bladder neck should support 50 cm of water pressure without leakage if the bladder neck plasty and suspension are adequate. Immediate revision is advisable when this degree of resistance is not obtained. Attempts are made to reduce the postoperative frequency and se-

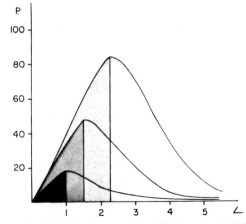

Figure 43–12. Urethral pressure profile measured with bladder open, before bladder neck reconstruction, after reconstruction, and with addition of bladder neck suspension. Each increases continence length and closure pressure.

verity of bladder spasms by the use of Pro-Banthine, Ditropan, Valium, or Tofranil. The patients are given urinary antibiotics to prevent infection, and little or no leakage through the urethra should occur during the 3 weeks of suprapubic drainage. Prior to removal of the suprapubic catheter, a clamp is applied to initiate voiding, and, if necessary, the urethra is calibrated using a soft catheter. Cultures are taken so that medication may be given to clear any bacterial contamination. In some patients a period of intermittent catheterization may be required if reasonable bladder emptying does not occur.

When the catheter is removed, we expect a short, dry interval to occur but bladder size and operative reaction may allow a capacity of no more than a few milliters initially. The patient has to learn to recognize bladder filling and to initiate detrusor contraction, which he may not previously have experienced. A readjustment period that may extend for many months or, in some patients, for years is required before a useful bladder volume and a long dry interval develop. Initially, the absence of stress incontinence or continuous urethral dribbling suggests that urethral resistance has been produced and that an increasing dry interval will occur. The patient can learn to use this interval profitably for daytime, and later for nighttime, continence.

URETHROPLASTY

Construction of the neourethra and further penile lengthening and dorsal chordee release are usually performed approximately 1 year following bladder neck reconstruction. We recommend that a modified Young urethroplasty be performed when there is sufficient penile skin for both construction of the urethra and coverage of the neourethra and when the dorsal urethral groove has sufficient length. The techniques for constructing the urethra from full-thickness grafts have been previously described (Hendren, 1979; Devine et al., 1980). These procedures are reserved for situations in which penile skin is unavailable to perform a modified Young urethroplasty. A pedicle tube constructed from ventral preputial tissue may also be used to bridge a defect between prostatic and glandular urethra (Duckett, 1981).

The modified Young urethroplasty (Fig. 43–13) is begun by placing a nylon suture through the glans, which provides for traction of the penis. Incisions are made over two parallel lines, previously marked on the dorsum of the penis, that outline an 18-mm strip of penile skin extending from the prostatic urethral meatus to the tip of the glans. Triangular areas of the dorsal glans are excised adjacent to the urethral strip, and glandular flaps are constructed. The lateral skin flaps are mobilized and a Z incision over the subpubic area permits exposure and division of suspensory ligaments and old scar tissue. The urethral strip is then

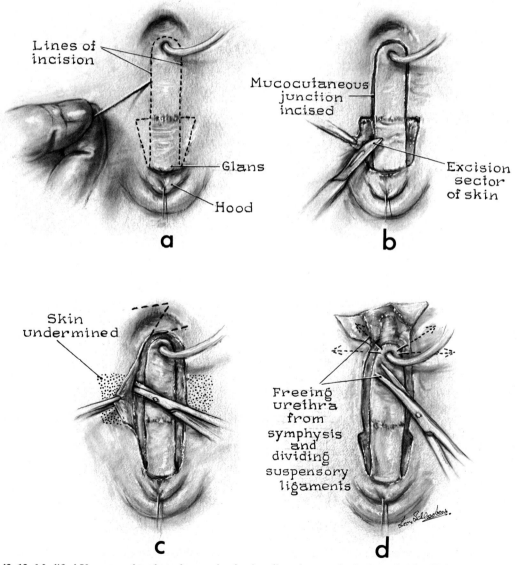

Figure 43–13. Modified Young urethroplasty for repair of epispadias when urethral groove is of sufficient length naturally or following prior lengthening procedures. (Drawings by Leon Schlossberg.)

Illustration continued on opposite page

closed in a linear manner from the prostatic opening to the glans over a No. 10 pediatric feeding tube with 6-0 polyglycolic acid suture. The subcutaneous tissue is closed with two separate continuous layers of 6-0 polyglycolic acid suture. The skin is reapproximated with interrupted 5-0 polyglycolic acid sutures. The glans is reapproximated with vertical mattress sutures of 4-0 proline; these sutures are removed in 10 days. The Z-plasty is closed with interrupted 6-0 polyglycolic acid suture. Several 6-0 polyglycolic acid sutures are inserted between the proline sutures in the glans. A pediatric feeding tube is left indwelling in the neourethra as a

stent. Urinary drainage occurs through the stent or may be further ensured by a percutaneous suprapubic tube.

RESULTS OF STAGED FUNCTIONAL CLOSURE

Recent reviews of functional bladder closure in bladder exstrophy have demonstrated dramatic improvement in the frequency of successful reconstructions. Secure abdominal wall closure and urinary continence with preservation of renal function have been achieved in greater than 40 per cent of patients reported by Mollard (1980), Chisholm (1979), Ansell (1983),

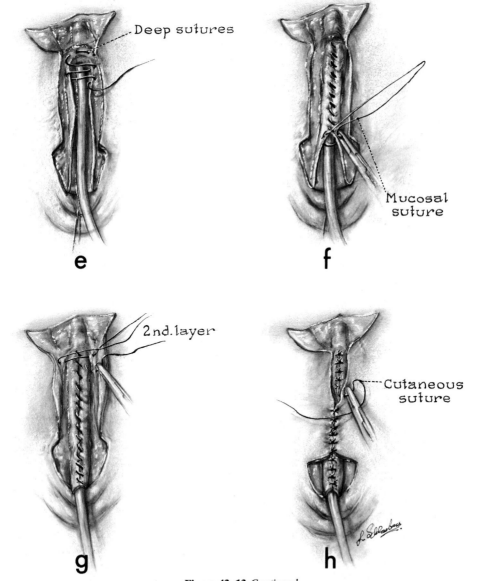

Figure 43–13 *Continued*

Illustration continued on following page

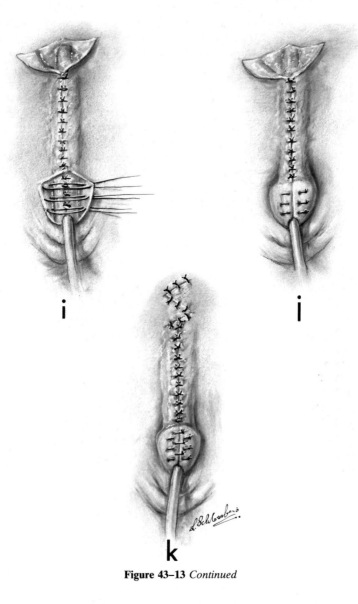

i

i

k

Figure 43–13 *Continued*

and Jeffs (1979) (Table 43–1). The recent experience (1975 to 1982) with functional bladder closure at our institution is reviewed in detail.

Primary Bladder Closure. Twenty-eight of 29 consecutive patients with bladder exstrophy (97 per cent) referred to our pediatric urology service prior to any surgical reconstruction between 1975 and 1982 underwent bladder closure (Lepor and Jeffs, 1983). Urinary diversion was initially performed in one child with a very small bladder patch. The complications following primary bladder closure and the additional surgical procedures required to correct these postoperative complications are presented in Table 43–2.

Bladder Neck Reconstruction (BNR). Twenty-five patients underwent initial BNR at our institution between 1975 and 1982 (Lepor and Jeffs, 1982). Urinary retention developed in eight cases postoperatively and resolved following dilatation or prolonged suprapubic catheter drainage in all cases.

The two parameters used to assess urinary continence were the average daytime dry interval and the frequency of incontinent episodes. Achievement of an average daytime dry interval exceeding 3 hours represented an excellent surgical result, a dry interval of greater than 1 hour and less than 3 hours a satisfactory result, and a dry interval of less than 1 hour a poor result. Another parameter used to assess urinary continence was the number of times the underclothes were soiled during the day. Soilage of

TABLE 43–1. Urinary Continence following Functional Bladder Closure

Series*	No. Closures Evaluated	Continent (No.)	Continent (%)
Chisholm (1979)	95	43	45
Mollard (1980)	16	11	69
Jeffs (1982)	55	33	60
Ansell (1983)	23	10	43
Lepor and Jeffs (1983)	22	19	86

*Only personal series reporting continence rates > 40 per cent are included.

TABLE 43–2. Complications in 28 Primary Bladder Closures

Complications	Number
Bladder prolapse	2
Outlet obstruction	2
Bladder calculi	3
Renal calculi	1
Wound dehiscence	0
CORRECTIVE SURGICAL PROCEDURES	
Repair of bladder prolapse	2
Cystolithopexy	3
Urethrotomy	1

From Lepor, H., and Jeffs, R. D.: J. Urol., *130*:1142, 1983.

underclothes less than once per day was considered an excellent surgical result, soilage one to two times per day a satisfactory result, and soilage greater than two times per day a poor result. Urinary continence according to average daytime dry interval and soilage of underclothing was achieved in 86 per cent and 80 per cent of cases, respectively (Table 43–3).

Forty-two renal units from 21 patients were evaluated by intravenous pyelography between 6 months and 6 years following BNR in order to assess the preservation of renal function following functional bladder closure. Only 10 per cent of these renal units showed significant hydronephrosis and deterioration of function.

Urethroplasty. Twenty-four patients with bladder exstrophy underwent initial urethral reconstruction at the Johns Hopkins Hospital between 1975 and 1982 (Table 43–4) (Lepor et al., 1984). A modified Young urethroplasty was performed in 22 patients, a distal urethral free graft in one patient and a ventral preputial pedicle graft in one patient. The average age at the time of urethral reconstruction was 4 years.

Fistulas developed in nine patients following epispadias repair. Four of the fistulas closed spontaneously, and five required surgical closure. Four of these five fistulas occurred near the corona, and one occurred at the midshaft. The corona is the area most deficient in circumferential penile skin, and multiple layered closure at this point over the tubularized urethra

is difficult to achieve. Proximally the skin is more redundant, and distally the glandular flaps cover the neourethra and heal quickly without fistulas. The coronal sulcus is, however, a weak spot in the repair. The fistulas were closed by excising a small rim of penile skin and urethra adjacent to the fistulas and closing the defect with 6–0 Vicryl suture in three layers. No persistent fistulas occurred.

We have assessed the effect of five parameters on the rate of fistula formation: (1) osteotomy, (2) sequence of bladder neck plasty and epispadias repair, (3) hospital of initial treatment, (4) total number of prior bladder closures performed, and (5) preoperative hormonal stimulation with testosterone application or HCG injections (Table 43–5). Eighty-three per cent of patients had bilateral osteotomies performed prior to epispadias repair. A prior osteotomy appeared to decrease the number of fistulas requiring surgical closure. Fistulas requiring surgical closure developed in 15 per cent of patients who had undergone prior bilateral osteotomies, whereas 67 per cent of patients who had not undergone prior osteotomy developed fistulas that required surgical closure. The fistula rate was found to be independent of the institution of pre-epispadias treatment, the sequence of bladder neck plasty and epispadias repair, the number of bladder closures performed, and the

TABLE 43–3. Urinary Continence following 22 Initial Bladder Neck Reconstructions

Result	Average Daytime Dry Interval (hrs)	Patients		Incontinent Episodes/Day	Patients	
		NUMBER	PER CENT		NUMBER	PER CENT
Excellent	>3	19	86	<1	16	80
Satisfactory	1–3	1*	5	1–2	1	5
Poor	<1	2*	9	>3	3*	15

*Includes patient's continence level prior to secondary reconstructive surgery.
From Lepor, H., and Jeffs, R. D.: J. Urol., *130*:1142, 1983.

TABLE 43–4. OPERATIVE COMPLICATIONS
FOLLOWING 24 INITIAL URETHRAL RECONSTRUCTIONS

Complication	Incidence	Per Cent
Fistulas		
Surgical closure	5	21
Spontaneous closure	4	17
Recurrent	0	0
Stricture	0	0

From Lepor, H., Shapiro, E., and Jeffs, R. D.: J. Urol., *131*:512, 1984.

use of preoperative hormonal stimulation of the genitalia.

All 24 patients who underwent epispadias repair are preadolescent, and a definitive assessment of their genital function cannot be made. An attempt was made to evaluate the current status of the genital reconstruction from parental interviews (Table 43–6). Eighteen parents were interviewed, four parents could not be contacted, and it is too early to evaluate the results in two children operated on within the last 3 months. The angulation of the flaccid penis when standing was directed downward to horizontally in 83 per cent of the boys. Erections were witnessed in 83 per cent of the youngsters; in these individuals the erect penis was directed upward in 47 per cent, horizontally in 47 per cent, and downward in 6 per cent. Every parent was extremely satisfied with the appearance of

TABLE 43–5. URETHROPLASTY: FACTORS AFFECTING
THE FISTULA RATE

| | Fistulas Surgically Closed | | |
	PATIENTS	NUMBER	PER CENT
Osteotomy			
Performed	20	3	15
Not performed	3	2	67
Unknown	1	0	0
Initial treatment			
Johns Hopkins	10	2	20
Elsewhere	14	3	22
Sequence of epispadias repair			
Prior to BNR*	10	2	20
Following BNR	10	2	21
During BNR	1	0	0
Urinary diversion	3	1	33
Number of bladder closures			
One	17	4	23
Multiple	5	1	10
Preoperative hormonal stimulation			
Received	9	2	22
Not received	15	3	20

*Bladder neck reconstruction
From Lepor, H., Shapiro, E., and Jeffs, R. D.: J. Urol., *131*:512, 1984.

TABLE 43–6. EVALUATION OF GENITAL
RECONSTRUCTION IN EXSTROPHY PATIENTS

	Number of Patients	Percentage of Patients
Parents surveyed		
Parents contacted	18	75
Parents not contacted	4	17
Too early to evaluate	2	8
Angulation of penis when standing		
Upward	3	17
Horizontal	9	50
Downward	6	33
Erections		
Documented	15	83
Not documented	3	17
Angulation of penis during erection		
Upward	7	39
Horizontal	7	39
Downward	1	1
No documented erection	3	7
Overall evaluation of penile reconstruction		
Very satisfied	18	100
Satisfied	0	0
Dissatisfied	0	0

From Lepor, H., Shapiro, E., and Jeffs, R. D.: J. Urol., *131*:512, 1984.

the penis, although some expressed concern about whether the penis would attain adequate size for sexual intercourse after puberty.

A review of staged functional closure for bladder exstrophy at the Johns Hopkins Hospital between 1975 and 1982 clearly demonstrated that secure abdominal wall closure, urinary continence with preservation of the upper urinary tracts, and a cosmetically acceptable penis can be achieved without wound dehiscence, with infrequent deterioration of renal function, and with occasional urethral fistulas that require surgical repair. Therefore, it is recommended that all neonates with bladder exstrophy be considered for staged functional bladder closure.

Management of Failed Bladder Closures

Urinary continence, defined as a 3-hour day interval, is usually achieved within one year following bladder neck reconstruction. Delayed achievement of urinary continence has been associated with puberty in the male (Kramer and Kelalis, 1982). The increase in urethral length associated with prostatic enlargement provides additional resistance to urinary outflow. In our experience, patients who do not achieve a 1-hour dry interval within 2 years following bladder neck reconstruction seldom develop a sufficient continence mechanism. These unfortunate individuals may be treated by the following means: repeat Young-Dees-Leadbetter bladder neck reconstruction; tubularization of the remaining bladder into a neourethra and bladder augmentation by colocystoplasty (Arap et al. 1976); anti-incontinence devices (Scott et al., 1974); or urinary diversion. If failed reconstruction efforts are associated with the development of renal insufficiency, renal transplantation into an intestinal segment (Marchioro and Tremann, 1974) or closed exstrophied bladder (Spees et al., 1984) may be considered. A patulous bladder neck with an adequate bladder capacity is managed by revising the Young-Dees-Leadbetter bladder neck plasty. Arap et al. (1976) manage bladder exstrophy by initially constructing a colon urinary conduit. The entire bladder is subsequently tubularized into a 5 to 6 cm neourethra, and the colon conduit is anastomosed to this urethrovesical tube. This technique is useful for the failed Young-Dees-Leadbetter bladder neck plasties with small contracted bladders, or for the initial treatment of bladder exstrophy when the bladder capacity is less than 5 ml. Hanna (1981) has inserted anti-incontinence devices to achieve continence in bladder exstrophy. The compromised blood supply to urethral and periurethral tissues from previous surgical manipulations increases the likelihood for erosion of the device. We have inserted only one anti-incontinence device in a patient with bladder exstrophy referred to our institution following failed bladder neck reconstruction. Despite insertion and activation of the device in two stages, erosion into the urethra occurred. Similar experiences with anti-incontinence devices in complete epispadias have been reported by others (Hanna, 1981; Kramer and Kelalis, 1982). The artificial sphincter may be useful in older children with well-vascularized bladder neck tissues or in those in whom the mature omentum can be interposed between the cuff and the reconstructed bladder neck.

Malignancy

In the 1920's it was estimated that 50 per cent of individuals with bladder exstrophy were dead by 10 years of age (Mayo and Hendricks, 1926). Development of operative techniques that preserved renal function, availability of broad-spectrum antibiotics, and understanding of the metabolic disorders associated with urinary diversion have resulted in 91 per cent of patients with this disorder surviving to age 30 years (Lattimer et al., 1979). This extended survival has uncovered two latent malignant processes that are associated with bladder exstrophy. Eighty per cent (45/57) of carcinomas identified in exstrophied bladders are adenocarcinomas (Kandzari et al., 1974). The incidence of adenocarcinomas in the exstrophied bladder is approximately 400-fold greater than in the normal population (Engel and Wilkinson, 1970). According to Mostofi (1954), chronic irritation, infection, and obstruction can induce a metaplastic transformation of the urothelium to cystitis glandularis, a premalignant lesion. Adenocarcinoma may also develop from the malignant degeneration of embryonic rests of gastrointestinal tissue that are incorporated in the exstrophied bladder (Engel and Wilkinson, 1970). The inherent malignant potential of the closed exstrophied bladder has not been determined, since long-term follow-up of a large number of bladder exstrophy cases without urinary tract infection, obstruction, and chronic irritation has not been done. Bladder abnormalities, including squamous metaplasia, acute inflammation, fibrosis, and epithelial submucosal inclusions, were observed in an exstrophied bladder at 2 weeks of age (Culp, 1964), suggesting that exstrophied bladders are inherently abnormal. On the other hand is the case of a 17-year-old male who underwent primary bladder closure at age 1 year and developed normal urinary control with preservation of the upper urinary tract. He was killed in an automobile accident, and serial sectioning of his bladder revealed no evidence of malignant or premalignant changes (Jeffs, 1979) (Fig. 43–14). Until the malignant potential of the noninfected, nonobstructed closed exstrophied bladder is determined, a high index of suspicion must be maintained for potential malignant degeneration. Only two epithelial malignancies have been reported in closed exstrophy patients, and these bladders were not closed at birth. Both bladder tumors were squamous in nature.

Exstrophied bladders that are left everted are predisposed to develop squamous cell carcinoma secondary to repeated trauma. Squamous cell carcinoma accounts for only 4 of 57 (7 per cent) of the carcinomas reported in exstrophied bladders (Kandzari et al., 1974). Rhabdomyosarcoma has been observed in three individuals with bladder exstrophy (Jeffs, unpublished data; Engel, 1973; Semerdjian et al., 1972).

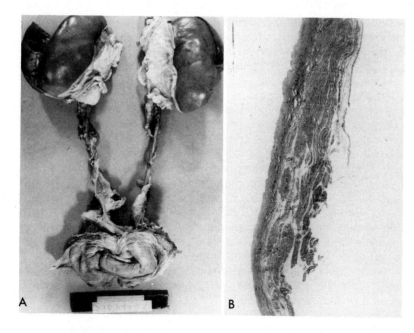

Figure 43–14. Gross *(A)* and microscopic *(B)* views of bladder of exstrophy patient who died accidentally after 17 years of normal bladder function.

Adenocarcinoma of the colon adjacent to the ureterointestinal anastomosis in an exstrophy patient was initially described by Dixon and Weisman (1948). The risk of adenocarcinoma of the colon in exstrophy patients following ureterosigmoidostomy is 100-fold that of the general population (Sooriyaarchchi et al., 1979). Spence et al. (1979) surveyed the literature to identify patients with bladder exstrophy who developed tumors following ureterosigmoid diversion. The mean latency interval from the time of ureterointestinal anastomosis to the diagnosis of intestinal tumor in these cases was 10 years, and the longest latent interval was 46 years. Twenty-eight of the 35 compiled tumors were malignant, 24 were adenocarcinomas, and approximately half the adenocarcinomas had metastasized at the time of diagnosis. Individuals with ureterosigmoidostomy, therefore, should undergo periodic barium enema examinations or sigmoidostomy, or both.

Fertility

Reconstruction of the male genitalia and preservation of fertility were not primary objectives of the early surgical management of bladder exstrophy. Sporadic accounts of pregnancy, or the initiation of pregnancy by males with bladder exstrophy, have been reported. In two large exstrophy series, male fertility was rarely documented, only 3 of 68 men (Bennett, 1973), and 4 of 72 men (Woodhouse et al., 1983) having successfully fathered children. Six of 26, and 7 of 27, women with bladder exstrophy in these respective studies successfully delivered offspring. Shapiro's (1984) survey of 2500 exstrophy and epispadias patients identified 38 males who had fathered children and 131 female patients who had borne offspring.

Hanna and Williams (1972) compared semen analyses of men who had undergone primary bladder closure and ureterosigmoidostomy. A normal sperm count was found in only one of eight men following functional bladder closures and in four of eight men with urinary diversions. The difference in the observed fertility potential is probably attributable to iatrogenic injury of the verumontanum during functional closure. Retrograde ejaculation may also account for the low sperm counts observed following functional bladder closure.

Libido in exstrophy patients is very high (Woodhouse et al., 1983). The erectile mechanism in patients who have undergone epispadias repair appears intact, since 87 per cent of young boys in our series have had witnessed erections following epispadias repair (Lepor et al., 1984).

Pregnancy

Clemetson's (1958) review of the literature identified 45 women with bladder exstrophy who successfully delivered 49 normal offspring. The main complications following pregnancy were cervical and uterine prolapse, which occurred in six of seven women (Krisiloff et al., 1978). Women must be informed of the likelihood of uterine prolapse following pregnancy. Spontaneous vaginal deliveries were performed in women who had undergone prior urinary diversion and cesarean sections were performed in women with functional bladder closures to alleviate stress on the pelvic floor and to avoid traumatic injury to the delicate urinary sphincter mechanism (Krisiloff et al., 1978).

Social Adjustment

Lattimer et al. (1978) assessed the social adjustment of 11 men and 6 women with bladder exstrophy who were more than 17 years of age. Sexual experiences were reported in 12 individuals, marriage in 6, college attendance in 13, and employment in 7. Overall, 13 of the patients were considered well adjusted. A similar review by Woodhouse et al. (1983) observed that 55 of 64 of their bladder exstrophy patients under personal review were strikingly normal and well adjusted.

The objectives of surgical intervention for bladder exstrophy are designed to enable individuals with this disorder to achieve normal social interactions in their community. It is gratifying that great progress toward this goal has been achieved.

CLOACAL EXSTROPHY

Cloacal exstrophy represents one of the most severe congenital anomalies that are compatible with intrauterine viability. Fortunately, the entity is exceedingly rare, occurring in approximately 1 in 200,000 live births (Gravier, 1968). The incidence in males and females is said to be similar (Soper and Kilger, 1965); however, a small personal series of 11 patients indicates a 2:1 male to female ratio. The inheritance pattern of cloacal exstrophy is unknown, since offspring have never been produced from individuals with this disorder.

Anatomically, owing to failure of the urorectal septum to partition the cloaca, there is exstrophy of the foreshortened hindgut or cecum, which displays its bulging mucosa between the two exstrophied hemibladders (Fig. 43–15A and B). The orifices of the terminal ileum, rudimentary tail gut, and a single (or paired) appendix are apparent on the surface of the everted cecum. The tail gut is blind-ending, and the ileum is usually prolapsed. The pubic symphysis is separated, the hips are externally rotated and abducted, and the phallus is separated into a right and left half with adjacent labium or scrotal half. Soper and Kilger (1965) described the anomalies associated with cloacal exstrophy in 57 cases reviewed in the literature. Forty-four of 74 renal units described were abnormal. The specific renal anomalies identified were: absent kidney, 4; hydronephrosis, 6; hydroureter, 11; multicystic kidney, 2; small kidney, 5; ptosis, 13; ureteral atresia, 6; and vascular anomalies, 4. The penis was absent in 8, single in 5, and bifid in 15. The clitoris was absent in 14, single in 1, and bifid in 7. In all genetic males, the testes were present and undescended in 24 of 26 individuals. Owing to the severity of the midline defect, disorders related to nonfusion of the müllerian ducts were frequently seen. The vagina was absent in 6, single in 2, and duplex in 14; the uterus was double in 22 of 23 described cases. In the male, the vas deferens may enter the bladder or distal ureter, an anatomic variant corresponding to a persistent mesonephric duct. Nongenitourinary anomalies were observed in 45 of 57 cases. The anomalies involved the extremities in 10; cardiovascular system in 9; small intestine in 4; ribs in 3; large intestine in 2; and diaphragm in 2. An omphalocele was described in 36 of 41 cases and a myelomeningocele in 24 cases.

Surgical Management

Steinbuchel (1900) described the first reported surgical reconstruction of cloacal exstrophy. The omphalocele was corrected at birth, and the atretic colon was pulled through the perineum; however, the neonate died at the age of 5 days. Until recently, surgical reconstruction of cloacal exstrophy was considered futile and untreated neonates frequently died from prematurity, sepsis, or short bowel syndrome or as a result of their renal and central nervous system deficits. Remigailo et al. (1976) reported the unusual case of an 18-year-old, well-adjusted patient with cloacal exstrophy who had never undergone surgical reconstruction. Rickham (1960) reported the first case of cloacal exstrophy to survive surgical reconstruction. The omphalocele was repaired, the intestinal strip was separated from the hemibladders and closed, and the blind-ending colon was pulled out through the perineum. The hemibladders were then reapproximated. A ureteroileal conduit was constructed at age 18 months, and a cystectomy was subsequently performed. Fecal contin-

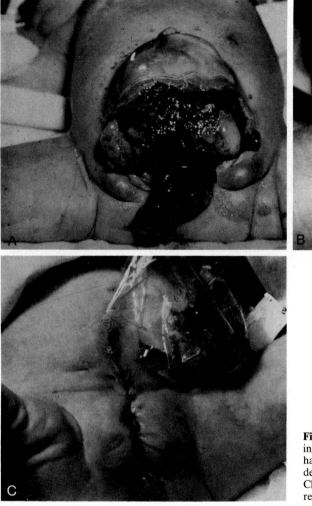

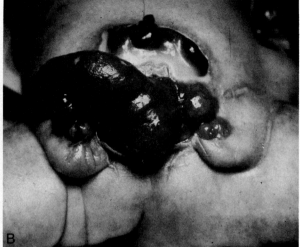

Figure 43–15. Cloacal exstrophy: *A,* Newborn female showing omphalocele, prolapsed ileum, and symmetric bladder halves. *B,* Male patient with similar appearance but also demonstrating orifice of small hindgut and bifid penis. *C,* Closure (patient shown in *B*) to conform to female sex of rearing. Left-sided ileostomy.

ence is rarely, if ever, achieved following perineal pull-through procedures. An alternative approach described by Fonkalsrud and Linde (1970) included terminal ileostomy at birth followed by cystectomy and ileal loop urinary diversion at age 2 years.

We approach reconstruction of cloacal exstrophy in staged surgical procedures (Table 43–7). The child's condition at birth may be critical, and attempts to reconstruct and repair may be futile or morally or ethically unwise. The more robust infant without serious spinal defects will survive, and reparative surgery is initiated at birth. Most individuals with cloacal exstrophy should be reared as females owing to the severe deformity and deficiency of the phallus. At birth the omphalocele is repaired, terminal ileostomy is performed or a colostomy is performed preserving as much of the hindgut as possible, including the rudimentary blind ter-

minal colon (Howell et al., 1983). The exstrophied bladder is closed, the bifid phallus is reapproximated in the midline, and osteotomies are performed when necessary. A gonadectomy is done when sexual reassignment is indicated. Figure 43–15C illustrates a surgical result following first-stage closure of cloacal exstrophy. Bladder closure may be delayed after omphalocele closure and ileostomy to reduce surgical risks in the weaker neonate. Intestinal absorptive problems are usually resolved at approximately 2 to 3 years of age, and the most advantageous type of urinary control can be considered. Urinary continence can be achieved in these individuals following a Young-Dees-Leadbetter bladder neck reconstruction or by tubularizing the bladder into a neourethra and augmenting the bladder capacity by a colocoloplasty as described by Arap (1976) for bladder exstrophy. We have achieved a continence interval of greater than 2

TABLE 43–7. STAGED FUNCTIONAL CLOSURE OF CLOACAL EXSTROPHY

Immediate Neonatal Assessment
  Evaluate associated anomalies
  Decide whether to proceed with reparative surgery
Functional Bladder Closure (immediately after neonatal assessment)
  Bilateral iliac osteotomies
  Gonadectomy in males with a duplicated or an absent penis
  Terminal ileostomy
  Closure of hemibladders
Anti-Incontinence and Anti-reflux Procedures (age 2–3 years)
  Bladder capacity > 50 m: Young-Dees-Leadbetter bladder neck plasty with Cohen ureteral reimplantations and Marshall-Marchetti-Krantz bladder neck suspension
  Bladder capacity < 50 m: Tubularize bladder into a urethrovesical tube. Ureters are reimplanted into a bladder or a bowel segment used to augment bladder capacity.
  Anti-incontinence devices: used for refractory incontinence
Vaginal Reconstruction (age 14–18 years)
  Vagina constructed or augmented using rudimentary colon

hours in four patients following functional closure of cloacal exstrophy. An ileal conduit is performed when there is insufficient bladder tissue available for functional bladder closure. The rudimentary colon is preserved and can be used for additional bowel length, bladder augmentation, or later vaginal reconstruction.

EPISPADIAS

In a combined study, Dees (1949) reported the incidence of complete epispadias to be 1 out of 117,000 males and 1 out of 484,000 females. The reported male to female ratio of epispadias varies between 3:1 (Des, 1949) and 5:1 (Kramer and Kelalis, 1982).

Epispadias in males is classified according to the position of the dorsally displaced urethral meatus. The degree of penile deformity and the occurrence of urinary incontinence are related to the extent of the dorsally displaced urethral meatus. In glandular epispadias, the glans is flattened and split dorsally and the urethral meatus located at the coronal sulcus. In penile epispadias, the urethral meatus is located between the pubic symphysis and coronal sulcus, the glans is splayed, and a dorsal groove extends from the urethral meatus to the glans. A varying amount of dorsal chordee is produced by the shortened urethral plate. In penopubic, or sub-symphyseal, epispadias, the urethral opening is located at the penopubic junction, the entire

penile urethra is opened, and the glans is splayed. The bladder outlet may be large enough to admit the examining finger, indicating obvious gross incompetence. The pubic symphysis is divergent and contributes to the deficiency of the external urinary sphincter. The divergence of the pubic symphysis and the shortened urethral plate result in a prominent dorsal chordee and a penis that appears short. The penile deformity is virtually identical to that seen in bladder exstrophy.

Kramer and Kelalis (1982) have reviewed their surgical experience of 82 males with epispadias. Penopubic epispadias occurred in 49 cases, penile epispadias in 21, and glandular epispadias in 12. Urinary incontinence was observed in 46 of 49 cases of penopubic epispadias, in 15 of 21 cases of penile epispadias, and in no case of glandular epispadias.

Epispadias in the female is characterized by a bifid clitoris, flattening of the mons, and separation of the labia. There are also three degrees of epispadias in females. In the least degree of epispadias, the urethral orifice merely appears patulous; in the intermediate degree of epispadias, the urethra is dorsally split along most of the urethra; and in the most severe degree of epispadias, the urethral cleft involves the entire length of the urethra and the sphincter mechanism is rendered incompetent.

The anomalies associated with complete epispadias are usually confined to deformities of the external genitalia, diastasis of the pubic symphysis, and deficiency of the urinary continence mechanism. The only renal anomaly observed in 11 cases of complete epispadias was the congenital absence of the left kidney (Campbell, 1952). The ureterovesical junction is inherently deficient and reflux occurs in 75 per cent of individuals with any degree of epispadias, the incidence being greater in cases of complete epispadias (Ambrose and O'Brien, 1974).

Surgical Management of Epispadias

The surgical objectives for penopubic epispadias include achievement of urinary continence with preservation of the upper urinary tract and reconstruction of functional and cosmetically acceptable genitalia. The surgical management of penopubic epispadias is virtually identical to that of closed bladder exstrophy.

Young (1922) reported the first cure of incontinence in a male with complete epispadias. A Young-Dees-Leadbetter bladder neck reconstruction is currently the preferred technique for reconstructing the bladder neck. Tanagho and Smith (1972) raise a pedicled flap of anterior bladder wall, based upward, that is formed into a tube.

The achievement of urinary continence following bladder neck reconstruction in patients with epispadias is summarized in Table 43–8 (Campbell, 1952; Gross and Cresson, 1952b; Burkholder and Williams, 1965; Dees, 1949; Kramer and Kelalis, 1982). The majority of these disorders were reconstructed by means of a Young-Dees-Leadbetter bladder neck plasty. Urinary continence was achieved in 65 per cent of males and 72 per cent of females following bladder neck reconstruction. Urinary diversion should not be considered in the initial management in complete epispadias.

Delayed achievement of urinary continence occurred in more than half the males with complete epispadias who eventually became continent following vesicoplasty (Kramer and Kelalis, 1982). The effect that urethral lengthening and prostatic enlargement have on increasing bladder outlet resistance is emphasized by these observations.

Reconstruction of glandular epispadias is simple and includes reapproximation of the splayed glans. Penile epispadias is usually repaired in one stage, which includes release of the dorsal chordee and urethroplasty. The ven-

tral prepuce is a potential source of additional skin coverage.

Techniques for genital reconstruction in males with bladder exstrophy and complete epispadias are virtually identical. Cantwell (1895) constructed the urethra in epispadias by completely mobilizing and tubularizing the dorsal penile skin and transplanting this urethral tube ventrally through the separated corpora. The dorsal skin defect was covered with lateral skin flaps. Young (1922) attributed the high fistula rate following the Cantwell urethroplasty to excessive mobilization of the urethra and recommended less mobilization during construction of the urethral tube. The Denis Browne technique of urethral regeneration was applied to epispadias repair by Michalowski and Modelski (1963).

Mays (1972) described a single-stage repair of epispadias. Release of the dorsal chordee and penile lengthening were performed by resecting the intercavernosal tissue and incising the suspensory ligaments. The prepuce was developed into a single layered epithelial flap, which was tubularized and then turned inward and anastomosed to the proximal urethra.

Khana (1973) repaired epispadias in three stages. In the first stage the dorsal curvature was corrected by mobilizing the entire urethral mucosa from the corpora cavernosa, dividing the bands of fibrous tissue, and covering the dorsum of the penis with a reversed Nesbit

TABLE 43–8. Urinary Continence Following Bladder Neck Reconstruction in Patients with Complete Epispadias

	Kramer and Kelalis (1982)	Campbell (1952)	Gross and Cresson (1952)	Burkholder and Williams (1965)	Dees (1949)	Total
Total patients with complete epispadias	53	11	12	27	6	109
Number of males with complete epispadias treated with BNR*	32†	3	8	17	5	65
Number of males with surgically corrected incontinence	22	1	6	8	5	45
Percentage of males with surgically corrected incontinence	69	33	75	47	100	65
Number of females with complete epispadias treated with BNR	8	7	3	10	1	29
Number of females with surgically corrected incontinence	7	5	1	7	1	21
Percentage of females with surgically corrected incontinence	88	71	33	70	100	72

*BNR = Bladder neck reconstruction.
†Male patients with penopubic epispadias and total incontinence included.

preputial flap. A dorsal strip was tubularized in the second stage, and the penis was covered using a bipedicled flap of scrotal skin. The penis was detached from the scrotum in the third stage of the repair.

The management of complete epispadias at our institution is virtually identical to that of a closed bladder exstrophy. Osteotomies are routinely not performed, since a firm intersymphyseal band bridges the divergent symphysis. A Young-Dees-Leadbetter bladder neck plasty, Marshall-Marchetti-Krantz bladder neck suspension, and Cohen ureteral reimplantations are performed when the bladder capacity reaches approximately 50 ml, which usually occurs by 3 years of age. Penile lengthening, release of the dorsal chordee, and a modified Young urethroplasty may be performed at the time of the anti-incontinence procedure, or preparation may be made for completion at a later stage. If penile skin is unavailable for tubularization into a neourethra, the urethra is constructed from a preputial free graft (Devine et al., 1980) or preputial pedicle graft similar to that used in hypospadias (Duckett, 1981).

The results following bladder neck reconstruction for complete epispadias are summarized in Table 43–8. Kramer and Kelalis (1982) have reviewed their experience following urethroplasty for epispadias. A Thiersch-Duplay procedure (modified Young urethroplasty) was selected in 49 of 67 cases (73 per cent), and various other reconstruction techniques were used in the remaining 18 cases. Urethral fistulas requiring surgical repair occurred in 21 per cent of these urethroplasties. A carefully considered and well-planned approach to the management of urinary incontinence and genital deformity associated with complete epispadias should provide gratifying results.

URACHAL ANOMALIES

ANATOMY AND HISTOLOGY

The urachus lies between the peritoneum and transversalis fascia and extends from the anterior dome of the bladder toward the umbilicus (Fig. 43–16). The urachus is encased between two layers of umbilicovesical fascia, which tend to contain the spread of urachal disease. The urachus is adjacent to the umbilical ligaments, the remnants of the umbilical arteries. When the urachus is present as a muscular tube, three distinct tissue layers are recognized: an epithelial canal of cuboidal or, more typically, transitional epithelium; a submucosal connective tissue layer; and an outer smooth muscle layer, thickest near the bladder. The central lumen is irregular and beaded, averaging 1 mm in diameter, and is plugged in areas with desquamated epithelial debris and epithelial islands. Where the upper urachus becomes a fibrous cord, there are generally no recognizable urachal elements (Begg, 1927; Hammond et al., 1941; Hector, 1961; Steck and Helwig, 1965).

EMBRYOLOGY

The allantois is an extraembryonic cavity located within the body stalk that projects onto the anterior surface of the cloaca, the future bladder. The descent of the bladder into the pelvis is associated with elongation of the urachus, a tubular structure that extends from the fibrotic allantois to the anterior bladder. During the fourth and fifth months of gestation, the urachus narrows to a small-caliber epithelial tube (Nix et al., 1958). Hammond et al. (1941) observed that continuity of the urachus with the posterior surface of the umbilicus and the apex of the bladder persisted in 50 per cent of fetal specimens. This tract subsequently obliterates, since patency was observed in only 2 per cent of adult specimens. The obliteration of the urachus results in different patterns of urachal termination: A well-defined urachal remnant may maintain an identifiable attachment to the umbilicus; at a variable distance above the bladder the urachal cord may merge with one or both of the obliterated umbilical arteries, resulting in a single common ligament to the umbilicus; or an atrophic extension from a short, tubular urachus may terminate within the fascia or blend into a plexus of fibrous tissue (the plexus of Luschka), formed by the urachus and umbilical arteries (Blichert-Toft and Nielson, 1971b; Hammond et al., 1941).

BENIGN DISORDERS OF THE URACHUS

Patent Urachus

Congenital patent urachus is a lesion that is usually recognized in the neonate. It is a rare anomaly, occurring in only 3 of more than 1

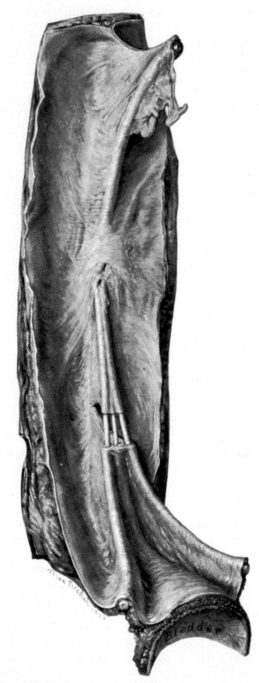

Figure 43–16. Posterior view of the umbilical region of the anterior abdominal wall, showing the relation of the urachus to the umbilical ligaments, peritoneum, and bladder dome. The urachus does not extend fully to the umbilicus. (The ligamentum teres is seen superior to the umbilicus.) (From Cullen, T. S.: Embryology, Anatomy and Diseases of the Umbilicus. Philadelphia, W. B. Saunders Co., 1916.)

million admissions to a large pediatric center (Nix et al., 1958). Two forms of congenital patent urachus are persistence of the patent urachus with a partially descended bladder; and

a vesicoumbilical fistula representing failure of the bladder to descend at all (Fig. 43–17). In the latter form, the bladder apex never forms a true urachal tract. The more common form of patent urachus results from the failure of obliteration of the urachal lumen. Persistence of the urachus has been attributed to intrauterine urinary obstruction; however, only 14 per cent of neonates born with a patent urachus have evidence of urinary obstruction (Herbst, 1937). It is unlikely that urinary obstruction is directly related to the development of a patent urachus, since the most severe cases of posterior urethral valves are not associated with this anomaly. Furthermore, urethral tubularization occurs after obliteration of the urachal lumen, suggesting that urinary obstruction is not the major factor producing the patent urachus (Schreck and Campbell, 1972).

Acquired patent urachus in the adult is usually a urinary umbilical fistula that results from bladder outflow obstruction. In these cases, the extravasation of infected urine into the periurachal space ultimately may result in erosion through the umbilical region, a relatively weak segment of the abdominal wall. Since the urachus can remain attached to the umbilicus in a minority of normal adults, at least some acquired umbilical urinary fistulas may drain through the existing urachal canal.

Patent urachus is readily diagnosed when there is free discharge of urine through the umbilicus. Patent urachus should be suspected when the umbilical cord is enlarged and edematous or when its normal slough is delayed. On occasion, the fistula is tiny and the discharge of urine may be minimal or intermittent.

The diagnosis of patent urachus is confirmed by catheterization or probing of the urachal tract, intravesical instillation of colored dye, and analysis of the discharged fluid for BUN and creatinine. Voiding cystourethrography is helpful in fully evaluating the lesion and any associated bladder outlet obstruction. Fistulography distinguishes the condition from a patent omphalomesenteric duct. Although cystoscopy is essential in the older patient, it is not necessary in the neonate, providing the urethra appears radiographically normal.

The differential diagnosis of a wet umbilicus in the infant includes patent urachus, omphalitis (an infection of the umbilical stump), simple granulation of the healing stump, a patent vitelline or omphalomesenteric duct (enteroumbilical fistula), an infected umbilical vessel, and an external urachal sinus. The presence of both urinary and enteric fistulas at the umbilicus is exceedingly rare (Davis and Nikhaus, 1926;

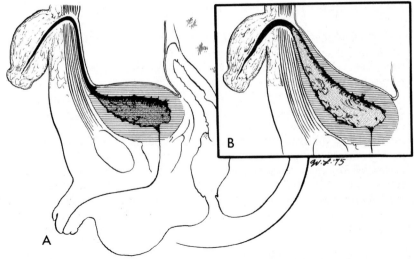

Figure 43–17. Forms of patent urachus. Note hydrops of the umbilical cord. *A,* Typical patent urachus. *B,* Vesicoumbilical fistula. (From Perlmutter, A. D.: Urachal anomalies. *In* Harrison, J. H., et al. (Eds.): Campbell's Urology. Philadelphia, W. B. Saunders Co., 1979.)

Herbst, 1937; Kenigsberg, 1975; Mendoza et al., 1968; Steck and Helwig, 1965).

Urachal Cyst

A cyst may form within the isolated urachal canal if the lumen enlarges from epithelial desquamation and degeneration. The tiny connection frequently present between the tract and the bladder may permit bacterial infection that seals the tract and remains loculated (Fig. 43–18*A*). Infected cysts occur most commonly in adults (Blichert-Toft and Nielson, 1971*b*; Sterling and Goldsmith, 1953); however, they have been reported in infants (Geist, 1952; Hinman, 1961). The cyst frequently manifests itself because infection has developed. The most common recoverable organism cultured in the cyst fluid is *Staphylococcus aureus* (MacMillan et al., 1973; Tauber and Bloom, 1951). Untreated, the infected cyst may drain into the bladder or through the umbilicus or may drain intermittently internally and externally, resulting in an "alternating sinus" (Sterling and Goldsmith, 1953; Hinman, 1961; Neidhardt et al., 1968; Blichert-Toft and Nielson, 1971*a*).

Serious complications of infected umbilical cysts include rupture into the preperitoneal tissues, rupture into the free peritoneal cavity with secondary peritonitis, and, rarely, inflammatory involvement of adjacent bowel with the formation of enteric fistulas (Nunn, 1952).

The symptoms and signs of a loculated, infected urachal cyst are lower abdominal pain, fever, voiding symptoms, midline hypogastric tenderness, often a palpable mass, and evidence of urinary infection. A urachal cyst should be suspected whenever localized suprapubic pain and tenderness are present with disturbed micturition, even when the urine remains clear. Useful diagnostic studies include excretory urography, cystography, cystoscopy, and B-scan ultrasound (Sanders et al., 1974).

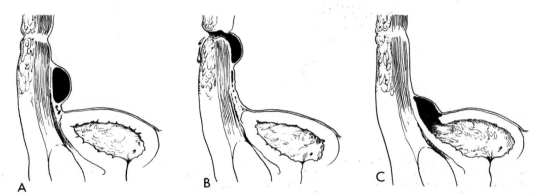

Figure 43–18. *A,* Urachal cyst. *B,* External urachal sinus. *C,* Urachal diverticulum. (From Perlmutter, A. D.: Urachal anomalies. *In* Harrison, J. H., et al. (Eds.): Campbell's Urology. Philadelphia, W. B. Saunders Co., 1979.)

External Urachal Sinus

Persistence of the urachal apex alone will result in a blind external sinus that opens at the umbilicus (Fig. 43–18B). This may become symptomatic at any age with an infected discharge. In the adult, umbilical pilonidal disease can mimic an external sinus (Steck and Helwig, 1965). Because the differential diagnosis also includes lesions listed in the previous section, probing and radiographic evaluation should be undertaken before surgery. A urachal sinus extends inferiorly, unlike an omphalomesenteric duct remnant, which extends inward toward the peritoneal cavity.

Urachal Diverticulum

A diverticulum of the bladder apex (Fig. 43–18C), or "blind internal sinus," may be an incidental finding on radiographic studies, not requiring treatment when small and minimally contractile. The large urachal divericula, typically seen with prune-belly syndrome (Lattimer, 1958) and occasionally associated with severe urethral obstruction will require resection. These may be poorly contractile or may expand paradoxically during voiding. Narrow neck urethral diverticula occasionally contain calculi (Bandler et al., 1942; Ney and Friedenberg, 1968).

TREATMENT

Adequate therapy for a patent urachus requires excision of all anomalous tissue with a cuff of bladder. Simple ligation or cauterization of a patent urachus is inadequate, as the tract is likely to recur. Similarly, simple drainage of a urachal cyst is associated with recurrent infection in 30 per cent of cases, and late occurrence of adenocarcinoma has been reported (Blichert-Toft and Nielson, 1971a).

In treatment of benign urachal lesions in children, it is rarely necessary to remove the umbilicus; whenever possible, cosmetic considerations should prevail. In infants, a small, curved, subumbilical incision is ample, for at this age the bladder dome is still high and readily accessible through this exposure.

A transverse midhypogastric incision is adequate exposure in older children and adults and allows for both superior and inferior dissection. Surgical management of umbilical anomalies is illustrated in Figure 43–19. The urachal stalk or fibrous urachal remnant should be detached from the dermis posterior to the umbilicus. A "buttonhole" in the umbilical skin is of

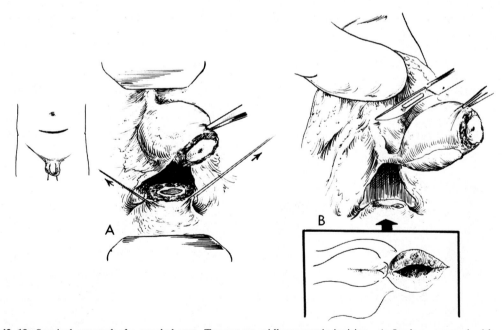

Figure 43–19. Surgical removal of a urachal cyst. Transverse midhypogastric incision. *A,* Lesion removed with a cuff of the bladder apex. *B,* Urachal stalk detached from the posterior umbilicus. A cuff of adherent peritoneum is excised with the specimen. (From Perlmutter, A. D.: Urachal anomalies. *In* Harrison, J. H., et al. (Eds.): Campbell's Urology. Philadelphia, W. B. Saunders Co., 1979.)

no consequence. Application of a small gauze pledget under the dressing obliterates dead space, maintains umbilical configuration, and allows the skin defect to close secondarily.

When peritoneum and umbilical ligaments are adherent to the inflammatory mass, these structures should be excised in continuity with the lesion. A vertical midline incision is the best approach for removal of an extensive inflammatory mass. Elliptical excision of the umbilicus may be necessary if it is involved in the inflammatory process, especially with an external urachal sinus or alternating sinus. A suppurating infection within a cyst or external sinus may require initial incision and drainage, and treatment as for an abscess. After healing is complete, an internal excision of urachal tissue should be done.

References

Exstrophy-Epispadias Complex

Ambrose, S. S., and O'Brien, D. P.: Surgical embryology of the exstrophy-epispadias complex. Surg. Clin. North Am., *54*:1379, 1974.

Ansell, J. E.: Exstrophy and epispadias. *In* Glenn, J. F. (Ed.): Urologic Surgery. Philadelphia, J. B. Lippincott Co., 1983, p. 647.

Arap, S., Giron, A., and Degoes, G. M.: Complete reconstruction of bladder exstrophy. Urology, *7*:413, 1976.

Bennett, A. H.: Exstrophy of the bladder treated by ureterosigmoidostomies. Urology, *2*:165, 1973.

Boyce, W. H.: A new concept concerning treatment of exstrophy of the bladder 20 years later. J. Urol., *107*:476, 1972.

Boyce, W. H., and Vest, S. A.: A new concept concerning treatment of exstrophy of the bladder. J. Urol., *67*:503, 1952.

Burkholder, G. V., and Williams, D. I.: Epispadias and incontinence: Surgical treatment of 27 children. J. Urol., *94*:674, 1965.

Campbell, M.: Epispadias: A report of fifteen cases. J. Urol., *67*:988, 1952.

Cantwell, F. V.: Operative technique of epispadias by transplantation of the urethra. Ann. Surg., *22*:689, 1895.

Chisholm, T. C.: Pediatric Surgery. Vol. 2. Chicago, Year Book Medical Publishers, 1962, p. 933.

Chisholm, T. C.: Exstrophy of the urinary bladder. *In* Kiesewetter, W. B. (Ed.): Long-Term Follow-up in Congenital Anomalies Pediatric Surgical Symposium. Vol. 6, p. 31. Pittsburgh, Pittsburgh Children's Hospital, 1979.

Clark, M., and O'Connell, K. J.: Scanning and transmission electron microscopic studies of an exstrophic human bladder. J. Urol., *110*:481, 1973.

Clemetson, C. A. B.: Ectopia vesicae and split pelvis. J. Obstet. Gynaecol. Br. Commonw., *65*:973, 1958.

Coffey, R. C.: Transplantation of the ureter into the large intestine in the absence of a functioning bladder. Surg. Gynecol. Obstet., *32*:383, 1921.

Cohen, S. J.: Ureterozysloneostomie eine neue Antirefluxtechnik. Aktuel. Urol., *6*:24, 1975.

Cracchiolo, A., III, and Hall, C. B.: Bilateral iliac osteotomy. Clin Orthop. Rel. Res., *68*:156, 1970.

Culp, D. A.: The histology of the exstrophied bladder. J. Urol., *91*:538, 1964.

Dees, J. E.: Congenital epispadias with incontinence. J. Urol., *62*:513, 1949.

Devine, C. J., Jr., Horton, C. E., and Scarff, J. E., Jr.: Epispadias: Symposium on pediatric urology. Urol. Clin. North Am., 7:465, 1980.

Dixon, C. F., and Weisman, R. E.: Polyps of the sigmoid occurring 30 years after bilateral ureterosigmoidostomies for exstrophy of the bladder. Surgery, *24*:6, 1948.

Duckett, J. W.: Use of paraexstrophy skin pedicle grafts for correction of exstrophy and epispadias repair. Birth Defects, *13*:171, 1977.

Duckett, J. W.: Epispadias. Symposium on congenital anomalies of the lower genitourinary tract. Urol. Clin. North Am., 5:107, 1978.

Duckett, J. W.: The island flap technique for hypospadias repair. Urol. Clin. North Am., 8:503, 1981.

Engel, R. M.: Bladder exstrophy: Vesicoplasty or urinary diversion. Urology, *2*:29, 1973.

Engel, R. M., and Wilkinson, H. A.: Bladder exstrophy. J. Urol., *104*:699, 1970.

Ezwell, W. W., and Carlson, H. E.: A realistic look at exstrophy of the bladder. Br. J. Urol., *42*:197, 1970.

Feinberg, T., Lattimer, J. K., Jetir, K., and Langford, W.: Questions that worry children with exstrophy. Pediatrics, *53*:242, 1974.

Fonkalsrud, E. C., and Linde, L. M.: Successful management of vesicointestinal fissure: Report of 2 cases. J. Pediatr. Surg., *5*:309, 1970.

Gravier, L.: Exstrophy of the cloaca. Am. Surg., *34*:387, 1968.

Gross, R. E., and Cresson, S. L.: Exstrophy of the bladder: Observations from eighty cases. JAMA, *149*:1640, 1952*a*.

Gross, R. E., and Cresson, S. L.: Treatment of epispadias: A report of 18 cases. J. Urol., *68*:477, 1952*b*.

Haller, J. A., Jr.: Pediatric surgery. *In* Schwartz, S. I., Lillehei, R. C., Shires, G. T., Spencer, F. C., and Starer, E. H. (Eds.): Surgery. New York, McGraw-Hill Book Co., 1974, p. 1513.

Hanna, M. K.: Artificial urinary sphincter for incontinent children. Urology, *18*:370, 1981.

Hanna, M. K., and Williams, D. J.: Genital function in males with vesical exstrophy and epispadias. Br. J. Urol., *44*:1969, 1972.

Harvard, B. M., and Thompson, G. J.: Congenital exstrophy of the urinary bladder: Late results of treatment by the Coffey-Mayo method of uretero-intestinal anastomosis. J. Urol., *65*:223, 1951.

Heitz-Boyer, M., and Hovelaque, A.: Creation d'une nouvelle vessie et d'une nouvelle uretre. J. Urol., *1*:237, 1912.

Hendren, W. H.: Exstrophy of the bladder: An alternative method of management. J. Urol., *115*:195, 1976.

Hendren, W. H.: Penile lengthening after previous repair of epispadias. J. Urol., *12*:527, 1979.

Higgins, C. C.: Exstrophy of the bladder: Report of 158 cases. Am. Surg., *28*:99, 1962.

Hinman, F., Jr.: A method of lengthening and repairing the penis in exstrophy of the bladder. J. Urol., *79*:237, 1958.

Howell, C., Caldamone, A., Snyder, H., Ziegler, M., and Duckett, J.: Optimal management of cloacal exstrophy. J. Pediatr. Surg., *18*:365, 1983.

Ives, E., Coffey, R., and Carter, C. O.: A family study of bladder exstrophy. J. Med. Genet., *17*:139, 1980.

Jeffs, R. D.: Exstrophy. *In* Harrison, J. H., Gittes, R. F., Perlmutter, A. D., Stamey, T. A., and Walsh, P. C. (Eds.): Campbell's Textbook of Urology. Philadelphia, W. B. Saunders Co., 1979, p. 1672.

Jeffs, R. D.: Exstrophy and cloacal exstrophy. Symposium on Congenital abnormalities of the lower genitourinary tract. Urol. Clin. North Am., *5*:127, 1978.

Jeffs, R. D., and Schwarz, G. R.: Ileal conduit urinary diversion in children: Computer analysis followup from 2 to 16 years. J. Urol., *114*:285, 1975.

Jeffs, R. D., Charrios, R., Many, M., and Juriansz, A. R.: Primary closure of the exstrophied bladder. *In* Scott, R. (Ed.): Current Controversies in Urologic Management. Philadelphia, W. B. Saunders Co., 1972, p. 235.

Jeffs, R. D., Guice, S. L., and Oesch, I.: The factors in successful exstrophy closure. J. Urol., *127*:974, 1982.

Johnston, J. H.: Lengthening of the congenital or acquired short penis. Br. J. Urol., *46*:685, 1974.

Johnston, J. H.: The genital aspects of exstrophy. J. Urol., *113*:701, 1975.

Johnston, J. H., and Kogan, S. J.: The exstrophic anomalies and their surgical reconstruction. Curr. Probl. Surg., August 1974, pp. 1–39.

Kandzari, S. J., Majid, A., Ortega, A. M., and Milam, D. F.: Exstrophy of the urinary bladder complicated by adenocarcinoma. Urology, *3*:496, 1974.

Kelly, J. H., and Eraklis, A. J.: A procedure for lengthening the phallus in boys with exstrophy of the bladder. J. Pediatr. Surg., *6*:165, 1971.

Khana, N. N.: A technique for epispadias repair. Plast. Reconstr. Surg., *52*:365, 1973.

Kramer, S. A., and Kelalis, P.: Assessment of urinary continence in epispadias: A review of 94 patients. J. Urol., *128*:290, 1982.

Krisiloff, M., Puchner, P. J., Tretter, W., MacFarlane, M. T., and Lattimer, J. K.: Pregnancy in women with bladder exstrophy. J. Urol., *119*:478, 1978.

Lattimer, J. K., and Smith, M. J. K.: Exstrophy closure: A followup on 70 cases. J. Urol., *95*:356, 1966*a*.

Lattimer, J. K., and Smith, M. J. K.: The management of bladder exstrophy. Surg. Gynecol. Obstet., *123*:1015, 1966*b*.

Lattimer, J. K., Beck, L., Yeaw, S., Puchner, P. J., MacFarlane, M. T., and Krisiloff, M.: Long-term followup after exstrophy closure—Late improvement and good quality of life. J. Urol., *119*:664, 1978.

Lattimer, J. K., Hensle, T. W., MacFarlane, M. T., Beck, L., Braun, E., and Esposito, X.: The exstrophy support team: A new concept in the care of the exstrophy patient. J. Urol., *121*:472, 1979.

Leadbetter, G. W., Jr.: Surgical correction of total urinary incontinence. J. Urol., *91*:261, 1964.

Leadbetter, W. F.: Consideration of problems incident to performance of uretero-enterostomy. Report of a technique. J. Urol., *73*:67, 1955.

Lepor, H., and Jeffs, R. D.: Primary bladder closure and bladder neck reconstruction in classical bladder exstrophy. J. Urol., *130*:1142, 1983.

Lepor, H., and Kuhar, M. J.: Characterization of muscarinic cholinergic receptor in genitourinary tissues of the rabbit. J. Urol., *132*:392, 1984.

Lepor, H., Shapiro, E., and Jeffs, R. D.: Urethral reconstruction in males with classical bladder exstrophy. J. Urol., *131*:512, 1984.

Lowe, F. C., and Jeffs, R. D.: Wound dehiscence in bladder exstrophy: An examination of the etiologies and factors for initial failure and subsequent closure. J. Urol., *130*:312, 1983.

MacFarlane, M. T., Lattimer, J. K., and Hensle, T. W.: Improved life expectancy for children with exstrophy of the bladder. JAMA, *242*:442, 1979.

Marchioro, T. L., and Tremann, J. A.: Ureteroileostomy in renal transplant patients. Urology, *3*:171, 1974.

Marshall, V. F., and Muecke, E. C.: Congenital abnormalities of the bladder. *In* Handbuch de Urologie, New York, Springer-Verlag, 1968, p. 165.

Marshall, V. F., and Muecke, E. C.: Functional closure of typical exstrophy of the bladder. J. Urol., *104*:205, 1970.

Marshall, V. F., Marchetti, A. A., and Krantz, K. E.: The correction of stress incontinence by simple vesicourethral suspension. Surg. Gynecol. Obstet., *88*:509, 1949.

Maydl, K.: Uber die radikaltherapie der ectopia vesical urinariae. Wien Med. Wochenschr., *25*:1113–1115, 1169–1172, 1209–1210, 1256–1258, 1297–1301, 1894.

Mayo, C. H., and Hendricks, W. A.: Exstrophy of the bladder. Surg. Gynecol. Obstet., *43*:129, 1926.

Mays, H. B.: Epispadias: A plan of treatment. J. Urol., *107*:251, 1972.

Michalowski, E., and Modelski, M.: The surgical treatment of epispadias. Surg. Gynecol. Obstet., *117*:476, 1963.

Mollard, P.: Bladder reconstruction in exstrophy. J. Urol., *124*:523, 1980.

Mostofi, R. K.: Potentialities of bladder epithelium. J. Urol., *71*:705, 1954.

Muecke, E. C.: The role of the cloacal membrane in exstrophy: The first successful experimental study. J. Urol., *92*:659, 1964.

Nisonson, I., and Lattimer, J. K.: How well can the exstrophied bladder work? J. Urol., *107*:668, 1972.

Perez Castro, E., and Martinez-Pineiro, J. A.: Enterotrigono urethroplasty—Surgical technique for correction of bladder exstrophy. Urol. Int., *23*:158, 1968.

Ransley, P. G.: Personal communication, 1984.

Remigailo, R. V., Woodard, J. R., Andrews, H. G., and Patterson, J. H.: Cloacal exstrophy: 18 year survival of an untreated case. J. Urol., *116*:811, 1976.

Rickham, P. P.: Vesico-intestinal fissure. Arch. Dis. Child., *35*:97, 1960.

Rickham, P. P.: The incidence and treatment of ectopia vesicae. Proc. R. Soc. Med., *54*:389, 1961.

Schultz, W. G.: Plastic repair of exstrophy of the bladder combined with bilateral osteotomy of the ilia. J. Urol., *92*:659, 1964.

Scott, F. B., Bradley, W. E., and Timm, G. W.: Treatment of urinary incontinence by an implantable prosthetic urinary sphincter. J. Urol., *12*:75, 1974.

Semerdjian, H. S., Texter, J. H., and Yawn, D. H.: Rhabdomyosarcoma occurring in repaired exstrophic bladder: Case report. J. Urol., *108*:354, 1972.

Shapiro, E., Jeffs, R. D., and Lepor, H.: Muscarinic cholinergic receptors in closed exstrophied bladders. In press.

Shapiro, E., Lepor, H., and Jeffs, R. D.: The inheritance of classical bladder exstrophy. J. Urol., *132*:308, 1984.

Shapiro, S. R., Lebowitz, R., and Colodny, A. H.: Fate of 90 children with ileal conduit urinary diversion a decade later. J. Urol., *114*:133, 1975.

Simon, J.: Ectopia vesicae. Lancet, *2*:568, 1852.

Sooriyaarchchi, G. S., Johnson, R. O., and Carbone, P. P.: Neoplasms of the large bowel following ureterosigmoidostomy. Arch. Surg., *112*:1174, 1979.

Soper, R. T., and Kilger, K.: Vessico-intestinal fissure. J. Urol., *92*:490, 1965.

Spees, E., Marshall, F., Lepor, H., Shapiro, E., Mostofi, F., and Jeffs, R. D.: Successful renal transplantation in closed bladder exstrophy. (AUA Seventy-ninth Annual Meeting Abstracts). J. Urol., *131*:935, 1984.

Spence, H. M., Hoffman, W. W., and Fosmire, P. P.: Tumors of the colon as a later complication of ureterosigmoidostomy of exstrophy of the bladder. Br. J. Urol., 51:466, 1979.

Spence, H. M., Hoffman, W. N., and Pate, V. A.: Exstrophy of the bladder: Long term results in a series of 37 cases treated by ureterosigmoidostomy. J. Urol., 114:133, 1975.

Steinbuchel: Ueber nabelschnurbruch und blasenbauchspalte mit clodken bildung von seiten des dunndormes. Arch. Gynaeckol., 60:465, 1900.

Sweetser, T. H., Chisholm, T. C., and Thompson, W. H.: Exstrophy of the urinary bladder: Discussion of anatomic principles applicable to its repair with a preliminary report of a case. Minn. Med., 35:654, 1952.

Taccinoli, M., Laurenti, C., and Racheli, T.: Sixteen years experience with the Heitz-Boyer Hovelacque procedure for exstrophy of the bladder. Br. J. Urol., 49:385, 1977.

Tanagho, E. A., and Smith, D. R.: Clinical evaluation of a surgical technique for the correction of complete urinary incontinence. J. Urol., 107:402, 1972.

Thiersch, C.: Ueber die ensstehuns weise und operative behandlung der epispadie. Arch. Heilkunde, 10:20, 1869.

Toguri, A. G., Churchill, B. M., Schillinger, J. F., and Jeffs, R. D.: Gas cystometry in cases of continent bladder exstrophy. J. Urol., 119:536, 1978a.

Toguri, A. G., Churchill, B. M., Schillinger, J. F., and Jeffs, R. D.: Continence in cases of bladder exstrophy. J. Urol., 119:538, 1978b.

Trendelenburg, R.: The treatment of ectopia vesicae. Ann. Surg., 44:281, 1906.

Walsh, P. C., and Donker, P. J.: Impotence following radical prostatectomy: Insight into etiology and prevention. J. Urol., 128:492, 1982.

Williams, D. I.: Urology in clinical childhood. In Handbuch der Urologie. New York, Springer-Verlag, 1974, p. 268.

Woodhouse, C. R. J., Ransley, P. C., and Williams, D. I.: The exstrophy patient in adult life. Br. J. Urol., 55:632, 1983.

Young, H. H.: An operation for the cure of incontinence associated with exstrophy. J. Urol., 7:1, 1922.

Young, H. H.: Exstrophy of the bladder: The first case in which a normal bladder and urinary control have been obtained by plastic operation. Surg. Gynecol. Obstet., 74:729, 1942.

Urachal Anomalies

Bandler, C. G., Milbed, A. H., and Alley, J. L.: Urachal calculus. N.Y. State J. Med., 42:2203, 1942.

Begg, R. C.: The urachus and umbilical fistulae. J. Anat., 64:170, 1927.

Blichert-Toft, M., and Nielson, O. V.: Diseases of the urachus simulating intra-abdominal disorders. Am. J. Surg., 112:123, 1971a.

Blichert-Toft, M., and Nielson, O. V.: Congenital patent urachus and acquired variants. Acta Chir. Scand., 137:807, 1971b.

Davis, H. H., and Nikhaus, F. W.: Persistent omphalomesenteric duct and urachus in the same case. JAMA, 86:685, 1926.

Geist, D.: Patent urachus. Am. J. Surg., 84:118, 1952.

Hammond, G., Yglesias, L., and Davis, J. E.: The urachus, its anatomy and associated fasciae. Anat. Rec., 80:271, 1941.

Hector, A.: Les vestiges de l'ouraque et leur pathologie. J. Chir. (Paris), 81:449, 1961.

Herbst, W. P.: Patent urachus. South. Med. J., 30:711, 1937.

Hinman, F., Jr.: Surgical disorders of the bladder and umbilicus of urachal origin. Surg. Gynecol. Obstet., 113:605, 1961.

Kenigsberg, K.: Infection of umbilical artery simulating patent urachus. J. Pediatr., 86:151, 1975.

Lattimer, J. K.: Congenital deficiency of the abdominal musculature and associated genitourinary anomalies: A report of 22 cases. J. Urol., 79:343, 1958.

MacMillan, R. W., Schullinger, J. N., and Santulli, V. T.: Pyourachus: An unusual surgical problem. J. Pediatr. Surg., 8:87, 1973.

Mendoza, C. B., Jr., Cueto, J., Payan, H., and Gerwig, W. H., Jr.: Complete urachal tract associates with Meckel's diverticulum. Arch. Surg., 96:438, 1968.

Neidhardt, J. H., Morin, A., Spay, G., Guelpa, G., and Chavvier, J.: Mise au point sur les kystes suppures de l'ouraque. J. Urol. Nephrol. (Paris), 74:793, 1968.

Ney, C., and Friedenberg, R. M.: Radiographic findings in the anomalies of the urachus. J. Urol., 99:288, 1968.

Nix, J. T., Menville, J. G., Albert, M., and Wendt, D. L.: Congenital patent urachus. J. Urol., 79:264, 1958.

Nunn, L. L.: Urachal cysts and their complications. Am. J. Surg., 84:252, 1952.

Sanders, R. C., Oh, K. S., and Dorst, J. P.: B-scan ultrasound: Positive and negative contrast material of congenital urachal anomaly. Am. J. Roentgenol., 120:448, 1974.

Schreck, W. R., and Campbell, W. A.: The relationship of bladder outlet obstruction to urinary umbilical fistula. J. Urol., 108:641, 1972.

Steck, W. D., and Helwig, E. B.: Umbilical granulomas, pilonidal disease, and the urachus. Surg. Gynecol. Obstet., 120:1043, 1965.

Sterling, J. A., and Goldsmith, R.: Lesions of urachus which appear in the adult. Ann. Surg., 137:120, 1953.

Tauber, J., and Bloom, B.: Infected urachal cyst. J. Urol., 66:692, 1951.

CHAPTER 44

Imperforate Anus, Persistent Cloaca, and Urogenital Sinus Outlet Obstruction

ERNEST H. AGATSTEIN, M.D.
RICHARD M. EHRLICH, M.D.

In practically every case, the future of a child so unfortunate as to be born with an imperforate anus is determined by the adequacy and skill of the first operation.

Willis Potts

Although congenital malformations of the anus, rectum, and urogenital sinus are seen commonly by pediatric surgeons, the urologist plays a crucial role in the diagnostic and therapeutic management of these complex and challenging clinical problems. Appropriate surgical management depends upon an understanding of normal and abnormal embryology, an ability to classify these disorders and associated clinical problems, and the application of diagnostic studies to determine the exact pathology. Prospects for superior long-term results are enhanced by the proper timing and choice of therapeutic options.

NORMAL EMBRYOLOGY

While a complete review of urogenital embryology is beyond the purview of this chapter, some salient points require emphasis. At 4 weeks (4 mm stage of gestation) the developing urogenital and digestive tracts empty into a common channel, the cloaca. This is followed promptly by downgrowth of mesoderm—the urorectal septum—dividing the cloaca into ventral and dorsal parts. The ventral part becomes the urogenital sinus, eventually forming the bladder and urethra, and the dorsal section becomes the rectum.

Two theories have been proposed to explain the final cloacal separation. In the classic theory postulated by Bill and Johnson (1958), the urorectal septum continues down to the cloacal membrane, which then ruptures, creating two separate excretory orifices. According to Stephens (1963), the urorectal septum divides the cloaca only as far down as the pubococcygeal line. Lateral ingrowth of mesoderm (Rathke's folds) moves toward the midline, completing the cleavage of the urinary tract from the rectum; this occurs during the 6- to 7-week stage.

Once the cloaca is divided and the cloacal membrane ruptures to create two excretory orifices, differentiation between male and female begins. In the male, the inner and outer genital ridges coalesce to form the urethra, whereas in the female, both sets of ridges form the labia minora and labia majora. The müllerian duct system initiates the development of the upper vagina and internal female genital system. As the müllerian elements descend, they separate

1922

the urinary and genital tracts, emptying into the open space between the genital ridges. Most varieties of anorectal malformation can be explained by these embryologic concepts.

IMPERFORATE ANUS

Imperforate anus is not an uncommon anomaly; most institutions report the incidence as being 1 in 5000 births (Kieswetter et al., 1964; Bradham, 1958). When the spectrum of cases seen only by the pediatric surgeon is considered, slightly less than 1 per cent of surgery is performed for malformations of the anus and rectum (Kieswetter, 1979).

A knowledge of the prior classifications of imperforate anus not only is historically valuable but also facilitates a better understanding of the present schema. The initial surgical classification was published by Ladd and Gross (1934), who divided the abnormality into four types: Type I (anal stenosis); Type II (persistent anal plate); Type III (anal atresia, implying imperforate anus with a blind-ending pouch); and Type IV (rectal atresia with an intact distal lumen and anus with atresia of a portion of the rectum) (Fig. 44–1).

The International Classification of anorectal abnormalities, first proposed in 1970 by Santulli et al., also divides anorectal anomalies into four major types, based primarily on the level of imperforation relative to the pelvic floor or puborectalis muscle: (1) low or translevator lesions, (2) intermediate lesions, (3) high or supralevator lesions, and (4) a miscellaneous group including imperforate anal membrane, cloacal exstrophy, and persistent urogenital sinus.

With increasing clinical adoption of the International Classification, a key determinant of therapeutic options has become whether or not the bowel has traversed the pelvic floor. This distinction also predicts the incidence of associated genitourinary and other organ system anomalies, in that patients with low lesions have a much lower incidence of sacral and urinary abnormalities than do those with high lesions.

Kieswetter (1979) modified Santulli's classification into a more workable form, taking into account the anatomic level of the imperforation; the presence or absence of a fistula from the rectum to the urinary tract, vagina, or perineum; and the gender of the patient (Table 44–1; Fig. 44–2).

Important facts to be emphasized are the following: (1) The most common type of low

infralevator lesion in this series was anal agenesis with the normal bowel descending through the levator sling, failing to reach the outside. (2) The most common supralevator lesion was rectal agenesis. (3) There is a relatively low incidence of fistulas in males with infralevator lesions. (4) In males with infralevator lesions, the fistula was rarely to the urethra but primarily to the perineum, and specifically to the midline posterior scrotal raphe. (5) Male infralevator lesions do present without fistulas, making it more difficult to differentiate this group of patients from those with supralevator lesions. (6) There is a relatively high incidence of fistulas in females who have infralevator lesions with the vulva as the major site. (7) In both males and females, supralevator lesions have a much higher incidence of fistulas than do infralevator lesions. (8) A significant number of males with supralevator lesions present without fistulas, making decompression of the bowel urgent. (9) Fistulas in females with supralevator lesions were rarely to the bladder and more commonly to the upper vagina. (10) Fistulas in males with supralevator lesions were almost exclusively to the prostatic urethra at the level of the verumontanum. (11) True rectal atresia is extremely rare.

The common types of fistulas seen in this disorder are illustrated in Figure 44–3.

Abnormal Embryology

Abnormal embryologic development explains the etiology of these lesions and some of the associated organ system anomalies. Insults early in embryologic life, at 4 weeks when the developing cloaca, spine, metanephros, and lower extremities are developing in close proximity, will result in a fetal monster. As described by Duhamel (1961), this results in fusion of the lower extremities, imperforate anus, sacral agenesis, and absence of the genitourinary tract. At the other end of the embryologic spectrum, failure of the posterior part of the cloacal membrane to rupture will result in imperforate anal membrane.

When the urorectal septum fails to descend completely, various anomalies will become manifest, depending on the level of the arrest. Arrest early and high will cause persistent cloaca seen in the female, with the urinary, genital, and intestinal tracts meeting in a common channel having a single perineal opening. Later failure of downgrowth of the urorectal septum will manifest itself in high supralevator lesions in the

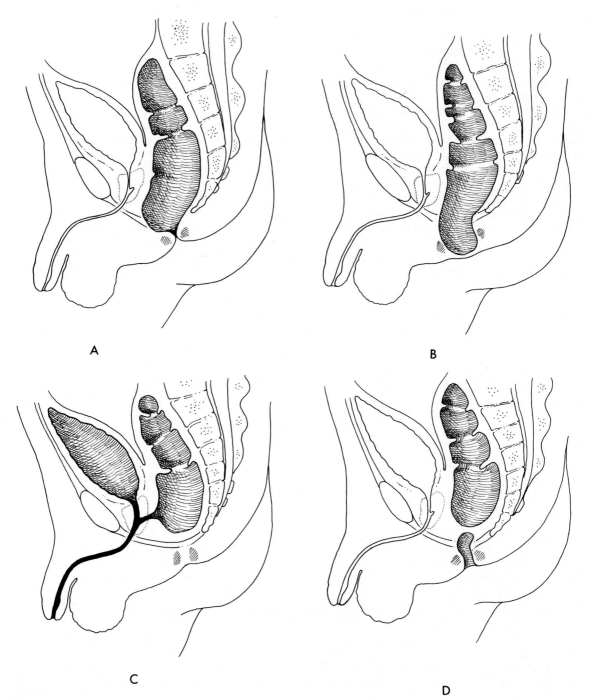

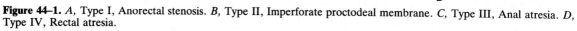

Figure 44–1. *A,* Type I, Anorectal stenosis. *B,* Type II, Imperforate proctodeal membrane. *C,* Type III, Anal atresia. *D,* Type IV, Rectal atresia.

male. A communication between posterior cloaca (rectum) and anterior cloaca (urogenital sinus) usually leads to a communication between the prostatic urethra and the rectum.

In the female, the rarity of rectovesical or rectourethral fistulas in high lesions can be explained by the interposition of the müllerian elements. The müllerian ducts fuse and meet the inferior urorectal septum when the vagina forms and interposes between the urinary and digestive tracts. Thus, females with high lesions will present with rectovaginal fistulas.

This further clarifies why high lesions have a high incidence of associated renal, sacral, and spinal abnormalities. The insult occurs early in embryologic life, when these organ systems are in close proximity. Failure of the ureteric bud to come off the wolffian duct, which inserts close to the urorectal septum, explains the high incidence of renal agenesis or hypoplasia in association with high imperforate anus. Faulty ureteral budding may explain vesicoureteral reflux as well (Churchill et al., 1978).

The low incidence of sacral and urinary tract anomalies with low imperforate anus suggests that the malformation stems from an insult later in fetal life, when other organ systems have already completed essential parts of their development. The rarity of rectourinary fistulas

TABLE 44–1. ANATOMIC CLASSIFICATION AND INCIDENCE OF ANORECTAL MALFORMATION

Type of Lesion		% of All Cases
LOW, INFRALEVATOR		
Anal stenosis		8
Imperforate anal membrane		6
Anal agenesis		36
Males		16
With fistula		9
Perineum	100%	
Urethra	0	
Without fistula		7
Females		20
With fistula		20
Vulva	68%	
Perineal body	32%	
Without fistula		0
HIGH, SUPRALEVATOR		
Rectal agenesis		47
Males		35
With fistula		20
Rectovaginal	95%	
Rectovesical	5%	
Without fistula		15
Females		12
With fistula		11
Rectovaginal	70%	
Rectovesical	30%	
Without fistula		1
Rectal atresia		1

Adapted from Kieswetter, W. B.: *In* Ravitch, M., et al. (Eds.) Pediatric Surgery. Chicago, Year Book Medical Publishers, 1979.

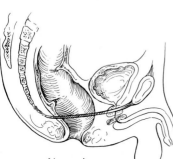

Anal Agenesis

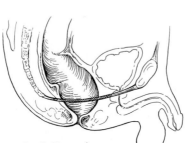

Rectal Agenesis

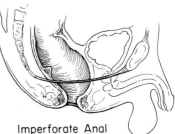

Rectal Atresia

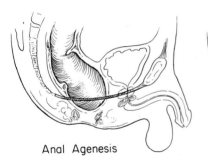

Normal

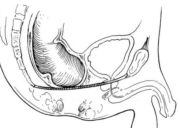

Anal Stenosis

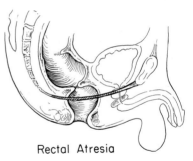

Imperforate Anal Membrane

Figure 44–2. Imperforate anus.

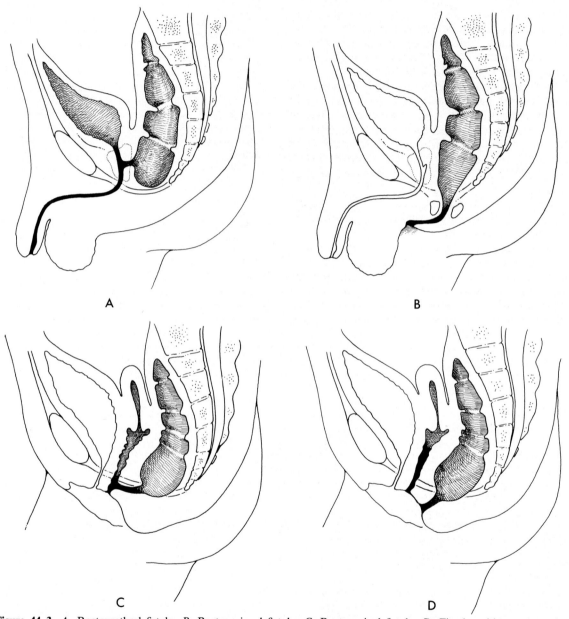

Figure 44–3. *A*, Rectourethral fistula. *B*, Rectoperineal fistula. *C*, Rectovaginal fistula. *D*, Fistula exiting at posterior fourchette.

in low lesions also implies completion of urorectal septal descent prior to these embryologic insults. In both sexes, perineal fistulas or ectopic openings in these low lesions can be explained by failure of the anus to migrate posteriorly to its normal position.

Associated Genitourinary Anomalies

To assess genitourinary anomalies, lesions must be adequately described with reference to the level of imperforation. Initially, all patients must undergo a thorough genitourinary radiologic evaluation, including an abdominal ultrasound study and a voiding cystourethrogram. (It should be noted that rectourethral fistulas are considered part of the anomaly itself and are not tabulated as an associated genitourinary anomaly. Incidence figures are listed in Table 44–2.)

Patients with supralevator lesions have a higher incidence of genitourinary anomalies than do those with infralevator lesions and tend to have more than one anomaly. When present, the genitourinary anomalies in supralevator lesions are more severe, commonly involving the upper tracts. In the review of Belman and King (1972), 30 per cent of patients with supralevator lesions had major upper tract anomalies, including renal agenesis, ureteropelvic junction obstruction, and renal dysplasia, as opposed to 10 per cent with low infralevator lesions who had upper tract anomalies. It was reported that renal agenesis is the most common single anomaly in patients with supralevator lesions, occurring in 12 per cent of that population. These data are supported by Wiener and Kieswetter (1973), who had reported 20 of 200 imperforate anus patients with renal agenesis, 5 of whom had bilateral renal agenesis. It was found that major genitourinary anomalies were present twice as often in supralevator lesions as in infralevator lesions. In a review by Munn and Schillinger

(1983), 21 per cent of 14 patients with infralevator lesions had a solitary kidney compared with 33 per cent of 14 patients with supralevator lesions, pointing out that severe upper tract anomalies may occur in patients with low lesions as well. Tables 44–3 to 44–5 list the spectrum of lesions that may be present with both high and low anomalies.

A 10 per cent incidence of neurogenic bladder due either to injury at anal pull-through or to concomitant lumbosacral anomalies has been reported (Hall et al., 1970; Belman and King, 1972). Because of the communication between the urinary and intestinal tracts, lower urinary tract infections may persist until a definitive rectal procedure is performed or if the fistula is not fully interrupted.

The incidence of vesicoureteral reflux in the series of Narasimharao et al. (1983) was 47 per cent, with higher rates and more severe reflux in supralevator lesions (Table 44–6). In this study, reflux tended to be mild and rarely progressed. Parrott and Woodard (1979) reported that reflux was the most common genitourinary anomaly found in 38 per cent of patients who had high imperforation and in 19 per cent of the entire group. Reflux was severe or moderate in 75 per cent of refluxing ureters. The high incidence of reflux in this population points out the necessity of obtaining a voiding cystourethrogram promptly after diagnosis.

Associated Anomalies in Other Organ Systems

Associated anomalies in other organ systems occur regularly in patients with imperforate anus. Lumbosacral spine abnormalities have been reported in as many as 38 per cent of patients, usually occurring with supralevator lesions (Denton, 1982). This association also explains the high incidence of neurogenic bladder. Cardiac anomalies, such as ventricular septal defects and pulmonary stenosis, occur in 7 per

TABLE 44–2. INCIDENCE OF ASSOCIATED GENITOURINARY ANOMALIES WITH IMPERFORATE ANUS

Series	No. of Patients	Overall Incidence (%)	Supralevator Lesions (%)	Infralevator Lesions (%)
Belman and King (1972)	143	31	52	16
Santulli et al. (1971)	1166	26	48 F	14 F
			40 M	21 M
Hoekstra et al. (1983)	150	50	70	34
			69 M	35 M
			73 F	33 F

TABLE 44–3. INCIDENCE OF UROGENITAL TRACT ABNORMALITIES IN CHILDREN WITH ANORECTAL ANOMALIES

	Supralevator		Infralevator	
	BOYS	GIRLS	BOYS	GIRLS
Total number of children	43	15	37	51
Urogenital tract abnormalities				
Agenesis two kidneys	1	3		
Agenesis one kidney	7			2
Hypoplastic kidney	4	1		
Polycystic disease	2			
Ectopic kidney	3	1	1	1
Ureteropelvic junction stenosis	1	1		1
Horseshoe kidney	4	2	1	1
Stenosis of ureter				1
Ectopic ureter	2	1		1
Ureterocele				1
Vesicoureteral reflux	13	4	5	12
Vesical exstrophy				1
Bladder duplication	1			
Segmented bladder		1		
Other bladder deformity	1			
Neurogenic bladder	1	1		2
Posterior urethral valves	2		2	
Urethral stenosis	4			
Urethral diverticula	2			
Hypospadias	6		4	
Penile duplication	2			
Micropenis	1			
Scrotal deformities	3			
Cryptorchidism	1		1	
Bicornuate uterus		1		1
Vaginal duplication		1		1
Hydrometrocolpos		1		
Total number of abnormalities (Total number of patients with lesions)	61(30)	18(11)	14(13)	25(17)

From Hoekstra, W. J., Scholtmeijer, J. C., Mocenaar, J. C., et al.: J. Urol., *130*:962, 1983.

cent of patients and central nervous system lesions in 4 per cent. The incidence of esophageal atresia associated with imperforate anus has been reported as 10 per cent (Kieswetter, 1979; Trusler and Wilkinson, 1962).

The VATER association, first described by Quan and Smith in 1973, has since been expanded to the acronym VACTERYL, denoting vertebral, anorectal, cardiac, tracheoesophageal, renal, and limb-associated anomalies. A genitourinary anomaly has been seen in 90 per cent of patients with this syndrome, consisting mainly of renal agenesis, ureteropelvic junction obstruction, vesicoureteral reflux, and crossed fused ectopia (Uehling et al., 1983).

TABLE 44–4. GENITOURINARY ANOMALIES WITH INFRALEVATOR LESIONS

Genitourinary Anomaly	Number of Patients
Dysplasia	1
UPJ obstruction	1
Duplication	2
Malrotation	2
Pelvic kidney	1
Reflux (cystograms not routine)	3
Lower urinary anomalies	2
Total numbers of patients with infralevator lesions	74

From Belman, A. B., and King, L. R.: J. Urol., *168*:823, 1972.

TABLE 44–5. GENITOURINARY ANOMALIES WITH SUPRALEVATOR LESIONS

Genitourinary Anomaly	Number of Patients
Unilateral agenesis	8
Hypoplasia or dysplasia	6
UPJ obstruction	2
Horseshoe kidney	1
Crossed ectopia	1
Midureteral stenosis	1
Single renal artery	1
Reflux (cystograms not routine)	2
Lower urinary anomalies	12
Total number of patients with supralevator lesions	65

From Belman, A. B., and King, L. R.: J. Urol., *168*:823, 1972.

TABLE 44–6. INCIDENCE OF VESICOURETERAL REFLUX ASSOCIATED WITH IMPERFORATE ANUS

Series	No. of Patients	Total Incidence (%)	Supralevator Lesions	Infralevator Lesions
Hoekstra et al. (1983)	150	40	47	3
Narasimharao et al. (1983)	36	47	66	10
Parrott and Woodard (1979)	51	19	38	8

Clinical Presentation and Diagnosis

The diagnosis of imperforate anus can be made within 24 hours of birth by visual inspection of the perineum. Irregular epithelium present at the anal site, which may represent anal stenosis, can be probed delicately and dilated with small Hegar dilators, in a search for meconium. If a veil of epithelium is found covering the normally positioned anal orifice with a bulging mass of meconium behind it, the diagnosis of imperforate anal membrane can be made.

Anal agenesis can present in both sexes, with no external opening at the normal anatomic site of the anus. In the female, the incidence of fistula is exceedingly high; therefore, inspection for meconium should be made along the vulva and perineum, where the fistula commonly exits. This orifice can be probed gently to determine if indeed it is a fistulous tract. Males with anal agenesis may also have a fistula located at the posterior scrotal raphe.

Males who have anal agenesis without a fistula may present a diagnostic problem in determining whether the lesions are of the low, infralevator or the high, supralevator type. The presence of meconium in the urine suggests a high lesion owing to the concomitant rectourethral fistula. Inverted radiographs to determine the position of the blind bowel relative to the pubococcygeal line have also been used to make this determination (Wangenstein and Rice, 1930). Some authors recommend direct aspiration through the perineum to confirm that the bowel is more or less than 2 cm from the skin (Kieswetter, 1979; Motovic et al., 1979). Others believe that when a male has no evident external opening there is a supralevator lesion that should be treated accordingly, reasoning that performing a temporary colostomy in a patient with an infralevator lesion is less risky than attempting a cutback procedure in a child who has a supralevator lesion (Asch and Sherman, 1983).

Rectal agenesis can present with or without fistula in both sexes. In females who have an orifice on the posterior wall of the vagina, vaginoscopy or insertion of a catheter into this orifice may be helpful. In males with a fistula, the opening is located at the level of the prostatic urethra or, less commonly, into the bladder. Thus, examination of the urine will usually show meconium. The use of indigo carmine may also be helpful. Cystoscopy either before or at the time of anal pull-through will differentiate between urethral and vesical fistulas.

If no fistula is present and diagnosis is delayed, abdominal distention and vomiting may occur inasmuch as the bowel has no avenue of decompression. In this setting, the inverted scout film will show the blind bowel to be located above the pubococcygeal line. On the plain film, air in the bladder may be seen, suggesting a rectourinary fistula.

Other initial radiographic studies should include abdominal ultrasonography and voiding cystourethrography because of the high incidence of upper tract abnormalities and reflux. Renal ultrasound can be used as well to determine the presence or absence of a kidney, acknowledging the high incidence of renal agenesis. There is a strong likelihood of finding an abnormality with high imperforations, but the significant number of upper tract abnormalities with low lesions makes imaging essential in all patients. Lumbosacral abnormalities can also be identified on these films. If vomiting or swallowing defects are noted, contrast studies of the upper intestinal tract may reveal a tracheoesophageal fistula or esophageal atresia, commonly found in association with this anomaly.

Treatment

These complex lesions are optimally managed by multidisciplinary specialists, always including a urologist. Although in-depth pediatric surgical considerations are beyond the scope of this chapter, certain points deserve emphasis. Treatment depends on the level of imperforation (Kieswetter, 1979). Anal stenosis is treated with dilatation and imperforate anal membrane with incision of the obstructing membrane. In male infants with infralevator lesions and fistulas, a perineal anoplasty is performed by enlarging the perineal fistula and cutting into the distal rectum with subsequent dilatation. Female infants with low lesions and fistulas may sometimes require only dilatation of the fistulous tract for the first few days of life, allowing good decompression of the bowel, followed by definitive anoplasty or fistula transfer.

Management of supralevator lesions is similar in both sexes. An initial diverting colostomy is performed to divert the fecal stream. Some authors use the transverse colon, leaving virgin bowel for the definitive pull-through and allowing the same colostomy to give protection after the pull-through procedure. Others prefer the sigmoid colon for a colostomy because the distal segment is shorter, can be cleansed with saline or antibiotics, and, in the presence of a rectourethral fistula, can prevent or lessen the incidence of urinary tract infection, urinary reflux, and hyperchloremic acidosis. Final reconstitution and pull-through of the bowel to the new external opening are currently being employed in the abdominoperineal approach at 1 year of age, with some authors utilizing a sacral approach. Interruption of the rectourinary fistula is accomplished at the same time as the pull-through.

Hyperchloremic acidosis due to retrograde urine flow across the fistula into the distal colon, with subsequent reabsorption during the interval between colostomy and definitive pull-through, is unusual and is generally managed with alkalinizing and antibacterial agents (Caldamone et al., 1979). This potential complication must be recognized and managed early inasmuch as profound acidosis and shock may ensue. If definitive fistula interruption cannot be undertaken because of the child's age or size, it is important to employ methods designed to decrease the amount of urine in contact with colonic mucosa. In this setting, cutaneous vesicostomy or intermittent catheterization of the bladder and/or distal colostomy are suggested until fistula interruption is performed.

Severe vesicoureteral reflux with concomitant urinary tract infection may lead to damage and scarring of the upper tracts. Both conservative management and ureteroneocystostomy have been used for this problem, depending upon the degree of reflux (Ehrlich, 1982a, b). Patients with neurogenic bladder or severe reflux often require early temporary cutaneous vesicostomy (Duckett, 1974). Long-term antibacterial prophylaxis is necessary in all instances of demonstrated reflux and rectourinary fistula. If long-term vesical drainage is anticipated, cutaneous vesicostomy is mandated and suprapubic cystostomy condemned.

Primary ureteropelvic junction obstruction should be corrected early in the neonatal period to prevent irreversible renal damage. Obstruction secondary to concomitant reflux will usually disappear after surgical correction of the primary problem.

Long-term urethral catheter drainage during the various operative procedures or urethral injury during anoplasty or pull-through often results in urethral stricture and stenosis. Other complications include prostatic urethral narrowing, urethral diverticula and calculus from an incompletely excised rectal stump, and chronic infection (Williams & Grant, 1969). Urethral damage can be avoided with appropriate use of a soft catheter gently placed in the urethra at the time of surgical pull-through. Persky et al. (1974), in reviewing urologic complications associated with correction of imperforate anus, emphasized the necessity for the urologist and pediatric surgeon to cooperate in order to reduce these unnecessary but devastating urologic complications. It cannot be overemphasized that frequent or prolonged urethral catheterization inexpertly performed is to be condemned. Early stricture formation in serious cases should be treated with cutaneous vesicostomy rather than with forced urethral dilatation, which in itself might prove harmful. Optical visual urethrotomy has been successfully performed but is best attempted in an older child and not in a neonate (Noe, 1983).

Bladder denervation can occur subsequent to correction of the rectourethral fistula and can lead to urinary incontinence but is fortunately rare. Concomitant sacral abnormalities and neuropathic bladder may, however, necessitate long-term management. Despite the fact that innovative pediatric surgical endorectal procedures have improved the gastrointestinal condition of these unfortunate children, long-term follow-up must be performed by the urologist. It is clear from the aforementioned genitourinary anomalies that both early and late urologic consultation is mandatory in the ongoing management of these children.

PERSISTENT CLOACA

Persistent cloaca in the female is an embryologically more complex lesion than imperforate anus and is much less common. Approximately 60 cases of such lesions have been reported in the literature.

Embryology

As noted earlier, the cloaca at 4 weeks' gestation serves as the common channel for the urinary, digestive, and reproductive tracts. Failure of the urorectal septum to divide the cloaca results in entry of the proximal urethra, upper two thirds of the vagina, and rectum into a common channel, the cloaca, with a single perineal opening.

In the female, the paired müllerian ducts fuse at the müllerian tubercle to form the uterovaginal canal, which eventually gives rise to the fallopian tubes, uterus, and vagina. The arrested descent of the urorectal septum interferes with fusion of the müllerian duct, causing duplication of the uterus and vagina, which is seen quite frequently with persistent cloaca (Johnson et al., 1972).

Associated Anomalies

Since persistent cloaca is a more severe form of high imperforate anus, with the embryologic insult occurring earlier in gestational life, there is a high incidence of associated anomalies. Upper urinary tract anomalies have been reported in as many as 75 per cent of patients with cloacal dysgenesis (Bartholomew and Gonzales, 1978; Kay and Tank, 1977) (Table 44–7). Abnormalities of the genital tract occur frequently, with uterovaginal duplications predominating (Table 44–8). Cardiac, respiratory, and upper alimentary tract anomalies may be present and should be evaluated.

Diagnosis

The presence of a single perineal opening in a female infant should alert the clinician to the diagnosis. An abdominal mass results from obstruction of the genitourinary or digestive tract. Plain films of the abdomen may help reveal these masses as well as a lumbosacral deformity. Initial studies should include ultrasonography and cystography to reveal urinary tract anomalies and to evaluate the obstruction that exists secondary to the hydrometrocolpos, if present. Injection of contrast dye into the perineal opening via a catheter, or a small Foley catheter with the balloon pulled against the perineum, helps define the anatomy.

TABLE 44–7. ASSOCIATED UPPER URINARY TRACT ANOMALIES WITH PERSISTENT CLOACA

Anomaly	No. of Patients
Renal dysplasia	5
Renal agenesis	3
Duplication	3
Ectopic ureter	2
Fused pelvic kidney	1
Crossed renal ectopia	1
Horseshoe kidney	1
Malrotated kidney	1
Total number of patients with persistent cloaca	39

From Kay, R., and Tank, E. S.: J. Urol., *117*:102, 1977.

Treatment

Decompression of the obstructed bowel, urinary tract, and genital tract is the first goal of treatment. A transverse loop colostomy is performed in the neonatal period. At this time, the urinary tract should be completely studied by means of endoscopy and by injection of all orifices with contrast so as to define the anatomy. Diversion or correction of the major upper tract urinary anomalies may be performed at

TABLE 44–8. GENITOURINARY ANOMALIES ASSOCIATED WITH PERSISTENT CLOACA

Anomaly	No. of Patients
URINARY	
Renal agenesis	7
Renal dysgenesis	8
Bilateral hydronephrosis	6
Unilateral hydronephrosis	7
Vesicoureteral reflux	9
Horseshoe kidney	3
Crossed renal ectopia	2
GENITAL	
Duplication of uterus	13
Duplication of vagina	9
Bicornuate uterus	6
Septate vagina	5
Ovarian cystic dysplasia	1
Hydrocolpos	12
OTHER	
Tracheoesophageal fistula	1
Malrotation of bowel	2
Duodenal atresia	2
Patent ductus arteriosus	3
Meningocele	3
Total number of patients with persistent cloaca	56

From Bartholomew, T. H., and Gonzales, E. T.: Urology, *11*:549, 1978.

the same time as the colostomy. Saline irrigation of the lower end of the colostomy serves to prevent urinary contamination with fecal contents.

Hydrometrocolpos may contribute to poor bladder drainage and upper tract dilatation. Thus, relief of hydrometrocolpos is essential. Dilatation of the stenotic perineal orifice is often adequate for decompression. Occasionally, transabdominal tube drainage is required. If urine preferentially enters the vagina, the hydrometrocolpos may continue to refill, leading to hydronephrosis. Temporary urinary diversion via intermittent catheterization or vesicostomy until a definitive operation can be performed is a simple and well-tolerated solution.

Definitive operative correction and immediate separation of the urinary, genital, and gastrointestinal tracts during the neonatal period have been advocated by some authors (Raffensberger and Ramenofsky, 1973), although minimal intervention during the neonatal period is suggested (Hendren, 1982). Once drainage has been established for the urinary, digestive, and genital tracts, the final reconstitution can be delayed until the child attains a weight of 25 pounds.

Rectal pull-through combined with vaginal pull-through for high vaginal lesions, or vaginoplasty at a later date for low vaginal lesions, completes the anatomic correction. However, urinary incontinence, neurogenic bladder, and vesicoureteral reflux are often present even after final anatomic correction.

UROGENITAL SINUS OUTLET OBSTRUCTION

A common urogenital sinus, in which the vagina and the urethra open into a common channel with a normal anus, may be obstructed by a persistent urogenital sinus membrane that fails to rupture at its normal time, i.e., 7 weeks of gestation. Patients with this disorder present with anuria and an abdominal mass representing hydrometrocolpos from stasis of urine in the uterus behind the persistent membrane. An imperforate anus may also coexist with this lesion.

Surgical rupture of the membrane can serve as definitive therapy when performed early. Plastic revision of the outlet is best performed after the child has reached 2 years of age (Tank et al., 1970).

References

Imperforate Anus

Asch, M. J., and Sherman, N. J.: Evaluation and management of anorectal malformation in the neonate. J. Calif. Perinatal Assn., 2:86, 1983.

Belman, A. B., and King, L. R.: Urinary tract abnormalities associated with imperforate anus. J. Urol., 168:823, 1972.

Bill, A. H., and Johnson, R. J.: Failure of migration of the rectal opening as the cause for most cases of imperforate anus. Surg. Gynecol. Obstet., 106:643, 1958.

Bradham, R. R.: Imperforate anus: report of 130 cases. Surgery, 44:578, 1958.

Caldamone, A. A., Emmens, R. W., and Rabinowitz, R.: Hyperchloremic acidosis and imperforate anus. J. Urol., 122(6):817, 1979.

Churchill, B. M., Hardy, B. E., and Stephens, C. A.: Urologic aspects of malformation and common abnormalities of the anus and rectum. Urol. Clin. North Am., 5:1, 1978.

Denton, J. R.: The association of congenital spinal anomalies with imperforate anus. Clin. Orthop., 162:91, 1982.

Duckett, J. W., Jr.: Cutaneous vesicostomy in childhood. Urol. Clin. North Am., 1:485, 1974.

Duhamel, B.: From the mermaid to anal imperforation: the syndrome of caudal regression. Arch. Dis. Childh., 36:152, 1961.

Ehrlich, R. M.: Success of the transvesical advancement technique for vesicoureteral reflux. J. Urol., 128:554, 1982a.

Ehrlich, R. M.: Vesicoureteral reflux: a surgeon's perspective. Symposium on pediatric nephrology. Pediatr. Clin. North Am., 29(4):827, 1982b.

Hall, J. W., Tank, E. S., and Lapides, J.: Urogenital anomalies and complications associated with imperforate anus. J. Urol., 103:810, 1970.

Hoekstra, W. J., Scholtmeijer, J. C., Mocenaar, J. C., et al.: Urogenital tract abnormalities associated with congenital anorectal anomalies. J. Urol., 130:962, 1983.

Kieswetter, W. B.: Malformations of rectum and anus. In Ravitch, M., et al. (Eds.): Pediatric Surgery. Chicago, Year Book Medical Publishers, 1979, pp. 1059–1072.

Kieswetter, W. B., Turner, C. R., and Sieber, W. K.: Imperforate anus: review of 16 year experience with 146 patients. Am. J. Surg., 107:412, 1964.

Ladd, W. E., and Gross, R. E.: Congenital malformation of anus and rectum: report of 162 cases. Am. J. Surg., 23:167, 1934.

Motovic, A., Kovalivker, M., Man, B., et al.: The value of transperineal injection for the diagnosis of imperforate anus. Ann. Surg., 190(5):662, 1979.

Munn, R., and Schillinger, J. F.: Urologic abnormalities found with imperforate anus. Urology, 21:260, 1983.

Narasimharao, K. L., Prasad, G. R., Mukhopadhyay, B., et al.: Vesicoureteral reflux in neonates with anorectal anomalies. Br. J. Urol., 55:268, 1983.

Noe, H. N.: Complications and management of childhood urethral stricture disease. Urol. Clin. North Am., 10:531, 1983.

Parrott, T. S., and Woodard, J. R.: Importance of cystourethrography in neonates with imperforate anus. Urology, 13:607, 1979.

Persky, L., Tucker, A., and Izant, R.: Urologic complications of correction of imperforate anus. J. Urol., 111:415, 1974.

Quan, L., and Smith, D. W.: The VATER association. Vertebral defects, anal atresia, T-E fistula with esophageal atresia, radial and renal dysplasia: a spectrum of associated defects. J. Pediatr., 82:104, 1973.

Santulli, T. V., Kieswetter, W. B., and Bill, A. H.: Anorectal anomalies: a suggested international classification. J. Pediatr. Surg., 5:281, 1970.

Santulli, T. V., Schullinger, J. N., Kieswetter, W. B., et al.: Imperforate anus: a survey from the members of the Surgical Section of the American Academy of Pediatrics. J. Pediatr. Surg., 6:484, 1971.

Stephens, F. D.: Congenital Malformations of the Rectum, Anus, and Genito-Urinary Tracts. Edinburgh, E & S Livingston, Ltd., 1963.

Trusler, G. A., and Wilkinson, R. H.: Imperforate anus: a review of 147 cases. Can. J. Surg., 5:269, 1962.

Uehling, D. T., Gilben, E., and Chesney, R.: Urologic implications of the VATER association. J. Urol., 129:352, 1983.

Wangensteen, O. H., and Rice, C. O.: Imperforate anus. Ann. Surg., 92:77, 1930.

Wiener, E. S., and Kieswetter, W. B.: Urologic abnormalities associated with imperforate anus. J. Pediatr. Surg., 8:151, 1973.

Williams, D. L., and Grant, J.: Urological complications of imperforate anus. Br. J. Urol., 41:660, 1969.

Persistent Cloaca and Urogenital Sinus Outlet Obstruction

Bartholomew, T. H., and Gonzales, E. T.: Urologic management in cloacal dysgenesis. Urology, 11:549, 1978.

Hendren, W. H.: Further experience in reconstructive surgery for cloacal anomalies. J. Pediatr. Surg., 17:695, 1982.

Johnson, R. J., Palken, M., Derrick, W., et al.: The embryology of high anorectal and associated genitourinary anomalies in the female. Surg. Gynecol. Obstet., 135:759, 1972.

Kay, R., and Tank, E. S.: Principles of management of the persistent cloaca in the female newborn. J. Urol., 117:102, 1977.

Raffensberger, J. G., and Ramenofsky, M. I.: The management of a cloaca. J. Pediatr. Surg., 8:647, 1973.

Tank, E. S., Konnak, J. W., and Lapides, J.: Urogenital sinus outlet obstruction. J. Urol., 104:769, 1970.

CHAPTER 45

Management of Intersexuality

A. D. PERLMUTTER, M.D.

INTRODUCTION

Intersex states present many complex management decisions, but an appropriate gender assignment is one of the most important. The time has long passed since sexual assignment has been made solely on a gonadal or chromosomal basis. Phallic inadequacy is now the single most important criterion used for female gender assignment, with certain exceptions. These include female pseudohermaphrodites with congenital adrenal hyperplasia, whose entirely normal internal female genital structures almost always dictate a female gender assignment regardless of phallic size, and an occasional true hermaphrodite with a morphologically normal ovary on one side who similarly might be potentially fertile.

The developmental, genetic, endocrinal, and other features of intersexual states are detailed in Chapter 41. Early neonatal sexual assignment is best, as soon as an appropriate evaluation is completed; evaluation and management of these infants and their families is generally a team effort, typically including a neonatologist, an endocrinologist, a psychiatrist, and a reconstructive surgeon. This chapter is limited to a discussion of the surgical approaches to genital reconstruction to achieve a genital appearance consistent with female sexual assignment; male genital reconstruction is covered in Chapter 47.

In clinical practice, the urologist will most commonly encounter the female pseudohermaphrodite as a manifestation of the adrenogenital syndrome (congenital adrenal hyperplasia). Despite variable virilization in these genetic females, the müllerian duct–derived structures (fallopian tubes, uterus, and proximal two thirds to four fifths of the vagina) are invariably present; in the absence of testes there is no inhibition of müllerian duct development by müllerian duct–inhibiting substance during early embryogenesis. The degree of phallic enlargement and of fusion and virilization of the urogenital sinus tissues is variable. A useful classification is that of Verkauf and Jones (1970), who described six degrees of virilization in girls with adrenogenital syndrome.

Group A: Normal female (rare).
Group B: Normal vulva with a degree of clitoral enlargement.
Group C: Mild labial fusion; traction on the posterior fourchette allows visualization of a separate vaginal orifice. The clitoris is enlarged.
Group D: Marked labial-scrotal fusion with urogenital sinus formation and a single orifice at the phallic base.
Group E: More marked fusion onto the ventral shaft of the phallus.
Group F: Fully masculine genitalia.

The degree of urogenital sinus fusion can be related to the time of onset of fetal androgen stimulation (Prader, 1958).

This chapter emphasizes reconstructive techniques to feminize female pseudohermaphrodites, using girls with congenital virilizing adrenogenital syndrome as the prototype. The same operative procedures are applicable for other forms of genital ambiguity, including exogenous virilization and true hermaphroditism. This chapter also outlines the creation of a vulva for male pseudohermaphrodites with phallic inadequacy. Because of the many surgical procedures and their modifications published through the years, this chapter presents selected techniques that the reader should find useful for most situations. Accordingly, the bibliography is representative; a complete review is not included.

PREOPERATIVE STUDIES RELEVANT TO PLANNING RECONSTRUCTIVE SURGERY

The diagnostic evaluation of intersexuality, including endocrinologic and genetic considerations, is covered in Chapter 41. With genital ambiguity, a rectal examination should permit identification of a cervix if it is present. Ultrasonography with the bladder filled can outline a uterus. When the vaginal orifice cannot be visualized owing to urogenital sinus fusion, a lateral urogenital sinogram will define the local anatomy. A syringe with a fistula tip adapter, a small plastic feeding tube, or a No. 8 F. Foley catheter with the tip amputated will serve the purpose. The tip of one of these instruments is inserted into the orifice of the urogenital sinus, and a retrograde instillation study is performed. The urethra, bladder, urogenital sinus, and vagina are filled, outlining the cervix (if present), and showing the relationships between these structures (Fig. 45–1).

When such studies are inadequate, or when the distal vaginal segment is very narrow and will not fill, endoscopic studies allow identification and localization of the vaginal opening. When done at the time of reconstruction, these studies permit placement of an indwelling vaginal catheter, such as a Fogarty balloon catheter, making dissection easier (Hendren and Crawford, 1969, 1972).

AGE FOR SURGICAL RECONSTRUCTION

After other appropriate diagnostic studies have been completed and after sex assignment, the appropriate time for surgery must be determined. The best time for genital reconstruction in female pseudohermaphrodites is not clearly established, but as a general rule early correction is desirable (Lewis and Money, 1977), preferably before the age of sexual awareness (3 or 3½ years); this is especially important for infants with severely virilized genitalia, so that parental and familial anxiety regarding the obvious genital deformities and the ambivalence this creates can be relieved. However, surgery in the first months of life may result in a higher than acceptable rate of complications (Jones et al., 1970). I have performed vaginoplasty and clitorectomy or clitoral recession on patients ranging in age from 6 months to 3 or 4 years,

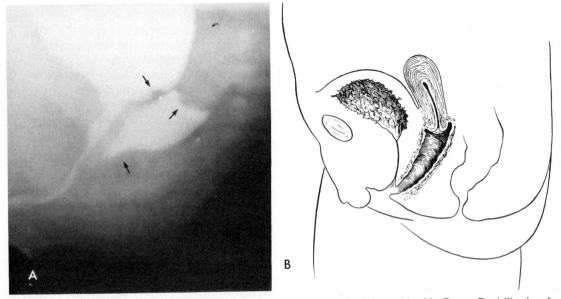

Figure 45–1. *A,* Retrograde injection of urogenital sinus, lateral view, in infant girl with Group D virilization from adrenogenital syndrome. Arrows point to interureteric ridge, cervix, and narrow lower vaginal segment. *B,* Line drawing to show entrance of urethra and hypoplastic lower vaginal segment into a common urogenital sinus.

and now prefer to wait until the patient is at least 12 months of age. Procedures before the first year of age may increase the difficulty of judging proportion and perspective; the procedure therefore should be postponed in chubby infants with a fatty mons, which is common in early infancy, until they lose this extra fat.

PSYCHOSEXUAL CONSIDERATIONS IN PLANNING SURGERY TO FEMINIZE FEMALE HERMAPHRODITES

All of the reconstructive techniques for correction of genital ambiguity should have both morphologic and functional goals. The procedure or procedures should restore, as far as possible, characteristic female morphology, with proportional size and position of the individual parts of the external genitalia. The length and size of the vaginal barrel must be adequate for later sexual function. Although genitopelvic eroticism is known to be present after clitoral amputation, preservation of the clitoris, or at least the glans with its neurovascular supply, may provide a more localized and intense focus for erotic sensation.

Hampson (1955) showed that clitoral amputation in girls with adrenogenital syndrome does not necessarily eliminate erotic responsiveness or the capacity for orgasm. Indeed, as Hampson pointed out, older children and young women with adrenogenital syndrome and an unduly large clitoris may be very troubled and discomfited by the inevitable experience of frequent, conspicuous erections, with all the sexual confusion and ambivalence such an experience can provoke, and they may be relieved of considerable anxiety by corrective surgery. Hampson's early, somewhat optimistic, report on clitorectomy involved only six women with sufficient sexual experience for evaluation, out of ten patients who had undergone genital repair at ages ranging from 4 to 37 years.

Money and Schwartz (1977) more recently studied 17 girls with adrenogenital syndrome who had been treated early; they were 16 to 25 years old at the time of follow-up, and all had had a prior clitorectomy. The authors noted four characteristics common to these girls during late adolescence and early adulthood: (1) relative diffidence in establishing friendships; (2) late onset of dating and romance; (3) possible bisexuality in imagery or experience; and (4) inhibition of erotic arousal or expression, or both. In their discussion, the authors suggested that these four characteristics might be related, possibly to the effects of prenatal androgen on developing brain pathways or perhaps to the unknown effects of long-term steroid replacement therapy.

It is known from animal studies that all fetuses have a dimorphic potential for sexual behavior, with the male gender role requiring the stimulation of prenatal androgen (hypothalamic imprinting); female fetuses exposed to androgen will develop male sexual behavioral traits. In the human, however, although infants with genital ambiguity may have had fetal androgen stimulation, early female gender assignment is associated with the appropriate behavioral influences on sexual function when it is accepted by the family and child. Therefore, although adrenogenital girls typically are tomboyish and have a tendency toward some bisexuality in imagery, which is perhaps related to prenatal androgen, they do have an appropriate female self-image, presumably owing to postnatal influences (Hurtig et al., 1983; Money and Schwartz, 1977). For a full discussion of sexual dimorphism and gender identity, the reader is referred to the work by Money and Ehrhardt (1972).

The sexual functioning of women who underwent reconstructive surgery in childhood by current innervation-sparing techniques of clitoral recession or reduction has not been compared directly with that of women who underwent early amputation. Although clitorectomy does not necessarily eliminate sexual responsiveness and gratification, erotic sensitivity may be altered. It is now the consensus from the literature that clitorectomy is rarely, if ever, indicated, since current techniques allow for an adequate cosmetic and functional reconstruction while sparing the clitoris or at least the innervated glans. Therefore, the following surgical descriptions do not include clitorectomy.

SURGICAL APPROACHES

Vaginoplasty

The amount of dissection required to create an adequate vaginal outlet will obviously vary according to the degree of urogenital sinus fusion. Vaginoplasty is unnecessary for Group B patients, but this minor degree of virilization is uncommon. Even in these patients, the vaginal orifice may be variably narrowed, as the lower vagina is derived from the urogenital sinus, and the inhibition of its development increases with increasing degrees of sinus virilization. If adequate distal vaginal enlargement and elasticity do not ensue at puberty in girls with a Group B deformity, vaginoplasty should be performed at that time. Alternatively, a small vaginal flap-plasty (as described later) can be performed initially at the time of clitoral surgery.

Most often vaginoplasty is required as part of the perineal reconstruction and should be done initially, regardless of the technique chosen to manage the clitoral enlargement. Some authors have favored treating only the clitoral enlargement early, postponing vaginoplasty until puberty to avoid possible postoperative stenosis (Allen et al., 1982; Sotiropoulos et al., 1976); others, including this author, prefer to perform the entire reconstruction in early childhood, thus ensuring a better relationship and proportion of the perineal structures. I feel that performing the vaginoplasty as the first step in a single-stage, total reconstruction procedure establishes the proper dimension for clitoral repair. Any rigidity or narrowing of the vaginal outlet that might occur can be revised after puberty. Another advantage of early reconstruction is to make the family's acceptance of the deformity easier; anxiety, ambivalence, and guilt will be diminished once repair is complete.

VAGINAL EXTERIORIZATION

Vaginal exteriorization is, in essence, a midline episiotomy of the perineal fusion. The incision is sutured into the inner urogenital sinus and vaginal mucosa as far as the incision in the perineal skin (Jones and Wilkins, 1960). Any redundant sinus or perineal tissue can be trimmed away prior to this closure. When the vagina is high, dissection limited to the posterior and lateral surfaces of the vaginal cuff will usually mobilize it sufficiently to be pulled down into the perineum. Many girls have been treated by vaginal exteriorization with good results, although vaginal stenosis can occur. In one series, 25 of 84 girls required treatment after puberty for vaginal stenosis. This, however, could be managed by simple techniques of revision (Jones et al., 1976). In another series, a second procedure was planned for 16 of 48 cases (33 per cent) during, or at the end of, puberty (Nihoul-Fekete et al., 1982). For both series, revisions were mainly in the more severely virilized girls with high vaginas. Vaginal exteriorization without flap-plasty is most suitable for milder degrees of urogenital sinus formation with minimal distal vaginal narrowing.

FLAP VAGINOPLASTY

Because distal vaginal narrowing and hypoplasia are related to the degree of virilization of the urogenital sinus but are present to some degree even with minor virilization, many authors, including this contributor, currently favor the use of a perineal skin flap, in most cases, to widen the vaginal outlet and to avoid overlapping incisions.

This author's technique is a modification of that described by Fortunoff et al. (1964). I use a shorter, widely based flap, taking care to preserve a good subcutaneous blood supply; the U-shaped tongue of the flap is inserted into a posterior midline vaginal incision extending through the narrowed lower vaginal segment into normal vaginal tissue. The results of a flap-plasty appear to be acceptable in the long term, although focal apical narrowing requiring dilatation or revision postpubertally is not uncommon. Ten of 13 girls from the original series of Fortunoff et al. (1964) had stenosis that required revision after puberty (Sotiropoulos et al., 1976). In this author's experience with a broadly based short flap, 4 of 24 girls had focal vaginal stenosis, but postpubertal assessment for the series is not completed. Only one of these four girls had adrenogenital syndrome.

The child is placed in the lithotomy position with exaggerated flexion of the thighs, but care should be taken not to abduct the thighs too widely, as this places undue traction on the monsplasty closure that is often done at the same time (Fig. 45–2A to C). Generally, the upper part of the dissection can be performed as a simple midline episiotomy into the urogenital sinus, with the skin incision extending posterolaterally as two diverging limbs 2 or 2.5 cm in length, creating a short, widely based, U-shaped flap involving the skin only (Fig. 45–2D). A thick subcutaneous layer of fat with its blood supply is left attached to the underside of the flap. After the flap is turned downward, lateral traction sutures will expose the deeper vulval tissues. A careful midline dissection will separate the deeper layers of the urogenital sinus and the narrow lower vaginal segment. Lateral dissection into the ischiorectal fossas is unnecessary. In patients with extreme virilization and a high and extremely narrow distal vaginal segment, preliminary endoscopic identification of the tract with placement of a Fogarty vascular balloon catheter will make subsequent dissection easier (Hendren and Crawford, 1969).

The anatomic structures encountered during this dissection in patients with greater degrees of virilization, such as those in Groups D

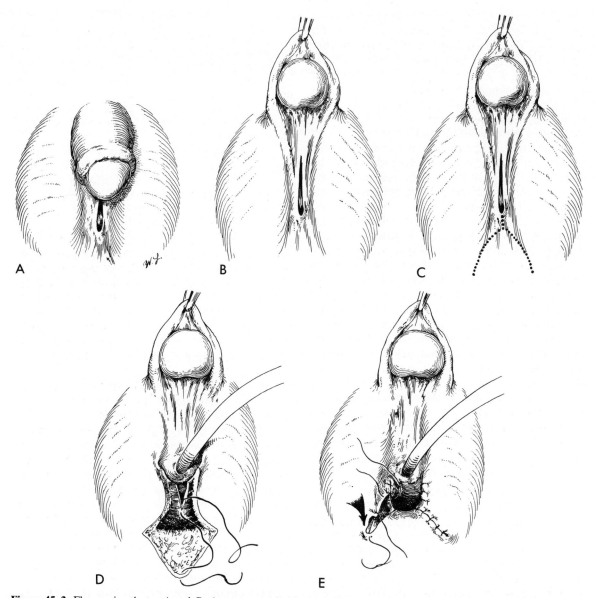

Figure 45–2. Flap vaginoplasty. *A* and *B,* Appearance of girl with Group D virilization from adrenogenital syndrome. *C,* Incisions for vaginal flap. *D,* Vaginal flap turned down. Flap tip should be rounded. Preservation of subcutaneous blood supply to flap. Posterior midline incision through hypoplastic distal vaginal segment. *E,* Completion of vaginoplasty. Flap secured. Rotation of labioscrotal skin during lateral closure.

and E, are those typically found in the male perineum—i.e., fused bulbocavernosus muscles covering a variably developed corpus spongiosum, and sometimes a bit of prostatic tissue surrounding the entrance of the narrowed vaginal segment into the urogenital sinus.

After incision of the urogenital sinus and its covering tissues in the midline to the level of the hymen, traction sutures should be inserted in the vaginal cuff to permit control during subsequent dissection. Gentle, mainly blunt, dissection directly on the posterior and poster-

olateral walls of the vagina will separate the vagina from the surrounding pelvic floor musculature and rectum, and allow it to be pulled outward a few millimeters, facilitating a clean midline incision through the posterior wall of the narrowed segment without injury to the surrounding structures (Fig. 45–2D). The perineal flap is then turned into this relaxing incision in the distal vagina, providing the vaginal barrel with an adequate caliber (Fig. 45–2D and E).

Closure of the labioscrotal skin to the lateral urogenital sinus mucosa can be accomplished in a variety of ways. When it is redundant, this labioscrotal skin can be trimmed before closure. When prominent rugation is present, rotation of the labia (Fig. 45–2E) stretches the rugae and reorients them more vertically, making the appearance of the labia majora less masculine.

SUPRASPHINCTERIC VAGINOPLASTY

Rarely, complete virilization is encountered in virilizing adrenogenital syndrome, and the genitalia have a totally male appearance (Group F). In these patients, the distal vaginal segment is often no larger than a narrow fistula and enters the urogenital sinus through, or proximal to, the external urethral sphincter. Here the type of vaginoplasty described earlier may result in urinary incontinence from urethral sphincter disruption. The alternative is a very elaborate procedure, described by Hendren and Crawford (1969), which involves endoscopic insertion of a Fogarty balloon catheter into the vagina, followed by detachment of the lower vaginal segment from the urethral wall (urogenital sinus), using a perineal approach. The transverse perineal muscles are left attached to the perineal body between the urethra and the future vaginal outlet instead of being located rectovaginally. Extensive lateral and posterior skin flaps are required to exteriorize the detached vaginal cuff. Readers should consult the literature (Hendren and Crawford, 1969; Hendren and Donahoe, 1980) for details of repair in this situation.

Clitoral Surgery

Because the clitoris will reduce in size to a definite, although limited, degree after the infant has been placed on an appropriate and adequate regime of steroid replacement, a decision about the type of clitoroplasty for clitorimegaly should not be made at the initial neonatal evaluation (Fig. 45–3).

CLITORECTOMY

Initially, clitorectomy was the most widely applied method for cosmetic repair of genital ambiguity. It is technically easier to achieve a satisfactory cosmetic appearance of the vulva by clitoral amputation than by clitoral preservation procedures. However, because of questions about altered erotic responsiveness after amputation, this option is now generally contraindicated and is rarely appropriate; it has been useful as a secondary procedure for progressive clitorimegaly in the occasional girl with adrenogenital syndrome who has been noncompliant with her medication program (Sotiropoulos et al., 1976).

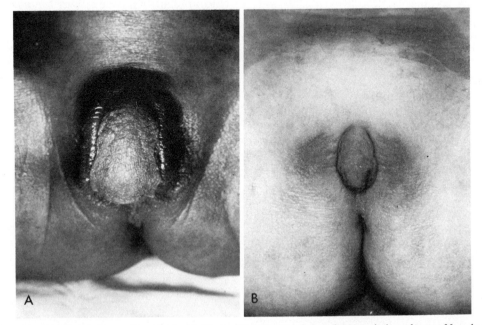

Figure 45–3. A, Appearance as neonate of girl with Group E virilization from adrenogenital syndrome. Note large size of phallus. B, Same girl at age 3½ years, immediately preceding reconstruction. Note relative reduction in phallic size with appropriate long-term steroid replacement. This phallus was easily managed by clitoroplasty and monsplasty at the time of vaginoplasty (see Fig. 45–8).

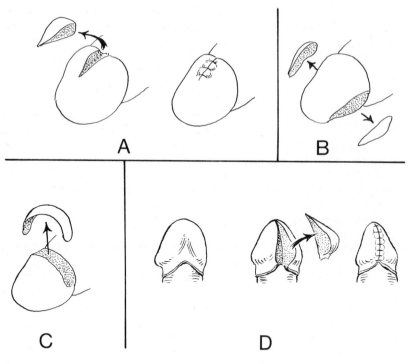

A

B

C

D

Figure 45–4. Options for glans reduction.

CLITORAL RECESSION

Current techniques emphasize preserving clitoral sensation by relocating the clitoris, using techniques designed to conceal it or make it less conspicuous. With recession of a very large, penis-sized phallus, however, bulging of the shaft under the mons tissues can occur during erections, making the clitoris fairly conspicuous. This problem may limit the choice of recession to a phallus that is not too large to be adequately concealed.

With the exception of Lattimer's (1961) technique for relocation of the shaft and glans, most recession procedures provide for relocation of the phallic body by attaching it more cephalad on the anterior periosteum of the symphysis and then closing the mons tissues over the shaft (Randolph and Hung, 1970). This is often combined with a reduction of glans size by trimming the lateral coronal margins and adjacent glans (Hendren and Crawford, 1972). For any form of clitoral recession or reduction, the glans too can be reduced to a suitable size by a variety of trimming or wedging techniques (Fig. 45–4).

CORPORAL PLICATION

Plication of the shaft is particularly suited to mild or moderate clitorimegaly. Heavy longitudinal through-and-through sutures on each side of the shaft, avoiding the neurovascular bundles, will shorten the shaft and obliterate the erectile spaces (Stefan, 1967) (Fig. 45–5). The use of multiple Nesbit wedges is an alternative to clitoral plication for shortening the clitoral shaft (Glassberg and Laungani, 1981), but this does not diminish corporal width or control bulging erections (Fig. 45–6).

In any form of clitoral revision involving a vaginoplasty, more than one stage may be re-

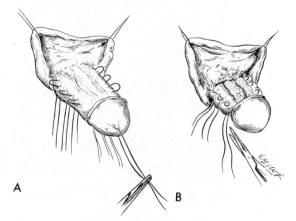

A

B

Figure 45–5. Technique for corporal plication. Heavy longitudinal through-and-through sutures shorten the phallus and obliterate the corporal cavities. The dorsal neurovascular bundles should be avoided.

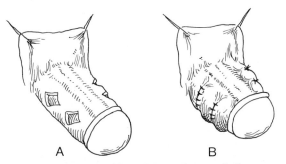

Figure 45–6. Nesbit wedges to shorten phallus.

quired to complete the clitoroplasty, especially the monsplasty and deeper mons dissection necessary for recession, because marked lymphedema may follow the extensive flap procedures used in the earlier steps of the operation. In such a situation it is better to complete the procedure at another sitting than to jeopardize tissue viability.

Figure 45–7 represents a follow-up after vaginoplasty and clitoroplasty by corporal plication. This is the same girl pictured in Figure 45–3.

CORPORAL REDUCTION (RESECTION)

To deal with a large phallic shaft, several authors have proposed shaft excision with preservation of the glans. Spence and Allen (1973) proposed total removal of the shaft and crura through a dorsal shaft degloving incision (dorsal circumcision incision) or, alternatively, after an elliptical transverse excision of excess dorsal midshaft skin. The glans is left attached to the midline vulval mucosa and is sutured to the pubic periosteum. Although the cosmetic results appear to be satisfactory, the authors do not describe preservation of the dorsal glans innervation.

Others have proposed excision of the shaft while identifying and preserving the dorsal neurovascular bundles. The glans is reattached to the proximal stump (Barinka et al., 1968; Kumar et al., 1974; Schmid, 1961) (Fig. 45–8). Here, too, the shaft and prepuce skin can be handled in a variety of ways for appropriate redistribution and creation of labia minora. When the midline mucosal strip is elongated, it can be detached from the glans, shortened, and then reattached to the ventral edge of the glans, provided the dorsal neurovascular bundle has not been compromised. Goodwin (1981) describes resection of the corpora from a ventral approach (Fig. 45–9).

The Toronto Sick Children's Hospital group has also performed dorsal shaft resection and dorsal glans wedging without regard to the dorsal nerves, relying on innervation to the residual glans tissue through an intact ventral mucosal strip. They report postoperative clitoral sensation (as tested by bielectrical stimulation), and the ability in the older patients to experience erotic gratification (Allen et al., 1982).

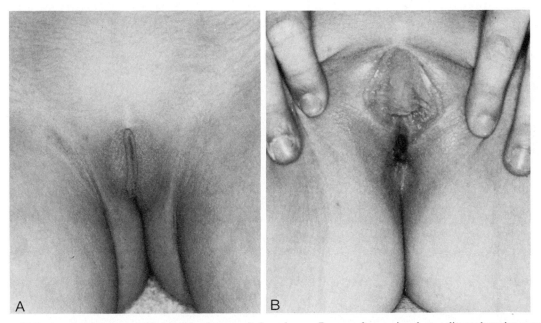

Figure 45–7. *A* and *B,* Ten-year-old girl with adrenogenital syndrome, 7 years after vaginoplasty, clitoroplasty by corporal plication, and monsplasty (see Fig. 45–3).

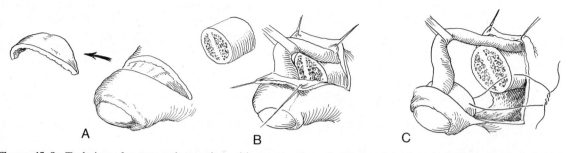

Figure 45–8. Technique for corporal resection with preservation of glans and its innervation. *A,* One method for approaching the phallic shaft and simultaneously trimming back the shaft skin by excising a transverse dorsal wedge. The shaft can also be exposed by dorsal degloving. *B,* Diagrammatic view of corporal excision with neurovascular preservation. *C,* Attachment of glans to phallic stump.

An alternative method to corporal resection for clitoral reduction has been described by Kogan et al. (1983). It involves subtunical resection of a segment of the erectile tissue within each corporal body. The midline mucosa is intentionally divided to mobilize the clitoral shaft and can be shortened, as appropriate, during reconstruction. The technique has the advantage of simplicity and of added safety, with little risk of superficial epithelial slough of the glans, which occurs at times with corporal resection. This technique is now the author's treatment of choice for management of the very large phallus. The steps are diagrammed in Figure 45–10.

Other Procedures

VULVOPLASTY (CREATION OF A VESTIBULE)

Male pseudohermaphrodites with ambiguous genitalia consisting of a micropenis with a fused perineum are best assigned a female gender role. The smallest size of a miniature penis that can develop into a sexually adequate adult penis is not known with certainty, but the responsiveness to growth of such an organ can be tested in early infancy with androgen. A phallus originally 2.5 cm or less in the full-term neonate is likely to be inadequate; in making decisions about altering sex assignment, it is helpful to

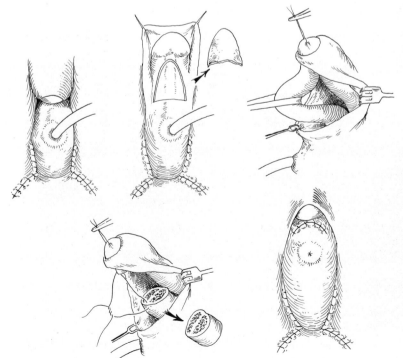

Figure 45–9. Corporal resection with preservation of neurovascular bundle, from a ventral approach. The midline ventral mucosal strip can be shortened, if necessary.

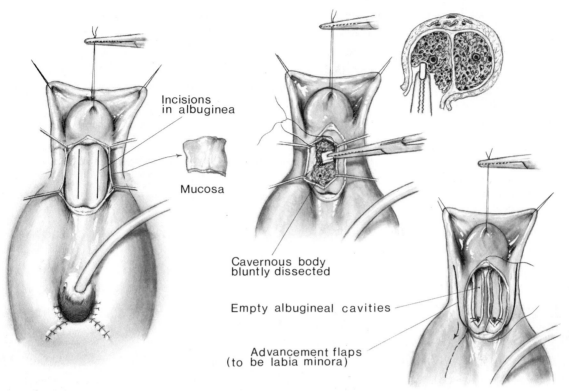

Incisions
in albuginea

Mucosa

Cavernous body
bluntly dissected

Empty albugineal cavities

Advancement flaps
(to be labia minora)

Wm. Loechel '83

Figure 45–10. Subtunical resection of tunica.

have a set of standards for normal ranges in penile size at all ages, including the newborn. Nomograms are available for this purpose (Feldman and Smith, 1975; Schonfeld, 1943).

In patients with micropenis, simple exteriorization of the penile and bulbar urethra (extended external urethrostomy) will simulate the appearance of a vulva. Lateral prepucial or shaft skin flaps can be advanced inferiorly on either side of the opened urethra to form labia minora. As in flap vaginoplasty, a small flap can be turned into the deep bulbar urethra to avoid perineal contracture during healing. When a short vaginal pouch from incomplete müllerian duct inhibition is also present, the flap can be turned into the vagina at the time of the urethral exteriorization. Orchiectomy, of course, should be done (Figs. 45–11 and 45–12).

VAGINAL REPLACEMENT

Some intersex patients have no vagina or at best a very shallow vaginal pouch. Vaginal augmentation or replacement procedures should not be attempted before puberty and are infrequently done by the urologist. The interested reader should consult the literature.

POSTOPERATIVE MANAGEMENT

Immediate postoperative management, aside from appropriate steroid replacement in cases of adrenogenital syndrome, consists primarily of wound care. It is usually possible to remove the urethral catheter inserted at surgery on the second or third postoperative day, but when excessive edema is present, the tube is best left in longer. At the completion of the vaginoplasty, I loosely pack the vaginal outlet with a strip of 1-inch Vaseline gauze, which keeps the suture lines apart and contributes to local hemostasis. This packing should be removed after 24 hours to avoid tissue maceration and to allow for drainage of serosanguineous intravaginal fluid.

The genitoplasty should be bandaged with a fluffy gauze dressing, using gentle compression to limit local edema. Dressings can generally be discontinued on the second or third day, at the time of catheter removal. Topical conjugated estrogen cream can be started after dressings are discontinued and applied twice daily for a period of up to 1 week at a time. This causes

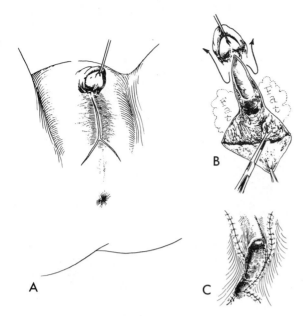

Figure 45–11. Technique for creating vulva ("vulvoplasty") in male pseudohermaphrodite with ambiguous genitalia or a micropenis. *A,* Urethotomy. Dorsal urethra becomes mucosa of created vestibule. *B,* Defatting of perineal portion of labia majora creates a flatter, more feminine contour of the genitalia. Development of V flaps for labia minora, outlined by arrows. Advancement of these flaps posteriorly on either side of new vestibule also pulls phallus downward. *C,* Completed repair. Flap plasty into deep bulb, or into small vaginal pouch when present, minimizes contracture of created vestibule during healing.

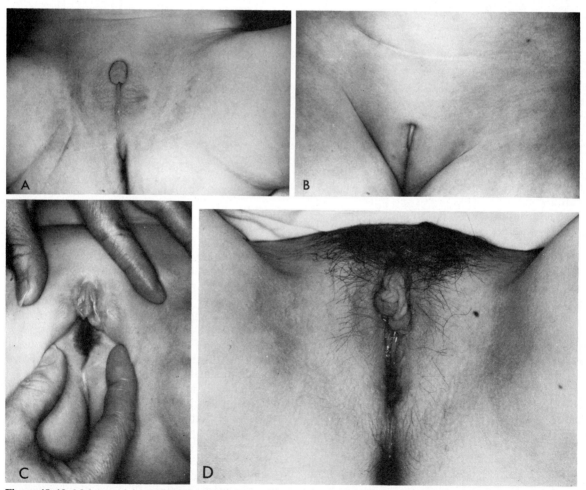

Figure 45–12. Male pseudohermaphrodite treated by vulvoplasty and vaginoplasty. *A,* One-year-old infant male, XY with dysgenetic testes. Phallus is tiny; scrotum is underdeveloped and empty. The infant was treated as in Figure 45–11. A small vaginal pouch was present. *B* and *C,* Appearance at age 5 years. *D,* Appearance at age 12 years, 11 years postoperatively, after beginning exogenous estrogen therapy. Hymen and vaginal orifice are visible. Appearance is appropriately female.

temporary local pubertal changes that are beneficial during healing. During the first few weeks postoperatively, gentle passage of a catheter or sound into the distal vagina may be helpful when focal vaginal outlet narrowing is suspected. However, overdilation can injure the repair and result in a dense scar.

RESULTS

Long-term results of multiple large series of children undergoing genital reconstruction for management of intersexuality are not yet available, and details about adult sexual functioning are still scanty. Several series have emphasized the generally good results obtained following female genital reconstruction. In some instances, vaginoplasty revision may be needed after puberty because of stenosis, regardless of the technique used for vaginoplasty. The articles listed in the References about clitoroplasty, with or without resection of the shaft, have reported generally favorable results, although an occasional revision is necessary.

Despite some tendency toward tomboy behavior during childhood, early sex assignment to a female gender role for girls with the adrenogenital syndrome, plus appropriate steroidal replacement, has resulted in a favorable outcome, and the patients have made a satisfactory adjustment in the sex of assignment. As Money (1973) has pointed out, "they experience romance, erotic attraction and marriage, usually concordantly with the sex of assignment and rearing. They experience genito-pelvic pleasure, not necessarily losing the orgasm even after extensive genital excision and reconstruction."

References

Allen, L. E., Hardy, B. E., and Churchill, B. M.: The surgical management of the enlarged clitoris. J. Urol., 128:351, 1982.

Barinka, L., Stavratjev, M., and Toman, M.: Plastic adjustment of female genitals in adrenogenital syndrome. Acta Chir. Plast., 10:99, 1968.

Barrett, T. M., and Gonzales, E. T., Jr.: Reconstruction of the female external genitalia. Urol. Clin. North Am., 7:455, 1980.

Feldman, K. W., and Smith, D. W.: Fetal phallic growth and penile standards for newborn male infants. J. Pediatr., 86:395, 1975.

Fortunoff, S., Lattimer, J. K., and Edson, M.: Vaginoplasty technique for female pseudohermaphrodites. Surg. Gynecol. Obstet., 118:545, 1964.

Glassberg, K. I., and Laungani, G.: Reduction clitoroplasty. Urology, 17:604, 1981.

Goodwin, W. E.: Partial (segmental) amputation of the clitoris for female pseudohermaphroditism. Soc. Pediatr. Urol. Newsletter, Jan. 21, 1981.

Gross, R. E., Randolph, J., and Crigler, J. F., Jr.: Clitorectomy for sexual abnormalities: Indications and technique. Surgery, 59:300, 1966.

Hampson, J. G.: Hermaphroditic genital appearance, rearing and eroticism in hyperadrenocorticism. Bull. Johns Hopkins Hosp., 90:265, 1955.

Hendren, W. H., and Crawford, J. D.: Adrenogenital syndrome: The anatomy of the anomaly and its repair. Some new concepts. J. Pediatr. Surg., 4:49, 1969.

Hendren, W. H., and Crawford, J. D.: The child with ambiguous genitalia. Curr. Probl. Surg., 1–64, Nov., 1972.

Hendren, W. H., and Donahoe, P. K.: Correction of congenital abnormalities of the vagina and perineum. J. Pediatr. Surg., 15:751, 1980.

Hurtig, A. L., Radhakrishnan, J., Reyes, H. M., and Rosenthal, I. M.: Psychological evaluation of treated females with virilizing congenital adrenal hyperplasia. J. Pediatr. Surg., 18:887, 1983.

Jones, H. W., Jr., and Jones, G. E. S.: The gynecological aspects of adrenal hyperplasia and allied disorders. Am. J. Obstet. Gynecol., 68:1330, 1954.

Jones, H. W., Jr., Facog, M. D., and Verkauf, B. S.: Surgical treatment in congenital adrenal hyperplasia. Age at operation and other prognostic factors. Obstet. Gynecol., 36:1, 1970.

Jones, H. W., Jr., Garcia, S. C., and Klingensmith, G. J.: Secondary surgical treatment of the masculinized external genitalia of patients with virilizing adrenal hyperplasia. Obstet. Gynecol., 48:73, 1976.

Jones, H. W., Jr., and Wilkins, L.: The genital anomaly associated with prenatal exposure to progestogens. Fertil. Steril., 11:148, 1960.

Kogan, S. J., Smey, P., and Levitt, S. B.: Subtunical total reduction clitoroplasty: a safe modification of existing techniques. J. Urol., 130:746, 1983.

Kumar, H., Kiefer, J. H., Rosenthal, I. E., and Clark, S. S.: Clitoroplasty: Experience during a 19-year period. J. Urol., 111:81, 1974.

Lattimer, J. K.: Relocation and recession of the enlarged clitoris with preservation of the glans: An alternative to amputation. J. Urol., 86:113, 1961.

Lewis, V. G., and Money, J.: Adrenogenital syndrome: The need for early surgical feminization in girls. In Lee, P. A., Plotnick, L. P., Kowarski, A. V., and Migeon, C. J. (Eds.): Congenital Adrenal Hyperplasia, pp. 463–466. Baltimore, University Park Press, 1977.

Mininberg, D. T.: Phalloplasty in congenital adrenal hyperplasia. J. Urol., 128:355, 1982.

Money, J.: Intersexual problems. Clin. Obstet. Gynecol., 16:169, 1973.

Money, J., and Ehrhardt, A. A.: Man and Woman, Boy and Girl: Differentiation and Dimorphism of Gender Identity from Conception to Maturity. Baltimore, Johns Hopkins University Press, 1972.

Money, J., and Schwartz, M.: Dating, romantic and nonromantic friendships, and sexuality in 17 early-treated adrenogenital females, aged 16–25. In Lee, P. A., Plotnick, J. P., Kowarski, A. V., and Migeon, C. J. (Eds.): Congenital Adrenal Hyperplasia. pp. 419–431. Baltimore, University Park Press, 1977.

Nihoul-Fekete, C., Philippe, F., Thibaud, E., Rappaport, R., and Pellerin, D.: Resultats à moyen et long terme de la chirurgie reparatrice des organes genitaux chez les filles atteintes d'hyperplasie congenitale virilisante des surrenales. Arch. Fr. Pediatr., 39:13, 1982.

Prader, A.: Vollkommen männliche äussere Genitalentwicklung und Salverlustsyndrom bei Mädchen mit kongenitalem androgenitalem Syndrom. Helv. Paediat. Acta, *13*:5, 1958.

Randolph, J. G., and Hung, W.: Reduction clitoroplasty in females with hypertrophied clitoris. J. Pediatr. Surg., *5*:224, 1970.

Schmid, M. A.: Plastiche Korrektur des äusseren Genitales bei einem männlichen Scheinzwitter. Arch. Klin. Chir., *298*:977, 1961.

Schonfeld, W. A.: Primary and secondary sexual characteristics. Am. J. Dis. Child., *65*:535, 1943.

Sotiropoulos, A., Morishima, A., Homsy, Y., and Lattimer, J. K.: Long-term assessment of genital reconstruction in female pseudohermaphrodites. J. Urol., *115*:599, 1976.

Spence, H. M., and Allen, T. D.: Genital reconstruction in the female with the adrenogenital syndrome. Br. J. Urol., *45*:126, 1973.

Stefan, H.: Surgical reconstruction of the external genitalia in female pseudohermaphrodites. Br. J. Urol., *39*:347, 1967.

Verkauf, B. S., and Jones, H. W., Jr.: Masculinization of the female genitalia in congenital adrenal hyperplasia. Relationship to the salt losing variety of the disease. South. Med. J., *63*:634, 1970.

CHAPTER 46

Congenital Anomalies of the Testis

JACOB RAJFER, M.D.

CRYPTORCHIDISM

Cryptorchidism means a hidden testis. This occurs when the testis fails to descend into its normal postnatal anatomic location, the scrotum. Since the testis originally develops in the abdominal region, its descent may be inhibited anywhere along its normal pathway or it may be diverted from this route into an ectopic location.

This apparently simple developmental anomaly represents one of the more common disorders of childhood. It affects all races, and there does not seem to be a geographic propensity. Although cryptorchidism may be associated with a number of chromosomal and hereditary disorders in which a specific defect can be identified, at the present time the majority of cases appear to be isolated. This is probably due to the fact that relatively little is known about what causes the testis to migrate from the abdomen into the scrotum. It seems certain that as technological and scientific advances continue to be made in the fields of genetics, biochemistry, and reproductive endocrinology, particularly involving the mechanisms that cause the testis to descend, more and more clinical cases of cryptorchidism will be identified as being the phenotypic expression of a more generalized systemic disorder.

Why the Testis Descends

For the production of viable and mature spermatozoa, the testis in most mammalian species must descend from the warmer intra-abdominal environment into the cooler scrotum (Moore and Quick, 1924; Cooper, 1929; Felizet

and Branca, 1902; Wangensteen, 1935; Pace and Cabot, 1936). The slight temperature difference of 1.5 to 2.0° C between these two locations is sufficient to inhibit spermatogenesis.

If the timing of testicular descent in various animal species is compared, interesting observations can be made regarding the thermoregulation of spermatogenesis. The primate is the only species in which the testis completely descends at or near the time of birth (Wislocki, 1933). In the monkey, the testes retract from the scrotum to the inguinal canal at about the fifth postnatal day only to return permanently to the scrotum between the third and fifth years of life, which is the normal time of puberty in this species. In certain hibernating animals, the testes, which are intra-abdominal during the winter months, descend into the scrotum only during the breeding season (Bishop, 1945). In other animals, the testes remain intra-abdominal except during copulation, when they descend into the scrotum. (Deming, 1936). In the whale, the testes are located intra-abdominally and are probably cooled by the animal's constant contact with cooler water (Huberman and Israeloff, 1935). The testes of birds are located in the lumbar region and presumably are cooled by the air stream that constantly flows over them during flight. Therefore, cooling of the testes via migration into the scrotum appears to be a phylogenetic mechanism that man has retained in order to propagate his species.

Embryology of Testicular Descent

In order to comprehend how the testis migrates into the scrotum, a knowledge of the embryology of testicular descent is essential

(Hamilton et al., 1957; Arey, 1965). In the human, by the sixth week of gestation the primordial germ cells have migrated from the wall of the embryonic yolk sac along the dorsal mesentery of the hindgut to invade the genital ridges (Witschi, 1948). At this stage of development, the gubernaculum first appears as a ridge of mesenchymal tissue extending from the genital ridge through a gap in the anterior abdominal wall musculature to the genital swellings that are the site of the future scrotum (Backhouse, 1964). This gap in the anterior abdominal wall is the future inguinal canal. By 7 weeks of gestation, possibly under the influence of the H-Y antigen that is secreted from the XY primordial germ cells, the indifferent gonad differentiates into the fetal testis (Wachtel et al., 1975; Ohno, 1979). During the eighth week of gestation in the male embryo, the fetal testis begins to secrete two hormones, testosterone and müllerian-inhibiting factor (Jost, 1953a and b). Testosterone, which is synthesized and secreted by the fetal Leydig cells (Siiteri and Wilson, 1974; Payne and Jaffe, 1975), is under the regulation of maternal chorionic gonadotropin (hCG) at this stage of development (Clements et al., 1976) and induces the ipsilateral wolffian duct to form the epididymis and vas deferens. Müllerian-inhibiting factor, which is secreted by the fetal Sertoli cells (Josso, 1972, 1973), causes regression of the müllerian ducts, leaving behind only the appendix testis, a remnant of the müllerian ductal system. At this time, the processus vaginalis, an outpouching of the peritoneum, may be seen ventral to the gubernaculum (Lemeh, 1960; Wyndham, 1943). The future muscle fibers of the cremaster may also appear at this time along the developing processus vaginalis. The processus vaginalis forms as a hernia in the weak triangle that consists of peritoneum backed only by the jelly of the gubernaculum (Gier and Marion, 1970). The margins of the triangle are formed dorsally by the internal iliac artery and vein and ventrolaterally by the most posterior bands of the transversus abdominis muscle.

Between the eighth and sixteenth weeks of gestation, the external genitalia develop (Jirasek et al., 1968). In the male embryo, testosterone, which is secreted systemically by the fetal testis, is picked up by the tissues of the external genitalia and converted to dihydrotestosterone (DHT) by the 5-alpha reductase enzyme within the tissues of the external genitalia (Siiteri and Wilson, 1974). DHT is the active androgen that induces differentiation of the external genitalia in the male embryo (Siiteri and Wilson, 1974).

After development of the testes, ductal system, and external genitalia, the testis lies on top of the conically shaped gubernaculum, awaiting descent (Backhouse, 1981). The gubernaculum can be seen running from the cauda epididymis distally through the inguinal canal toward the genital swellings. Under continued androgenic stimulation the genital swellings are transformed into the scrotum. The testis has now assumed an intra-abdominal position right behind the internal inguinal ring. In reality, the testis is never more than 1.3 mm from the internal inguinal ring at any time during its development (Wyndham, 1943).

The process of testicular descent remains relatively dormant between the twelfth week and the seventh month of gestation. During this time, the processus vaginalis, an outpouching of the peritoneum, slowly extends into the scrotum (Wyndham, 1943). At about the seventh month of gestation, just prior to actual descent of the testis, rapid alterations occur simultaneously in the gubernaculum, processus vaginalis, and other surrounding structures. There is an increase in the size of the vasa deferentia and testicular vessels, the gubernaculum begins to swell, and the processus vaginalis now extends rapidly into the scrotum (Backhouse, 1964; Backhouse and Butler, 1960). A separation now occurs between the gubernaculum and the scrotal wall. As the scrotum and inguinal canal are stretched by the developing gubernaculum, the gonad, which sits on top of the gubernaculum, slips very rapidly through the inguinal canal into the scrotum (Wyndham, 1943; Backhouse, 1981; Schechter, 1963). During descent, the epididymis precedes the testis in its journey into the scrotum. After descent occurs, the scrotal part of the processus vaginalis persists as the tunica vaginalis, while the upper part obliterates, and the gubernaculum subsequently atrophies. If the processus vaginalis fails to obliterate, a hernia may form.

Mechanisms of Testicular Descent

Since Hunter's (1841) treatise on testicular descent, various mechanisms have been proposed to be responsible for the final placement of the testes into the scrotum. Foremost are certain physical factors, which include (1) traction on the testis by the gubernaculum and/or cremaster muscle; (2) differential growth of the body wall in relation to a relatively immobile gubernaculum; (3) intra-abdominal pressure pushing the testis through an inguinal canal that is engorged by the swollen gubernaculum; and (4) development and maturation of the epididymis being responsible for testicular migration. The traction theory adheres to the concept that the gubernaculum, or the cremaster muscle, or both, pull the testis into the scrotum (Sonneland, 1925; Curling, 1840). Support for this concept comes from the observation that severance of the genitofemoral nerve, which innervates the gubernaculum, prevents testicular descent in rodents (Tayakkononta, 1963). However, severance of the gubernaculum in a variety of animal species did not prevent the testis from descending into the scrotum (Wells, 1944; Bergh et al., 1978). In addition, in the human fetus there is only a weak attachment between the gubernaculum and the scrotum and this is probably insufficient to support any traction on the testis (Wyndham, 1943; Tayakkononta, 1963; Bergh et al., 1978). Regarding the cremaster, it is well established that the sole function of this muscle is to retract the testis; consequently, traction of the testis into the scrotum by the cremaster muscle is unlikely.

The differential growth theory adheres to the concept that as the body wall grows, the testis is kept in proximity to the internal inguinal ring. It is then pulled into the scrotum by the relatively immobile gubernaculum as a result of rapid growth of the body wall during the last trimester of pregnancy (McMurrich, 1923; Hunter, 1927). However, it has been demonstrated that the gubernaculum actually increases in size prior to descent and that it actually grows faster than the body as a whole (Lemeh, 1960; Hunter, 1927), thereby casting doubt on the validity of this theory.

The intra-abdominal pressure theory states that an increase in intra-abdominal pressure is the primary force that causes the testis to leave the abdomen and enter the inguinal ring (Gier and Marion, 1970; Schechter, 1963; Bergin et al., 1970). Recently, a number of investigators have provided theoretical and experimental evidence that appears to support the concept of intra-abdominal pressure (Elder et al., 1982; Frey and Rajfer, 1984; Frey et al., 1983).

The epididymal theory of testicular descent, which is based on the assumption that differentiation and maturation of the epididymis induce testicular descent (Frey and Rajfer, 1984), has been refuted and may not be as important as initially thought (Frey and Rajfer, 1982).

Although it is difficult to refute unequivocally the aforementioned mechanical theories of testicular descent, and indeed all may play some role in testicular descent, it is generally accepted that endocrine factors somehow play the major role in promoting the descent of the testis into the scrotum. The endocrine regulation of testicular descent was initially inferred by Engle (1932) who induced premature testicular descent in the monkey by the use of gonadotropins. Very soon after, testosterone was found to be as efficacious as gonadotropins in inducing testicular descent in humans (Arnheim, 1938; Thompson et al., 1937; Bigler et al., 1938; Goldman et al., 1938; Hamilton and Hubert, 1938; Hamilton, 1938). More recently, it has been demonstrated that dihydrotestosterone, the 5-alpha reduced product of testosterone, appears to be the active androgen involved in testicular descent in at least two animal species (Rajfer and Walsh, 1977; Rajfer, 1982).

Endocrine Aspects of Cryptorchidism

If gonadotropins and androgens are necessary for testicular descent to occur, it follows that abnormalities in the hypothalamic-pituitary-testicular axis will result in cryptorchidism. Indeed, in a variety of clinical syndromes characterized by defects in gonadotropin production, androgen synthesis, or androgen action, cryptorchidism may be observed (Fig. 46–1). In Kallmann's syndrome, in which there exists a deficiency in gonadotropin-releasing hormone (GnRH) secretion from the hypothalamus, cryptorchidism may be a presenting feature (Bardin et al., 1969; Santen and Paulson, 1972). In anencephaly or developmental abnormalities of the pituitary gland, such as hypoplasia or aplasia, undescended testes are very common (Ch'in, 1938; Sadeghi-Nejad and Senior, 1974; Steiner and Boggs, 1965). In disorders of androgen synthesis or androgen action, cryptorchidism may also be a presenting feature (Grumbach and Van Wyk, 1974). And finally, in pseudovaginal perineoscrotal hypospadias, a condition in which there is an absence of the 5-alpha reductase enzyme that converts testosterone into dihydrotestosterone, cryptorchidism is frequent (Opitz et al., 1972; Walsh et al., 1974).

Although hormonal involvement in testicular descent appears clear-cut, there is, nevertheless, some discrepancy in the literature as to whether patients with cryptorchidism have discernible abnormalities in their hypothalamic-pituitary-testicular axis. Walsh et al. (1976) found no difference in basal plasma testosterone levels between cryptorchid and normal children. In contrast, Cacciari et al. (1976) found a sub-

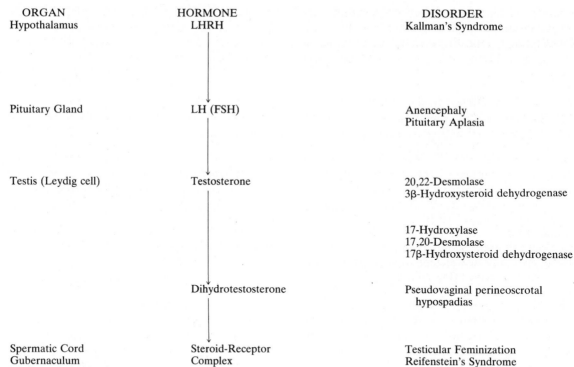

ORGAN	HORMONE	DISORDER
Hypothalamus	LHRH	Kallman's Syndrome
Pituitary Gland	LH (FSH)	Anencephaly Pituitary Aplasia
Testis (Leydig cell)	Testosterone	20,22-Desmolase 3β-Hydroxysteroid dehydrogenase
		17-Hydroxylase 17,20-Desmolase 17β-Hydroxysteroid dehydrogenase
	Dihydrotestosterone	Pseudovaginal perineoscrotal hypospadias
Spermatic Cord Gubernaculum Processus Vaginalis	Steroid-Receptor Complex	Testicular Feminization Reifenstein's Syndrome

Figure 46–1. Disorders of the hypothalamic-pituitary-testicular axis in the presence of cryptorchidism. (From Rajfer, J., and Walsh, P. C.: J. Urol., *118*:985, 1977. Used by permission.)

normal testosterone response to gonadotropin in the cryptorchid children. When Cacciari et al. (1976) used GnRH to stimulate the hypothalamic-pituitary axis, they did not find any difference in pituitary LH and FSH secretion between the cryptorchid and normal children. This was confirmed by Sizonenko et al. (1978) and Van Vliet et al. (1980). On the other hand, the data of Hadziselimovic (1983) and Job and Gendrel (Job et al., 1977; Gendrel et al., 1977, 1978, 1980*a* and *b*) suggest that cryptorchid infants and children do indeed have abnormalities in their hypothalamic-pituitary-testicular axis, as evidenced by a decrease in their basal LH and testosterone levels and a blunted response of LH and testosterone to GnRH stimulation (Fig. 46–2). This deficiency in the secretion of LH and testosterone found in the cryptorchid infant persists through early puberty but disappears at midpuberty. There was no significant abnormality seen in the FSH levels of these cryptorchid patients, although an occasional patient did demonstrate elevated basal FSH levels indicative of seminiferous tubular damage.

In spite of these data, the exact mechanism by which androgens act to promote testicular descent is still unknown. It is apparent, based on embryologic observations and some experimental data, that the gubernaculum is intimately

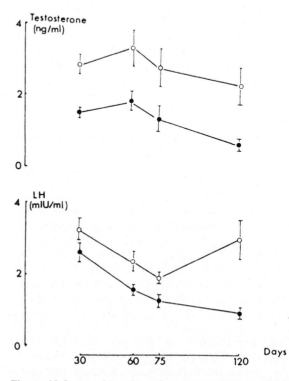

Figure 46–2. Age-dependent plasma testosterone and LH (mean ± SEM) in newborn infants who presented at birth with undescended testes. One group (○) had spontaneous descent by 4 months, whereas in the other group (●) there was no testicular descent. (From Gendrel, D., et al.: J. Pediatr., *97*:217, 1980. Used by permission.)

involved with this important physiologic event. However, to date, no investigator has been able to detect the presence of an androgen receptor, a necessary prerequisite for any androgen-induced response, in the gubernaculum of any animal species.

Classification of Undescended Testis

Based on its location, the cryptorchid testis can be classified as either being (1) abdominal, located inside the internal inguinal ring; (2) canalicular, located between the internal and external inguinal rings; (3) ectopic, located away from the normal pathway of descent between the abdominal cavity and the bottom of the scrotum, or (4) retractile, in which the fully descended testis moves freely between the bottom of the scrotum and the groin, where it enters the superficial inguinal pouch of Denis Browne (Browne, 1949). This pouch is actually a subcutaneous pocket lined by thin fibrous tissue situated in front of and lateral to the external inguinal ring.

The intra-abdominal testis, by definition, is impalpable. Very commonly, the testis is located just at the internal inguinal ring, and at the time of surgical exploration slight abdominal pressure will usually cause the testis to pop into the inguinal canal. The canalicular testis is farther along the pathway of descent than the intra-abdominal testis. It may be located within the canal or may become emergent from within the canal to lie at the top of the scrotum. When it is located in the inguinal canal, the tension of the aponeurosis of the external oblique muscle may be too firm a barrier to allow the testis to become palpable (Scorer and Farrington, 1971).

On rare occasions, the testis may migrate from its normal pathway of movement between the abdominal cavity and the bottom of the scrotum and become located in an ectopic position. There are five major sites of testicular ectopia: the perineum, the femoral canal, the superficial inguinal pouch, the suprapubic area, and the opposite scrotal compartment (Fig. 46–3). Testicular ectopia is believed to be directly related to the development of the gubernaculum. The gubernaculum is known to be divided into five branches, one each going to the aforementioned areas (Schechter, 1963; Lockwood, 1888). The scrotal area normally contains the bulk of the gubernaculum, and the testis normally follows this path during its descent. It has been suggested that when one of the other four

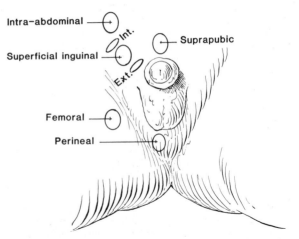

Figure 46–3. Schematic representation of sites of ectopic testes (Int = internal inguinal ring; ext = external inguinal ring). (Reproduced with permission from Rajfer and Frey, 1981, The Williams & Wilkins Co.)

branches contains the bulk of the gubernaculum, the testis is misdirected from its normal pathway of descent into the ectopic location. The most common ectopic location is in the superficial inguinal pouch. Transverse testicular ectopia is the rarest of all ectopic conditions but should also be considered in any patient with an empty hemiscrotum and an additional mass in the contralateral hemiscrotum (Davis, 1957; Mukerjee and Amesur, 1965; Dajani, 1969).

The single most common factor that leads to inaccurate diagnosis of an undescended testis is the presence of testicular retraction. Testicular retraction results from the spontaneous or provoked activity of the cremaster muscle. It is most apparent in prepubertal males of 5 to 6 years of age. In a survey of some 600 normal boys, Farrington (1968) found that in those under the age of 12 years up to 20 per cent of the testes were in the superficial inguinal pouch at an initial inspection. Between 6 months and 11 years of age, deliberate stimulation of the cremasteric reflex would result in withdrawal of up to 80 per cent of fully descended testes from their scrotal positions, leaving a seemingly empty hemiscrotum. Some 25 per cent of these testes will retract fully into the superficial inguinal pouch, and the remainder will retract into the neck of the scrotum. From the fifth to the sixth year of age until puberty, there is a gradual decline in the number of testes that will fully retract out of the scrotum. At 11 years of age, with half of the boys who were showing evidence of the onset of puberty, only half of the testes retracted upon stimulation of the cremasteric reflex. At 13 years of age, the testis was usually found to be no longer retractile.

This retraction of the normal testis into the upper part of the scrotum or the superficial inguinal pouch during boyhood seems to be a protective reflex. Why this reflex appears to dissipate at the time of puberty is unknown. Therefore, it is of paramount importance to determine and record in the infant's chart whether the testes are palpable in the scrotum at birth or within the first year of life. In order to differentiate a retractile from a true cryptorchid testis, more than one visit to the physician may be necessary.

If a testis is not palpable, it is intracanalicular, intra-abdominal, or absent (Scorer and Farrington, 1971). The diagnosis of bilateral anorchia should always be considered in the presence of bilateral nonpalpable testes (Goldberg et al., 1974). Human chorionic gonadotropin stimulation tests are frequently applied to distinguish bilateral anorchia from bilateral nondescent (Grant et al., 1976; Winter et al., 1972). A 3-day short course of hCG (2000 IU daily for 3 days) may be used to distinguish bilateral anorchia from bilateral cryptorchidism. In bilateral anorchia, basal gonadotropin levels are extremely high and there is no response by testosterone to exogenous hCG.

The unilateral impalpable testis itself presents a unique diagnostic problem. Its presence must be verified and appropriate therapy taken either to make it palpable or to remove it. A variety of tests have recently found their way into clinical practice in the search for the impalpable testis. These include herniography, ultrasound, CT scanning, and testicular arteriography or venography. Herniography is the oldest and least commonly practiced of these tests (White et al., 1973, 1970). It involves placement of contrast material intra-abdominally through a percutaneous catheter and x-ray demonstration of the presence of a hernia. Sometimes it is possible to outline an undescended testis near the hernia sac, but, as can be expected, this procedure has an unacceptably high incidence of false positive and false negative results. For this reason, it is rarely used in routine clinical practice today. Ultrasound scanning has been helpful in locating the testis only if it is located within the inguinal canal (Madrazo et al., 1979). If the testis is intra-abdominal, ultrasound is not very reliable. CT scanning of the child is especially useful in bilateral impalpable testes (Fig. 46–4) to document their location, but the test is expensive and sometimes difficult to perform in the very young individual (Lee et al., 1980; Walverson et al., 1980; Pak et al., 1981; Rajfer et al., 1983). It is, however, the least invasive of all the currently used procedures. Angiography of the testicular vessels is

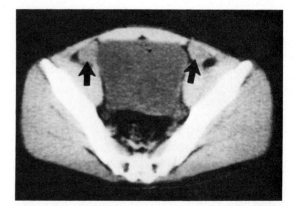

Figure 46–4. CT scan of pelvis demonstrating bilateral undescended testes (arrows) at the internal inguinal rings (B = bladder) (From Rajfer, J., et al.: J. Urol., *129*:978, 1983. Used by permission.)

technically difficult, and its complications (e.g., femoral thrombosis) may have disastrous consequences (Ben-Menachem et al., 1974; Vitale et al., 1974). Testicular venography has less morbidity than arteriography but is still an invasive procedure. Venography relies on the fact that when the pampiniform plexus of veins is present (Fig. 46–5), the testis presumably is

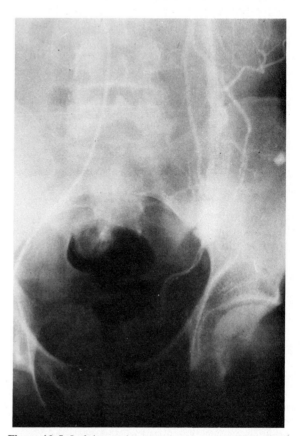

Figure 46–5. Left internal spermatic vein venography, demonstrating pampiniform plexus at termination of internal spermatic veins in pelvis.

TABLE 46–1. INCIDENCE OF CRYPTORCHIDISM FROM
BIRTH TO ADULTHOOD

Age	Incidence (%)
Preterm infant	30.3
Full-term infant	3.4
One year	0.8
Adulthood	0.8

Adapted from Scorer, G., and Farrington, G. H.:
Congenital Deformities of the Testis and Epididymis. New
York, Appleton-Century-Crofts, 1971.

always present (Amin and Wheeler, 1976; Weiss
et al., 1979). However, if the plexus is not
visualized for one reason or another or if the
testicular vein is blind-ending, one cannot unequivocally state that the testis is absent on that
side (Weiss et al., 1979). For this reason, the
test has its drawbacks. In the future, it is possible that pediatric laparoscopy may be used
more frequently in the search for the impalpable
testis (Silber and Cohen, 1980). Although this
procedure requires an anesthetic in the young
individual, it may be performed just prior to
surgical exploration so that only one anesthetic
is used.

Incidence of Cryptorchidism

Cryptorchidism represents one of the most
common disorders in man. Indeed, it is not
unusual to see the genitourinary system well
represented by the cryptorchid state in a multitude of congenital and hereditary abnormalities
(Frey et al., 1981). In some premature babies,
birth may occur prior to the onset of normal
testicular descent during the last trimester of
gestation. Indeed, Scorer and Farrington (1971)
found that of 1500 full-term (birth weight
greater than 2500 gm) infants examined at birth,
3.4 per cent had true undescended testes, while
30.3 per cent of 142 premature infants had
undescended testes (Table 46–1). This discrepancy in the incidence of testicular descent in
full-term and premature infants has also been
reported by other investigators (Buemann et
al., 1961).

Furthermore, the smaller the birth weight
of the infant, the greater the incidence of cryptorchidism. For example, 68.5 per cent of infants
weighing less than 1800 gm had undescended
testes, while almost 100 per cent of infants
weighing less than 900 gm showed bilateral
cryptorchidism (Scorer, 1964). However, once
these babies, particularly the premature ones,
begin to gain weight and advance in age, the
undescended testes begin to descend postnatally. Indeed, by 1 year of age, the incidence of
testicular descent is approximately 0.8 per cent,
a marked decrease during this short time period
of 1 year (Scorer and Farrington, 1971; Villumsen and Zachau-Christiansen, 1966). Scorer and
Farrington's data (1971) show that approximately 75 per cent of full-term cryptorchid testes
and up to 95 per cent of premature cryptorchid
testes will spontaneously descend by 1 year of
age. What is more amazing is that most of these
testes that descend during the first year of life
actually do so within the first 3 months after
birth. If descent had not occurred by this time,
the testis never descended completely and remained relatively smaller than the contralat-
erally descended testis.

It is assumed, although not proved, that
the reason the testis may descend within the
first year is the elevated level of androgens in
the plasma of the male infant during the first 3
months of life (Table 46–2) (Scorer, 1964; Forest et al., 1974). This rise in the plasma testosterone during the first 3 months in the male
gradually drops to prepubertal levels (Forest et
al., 1974; Winter et al., 1976), and the Leydig
cells, the source of the testosterone, become
inactive and remain so until puberty. Despite
the fact that the Leydig cells are inactive during
the prepubertal years, they nevertheless retain
the potential to respond to hCG stimulation.
This response to gonadotropin has been amply
demonstrated in both prepubertal normal testes
and prepubertal cryptorchid testes (Grant et al.,
1976; Winter et al., 1972).

The cryptorchid state is most easily determined at birth, when the scrotum is relatively
large, minimal subcutaneous fat exists, and the
cremasteric reflex is absent (Scorer and Farrington, 1971). However, the cremasteric reflex is
most active between the second and seventh
years of age, and, as a result, a falsely high
incidence of cryptorchidism may be obtained
during childhood (McCutcheon, 1938; Ward and

TABLE 46–2. PLASMA TESTOSTERONE (ng%) IN HUMANS

	1–15 days	1–3 months	1 year	Prepuberty	Adulthood
Male	68 ± 60	208 ± 68	6.6 ± 4.6	6.6 ± 2.5	572 ± 135
Female	12 ± 6	9 ± 4	5.5 ± 2.8	6.6 ± 2.5	37 ± 10

Adapted from Forest, M. G., et al.: J. Clin. Invest., 53:819, 1974.

Hunter, 1960). In fact, in a number of studies the incidence of cryptorchidism at or about the fifth year of age was estimated at about 10 per cent (Farrington, 1968). This high percentage was probably due to the inclusion of unrecognized cases of retractile testes, and there is ample evidence to support this assumption. For example, if the incidence of cryptorchidism is the same at 1 year and at adulthood (0.8 per cent), this incidence cannot change at any time between these ages because human testes do not ascend permanently in the postnatal period. Consequently, if there appears to be an increase in the incidence of cryptorchidism beyond 0.8 per cent at other ages, it must certainly be due to testes that retract and then descend at a later date. When Cour-Palais (1966) re-examined those cases of undescended testes of various age groups, the majority were indeed found to be retractile testes. In Cour-Palais's series, the true incidence of cryptorchidism was 0.76 per cent at age 5 years, 0.95 per cent at age 8 years, and 0.64 per cent at age 11 years or thereafter.

In adults, Cour-Palais found the incidence of cryptorchidism to be slightly less than 1 per cent of the male population. In addition to this careful study, other studies attest to the fact that the incidence of cryptorchidism at adulthood is less than 1 per cent. Baumrucker (1946) determined that the incidence of cryptorchidism in 10,000 consecutive U.S. Army inductees was 0.8 per cent. Others have noted similar incidences: 0.5 per cent in 10,000 Scottish recruits (Southam and Cooper, 1927), 0.7 per cent in male autopsies, and 0.55 per cent in almost 3 million U.S. Selective Service registrants between 1940 and 1944 (Campbell, 1959). It is clear from the aforementioned data that the true incidence of cryptorchidism remains relatively constant from age 1 year until adulthood.

In surgical explorations for cryptorchidism, absence of one or both testes may be encountered in 3 to 5 per cent of cases (Goldberg et al., 1974). In 10 per cent of patients with cryptorchidism, the defect is bilateral; in 3 per cent, one or both of the testes are absent (Scorer and Farrington, 1971). There also appears to be a familial incidence in certain patients with cryptorchidism: Approximately 14 per cent of boys with undescended testes have family members with the same condition (Bishop, 1945; Wiles, 1934; Brimblecomb, 1946).

Histology

In 1929, Cooper published her classic paper on the histology of the cryptorchid testis. She noted that the longer a testis remained cryptorchid, the more likely it was to be histologically abnormal; and that the higher the testis resided away from the bottom of the scrotum, the more pronounced was the histologic abnormality. These histologic alterations in the cryptorchid testis appear by 2 1/2 years of age and include smaller seminiferous tubules, fewer spermatogonia, and an increase in the peritubular tissue. Since Cooper's work, a multitude of papers have appeared confirming these histologic alterations in the cryptorchid testis (Scorer and Farrington, 1971; Mack et al., 1961; Sohval, 1954; Mengel et al., 1974). While the seminiferous tubules are definitely altered by the cryptorchid state, there is conflicting histologic evidence as to whether the Leydig cells are affected.

More recently, the electron microscope has been used to document certain ultrastructural changes in the seminiferous tubules as early as the second year of life (Hadziselimovic, 1977; Hadziselimovic and Seguchi, 1973; Zanzycki et al., 1977; Mengel et al., 1981). These changes include (1) degeneration of the mitochondria, (2) loss of ribosomes in both the cytoplasm and the smooth endoplasmic reticulum, and (3) increase in collagen fibers in the spermatogonia and Sertoli cells. Again, there is conflicting ultrastructural data as to whether there are changes in the Leydig cells. It is still uncertain whether the known changes in the cryptorchid testis represent a primary defect or just reflect an alteration secondary to the cryptorchid state. Support for the idea that the testis itself is defective lies in the observation that some of these histologic changes may also occur in the contralateral scrotal testis of the unilateral cryptorchid male (Mengel et al., 1974).

Complications

NEOPLASIA

The association between neoplasia and cryptorchidism continues to be controversial. Approximately 10 per cent of testicular tumors arise from an undescended testis (Campbell, 1959; Gilbert, 1941; Gordon-Taylor and Wyndham, 1947). Statistically, the undescended testis is reported to be 35 to 48 times more likely to undergo malignant degeneration than the normal testis (Johnson et al., 1968; Jones and Scott, 1971; Martin and Menck, 1975). The fact that neoplastic degeneration of an undescended testis is in itself a rare entity allows some surgeons to state that orchiectomy may not be the only choice of therapy in the postpubertal patient with a cryptorchid testis (Welvaart and Tijssen, 1981).

With regard to location, an abdominal testis is four times more likely to undergo malignant degeneration than an inguinal testis (Campbell, 1959). Tumors in undescended testes occur mainly at the time of puberty or after, although some neoplasias have occurred in children and infants (Gordon-Taylor and Wyndham, 1947). For this additional reason, if surgical correction is to be done, it should preferentially be carried out prepubertally.

In 1972, Skakkebaek reported the finding of carcinoma in situ in the testis of an infertile man with an undescended testis who developed a germ cell tumor 16 months later. In a follow-up study of 50 patients with a history of cryptorchidism treated by surgery who subsequently agreed to have a testicular biopsy, 4 (8 per cent) were found to have carcinoma in situ (Krabbe et al., 1979). Two of these four patients were also found to have unsuspected frank carcinomas as well, and one was then found to have 45,XO/46,XY karyotype, which is characteristic of an intersex disorder known to have a very high incidence of testicular cancer. Although these data suggest that cryptorchidism may be associated with testicular carcinoma in situ, the exact magnitude of that risk is unknown. However, Skakkebaek et al. (1982) recommend diagnostic testicular biopsies in postpubertal patients with a documented history of a unilateral germ cell tumor and a history of maldescent.

Since testicular tumors have occurred in patients who have undergone orchiopexy as early as 5 years of age (Altman and Malament, 1967), most authors currently recommend surgical correction sometime around 2 years of age, especially in light of the fact that ultrastructural changes begin to occur in the undescended testis at this early age (Mengel et al., 1974, 1981; Hadziselimoric, 1977) Whether this earlier surgical correction will deter the subsequent development of neoplasias in the undescended testis remains to be seen. Further support for the concept that there is an underlying pathologic process that affects both testes in the unilateral cryptorchid patient comes from the data of Johnson et al. (1968), who showed that one in five testicular tumors occurring in patients with cryptorchidism has developed in the contralateral, supposedly normal, scrotal testis.

In bilateral cryptorchidism, there is a 15 per cent chance of developing a tumor in the opposite testis if one of the testes becomes involved with a tumor (Gilbert and Hamilton, 1970). If both the testes are intra-abdominal and one testis becomes malignant, there is a 30 per cent chance of the other testis becoming malignant. Seminomas are the two most frequent neoplasms encountered in cryptorchid testes, followed by embryonal cell carcinomas (Gilbert and Hamilton, 1970; Batala et al., 1930; Martin, 1979). In patients with certain intersex disorders in which cryptorchidism is a presenting feature, gonadoblastoma is the most common tumor seen (Scully, 1970).

TORSION

The increased susceptibility of the testis to undergo torsion is due to an anatomic abnormality between the testis and its mesentery. If the testis is broader than its mesentery, it is more likely to twist on its stalk (Scorer and Farrington, 1971). Therefore, it is not surprising that the incidence of torsion is greatest in the postpubertal period; when the testis usually increases in size. Similarly, the undescended testis is more susceptible to torsion by any mechanism causing an increase in testicular size, e.g., a tumor. In a review of the literature, Rigler (1972) found that 64 per cent of adults with torsion in an undescended testis had an associated germ cell tumor. The presentation of a patient with abdominal pain and an ipsilateral empty hemiscrotum should alert the physician to the possibility of torsion of a cryptorchid testis.

HERNIA

As stated earlier in the section on embryology, the processus vaginalis is intimately associated with the structures involved in testicular descent. Following descent (which occurs at or about the seventh month of fetal life), the processus vaginalis, which connects the peritoneal cavity to the tunica vaginalis, closes sometime between the eighth month of fetal life and the first month after birth. However, when the testis fails to descend, the processus vaginalis remains patent; this may permit some of the intra-abdominal contents to enter the tunica vaginalis through the processus vaginalis and present clinically as a hernia or a hydrocele. Although the true incidence is unclear, hernia sacs may be found in greater than 90 per cent of cryptorchid patients (Scorer and Farrington, 1971).

INFERTILITY

Testicular maldescent retards the production of spermatozoa. Therefore, it is not surprising that the fertility of patients with bilaterally retained testes is generally very poor (Hansen, 1949; Mack, 1953; Scott, 1962; Scorer, 1967; Albescu et al., 1971; Walloch et al., 1980).

The higher and longer the testis resides away from the bottom of the scrotum, the greater the likelihood of damage to the seminiferous tubules; the earlier the testis is brought down into the scrotum, the greater the potential for recovering spermatogenic activity. Consequently, it would seem prudent to perform orchiopexy at an age prior to degeneration of the seminiferous tubules (Ludwig and Potempa, 1975).

It has been demonstrated that there may be a defect in the spermatogenic activity of the contralateral scrotal testis in the unilateral cryptorchid patient (Scorer, 1967; Hecker and Heinz, 1967; Woodhead et al., 1973). By comparing the sperm density of normal adult patients with that of adults who had undergone successful unilateral orchipexy during childhood, Lipschultz et al. (1976) discovered that unilateral cryptorchid men had a much lower than expected sperm count. This observation further supports the hypothesis that there may be an inherent defect in both testes of the unilateral cryptorchid males.

Besides the defect in spermatogenesis, there is clinical and experimental evidence to suggest that cryptorchidism may also affect the interstitial compartment of the testis. In cryptorchid animals, sex accessory tissue weight has been shown to be retarded, and the testicular enzymes necessary for testosterone synthesis may be inhibited (Korenchevsy, 1931; Clegg, 1960). In addition, it has been demonstrated that the testosterone response of prepubertal cryptorchid children to exogenous hCG stimulation is retarded (Job et al., 1977; Gendrel et al., 1977, 1978, 1980a and b). Postpubertally, however, there is no difference in the hCG response between cryptorchid and normal children. If, indeed, cryptorchidism does have an adverse effect on testosterone synthesis, the defect is probably not clinically significant because most patients with bilateral cryptorchidism are normally androgenized both in utero and at adulthood.

Associated Anomalies

There is some question in the literature regarding the incidence of chromosomal abnormalities in patients with uncomplicated unilateral cryptorchidism (Mininberg and Bragol, 1973; Dewald et al., 1977). The genetic syndromes that are associated with the undescended testis are extremely rare and are associated with poor survival. Of these, the best known are the Klinefelter, Noonan, and Prader-Willi syndromes. Most patients with Klinefelter's syndrome are sterile, and the disease is therefore self-limited. However, there is an occasional patient with a mosaic chromosomal constitution who may be potentially fertile. Noonan's syndrome, or male Turner's syndrome, is an endocrine disorder in which cryptorchidism is commonly seen (Redman, 1973). As in Klinefelter's syndrome, a patient may occasionally be fertile, but the disorder is usually self-limiting. Patients with the Prader-Willi syndrome, which is believed to be secondary to a hypothalamic defect, are usually obese, mentally retarded, hypotonic, and of short stature (Laurence, 1967). Treatment is currently directed at replacement of hypothalamic hormones.

Vasal and epididymal abnormalities have long been recognized as being associated with the undescended testis (Marshall, 1982). The epididymis may be extended in length, may undergo partial or total atresia, or may be totally disassociated from the testis (Scorer and Farrington, 1971). The same abnormalities may be seen with the vas deferens. Indeed, in the disorder cystic fibrosis, in which there is a very high incidence of congenital absence of the vasa deferentia, cryptorchidism is frequently seen (Schwachman et al., 1977; Landing et al., 1969; Holschaw et al., 1971; Touesig et al., 1972).

Epididymal defects have also been described in the male offspring of women exposed to diethylstilbestrol during pregnancy (McLachlan et al., 1975; Cosgrove et al., 1977; Bibbo et al., 1975). The most common abnormalities in these patients are cryptorchidism and cystic dilatations of the epididymis. This may suggest that some cases of cryptorchidism may be due to elevated in utero levels of estrogen, which may act either via the hypothalamic-pituitary-testicular axis or via a direct effect on the tissues themselves.

Treatment

The reasons for correcting the undescended testis are as follows: (1) A defect that is obvious and visible to both parents and patient is permanently corrected; (2) certain psychopathologic tendencies that surface initially around the fifth year of age, when the cryptorchid child enters school, may be prevented or reversed (Cytryn et al., 1967); (3) the undescended testis has an increased susceptibility to malignant degeneration, and, consequently, it seems wise to place the testis in a site where it can be palpated easily; and (4) fertility is improved. Since the prognosis for fertility in patients with bilateral cryptorchidism is extremely poor, every conceivable effort should be expended to salvage at least one, or preferably both, of the testes and place them into the scrotum. The placement of the testis within the scrotum should be accomplished as early as possible during childhood. In the unilateral cryptorchid male, a determined effort should be made to deliver the retained testis into the scrotum, in light of recent reports that suggest that fertility may be impaired in these patients also. It is our policy at the present time to salvage all testes, if at all possible, and position them at a site where they are readily palpable. Otherwise, an orchiectomy is performed. Orchiectomy is also reserved for the late postpubertal male patient and for those patients with certain intersex disorders in which the testis is dysgenetic and prone to malignant degeneration (Scully, 1970).

There are two avenues of therapy available for placing the cryptorchid testis into the scrotum—hormonal and surgical. The method selected depends on the pathogenesis of maldescent for the individual patient. Although the optimal time for attempting to place the retained testis into the scrotum is debatable, it appears, from the data concerning the changes in the seminiferous tubules by the second year of age and the observation that a testis not descended by 1 year of age will probably remain undescended, that treatment should be rendered as early as possible, preferably during or prior to the second year of life.

HORMONAL THERAPY

Hormonal therapy is the only medical therapy available for the undescended testis. At present, there are two types of hormonal therapy: hCG and GnRH (LHRH). hCG is given under the premise that stimulation of the Leydig cells will result in an increase in plasma testosterone, which will promote testicular descent. GnRH is used under the premise that cryptorchid children have an abnormality in the secretion of GnRH (LHRH) from the hypothalamus, as evidenced by a decrease in their basal LH levels, and replacement therapy with exogenous GnRH should reverse this defect.

Over the past two decades, there have been a number of studies in which hCG has been used parenterally to induce testicular descent in cryptorchid children, and the success rate has varied between 14 per cent and 50 per cent (Bigler et al., 1938; Ehrlich et al., 1969; Job et al., 1982). hCG has been given in a total dose varying from 3000 IU to more than 40,000 IU, the frequency of injection ranging from daily to weekly, and the duration of treatment being from a few days to several months.

Job et al. (1982) have demonstrated that in order to get a maximal stimulation of the Leydig cells from hCG, a total dose of at least 10,000 IU is needed; however, above 15,000 IU of hCG, potential side effects may occur. Under 15,000 IU of hCG, testicular histology does not change and bone age is not affected. Rarely, there is a transient increase in the size of the penis, which regresses following cessation of therapy.

The less than ideal results with exogenous hCG and the fact that it has to be given parenterally led European investigators to initiate studies using exogenous GnRH as a form of therapy for cryptorchidism (Bartsch and Frick, 1974). The initial excellent results using this form of therapy were believed to be due to the fact that retractile, but not truly cryptorchid, testes were responding to therapy. Since then, however, a number of investigators have demonstrated the efficacy of this form of hormonal therapy in cryptorchidism, reporting a success rate of up to 70 per cent (Bartsch and Frick, 1974; Happ et al., 1975, 1978a; Illig et al., 1977, 1980; Pirazzoli et al., 1978; Spona et al., 1979; Zabransky, 1981; Hadziselimovic, 1982; Job et al., 1974). The dosage of native GnRH that has been used is 1.2 mg per day given as a pernasal spray for about 4 weeks. Synthetic, long-lasting analogs have also been used, but their results are not as good as those of native GnRH (Happ et al., 1978b; Frick et al., 1980). No side effects, such as precocious growth, have been reported, although the relapse rate after 6 months of therapy approximates 10 per cent. In addition, there does not appear to be a difference in the success rate between treated unilateral and bilateral cryptorchid patients. There is some evidence to suggest that hCG injections subsequent to GnRH therapy may have an additional effect in promoting descent of the testes (Hadziselimovic, 1982).

SURGICAL THERAPY

The surgical placement of the undescended testis into the scrotum is one of the most common procedures. This is related to the relatively high incidence of cryptorchidism in the male population and the fact that the results of nonsurgical therapy, at least in the United States, are less than ideal. Over the past century, great strides have been made in pediatric surgical technique to allow the safe placement of the

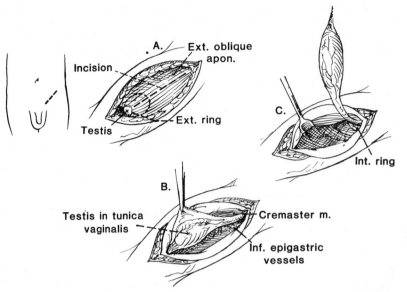

Figure 46–6. Technique of standard orchiopexy. *A* and *B,* After incision in skin crease, the aponeurosis of the external oblique muscle is incised in the direction of its fibers to expose underlying spermatic cord and testis. *C,* The internal oblique muscle may be incised laterally to clearly expose the internal inguinal ring.

small, prepubertal testis, with its tenuous blood supply and fragile excretory system, into the scrotum. These patients with undescended testes present to the surgeon at a much younger age than even 5 or 10 years ago. Therefore, there is less complacency regarding some of the technical aspects of orchiopexy because of the potential long-term damage to the testis or vas deferens that may ensue from a less than ideally performed surgical procedure.

Principles of Orchiopexy. The first orchiopexy was performed in 1820 (Rosenmerkel, 1820), but because of the initial poor results, the procedure was not accepted until the turn of the century, when Bevan (1899) described his technique for a successful orchiopexy. Since then, a number of surgeons have expanded on the principles that Bevan considered important in the performance of a successful orchiopexy: (1) mobilization of the testis; (2) sufficient dissection to obtain adequate length of the spermatic vessels, allowing placement of the organ into the scrotum; (3) retention of the testis in the scrotum; and (4) repair of an associated hernia. Eight decades later, the performance of a successful orchiopexy still requires adherence to these four principles (Figs. 46–6 to 46–8).

An orchiopexy is usually indicated in the ectopic, mechanically obstructed, or impalpable testis; in the majority of cases, the testis can be advanced successfully into the scrotum. Although the standard orchiopexy technique will

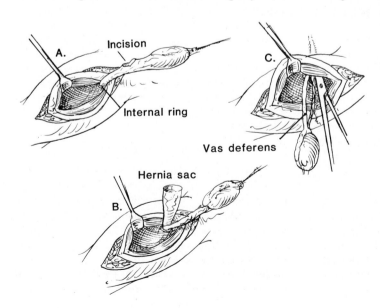

Figure 46–7. Technique of standard orchiopexy. *A* and *B,* Hernia sac is dissected off spermatic cord and ligated. *C,* Lateral spermatic fascia is incised to gain length of vessels.

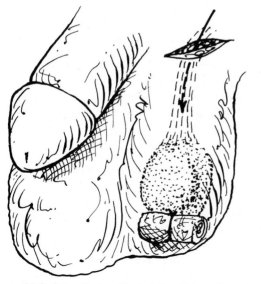

Figure 46–8. Subcuticular skin incision at top of scrotum, where subdartos pouch is created.

allow the testis to be brought down into the scrotum in most cases, there are those testes in which adequate length of the spermatic vessels cannot be obtained by this method. This occurs more often in the impalpable testis, which constitutes approximately 20 per cent of all undescended testes (Levitt et al., 1978). In these cases, there are other techniques that will help deliver the testis without tension into the scrotum. If, during a standard orchiopexy, adequate length of the spermatic vessels cannot be obtained, the first alternative is to incise the floor of the inguinal canal, ligating the inferior epigastric vessels, and bringing the testis into the scrotum in a straight line. With this technique, initially popularized by Prentiss et al., (1960), 2 or 3 cm of extra length may be obtained by bypassing the normal course of the spermatic cord that runs through the inguinal canal.

While the Prentiss technique may add a few centimeters to the length of the testicular vessels, it is sometimes not very helpful in the high intra-abdominal testis. The most widely used technique for such a situation is the Fowler-Stephens procedure (Scorer and Farrington, 1971; Fowler and Stephens, 1959); although Bevan (1903) was the first to perform this at the turn of the century. In this procedure, the testicular artery and veins in the spermatic cord are sacrificed. This technique rests on the assumption that collateral blood supply, primarily from the artery of the vas deferens, will prevent infarction of the testis. Therefore, if this operation is contemplated, the dissection to the vas should be minimized. The testicular vessels are clamped atraumatically for 5 minutes, and then the tunica albuginea of the testis is incised. If there is brisk bleeding from the testis, we assume that the collateral blood supply is sufficient to obtain a viable organ. The spermatic vessels are then sacrificed, and the testis is placed into the scrotum. The nuclear perfusion studies of Datta et al. (1977) appear to confirm the efficacy of this procedure, and the success rate is approximately 50 to 75 per cent (Gibbons et al., 1977).

Besides the Fowler-Stephens procedure, the two-stage orchiopexy may be utilized for the high undescended testis (Corkery, 1975; Firor, 1975; Zer et al., 1975). In the first stage, the testis is mobilized as much as possible. It is then either anchored to the pubis or inguinal canal by a suture ligature or encased in a Silastic sheet to prevent formation of adhesions that may make a second operation hazardous. The second stage is attempted 1 to 2 years after the first stage. Success has been reported as high as 77 per cent.

It should be mentioned that in certain instances, the high testis may be atrophic; with clamping of the testicular vessels, the viability of the organ would be compromised. In such a situation, orchiectomy may have to be considered, with either simultaneous or subsequent placement of a testicular prosthesis. A prosthesis placed in a prepubertal individual may need to be replaced with one of a bigger size at a later date. If a larger than acceptable prosthesis is placed into the scrotum at any age, erosion through the scrotal skin may occur.

Orchiectomy for the high undescended testis may seem too radical a course to those surgeons capable of performing a microvascular anastomosis of the testicular vessels. Silber introduced this technique, in which the testicular artery is anastomosed to the inferior epigastric artery and the testicular vein to the epigastric vein, but the vas and vasal artery are left undisturbed (Silber and Kelly, 1976). Experience in using a microscope is necessary to perform this procedure (MacMahon et al., 1980; Martin and Salikian, 1980). If this technique is used, it is difficult to determine postoperatively whether testicular viability is secondary to perfusion through the new anastomosis or through the collateral circulation.

In patients with bilateral palpable undescended testes, separate inguinal incisions may be made on each side to approach each testis individually. If bilateral impalpable testes are present, an alternative choice is to make a solitary incision that will allow an intra-abdominal approach, if necessary (Hunt et al., 1981). This may be made either in the midline or through a Pfannenstiel incision. With this exposure, both testes can be approached through a single incision and the testes can be brought into the scrotum in a straight line, a modification of the Prentiss procedure. But, unlike the Prentiss procedure, the floor of the inguinal canal is not disturbed.

The prospects for future spermatogenesis and fertility after orchiopexy are extremely variable. In a review of six collected series of untreated unilateral cryptorchid males, Hecker and Heinz (1967) calculated a 35 per cent incidence of fertility in 346 patients. Scott (1961) reported that approximately two thirds of untreated unilateral cryptorchid men were infertile, whereas 74 per cent of 119 patients who underwent orchiopexy prior to puberty were fertile. Similarly, after unilateral orchiopexy Gross and Replogle (1963) reported an 80 per cent incidence of fertility. Yet the sperm concentration from the unilateral cryptorchid testis that had been brought down surgically was extremely poor (Eldrup and Steven, 1980). Although paternity has been reported in patients who have undergone bilateral orchiopexies, in the majority of cases the results are uniformly poor, regardless of whether the procedure is performed prepubertally or postpubertally (Hohenfeller and Eisenhut, 1964; MacCollum, 1935; Rea, 1951; Scheiber et al., 1981).

Kiesewetter et al. (1969) performed repeat biopsies in 29 patients who originally had bilateral cryptorchidism and had undergone initial unilateral orchiopexy 1 to 11 years previously. In approximately one half of these patients, the subsequent biopsy demonstrated marked to moderate improvement in the histology of the testis when compared with the original biopsy. The higher the testis was away from the bottom of the scrotum and the longer it remained undescended, the poorer the results were both anatomically and physiologically. It remains to be determined whether the disappointing results of orchiopexy are a function of the length of time the testis remains undescended or are secondary to an intrinsic abnormality in the testis itself.

INGUINAL HERNIA IN INFANCY AND CHILDHOOD

In clinical practice, the large majority of infantile inguinal hernias appear in the first year, the diagnosis being made most commonly in the first month after birth and new cases being less frequent as childhood advances.

The overall incidence in the pediatric population has been variously reported as being from 1.0 to 4.4 per cent. In immature infants, those weighing less than 2000 gm at birth, the incidence rises to over 13 per cent. The condition affects boys nine times more frequently than it does girls.

Bilateral Inguinal Hernias

In recent years, controversy has arisen with regard to the desirability of routine bilateral exploration in cases of apparent unilateral inguinal hernia. For instance, Gunnlaugsson and colleagues (1967) reported that 60 per cent of such patients were found, on surgical exploration, also to have a clinically undiagnosed hernial sac on the contralateral side.

While accepting that these and other authors have shown it to be likely that a patent sac is present on the opposite side in early childhood, it seems pertinent to inquire whether this is of practical significance, as long as the sac does not accept abdominal viscera. A follow-up study performed by Hamrick and Williams (1962) on 229 patients showed that only 15 patients (6.55 per cent) developed a clinical hernia on the contralateral, unexplored side. The majority of these appeared in patients operated upon under the age of 6 years, of whom only one child in ten developed a second hernia. Hence, it may reasonably be argued that routine operation on the second side of the younger child may be unnecessary in up to 90 per cent of cases. When additional consideration is given to the close association of the spermatic vessels and vas deferens to the patent processus vaginalis, it will be appreciated that routine exploration cannot be said to be without risk to the testicular apparatus. Indeed, there is an incidence of testicular atrophy of approximately 0.5 per cent following infantile hernia repair.

DIAGNOSIS

The majority of infantile inguinal hernias present to the physician within the first 3 months of life. The mother describes the sudden appearance of a bulge in the child's groin, often after a period of crying, coughing, or straining at stool. The swelling is generally absent in the morning, becoming more noticeable in the latter part of the day.

The diagnosis is sometimes easy—a fullness is visible in one groin as compared with the other, a cough or cry making the swelling briefly more obvious. Gentle pressure on the abdomen may provoke the child to grunt and cause the swelling to reappear. Palpation reveals an indistinct swelling in the area, accompanied by an impulse on coughing or crying. On occasion there is no immediately visible abnormality, yet the child's mother is convinced that she has seen a swelling, that the child was distressed at the time, but that the swelling has since disappeared. Careful synchronous palpation, in which both spermatic cords are rolled gently over the pubic tubercles, may reveal that the cord on the suspected side is more bulky and more tangible than the delicate structure on the other side. The presence of a patent processus does seem to impart a palpable thickness and substance to the spermatic cord, and such a finding gives reliable confirmation to the mother's story. To complete the examination, it is important to inspect the scrotum, ensuring that both testes are fully descended, since up to 6 per cent of congenital inguinal hernias are associated with incomplete descent.

Inguinal Hernia in Girls

Some 1.6 per cent of girls with inguinal hernias prove to be of male nuclear sex, with intra-abdominal testes but with female external genitalia and female endocrine function (the testicular feminization syndrome). Buccal smears should routinely be performed on all female infants presenting with inguinal hernias, particularly if these are bilateral. The importance lies in the realization that the hernial sac may contain not an ovary (as is commonly the case in girls with inguinal hernias) but a testis. If a testis is found, it must not be excised during childhood. A simple herniotomy should be performed, with excision of the processus vaginalis but return of the testis to the abdomen. Once the patient has passed puberty and growth and feminization are complete, these testes should be excised, as they are liable to malignant change. In adult life these patients become normal women in build, with anatomically normal female external genitalia (although the vagina tends to be hypoplastic). They have normal breast development and female social behavior. As the uterus and ovaries are absent, there is a consequent primary amenorrhea.

INFANT HYDROCELE

A hydrocele is a collection of fluid between the parietal and visceral layers of the tunica vaginalis. Hydroceles usually occur during infancy or at adulthood. During infancy, it is believed that a patent processus vaginalis contributes to the collection of peritoneal fluid in the tunica vaginalis (Fig. 46–9). In adulthood, there is some theoretical evidence that an imbalance in the secretory and absorptive capacities of the parietal and visceral layers of the tunica vaginalis is responsible for the collection of fluid within the tunic (Rinker and Allen, 1951; Ozdilek, 1957).

Clinical Presentation

A hydrocele is very common after birth, occurring in about 6 per cent of full-term boys (Scorer and Farrington, 1977). It presents as a transilluminating, painless, oval, scrotal swelling that may extend along the spermatic cord (Fig. 46–9). Because a hydrocele at birth is almost

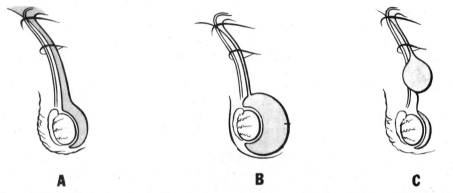

A   **B**   **C**

Figure 46–9. Causes of infantile hydrocele. *A,* Completely open processus vaginalis, which may also allow herniation of bowel contents. *B,* Incomplete closure of the processus vaginalis, which allows peritoneal fluid, but not bowel contents, to enter. *C,* Hydrocele of spermatic cord as a result of complete closure of lower end of processus vaginalis.

universally secondary to a patent processus vaginalis, therapy should be delayed until after the processus closes, which may occur spontaneously within the first year of life. The patent processus vaginalis also explains why the size of the infant hydrocele may vary in size daily. While this would suggest that the hydrocele fluid can be manually reduced back into the peritoneal cavity, this is usually not the case. The presence of mesenteric adenitis may also accentuate the size of a hydrocele.

Occasionally, an inguinal hernia or a torsion (if the testis cannot be palpated) may be suspected in a patient with a hydrocele, but a history of no previous scrotal pain or swelling and an adequate physical examination will usually rule out torsion or an inguinal hernia.

Therapy involves observation during the first year of life, but thereafter surgical intervention is necessary. In the pediatric age group, surgery involves ligation of the patent processus vaginalis (McKay et al., 1958). Sclerosing agents are not to be used in children because the patent processus vaginalis will allow the agent to pass freely into the peritoneal cavity and produce a chemical peritonitis. Aspiration of the hydrocele fluid from the tunic is usually an unsuccessful procedure, since the fluid recollects owing to the patency between the peritoneum and the tunic. Occasionally, aspiration is necessary in order to carefully palpate the testis. However, it should be noted that there is a risk of introducing infection and possible peritonitis when this is performed.

TESTICULAR TORSION

Torsion or twisting of the testis is considered a surgical emergency because it places the gonad at risk. When torsion occurs, obstruction to the venous blood supply, with secondary edema and hemorrhage and subsequent arterial obstruction, results. This ultimately leads to necrosis of the entire gonad. While testicular torsion is possible at any age, it is most common during adolescence (between the ages of 12 and 18 years), after which the incidence slowly decreases (Scorer and Farrington, 1971). A few cases also present during the neonatal period (Scorer and Farrington, 1971).

Although a variety of predisposing factors have been mentioned as an etiology for testicular torsion, Scorer and Farrington believe that torsion occurs because of a short mesenteric attachment from the cord onto the testis and epididymis (Fig. 46–10). This short mesenteric attachment allows the testis to fall forward. Within the vaginal cavity, the testis is then free

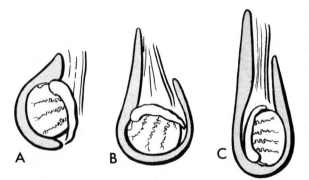

Figure 46–10. Attachment of testicular mesentery to testis. *A,* The normal peritoneal disposition around the testis. *B,* A capacious tunica vaginalis surrounding the cord; the testis lies horizontally. *C,* The inverted testis, which most easily twists because of its narrow attachment.

to rotate like a bell in a clapper. When the mesenteric attachment to the testis and epididymis is broad the testis does not fall forward but attains a more upright position, thereby making it less likely to rotate on its axis. This explains why the pubertal testis has more of a propensity for undergoing torsion than its prepubertal counterpart, for at puberty the testis increases in volume approximately five- to six-fold (Marshall and Tanner, 1980). This also explains why the onset of torsion in an undescended testis may signal the development of a testicular tumor, since this will also increase the size of the testis in relation to its mesentery (Rigler, 1972).

Differential Diagnosis of Testicular Torsion

The classic presentation of testicular torsion is pain and swelling on the affected side. In order to make the diagnosis, one must first be aware of the disorder. In the infant, symptoms may be absent such that the patient may present only with irritability, restlessness, and a lack of appetite (Scorer and Farrington, 1971). Usually the temperature is normal and the urinalysis is clear.

The most common misdiagnosis of testicular torsion is acute epididymitis. Acute epididymitis may present with similar symptoms except that the patient may have a temperature or a urethral discharge and the urinalysis demonstrates pyuria or bacteriuria. Strangulated hernias, hematoceles, hydroceles, testicular tumor, and idiopathic scrotal edema are to be considered in the differential diagnosis. Usually the history and physical examination will help in arriving at the correct diagnosis. However, in those instances when the diagnosis is in doubt, a Doppler study (Thompson et al., 1975; Levy, 1975) or a nuclear perfusion study (Datta and Mishkin, 1975; Holder et al., 1977) (Fig. 46–11) may be helpful.

Neonatal Testicular Torsion

In the newborn period, the testis has just descended into the scrotum and the gubernaculum has still not become completely attached to the scrotal wall (Backhouse, 1982). Therefore, the testis and gubernaculum are free to rotate within the neonatal scrotum; in this age group the entire testis, epididymis, and tunica vaginalis may twist together in a vertical axis on the spermatic cord above. Clinically, the neonate presents with a firm, hard, and large scrotal mass that does not transilluminate. Usually, the mass is not tender and the child does not appear to be disturbed. Occasionally, the child may appear restless and may be reluctant to take feedings. Although early exploration has been the rule in this situation, most testes are gangrenous at the time of exploration. Logic would then dictate that unless a pyogenic infection is present, surgical exploration need not be undertaken in the newborn with testicular torsion because the testis is already necrotic and there is no basis for contralateral orchiopexy at this time. However, clinical and experimental evidence suggests that immunologic damage to the contralateral testis may occur if a necrotic testis that has undergone torsion is left in situ (Khorup, 1978).

Pubertal Testicular Torsion

It is a wise axiom that an acutely painful, swollen testis in an adolescent is due to torsion until proved otherwise at surgery. In this form of torsion, the testis twists intravaginally, since the gubernaculum is fixed to the scrotal wall. The testis is therefore free to rotate because of its short peritoneal attachment (see Fig. 46–10). The onset of pain is sudden, and scrotal edema occurs very soon thereafter. Scrotal exploration should be performed if the diagnosis is considered at all, and contralateral orchiopexy is done simultaneously because of the propensity for the disorder to occur bilaterally (Burton, 1972; Chapman and Walton, 1972; Macnicol, 1974). If a torsion is reduced manually, surgical fixation should be performed because recurrent torsion and testicular loss may occur even before the patient leaves the hospital (Sparks, 1972; Korbel, 1974).

Torsion of Testicular Appendages

The most common testicular appendage involved in torsion is the appendix testis, which is a remnant of the müllerian duct. The clinical picture is not different from that seen in a patient with true testicular torsion. Usually the patients are adolescents, and they present with the sudden onset of testicular pain. Scrotal swelling may occur, and careful physical examination may allow one to palpate the distended appendage. Occasionally, Xylocaine may be ad-

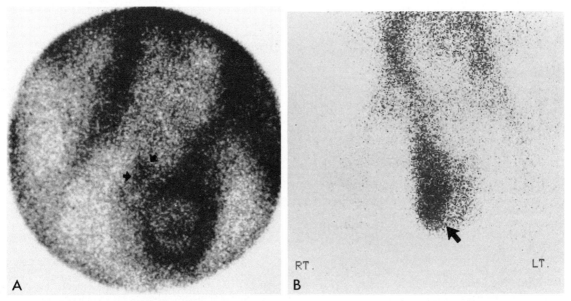

Figure 46–11. Radionuclide testicular scan, demonstrating *(A)* increased flow to left testis and epididymis, indicative of acute epididymitis. Arrows point to normal right testis next to large left testis. *B,* Absence of testicular flow is characteristic of a right testicular torsion. Left testis (arrow) is normally perfused.

ministered to the cord near the external inguinal ring to allow a more definitive examination. Again, if any doubt exists as to the reason for the testicular pain and swelling, scrotal exploration is recommended.

Prognosis

The prognosis for torsion is good if the patient is operated on within 4 to 6 hours and contralateral orchiopexy is performed (Krorup, 1978). In the operating room, an injection of fluorescein may be given and the testis may be observed under the Wood's ultraviolet lamp if testicular viability is in doubt. If the fluorescein is seen to perfuse the testis, then testicular viability is almost certain and the testis is left in situ. If a necrotic testicular mass is found, the testis should be removed. A testicular prosthesis may be inserted at the same time or at a later date.

In the past few years there have been some data to suggest that if testicular torsion occurs and the testis is left in situ, an abnormal sperm count at adulthood is more common than if the affected testis had been excised (Krorup, 1978; Bartsch et al., 1980). It is believed that when the testis undergoes torsion, certain proteins may be liberated within the systemic circulation, with the development of antitesticular antibodies that theoretically may damage the normal contralateral testis. This autoimmune theory of torsion is at present hypothetical, and further investigation must be conducted to verify this assumption.

References

Cryptorchidism

Albescu, J. Z., Bergada, C., and Cullen, M.: Male fertility in patients treated for cryptorchidism before puberty. Fertil. Steril., *22*:829, 1971.

Altman, B. L., and Malament, M.: Carcinoma of the testis following orchiopexy. J. Urol., *97*:498, 1967.

Amin, M., and Wheeler, C. S.: Selective testicular venography in abdominal cryptorchidism. J. Urol., *115*:760, 1976.

Arey, L. B.: The genital system. *In* Arey, L. B. (Ed.): Developmental Anatomy. 7th ed. Philadelphia, W. B. Saunders Co., 1965, pp. 315–341.

Arnheim, R. E.: The treatment of undescended testes with gonadotropic horomones. J. Mt. Sinai Hosp., *4*:1036, 1938.

Backhouse, K. M.: Embryology of the normal and cryptorchid testis. *In* Fonkalsrud, E. W., and Mengel, W. (Eds.): The Undescended Testis. Chicago, Year Book Medical Publishers, 1981, p. 5.

Backhouse, K. M.: The gubernaculum testis Hunteri: testicular descent and maldescent. Ann. R. Coll. Surg. (Engl.), *35*:15, 1964.

Backhouse, K. M., and Butler, H.: The gubernaculum testis of the pig (sus scropha). J. Anat., *94*:107, 1960.

Bardin, C. W., Ross, G. T., Rifkind, A. B., Cargille, C. M., and Lipsett, M. B.: Studies of the pituitary–Leydig cell axis in young men with hypogonadotropic hypogonadism and hyposmia: comparison with normal men, prepubertal boys and hypopituitary patients. J. Clin Invest., *48*:2056, 1969.

Bartsch, G., and Frick, J.: Therapeutic effects of luteinizing hormone–releasing hormone (LH-RH) in cryptorchidism. Andrologia, *6*:197, 1974.

Batala, M. A., Whitmore, W. F., Jr., Chu, F. C. H., Hilaris, B., Loh, J., Grabstald, H., and Golbey, R.: Cryptorchidism and testicular cancer. J. Urol., *124*:382, 1980.

Baumrucker, G. O.: Incidence of testicular pathology. Bull. U.S. Army Med. Dept., *5*:312, 1946.

Ben-Menachem, Y., deBerardinis, M. D. C., and Salinas, R.: Localization of intraabdominal testes by selective testicular arteriography: a case report. J. Urol., *112*:493, 1974.

Bergh, A., Helander, H. F., and Wahlquist, L.: Studies on factors governing testicular descent in the rat—particularly the role of the gubernaculum testis. Int. J. Androl., *1*:342, 1978.

Bergin, W. C., Gier, H. T., Marion, G. B., and Coffman, J. R.: A developmental concept of equine cryptorchidism. Biol. Reprod., *3*:82, 1970.

Bevan, A. D.: Operation for undescended testicle and congenital inguinal hernia. JAMA, *33*:773, 1899.

Bevan, A. D.: The surgical treatment of the undescended testicle. JAMA, *41*:718, 1903.

Bibbo, M., Al-Nageeb, M., Baccarini, L., Gill, W., Newton, M., Sleeper, K. M., Sonek, M., and Wied, G.: Follow-up study of male and female offspring of DES-treated mothers. A preliminary report. J. Reprod. Med., *15*:129, 1975.

Bigler, J. A., Hardy, L. M., and Scott, H. V.: Cryptorchidism treated with gonadotropic principle. Am. J. Dis. Child., *55*:273, 1938.

Bishop, P. M. F.: Studies in clinical endocrinology vs. the management of the undescended testicle. Guys Hosp. Rep., *94*:12, 1945.

Brimblecomb, S. L.: Bilateral cryptorchidism in three brothers. Br. Med. J., *1*:526, 1946.

Browne, D.: Treatment of undescended testicle. Proc. R. Soc. Med., *42*:643, 1949.

Buemann, B., Henriksen, H., and Villumsen, A. L.: Incidence of undescended testis in the newborn. Acta Chir. Scand. (Suppl.), *283*:289, 1961.

Cacciari, E., Cicognani, A., Pirazzoli, P., Zappulla, F., Tassoni, P., Bernardi, F., and Salardi, S.: Hypophysogonadal function in the cryptorchid child: differences between unilateral and bilateral cryptorchids. Acta Endocrinol., *83*:182, 1976.

Campbell, H. E.: The incidence of malignant growth of the undescended testicle: a reply and re-evaluation. J. Urol., *81*:653, 1959.

Ch'in, K. Y.: The endocrine glands of anencephalic foetuses. Chin. Med. J., *2*:63, 1938.

Clegg, E. J.: Some effects of artificial cryptorchidism on the accessory reproductive organs of the rat. J. Endocrinol., *10*:210, 1960.

Clements, J. A., Reyes, F. I., Winter, J. S. D., and Faiman, C.: Studies on human sexual development. III. Fetal pituitary and amniotic fluid concentration of LH, CG and FSH. J. Clin. Endocrinol. Metab., *42*:9, 1976.

Cooper, E. R.: The histology of the retained testis in the human subject at different ages and its comparison with the testis. J. Anat., *64*:5, 1929.

Corkery, J. H.: Staged orchiopexy—a new technique. J. Pediatr. Surg., *10*:515, 1975.

Cosgrove, M. D., Benton, B., and Henderson, B. W.: Male genitourinary abnormalities and maternal diethylstilbestrol. J. Urol., *117*:220, 1977.

Cour-Palais, I. J.: Spontaneous descent of the testicle. Lancet, *1*:1403, 1966.

Curling, J. B.: Observations on the structure of the gubernaculum and on the descent of the testis in the foetus. Lancet, *2*:70, 1840.

Cytryn, L., Cytryn, E., and Reger, R. E.: Psychological implications of cryptorchidism. J. Am. Acad. Child Psychiatr., *6*:131, 1967.

Dajani, A. M.: Transverse ectopia of the testis. Br. J. Urol., *41*:80, 1969.

Datta, N. S., Tanaka, T., Zinner, N. R., and Mishkin, F. S.: Division of spermatic vessels in orchiopexy: radionuclide evidence of preservation of testicular function. J. Urol., *118*:447, 1977.

Davis, J. E.: Transverse aberrant testicular maldescent. U.S. Armed Forces Med. J., *8*:1046, 1957.

Deming, C. L.: The gonadotropic factor as an aid to surgery in the treatment of the undescended testicle. J. Urol., *36*:274, 1936.

Dewald, G. W., Kelalis, P. P., and Gordon, H.: Chromosomal studies in cryptorchidism. J. Urol., *117*:110, 1977.

Ehrlich, R. M., Dougherty, L. M., Tomashefsky, P., and Lattimer, J. K.: Effect of gonadotropin in cryptorchidism. J. Urol., *102*:793, 1969.

Elder, J. S., Issacs, J. T., and Walsh, P. C.: Androgenic sensitivity of the gubernaculum testis: evidence for hormonal/mechanical interactions in testicular descent. J. Urol., *127*:170, 1982.

Eldrup, J., and Steven, K.: Influence of orchiopexy for cryptorchidism on subsequent fertility. Br. J. Surg., *67*:269, 1980.

Engle, E. T.: Experimentally induced descent of the testis in the Macacs monkey by hormones from the anterior pituitary and pregnancy urine. Endocrinology, *16*:513, 1932.

Farrington, G. H.: The position and retractability of the normal testis in childhood, with reference to the diagnosis and treatment of cryptorchidism. J. Pediatr. Surg., *3*:53, 1968.

Felizet, G., and Branca, A.: Sur le testicule en ectopie. J. L'Anat., *38*:329, 1902.

Firor, H. V.: Two-stage orchiopexy. Arch. Surg., *102*:598, 1971.

Forest, M. G., Sizonenko, P. C., Cathard, A. M., and Bertrand, J.: Hypophysogonadal function in humans during the first year of life. J. Clin. Invest., *53*:819, 1974.

Fowler, R., and Stephens, F. D.: The role of testicular vascular anatomy in the salvage of the high undescended testes. Aust. N.Z. J. Surg., *29*:92, 1959.

Frey, H. L., and Rajfer, J.: The role of the gubernaculum and intraabdominal pressure in the process of testicular descent. J. Urol., *131*:574, 1984.

Frey, H. L., and Rajfer, J.: Epididymis does not play an important role in the process of testicular descent. Surg. Forum, *23*:617, 1982.

Frey, H. L., Blumberg, B., and Rajfer, J.: Genetics for the urologist. In Goldsmith, H. S. (Ed.): Practice of Surgery. Vol. 1. New York, Harper & Row, 1981, p. 1.

Frey, H. L., Peng, S., and Rajfer, J.: Synergy of androgens and abdominal pressure in testicular descent. Biol. Reprod., *29*:1233, 1983.

Frick, J., Danner, C., Kunit, G., Glavan, G., and Bernroider, G.: The effect of chronic administration of a synthetic LH-RH analogue intranasally in cryptorchid boys. Int. J. Androl., *3*:469, 1980.

Gendrel, D., Chaussain, J. L., Roger, M., and Job, J. C.: Simultaneous postnatal rise of plasma LH and testosterone in male infants. J. Pediatr., *97*:600, 1980*a*.

Gendrel, D., Job, J. C., and Roger, M.: Reduced postnatal rise of testosterone in plasma of cryptorchid children. Acta Endocrinol., *89*:372, 1978.

Gendrel, D., Roger, M., and Job, J. C.: Plasma gonadotropin and testosterone values in infants with cryptorchidism. J. Pediatr., *97*:217, 1980*b*.

Gendrel, D., Roger, M., Chaussain, J. L., Canlorbe, P., and Job, J. C.: Correlation of pituitary and testicular responses to stimulation tests in cryptorchid children. Acta Endocrinol., *86*:641, 1977.

Gibbons, M. D., Cromie, W. J., and Duckett, J. W., Jr.: Management of the abdominal undescended testicle. J. Urol., *122*:76, 1977.

Gier, H. T., and Marion, G. B.: Development of the mammalian testis. In Johnson, A. D., and Gomes, W. R. (Eds.): The Testis. New York, Academic Press, 1970, pp. 1–45.

Gilbert, J. B.: Studies in malignant testis tumors. V. Tumors developing after orchiopexy. J. Urol., *46*:740, 1941.

Gilbert, J. B., and Hamilton, J. B.: Incidence and nature of tumors in ectopic testes. Surg. Gynecol. Obstet., *71*:731, 1970.

Goldberg, L. M., Skaist, L. B., and Morrow, J. W.: Congenital absence of testis: Anorchia and nonorchism. J. Urol., *111*:840, 1974.

Goldman, A., Stein, L., and Lapin, J.: The treatment of undescended testes by the anterior pituitary–like principle. N. Y. State J. Med., *36*:15, 1936.

Gordon-Taylor, G., and Wyndham, N. R.: On malignant tumors of the testis. Br. J. Surg., *35*:6, 1947.

Grant, D. B., Laurence, B. M., Atherden, S. M., and Ryness, J.: hCG stimulation test in children with abnormal sexual development. Arch. Dis. Child., *51*:596, 1976.

Gross, R. E., and Replogle, R. L.: Treatment of the undescended testis. Postgrad. Med., *34*:266, 1963.

Grumbach, M. M., and Van Wyk, J. J.: Disorders of sex differentiation. In Williams, R. H., (Ed.): Textbook of Endocrinology. 4th ed. Philadelphia, W. B. Saunders Co., 1974, p. 481.

Hadziselimovic, F.: Cryptorchidism. Management and Implications. Heidelberg, Springer-Verlag, 1983.

Hadziselimovic, F.: Cryptorchidism: ultrastructure of cryptorchid testes development. Adv. Anat. Embryol. Cell Biol., *53*:3, 1977.

Hadziselimovic, F.: Pathogenesis of cryptorchidism. Clin. Androl., *7*:147, 1981.

Hadziselimovic, F.: Treatment of cryptorchidism with GnRH. Urol. Clin. North Am., *9*:413, 1982.

Hadziselimovic, F., and Seguchi, H.: Electron microscopic investigations in cryptorchidism (elektronen mikroskopische untersuchungen beim kryptorchismus). Z. Kinderchir., *12*:376, 1973.

Hamilton, J. B.: The effect of male hormone upon the descent of the testes. Anat. Rec., *70*:533, 1938.

Hamilton, J. B., and Hubert, G.: Effect of synthetic male hormone substance on descent of testicles in human cryptorchidism. Proc. Soc. Exp. Biol. Med., *39*:4, 1938.

Hamilton, W. J., Boyd, J. D., and Mossman, J. D.: Human Embryology. Cambridge, England, W. Heffer and Sons, 1957, pp. 255–256.

Hansen, T. S.: Fertility in operatively treated and untreated cryptorchidism. Proc. R. Soc. Med., *42*:645, 1949.

Happ, J., Kollmann, F., Krawehl, C., Neubauer, M., and Beyer, J.: Intranasal GnRH therapy of maldescended testes. Horm. Metab. Res., *7*:440, 1975.

Happ, J., Kollmann, F., Krawehl, C., Neubauer, M., Krause, U., Demisch, K., Sandow, J., Von Rechenberg, W., and Beyer, J.: Treatment of cryptorchidism with pernasal gonadotropin-releasing hormone therapy. Fertil. Steril., *29*:546, 1978*a*.

Happ, J., Weber, T., Callensee, W., Ermert, J. A., Eshkol, A., and Beyer, J.: Treatment of cryptorchidism with a potent analog of gonadotropin-releasing hormone. Fertil. Steril., *29*:552, 1978*b*.

Hecker, W. C., and Heinz, H. A.: Cryptorchidism and fertility. J. Pediatr. Surg., *2*:513, 1967.

Hohenfeller, R., and Eisenhut, L.: Evaluation of fertility in cryptorchidism. Int. J. Fertil., *9*:575, 1964.

Holschaw, D. S., Perlmutter, A. D., Joclin, H., and Shwachman, H.: Genital abnormalities in male patients with cystic fibrosis. J. Urol., *106*:568, 1971.

Huberman, J., and Israeloff, H.: The application of recent theories in the treatment of undescended testes. J. Pediatr., *7*:759, 1935.

Hunt, J. B., Witherington, R., and Smith, A. D.: The midline approach to orchiopexy. Am. Surg., *47*:184, 1981.

Hunter, J. A.: A description of the situation of the testis in the fetus with its descent into the scrotum. *In* Observations on Certain Parts of the Animal Oeconomy. New Orleans, John J. Haswell and Co., 1841, pp. 42–50.

Hunter, P. A.: The etiology of congenital inguinal hernia and abnormally placed testes. Br. J. Surg., *14*:125, 1927.

Illig, R., Bucher, H., and Prader, A.: Success, relapse and failure after intranasal LH-RH treatment of cryptorchidism in 55 perpubertal boys. Eur. J. Pediatr., *133*:147, 1980.

Illig, R., Kollmann, F., Borkenstein, M., Kuber, W., Exner, G. U., Kellerer, K., Lunglmayr, L., and Prader, A.: Treatment of cryptorchidism by intranasal synthetic luteinising-hormone releasing hormone. Lancet, *2*:518, 1977.

Jirasek, J. E., Raboch, J., and Uher, J.: The relationship between the development of the gonads and external genitals in human fetuses. Am. J. Obstet. Gynecol., *101*:803, 1968.

Job, J. C., Canlorbe, P., Garagorri, J. M., and Toublanc, J. E.: Hormonal therapy of cryptorchidism with human chorionic gonadotrophin (hCG). Urol. Clin. North Am., *9*:405, 1982.

Job, J. C., Garnier, P. E., Chaussain, J. L., Toublanc, J. E., and Canlorbe, P.: Effect of synthetic luteinizing hormone–releasing hormone on the release of gonadotropins in hypophyseal disorders of children and adolescents. IV. Undescended testes. J. Pediatr., *84*:371, 1974.

Job, J. C., Gendrel, D., Safar, A., Roger, M., and Chaussain, J. L.: Pituitary LH and FSH and testosterone secretion in infants with undescended testes. Acta Endocrinol., *85*:644, 1977.

Johnson, D. E., Woodhead, D. M., Pohl, D. R., and Robinson, J. R.: Cryptorchidism and testicular tumorigenesis. Surgery, *63*:919, 1968.

Jones, H. W., and Scott, W. W.: Cryptorchidism. *In* Jones, H. W., and Scott, W. W. (Eds.): Hermaphroditism, Genital Anomalies and Related Endocrine Disorders. 2nd ed. Baltimore, Williams & Wilkins Co., 1971, p. 363.

Josso, N.: Evolution of the Mullerian-inhibiting activity of the human testis. Biol. Neonate, *20*:368, 1972.

Josso, N.: In vitro synthesis of mullerian-inhibiting hormone by seminiferous tubules isolated from the calf fetal testis. Endocrinology, *93*:829, 1973.

Jost, A.: A new look at the mechanisms controlling sex differentiation in mammals. Johns Hopkins Med. J., *130*:8, 1953*a*.

Jost, A.: Problems of fetal endocrinology: the gonadal and hypophyseal hormones. Rec. Prog. Horm. Res., *8*:379, 1953*b*.

Kieswetter, W. B., Shull, W. R., and Fetterman, G. H.: Histologic changes in the testis following successful orchiopexy. J. Pediatr. Surg., *4*:59, 1969.

Korenchevsky, V.: The influence of cryptorchidism and of castration on body-weight, fat deposition, the sexual and endocrine organs of male rats. J. Pathol. Bacteriol., *33*:607, 1931.

Krabbe, S., Skakkebaek, N. E., Berthelsen, J. G., Eyken, F. V., Volsted, P., Mauritzen, K., Eldrup, J., and Nielsen, A. H.: High incidence of undetected neoplasia in maldescended testes. Lancet, *1*:999, 1979.

Landing, B. H., Wells, T. R., and Wong, C. I.: Abnormality of the epididymis and vas deferens in cystic fibrosis. Arch. Pathol., *88*:569, 1969.

Laurence, B. M.: Hypotonic, mental retardation, obesity, cryptorchidism associated with dwarfism and diabetes in children. Arch. Dis. Child., *42*:126, 1967.

Lee, J. K., McClennan, B. L., Stanley, R. J., and Sagel, S. S.: Utility of computed tomography in the localization of the undescended testis. Radiology, *135*:121, 1980.

Lemeh, C. N.: A study of the development and structural relationships of the testis and gubernaculum. Surg. Gynecol. Obstet., *110*:164, 1960.

Levitt, S. B., Kogan, S. J., Engel, R. M., Weiss, R. M., Martin, D. C., and Ehrlich, R. M.: The impalpable testis: a rational approach to management. J. Urol., *120*:515, 1978.

Lipschultz, L. I., Caminos-Torres, R., Greenspan, C. S., and Snyder, P. J.: Testicular function after orchiopexy for unilaterally undescended testis. N. Engl. J. Med., *195*:15, 1976.

Lockwood, C. G.: Development and transition of the testis, normal and abnormal. J. Anat. Physiol., *22*:505, 1888.

Ludwig, G., and Potempa, J.: Der optimale Zeitpunkt der Bahandlung des Kryptorchismus. Dtsch. Med. Wochenschr., *100*:680, 1975.

MacCollum, D. W.: Clinical study of the spermatogenesis of undescended testicles. Arch. Surg., *31*:290, 1935.

MacMahon, R. A., O'Brien, B., Aberdeen, J., Richarson, W., and Cussen, L. J.: Results of the use of autotransplantation of the intraabdominal testis using microsurgical vascular anastomosis. J. Pediatr. Surg., *15*:92, 1980.

Mack, W. S.: Discussion on male infertility. Proc. R. Soc. Med., *46*:840, 1953.

Mack, W. S., Scott, L. S., Ferguson-Smith, M. A., and Lennox, B.: Ectopic testis and true undescended testis: a histological comparison. J. Pathol. Bacteriol., *82*:439, 1961.

Madrazo, B. L., Klugo, R. C., Parks, J. A., and DiLoreto, R.: Ultrasonographic demonstration of undescended testes. Radiology, *123*:181, 1979.

Marshall, F. F.: Anomalies associated with cryptorchidism. Urol. Clin. North Am., *9*:339, 1982.

Martin, D. C.: Germinal cell tumors of the testis after orchiopexy. J. Urol., *121*:422, 1979.

Martin, D. C., and Menck, H. R.: The undescended testis: Management after puberty. J. Urol., *114*:77, 1975.

Martin, D. C., and Salikian, A. H.: Orchiopexy using microvascular surgical technique. J. Urol., *123*:435, 1980.

McCutcheon, A. B.: Further observations on delayed testis. Med. J. Aust., *1*:654, 1938.

McLachlan, J. A., Newbold, R. R., and Bullock, B.: Reproductive tract lesions in male mice exposed prenatally to diethylstilbestrol. Science, *90*:991, 1975.

McMurrich, J. P.: The Development of the Human Body. A Manual of Human Embryology. 7th ed. Philadelphia, P. Blakiston's Son and Co., 1923, pp. 374–376.

Mengel, W., Heinz, H. A., Sippe, W. G., and Hecker, W. C. H.: Studies on cryptorchidism: A comparison of histological findings in the germinal epithelium before and after the second year of life. J. Pediatr. Surg., 9:445, 1974.

Mengel, W., Wronecki, K., and Zimmerman, F. A.: Comparison of the morphology of normal and cryptorchid testes. In Fonkalsrud, E. W., and Mengel, W., (Eds.): The Undescended Testis. Chicago, Year Book Medical Publishers, 1981, p. 72.

Mininberg, D. T., and Bragol, N.: Chromosomal abnormalities in undescended testis. Urology, 1:98, 1973.

Moore, C. R., and Quick, W. J.: The scrotum as a temperature regulator for the testes. Am. J. Physiol., 68:70, 1924.

Mukerjee, S., and Amesur, N. R.: Transverse testicular ectopia with unilateral blood supply. Ind. J. Surg., 27:547, 1965.

Ohno, S.: Major sex determining genes. Monogr. Endocrinol., 11:1, 1979.

Opitz, J. M., Simpson, J. L., Sarto, G. E., Summitt, R. L., New, M., and German, J.: Pseudovaginal perineoscrotal hypospadias. Clin. Genet., 3:1026, 1972.

Pace, J. M., and Cabot, M.: A histological study in 24 cases of retained testes in the adult. Surg. Gynecol. Obstet., 63:16, 1936.

Pak, K., Sakaguchi, N., Takeuchi, H., and Tomoyoshi, T.: Computed tomography of carcinoma of the intraabdominal testis: a case report. J. Urol., 125:253, 1981.

Payne, A. H., and Jaffe, R. B.: Androgen formation from pregnenolone sulfate by fetal neonatal and adult human testes. J. Clin. Endocrinol. Metab., 40:102, 1975.

Pirazzoli, P., Zappulla, F., Bernardi, F., Villa, M. P., Aleksandrowitz, D., Scandola, A., Stancari, P., Cicognani, A., and Cacciari, E.: Luteinising hormone–releasing hormone nasal spray as therapy for undescended testicle. Arch. Dis. Child., 53:235, 1978.

Prentiss, R. J., Weickgenant, C. J., Moses, J. J., and Frazier, D. B.: Undescended testis: surgical anatomy of spermatic vessels, spermatic surgical triangles and lateral spermatic ligament. J. Urol., 83:686, 1960.

Rajfer, J.: An endocrinological study of testicular descent in the rabbit. J. Surg. Res., 33:158, 1982.

Rajfer, J., and Walsh, P. C.: Hormonal regulation of testicular descent: experimental and clinical observations. J. Urol., 118:985, 1977.

Rajfer, J., Tauber, A., Zinner, N., Naftulin, E., and Worthen, N.: The use of computerized tomography scanning to localize the impalpable testis. J. Urol., 129:978, 1983.

Rea, C. E.: Fertility in cryptorchids: Minn. Med., 34:216, 1951.

Redman, J.: Noonan's syndrome and cryptorchidism. J. Urol., 109:909, 1973.

Rigler, H. C.: Torsion of intraabdominal testes. Surg. Clin. North Am., 52:371, 1972.

Rosenmerkel, J. F.: Veberdie Radiculur des in der Weiche liegenden Testikels bei necht Descensus Desselben. Munich, J. Lindauer, 1820.

Sadeghi-Nejad, A., and Senior, B.: A familial syndrome of isolated aplasia of the anterior pituitary. J. Pediatr., 84:79, 1974.

Santen, R. J., and Paulsen, C. A.: Hypogonadotropic eunuchoidism. Gonadal responsiveness to exogenous gonadotropins. J. Clin. Endocrinol. Metab., 36:47, 1972.

Schechter, J.: An investigation of the anatomical mechanisms of testicular descent. Thesis for Master of Arts degree. Baltimore, Johns Hopkins University, 1963.

Scheiber, K., Menardi, G., Marberger, H., and Bartsch, G.: Late results after surgical treatment of maldescended testes with special regard to exocrine and endocrine testicular function. Eur. Urol., 7:268, 1981.

Scorer, C. G.: Early operation for the undescended testis. Br. J. Surg., 54:694, 1967.

Scorer, C. G.: The descent of the testis. Arch. Dis. Child., 39:605, 1964.

Scorer, G., and Farrington, G. H.: Congenital Deformities of the Testis and Epididymis. New York, Appleton-Century-Crofts, 1971.

Scott, L. S.: Fertility in cryptorchidism. Proc. R. Soc. Med., 55:1047, 1962.

Scott, L. S.: Unilateral cryptorchidism; subsequent effects on fertility. J. Reprod. Fertil., 2:54, 1961.

Scully, R. E.: Gonadoblastoma. A review of 74 cases. Cancer, 25:1340, 1970.

Shrock, P.: The processus vaginalis and gubernaculum. Surg. Clin. North Am., 51:1263, 1971.

Shwachman, H., Kowlski, M., and Khaw, K.: Cystic fibrosis: a new outlook. Medicine, 56:129, 1977.

Siiteri, P. K., and Wilson, J. D.: Testosterone formation and metabolism during male sexual differentiation in the human embryo. J. Clin. Endocrinol. Metab., 38:113, 1974.

Silber, S. J., and Cohen, R.: Laparoscopy for cryptorchidism. J. Urol., 124:928, 1980.

Silber, S. J., and Kelly, J.: Successful auto-transplantation of an intra-abdominal testis to the scrotum by microvascular technique. J. Urol., 115:452, 1976.

Sizonenko, P. C., Schindler, R. A., Roland, W., Paunier, L., and Cuendet, A.: FSH III: evidence for a possible prepubertal regulation of its secretion by the seminiferous tubules in cryptorchid boys. J. Clin. Endocrinol. Metab., 46:301, 1978.

Skakkebaek, N. E.: Possible carcinoma-in-situ of the testis. Lancet, 1:516, 1972.

Skakkebaek, N. E., Berthelesen, J. G., and Muller, J.: Carcinoma-in-situ of the undescended testis. Urol. Clin. North Am., 9:377, 1982.

Sohval, A. R.: Histopathology of cryptorchidism. Am. J. Med., 16:346, 1954.

Sonneland, C. G.: Undescended testicle. Surg. Gynecol. Obstet., 40:535, 1925.

Southam, A. H., and Cooper, E. R. A.: Hunterian lecture on the pathology and treatment of the retained testis in childhood. Lancet, 1:805, 1927.

Spona, J., Gleispach, H., Happ, J., et al.: Changes of serum testosterone and of LH-RH test after treatment of cryptorchidism by intranasal LH-RH. Endocrinol. Exp., 13:204, 1979.

Steiner, M. D., and Boggs, J. D.: Absence of the pituitary gland, hypothyroidism, hypoadrenalism and hypogonadism in a 17 year old dwarf. J. Clin. Endocrinol. Metab., 25:1591, 1965.

Tayakkononta, K.: The gubernaculum testis and its nerve supply. Aust. N.Z. J. Surg., 33:61, 1963.

Thompson, W. D., Bevan, A. D., Heckel, N. J., McCarthy, E. R., and Thompson, P. K.: The treatment of undescended testes with anterior pituitary–like substance. Endocrinology, 21:220, 1937.

Toussig, L. M., Lobeck, L. C., DiSant'Aznese, P. A., Ackerman, D. R., and Kattwinkel, J.: Fertility in males with cystic fibrosis. N. Engl. J. Med., 287:586, 1972.

Van Vliet, G., Caufriez, A., Robyn, C., and Wolter, R.: Plasma gonadotropin values in prepubertal cryptorchid boys: Similar increase of FSH in uni- and bilateral cases. J. Pediatr., 97:253, 1980.

Villumsen, A. L., and Zachau-Christiansen, B.: Spontaneous alterations in position of the testis. Arch. Dis. Child., 41:198, 1966.

Vitale, P. J., Khademi, M., and Seebode, J. H.: Selective gonadal angiography for testicular localization in patients with cryptorchidism. Surg. Forum, 25:538, 1974.

Wachtel, S. S., Ohno, S., Koo, G. C., and Boyse, E. A.: Possible role for H-Y antigen in the primary determination of sex. Nature, 257:235, 1975.

Walsh, P. C., Curry, N., Mills, R. C., and Siiteri, P. K.: Plasma androgen response to hCG stimulation in pre-pubertal boys with hypospadias and cryptorchidism. J. Clin. Endocrinol. Metab., *42*:52, 1976.

Walsh, P. C., Madden, J. D., Harrod, M. J., Goldstein, J. L., MacDonald, P. C., and Wilson, J. D.: Familial incomplete male pseudohermaphroditism, type 2. De-creased dihydrotestosterone formation in pseudova-ginal perineoscrotal hypospadias. N. Engl. J. Med., *291*:944, 1974.

Wangensteen, O. H.: The undescended testis. Ann. Surg., *102*:875, 1935.

Ward, B., and Hunter, W. M.: The absent testicle, a report on a survey carried out among schoolboys in Not-tingham. Br. Med. J., *1*:2220, 1960.

Weiss, R. N., Glickman, M. G., and Lytton, B.: Clinical implications of gonadal venography in the management of the non-palpable undescended testis. J. Urol., *121*:745, 1979.

Wells, L. J.: Descensus testiculorum: descent after sever-ance of the gubernaculum. Anat. Rec., *88*:465, 1944.

Wells, L. J.: Descent of the testis. Anatomical and hormonal considerations. Surgery, *14*:436, 1943.

Welvaart, K., and Tijssen, J. P. G.: Management of the undescended testis in relation to the development of cancer. J. Surg. Oncol., *17*:218, 1981.

White, J. J., Haller, J. A., Jr., and Dorst, J. P.: Congenital inguinal hernia and inguinal herniography. Surg. Clin. North Am., *50*:823, 1970.

White, J. J., Shaker, I. J., and Oh, K. S.: Herniography: a diagnostic refinement in the management of cryptor-chidism. Ann. Surg., *39*:624, 1973.

Wiles, P.: Family tree showing hereditary undescended right testis and associated deformities. Proc. R. Soc. Med., *28*:157, 1934.

Winter, J. S. D., Hughes, I. A., Reyes, F. I., and Faiman, C.: Pituitary-gonadal relations in infancy: 2. Patterns of serum gonadal steroid concentrations in man from birth to two years of age. J. Clin. Endocrinol. Metab., *42*:679, 1976.

Winter, J. S. D., Taraska, S., and Farman, C.: The hor-monal response to hCG stimulation in male children and adolescents. J. Clin. Endocrinol. Metab., *34*:348, 1972.

Wislocki, G. B.: Observation on the descent of the testes in the macaque and in the chimpanzee. Anat. Rec., *57*:133, 1933.

Witschi, E.: Migration of the germ cells of human embryos from the yolk sac to the primitive gonadal folds. Con-trib. Embryol. Carnegie Inst., *32*:67, 1948.

Wolloch, Y., Shaher, E., Schachter, A., and Dintsman, M.: Fertility and sexual development after bilateral orchiop-exy for cryptorchidism. Isr. J. Med. Sci., *16*:707, 1980.

Wolverson, M. K., Jagannadharao, B., Sundaram, M., Riaz, M. A., Nalesnik, W. J., and Houttiun, E.: CT localization of impalpable cryptorchid testes. Am. J. Roentgenol. *134*:725, 1980.

Woodhead, D. M., Pohl, D. R., and Johnson, D. E.: Fertility of patients with solitary testes. J. Urol., *100*:66, 1973.

Wyndham, N. R.: A morphological study of testicular descent. J. Anat., *77*:179, 1943.

Zabransky, S.: LH-RH-Nasal spray (Kryptocur), ein neur Aspekt in der hormonellen Behandlung des Hoden-hoch-Standes. Klin. Paediatr., *193*:382, 1981.

Zarzycki, J., Szroeder, J., and Michaelowski, W. L.: Ultra-structure of seminiferous tubule cells and interstitial cells in cryptorchid human testicles. Acta Med. Pol., *18*:38, 1977.

Zer, M., Yolloch, Y., and Dintsman, M.: Staged orchior-rhaphy. Therapeutic procedure in cryptorchid testicle with a short spermatic cord. Arch. Surg., *110*:387, 1975.

Inguinal Hernia in Infancy and Childhood

Gunnlaugsson, G. H., Dawson, B., and Lynn, H. B.: Treatment of inguinal hernia in infants and children: Experience with contralateral exploration. Mayo Clin. Proc., *42*:129, 1967.

Hamrick, L. C., and Williams, J. O.: Is contralateral exploration indicated in children with unilateral in-guinal herniae? Am. J. Surg., *104*:52, 1962.

Infant Hydrocele

McKay, D. G., Fowler, R., and Barnett, J. S.: The patho-genesis and treatment of primary hydroceles in infancy and childhood. Aust. N.Z. J. Surg., *28*:2, 1958.

Ozdilek, S.: The pathogenesis of idiopathic hydrocele and a simple operative technique. J. Urol., *77*:282, 1957.

Rinker, J. R., and Allen, L.: Lymphatic defect in hydrocele. Am. Surg., *17*:681, 1951.

Scorer, G. C., and Farrington, G. H.: Congenital anomalies of the testis. *In* Harrison, J. H., Gittes, R., Perlmutter, A., Stamey, T. A., and Walsh, P. C. (Eds.). Campbell's Urology. Vol. 2. Philadelphia, W. B. Saunders Co., 1977, p. 1564.

Testicular Torsion

Backhouse, K. M.: Embryology of testicular descent and maldescent. Urol. Clin. North Am., *9*:315, 1982.

Bartsch, G., Frank, S., Marberger, H., and Mikuz, G.: Testicular torsion: late results with special regard to fertility and endocrine function. J. Urol., *124*:375, 1980.

Burton, J. A.: Atrophy following testicular torsion. Br. J. Surg., *59*:422, 1972.

Chapman, R. H., and Walton, A. J.: Torsion of the testis and its appendages. Br. Med. J., *1*:164, 1972.

Datta, N. S., and Mishkin, F.: Radionuclide imaging in intrascrotal lesions. JAMA, *231*:1060, 1975.

Holder, L. E., Martine, J. R., Holmes, E. R., and Wagner, H. N.: Testicular radionuclide angiography and static imaging: Anatomy, scintigraphic interpretation, and clinical indications. Radiology, *125*:739, 1977.

Korbel, E. I.: Torsion of the testis. J. Urol., *111*:521, 1974.

Krorup, T.: The testes after torsion. Br. J. Urol., *50*:43, 1978.

Levy, B. J.: The diagnosis of torsion of the testicle using the Doppler ultrasonic stethoscope. J. Urol., *113*:63, 1975.

Macnicol, M. F.: Torsion of the testis in childhood. Br. J. Surg., *61*:905, 1974.

Marshall, J. C., and Tanner, J. M.: Variations in pattern of pubertal changes in boys. Arch. Dis. Child., *45*:13, 1980.

Rigler, H. C.: Torsion of intraabdominal testes. Surg. Clin. North Am., *52*:371, 1972.

Scorer, C. G., and Farrington, G. H.: Congenital Deform-ities of the Testis and Epididymis. London, Butterworth and Co., 1971.

Sparks, J. P.: Torsion of the testis in adolescents and young adults. Clin. Pediatr., *11*:484, 1972.

Thompson, I. M., Latourette, H., Chadwick, S., Ross, G., and Lichti, E.: Diagnosis of testicular torsion using Doppler ultrasonic flowmeter. Urology, *6*:706, 1975.

CHAPTER 47

Hypospadias

JOHN W. DUCKETT, M.D.

Hypospadias is a congenital defect of the penis resulting in incomplete development of the anterior urethra. The abnormal urethral opening may be any place along the shaft of the penis, or it may open into the perineum. The more proximal the meatus, the more likely that the ventral aspect of the penis will be shortened and curved from chordee.

The normal anatomy of the penis consists of paired corpora cavernosa covered by a thick, fibrous tunica albuginea with a midline septum. The urethra traverses the penis within the corpus spongiosum, which lies in a ventral position in the groove between the two corpora cavernosa. The urethra emerges at the distal end of the conical glans penis. The spermatic fascia, or dartos fascia, is the loose layer of connective tissue immediately beneath the skin. Superficial lymphatics and the dorsal veins of the penis are located in this fascia. Beneath the dartos fascia is the Buck's fascia, which surrounds the corpora cavernosa and splits to contain the corpus spongiosum separately. The dorsal neurovascular bundle lies deep to Buck's fascia in the groove between the corpora cavernosa.

Hypospadias results in various degrees of urethral and corpus spongiosum deficiency. The fibrous tissue that causes chordee replaces Buck's fascia and the dartos fascia. The skin on the ventral surface is thin, and the prepuce is deficient ventrally and forms a dorsal hood over the glans.

CLASSIFICATION

The most commonly used classification of hypospadias relates to the location of the meatus (glanular, distal penile, proximal penile, penoscrotal junction, and perineal hypospadias). However, the type of hypospadias cannot always be defined by the original site of the meatus. The meatus may be close to the tip of the glans yet may have significant chordee. We, therefore, prefer the classification proposed by Barcat (1973) (Table 47–1), which uses the location after correction of the associated chordee (orthoplasty)* instead of the original site.

EMBRYOLOGY

Formation of the genital and lower urinary structures in the male centers around the cloaca and its surrounding mesoderm. During the fourth week of gestation, the urorectal septum begins its descent. This wedge of mesenchyme advances gradually toward the cloacal membrane, forming an anterior urogenital sinus and posterior rectum. The location of the cloacal membrane at the caudal end of the primitive streak provides the surrounding mesoderm with vast developmental potential. During the fourth week, paired swellings anterolateral to the membrane appear, and these swellings fuse into the midline genital tubercle by the sixth week of gestation. Simultaneously, the posterolateral anal tubercles form and the lateral mesoderm heaps up to form the urethral and genital folds. All of these mesodermal components retain the capacity to convert testosterone to dihydrotestosterone, thus heralding the first signs of sexual differentiation.

As the urorectal septum completes its descent and fuses with the cloacal membrane, the perineal body is formed. The urogenital sinus then begins to elongate onto the ventral surface of the phallus to the level of the corona, forming

---

*Orthoplasty (orthus = Greek, straighten) is a term used in Europe referring to chordee excision and penile straightening.

TABLE 47–1. CLASSIFICATION OF HYPOSPADIAS ACCORDING TO MEATAL LOCATION AFTER RELEASE OF CHORDEE

Anterior Hypospadias (70 Per Cent of Cases)	Middle Hypospadias (10 Per Cent of Cases)	Posterior Hypospadias (20 Per Cent of Cases)
Glanular (meatus situated on the inferior surface of the glans) Coronal (meatus situated in the balanopenile furrow) Anterior penile (meatus situated in the distal third of the shaft)	Middle penile (meatus situated in the middle third of the shaft)	Posterior penile (meatus situated in the posterior third of the shaft) Penoscrotal (meatus situated at the base of the shaft in front of the scrotum) Scrotal (meatus situated on the scrotum or between the genital swellings) Perineal (meatus situated behind the scrotum or behind the genital swellings)

the urethral groove, which is flanked laterally by mesoderm. Conversion of the anterior walls of the urogenital sinus results in the formation of an endodermal urethral plate on the floor of the urethral groove. This soon disintegrates, deepening the groove and facilitating the formation of the anterior urethra. At this time, the urethral and cloacal membranes rupture.

From the indifferent state, the external genital structures develop a typically male configuration under the influence of testosterone. As the phallus elongates, the urethral groove extends to the level of the corona. Gradually, the urethral folds coalesce in the midline, closing the urethra and forming the median raphe of the scrotum and penis. Dorsal to the urethra, mesenchyme coalesces to form the corporal bodies, vascular channels, and nerves. The glanular urethra may form by an identical mechanism, though there is controversy surrounding this premise. Glenister (1954) believes that the distal glans channel, which is most likely induced by hormonal and local factors, forms a solid core that tunnels to join the proximal urethra, which is created by closure of the urethral groove. This core later undergoes canalization, forming a complete urethra (Fig. 47–1). Anomalous canalization of this distal channel may be responsible for the blind-ending lacuna magna commonly found in young boys (Sommer and Stephens, 1980).

The prepuce forms as a ridge of skin that gradually grows to enclose the glans circumferentially with fusion to the glans epithelium. The preputial defect associated with hypospadias has a deficient ventral segment and resultant dorsal hood. The normal scrotal and penile raphe divides in hypospadias into a "Y" running onto the dorsal preputial hood around the glans in varying configurations. Even with the severe scrotal meatus, this defect of the raphe is ap-

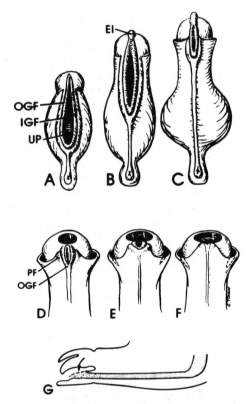

Figure 47–1. Embryology of penile and glanular urethra. *A* to *C,* The inner and outer genital folds cover the urethral plate (UP) and form the raphe. The glanular urethra is a compound of ectodermal pit at tip of glans and open end of the urethral groove. *D* to *F,* Further closure of the groove by outer genital and preputial folds, and orifice of the central pit in the glans. *G,* Breakdown (arrow) of the intervening septum to create one orifice, the fossa navicularis and the lacuna magna. Arrow indicates site of "anastomosis" between the ectodermal pit and the urethral groove. (OGF, outer genital folds; IGF, inner genital folds; PF, preputial folds; UP, urethral plate; EI, ectodermal tag marking site of ectodermal ingrowth. (From Sommer, J. T., and Stephens, F. D.: Dorsal urethral diverticulum of the fossa navicularis: symptoms, diagnosis and treatment. J. Urol., *124*:94, 1980. © The Williams & Wilkins Co., Baltimore. Used by permission.)

parent, fusing the penis into a vulviform appearance; even a penoscrotal transformation may occur. A glanular cleft may exist with a normal intact foreskin (Kumar, in press).

Chordee is the abnormal ventral curvature of the penis, an entity that is poorly understood. Apparently, the mesenchyme that would normally form the corpus spongiosum and fascial layers distal to the hypospadias meatus in the normal urethra persists as chordee tissue (Kaplan and Lamm, 1975; Kaplan and Brock, 1981). Alternatively, the abnormal disintegration of the urethral plate and the missing mesenchymal ingrowth distal to the hypospadias opening may give rise to fibrous tissue, which causes the downward curvature. It seems unlikely that the mere presence of this tissue is responsible for all cases of penile curvature. Rather, during penile development, a growth differential between normally formed dorsal tissue (corporal bodies and deficient ventral tissue and urethra) may result in curvature in some cases (Bellinger, 1981).

INTERSEX*

The presence of hypospadias is thought by some to be a form of intersex. Certainly intersex must be ruled out in the more severe forms of hypospadias, but in general the majority of hypospadias cases should not be considered as an intersex condition.

Genetic sex is established at the moment of fertilization and determines the gonadal sex, which, in turn, determines the phenotypic sex. The genetic endocrine and molecular levels in the overall process are well understood. However, the pathophysiology of the embryonic development is still not clear. The mechanisms by which genetic and developmental determinants influence differentiation of tissues during the initial phases of embryogenesis, and the specific transformation of cell types to initiate specific anatomic development, will be further clarified in the future (Wilson and Walsh, 1979).

Proper investigation of patients with ambiguous genitals includes a history, determination of genetic sex with karyotyping, biochemical evaluation of plasma and urinary steroid levels, evaluation of the urogenital sinus with a genitogram, assessment of androgen action in cultured fibroblasts when possible, and laparotomy and gonadal biopsy, if necessary.

---

*A more detailed discussion of disorders of sexual differentiation can be found in Chapter 41.

The following intersex states must be ruled out in a child with hypospadias:

1. Adrenogenital syndrome: Clearly, if a baby has nonpalpable testes, she is a girl until proved otherwise, no matter how masculinized she may be.

2. Mixed gonadal dysgenesis: This is considered the second most frequent cause of ambiguous genitals in the neonate. With a testis on one side and a streak gonad on the other, the most frequent karyotype is 45XO/46XY. However, the clinical entity is by no means confined to that chromosomal pattern. A uterus, vagina, and at least one fallopian tube are almost invariably present. The prepubertal testis appears relatively normal histologically, whereas postpubertally it does not develop germinal elements and contains only Sertoli cells. Because of the high incidence of gonadal neoplasms (25 per cent), streak gonads should be removed. Scrotal testes should be preserved, and intra-abdominal testes should be excised unless they can be relocated in the scrotum and are not associated with ipsilateral müllerian duct structures (Aarskog, 1970).

3. Incomplete male pseudohermaphroditism, type I, Reifenstein syndrome: Boys with this condition have perineal scrotal hypospadias with azoospermia, infertility, incomplete virilization at puberty, and gynecomastia that develops at or after puberty. Severe manifestations may include a vagina with small testes that are cryptorchid. The etiology of this syndrome can be demonstrated by fibroblast culture to be a defect in androgen binding of a varying degree. If detected early, severely affected males should have their gender converted to female, whereas in the majority of cases, the milder forms are phenotypic and physiologic males, and their hypospadias can be repaired. Supplemental testosterone, unfortunately, is not effective.

4. Incomplete male pseudohermaphroditism, type II (pseudovaginoperineoscrotal hypospadias—5 α-reductase deficiency): These perineoscrotal hypospadias patients have a blind vaginal pouch of variable size, which opens either into the urogenital sinus or, more frequently, into the urethra immediately behind the urethral orifice (Opitz et al., 1972; Walsh et al., 1974). Unlike incomplete pseudohermaphroditism, type I, these patients have well-developed and histologically normal testes, as well as normal epididymis, vasa, and seminal vesicles that terminate in the blind-ending vagina. Most patients are raised as females. Because of an enlarged clitoris, they are diagnosed early, and castration is performed early. If the

natural history is allowed, they will develop profound masculinization at puberty with muscle development, phallomegaly, ejaculation, and erections. In some, the sperm count has even been normal. Such a population has been studied in the Dominican Republic (Peterson et al., 1977).

5. True hermaphroditism: In these rare cases, both an ovary and a testis or ovotestis are present. The external genitalia display all gradations from male to female, but most are masculinized to some degree. For that reason, 75 per cent of patients are reared as males. Twenty-five per cent of the patients have bilateral ovotestes, 35 per cent have unilateral ovotestes, 25 per cent have a testis on one side and an ovary on the other, and 10 per cent are indeterminate (Butler et al., 1969). Fifty per cent have a 46XX karyotype, whereas 20 per cent have an XY karyotype, and 30 per cent are mosaics. Abdominal exploration with biopsy of both gonads is appropriate in these cases. In a patient who is sufficiently virilized to warrant male gender assignment, inappropriate ovarian tissue and müllerian structures should be removed. Repair of the hypospadias is indicated.

Micropenis is a miniature penis unaffected with hypospadias. Most often, it is due to a central defect consisting of gonadotropin deficiency, but a large number of cases are idiopathic.

Allen and Griffin (1984) have recently presented evidence in support of the concept that hypospadias is not just a local dysmorphic problem but rather is a local manifestation of a systemic endocrinopathy. A variety of endocrine abnormalities were seen in 11 of 15 patients studied in their series. They failed to confirm the impression that the principle defect lies in the inability of the target tissues to respond to androgen, either because of the numbers of androgen receptors or because of the inability to convert testosterone to dihydrotestosterone. Only one of the patients studied had abnormally low numbers of receptors. Half of 14 patients studied exhibited a substandard response to human chorionic gonadotropin (HCG) injections, suggesting a primary testicular defect. In four patients, there was an improved response at a later date, further complicating the picture and calling HCG stimulation into question unless it is an age-related response. Poor phallic development at an early age may indeed improve considerably with time and testosterone stimulation. For this reason, gender reassignment in the neonatal period for a small penis and severe hypospadias remains a very difficult

decision. Perhaps testosterone stimulation and observation for phallic enlargement may prove helpful in this regard (Allen and Griffin, 1984; Meyer et al., 1984). A substantial rise in testosterone after a 5-day stimulus of HCG is thought to indicate not only normal testes but also an intact hypothalamic-pituitary-gonadotropin axis. Meyer et al. (1984) presented two cases of hypospadias with adequate response to HCG at 2 months of age. However, when these patients were retested at 3 and 4 years of age, neither showed an adequate response to a short course of HCG, though both responded to a 6-week stimulus. This latter response is typical of gonadotropin deficiency. They also showed that 13 children with third-degree hypospadias responded normally to HCG stimulation, as did normal 2-month-old infants. This normal response in the neonatal period is probably the result of maternal chorionic gonadotropin priming of the fetal testis in utero, indicating that HCG testing is an unreliable method of identifying gonadotropin deficiency in the neonatal period.

ASSOCIATED ANOMALIES

The most common anomalies associated with hypospadias are undescended testes and inguinal hernia. Khuri et al. (1981) found an incidence of 9.3 per cent of undescended testes overall in patients with hypospadias. Third-degree hypospadias had a 31.6 per cent incidence, second-degree hypospadias had a 6.2 per cent incidence, and first-degree hypospadias had a 4.8 per cent incidence. They also found the incidence of inguinal hernia to be 9.1 per cent in the total group, with 17 per cent in the third-degree group, 8.5 per cent in the second-degree group, and 7.1 per cent in the first-degree group.

There have been conflicting reports as to the significance of anomalies of the upper urinary tract associated with hypospadias, and the question of obtaining routine intravenous urography or voiding cystography has been debated (Fallon et al., 1976; McArdle and Lebowitz, 1975). Khuri et al. (1981) grouped the patients according to the degree of their hypospadias and also subdivided them according to whether the hypospadias was isolated, whether it was associated with cryptorchidism, or whether it was associated with other system anomalies, such as cardiac, gastrointestinal, skeletal, neurologic, ophthalmologic, otorhinolaryngologic, and hematologic abnormalities. Another group included hypospadias with imperforate anus, and the final group included hypospadias with myelomeningocele and sacral agenesis. Significant upper tract anomalies were considered to be ureteropelvic junction obstruction, severe reflux, renal agenesis, Wilms tumor, pelvic kidney, and, finally, renal ectopia or fusion. The incidence was low (5.5 per cent) unless other system anomalies were associated. If one other system was present, the incidence was 12.2 per cent; with two other systems, the incidence was 16.7 per cent, whereas three other system anomalies increased the incidence to 50 per cent. With imperforate anus, the incidence was 46 per cent. With myelomeningocele, the incidence was 33 per cent. They concluded that all patients having hypospadias of any degree with associated anomalies should have the urinary tract screened, whereas such screening is unnecessary for hypospadias alone, with or without undescended testis or hernia.

FAMILIAL INCIDENCE

Bauer et al. (1981) found a 14 per cent incidence of hypospadias in siblings of the index child, whereas a 21 per cent incidence was found in a second individual in the families. Fathers were found to have hypospadias in 8 per cent of the cases.

The incidence of hypospadias has been calculated to be between 1 and 8 per 1000 live births, with an average of 3.2 or 0.32 per cent. Thus 1 out of every 300 live male births will have hypospadias (Sweet et al., 1974).

A multifactorial mode of inheritance for hypospadias has been implicated as a more logical explanation than a single factorial or sex-linked explanation.

HISTORY OF SURGICAL PROCEDURES*

The first account of hypospadias surgery was by Heliodorus and Antyllus (100 to 200 AD). The repair consisted of amputation of the shaft distal to the existing meatus. In 1838, Dieffenbach pierced the glans to the normal urethral meatus, allowing a cannula to remain in position until the channel became lined with epithelium, an unsuccessful procedure. In 1842, Mettauer suggested that the "organ be liberated by multiple subcutaneous incisions," whereas in

1861, Bouisson was the first to suggest a transverse incision at the point of greatest curvature. He also reported the use of scrotal tissue to reconstruct the urethra. In 1869, Thiersch described the use of local tissue flaps to repair epispadias, a technique he later used in hypospadias. He suggested that perineal urinary diversion be done to temporarily divert the urine away from the urethral reconstruction. He also did the first button-hole flap in the prepuce to allow the ventrum of the penis to be resurfaced with the prepuce.

In 1874, Duplay used Bouisson's technique to release chordee and at a later stage he formed a central flap, which was tubed and then covered with lateral penile flaps. He also stated that it did not matter if the central tube was incompletely formed, as he believed epithelialization would occur to form a channel if the tube was buried under lateral flaps, as was later popularized by Denis Browne in 1950. In 1875, Wood described a meatal-based flap to form the urethral channel and combined this with the Thiersch-type button-hole flap to cover the raw surface, a technique quite similar to Ombredanne's (1932) or Mathieu's (1932).

Rosenberger in 1891, Landerer in 1891, Bidder in 1892, and Bucknall in 1907 all used scrotal tissue for urethroplasty and described burying the penis in the scrotum to obtain skin coverage, similar to the technique used by Leveuf in 1936 and by Cecil-Culp in 1951.

In 1896, Hook described a vascularized preputial flap for urethroplasty, which was similar to the procedure Davis used in 1950. Hook further suggested the use of a lateral oblique flap from the side of the penis, which was later popularized by Broadbent in 1951.

In 1897, Beck and Hacker undermined and advanced the urethra onto the glans for subcoronal cases, similar to the technique used by Waterhouse and Glassberg in 1975. Beck in 1897 and White and Martin in 1917 used adjacent rotation flaps from the scrotum for resurfacing after a Duplay-type urethroplasty, similar to the procedure used by Marberger in 1981 and Turner-Warwick in 1979. In 1897 and again in 1914, Nove-Josserand reported attempts to repair hypospadias with split-thickness grafts, similar to the technique used by McIndoe in 1937. In 1899 Rochet used a large distally based scrotal flap for urethroplasty and buried it in a tunnel on the ventral surface of the penis. In 1913, Edmunds was the first to transfer the skin of the prepuce to the ventral surface of the penis at the time of chordee release. This abundant ventral skin was then used in a Duplay-type

---

*References for this historical review are found in Horton et al., 1973.

urethroplasty at a later stage, similar to what Blair accomplished in 1933 and later Byars in 1955. In 1917, Bevan used a urethral meatal-based flap, channeled through the glans for distal repair, similar to that used by Mustarde in 1965.

MULTISTAGE REPAIRS

In the standard two-stage repair, the chordee release (orthoplasty) was accomplished by dividing the urethral plate distal to the meatus, straightening the penis, and allowing the meatus to retract to a more proximal position. Skin cover of the ventrum was achieved by mobilizing the dorsal preputial and penile skin around to the ventrum to be used in a later urethroplasty. Since the technique of artificial erection (Gittes and McLaughlin, 1974) was not used, residual chordee was not an unusual result of this orthoplasty. Secondary chordee releases were required before moving to form the urethra.

Browne (1953) was very influential in promoting his "buried strip" principle for hypospadias repair. A ventral strip of skin was covered by generous mobilized skin flaps brought together in the midline with "beads and stops." The channel under the skin flaps would epithelialize around a stenting catheter that was left for 3 to 6 weeks. Results were never very satisfactory until Van der Meulen (1964) demonstrated that a rotated skin cover from the dorsum with an eccentric suture line would offer more successful healing. In fact, he uses no stenting or diversion of urine and has the patient void through the repair, leaving only subcutaneous drains for several days. His recent results are dramatic—no fistulas! (Van der Muelen, 1982).

Byars (1955) further developed the two-stage method by extending the foreskin onto the glans in the first stage and rolling a complete tube in the second. Smith (1981) refined the Byars approach by denuding the epithelium on one skin edge to allow "double-breasting" of raw surfaces. His review of 285 repairs with only a 2.8 per cent incidence of fistulas is commendable.

In 1955, Belt devised a technique that he never published but that gained acclaim after Fuqua (1973) published his series. Hendren (1981) had the largest series with excellent results. Of the two-stage methods, the Belt-Fuqua is popular today (Fig. 47–2).

Numerous more modern methods have been introduced to repair hypospadias. Creevy (1958) and Backus and DeFelice (1960) provide excellent reviews of the multistaged procedures performed up to 1960. All of these methods must be studied to understand the pitfalls of this difficult surgery. However, emphasis in this chapter is placed on the one-stage methods that are currently popular.

ONE-STAGE REPAIRS

In the late 1950's when surgeons were more confident of their ability to remove chordee tissue in its entirety, one-stage hypospadias procedures became popular. In 1900, Russell described a procedure for one-stage repair of hypospadias, using a urethral tube constructed from a flap that was developed on the ventral surface of the penis. This flap extended around the entire circumference of the corona to include a cuff of the prepuce. This new urethra was placed through a tunnel in the glans and secured to the tip of the glans. Broadbent et al. (1961) created a urethral tube from the skin of the penis and prepuce and laid this tube into the split glans. DesPrez et al. (1961) developed a one-stage procedure similar to that of Broadbent and colleagues. In 1954, McCormack reported a two-stage procedure in which a full-thickness tube graft urethroplasty was placed at the first procedure, but the proximal anastomosis closure was delayed. In 1955, Devine and Horton (1961) developed this technique further by utilizing a free graft of preputial skin to replace the urethra after release of chordee; they then closed this McCormack procedure in one stage. In 1970 and in 1972, Hodgson described three different procedures that utilized vascularized flaps from the dorsal prepuce, as well as penile skin. This urethral flap was brought to the ventral aspect with a button-hole transposition (Hodgson, 1975).

One-stage hypospadias repair has had the test of time, supporting the feasibility of this type of surgery. Besides the desirability of completing the reconstruction in one operation, a one-stage procedure has the additional advantage of using skin that is unscarred from previous surgical procedures, the normal blood supply of which has not been disrupted. The main impediment to the success of this procedure, inadequate chordee release, has been nearly eliminated since the introduction of the artificial erection technique (Gittes and McLaughlin, 1974).

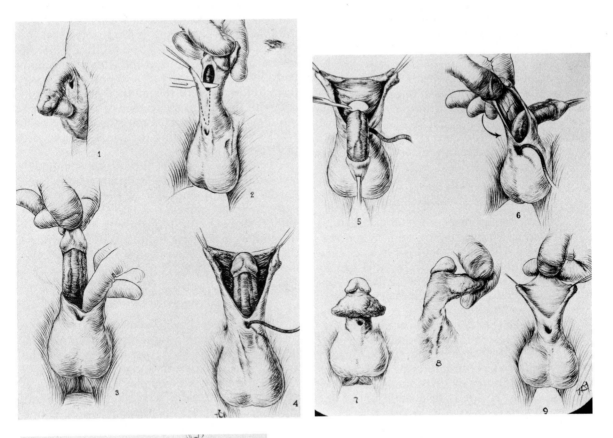

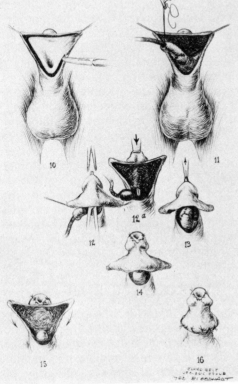

Figure 47–2. Belt-Fuqua repair. *1* to *6*, First stage. Exaggerated button-hole transposition of dorsal preputial skin to the ventrum after chordee release. *7* to *16*, Second stage. Both inner and outer preputial surfaces are transposed to the ventrum. *9* to *11*, Inner preputial skin is mobilized into a vascularized urethra. *12* to *14*, The channel is made next to the corporal bodies beneath the subcutaneous tissues and is channeled through the glans to the tip of the penis. *15* and *16*, Outer preputial skin covers as an apron to surface the ventrum. The bulky tissue may be excised at a later date. (Original drawings courtesy of Willard Goodwin.)

CONGENITAL CURVATURE OF THE PENIS (CHORDEE WITHOUT HYPOSPADIAS)

Congenital curvature of the penis without hypospadias is quite rare. Secondary curvatures associated with Peyronie disease or periurethral sclerosis associated with urethral stricture are much more common in adults. There are two kinds of primary curvatures, those associated with a normal urethral spongiosum and those with a hypoplastic urethra.

PRIMARY CURVATURE WITH A NORMAL CORPUS SPONGIOSUM

Two thirds of primary congenital curvatures have a normal corpus spongiosum. When flaccid, the penis looks normal with a circular prepuce. During erection, the penis is usually curved downward but may have a lateral curvature of as much as 90 degrees. An upward curvature (without epispadias) is exceptional (Udall, 1980). This deformity becomes noticeable to the adolescent or young adult. However, many with this condition find little difficulty having intercourse. The lateral deviations seen in about one third of cases is almost always to the left. With erection, disproportion of the corpora cavernosa is usually apparent.

Physiologic ventral curvature of the penis in the fetus has been noted at different stages of development (Kaplan and Lamm, 1975; Kaplan and Brock, 1981). It usually disappears by the time of birth, yet it may be found more commonly in premature infants. Within the first several years of life, this condition slowly disappears (Cendron and Melin, 1981).

Treatment. In cases in which the urethra is normal, treatment varies with the direction of the deviation and whether one believes that true chordee tissue is responsible for the ventral bend (Devine and Horton, 1975). Good results have been reported by Devine and Horton with resection of fibrous dartos fascia beneath and beside the mobilized normal urethra. However, this rather extensive dissection does not offer consistent results (Kramer et al., 1982). There has been greater acceptance of the concept Nesbitt described in 1965 of taking tucks in or plicating the disproportionally large tunica albuginea. This technique was first described by Syng Physick, the "Father of American Surgery," in the early nineteenth century. He treated chordee by shortening the dorsal tunica albuginea (Pancoast, 1844). When the arc of maximum curvature is located with artificial erection, wedges of tunica albuginea are excised in a stepwise fashion. These diamond wedges are closed transversely with permanent sutures until the penis is straight. It is possible to plicate the fascia without cutting the tunica by placing several rows of sutures at the site of maximum convexity. Nesbit, however, reported his long-term follow up with this method as disappointing, with significant recurrence of chordee (Nesbit, 1966). Exposure for the surgical approach is achieved by retracting the penile skin toward the base as a sleeve.

The age at which this defect should be corrected is important. Cendron feels it should not be done too early for two reasons: (1) the curvature may spontaneously improve with age and (2) there is risk of disturbing the growth of the phallus by altering the tunica of the corpora. Both of these reasons suggest it is better to do the repair after puberty.

PRIMARY CURVATURE WITH A HYPOPLASTIC URETHRA

About one third of congenital curvature cases have a hypoplastic urethra (Cendron and Melin, 1981). In this type of curvature, the urethral meatus is well situated on the glans, but the foreskin is incomplete and the ventral penis is not normal. The skin covering the urethra is very thin and there is no spongiosal tissue for a long portion. Chordee is present with erection. Lengthening the frenulum and eliminating the penoscrotal web does not alter the curvature. Since the segment of urethra is hypoplastic, it may be considered a "concealed" hypospadias. Congenitally short urethra may be a variant of this condition.

Treatment. For the hypoplastic urethra or short urethra variant of congenital curvature, a chordee release with division of the midportion of the hypoplastic urethra is required. Urethroplasty using the same techniques that are applicable to the usual hypospadias anomaly will follow. The author prefers to replace the midurethral segment with an island flap from the ventral prepuce, making two oblique anastomoses with the remaining good proximal and distal urethral segments, leaving the meatus naturally on the glans.

FIBROUS CHORDEE

When associated with hypospadias, chordee has commonly been attributed to hypoplasia of the corpus spongiosum distal to the hypospadias meatus. This results in a midline fibrous band or fan-shaped area of fibrosis, tethering the penis ventrally. When this tissue is excised (*or-*

thoplasty), the penis straightens. This simplified explanation is not altogether applicable to the variety of expressions of hypospadias or pure chordee without hypospadias. Certainly the concept of a "bow string" tethering that requires a simple incision is not true.

Kaplan and Lamm (1975) put forth a convincing case that chordee may indeed be an arrest of normal embryologic development analogous to failure of testicular descent. Thus, it is no surprise that fibrosis is conspiciously absent in some clinical cases of chordee. Chordee may also result from differential growth of the dorsal and ventral aspects of the corpora (Bellinger, 1981), which is best corrected by shortening the dorsal tunica albuginea. Some have suggested that occasionally adherence of skin to the distal hypoplastic urethra is the element that causes chordee and that correction of the bend may be achieved simply by freeing the skin attachments. This may be so rarely if associated with a marked skin deficiency on the ventrum (Allen and Spence, 1968).

CLASSIFICATION

Devine and Horton (1973) proposed three types of chordee. Class I consists of chordee without hypospadias and is the most severe defect. The corpus spongiosum is deficient from the site at which the chordee begins to the glans penis. The urethra consists of a thin tube of mucous membrane located just beneath the skin and ending in the glans in the normal meatus. The chordee is caused by dense fibrous tissue lying beneath the urethra, similar to the tissue causing the chordee in hypospadias with chordee. In Class II, the urethra is surrounded by normal corpus spongiosum with Buck's fascia and the dartos fascia layers being abnormal. In Class III, the urethra, corpus spongiosum, and Buck's fascia are normal, with the abnormal dartos fascia holding the penis curved in chordee. Forty per cent of Devine and Horton's patients were Class I, 40 per cent were Class II, and 20 per cent were Class III. They have claimed that chordee without hypospadias can be corrected without severing the urethra, and they were able to straighten all of the bend. These claims have not been generally verified. Their Class III group may be what some call "skin chordee." As the reader will see, there is considerable debate regarding chordee, its origin, and its treatment.

ORTHOPLASTY

Artificial erection, introduced in 1974 by Gittes and McLaughlin, has been a very signif-

icant contribution to orthoplasty. By placing a tourniquet at the base of the penis and injecting a corpus cavernosum with saline, both corporal bodies fill and it is possible to determine both the extent of chordee and the success of chordee correction. The assurance of complete correction is essential in order to proceed on to a one-stage repair with urethroplasty. So far, there has been no report of damage to the cavernous tissue from this technique. It has also been used extensively in adults with no untoward effects. Care must be taken to assure that normal saline is used. Penile necrosis occurred when 50 per cent saline was injected inadvertently.

For true fibrous chordee, the penis is curved ventrally with only a short distance between the location of the meatus and the glans. An incision is made in a circumferential manner around the corona and is carried well below the glans cap just distal to the urethral meatus and down to the tunica albuginea of the corpora cavernosa. Proximal dissection is then achieved, freeing the fibrous plaque of tissue closely adherent to the tunica albuginea with sharp dissection, moving from side to side as the ventral curvature is released. The urethra is elevated from the corpora in this en bloc dissection. In most cases, the chordee tissue surrounds the urethral meatus and extends proximally along the urethra for a distance. This tissue should all be freed well down to the penoscrotal junction and many times into the perineoscrotal area. Once this urethral mobilization is accomplished, the shaft of the penis should be stripped of any fibrous tissue, extending out to the lateral shaft of the penis and distally below the glans. Artificial erection is used to check the success of the excision.

Several further maneuvers have been offered for releasing the last bit of bend. A midline incision along the septum between the two corpora cavernosa has, in some cases, been effective (Devine, 1983). Lateral incisions in a stepwise manner may be effective in the groove between the dorsal corpora and the ventral segment.

If after adequate excision of all abnormal fibrous tissue, artificial erection continues to demonstrate chordee, corporal disproportion is present. This should be corrected by dorsal plication as discussed in the section on Congenital Curvature, and permanent sutures should be used. A glans "tilt" is also effective to get the last little bit of bend from the glans area. The sutures should be placed laterally to avoid injuring the midline neurovascular structures (Hodgson, 1981).

In the rare case, there is so much deficiency of the tunica albuginea on the ventrum that excision of the tunica albuginea is required with replacement by dermal graft or with tunica vaginalis. Tunica vaginalis is obtained by exposing the testis and removing a patch of the tunica from around the testis.

Once the chordee has been released, a urethroplasty may proceed in the one-stage repair. Some still prefer to re-surface the ventrum of the penis with preputial skin to await a second-stage urethroplasty. There are several disadvantages with this approach, and the one-stage techniques are much preferred today.

MEATUS

Considerable controversy surrounds the need for the meatus to be at the tip of the glans versus the subcoronal area. For many years, the two-stage techniques (Byars, 1955; Browne, 1953) left the meatus just beneath the glans. In more recent years, an effort has been made to move the meatus to the tip, particularly in the more extensive one-stage repairs (Devine and Horton, 1961; Duckett, 1981a). Even with distal hypospadias, the trend seems to be to strive to achieve the same goal in patients with relatively minor defects. However, Mills et al. (1981) reviewed 23 cases of distal hypospadias repaired by the Devine-Horton flip-flap procedure or the Ombredanne flip-flap technique and found a 25 per cent complication rate with fistula formation or meatal stenosis. Compared with their 11 cases without complications using the Allen and Spence (1968) procedure, in which the meatus is not moved from its subcoronal position, their conclusion was obvious—at what price perfection!

There are several different techniques to achieve an apical meatus, depending on the variation of the proximal meatus (Gibbons and Gonzales, 1983). The triangularized glans (Devine and Horton, 1961) achieves a flap meatoplasty and avoids a circumferential meatal closure. Although this may prevent meatal stenosis, the glans is flattened with distortion of the normal configuration. Extension of the meatus onto the ventral glans may be effected with either a meatal-based flap or onlay vascularized flap, as described later. The glans fillet described by Turner-Warwick (1979) and Cronin and Guthrie (1973) is a two-stage procedure that lays preputial skin onto the ventrum of the spatulated glans. The meatus can later be tubularized and the glans can be closed over it to achieve a quite normal-appearing glans with an apical meatus. This technique is more applicable to the adult penis.

The glans channel technique to deliver the urethra to the apex is another method. Bevan (1917) devised a technique that created a proximal penile flap that was converted into a urethral tube and was pulled through a tunnel in the glans. Mays (1951) employed a staged technique that straightened the penis, bringing the prepuce over the glans to cover the ventral defect and constructing a glanular urethra that was carried through a tunnel to the tip of the glans. Both Ricketson (1958) and Hendren (1981) have channeled a full-thickness skin tube through the glans. Hinderer (1971) uses a trocar to tunnel, entering the glans at the tip and emerging a few millimeters below the coronal sulcus through a "trap door" flap of albuginea.

We have combined the glans channel technique with the creation of a vascularized island flap neourethra (Duckett, 1980a). This procedure requires a generous channel through the glans tissue, allowing the vascularized skin flap to be placed through the glans without compression of the blood supply. Because the rigid tissue of the glans may be predisposed to stricture formation, the glans channel technique must avoid too timid a channel. However, if attention to the details of the technique are followed, the incidence of meatal stenosis is quite low. In the Mustarde procedure (1965), a dorsal "V" flap is used with the glans channel; we have not felt this necessary.

In the more distal cases of hypospadias, the configuration of the glans may dictate the type of meatoplasty. If the glans furrow is deep, a Mathieu procedure may be preferred. If the glans is broad and flat, a Hodgson II or an onlay island flap technique will allow the glans to be rolled around the glanular vascularized two-faced tube.

TECHNIQUES FOR ANTERIOR HYPOSPADIAS

MAGPI (MEATOPLASTY AND GLANULOPLASTY) (Fig. 47–3)

The majority of boys with hypospadias (65 to 75 per cent) have the meatus situated on the inferior surface of the glans in the balanopenile furrow, or on the distal 1 cm of the shaft. When not associated with chordee, such a meatal location may cause little functional handicap in regard to voiding or sexual activity aside from

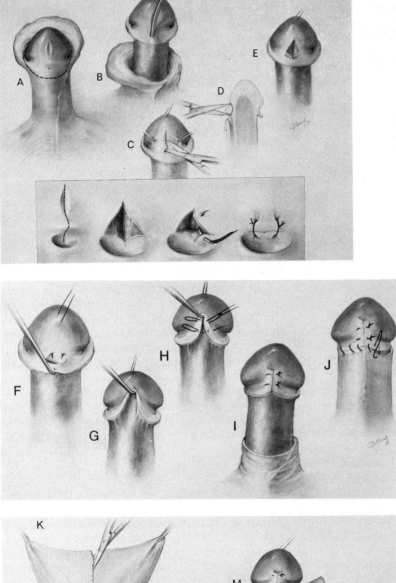

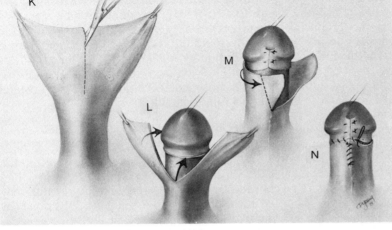

Figure 47–3. MAGPI Procedure. *A,* Subcoronal meatus. *B,* Circumferential subcoronal incision 8 mm proximal to meatus and corona. *C to E,* Incision of bridge of tissue between meatus and glanular groove. Note the extent and depth of the incision *(inset). Inset,* Transverse Heineke-Mikulicz closure of dorsal meatal edge to distal glanular groove. *F and G,* Traction toward the glans conforms the lateral glans edges into a "V". *H and I,* Vertical mattress approximation brings the glans beneath the meatus. *J,* Sleeve re-approximation of the penile skin, with excision of excess foreskin, completes the repair. *K to N,* A Byars' flap closure is used if a ventral skin defect exists. (From Duckett, J. W.: MAGPI (Meatoplasty and Glanuloplasty). Urol. Clin. North Am. *8:*513, 1981. Used by permission.)

deflection of the stream. For this reason, reconstructive surgery has been denied many of these patients in the past. An operation that can be accomplished with minimal complications and a short hospital stay and that improves the cosmetic appearance, resulting in considerable patient and parental satisfaction, has recently become popular. This plastic surgical rearrangement incorporates a meatal advancement and glanuloplasty and is called the MAGPI procedure (Duckett, 1981a).

The MAGPI procedure may be performed as a day surgical case without urinary diversion. It is helpful to instill 1:100,000 epinephrine solution, particularly in the glans tissue, to assist in hemostasis. For the meatal advancement, a generous longitudinal incision is made from inside the dorsal edge of the meatus to the distal glans groove. This effectively obliterates the bridge of tissue, which deflects the urinary stream ventrally. The dorsal meatal edge is left with a "V" configuration, which enlarges it, correcting any stenosis. A diamond-shaped defect results. The dorsal wall of the urethra is advanced to the apex of the glanular groove in a transverse fashion and is closed using 6-0 chromic suture. This effects a Heineke-Mikulicz transverse closure of a vertical incision. The dorsal meatal edge is now flattened into the glanular groove so that the stream is not deflected, and the meatus is enlarged and advanced.

A drop-back of the penile skin is accomplished with a circumferential incision made approximately 6 to 8 mm from the coronal edge and proximal to the meatus. Extreme care must be taken in dissecting the thin skin from over the thin urethra, because it is easy to injure the urethra, thereby increasing the risk of fistula formation. The dissection is carried out in a sleeve fashion between Buck's fascia and the layer of subcutaneous tissue of the prepuce. Torsion will also be corrected in many cases if the dissection is carried back to the base of the penis.

The glanuloplasty portion of the procedure is accomplished by placing a small holding stitch on the ventral meatal edge and retracting it toward the glans. The lateral edges of the glans form an inverted "V" in this fashion and can be brought together in the midline. This effectively brings glanular tissue beneath the meatus to advance and support it. Mobilization of the lateral glanular tissue is not necessary. The glanular tissue is approximated with polyglycolic sutures and chromic sutures to the skin edge. Sleeve re-approximation of the skin is usually accomplished; however, a limited Byars type of rotation of preputial skin to the ventrum may be necessary to cover a ventral skin defect and permit a more normal location of the penoscrotal junction.

In some cases, a meatus located 1 to 2 cm from the corona may be advanced onto the glans with the MAGPI technique. The feasibility of this maneuver can be determined by lifting the skin beneath the meatus and moving it and the urethra forward. This can usually be done with a relatively long penis that is not deficient in ventral skin. We have been surprised at this extended use of the MAGPI procedure.

Occasionally, if there is a slight ventral tilt to the glans, we have been able to correct this by tucking the coronal edge of the glans dorsally onto the tunica albuginea using nonresorbable sutures, as described by Hodgson (1981). Care must be taken not to place these sutures near the midline in order to avoid injury to the dorsal arteries and nerves that supply the glanular tissue.

We have done more than 500 of these procedures with the occurrence of only two fistulas, which resulted from injury to the underlying urethra while the ventral skin was being incised. In 11 cases, we have had breakdown of the meatal advancement. This was caused by failure to recognize the occasional duplicated epithelialized channel dorsal to the meatus. If this is not removed or incorporated into the meatal advancement, healing may be compromised. All of these cases required repeat surgery.

URETHRAL MOBILIZATION

Another method of dealing with the subcoronal meatus is by urethral mobilization. Reported as far back as Beck and Hacker in 1897 and Beck in 1917, urethral mobilization was recently revived by Belman (1977), Waterhouse and Glassberg (1981), Koff (1981), and Nasrallah and Minott (1984). This technique offers very little advantage over the MAGPI and requires a more extensive procedure. The meatal stenosis rate is significant.

PERIMEATAL-BASED FLAP (MATHIEU PROCEDURE) (Fig. 47–4)

When the meatus is too proximal on the shaft to achieve a MAGPI and there is no chordee by artificial erection, the meatus may be advanced onto the glans as described by Mathieu (1932) and more recently reported by Hoffman and Hall (1973), Kim and Hendren (1981), Wacksman (1981), Gonzales et al.

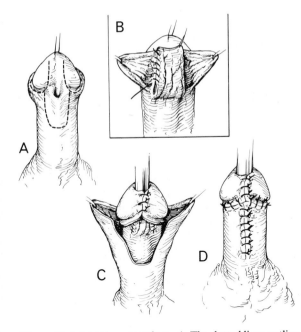

Figure 47–4. Mathieu procedure. *A,* The dotted lines outline the skin flaps. *B,* The proximal flap is rotated, and the lateral glans flaps are developed. *C,* The glans flaps cover the neourethra, and preputial skin is moved if necessary. *D,* Completed repair.

(1983), and Devine (1983). A flap of perimeatal skin is raised from tissue proximal and adjacent to the meatus, taking care to preserve the vascular subcutaneous tissue. Parallel incisions are made on either side of the glanular groove, developing the lateral glans as wings. The proximal flap closes into the glans groove as leaves of a book, and two suture closures are made on either side of the flap, extending the meatus to the tip of the glans. Preserving the vasculature to the flap is important. The lateral glans wings will come together for closure over the urethral advancement. Appropriate skin cover is achieved. In this procedure, diversion of urine is used for 5 to 7 days.

Gibbons and Gonzales (1983) have described three subcoronal meatal variants and have suggested creating a perimeatal based flap to ascertain whether MAGPI or an alternative procedure is applicable.

ONLAY FLAP URETHRAL EXTENSION

If there is no chordee by artificial erection, but the meatus is too proximal for a Mathieu procedure or the ventral skin too thin to use, a procedure to replace the ventral urethra is required. The urethral plate in this situation may be left intact. The Hodgson II procedure (Hodgson, 1975) (Fig. 47–5) incorporates a parallel

strip of urethral plate skin onto the glans to serve as the dorsal urethral wall, and the ventral urethral wall is created by a vascularized flap of tissue from the dorsal prepuce. This is outlined in a fashion longitudinal to the axis of the penis using the outer preputial layer and is transposed to the ventrum with a buttonhole technique. A U-shaped closure extends the meatus to the glans tip. We have wrapped the glanular tissue around the new urethral tube in such a way that a suitable conical glans will be attained. The Hodgson technique (1975) uses penile skin on the ventrum of the glans for cover. Because of the adequate vasculature of the flap, healing is better assured. This procedure is distinctly different from the other techniques described by Hodgson, which required a tubularization of the ventral or dorsal preputial skin "flip-flopped" over with a proximal anastomosis made with the old urethral meatus. In the Hodgson II technique, the urethral meatus is continuous with the ventral penile skin, covered by the onlay flap (Hodgson, 1979). A procedure similar to the Hodgson II was described by Nesbit (1966).

ISLAND FLAP ONLAY (Fig. 47–6)

We have modified the island flap onlay technique by using an island flap of transverse

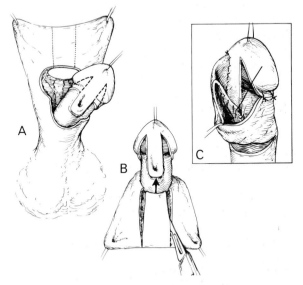

Figure 47–5. Hodgson II procedure. Used when no chordee exists and smooth ventral skin is present distal to a midshaft meatus. *A,* Mobilization of prepuce with outline of vertical dorsal strip for onlay to ventrum. *B,* Buttonhole transposition of vascularized outer preputial flap. *C,* Parallel closure onto glans. (From Hodgson, N. B.: Use of vascularized flaps in hypospadias repair. Urol. Clin. North Am. 8:471, 1981. Used by permission.)

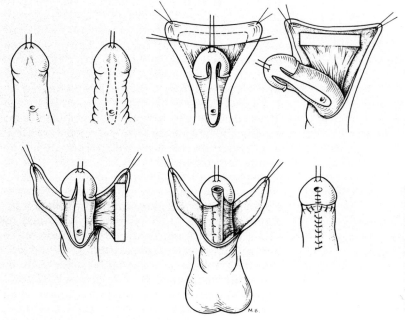

Figure 47–6. Island flap onlay. Used for cases without chordee with a meatus too proximal for a flip-flap. Urethral plate left intact. Onlay of inner preputial island flap with two parallel suture lines. Meatus is extended to the apex of the glans. Skin cover by Byars' flaps. (Used with permission of Department of Medical Illustration, Institute of Urology, London WC2. Reference No. 10521.)

ventral preputial skin to construct the onlay flap. This allows more mobility of the strip for urethroplasty, avoiding the buttonhole transposed apron of penile skin. The skin cover stage is more flexible also. Such a technique will cover a rather long strip on the ventrum if the proximal urethra is deficient. Even though the proximal meatus may be located near the corona, the dorsal urethra should be opened back to good spongiosum tissue, discarding the thin ventral urethra. However, it can be used only if there is no chordee. A glanular meatus may also be achieved by bringing the glanular wings around the extension into the glans groove (Duckett, 1980c).

OTHER METHODS FOR ANTERIOR HYPOSPADIAS

Other techniques to extend the distal meatus without hypospadias include tubularization of the distal urethral plate into a full tube with skin coverage by various means (Belman and King, 1979). Nesbit (1966) described this method, as did King (1970, 1981) and Perlmutter and Vatz (1975).

TECHNIQUE FOR MIDDLE HYPOSPADIAS WITH CHORDEE

When the meatus is in a distal position but there is significant chordee, an incision must be made dividing the urethra distal to the meatus to free the chordee. If the urethral meatus does not retract more than 1 cm proximally, the Horton-Devine flip-flap procedure (Fig. 47–7) is a good choice for repair. A proximal flap of penile skin is made, and three triangular flaps of glans tissue are mobilized to form a meatus (Devine, 1983). The middle dart of glanular skin is fixed to the ventral surface and serves as the dorsal wall of the new urethra. The apex of the dart is placed into the dorsal urethral meatus, and the flap of proximal skin is brought up as the ventral urethral layer. The glanular wings are brought around and are closed ventrally as a cover for the urethra. This technique is effective but has limited usage, since the particular association of a distal meatus with chordee is rare now that artificial erection is available.

The creation of a rolled urethra from the proximal penile skin with subsequent tunneling through the glans has been around since Bevan (1917). More recently, it carries the eponym of Mustarde (1965).

THE MUSTARDE PROCEDURE (Fig. 47–8)

The Mustarde technique is applicable for cases in which mild chordee exists with a distal meatus or when the glans has a conical configuration, lending better to a tunneling procedure. An incision is made distal to the meatus, and chordee is released. A proximal flap of perimeatal skin is outlined and rolled into a completed tube of 1 to 2 cm, which is flipped forward, and a glans channel is created to de-

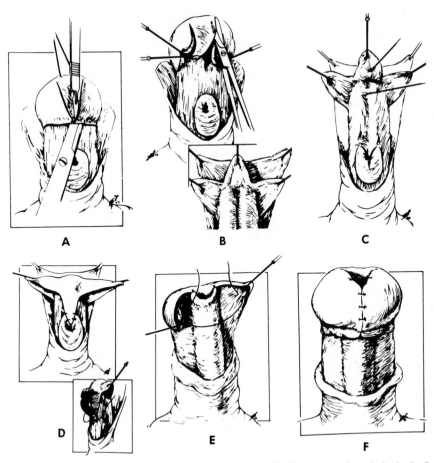

Figure 47–7. Horton-Devine flip-flap repair of distal hypospadias. *A*, Epithelium of glans is incised. *B*, Glans flap is thinned as it is being cut. When it is retracted upward, bulge of tissue at its base will be excised. *C*, Suture is placed to secure flap to tunica of corpora. Dorsal wall of urethral meatus has been incised. *D*, Tip of glans flap is approximated to urethra and flip-flap to construct neourethra. *E*, Suture in erectile tissue of glans to approximate lateral wings without tension. *F*, Glans is closed with new meatus at tip. (From Devine, C. J., Jr., and Horton, C. E.: J. Urol., *118*:188, 1977. Used by permission.)

Figure 47–8. Mustarde procedure. Used for cases in which an incision is required distal to the meatus, yet the proximal meatus remains near the glans (also for cases with residual chordee). *A*, Peri-meatal skin flap outlined. *B*, Skin flap rolled into complete tube and channeled through glans to the apex. *C*, Skin cover depicted here with button-hole transposition. (From Mays, H. B.: Utilization of the prepuce for repair. *In* Horton, C. E. (Ed.): Plastic and Reconstructive Surgery of the External Genitalia. Little, Brown & Co., 1973, p. 333. Used by permission.)

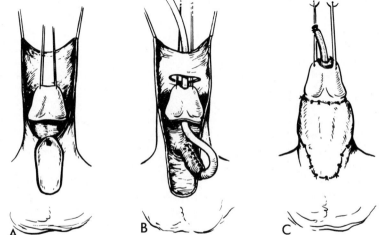

liver the meatus to the tip. Care must be made to keep the subcutaneous tissue attached to the skin flap to preserve the vasculature. Ballesteros (1977) uses two skin strips circumferential to the corona, and these strips are folded together as a tube and extended through the glans similar to the Mustarde technique. Belman (1982) has modified the method simply by a different skin cover. Use of this technique is appropriate for secondary cases combining residual chordee and a retrusive meatus. The proximal ventral skin next to the meatus should not be scarred as a result of previous operations.

TECHNIQUES FOR POSTERIOR HYPOSPADIAS

Urethroplasty techniques for the more difficult 20 per cent of hypospadias cases with the proximal meatus near or below the penoscrotal junction fall into three basic categories: (1) adjacent skin flaps, (2) free skin grafts, and (3) mobilized vascularized flaps.

Skin adjacent to the meatus may be tubularized for the neourethra as performed by Broadbent et al. (1961) and Des Prez et al. (1961) in their one-stage procedures. Hinderer (1971) used a similar neourethra, which he tunneled through the corporal bodies. He has since abandoned this method in favor of an island flap method (Hinderer, 1978). Transfer of dorsal skin to the ventrum in a previous stage will also provide skin that is adjacent to the meatus for urethroplasty. Less than optimum vascularity to these thin rotational flaps makes results with these methods more prone to complications.

Free skin grafts should be full thickness rather than split thickness. Devine and Horton (1983) have had successful experiences for more than 25 years using the inner preputial skin detached and defatted as a thin, full-thickness graft to form the neourethra (Fig. 47–9). Their good results have not been reproducible in a uniform manner in the hands of others, however (Filmer et al., 1977; Woodard and Cleveland, 1982; Redman, 1983). Since the free graft must be revascularized, the key element to success is a perfect skin cover of the graft with well-vascularized dorsal preputial and penile skin.

Vascularized flaps of the preputial or penile

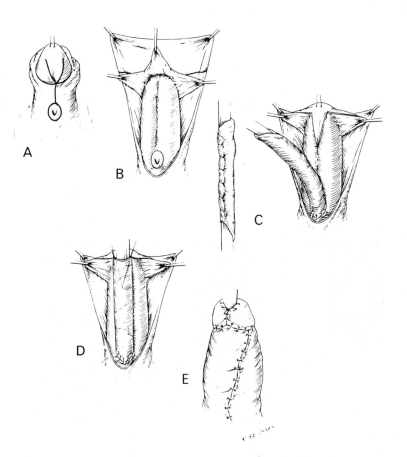

A

B

C

D

E

Figure 47–9. Devine-Horton free graft. *A,* Glans "V" incision; chordee resection after mobilization of penile skin. *B,* Triangularized glans wings developed; ventral preputial skin used for full-thickness free graft; free graft formed into neourethra over stent. *C,* Proximal anastomosis; middle glans dart fixed to corpora; suture line of tube against corpora. *D,* Meatoplasty with dorsal glans dart. *E,* Completed repair. (From Devine, C. J.: *In* Urologic Surgery. 3rd ed. Philadelphia, J. B. Lippincott Co., 1983, p. 788. Used by permission.)

skin may be mobilized to the ventrum for urethroplasty either by attaching them to the outer face of the prepuce or as an island flap unrestricted by the limitations of the skin of the outer face. Hodgson (1970) used the inner-faced prepuce in a vertical orientation with the tumble-flap technique he first described (the Hodgson I technique). He later added the vertically oriented dorsal penile skin neourethra (the Hodgson II and III techniques), which was transposed to the ventrum with a button-hole maneuver (Hodgson, 1975). Asopa et al. (1971) used a vascularized flap attached to the outer prepuce. In the Asopa technique, the ventral preputial skin is used for the new urethra, but it is left attached to the penile skin and is spiraled around to the ventrum. The final result is asymmetric and bulky. A similar procedure is now preferred by Hodgson, which he calls an inner preputial tangential tube (Hodgson XX, 1981) (Fig. 47–10). Standoli (1979, 1982) has reported an island flap procedure utilizing the outer preputial skin to form the neourethra. Healing of these neourethras was more assured than with the free graft techniques. We now prefer the transverse preputial island flap neourethra with a glans channel positioning for the meatus (Duckett, 1980c).

TRANSVERSE PREPUTIAL ISLAND FLAP AND GLANS CHANNEL (Figs. 47–11 to 47–13)

We have developed this technique over the last 10 years as a modification of the Hodgson III (Hodgson, 1975) and Asopa (Asopa et al., 1971) procedures. In contrast with Devine and Horton's preference for a free full-thickness skin graft, we have concluded that a vascularized urethral tube is preferable for the construction of a neourethra. However, it seems inappropriate to utilize the penile skin on the dorsum for the new urethra, as Hodgson has done, while discarding the delicate ventral preputial skin.

We have found that the blood supply to the hypospadias preputial tissue is reliable and quite easily delineated. The abundant subcutaneous tissue on the dorsum of the penis is vascularized in a longitudinal fashion (Quartey, 1983). This tissue may be dissected free from the penile skin, creating an island flap from the inner layer of the prepuce. The blood supply to the dorsal skin of the foreskin and the penile skin comes from its broad base and is not dependent on the

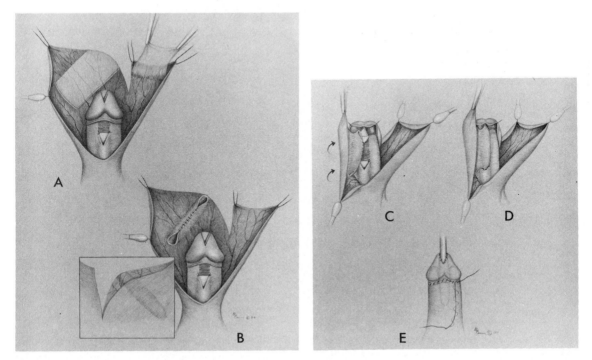

Figure 47–10. Hodgson XX procedure. *A,* An asymmetric split of the preputial skin allows the inner surface of the prepuce to remain attached to the outer preputial layer. The thin inner preputial layer is removed from the opposite smaller preputial flap. *B,* The inner preputial strip is tubularized and the distal portion is mobilized enough to tunnel the strip through the glans. *C,* The tubularized inner preputial flap is brought to the ventrum with its dorsal preputial skin attached. *D,* Appropriate anastomoses are made to the proximal and distal urethra. *E,* The eccentric skin flap is closed with the suture line off the midline. (Courtesy of N. B. Hodgson.)

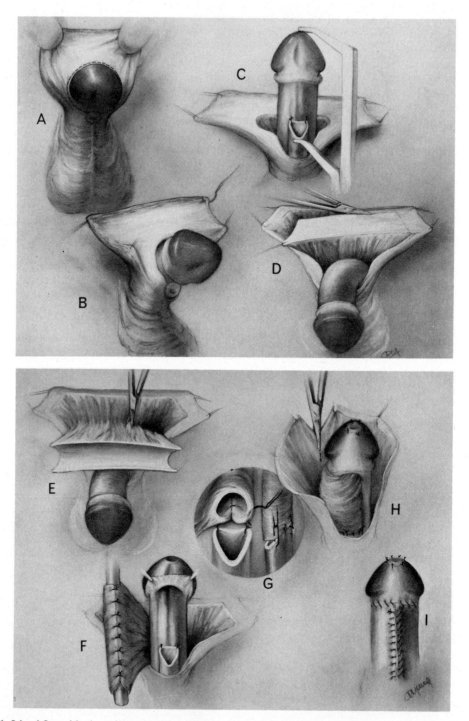

Figure 47–11. Island flap with glans channel hypospadias repair. *A*, Release of chordee. *B*, Fanning out of ventral preputial shiny skin. *C*, Measurement of rectangle of skin rolled into neourethra. *D* and *E*, Development of island flap by dissecting subcutaneous tissue from dorsal penile skin. *F*, Development of glans channel with plastic scissors in plane just above corpora removing glans tissue with channel (16 to 20 Fr); fixation of proximal urethra to corpora; spiraling of island flap urethra to ventrum. *G*, Anastomosis to proximal urethra. *H*, Delivery to the tip of the glans. *I*, Lateral transposition of Byars' flaps of dorsal penile skin to midline; excision of the tips.

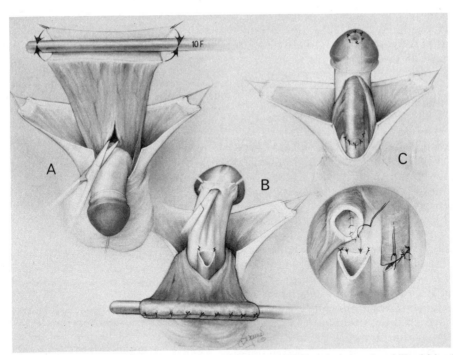

Figure 47–12. Island flap with button-hole transposition of pedicle. *A,* Window in base of mobilized island flap for very proximal meatus. *B,* Transposition to ventrum; also glans channel developed. *Insert,* Fixation of proximal urethra to corpora; oblique anastomosis. *C,* Neourethra channeled to apex of glans. (From Duckett, J. W.: The island flap technique for hypospadias repair. Urol. Clin. North Am. *8:*503, 1981. Used by permission.)

Figure 47–13. Perineal hypospadias with bifid scrotum; Island flap repair. *A,* Outline of initial incisions allowing generous paraurethral flap of non–hairbearing skin. *B,* Tubularization of proximal skin tube to penoscrotal junction; outline of transverse preputial island. *C,* Island flap neourethra transposed to ventrum; glans channel created; anastomosis to proximal skin tube and to distal meatoplasty. *D,* Completed repair.

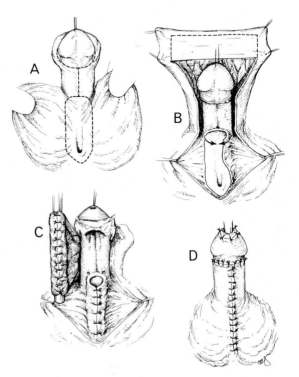

subcutaneous tissues, except at the remote edges of the dorsal preputial skin. The tips of the distal portions of the penile skin flaps are excised and are not used in the repair.

In plastic surgical principles, an island flap is an isolated segment of skin, the viability of which is maintained by an intact vascular pedicle. Certainly, the transverse, ventral, preputial rectangle of skin we have isolated with its own vascular pedicle qualifies as an island flap (Duckett, 1980a, 1980b, 1980c, 1981; Standoli, 1979, 1982; DeSy and Oosterlinck, 1981).

The viability of an arterialized island flap may be tested by systemic injection of fluorescein (15 to 20 mg per kg) and then evaluating the fluorescence of the flap with an ultraviolet light in a dark room 10 to 15 minutes later. The intensity of the skin fluorescence is a function of the amount of extracellular or interstitial deposition of fluorescein and is dependent on the functional microcirculation (McCraw et al., 1977). We have used this technique to demonstrate viability of the preputial island flap and of the dorsal penile skin from which the underlying subcutaneous tissue was mobilized for the island flap. In 35 cases utilizing fluorescence, all island flaps demonstrated excellent microcirculation.

The viability of the neourethral flap is further demonstrated in situations in which ventral skin loss occurred without the development of urethral fistulas or the formation of stricture. In these cases, secondary epithelialization has occurred without scar formation.

The addition of the glans channel technique has been most satisfactory. We prefer using the glans channel rather than leaving the meatus at the corona, using the triple glans flap (Devine and Horton, 1977), or splitting the glans (Barcat, 1973). Hinderer (1971) described a technique of "penis tunnelization" very similar to our glans channel. He has used a trocar for the tunnel. Hendren (1981) has used the glans channel technique in a large number of patients with success. His experience encouraged us in its use. Certainly, it is not a new procedure, as it has been described by others (Bevan, 1917; Davis, 1940; Mays, 1951; Mustarde, 1965; Ricketson, 1958).

Technique for Transverse Preputial Island Flap (Duckett, 1980a). A circumferential incision is made well proximal to the corona and around the meatus. A generous cuff of ventral glanular tissue is preserved and the dorsal penile skin with the attached prepuce is dissected free of the penis at the level of Buck's fascia. The ventral chordee tissue is excised. This frequently extends around the lateral aspects of the shaft of the penis and distally beneath the glans.

Mobilization of the urethra is generally required to free the proximal chordee. This will drop the meatus back to the penoscrotal junction or into the scrotum. Adequate resection of the tissue causing the chordee is tested by the artificial erection technique.

To create the neourethra, the ventral surface of the prepuce (the shiny undersurface) is placed on tension with holding sutures in the skin of the dorsal prepuce. The measured urethra is outlined with a marking pencil; usually 3 to 4 cm in length and 12 to 15 mm in width. A neourethra as long as 6 cm has been created with this technique in a two-year-old. The outlined rectangle is incised and rolled into a tube over a 10 or 12 French (Fr) catheter. Fine chromic or polyglycolic 6- or 7-0 sutures are used with a cutting needle. Interrupted sutures are used on the ends so that excision of excess length may be accomplished. A plane is then developed between the dorsal skin and the island flap, leaving a generous pedicle to the new urethra. Mobilization is achieved about two thirds of the way down the dorsal skin so that the tube may be rotated around the ventrum without distorting the penile skin. Careful dissection is required to preserve the pedicle to the flap, yet leaving enough vascularization of the penile skin.

The stent around which the urethra was created is replaced with a smaller 8 Fr polyethylene feeding tube. The flap is usually rotated so that the right side of the transverse flap is attached to the proximal urethra. An oblique anastomosis is made, freshening up the proximal urethra so that good tissue along with spongiosum is anastomosed to the tube. Excessive epithelium is excised. The neourethra is gently pulled distally toward the glans to avoid kinking of the proximal anastomosis. We had this as a complication early on and now avoid the problem by fixing the proximal anastomosis to the tunica albuginea of the corpora.

The glans channel is created with fine plastic scissors flat against the corpora cavernosa and snipping into the glanular tissue in the plane between the cap of the glans and the corpora. This plane is readily identified. The points of the scissors are taken up to the apex of the glans just superior to the dimple of the blind ending fossa. A button of glans epithelium is excised. Glanular tissue may need to be excised within this new channel to make a generous lumen. The channel should not be simply dilated as this will later constrict. Once a free channel is created that will calibrate at 16 to 18 Fr, the distal portion of the graft may be delivered through the channel. This is pulled up so that the suture line of the neourethra lies adjacent to the corporal tissue. The excess tip of the graft is excised so that no redundancy exists. Interrupted fine chromic sutures used circumferentially fix the edge of the tube to the glanular tissue. No glanular darts have been used.

The dorsal penile skin is fanned out, and a vertical incision is made in the midline down to the point where the dorsal skin of the penis can be drawn comfortably up to the subcoronal incision. The Byars' flaps are brought around to the ventrum either symmetrically or one above the other. A midline closure is made from the glans down to the scrotum and the excessive lateral triangles of the two Byars' flaps are excised (Byars, 1955). A running mattress suture is used to avoid inversion of epithelial surfaces. The proximal anastomosis is covered with adjacent subcutaneous tissue.

A pressure dressing using fine mesh gauze, coarse gauze, and Elastoplast is applied and a suprapubic catheter is placed for urinary diversion to make home care less complicated. The dressing is first changed in four to five days and the urethral stent is removed at that time. The meatus is dilated daily by the family using an ophthalmic ointment tube tip (Lacrilube). The suprapubic diversion is used for 10 to 14 days, then removed in the office.

Results with the island flap technique have been quite acceptable with a secondary surgery rate of 10 to 15 per cent (Duckett, 1981; Monfort et al., 1983; DeSy and Oosterlinck, 1981; Belman, 1982). The method is transferable in the hands of other surgeons, with improved results from their previous techniques.

DOUBLE-FACED PREPUTIAL ISLAND FLAP
(Fig. 47–14)

Recently, we became enamored of a technique that combines the inner and outer preputial skin layers as an island flap. It utilizes the outer preputial flap, as Standoli reported (1982), leaving it attached to the inner layer, which is rolled into a neourethra. When the combined preputial island flap is mobilized to the ventrum, the new urethra is channeled through the glans as before. The outer skin serves as a skin cover for the ventral one third of the penile cylinder, the dorsal two thirds being covered by the remaining penile skin. This procedure redistributes better vascularity to the penile and outer preputial skin that is required for shaft coverage. Our results with the first ten cases have been most gratifying cosmetically and functionally (May 1984).

This technique is a combination of ideas resulting from recent personal communications with Standoli, Hinderer, Van der Meulen, Horton, Devine, Hodgson, and indirectly with Asopa. It combines the Asopa-Hodgson tangential flap with the Standoli use of the outer prepuce as an island flap with the inner preputial neourethra.

SKIN COVER

Once the urethroplasty has been accomplished, the ventral surface of the penis must be resurfaced with skin. Because of the abundant dorsal foreskin, coverage may be achieved by mobilizing the penile and preputial skin to the ventrum in most cases. The skin may be transferred by one of several techniques.

The preputial tissue may be transposed by opening a small buttonhole in the midline, spreading the vasculature laterally, and bringing the glans penis through the buttonhole (see Fig. 47–8). The well vascularized dorsal preputial tissue will re-surface the ventrum. The major drawback, however, is the lateral edges, which are difficult to fashion without leaving bulky wedges of skin. One must be cautious not to trim these lateral pedicles too much at this stage and risk devascularizing the flap. A secondary procedure may be required to remove these extra bits of skin. Transposition in this manner is first credited to Thiersch, who used it in 1869. However, Ombredanne in 1930 and Nesbit in 1941 also used this method (Horton et al., 1973).

The prepuce may be split vertically, taking care not to disturb the vertically oriented vessels. The bipedicled preputial skin may be brought around to the ventrum for resurfacing (Fig. 47–3K to N). If this is done in a symmetric fashion as the first stage of a two-stage procedure (as in the Blair-Byars technique), redundant preputial skin is relocated on the distal shaft and glans (Smith, 1981). If, however, this technique is used to cover a urethroplasty in a one-stage technique, there is sometimes difficulty in overlapping these flaps to make the symmetry acceptable. The "bear hug" arrangement of the two flaps above and below each other avoids midline suturing (Devine, 1983) (Fig. 47–7). Likewise, an eccentric preputial split that is transposed to the ventrum will avoid a midline suture line, as described by King (1981) and Marberger and Pauer (1981).

Ventral skin cover may also be achieved by rotation of the entire penile and preputial skin in a spiral method around to the ventrum. Van der Muelen (1971, 1982), Asopa (1971), and Hodgson (1981) (Fig. 47–10) utilize this technique. In the Hodgson XX and the Asopa techniques, the neourethra is attached to the dorsal preputial or penile skin.

Fortunately, the healing of the penile skin and preputial layers is generally quite satisfactory, without unsightly scarring or hypertrophic thickening. The scars usually blend in with the coloring of the penile skin and are quite unnoticeable. It is possible, for instance, as Denis-Browne (Browne, 1953) has demonstrated, to incise the dorsal penile skin down the midline, relaxing the tension on the ventral skin. It will epithelialize with very little scarring. Although this technique is rarely needed, the results from

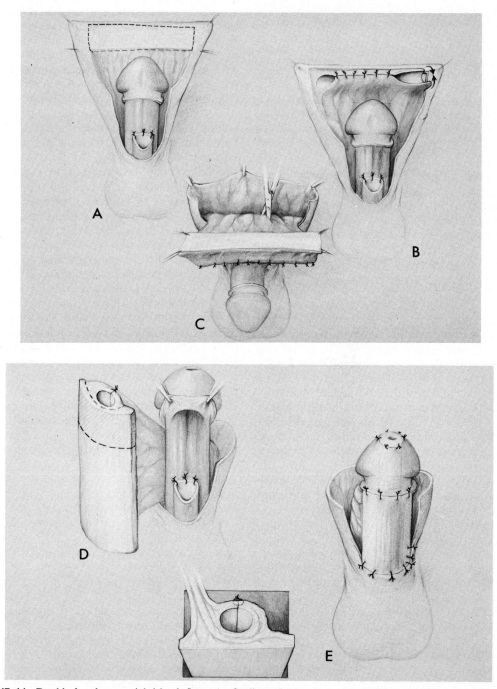

Figure 47–14. Double-faced preputial island flap. *A,* Outline of transverse island flap of inner preputial skin. *B,* Tubularization of inner preputial flap without mobilization. *C,* Outer preputial skin left attached to tubularized inner surface island flap as a double-faced pedicle. *D,* Mobilization of double-faced island flap to ventrum; hatched area will be discarded so that the distal tube may be channeled through the glans. *E,* Outer preputial island flaps serve as ventral skin cover, whereas penile skin covers the dorsum.

its use have been helpful in understanding penile scarring. There is no need to skin graft such a defect.

When an inner preputial island flap is developed, the lateral tips of the outer preputial skin may be devascularized to a certain degree. Although the edges of these flaps are discarded in most cases, sometimes the poor vascularization extends further than anticipated. There may be a slough of this ventrally positioned preputial skin. In our experience, when this has occurred the neourethra is well vascularized and does not suffer. When the eschar is removed, this area epithelializes in a manner similar to the Denis-Browne experience on the dorsum.

Utilizing the double-faced preputial island flap technique provides, we think, the best symmetric skin cover with well-vascularized skin (Fig. 47–11). The outer preputial skin, the distal edges of which may have a precarious blood supply in the island flap technique, is left attached to the joint blood supply of the inner prepuce. Thus, when transposed to the ventrum, the thicker outer preputial skin serves as a skin cover of the ventral midportion of penile shaft, whereas the dorsal penile skin covers the rest.

The older technique of burying the ventral penis in the scrotum for skin coverage, as exemplified by the Cecil-Culp technique (introduced in 1959), is helpful on occasion. A midline incision is made into the scrotum. The subcutaneous tissue of the dartos fascia of the scrotum is fixed to the dartos fascia on the penis in one layer. The skin edges are then closed. Two layers must be closed in order to prevent the penis from pulling on the skin edges too much. At a later time (3 to 6 months), the penis is lifted from the scrotal trough. The penile skin is sufficiently mobile to bring together on the penile surface in the midline. No scrotal skin is transposed to the penis in this fashion. It is used only for healing purposes. Marberger and Pauer (1981) and Turner-Warwick (1972) have utilized scrotal flaps to cover penile deficiencies, but they are mainly in adults and for secondary procedures. Marberger and Pauer showed the usefulness of asymmetric rotational scrotal flaps (1981).

MATERIALS

The development of fine delicate instruments and fine suture material, along with the precise delicate tissue handling taught by plastic surgeons, have advanced the principles of hypospadiology over the years. Instruments may be borrowed from the ophthalmologic or plastic surgery cabinets, or even microsurgical instruments may be used (Carmignani et al., 1982; Monfort, 1983). Fine iris scissors with delicate tooth forceps are the principal tools. Bishop-Harmon forceps and Castroviejo needle holders are useful for the very delicate maneuvers. Skin hooks are helpful to prevent overhandling of the tissues, though we prefer fine chromic stay sutures.

SUTURE MATERIAL

Removal of permanent sutures such as Prolene or nylon will usually require an anesthetic. Therefore, most surgeons use absorbable material. Chromic catgut is a favorite for the skin, because it absorbs rapidly and will be gone in 10 to 20 days. Polyglycolic sutures stay around longer and are ill-advised for skin closure. The 6- or 7-0 polyglycolic material is quite satisfactory for constructing the neourethra and for buried sutures. The new polydioxanone (PDS) remains for a much longer period of time and may therefore cause more reaction. Pull-out nylon sutures are less reactive and are used by some to close the urethra and also for skin suture lines in several layers (Belman, 1982). By cutting one end of the suture, the other may be wrapped around a hemostat and removed easily. It is embarrassing, however, for one to break beneath the skin, so 4-0 nylon, which is less likely to break, is used.

Hemostasis may be achieved in a number of ways. Placing a tourniquet at the base of the penis has been used (Ossandon and Ransley, 1982). It is generally recommended that the tourniquet be removed every 20 to 30 minutes to make sure the tissue is not devascularized for too long a period. Sponges soaked in epinephrine will aid vasoconstriction. We have preferred the injection of 1:100,000 epinephrine in 1 per cent Xylocaine (lidocaine) using a 26-gauge needle. Infiltration around the proximal urethra, into the chordee tissue, and into the glans for creation of a glans channel is helpful. Usually only 1.5 to 2 ml is required. There is a wide range of safety before epinephrine will sensitize the myocardium to arrhythmias with inhalational anesthetics (Karl et al., 1983). A study done at Children's Hospital of Philadelphia determined that at least 10 mg per kg of epinephrine may be used safely for cutaneous infiltration. As a 1:100,000 dilation, that safety dose is 1 ml per kg. At no time have we felt the use of epinephrine compromised the vasculature of our flaps. Various methods of coagulation have been recommended; we prefer a low-current Bovie.

Bipolar electrodes stick to the tissue too much. Battery supplied hot wires are probably more prone to excessive tissue damage. With epinephrine, the need for electrocoagulation is diminished.

Optical magnification has been clearly demonstrated to be a significant advance. The more expensive Loupes are generally supplied in 3 1/2 to 6 1/2 power. They give a very narrow field of vision. When one is familiar with their use, they are indispensable. We prefer an Optivisor, which allows a broader field of vision but lower magnification at 1 1/2 to 2 1/2. The focal length is 14 to 20 in (35 to 50 cm), which is quite satisfactory for this type of surgery. The major drawback is the bulk of the Optivisor and the likelihood of contaminating instruments and sutures. Some operating microscopes will go down to 3 1/2 power, but most of those in the standard operating rooms are 10 power, which is too great a magnification. Each surgeon must try all of these forms of magnification and pick the one best suited for his purposes.

DRESSING

The most significant factors contributed by the proper dressing is to provide immobilization with prevention of hematoma and edema. Protection of the suture lines from contamination is the least important factor. It is unlikely that dressings contribute to skin slough or subsequent fistula formation (Cromie and Bellinger, 1981).

The partially concealed dressing seems the most popular, with an impregnated gauze next to the repair, followed by fluff gauze and elastic tape, which sticks to the abdominal wall. Generally, the glans is exposed in this type of dressing. The totally concealed type of dressing allows more diffuse pressure to be applied by placing the penis onto the abdominal wall for compression. An unconcealed dressing was promoted by Devine and Horton recently, gently wrapping the penis in bleached cotton for intermittent irrigation with cold saline in order to reduce edema. This requires hospitalization and immobilization. Many modifications have been utilized, such as polyurethane foam and recently an adhesive membrane (Vordermark, 1982). In some cases, after fistula closure, collodion or "super glue" is used for cover (Duckett et al., 1980).

DIVERSIONS

The perineal urethrostomy has gradually been replaced by the suprapubic cystostomy for more long-term diversions. Bladder spasms, caused by irritation of the trigone with the catheter, remain the most aggravating complication in the postoperative period. Therefore, the least amount of tubing within the bladder is best.

Tiny silastic tubing of 6 F placed through the repair and into the bladder with several holes along the tubing allow a constant drip of urine from the catheter into a diaper, along with stenting the repair. They must be well sutured to the glans (Snyder and Duckett, 1984). Delicate silicon Foley catheters still have their place. Silicone tubing is less reactive than polyethylene. Theoretically, stenting will keep the neourethra from sealing and will allow adequate drainage of tissue fluids. However, the stent may also tend to irritate the bulb or trigone and create spasms. The stents vented all the way along the tubing allow tissue fluids to diffuse out freely. It is clear that the simplest form of dressing and diversion generally works the best.

Bladder spasms are most aggravating to the patient and his family. Since they occur without warning, medication as needed will not likely help. We use Banthine (methantheline bromide) and opium suppositories (B & O), cut into thirds, for several days. Oral Pro-Banthine (propantheline bromide) or oxybutynin also may help. As long as the meatus is kept open from crusting, occasional passage of urine with a spasm through the newly repaired urethra should not be harmful.

ANALGESIA

In anticipation of postoperative discomfort leading to dislodging of penile dressing or diversion tubes, it is probably worthwhile to add a supplemental local block (Jensen, 1981) with bupivacaine (Marcaine) at the end of the procedure. Bupivacaine 0.5 per cent was used as a caudal block or a penile block in two groups of children having circumcision (Yeoman, 1983). Duration and degree of analgesia were compared and were found to be equal. However, 30 per cent of those with caudal blocks were unable to walk at 6 hours. A penile block seems the better choice and should be a supplement to hypospadias surgery.

OTHER CONSIDERATIONS

The age for repair of hypospadias has continually decreased since Culp (1959) first advocated "the inalienable right of every school-age child to be a pointer instead of a sitter." Comparison of normal penile size with age indicates some growth in the first 2 years followed by a relative plateau until puberty. Thus, 2 to 5 years was usually the age selected for staged repairs. However, the psychological effects of maternal-child separation with hospitalization at this difficult age became apparent. Schultz et al. (1983) pointed out an ideal window might be age 6 to 18 months to minimize the emotional effect of this traumatic insult.

In addition, the advantage of improved optical magnification has made surgical correction at an earlier age more successful. Currently, many hypospadiologists using a one-stage repair chose 6 to 18 months as an optimal time (Manley and Epstein, 1981; Belman, 1982). Anesthesia risks are minimized after 6 months of age, when the chance of sudden infant death syndrome (SIDS) is diminished. Day surgical cases may be performed after the patient reaches 6 months of age; if younger than 6 months, the patient should remain hospitalized overnight. Generally, the penis with hypospadias is of sufficient size at 6 to 18 months to accomplish this delicate surgery with the aid of optical magnification.

Enlargement of the infant penis is possible by testosterone stimulation. A 5 per cent testosterone cream rubbed on the genitals daily for 3 weeks works by local absorption. Blood levels of testosterone reach pubertal levels quickly. Dihydrotestosterone (DHT) is also used (Monfort and Lucas, 1982). Equally as effective is testosterone proprionate, 25 mg intramuscularly (IM) once a week for 3 weeks (Villee, 1984). The IM dosage is better controlled and is preferable to the esthetically displeasing request of the parents to rub cream on the penis to make it bigger. We have not found use of testosterone stimulation to be beneficial.

With the continued escalation of health care cost, maximal hospital benefit has become a concept of economic necessity today. The postoperative management of hypospadias surgery is concerned mainly with the difficulties associated with diversion and dressings. These children are usually healthy, elective surgical candidates requiring little in the way of medication or wound care that cannot be offered by the mother. It, therefore, obligates the surgeon to coordinate postoperative care by adequate preoperative education, simplification of instructions, and ready accessibility to the telephone in order to accomplish most of the care on an outpatient basis. A day surgical procedure or an overnight hospital stay should be the goal.

Psychosocial support should be offered by the surgeon or a well-trained nurse to alleviate the parental guilt frequently accompanying this genital anomaly. Unexpressed anxieties as to the cause for hypospadias and the later sexual capabilities must be anticipated and discussed. The child's future positive body image may well depend on his parents' thorough understanding of his condition. The surgeon must be certain these issues are made clear to the parents.

Follow-up care depends on the complexity of the procedure required. Dressing changes, catheter or tube removals, and wound care may be done in the office or outpatient clinic without the need for general anesthetic support. Bougienage of the meatus or urethroplasty may be accomplished deftly and with minimal discomfort if small-caliber, straight sounds or bougie à boules are used. Care should be taken not to force through a narrowing. A kink at the proximal anastomosis is more likely than a stricture in the early postoperative period.

Probing of the meatus using the nozzle tip of an ophthalmic ointment tube will prevent the meatus from crusting. Soaking the healing wound edges with sitz baths three to four times a day or using gauze soaks in the diaper will keep the area clean. Follow-up visits are at 1, 2, 4, and 6 weeks, 3- and 6-month intervals, and thereafter as needed, which is usually once a year for several years. The follow-up visits are discontinued after puberty. Observation of the voided stream, voiding cystourethrography, or uroflowmetry are techniques preferred to sounding the urethra as the child grows.

COMPLICATIONS

Acute. Attention to the details that will avoid complications is paramount. Diversion of urine either by suprapubic or urethral tube or perineal urethrostomy is intended to allow sealing of the suture lines and sufficient healing to avoid leakage of urine into the tissues outside the neourethra. A few squirts of urine out the new urethra with bladder spasms will cause little harm as long as the meatus is patent. Therefore, meatal probing to dislodge crusting is required periodically. A stent used for 5 to 7 days accomplishes the same goal.

Placement of a Cystocath tube within the bladder is usually done with a trocar. Leaving too much silicone tubing in the bladder may cause bladder spasms or extrusion out through the urethra. Too short a length of tube in the bladder may pull out as the bladder empties. Before fixation to the skin, one should ascertain proper tube placement. A flange glued to the skin for fixation will not remain adherent for the desired 10 days, and sutures to hold it are unsightly when healed. Therefore, direct suture fixation of the tubing is advisable.

To avoid wound infection, well-prepared skin should be assured. Separation of the foreskin adherence with removal of the desquamated epithelial debris should be done under anesthesia prior to application of a satisfactory skin preparation, which, in the postpubertal male, should commence several days before surgery with cleansing. Infection seems more of a problem in this age group. Prophylactic antibiotics should have little value in avoiding wound infection. Sulfonamide or nitrofurantoin suppression may be useful to prevent cystitis, particularly if the tube is left to drain in the diaper.

Poor wound healing is primarily due to ischemic flaps. If a technique is used in which preputial skin and its arterial pedicle are separated from the penile skin, it may be more likely that the covering tissue will be less vascularized. If, however, the neourethra is well vascularized, healing should occur per primam in this layer, and the sloughed covering skin will granulate and re-epithelialize without a noticeable scar. A technique to avoid this complication is the use of fluorescein to demonstrate the viability of the skin flaps. Systemic injection of fluorescein, 15 to 20 mg per kg, and the subsequent evaluation of the fluorescence of the flap with an ultraviolet light in a dark room 10 to 15 minutes after administration, will clearly demonstrate the viability of an arterialized flap. The intensity of skin fluorescence is a function of the amount of extracellular or interstitial deposition of fluorescein and seems to be dependent upon the functional microcirculation. We have used this technique to demonstrate the viability of the preputial island flap, as well as the dorsal penile skin, from which the underlying subcutaneous tissue has been mobilized for the island flap.

Edema occurs to some degree in most hypospadias repairs. A compression dressing has been the standard method in an attempt to diminish this effect on healing. It is, of course, difficult to get a diffuse compression effect, and many different dressing methods have been attempted. The use of cold saline soaks immediately after surgery, which is similar to the technique used in blepharoplasties, has been effective in some hands (Devine, 1983); however, it requires rather attentive nursing care and extended stays in the hospital. A compression dressing left for 5 to 7 days seems effective, not only for edema formation but also for controlling hemorrhage or hematoma formation.

Intraoperative bleeding can be controlled in various ways. A tourniquet is useful with release every 20 minutes (Ossandon and Ransley, 1982). We have preferred the use of 1:100,000 epinephrine in 1 per cent lidocaine for instillation with a 26-gauge needle at the start of the procedure. Maximum hemostasis is achieved in about 7 minutes. Epinephrine negates the effective use of fluorescein.

Drainage tubes used as wicks underneath the repair are important if a free full-thickness graft is used so that the interface between the graft and the overlying skin is perfectly approximated. A vacuum suction on the tubing can be created with a mini-Hemovac utilizing vacuum tubes and scalp vein needles (Devine, 1983). Firm compression should be applied at the end of the procedure in order to evacuate all subcutaneous blood clots and control the immediate postoperative ooze.

Postoperative erections are a problem in the postpubertal patient. Various medications have been tried without much success. The best is probably amylnitrate pulvules.

Chronic. Urethrocutaneous fistulas are likely to remain an inherent risk of hypospadias repair for years to come. The fistula rate after a particular procedure is often used as a measure of the effectiveness of that surgical repair. Currently, an expected complication rate of 10 to 15 per cent (mostly fistulas) exists for one-stage hypospadias surgery.

The second procedure required to close a hypospadias fistula may unfortunately carry a rather significant failure rate of up to 40 per cent. Details of various techniques of fistula closure in the literature emphasize wide mobilization, adjacent skin flaps, multilayered closures, and the use of urinary diversion by urethral catheter or suprapubic cystotomy, including several days to weeks in the hospital (Horton et al., 1980).

We recommend a microtechnique using magnification and delicate instruments. A properly sized lacrimal duct probe placed in the fistulous tract assists in the identification of the epithelial-lined tract while careful dissection is made down to the urethra. Fine catgut suture is used to close the urethral edge with Lembert-type sutures. A watertight closure is assured by distending the distal urethra with saline while compressing the bulbar urethra in the perineum. The skin is approximated loosely with vertical mattress sutures. No diversion of urine is needed. The patient is allowed to void by the fistula repair and goes home the same day.

In a 3 1/2-year period we repaired 32 fistulas. In three cases, suprapubic urinary diversion was elected for added safety. In all three patients, the fistula was considered large, and all healed per primam. Of the remaining 29 cases, there were three with recurrence of the fistula (10 per cent). These three fistulas were successfully closed in one subsequent procedure, using the same method. The intervals in these cases were 6 to 9 months in 13 patients, 10 to 14 months in 13 patients, 15 to 18 months in two patients, and 3 years in 1 patient.

We have concluded from our experience that extensive flaps and diversion are not necessary for closure of the usual pinpoint to moderate sized fistula. The most common error in fistula closure is failure to recognize a concomitant diverticulum or distal stricture. A diverticulum can be demonstrated either by probing with a bougie à boule or with urethrograms prior to fistula closure. Diverticula should be excised along with the fistula in order to assure adequate repair. Meatal stenosis may also need enlarging with the fistula repair.

Residual chordee is another complication, particularly in those cases that were repaired many years ago prior to artificial erection techniques. They may be resolved with a circumferential incision around the corona, dissecting the urethral meatus and urethra along with the sleeve of skin cover down to the penoscrotal junction. Residual chordee tissue is excised, and artificial erection is utilized to ascertain this proper correction. The sleeve of penile skin and urethra is then brought back as far as possible and is fixed onto the tunica albuginea. A further extension of the urethroplasty is usually required and may be done by mobilizing a flap of skin on the ventrum in a manner similar to a Mustarde procedure. When this is done, a glans channel can be created, placing the meatus on the tip. Otherwise, innovative techniques for a more extensive urethroplasty may be required (Stecker et al., 1981). If slight ventral chordee remains, dorsal suture plication with permanent sutures may achieve adequate penile straightening (Livne et al., in press).

Rarely, extensive scarring on the ventrum of the penis or ventral tunical deficiency requires excision of a patch of the tunica albuginea with replacement with a strip of tunica vaginalis obtained from the paratesticular tunica (Duckett, 1981a). Dermal grafts have also been used for this tunica albuginea replacement (Devine and Horton, 1975). If dermal grafts are used, care must be taken to make sure all the epithelial elements are removed. Otherwise, dermal cysts will develop. Woodhouse and Ransley

(1984) have successfully replaced the tunica with lyophilized dura mater.

Urethroplasty problems may occur with a stricture at the proximal anastomosis. This may be due to "angulation" of the anastomosis and may be avoided by lateral fixation of the anastomosis to the tunica albuginea so that the back wall will not overlap the front. Strictures may be repaired by excision and re-anastomosis, use of a patch graft, or, occasionally, optical cold knife urethrotomy.

The neourethra may inadvertently be made too wide, resulting in diffuse diverticulum formation. If meatal stenosis occurs, further dilatation may occur. Reduction of such a diverticulum in a longitudinal fashion is necessary. Anastomotic urinary extravasation may epithelialize in such a way that a bulbous diverticulum results at the penoscrotal junction. This too must be excised. A diverticulum and fistula may occur simultaneously, and excision of both is necessary.

Use of hair-bearing skin for urethroplasty has been criticized for many years. If scrotal tissue is incorporated, a hairy urethra may occur after puberty with stone formation and encrustation. Excision of the hairy urethra may be required with replacement with non–hair-bearing skin.

Persistent hypospadias with a retrusive meatus that deflects the stream downward is a common complaint with the older procedures. They may be improved using a Mustarde-type flap and a glans channel or with a Mathieu flip-flap technique. Occasionally, the Devine-Horton triangularization procedure may be beneficial (Stecker et al., 1981).

If persistent chordee along with a proximal meatus is present, a vascularized flap from some of the remaining dorsal penile skin may be an option. Adjacent skin with its vasculature may be utilized. In the severe case in which there is no adjacent skin or vascularized flap available, a free graft from the inner surface of the arm may be used, and tunneled beneath the penile skin and through the glans channel. Results using this technique have varied. Some have advocated a very thick split-thickness graft with long-term stenting (Hendren and Crooks, 1980). Bladder mucosa has also been used as a free graft, especially good for long urethral replacement (Coleman et al., 1981).

Meatal stenosis should be avoided by a generous channel through the glans, excising tissue in order to lay the neourethra and pedicle in place without compromising its blood supply. If flap loss should occur through the glans, a dense intraglanular stricture may appear. This generally requires excision and reconstruction. Occasionally, a V-flap meatoplasty may widen the more restricted distal meatal stenosis.

Balanitis xerotica obliterans (BXO) is a late complication resulting from chronic inflammation. Short-term diminution of the inflammation may be achieved with steroid injection, but we have not been able to control this process for more than several years. Excision of the BXO lesion is then required with a meatoplasty as indicated. The use of the Brannen meatoplasty in adults is useful (Brannen, 1976). The DeSy meatoplasty may be applicable in the future (DeSy, 1984).

Scars of the penile skin are rarely a problem. Excision with Z-plasties, scrotal flaps, or replacement with a free split-thickness graft are various options.

ADULT FOLLOW-UP

Long-term follow-up is available on patients undergoing previous repair (Berg et al., 1981; Berg and Berg, 1983; Svensson and Berg, 1983). Discouraging outcomes reported by some may reflect the difficulty of hypospadias surgery in the past, as well as the older ages at which repair was carried out, and therefore, may not be a true reflection of our modern methods (Kenawi, 1975).

Cosmetic and functional results are far better today than in the past. The concept of one-stage hypospadias repair accomplished at an early age, coupled with low complication potential, reinforces the current positive approach to this problem. Correction of chordee is extremely important and is crucial for assuring satisfactory sexual function. With a distal meatus, there appears to be no increase in infertility, unless cryptorchidism or another testiculopathy coexists. Evidence supports the fact that urethral growth with free grafts, as well as with vascular flaps, occurs. Psychologically, early hypospadias repair (with maternal rooming in) avoids castration anxiety, as well as separation anxiety. It is comforting to be able to counsel parents that there is optimism in striving for an excellent cosmetic and functional result in boys with all degrees of hypospadias.

CONCLUSION

"Hypospadias is a grievous deformity which must ever move as to the highest surgical endeavor. The refashioning of the urethra offers a problem as formidable as any in the wide field of our art" (Higgins, 1947). Hypospadiology requires an in-depth study of the contributions of our predecessors, as well as a thorough knowledge of the methods and maneuvers of the current experts. To study with or precept onself at a center in which large numbers of hypospadias cases are managed will prove more beneficial than the anguish of learning through one's mistakes. The minor complications of a properly executed one-stage procedure in a fresh case are far easier to manage to a successful outcome than the poorly conceived failures of the inexperienced surgeon. It is to be hoped that the hypospadias cripple (Stecker et al., 1981) will be of historical interest only.

It is difficult to be truly objective in writing such a chapter, so I have not tried to restrain my bias. Clearly, some of my colleagues will have differing opinions. Hypospadiology will continue to evolve innovative new methods as we refine the old ones. Look at the dramatic improvement over the past 25 years. Much of our current success should be attributed to the delicate and precise methods of tissue handling, as well as to the principles of flaps and grafts learned in conjunction with our plastic surgery colleagues. The delicate ophthalmic instruments and optical magnification are also significant improvements.

Although we have made great advances, more progress may be anticipated in this fascinating, challenging field of hypospadiology.

References

Aarskog, D.: Clinical and cytogenetic studies in hypospadias. Acta Paediatr. Scand. (Suppl.), *203*:7:1970.

Allen, T. D., and Griffin, J. E.: Endocrine studies in patients with advanced hypospadias. J. Urol., *131*:310, 1984.

Allen, T. D., and Spence, H. M.: The surgical treatment of coronal hypospadias and related problems. J. Urol., *100*:504, 1968.

Asopa, H. S., Elhence, E. P., Atria, S. P., et al.: One-stage correction of penile hypospadias using a foreskin tube. A preliminary report. Int. Surg., *55*:435, 1971.

Backus, L. H., and DeFelice, C. A.: Hypospadias: Then and now. Plast. Reconstr. Surg., *25*:146, 1960.

Ballesteros, J. J.: Personal technique for surgical repair of balanic hypospadias. J. Urol., *118*:983, 1977.

Barcat, J.: Current concepts of treatment. *In* Horton, C. E. (Ed.): Plastic and Reconstructive Surgery of the Genital Area. Boston, Little, Brown & Co., 1973, pp. 249–263.

Bauer, S. B., Retik, A. B., and Colodny, A. H.: Genetic aspects of hypospadias. Urol. Clin. North Am., *8*:559, 1981.

Beck, C.: Hypospadias and its treatment. J. Gynecol. Obstet., *5*:511, 1917.

Bellinger, M. F.: Embryology of the male external genitalia. Urol. Clin. North Am., *8*:375, 1981.

Belman, A. B.: Urethroplasty. Soc. Pediatr. Urol. Newsletter, December 1977.

Belman, A. B.: The Broadbent hypospadias repair. Urol. Clin. North Am., *8*:483, 1981.

Belman, A. B.: The modified Mustarde hypospadias repair. J. Urol., *127*:88, 1982.

Belman, A. B., and Kass, E. J.: Hypospadias repair in children less than 1 year old. J. Urol., *128*:1273, 1982.

Belman, A. B., and King, L. R.: The urethra. *In* Kelalis, P., and King, L. R. (Eds.): Clinical Pediatric Urology. Philadelphia, W. B. Saunders Co., 1979, pp. 576–594.

Berg, R., and Berg, G.: Penile malformation, gender identity and sexual orientation. Acta Psychiatr. Scand., *68*: 154, 1983.

Berg, R., Svensson, J., and Astrom, G.: Social and sexual adjustment of men operated for hypospadias during childhood: a controlled study. J. Urol., *125*: 313, 1981.

Bevan, A. D.: A new operation for hypospadias. JAMA, *68*:1032, 1917.

Brannen, G. E.: Meatal reconstruction. J. Urol., *116*:319, 1976.

Broadbent, T. R. Woolf, R. M., and Toksu, E.: Hypospadias: one-stage repair. Plast. Reconstr. Surg., *27*:154, 1961.

Browne, D.: A comparison of the Duplay and Denis Browne techniques for hypospadias operation. Surgery, *34*:787, 1953.

Butler, L. J., Snodgrass, G. J. A., France, N. E., Russell, A., and Swain, V. A. J.: True hermaphroditism or gonadal intersexuality. Arch. Dis. Child., *44*:666, 1969.

Byars, L. T.: Technique of consistently satisfactory repair of hypospadias. Surg. Gynecol. Obstet., *100*:184, 1955.

Carmignani, G., Belgrande, E., Gaboardi, F., and Farina, F. P.: Microsurgical one-stage repair of hypospadias with a rectangular transverse dorsal preputial vascularized skin flap. J. Microsurg., *3*:222, 1982.

Cendron, J., and Melin, Y.: Congenital curvature of the penis without hypospadias. Urol. Clin. North Am., *8*:389, 1981.

Coleman, J. W., McGovern, J. H., and Marshall, V. F.: The bladder mucosal graft technique for hypospadias repair. Urol. Clin. North Am., *8*:457, 1981.

Creevy, C. D.: The correction of hypospadias: a review. Urol. Surv., *8*:2, 1958.

Cromie, W. J., and Bellinger, M. F.: Hypospadias dressings and diversions. Urol. Clin. North Am., *8*:545, 1981.

Cronin, T. D., and Guthrie, T. H.: Method of Cronin and Guthrie for hypospadias repair. *In* Horton, C. E. (Ed.): Plastic and Reconstructive Surgery of the Genital Area. Boston, Little, Brown & Co., 1973.

Culp, O. S.: Experience with 200 hypospadias: evaluation of therapeutic plans. Surg. Clin. North Am., *39*:1007, 1959.

Davis, D. M.: Pedicle tube graft in surgical management of hypospadias, male, with new method of closing small urethral fistulas. Surg. Gynecol. Obstet., *71*:709, 1940.

Des Prez, J. D., Persky, L., and Kiehn, C. L.: A one-stage repair of hypospadias by island-flap technique. Plast. Reconstr. Surg., *28*:405, 1961.

DeSy, W. A.: Aesthetic repair of meatal stricture. J. Urol., In press.

DeSy, W. A., and Oosterlinck, W.: One-stage hypospadias repair by free full-thickness skin graft and island flap techniques. Urol. Clin. North Am., *8*:491, 1981.

Devine, C. J., Jr.: Chordee and hypospadias. *In* Glenn, J. F., and Boyce, W. H. (Eds.): Urologic Surgery, 3rd ed. Philadelphia, J. B. Lippincott, 1983, pp. 775–797.

Devine, C. J., Jr., and Horton, C. E.: A one-stage hypospadias repair. J. Urol., *85*:166, 1961.

Devine, C. J., Jr., and Horton, C. E.: Chordee without hypospadias. J. Urol., *110*:264, 1973.

Devine, C. J., Jr., and Horton, C. E.: Use of dermal graft to correct chordee. J. Urol., *113*:56, 1975.

Devine, C. J., Jr., and Horton, C. E.: Hypospadias repair. J. Urol., *118*:188, 1977.

Duckett, J. W.: Transverse preputial island flap technique for repair of severe hypospadias. Urol. Clin. North Am., *7*:423, 1980*a*.

Duckett, J. W.: Hypospadias. Clin. Plastic Surg., *7*:149, 1980*b*.

Duckett, J. W.: Repair of hypospadias. *In* Hendry, W. F. (Ed.): Recent Advances in Urology/Andrology. Vol. 3. London, Churchill Livingstone, 1980*c*, pp. 279–290.

Duckett, J. W.: MAGPI (Meatoplasty and Glanuloplasty): A procedure for subcoronal hypospadias. Urol. Clin. North Am., *8*:513, 1981*a*.

Duckett, J. W.: The island flap technique for hypospadias repair. Urol. Clin. North Am., *8*:503, 1981*b*.

Duckett, J. W., Kaplan, G. W., Woodard, J. R., et al.: Panel: Complications of hypospadias repair. Urol. Clin. North Am., *7*:443, 1980.

Fallon, B., Devine, C. J., Jr., and Horton, C. E.: Congenital anomalies associated with hypospadias. J. Urol., *11*:585, 1976.

Filmer, R. B., Duckett, J. W., and Sowden, R.: One-stage correction of hypospadias/chordee. Birth Defects, *13*:267, 1977.

Fuqua, F.: Belt technique. *In* Horton, C. E. (Ed.): Plastic & Reconstructive Surgery of the Genitalia. Boston, Little, Brown & Co., 1973, pp. 321–326.

Gibbons, A. U., and Gonzales, E. T., Jr.: The subcoronal meatus. J. Urol., *130*:737, 1983.

Gittes, R. F., and McLaughlin, A. P., III: Injection technique to induce penile erection. Urology, *4*:473, 1974.

Glenister, T. W.: The origin and fate of the urethral plate in man. J. Anat., *288*:413, 1954.

Gonzales, E. T., Jr., Veeraraghavan, K. A., and Delaune, J.: The management of distal hypospadias with meatal-based, vascularized flaps. J. Urol., *129*:119, 1983.

Hendren, W. H.: The Belt-Fuqua for repair of hypospadias. Urol. Clin. North Am., *8*:431, 1981.

Hendren, W. H., and Crooks, K. K.: Tubed free skin graft for construction of male urethra. J. Urol., *123*:858, 1980.

Higgins, C. C.: Hypospadias. Cleveland Clin. Quart., *14*:176, 1947.

Hinderer, U.: New one-stage repair of hypospadias (technique of penis tunnelization). *In* Hueston, J. T. (Ed.): Transactions of the 5th International Congress of Plastic and Reconstructive Surgery. Sydney, Butterworth Co., 1971, p. 283.

Hinderer, U.: Hypospadias repair in long term results. *In* Goldwyn, R. M. (Ed.): Plastic and Reconstructive Surgery. Boston, Little, Brown & Co., 1978.

Hodgson, N. B.: A one-stage hypospadias repair. J. Urol., *104*:281, 1970.

Hodgson, N. B.: Hypospadias. *In* Glenn, J. F., and Boyce, W. H. (Eds.): Urologic Surgery. 2nd ed. Hagerstown, Harper & Row, 1975, pp. 656–667.

Hodgson, N. B.: Hypospadias and urethral duplication. *In* Harrison, J. H., Gittes, R. F., Perlmutter, A. D., Stamey, T. A., and Walsh, P. C. (Eds.): Campbell's Urology. W. B. Saunders Co., Philadelphia, 1979.

Hodgson, N. B.: Use of vascularized flaps in hypospadias repair. Urol. Clin. North Am., *8*:471, 1981.

Hoffman, W. W., and Hall, W. V.: A modification of Spence's hood for one-stage surgical correction of distal shaft penile hypospadias. J. Urol., *109*:1017, 1973.

Horton, C. E., Devine, C. J., and Baran, N.: Pictoral history of hypospadias repair techniques. *In* Horton, C. E. (Ed.): Plastic and Reconstructive Surgery of the Genital Area. Boston, Little, Brown & Co., 1973.

Horton, C. E., Devine, C. J., and Graham, J. K.: Fistulas of the penile urethra. Plast. Reconstr. Surg., 66:407, 1980.

Jensen, B. H.: Caudal block for post-operative pain relief in children after genital operations. A comparison between bupivacaine and morphine. Acta Anesthesiol. Scand., 25:373, 1981.

Kaplan, G. W., and Brock, W. A.: The etiology of chordee. Urol. Clin. North Am., 8:383, 1981.

Kaplan, G. W., and Lamm, D. L.: Embryogenesis of chordee. J. Urol., 114:769, 1975.

Karl, G. W., Swedlon, D. B., Lee, K. W., and Downes, J. J.: Epinephrine-halothane interaction in children. Anesthesiology, 58:142, 1983.

Kenawi, M. M.: Sexual function in hypospadias. Br. J. Urol., 47:883, 1975.

Khuri, F. J., Hardy, B. E., and Churchill, B. M.: Urologic anomalies associated with hypospadias. Urol. Clin. North Am., 8:565, 1981.

Kim, S. H., and Hendren, W. H.: Repair of mild hypospadias. J. Pediatr. Surg., 16:806, 1981.

King, L. R.: One-stage repair without skin graft based on a new principle: chordee is sometimes produced by skin alone. J. Urol., 103:660, 1970.

King, L. R.: Cutaneous chordee and its implications in hypospadiasias. Urol. Clin. North Am., 8:397, 1981.

Koff, S. A.: Mobilization of the urethra in the surgical treatment of hypospadias. J. Urol., 125:394, 1981.

Kramer, S. A., Aydin, G., and Kelalis, P. P.: Chordee without hypospadias in children. J. Urol., 128:559, 1982.

Kumar, S.: Hypospadias with normal prepuce. J. Urol., In press.

Livne, P. M., Gibbons, M. D., and Gonzales, E. T.: The correction of disproportion of the corpora cavernosa as a cause for chordee in hypospadias. J. Urol. In press.

Manley, C. B., and Epstein, E. S.: Early hypospadias repair. J. Urol., 125:698, 1981.

Marberger, H., and Pauer, W.: Experience in hypospadias repair. Urol. Clin. North Am., 8:403, 1981.

Mathieu, P.: Traitement en un temps de l'hypospadias balanique et juxta-balanique. J. Chir., 39:481, 1932.

Mays, H. B.: Hypospadias: a concept of treatment. J. Urol., 65:279, 1951.

McArdle, F., and Lebowitz, R.: Uncomplicated hypospadias and anomalies of upper urinary tract. Need for screening? Urology, 5:712, 1975.

McCormick, R. M.: Simultaneous chordee repair and urethral reconstruction for hypospadias. Plast. Reconst. Surg., 60:710, 1977.

McCraw, J. B., Myers, B., and Shanklin, K. D.: The value of fluorescein in predicting the viability of arterialized flaps. Plast. Reconstr. Surg., 60:710, 1977.

Meyer, W. J., Brosman, P. G., and Matustik, M. C.: Human chorionic gonadotrophin testing. Am. J. Dis. Child., 138:181, 1984.

Mills, C., McGovern, J., Mininberg, D., Coleman, J., Muecke, E., and Vaughan, E. D., Jr.: An analysis of different techniques for distal hypospadias repair: the price of perfection. J. Urol., 125:701, 1981.

Monfort, G., and Lucas, C.: Dehydrotestosterone penile stimulation in hypospadias surgery. Eur. Urol., 8:201, 1982.

Monfort, G., Jean, P., and Lacoste, M.: One-stage correction of posterior hypospadias using a transverse pedi-

culed flap (Duckett's operation). Chir. Pediatr., 24:71, 1983.

Mustarde, J. C.: One-stage correction of distal hypospadias and other people's fistulae. Br. J. Plast. Surg., 18:413, 1965.

Nasrallah, P. F., and Minott, H. B.: Distal hypospadias repair. J. Urol., 131:928, 1984.

Nesbit, R. M.: Congenital curvature of the phallus: report of three cases with description of corrective operation. J. Urol., 93:230, 1965.

Nesbit, R. M.: Operation for correction of distal penile ventral curvature with and without hypospadias. Trans. Am. Assoc. Genitourin. Surg., 58:12, 1966.

Opitz, J. M., Simpson, J. L., Sarto, G. E., Summitt, R. L., New, M., and German, J.: Pseudovaginal perineoscrotal hypospadias. Clin. Genet., 3:1, 1972.

Ossandon, F., and Ransley, P. G.: Lasso tourniquet for artificial erection in hypospadias. Urology, 19:656, 1982.

Pancoast, J. A.: Treatise on Operative Surgery. Philadelphia, Carrey and Hart, 1844, pp. 317–318.

Perlmutter, A. D., and Vatz, A. D.: Meatal advancement for distal hypospadias without chordee. J. Urol., 113:850, 1975.

Peterson, R. E., Imperato-McGinley, J., Gautier, T., and Sturla, E.: Male pseudohermaphroditism due to steroid 5 alpha reductase deficiency. Am. J. Med., 62:170, 1977.

Quartey, J. K. M.: One stage penile/preputial cutaneous island flap urethroplasty for urethral stricture: a preliminary report. J. Urol., 129:284, 1983.

Redman, J. F.: Experience with 60 consecutive hypospadias repairs using the Horton-Devine techniques. J. Urol., 129:115, 1983.

Ricketson, G.: A method of repair for hypospadias. Am. J. Surg., 95:279, 1958.

Russell, R. H.: Operation for severe hypospadias. Br. J. Med., 2:1432, 1900.

Schultz, J. R., Klykylo, W. M., and Wacksman, J.: Timing of elective hypospadias repair in children. Pediatrics, 71:342, 1983.

Smith, E. D.: Durham Smith repair of hypospadias. Urol. Clin. North Am., 8:451, 1981.

Snyder, H. M., and Duckett, J. W.: Hypospadias 'pearls.' Soc. Ped. Urol. Newsletter, May 1984.

Sommer, J. T., and Stephens, F. D.: Dorsal ureteral diverticulum of the fossa navicularis: symptoms, diagnosis and treatment. J. Urol., 124:94, 1980.

Standoli, L.: Correzione Dell'ipospadias in tempo unico: technica dell'ipospadias con tempo ad isola prepuziale. Rass. Italia Chir. Pediatr., 21:82, 1979.

Standoli, L.: One-stage repair of hypospadias: preputial island flap technique. Ann. Plast. Surg., 9:81, 1982.

Stecker, J. F., Horton, C. E., Devine, C. J., and McCraw, J. B.: Hypospadias cripples. Urol. Clin. North Am., 8:539, 1981.

Svensson, J., and Berg, R.: Micturition studies and sexual function in operated hypospadiacs. Br. J. Urol., 55:422, 1983.

Sweet, R. A., Schrott, H. G., Kurland, R., et al.: Study of the incidence of hypospadias in Rochester, Minnesota 1940–1970, and a case control comparison of possible etiologic factors. Mayo Clin. Proc., 49:52, 1974.

Turner-Warwick, R.: The use of pedicle grafts in the repair of urinary tract fistulae. Br. J. Urol., 44:644, 1972.

Turner-Warwick, R.: Observations upon techniques for reconstruction of the urethral meatus, the hypospadiac glans deformity and the penile urethra. Urol. Clin. North Am., 6:643, 1979.

Udall, A.: Correction of three types of congenital curvature of the penis including the first reported case of dorsal curvature. J. Urol., *124*:50, 1980.

Van der Meulen, J. C.: Hypospadias monograph. Leiden, The Netherlands, A. G. Stenfert, Kroese, N. V., 1964.

Van der Meulen, J. C.: Hypospadias and cryptospadias. Br. J. Plast. Surg., *24*:101, 1971.

Van der Meulen, J. C.: Correction of hypospadias, Types I and II. Ann. Plast. Surg., *8*:403, 1982.

Villee, D.: Micropenis. Dialogues Pediatr. Urol., *7*(1):2, 1984.

Vordermark, J. S.: Adhesive membrane: a new dressing for hypospadias. Urology, *20*:86, 1982.

Wacksman, J.: Modification of the one-stage flip-flap procedure to repair distal penile hypospadias. Urol. Clin. North Am., *8*:527, 1981.

Walsh, P. C., Madden, J. D., Harrod, M. J., Goldstein, J. L., MacDonald, P. C., and Wilson, J. D.: Familial incomplete male pseudohermaphroditism, Type 2. Decreased dihydrotestosterone formation in pseudovaginal perineoscrotal hypospadias. N. Engl. J. Med., *291*:18, 944, 1974.

Waterhouse, K., and Glassberg, K. I.: Mobilization of the anterior urethra as an aid in the one-stage repair of hypospadias. Urol. Clin. North Am., *8*:521, 1981.

Wilson, J. D., and Walsh, P. C.: Disorders of sexual differentiation. *In* Harrison, J. H., Gittes, R. F., Perlmutter, A. D., Stamey, T. H., and Walsh, P. C. (Eds.): Campbell's Urology. Philadelphia, W. B. Saunders Co., 1979, pp. 1484–1524.

Woodard, J. R., and Cleveland, R.: Application of Horton-Devine principles to the repair of hypospadias. J. Urol., *127*:1155, 1982.

Woodhouse, C., and Ransley, P. R.: Personal communication, 1984.

Yeoman, D. M., Cooke, R., and Hain, W. R.: Penile block for circumcision? A comparison with caudal block. Anesthesia, *38*:862, 1983.

CHAPTER 48

Disorders of the Urethra and Penis

JOHN W. DUCKETT, M.D.
BRENT W. SNOW, M.D.

Anomalies of the urethra include both congenital and acquired lesions, which are manifested by voiding abnormalities, daytime and nighttime wetting, or urinary tract infections. Radiographic techniques with the use of excretory urography and voiding cystourethrography allow better visualization of most urethral anomalies and obstruction. In addition, the refined optics and miniaturization of pediatric endoscopic instruments have dramatically improved diagnostic and therapeutic efficacy, particularly in the primary ablation of posterior urethral valves.

Obstruction of the urethra occurs predominantly in the male and is most frequently attributed to posterior urethral valves. Other causes include urogenital membranes at the bulbomembranous junction, polyps attached to the verumontanum, anterior urethral diverticula, strictures, and ureteroceles. "Primary bladder neck obstruction" as a cause of bladder outlet obstruction in children is an exceedingly rare occurrence in spite of the emphasis placed upon it in the past.

In the female child, urethral obstruction is quite uncommon and is usually attributable to a ureterocele, diverticulum, hypospadias, prolapse, or those obstructions associated with a persistent urogenital sinus or with high anorectal malformations. The concept of obstructive "distal urethral stenosis" is no longer valid but may be a cause of functional disturbances of micturition.

CONGENITAL VESICAL NECK CONTRACTURE

The entity of bladder neck contracture in children, first described in 1933 by Marion, became a popular diagnosis in the 1950's and 1960's. Various operative procedures were devised to improve the flow through the vesicourethral junction; they included posterior wedge resection (Lich et al., 1950), anterior Y-V vesicourethroplasty (Andreassen, 1953; Young, 1953), and combinations of both anterior and posterior resections (Young and Goebel, 1954).

Pathologic findings in patients with bladder neck obstruction have been variable. Marion (1933) suggested that the cause might be primary hypertrophy of the smooth muscles at the vesical neck. He also implicated fibrosis and sclerosis in acquired lesions. Bodian (1957) described a condition of fibroelastosis of the posterior urethral wall in infant males that he believed to be responsible for the disease described by Marion. Bodian reported an increase in fibroelastic tissue associated with prostatic elongation and a decrease in the prostatic glands and smooth muscle. Although the changes he demonstrated occurred predominantly below the verumontanum, they extended from the bladder neck into the bulbous urethra. However, no satisfactory clinical correlation between Bodian's fibroelastosis and obstruction at the bladder neck was established. Young (1972) reported a dense fibroelastosis of the vesical neck as the principal histologic finding in eight carefully selected cases of idiopathic congenital vesical neck obstruction. However, because the elastosis was conspicuously absent from the tunica propria and because it was quite unlike the primary fibroelastosis seen in the hearts of babies with severe congenital heart disease, the authors suggest that this might be a secondary phenomenon.

Varying degrees of vesical neck hypertrophy occur in association with more distal urethral obstructions such as valves, membranous diaphragms, polyps, and especially neuropathic dysfunction. The enigmatic condition of occult neuropathic bladder (Williams, 1974) and the condition of dyssynergia of the detrusor and sphincter muscles (Turner-Warwick et al., 1973) are only two of many explanations for vesical neck hypertrophy as a secondary phenomenon.

Primary congenital bladder neck obstruction remains a diagnosis of exclusion (Spence et al., 1964). With a better understanding of neuropathic vesical dysfunction and improved diagnostic techniques, including voiding cystourethrography and physiologic pressure and flow measurements, the entity of congenital vesical neck contracture has become obsolete (Smith, 1969). There may be convincing case reports in which surgical revision of the bladder neck has improved both the urodynamics of voiding and the clinical symptoms in children whose condition did not correspond with any other diagnosis (Kaplan and King, 1976). These cases, however, are quite rare. The authors believe that vesical neck contracture does not exist independently. Before Y-V-plasties are undertaken in male children, careful consideration should be given to the significant incidence of retrograde ejaculation that occurs in adult life as a result of such procedures (Ochsner et al., 1970).

CONGENITAL VALVES OF THE POSTERIOR URETHRA

Posterior urethral valves represent the most common cause of bladder outlet obstruction in children. In many patients, these valves are diagnosed in the newborn period because of abdominal masses, infection, or voiding difficulties. Patients may have severe fluid and electrolyte disorders and renal insufficiency. Bladder outlet obstruction may be so severe as to cause trabeculation, detrusor hypertrophy, formation of diverticula, and secondary bladder neck hypertrophy. Chronic distension and elevated intravesical pressure leads to severe hydroureteronephrosis. In some patients, this obstruction may be almost complete, resulting in oligohydramnios and renal dysplasia (Type IV of Potter's classification) of both kidneys (Osathanondh and Potter, 1964).

With refined radiographic techniques and smaller endoscopic instruments, the diagnosis and treatment of posterior urethral valves has made great progress.

Anatomy and Classification

Young et al. (1919) proposed a classification of congenital posterior urethral valves based on their anatomic appearance.

Type I consists of posterior mucosal folds distal to the verumontanum. In the normal urethra, the inferior crest (crista urethralis) arises as a continuation of the caudal end of the verumontanum. It appears as a straight tapering ridge that terminates in two fins (plicae colliculi), which diverge laterally and distally in the membranous urethra, disappearing at the level of the urogenital diaphragm. The accentuation of these normal folds is characteristic of obstructive urethral valves. Usually the two cusps fuse anteriorly, creating an oval, oblique diaphragm with an elliptical opening that is widest proximally (Fig. 48–1). This is by far the most common type of posterior urethral valve.

Type II valves are folds that diverge from the verumontanum toward the bladder neck. These folds have been seen in conjunction with Type I valves and have been confused with the more distal obstructing element. The authors' opinion is that this type of fold is not an obstructing lesion, though others have reported its obstructing characteristics (Hendren, 1976).

Type III valves involve either a marked fusion of the anterior folds (severe Type I) or the congenital urethral membrane, which will be discussed later in this chapter.

Stephens (1983) described a Type IV urethral valve in the posterior urethra. This valve is unrelated to the valves previously described by Young on the posterior wall. A Type IV valve is characterized as a deep infold of the anterior and anterolateral walls that overrides the lumen of the membranous urethra, and is noted rarely in conjunction with the prune belly syndrome. It is not seen except with voiding urethrography. The dynamics of distension of the lax prostatic urethra may act as an anterior diverticulum, creating a lip or valvelike obstruction.

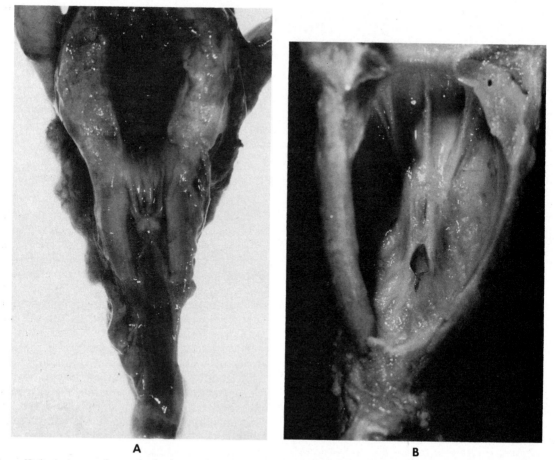

A   **B**

Figure 48–1. *A,* A posterior urethral valve specimen unfolded after an anterior urethra midline incision gives the impression of two folds coapting in the midline. *B,* Another specimen opened by unroofing rather than incising anterior urethral wall shows the folds to be an oblique diaphragm fused anteriorly. Note also the proximal folds confused as Type II valves. (From Robertson, W. B., and Hayes, J. A.: Br. J. Urol., *41*:592, 1969.)

After describing four types of valves, it is the authors' opinion that the term *posterior urethral valve* should be applied to Young's Type I valve only.

Embryology

In embryogenesis, after the mesonephric (wolffian) ducts fuse with the urogenital sinus, they regress before terminating in the verumontanum as ejaculatory ducts. Their path of regression may be noted via the plicae colliculi into the crista urethralis. Incomplete regression results in residual or substantive folds that act as urethral valves (Stephens, 1963; 1983) (Fig. 48–2). Young (1972) suggested that possibly the anterior portion of the hymenal ring derived from the urethrovaginal folds as a Müllerian derivative is the origin of the inferior crest and the more prominent urethral valves.

Endoscopic Appearance

Since valve cusps coapt only during antegrade flow, they usually cannot be demonstrated during the retrograde passage of an instrument or irrigation. The changing configuration of these valves is best observed with the bladder filled and the endoscope placed well distal to the verumontanum with the water source removed and the connection open. This allows irrigant to flow from the bladder through the instrument, ballooning the cusps and demonstrating their coapting margins (Cendron et al., 1969; Cornil and Bakker, 1971). Initially, the valve margins appear as a V similar to the vocal cords. With antegrade flow, these valve leaflets are observed to coapt in the midline.

Radiographic Findings

The cornerstone of diagnosing congenital posterior urethral valves is voiding cystoure-

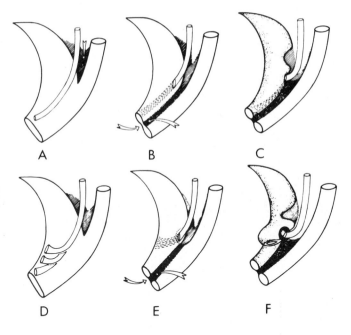

Figure 48–2. Development of Type I valves. *A–C,* Development of the normal urethral crest. Migration of the orifice of the wolffian duct from its anterolateral position in the cloaca to the site of the Müller tubercle on the posterior wall of the urorectal septum occurs synchronously with cloacal division. (Dots denote pathway of migration.) This wolffian remnant is more lateral and posterior and remains as the normal inferior crest and the plicae colliculi. *D,* Abnormal anterior positions of the wolffian duct orifices. *E,* Abnormal migration of the terminal ends of the ducts. *F,* Circumferential obliquely oriented ridges that compose the valve. (From Kelalis, P. P., and King, L. R. (Eds.): Clinical Pediatric Urology. Philadelphia, W. B. Saunders Co., 1976.)

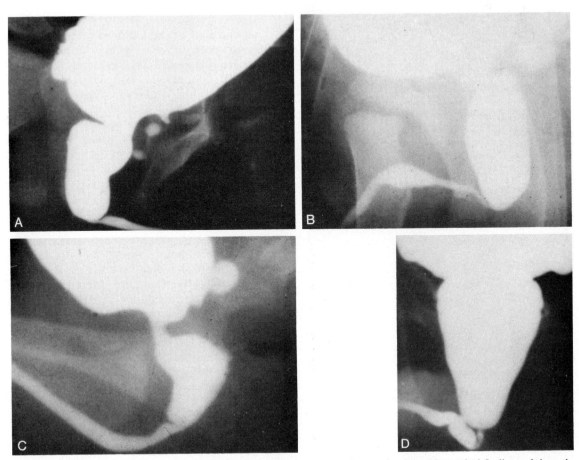

Figure 48–3. Posterior urethral valves demonstrated by voiding cystourethrography. Note the typical findings of the valve leaflets (*A*), dilated posterior urethra (*A* to *D*), hypertrophied bladder neck (*A* to *C*), and trabeculated bladder (*A* and *C*).

thrography (Fig. 48–3). Some authors, however, have presented cases with apparently normal voiding cystourethrograms and excretory urograms, but with cystoscopic photographs indicating urethral valves (Arnold and Ginsburg, 1974; Mahony, 1971). The authors consider such demonstrations to be evidence of prominent plicae colliculi that should not be classified as posterior urethral valves (Fig. 48–4). Care must also be taken not to confuse the radiographic picture of the urethra associated with the prune belly syndrome (Fig. 48–5) with valves. Prominent folds may cause flow disturbances and may be associated with wetting problems, but it is difficult to accept these as obstructing lesions. Certainly, more harm than benefit results from unnecessary endoscopy of enuretic boys looking for valvular obstruction in the face of normal radiographs. As the relative diameter of the urethral lumen increases with age, these folds become less prominent, as proved by their low incidence in the adult male population. Certainly, there is a spectrum of valvular obstruction, but significant obstruction can always be demonstrated with proper voiding cystourethrography. When congenital posterior urethral valvular obstruction exists, ultrasonography, excretory urography, and nuclear scanning techniques have all been used effectively to image the upper urinary tracts. The choice is individualized to each patient as well as the information desired.

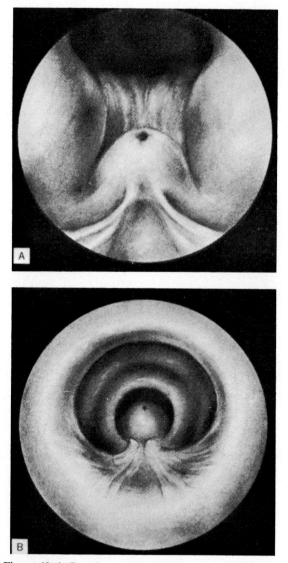

Figure 48–4. Drawings of the cystoscopic appearance of excessively prominent plicae colliculi arising from the base of the verumontanum *(A)*. The panendoscope has been withdrawn into the bulbous urethra. *B,* The plical folds (false valves) can be seen extending through the distal limit of the external sphincter. (From Young, B. W.: Lower Urinary Tract Obstruction in Childhood. Philadelphia, Lea & Febiger, 1972.)

Clinical Presentation in the Newborn

About half of the children presenting with significant obstructive uropathy due to urethral valves are diagnosed in the neonatal period (Cass and Stephens, 1974; Duckett, 1974a; Atwell, 1983). On careful examination, bilateral flank masses or a distended bladder may be found, suggesting the presence of urethral valves. A dribbling or weak urinary stream may be noted; however, a full urinary stream does not preclude significant urethral obstruction. Naturally, valves should be suspected in a sickly boy with sepsis or urinary tract infection. With renal failure and its associated electrolyte abnormalities, it is not unusual for such sick infants to be treated for respiratory distress syndrome for several days before the correct diagnosis is made. Babies with respiratory distress syndrome are predominantly premature. Most babies with valves are full-term infants, though an acutely ill baby with posterior urethral valves may have rapid respirations resulting from acidosis.

It should be noted that accompanying congenital anomalies not related to the urinary tract are infrequently seen (Cornil, 1975).

Neonatal urinary ascites or extravasation associated with an abdominal mass can be caused by lower urinary tract obstruction. Posterior urethral valves are the most common cause (Cendron and Lepinard, 1972; Mitchell and Garrett, 1980; Greenfield et al., 1982). Urinary extravasation from the kidney is usually

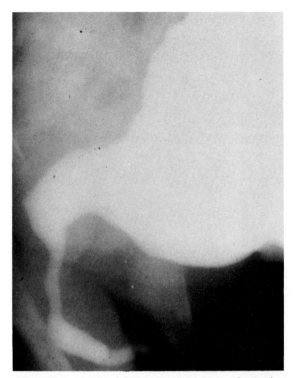

Figure 48–5. Voiding with cystourethrogram of a patient with the prune belly syndrome. (Compare with Figure 48–3.) Note the well-filled distal urethra and the absence of bladder neck hypertrophy and trabeculation.

considered to be a pressure-related phenomenon. Since the urinary tract has been "vented," frequently renal function has been preserved. With prompt, early effective drainage and support, these infants may do well.

Treatment in the Newborn

In infants with posterior urethral valves, electrolyte and fluid imbalance, acidosis, and sepsis should be promptly and aggressively treated. Effective management and bladder drainage, which can be achieved with a No. 8 French feeding tube or suprapubic Intracath or Cystocath, may dramatically reverse the clinical course. Once drainage has been established, a postoperative diuresis may occur with considerable salt and water loss. Careful management and replacement of electrolytes, with monitoring of body weight, urinary and serum electrolytes, and serum osmolality, is necessary. Occasionally, sodium polystyrene sulfonate (Kayexalate) resin may be needed for potassium control. Some feel that prompt bilateral nephrostomy drainage may occasionally be required, but the authors have not found this necessary.

Regardless of the severity of the upper tract dilatation, the primary surgical approach should be directed toward the relief of the urethral valvular obstruction. Smaller endoscopic instruments and improved optics now permit satisfactory valve ablation with only minimal risks of urethral trauma. A No. 10 French panendoscope will usually pass transurethrally without resistance in a male infant. The small sheath of the instrument must pass with ease, and no dilatation of the anterior urethra should be performed for fear of stricture formation. A Bugbee electrode may be used beside the telescope for fulguration of the valve cusps (Hendren, 1971). A perineal urethrotomy has been used in the past to permit access to the posterior urethra but is now seldom necessary. Williams (1973) and Parkkulainen (1977) have advocated valve ablation at the anterior junction at the 12 o'clock position, and this procedure is now our preference. Others have advocated destruction of the valve cusps at the 5 and 7 o'clock positions. Care should be exercised so that the sphincteric mechanism of the posterior urethra is not destroyed (Whitaker et al., 1972). Incomplete incision occurs in 20 to 30 per cent of the neonates managed this way (Cass and Stephens, 1974; Johnston and Kulatilake, 1972; Perlmutter, 1974). It is, however, preferable to err in undercutting rather than in overcutting. Strictures have occurred after transurethral valvular ablation in neonates (Fig. 48–6) (Myers and Walker, 1981). Use of the infant resectoscope cutting loops may be responsible for many of the strictures formed (Crooks, 1982). Therefore, we have bent this loop together to form a hook, which we use successfully to ablate the valves at the 12 o'clock position.

An alternative to primary valve resection is the creation of a temporary cutaneous vesicostomy (Duckett, 1974b). This procedure is done with a transverse lower abdominal incision midway between the umbilicus and the symphysis pubis. The bladder dome is mobilized and brought out as a cutaneous vesical fistula (Blocksom, 1957). Bladder or skin tubes used with the Lapides vesicostomy are not necessary in children. To avoid prolapse, it is important that the dome be brought to the skin, not the anterior bladder wall. We have used this method of diversion in 23 children with urethral valves and have found it to be a quite satisfactory method of drainage. When increased intravesical pressure is relieved by cutaneous vesicostomy, the functional ureteral obstruction observed at the ureterovesical junction will also decompress (Fig. 48–7). This cannot be achieved

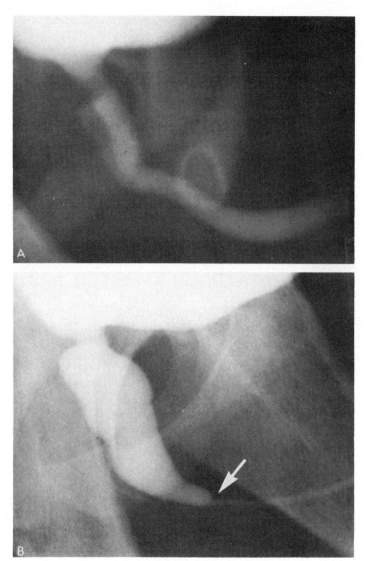

Figure 48–6. *A,* Voiding study of a 7-year-old patient taken before transurethral resection of "small valves" was performed elsewhere. Note the slight dilatation and elongation of the prostatic urethra, interpreted as valves both radiographically and endoscopically. *B,* Voiding study performed at time of referral at age 14 years. Patient presented with a stricture. Note that the stricture is in bulbous urethra 2 to 3 cm distal to the point at which valves were resected. This was managed by patch graft urethroplasty. (From Hendren, W. H.: *In* Smith, R. B., and Skinner, D. G.: Complications of Urologic Surgery: Prevention and Management. Philadelphia, W. B. Saunders Co., 1976.)

with a suprapubic cystostomy, since prolonged tube drainage is associated with infection, bladder inflammation, and continued functional obstruction at the ureterovesical junction. Vesicostomy as a form of tubeless drainage is unassociated with infection and should not be compared with tube drainage of the bladder. It should be emphasized that the authors' preference is for primary valve resection without vesicostomy. However, vesicostomy is certainly an adequate means of temporization for the newborn with a narrow urethra and for the surgeon who is inexperienced in urethral valve resection or is without the proper endoscopic instruments.

Another effective alternative when endoscopic instruments are not available was described by Johnston (1966). He used an otoscope through a perineal urethrotomy for direct vision of the valve cusps, which were destroyed with a skin hook and cautery.

Once the valves have been resected, the patient should thrive and maintain a sterile urinary tract with the aid of suppressive medication (Fig. 48–8). If, within the following weeks, azotemia progresses or uncontrollable infection occurs, higher urinary diversion may be necessary. For this we advise flank approaches to each kidney to obtain a biopsy and to establish either a cutaneous pyelostomy or ureterostomy. In our experience (Duckett, 1974*a*), when this step is necessary the kidneys are severely dysplastic and the prognosis is grave

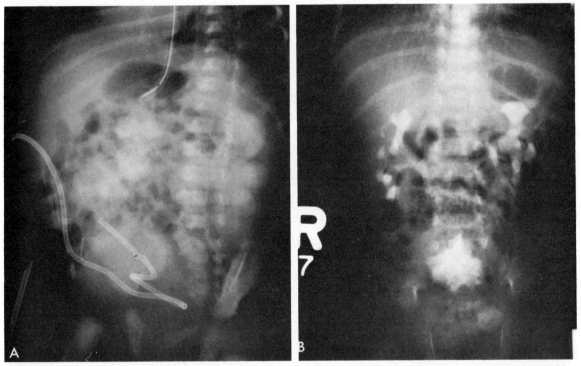

Figure 48–7. *A,* A premature newborn with valves had a cutaneous vesicostomy performed to decompress the bladder. An Intracath is in place in this picture. *B,* Excretory urogram 1 month later shows excellent drainage. His valves were resected at age 2 years and the vesicostomy was closed.

(Milliken, 1972). By this stepwise approach, unnecessary ureterostomies or nephrostomies can be avoided.

UPPER URINARY TRACT DIVERSIONS

When upper urinary tract diversion is deemed necessary, temporary loop ureterostomy has proved to be satisfactory in babies with urethral valves (Johnston, 1963). This creates a tubeless high drainage that is preferable to nephrostomy diversion (Perlmutter and Tank, 1968).

The Sober ureterostomy (Sober, 1972) makes use of *pelvio-ureterostomy-en-y* in which the proximal ureter is divided and brought to the skin in the flank, and the distal ureter is then anastomosed to the renal pelvis. This allows part of the urine to enter the bladder and keep it functional, whereas the ureterostomy acts as a vent for the system. When this procedure is combined with primary resection of the valves, the function of the venting limb of the ureterostomy gradually lessens until the ureter regains efficient peristalsis, dilatation decreases, and the tortuosity resolves. A procedure to close off the high ureterostomy is then quite simple.

Cromie and Williams (1975) modified the loop ureterostomy by connecting the internal portion of the loop, creating a *ring ureterostomy*. Urine is directed into the bladder and this procedure is less likely to compromise ureteral blood supply than is the Sober technique.

Pyelostomy is also an efficient high diversion when the renal pelvis is sufficiently large to be brought to the skin without tension. This vent is easier to close and also preserves upper ureteral blood supply (Immergut et al., 1969).

Problems with Undiversion in Valves

Several problems may arise with later reconstruction of the urinary tract. There has been fear of causing a defunctionalized bladder that would become contracted and fibrotic, resulting in a small capacity (Lome et al., 1972) after upper tract diversion or vesicostomy. In our institution, Snyder et al. (1983) demonstrated that in 16 myelodysplastic children, vesicostomy diversion is reversible without loss of bladder volume.

Another problem has been vesicoureteral reflux. Ureteroneocystostomy in these difficult

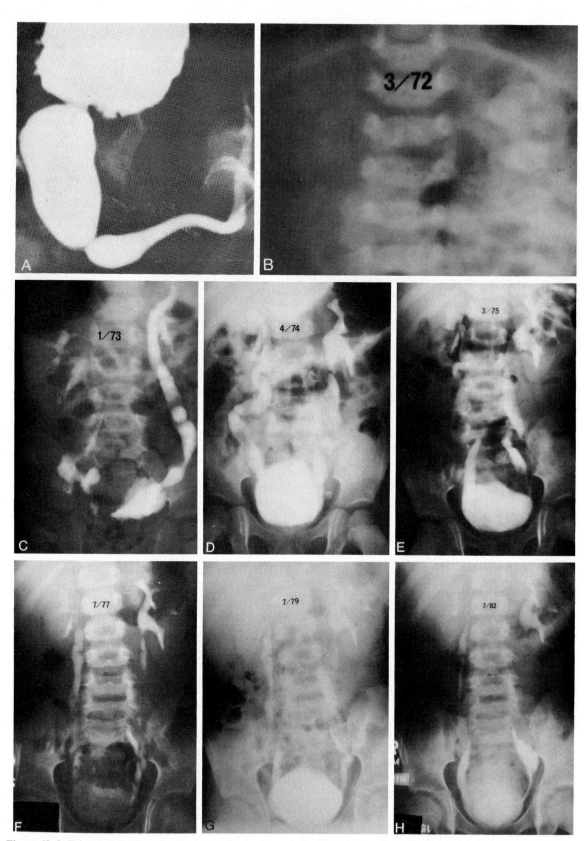

Figure 48–8. Primary resection of posterior urethral valves. *A,* Voiding cystourethrogram with typical finding of valves. *B,* Initial excretory urogram with hydronephrosis. *C–H,* Initial improvement was observed, and long-term follow up shows good results. Vesicoureteral reflux to the right kidney ceased within 3 years. Note the straightening of the ureters with time.

bladders has been fraught with complications. Unfortunately, many surgeons have felt that vesicoureteral reflux needs correction prior to reversing the diversion. This concept has led to many problems with ureteral obstruction at the bladder hiatus, resulting in permanent diversion for some children after failure of several reconstructive efforts. Avoiding ureterovesical reconstruction at the time that urinary continuity is re-established is preferred. Reflux demonstrated in a defunctionalized bladder will often resolve when urine flow is re-established. Pre-existing reflux may still resolve spontaneously with growth. After the dormant bladder has regained capacity, ureteroneocystostomy is easier to perform and is more likely to succeed. Whenever these partial high diversions are used in the management of urethral valves, it is preferable that the valvular obstruction be relieved. This allows the bladder to decompress and begin to function at lower pressures, thus relieving the functional ureterovesical obstruction and permitting the ureter to regain its normal capabilities.

Although most patients with congenital posterior urethral valves currently can be treated without upper urinary tract diversion, these treatment options still have occasional clinical value. Krueger et al. (1980) and Churchill et al. (1983) reported that somatic growth was significantly improved in nine infants treated with upper urinary tract diversion as compared with ten infants treated with primary valvular ablation. Their supposition was that high diversion immediately relieved obstruction and allowed for continued nephrogenesis during the first few months of life. This data is contrary to the authors' experience with 38 patients treated in a contemporary time period. By plotting each patient's height and weight against a logarithm of time, an individual's growth could be evaluated. Only three patients had poor growth, two of whom had abnormal renal function prior to treatment and thereafter. The other patient had early supravesical diversion with bilateral renal biopsies consistent with renal dysplasia.

TOTAL RECONSTRUCTION

In the past, some authors (Hendren, 1970; Rabinowitz et al. 1979; Monfort, 1976) have performed total urinary tract reconstruction in the newborn period. This procedure was reserved for patients with severe obstructive uropathy due to their posterior urethral valves and included ureteral tapering and reimplantation. With the approach advocated by the authors of early valve ablation and careful follow-up, total reconstruction in the newborn period has not been necessary.

Management in Older Children

Obstructive uropathy is not detected in the neonatal period in about half of boys with urethral valves (Ericsson, 1977; Crooks, 1981). The later clinical signs may include urinary infections, failure to thrive, daytime wetting, straining, a weak voiding stream, signs of renal failure, or a flank mass detected on physical examination. In this age group, primary resection of the urethral valves initially is preferred. Further reconstructive surgery is performed as indicated.

URETEROVESICAL JUNCTION

The severely dilated and tortuous ureter typical of urethral valves may demonstrate impaired emptying at the ureterovesical junction. Once intravesical pressure is diminished by relieving the obstruction, the hydroureteronephrosis generally improves, though not as dramatically as in the infant. Decompensation of the ureteral musculature may have caused chronic changes, which, in turn, allow persistent ureteral dilatation. Ureteral dilatation may not necessarily indicate an obstructing factor at the ureterovesical junction.

This clinical impression has been supported by direct measurements made by Whitaker (1973a and b) on patients with urethral valves. He recorded ureteral pressures in dilated systems under constant saline infusion of 10 ml per minute and found that most ureters in urethral valve patients do not have obstructive pressures. Other studies over the next 10 years confirmed this finding. If the bladder is filled to capacity, the intraureteral pressure must be greater than the intravesical pressure for urine to flow into the bladder. It is at this stage of increased intravesical pressure that an obstructive pattern appears in the ureter.

It is not uncommon to find a moderate hydronephrosis and hydroureter in the early phases of excretory urography that improves significantly after the bladder has been emptied. The persistence of gross dilatation in the absence of obstruction is a fact not easily accepted by clinicians who do not regularly deal with upper urinary tract abnormalities in children. The typically dilated upper urinary system of prune belly syndrome is another example of primary ureteral abnormalities unassociated with obstruction in most cases.

A continuous period of increased bladder

pressure with obstructing urethral valves prevents the ureters from emptying properly. This back-pressure causes overstretching and fibrosis of the ureteral walls. It is not surprising, therefore, that many of these ureters remain wide and atonic after release of the obstruction. In the older age group, about half of the renal units will show persistent dilatation after relief of the urethral obstruction (Cass and Stephens, 1974; Eklof and Ringertz, 1975).

The decision to reconstruct dilated ureters in these patients may be extremely difficult. Antegrade perfusion studies may be of assistance, provided that care is taken to be sure the entire system is full and that the bladder is simultaneously evaluated (Whitaker, 1973a).

An attractive alternative is the diuretic radioisotope nuclear scan. This, unlike the antegrade perfusion test, requires no invasive technique and can yield very accurate data. Computer calculations of the isotope washout curves may aid in differentiating dilated unobstructed ureters from obstructed ureters that would benefit from surgical correction.

VESICOURETERAL REFLUX

Between 40 and 66 per cent of posterior urethral valve patients have reflux before treatment (Cass and Stephens, 1974; Johnston and Kulatilake, 1972; Williams, 1973; Johnston, 1978; Hoover and Duckett, 1982; Egami and Smith, 1982). At presentation, approximately half of the patients with reflux have bilateral reflux (Table 48–1). This has been shown to carry a worse prognosis (Johnston, 1978). When these patients have their valves resected and their reflux followed (Williams, 1977; Johnston, 1978; Hoover and Duckett, 1982), approximately one quarter of the refluxing units will cease to reflux. The cessation of reflux usually occurs within 1 year from the time of valve ablation. Persistent unilateral reflux after valve ablation in the majority of patients is associated with a functionless kidney. The great majority of these functionless kidneys with persistent reflux are found to have renal dysplasia (Johnston, 1978; Hoover and Duckett, 1982). This substantiates the data of Henneberry and Stephens (1980) in their post-mortem study of posterior urethral valve patients relating reflux to renal dysplasia.

It is the authors' opinion that after valve ablation, reflux should be followed carefully. If spontaneous improvement does not occur after waiting an adequate period of time, careful assessment of renal function should be done. Nephroureterectomy of the refluxing unit should

TABLE 48–1. REFLUX DATA IN POSTERIOR URETHRAL VALVE PATIENTS

	Williams	Johnston	Hoover and Duckett
Study period	1966–1975	1956–1977	1970–1979
Total patients	100	66	82
Patients with reflux	46	44	38
unilateral	21	23	20
bilateral	25	21	18
Patient deaths	5	18	3
unilateral reflux	0	5	—
bilateral reflux	5	13	3
Cessation of reflux			
unilateral	5	7	6
bilateral	1	4	6
one side resolved	—	5	3
Number of refluxing units with function	25	5	17
Number of refluxing units without function	16	18	12
Dysplasia in nonfunctioning kidneys removed	—	14 of 18 (9 of 14)	10 of 12 (6 of 6)
Abnormal renal function in refluxing patients	20	2	3
( ) Autopsy data			

be considered if no function can be demonstrated. If function is found, ureteral reimplantation should be considered on an individual basis. If this course of action is followed only a small number of patients will require reimplantation, and reflux should not be of immediate concern during the early management of these patients.

UNILATERAL REFLUX AND DYSPLASIA

Vesicoureteral reflux and renal dysplasia in patients with posterior urethral valves has been noted previously (Williams, 1977; Johnston, 1978). In 82 patients, Hoover and Duckett (1982) found 17 with persistent unilateral reflux, 11 of which (65 per cent) had a nonfunctioning dysplastic kidney. This dysplasia and reflux was noted on the left side in 92 per cent. These findings are thought to occur because of abnormal ureteral bud embryogenesis as described by Mackie and Stephens (1975) and Henneberry and Stephens (1980). In order for the infant to establish more normal voiding dynamics and to reduce the likelihood of infection, a nephroureterectomy is recommended for the refluxing, nonfunctioning, dysplastic kidney.

BLADDER DYSFUNCTION

Many authors have noted persistent upper urinary tract dilatation after posterior urethral valve ablation (Rabinowitz et al., 1979; Glassberg et al., 1982; Mitchell, 1982; Churchill et al., 1983). Whether this dilatation represents ureterovesical junction obstruction or bladder dysfunction has been the subject of much discussion. The severely dilated and tortuous ureter typical of urethral valves frequently demonstrates impaired emptying at the ureterovesical junction. Once the intravesical pressure is diminished by relieving the bladder outlet obstruction, the hydroureteronephrosis generally improves. This frequently is more dramatic in infants than in older children. Occasionally, decompensation of the ureteral musculature precludes complete resolution of the ureteral dilatation. Thus, dilatation may not necessarily indicate an obstruction at the ureterovesical junction. This clinical impression has been supported by direct measurements made by Whitaker (1973a and b) on patients with urethral valves. He recorded ureteral pressures in dilated systems under constant saline infusion of 10 ml per minute and found that most ureters in urethral valve patients do not have obstructive pressures. He is also careful to note, as has Mitchell (1982), that bladder pressures should be simultaneously measured. In some patients, the upper tract dilatation is aggravated by incomplete bladder emptying or persistent bladder hypertonicity. In evaluating incomplete bladder emptying, it should be remembered that children of this age group may not void to completion each time. Incomplete bladder emptying may also be secondary to incomplete valve ablation, which may occur in 20 to 30 per cent of patients. After endoscopic valve ablation, stricture formation may occur (Myers and Walker, 1981), which may also cause incomplete bladder emptying. Unfortunately, in the past some have thought the incomplete bladder emptying was due to the secondarily hypertrophied bladder neck, and have performed posterior wedge resections of the bladder neck. This operation has frequently led to incontinence and subsequently to retrograde ejaculation.

FULL VALVE BLADDER SYNDROME

In some patients, upper tract dilatation may progress in spite of adequate valvular ablation. This may result from elevated intravesical pressures at relatively low bladder volumes. This lack of bladder compliance may lead to a functional obstruction of the ureter at the level of the bladder. Sensation of a full bladder in these boys seems to be diminished, which further compounds this problem. Double and triple voiding may demonstrate rapid bladder refilling from the large volume of urine stored in the upper urinary tract.

In patients with the full valve bladder syndrome, in which the bladder remains noncompliant, intermittent catheterization may be of benefit. This allows the bladder to empty completely at regular intervals and may reduce the intravesical pressure sufficiently to allow resolution of upper tract dilatation.

Mitchell (1982) reviewed 11 patients with severe upper tract dilatation and bladder dysfunction and found an associated concentrating defect in the kidney, with a high urinary output. Urodynamic studies showed that intravesical pressure rose significantly in a linear fashion and that sensation of fullness was delayed. He and others (McGuire and Weiss, 1975) have suggested anticholinergics to improve vesical compliance. In a selected few patients, Mitchell (1982) has also recommended bladder augmentation with colonic segments. Unfortunately, long-term follow up to judge the efficacy of this treatment approach is not available. The management of patients with the full valve bladder syndrome remains a dilemma.

Congenital Urethral Membranes

Rarely, urethral obstruction in boys is caused by a transverse membrane in the urethra distal to the verumontanum. This membrane differs in many respects from the more common Young's Type I posterior urethral valve. The attachment of a congenital urethral membrane occurs in the membranous urethra or proximal bulbous urethra. Variants have been described, as either a rather firm diaphragm with a central orifice or a soft redundant membrane that acts as a "wind-sock," prolapsing into the bulbous urethra. A multiloculated variant of the membrane has been noted as well. In contrast, a posterior urethral valve courses in an oblique manner, arising posteriorly from the crista urethralis, extending from the verumontanum, and attaching anteriorly to the urethral wall; the two cusps are fused at the anterior aspect, creating a complete annulus.

On voiding urethrography, it may be difficult to distinguish this lesion from a Type I valve of the posterior urethra (Fig. 48–9). The urethral valve usually has characteristic linear filling defects along the posterior urethral wall (see Fig. 48–3A) and an elliptical opening in the diaphragm, through which the main flow is eccentric just below the verumontanum. However, there is a concentric opening in the mid-

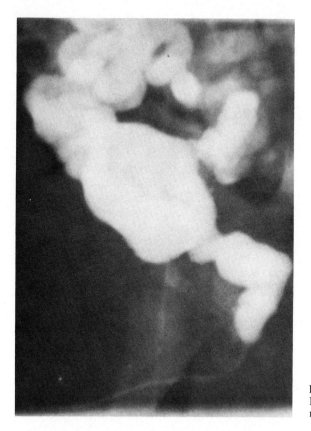

Figure 48–9. Congenital urethral membrane (Young's Type III urethral valve) causing severe obstruction with bilateral renal dysplasia; a retrograde catheter could not be passed.

portion of the obstructing urethral membrane that may be demonstrated with retrograde urethrography. The "wind-sock" variant, which prolapses into the bulbous urethra, may be difficult to differentiate from an anterior urethral diverticulum (Fig. 48–10).

The etiology of this congenital urethral membrane has been attributed to persistence of the urogenital portion of the cloacal membrane. Its diaphanous quality and regular occurrence in the membranous urethra favor this explanation (Fig. 48–11) (Field and Stephens, 1974).

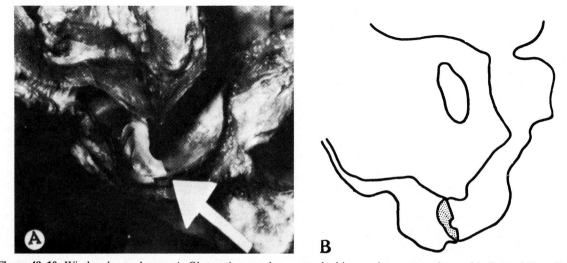

Figure 48–10. Wind sock membrane. *A,* Obstructing membrane attached in membranous urethra and ballooned like wind sock into expanded bulbous urethra (autopsy specimen). *B,* Diagram of the anatomic findings. (From Field, P. L., and Stephens, F. D.: J. Urol., *111*:250, 1974.)

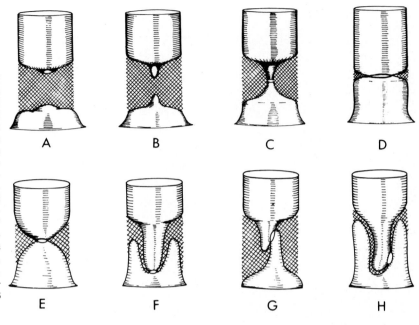

Figure 48–11. Development of congenital urethral membranes (Type III valves). *A–D,* Normal canalization of the urogenital membrane. *D* shows normal slight constriction at the level of the perineal membrane. *E,* Stricture formation. *F,* Canalization by central downgrowth and circumferential ingrowth resulting in bulging membrane with a central stenotic orifice. *G–H,* Side openings creating valvular "wind sock" membranes. (Drawings and descriptions supplied through the courtesy of Dr. F. D. Stephens. From Kelalis, P. P., and King, L. R. (Eds.): Clinical Pediatric Urology. Philadelphia, W. B. Saunders Co., 1976.)

These urethral membranes may correspond to the Type III lesion in Young's classification of urethral valves, and they may also be the explanation for some of the lesions previously classified as congenital urethral strictures (Cobb et al., 1968).

CLINICAL PRESENTATION

Boys with congenital membranes may present in the neonatal period with severe obstruction and dysplastic kidneys. The degree of obstruction from this lesion varies greatly, and milder manifestations are occasionally seen. Mild obstruction may not be discovered until later in childhood and then only because of persistent daytime and nighttime wetting.

TREATMENT

As with management for urethral valves, precise transurethral fulguration with infant endoscopic instruments can usually be performed. If the lesion is mild, an instrument can be passed through the opening in the membrane and gradual dilatation can be performed, which ruptures the membrane, thereby relieving the obstruction. The "wind-sock" type of lesion may produce dilatation in the bulbous urethra from the "toe" of the long sock. The bulbous urethra at the site of a urethrostomy, therefore, may appear capacious yet free of obstruction. When relieved of the distending forces of voiding, the membrane will be found in the posterior urethra endoscopically. The membrane may also be accessible to excision by a retropubic approach, but this is seldom indicated.

CONGENITAL URETHRAL STRICTURE

Rarely, segmental urethral stenosis or complete urethral agenesis is found. These conditions are usually associated with severe cases of prune belly syndrome (Fig. 48–12). However, the diagnostic entity of congenital urethral stricture has been most confusing in the pediatric urologic literature. Campbell (1970), in previous editions of this text, has used the term to describe meatal stenosis and urethral strictures in the anterior urethra that were most likely acquired rather than congenital. Likewise, the term *congenital urethral stenosis* has been used to designate narrowings in the membranous urethra that probably are congenital urethral membranes. If the embryologic explanation for canalization of the urogenital membrane is correct, pathologic lesions of urethral membranes and congenital urethral stricture may be variations of the same defect. These strictures or membranes are located at the point at which the bulbous urethra, which arises from genital folds (ectoderm), joins the posterior or membranous urethra, which arises from the cloaca (entoderm). Therefore, true congenital urethral strictures, defined as localized narrowings of the bulbous or pendulous urethra, probably do not exist except at the juncture of the posterior and anterior urethra. The use of the diagnosis congenital urethral stricture should apply only to the extremely rare lesions that meet the described criteria. Avoiding this diagnosis for nonspecific voiding symptoms in young boys will prevent unnecessary urethral dilatations.

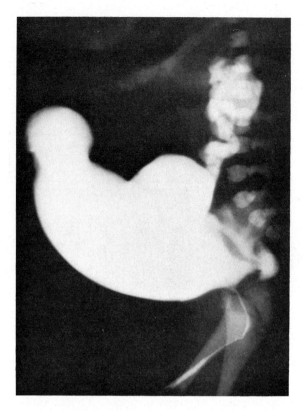

Figure 48–12. Urethral stenosis in a stillborn baby with renal dysplasia, prune-belly syndrome, fusiform megalourethra (see Fig. 48–22) and anorectal malformation. (From Kelalis, P. P., and King, L. R. (Eds.): Clinical Pediatric Urology. Philadelphia, W. B. Saunders Co., 1976.)

Although efforts have been made to simplify the classification of obstructing lesions of the urethra by using the same embryologic explanation for urethral membranes and congenital urethral strictures, others prefer to keep these entities distinct (Kelalis, 1976).

ACQUIRED URETHRAL STRICTURE

Urethral strictures may develop as acquired lesions secondary to inflammation or trauma. The most common cause of urethral stricture in male children remains hypospadias repair, which is discussed in detail elsewhere.

Studies in children (Devereaux and Williams, 1972; Harshman et al., 1981; Kaplan and Brock, 1983) have shown that posterior urethral strictures most commonly are secondary to trauma. As in adults, these strictures develop with severe pelvic trauma resulting in rupture of the prostatomembranous junction and dislocation of the prostate. Strictures of the anterior urethra are often due to inappropriate urethral dilations or cystoscopy with too large an instrument (Fig. 48–13). Foley catheters are also noted as a cause of urethral stricture. It should be observed that all strictures reported in these large series were acquired and that no congenital strictures were found. It is possible that insignificant trauma, such as straddle injuries that occur in active boys, may go unnoticed until subsequent strictures appear. When discovered, these strictures are falsely termed *congenital urethral strictures*, though they do not fit the described criteria. A meatal stenosis should also generally be considered acquired and is usually a result of meatitis after circumcision.

Treatment of these acquired urethral strictures, as in adults, is individualized. In cases of severe pelvic trauma with urethral disruption, suprapubic bladder drainage and delayed urethral repair is usually the treatment of choice. This treatment is most appropriate in the pediatric age group because of the smaller caliber of the urethra and the difficulty of its repair. Treatment of the anterior urethral stricture is also similar to that in adults. Excision and reanastomosis patch grafts, island flap urethral replacements, and internal urethrotomy are techniques in use.

CONGENITAL POLYPS OF THE PROSTATIC URETHRA

Pedunculated polyps of the verumontanum may partially and intermittently obstruct the posterior urethra (Fig. 48–14). These lesions have been considered by Downs (1970) to be congenital in origin, since they occur predominantly in infants and children. Micropathologic

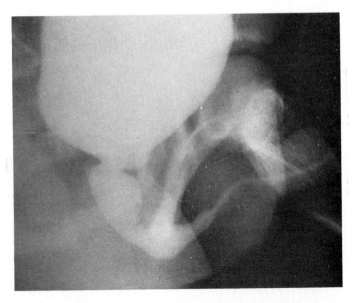

Figure 48–13. Iatrogenic anterior urethral stricture in bulbous urethra in 10-year-old boy 2 years after instrumentation for enuresis.

examination indicates that they are hamartomatous protrusions of the urethral wall rather than neoplasms. The membranous covering of the polyp is composed of transitional cell epithelium. The core is predominantly fibrous connective tissue with cellular constituents of the tunica propria from which it arises. Smooth muscle, islets of glandular cells, and even nerve tissue have been reported within a polyp. Squamous metaplasia and glandular nests may develop.

Patients usually present with obstructive symptoms and about half are found to have upper tract changes. Reflux and bladder diverticula may also be present. The polyp clinically acts as a ball valve that obstructs the prostatic area and can be seen floating freely in various positions during voiding studies. Surgical exci-

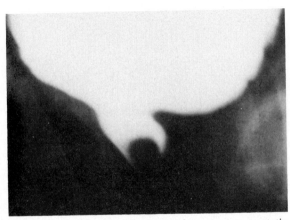

Figure 48–14. Congenital urethral polyp seen as a prostatic urethral filling defect.

sion can be accomplished quite easily suprapubically, with smaller lesions being accessible by transurethral resection.

DIVERTICULA OF THE URETHRA

Diverticulum of the Anterior Urethra (Anterior Urethral Valves)

The most common type of anterior urethral diverticulum that causes significant obstruction is a saccular diverticulum at the penoscrotal junction. These diverticula occur in the proximal part of the penile urethra, expanding within the developing tunica albuginea of the corpus spongiosum. The dorsal wall of the urethra remains intact, but the ventral wall is thinned and distended by 2 to 4 cm. The diverticulum has an oval shape, and its distal lip is thin and valvular in appearance. As the wide mouth of the diverticulum becomes distended with urine, the pocket fills and the distal lip presses against the dorsal wall of the urethra, obstructing outflow. The proximal lip may be less clearly defined. Thus, this distal lip of the diverticulum has been called an anterior urethral valve. Generally, they cause less damage from obstruction than do posterior urethral valves. They can, however, cause marked dilatation (Firlit and King, 1972) (Fig. 48–15). It is possible that the degree of obstruction increases as the mouth of the diverticulum is narrowed. Milder forms of anterior urethral valves are probably caused by smaller

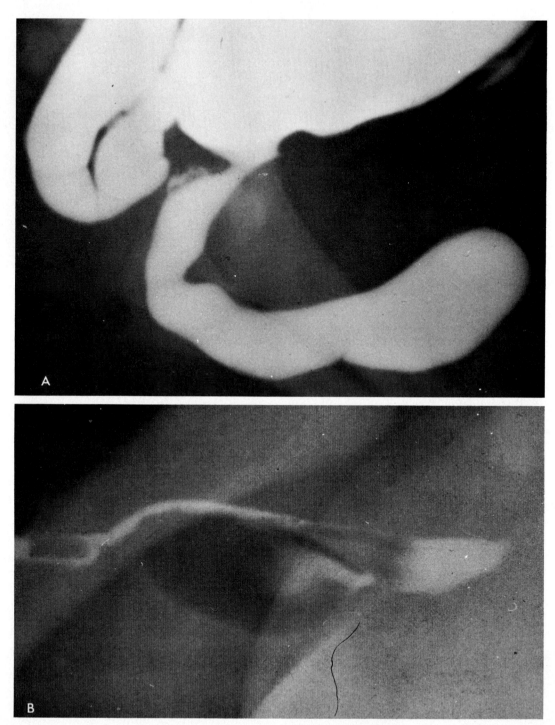

Figure 48–15. *A,* Anterior urethral diverticulum (valve). This voiding cystourethrogram in a newborn boy shows severe obstruction associated with reflux into a dysplastic left kidney and compromised right renal function. *B* and *C,* Demonstration of anterior diverticulum, using air injected retrograde with compression of urethra in perineum followed by contrast injection, showing neck of diverticulum and mechanism of obstruction.

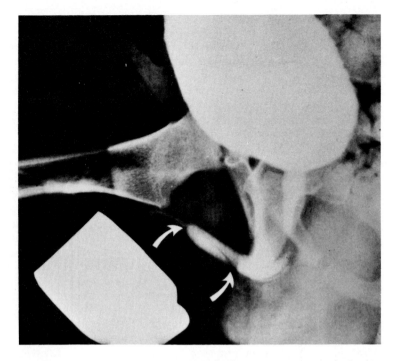

Figure 48–16. Anterior urethral diverticulum (valve) demonstrated by voiding cystourethrogram in 4-year-old boy with symptoms of straining to void and a fine stream.

anterior diverticula (Fig. 48–16) (Rudhe and Ericsson, 1970; Williams and Retik, 1969).

Stephens (1963) considers these diverticula to be the result of incomplete migration of the spongy tissue and its vascular network. This results in the defective closing of the bulbous urethra and causes outpouchings of urethral epithelium within the confines of the tunica albuginea. Others (Cooke and Shaw, 1961; Edling, 1953; Kjellberg et al., 1957; Currarino and Fuqua, 1972) believe that the origin of diverticula arising in the bulbous urethra is related to cystic dilatations of the ducts of the Cowper glands. Maizels et al. (1983) have called these cystic dilatations of the Cowper ducts syringoceles. The Cowper duct dilatations are seldom obstructing. They usually originate in the proximal half of the bulbous urethra and course in a cephalad direction. Anterior diverticula originate in the distal half of the bulbous urethra and may have their orifice at any point along the diverticulum causing obstruction.

The symptoms and signs of urinary obstruction generally prompt the parents to present the child for treatment. In addition, some patients have a palpable swelling in the perineal or scrotal area that becomes enlarged during voiding (Fig. 48–17).

The obstructing distal lip can be clearly demonstrated by voiding cystourethrograms. For accurate diagnosis, it is imperative that the area between the membranous urethra and the external urethral meatus be included in all these radiographic studies. Unfortunately, it is a com-

mon error to omit this portion of the male urethra from the voiding radiographic studies.

TREATMENT

A primary one-stage repair can usually be accomplished (Gross and Bill, 1948). Anterior

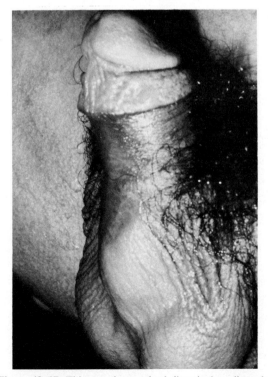

Figure 48–17. This anterior urethral diverticulum distended during voiding, revealing a palpable penoscrotal mass.

urethral diverticula that cause severe obstruction in infancy may be best treated by laying the urethra open onto the skin, as in a Johanson urethroplasty for stricture, so that the upper tract dilatation will be decompressed. Subsequently, at the time of closure the obstructing distal lip may be removed and the excess urethral mucosa excised. Minor lesions in children may be treated by simple transurethral resection of the distal lip (Firlet et al., 1978); however, subsequent stricture is a considerable risk with fulguration procedures in the anterior urethra.

Other Diverticula of the Urethra

Narrow-necked diverticula are round and communicate with the bulb of the urethra through a thin channel. The etiology of these diverticula is thought to be similar to other anterior urethral diverticula. Since the diverticular neck is narrow, the lip does not act like a valve or cause obstruction. However, stasis within the diverticulum may lead to infection or stone formation. The symptoms include local pain and dysuria, and simple excision is sufficient treatment.

Inflammatory diverticula may develop subsequent to the presence of an indwelling catheter; this causes damage to the ventral wall of the urethra at the penoscrotal junction. Similar lesions occur after hypospadias repair.

An *acquired diverticulum of the prostatic urethra* may result from incomplete excision of a rectourethral fistula associated with anorectal malformations (Currarino, 1969). Such a stump usually causes little trouble despite the considerable degree of dilatation that often accompanies it (Fig. 48–18). Excision may be necessary for stones or infection and can be done by a retrovesical dissection through a transperitoneal approach. A parasacral approach may be preferable in some cases (Kaplan et al., 1977).

A *diverticulum of the bladder* rarely may expand caudally, compressing the urethra and causing urinary retention (Fig. 48–19).

Congenital diverticulum of the posterior urethra has rarely been described (Williams, 1974).

An enlarged *utriculus masculinus* of müllerian origin may appear as a diverticulum arising in the posterior urethra. They are usually associated with intersex states or hypospadias and rarely require excision.

Cystic Anomalies of the Ducts of the Cowper Glands

The bulbourethral, or Cowper, glands are paired 5-mm glands located within the urogenital membrane. The Cowper glands' ducts are directed distally through the substance of the bulb of the corpus spongiosum, entering the ventral wall of the proximal bulbous urethra as

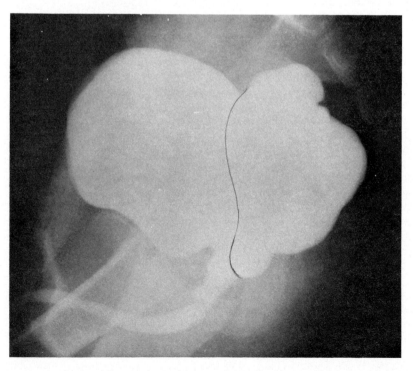

Figure 48–18. Posterior urethral diverticulum with no sequelae or symptoms caused by a rectourethral fistula remnant after "pull through" surgery (voiding cystourethrogram).

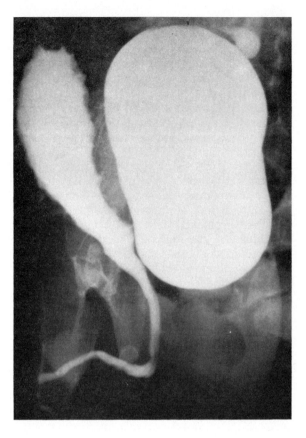

Figure 48–19. Giant bladder diverticulum (paraureteral) may cause outflow obstruction by compression of urethra and bladder neck.

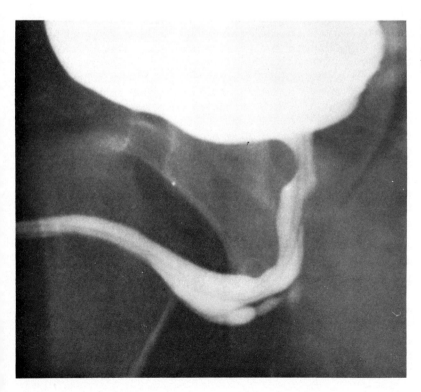

Figure 48–20. The Cowper gland duct filled on voiding cystourethrogram. Note the fuzzy contrast in the gland proper and the cystic dilatation of the distal duct.

two very small openings. They are the homolog of the Bartholin glands in the female and are considered accessory male sex glands that contribute a clear fluid that acts as a lubricant for spermatozoa and as a coagulation factor during ejaculation.

Opacification of the Cowper ducts by retrograde or voiding urethrography has become more prevalent with the increasing use of these diagnostic techniques (Fig. 48–20). Colodny and Lebowitz (1978) noted the more frequent documentation of the Cowper duct abnormalities and reviewed their radiographic findings. Edling (1953) reported 24 patients, mostly children, who had a channel or pouch originating from the floor of the bulbous urethra, which he interpreted as dilated Cowper ducts and glands. He divided the lesions into two main groups with transitional forms. The *globular type* consisted of rounded or oval cavities originating from the ventral surface of the bulbous urethra. The *tubular type* consisted of tubular structures or channels that originated from the same area of the urethra and coursed backward directly below and parallel to the urethra. Some were only slightly larger than normal Cowper ducts, but others reached considerable size. Kjellberg et al. (1957) described seven children with urethrographic findings similar to those of Edling's series and concluded that the diverticula formed on the ventral surface of the bulbous urethra were congenitally dilated Cowper ducts. Cooke and Shaw (1961) agreed that these diverticula were cystic dilatations of Cowper ducts. Currarino and Fuqua (1972) presented ten cases that proved to be transitional diverticula formations. Maizels et al. (1983) categorized lesions of the ducts of the Cowper glands, which they called syringoceles, into four groups, depending upon their dilatation and drainage. This subclassification in this unusual entity serves little purpose, since treatment must be individualized.

These anomalies usually do not have a profound effect on urination, but their discovery does explain some symptoms and signs, such as terminal hematuria. Those symptomatic lesions can be drained transurethrally. Excision is usually not necessary.

MEGALOURETHRA

Megalourethra is a rare congenital disorder of which there are two basic types: scaphoid and fusiform. These two types are separated both in appearance and embryology. Most of these patients present with nonobstructed enlargement of the phallus and urethra with associated congenital anomalies. Megalourethra has been noted with prune belly syndrome and with other urologic, as well as nonurologic, congenital anomalies.

The scaphoid variety is the most common and, fortunately, the least severe form of this anomaly (Fig. 48–21). In its development, the penile urethra forms by closure of the urethral groove from the urogenital diaphragm to the distal confluence with the ectodermal ingrowth of the glans penis. Under normal conditions, this urethra is then invested with vascular sinusoids and connective tissues, forming the corpus spongiosum. It is thought that failure of these mesenchymal elements to invert the urethra produces the defect seen in scaphoid megalourethra. Histopathologic specimens have revealed normal but attenuated urethral tissue, Buck fascia, and penile skin, but no sinusoidal tissue (Stephens, 1963).

The fusiform type of megalourethra is a more severe defect caused by failure of the mesoderm in the urethral folds to form erectile tissue (Fig. 48–22), which results in urethral epithelium being laid upon a fibrous wall of tunica albuginea (Dorairajan, 1963). This type of fusiform defect has been reported to occur with the severe forms of prune belly syndrome (Duckett, 1976) and in stillborns with cloacal anomalies (Stephens, 1963).

Shrom et al. (1981) presented five cases and a review of the literature that amply demonstrated that many of these patients had associated urologic anomalies. The most common was prune belly syndrome, whereas others included megaureter, megacystis, reflux, bladder diverticula, and renal hypodysplasia.

In the authors' experience, sepsis following radiographic instrumentation can occur, and therefore an excretory urography with a follow-up voiding film should be the first diagnostic test. Because of the risk of urethral contamination, retrograde urethrography should be avoided. A percutaneous bladder puncture with an antegrade voiding study offers a reasonable alternative. Systemic antibiotics are recommended during the diagnostic evaluation, and suppressive antibiotics are indicated for the long-term management of these patients. This is especially important in those patients who have associated urologic anomalies.

The repair of megalourethra can be satisfactorily achieved using a variety of hypospadias techniques in a one-stage repair as has been described by Nesbitt (1955). This frequently entails a circumscribing incision around the co-

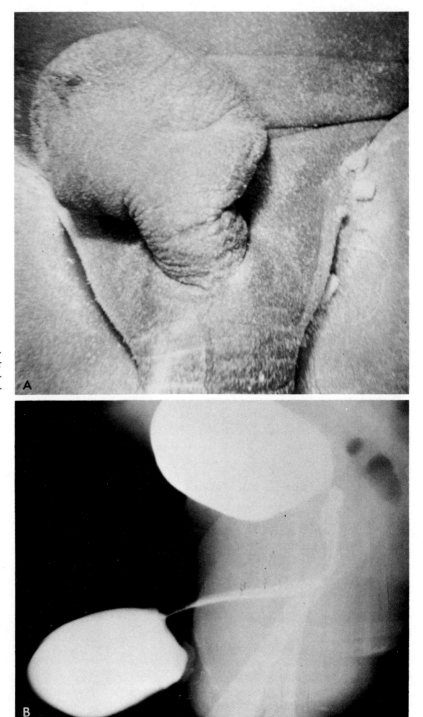

Figure 48–21. *A,* Scaphoid megalourethra in a baby with no other anomalies. *B,* Voiding cystourethrogram demonstrates large diverticulum without obstruction.

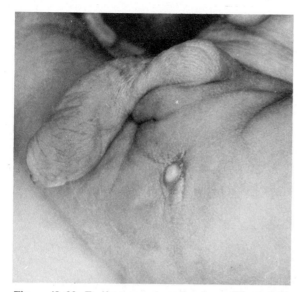

Figure 48–22. Fusiform megalourethra in a stillborn baby with the prune-belly syndrome and anorectal malformation. (From Kelalis, P. P., and King, L. R. (Eds.): Clinical Pediatric Urology. Philadelphia, W. B. Saunders Co., 1976.)

rona and degloving the penile skin to the base of the phallus. The redundant urethra is excised, and a new urethral tube is formed around a catheter using fine absorbable suture. The redundant penile skin is then excised and tailored to the cylindrical form of the phallus. Proximal diversion may be used. An alternative approach of marsupialization of the megalourethra with a subsequent second-stage procedure when the child is older may be considered.

URETHRAL GLANDS

Male

Numerous follicles situated in the submucosal tissues of the cavernous portion of the urethra are the glands of Littre. They generally serve to lubricate the urethra, especially during ejaculation. Occasionally, an orifice of the gland of Littre may become obstructed and form a small submucosal cyst, which is seldom obstructive but may cause voiding symptoms.

Along the urethra are a number of small recesses called lacunae, the largest of which, the lacuna magna, is in the fossa navicularis (valve of Guérin). Bellinger et al. (1983) reported 12 patients in whom this embryologic remnant was found who had dysuria and blood spotting occasionally. These symptoms were usually transient and subsided spontaneously. Occasionally, a minor surgical excision is necessary.

Female

The periurethral glands of Skene, which are the homolog of the male prostate, have their ducts open just inside the urethral meatus. Occasionally, ductal obstruction will lead to cyst formation, which may present at the urinary meatus. These cysts are seldom obstructive, and with drainage they may resolve. In the newborn, periurethral glands infrequently respond to maternal estrogens, enlarging at the urinary meatus (Fig. 48–23). They require no drainage and will resolve with time.

The Bartholin glands are on either side of the vaginal orifice and are the homolog of the bulbourethral glands in the male. Cyst or abscess formation can develop, especially in patients beyond the pediatric age group.

DISTAL URETHRAL STENOSIS IN YOUNG GIRLS

Therapy for girls with urinary tract infections has changed radically over the past three decades. At one time, bladder neck obstruction was the major point of concern, primarily because of the appearance of the urethra in radiographic voiding studies. Voiding radiographs frequently demonstrated a narrow collar at the bladder neck with ballooning of the urethra, known as the spinning top deformity. This was explained as poststenotic dilatation similar to that seen in vascular disease. Surgery on the bladder neck with Y-V plasties offered a cure rate of approximately 50 per cent.

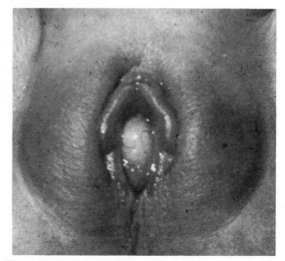

Figure 48–23. Enlarged periurethral gland bulging from the urethral meatus in a newborn.

As this explanation fell into disrepute, the dilatation seen on urethrography was explained as distal urethral stenosis. With recognition of a distal urethral ring (Lyon and Smith, 1963), this explanation seemed reasonable. The distal urethral ring, composed of collagen, is described as the narrowest segment of the lower urinary tract in the female child. Because of its relatively small diameter and its inflexibility, the ring has been thought to represent distal urethral stenosis. There is histologic support for this segment being the location at which both smooth and striated inner and outer layers of urethral musculature appear to insert into a dense, collagenous tissue ring situated just proximal to the external meatus (Lyon, 1974). However, as this concept was extensively studied, most radiologists and pediatric urologists concluded that it was impossible to identify urethral obstruction in the female on the basis of a urethrogram (Shopfner, 1967; Uehling and King, 1966).

Great emphasis has been placed on calibration of the female urethra. Immergut and Wahman (1968) calibrated urethras in a group of girls without urinary tract disease and established normal urethral measurements (the mean at 0 to 4 years was 15 F; at 5 to 9 years it was 17 F; at 10 to 14 years it was 21 F). In a further study (Graham et al., 1967), it was found that girls with urinary tract infections generally had average or even larger than average distal urethral rings on calibration. In the majority of cases, initial calibration has not been correlated with the degree of postoperative improvement in the child's symptoms following meatotomy, dilatation, or urethrotomy. The current consensus is that no "stenosis" comparable to a stricture exists.

Why, then, have the proponents of meatotomy, intermittent or single wide urethral dilatation, and urethrotomy all made similar claims of improvement in the incidence of infection, daytime and nighttime wetting, and voiding patterns (Halverstadt and Leadbetter, 1968; Kerr, 1969; Lyon, 1974; Vermillion et al., 1971)? Reports of smaller controlled studies generally do not support this claim (Forbes et al., 1969; Hendry et al., 1973; Kaplan et al., 1973). Kaplan et al. (1973) made a comparison of patients treated by dilatation, urethrotomy, and medication alone and found no difference among treatment methods. It is possible that some of those with longstanding recurrent infections were improved by dilatation techniques. Hendry et al. (1973) found no difference between children treated with medication alone and those treated by urethral dilatation plus medication. His group found that if some benefit from dilatation might be claimed, it would be for the group of children with uninhibited bladder contractions as determined by cystometric procedures.

It is evident from cystometric and pressure flow measurements that some bladder function abnormalities may be found in children with recurrent infections (Allen, 1978; Firlit et al., 1977). Whether these abnormalities are a consequence of the infection or a contributory cause is still uncertain. Some believe that measurement of the urethral pressure profile is more valuable than cystometry or flow studies. Tanagho et al. (1971) have shown that the high point of the pressure profile in the midurethra can be lowered by general anesthesia and abolished by curare. They postulate that an asynchronous contraction of the external sphincter occurs during detrusor contraction, causing an interruption of the stream. Local inflammation in the region of the external meatus could result in tenderness and spasm of the external sphincter. This would cause turbulent flow within the urethra, flushing bacteria from the region of the external meatus into the bladder. Minor external meatal inflammation might perpetuate recurrent infections, and overstretching of the sphincter would eliminate this spasm. This is analogous to dilatation of the anal sphincter, which generally improves spasm arising from anal fissures and proctitis.

Regardless of this continuing controversy over the treatment of young girls with recurrent infections and voiding problems, no appreciable harm has been noted from urethral dilatations up to 32 F. In addition, it is possible that some benefit may be derived from this procedure; however, repeated dilatations do not seem to have significant effect. Conversely, urethrotomy has led to incontinence in some cases and it is certainly more hazardous. Further, it generally requires a more lengthy hospitalization because of bleeding and does not seem to offer any greater benefit than urethral dilatation. Bladder neck surgery is rarely, if ever, needed. Lyon (1974) now refers to this condition as "symptomatic distal urethral ring" as opposed to "stenosis," which implies an organic abnormality.

It seems fair to conclude that the obstructive concept of distal urethral stenosis is no longer valid, but it may still be a cause of functional voiding disturbances. As Stephens (1972) has concluded, urethral dilatation in female children should be withheld from all except a small selected group who are refractory to other forms of medical treatment.

Ureteroceles Obstructing the Urethra

Occasionally, a ureterocele may act as an obstruction to the bladder outlet by prolapsing either into the posterior urethra in boys or through the urinary meatus in girls (Williams and Woodard, 1964). Cecoureteroceles, as described by Stephens (1971), may fill during voiding through their more proximal orifice and distend the suburethral portion of the ureterocele, causing urethral obstruction. It is more common to see urethral obstruction caused by a flap of residual mucosa following incomplete ureterocele excision. This can be ablated with transurethral resection.

Urethral Prolapse

Urethral prolapse is a circular eversion of the mucosa at the urethral meatus (Fig. 48–24). It occurs in premenarchal and postmenopausal patients. In the younger age group, a large majority of these patients are black. The prolapse is usually painless and presents as bloody vulval spotting. If urinary symptoms exist, they usually consist of mild frequency and slight dysuria. Suggested predisposing factors include

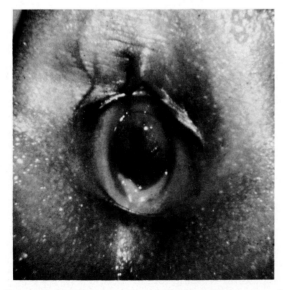

Figure 48–24. Urethral prolapse. Note the circular mucosal eversion.

increases in abdominal pressure as a result of coughing, straining to void, constipation, and trauma. The differential diagnosis includes prolapse of the bladder, ureterocele, ectopic ureter, urethral cysts, hydrometrocolpos, and sarcoma. Urethral prolapse is the only lesion in which a soft circular mass of tissue completely surrounds the urethral meatus.

Many treatments have been proposed for urethral prolapse (Richardson et al., 1982; Venable and Markland, 1982). In the past, a catheter has been placed and a ligature has been tied around the prolapsing tissue, which has been allowed to slough. This method is not recommended because of prolonged catheterization. Surgical excision with a circumscribing incision approximating normal mucosa to normal mucosa is still employed (Venable and Markland, 1982). In premenarchal children, conservative management consisting of antibiotics, estrogen cream, and sitz baths has been shown to be effective (Richardson et al., 1982). At this time, we recommend that this conservative treatment be instituted initially, with surgical intervention only if conservative measures fail.

Female Hypospadias

Hypospadias in girls is an uncommon abnormality. Generally, the vaginal introitus appears normal upon initial inspection, but the urethra is noted to be further recessed on the anterior vaginal wall. Frequently, this is first noticed when attempts are made to catheterize the patient. Symptoms are related to urinary tract infection and dribbling after urination secondary to vaginal pooling. Occasionally, more severe meatal stenosis and obstruction can occur. Normally, continence is maintained, though an infrequent patient with an extremely short urethra may have urinary leakage.

MEATAL STENOSIS IN THE MALE

For many years, stenosis of the external meatus in the male has carried grave implications in both pediatric and urologic disciplines. It is the authors' impression that congenital meatal stenosis is grossly overrated as a cause of obstructive uropathy in childhood.

Allen and Summers (1974) reported a 32 per cent incidence of meatal stenosis in 1800 boys 6 to 10 years of age who were diagnosed by clinical inspection alone. Morton (1963) reported on meatal size in 1000 circumcised boys using calibration by bougie à boule. Litvak et al. (1976) confirmed these results, in the same manner, in 200 boys with no urinary complaints. There was little correlation between visual observation and actual calibration.

It seems apparent that adequate criteria for the diagnosis of meatal stenosis are lacking. Congenital meatal stenosis in the uncircumcised boy is extremely rare; however, the meatus associated with all degrees of hypospadias often appears to be pinpoint. Acquired stenosis in the circumcised male comprises a membranous web running across the ventral portion of the meatus. It is frequently associated with a history of meatitis and perimeatal balanitis attributable to diaper irritation. Obstruction, with dorsal deflection of urinary flow, is noted in true meatal stenosis caused by this ventral web of tissue. A very forceful, fine stream, with a great casting distance, is characteristic. Mothers may complain of poor aim, wet bathrooms, and prolonged voiding times. The child may have to hold his penis down to direct the stream properly; the pendulous urethra may bulge ventrally. Burning, frequency, terminal hematuria or bloody spotting, and day and night wetting are complaints that may lead to the discovery of a small meatus, but they are not necessarily attributable to meatal stenosis.

Severe constrictions can be associated with hypospadias. At times, vesicoureteral reflux is found on cystourethrography (Mowad and Michaels, 1974). However, the previous implications that severe hydroureteronephrosis may be caused by congenital meatal stenosis (Campbell, 1951) are not upheld by current studies. Previously reported cases of such a cause-and-effect relationship can now be more properly evaluated with cystourethrography, urodynamics, and improved miniature endoscopic instruments.

Evaluation

The report on the extent of evaluation needed for meatal stenosis by Noe and Dale (1975) helps put it into logical perspective. Over a 5-year period, 280 male children with meatal stenosis were admitted to the hospital. An excretory urogram and cystoscopy were done on all patients, and 245 had a voiding cystourethrogram. When the diagnosis of meatal stenosis was made on visual inspection and not by calibration, less than 1 per cent of the total patients studied were found to have a surgically significant finding such as reflux or hydronephrosis. Five per cent of the total number of patients (13) had lesions of surgical significance on voiding cystourethrography. In all 13 patients, however, evidence of urinary tract infection was present. Only three patients had abnormalities detected on excretory urography and all three had urinary tract infections. Some investigators would say that these infections are the results of the meatal stenosis (Mahony, 1971).

This is not to say that the evaluation of meatal stenosis should be abandoned. A careful history, periodic assessment of urine cultures, and observation of the urinary stream by the urologist would, however, avoid a great number of unnecessary x-ray studies, hospitalizations, anesthesias, and cystoscopies with their attendant risks. Neither cystoscopy nor radiographic assessment is required for simple meatal stenosis.

Treatment

Meatotomy can usually be done very easily in the office with a cooperative boy, using 1 per cent lidocaine with 1:100,000 epinephrine as anesthetic placed into the ventral web with a 26-gauge or finer needle. Simple meatotomy is accomplished by crushing the ventral web with a hemostat to prevent the edges from bleeding. An incision is then made two thirds of the distance to the frenulum. The mother is instructed to separate the meatal edges twice daily to prevent them from healing back and to apply ointment to keep the edges from crusting and sticking. Sutures are occasionally required for bleeding but are not used routinely. Preliminary sedation or even general anesthesia may be required for the extremely apprehensive patient.

PHIMOSIS

Embryologically, the foreskin begins development during the eighth week of gestation as a thickening of the epidermis which eventually grows forward over the base of the glans penis. This process is completed by the 16th week of gestation, and the inner surface of the prepuce and the surface of the glans are adherent. For this reason, only 4 per cent of newborns have a fully retractable foreskin (Gairdner, 1949). As the child grows, the space between the glans and the foreskin develops such that by 6 months of age, 20 per cent can be retracted, and half of males 1 year of age have fully retractable foreskins. However, by age three years, 10 per cent of boys still have "physiologic" phimosis.

Since, in childhood, the foreskin cannot usually be retracted, it is important that parents learn to cleanse this area, as with all other areas. There is no need to forcibly retract the foreskin, and this practice should be condemned. Aside from unnecessary discomfort, it may lead to paraphimosis and balanitis and it can tear the prepuce, resulting in fibrosis and thickening. As the child grows, the foreskin will gradually become retractable and then the glans and foreskin should be cleansed on a routine basis. When symptomatic phimosis occurs after childhood, it generally presents with a thickened distal ring of foreskin that cannot be retracted. This can cause discomfort with voiding or sexual activity. Sometimes, fissures develop that are also painful. The treatment of choice is circumcision. Symptomatic phimosis occurs in approximately 10 per cent of all uncircumcised males.

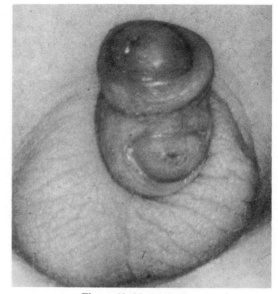

Figure 48–25. Diphallia.

CIRCUMCISION

The topic of nonritual circumcision has gained a great deal of attention. The American Academy of Pediatrics has stated that there is no valid medical indication for circumcision in the newborn period. Yet in the United States, an estimated 80 per cent of newborns are circumcised. Circumcision is not without complications. Gee and Ansell (1976) reviewed inpatient circumcision complications and found the overall incidence to be 0.2 per cent.

In the authors' opinion, there is no indication for neonatal circumcision, and further emphasis should be placed on the care of the normal foreskin.

DIPHALLIA

Duplications of the penis unassociated with exstrophy are extremely rare occurrences. A wide spectrum of this anomaly, including duplication of the glans (Johnson et al. 1974) to complete duplication of the phallus (Remzi, 1973) has been reported. Further, the penises may be equal or unequal in size and usually lie side by side, but they may lie one above the other (Fig. 48–25). Both may have a patent urethra or one may have a blind duct. Urine and semen may be expelled through one or both urethras. Either or both may be capable of erection. Varying degrees of hypospadias have been noted. Associated anomalies are common, including a bifid scrotum, a double bladder, renal and ureteral agenesis, ectopic kidney, supernumerary kidney, and occasionally diastasis of the symphysis pubis. Nonurologic anomalies may include imperforate anus, colon duplica-

tions, congenital heart disease, and myelomeningocele.

Embryologically, this deformity arises from either separation of the pubic tubercles, wherein each phallus will have only one corporal body and urethra, or cleavage of the pubic tubercle, wherein each phallus will have two corporal cavernosus bodies and urethras.

The treatment should be individualized to attain a good functional and cosmetic result.

CONCEALED (BURIED) PENIS

Occasionally, in obese infants or boys, the penis appears extremely short or absent because of fat deposits in the pubic area. Further inspection shows the penis to be of adequate length. Phimosis may coexist. Weight reduction is the treatment of choice. A concealed penis, as described by Johnston (1978), is a congenital abnormality wherein the skin is unattached to the penile shaft. Its treatment is effected by fixing the skin in the pubic area to the base of the penis.

WEBBED PENIS

Webbed penis is a condition in which a thin strip of scrotal skin extends well onto the ventrum of the penis (Fig. 48–26). It is asymptomatic except for its unacceptable cosmetic appearance and can be corrected by a simple division and closure.

PENILE AGENESIS

This very rare anomaly is usually associated with a normal scrotum and descended testes

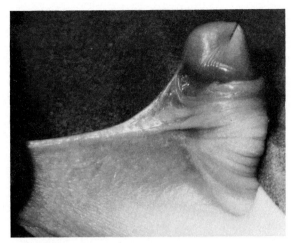

Figure 48–26. Webbed penis. Note the scrotal skin that extends to the frenulum.

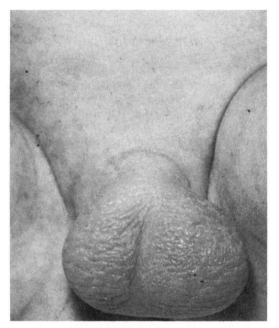

Figure 48–27. Penile agenesis.

(Fig. 48–27). It results from abnormal or absent development of the genital tubercle. Most cases have XY chromosomes, though Soderdahl et al. (1972) reported an XX-XY mosaic pattern. It frequently is associated with other coexisting congenital malformations, some of which are incompatible with life. The urethra generally opens on the perineum or just inside the anus and there may be associated anal skin tag.

Female gender assignment is recommended in the newborn period and elective orchiectomy should be performed prior to puberty.

CYSTS OF THE PENIS

The most common cause of cysts of the penis is entrapment of smegma beneath the nonretractable foreskin. Since the foreskin in young boys will naturally separate from the glans in time, there is no reason to express the smegma or forcibly retract the foreskin.

Mucoid cysts of the penis are rare lesions and have been reviewed by Cole and Helwig (1976). These lesions are generally found in the 15 to 35-year-old age group and most are asymptomatic. Cole and Helwig suggest that these mucoid cysts arise from ectopic urethral tissue, specifically within the periurethral glands. Most often, simple surgical excision is the recommended treatment.

Other types of cysts occurring on the penis include epidermal inclusions and sebaceous and dermoid cysts. Epidermal inclusion cysts are the most common, resulting from trapped epithelium secondary to penile surgery and circumcision. Sebaceous cysts can occur and are most prominent in the Tyson glands at the coronal margin. Dermal cysts are least common and represent congenital squamous rests. Each of these cysts can be treated with simple excision.

URETHRAL DUPLICATIONS

Classifications

A wide variety of urethral duplications occur. In general, they can be divided into cases in which the accessory channel presents on the dorsum of the penis, the ventrum of the penis, or the perineum. These can be further divided into those that are in the sagittal plane, which is most common, and those that occur side by side. In some cases, the accessory channel is complete, having a separate bladder opening and no communication with the more normal ventral urethra. In other circumstances, the accessory urethra is incomplete, either ending blindly or communicating with the urethra distal to the bladder neck (Gross and Moore, 1950; Das and Brosman, 1977; Woodhouse and Williams, 1979). On rare occasions, trifurcation of the urethra has been reported (Forgaard and Ansell, 1966; Wirtshafter et al., 1980).

Embryology

Effmann et al. (1976) noted along with others that dorsal duplications may have a widened symphysis pubis separation. This suggests that this may be a variant of epispadias, sharing its embryologic background. Stephens (1983) suggests that dorsal duplications may be a result of a shortfall of the mesoderm of the abdominal wall in its medial migration.

Ventral channel duplications originate from fusion errors of the genital folds and urethra plate (Stephens, 1983).

The ventral duplications in which a perineal urethra is present is known as a H-type fistula. Generally, both urethras are patent, though the majority of the urine passes through the perineal channel (Williams and Bloomberg, 1976). This H-type fistula results in the misalignment of the Tourneux fold and the Rathke component (Stephens, 1983).

Treatment

The treatment of these patients must be tailored to the individual and their specific complaints. A functional urethra should be the goal of the surgical therapy. Some cases of complete duplication with urinary incontinence require complete surgical excision, whereas milder cases of blind-ending duplications may require no treatment at all.

Female Urethral Duplications

Duplications of the female urethra are extremely uncommon. They present with a short phallus without chordee and a patent phallic urethra along with a patent vaginal urethral meatus. This is thought to result from posterior displacement of the müllerian duct termination in relationship to the urogenital sinus (Bellinger and Duckett, 1982). The treatment includes clitoral relocation and vaginoplasty with or without excision of the accessory urethra.

References

Allen, J. S., and Summers, J. L.: Meatal stenosis in children. J. Urol., 112:526, 1974.

Allen, T. D.: Urodynamic patterns in children with dysfunctional voiding problems. Trans. Am. Assoc. Genitourin. Surg., 69:12, 1978.

Andreassen, M.: Vesical neck obstruction in children. Acta Chir. Scand., 105:398, 1953.

Arnold, S. J., and Ginsburg, A.: Radiographic and photoendoscopic studies in posterior urethral valves in enuretic boys. Urology, 4:145, 1974.

Atwell, J. D.: Posterior urethral valves in the British Isles: a multicenter. B.A.P.S. Review. J. Pediatr. Surg., 18:70, 1983.

Bellinger, M. F., and Duckett, J. W.: Accessory phallic urethra in the female patient. J. Urol., 127:1159, 1982.

Bellinger, M. F., Purhoit, G. S., Duckett, J. W., and Cromie, W. J.: Lacuna magna: a hidden cause of dysuria and bloody spotting in boys. J. Pediatr. Surg., 18:163, 1983.

Blocksom, B.: Bladder pouch for prolonged tubeless cystostomy. J. Urol., 78:398, 1957.

Bodian, M.: Some observations of the pathology of congenital idiopathic bladder neck obstruction. Br. J. Urol., 29:393, 1957.

Campbell, M.: Clinical Pediatric Urology. Philadelphia, W.B. Saunders Co., 1951.

Campbell, M., and Harrison, J. H.: Urology. Vol. 1. Philadelphia, W.B. Saunders Co., 1970.

Cass, A. S., and Stephens, F. D.: Posterior urethral valves; diagnosis and management. J. Urol., 112:519, 1974.

Cendron, J., and Lepinard, V.: Maladie du col vésical chez l'enfant. Urol. Int., 27:355, 1972.

Cendron, J., Deburge, J. P., and Karlaftis, C.: Valvulae of the posterior urethra. J. Urol. Nephrol., 75:15, 1969.

Churchill, B. M., Fleisher, M. H., Kreuger, R., and Hardy, B. E.: Posterior urethral valves management. Dialogues Pediatr. Urol., 6:3, 1983.

Cobb, B. G., Wolf, J. A., Jr., and Ansell, J. S.: Congenital stricture of the proximal urethral bulb. J. Urol., 99:629, 1968.

Cole, L. A., and Helwig, E. B.: Muccoid cysts of the penile skin. J. Urol., 115:397, 1976.

Colodny, A. H., and Lebowitz, R. L.: Lesions of Cowper's ducts and glands in infants and children. Urology, 11:321, 1978.

Cooke, F. E., and Shaw, J. L.: Cystic anomalies of ducts of Cowper's glands. J. Urol., 85:659, 1961.

Cornil, C.: Urethral Obstruction in Boys. Amsterdam, Excerpta Medica, 1975.

Cornil, C.: Endoscopic diagnosis of posterior urethral valves. In Bergsma, D., and Duckett, J. W. (Eds.): Urinary System Malformations in Children. New York, Alan R. Liss, 1977.

Cornil, C., and Bakker, N. J.: Treatment of congenital valves of the posterior urethra in children. Ann. Chir. Inf., 12:215, 1971.

Cromie, W. J., and Williams, D. I.: "Ring" ureterostomy. Br. J. Urol., 47:789, 1975.

Crooks, K. K.: The protean aspects of posterior urethral valves. J. Urol., 126:763, 1981.

Crooks, K. K.: Urethral strictures following transurethral resection of posterior urethral valves. J. Urol., 127:1153, 1982.

Currarino, G.: Diverticulum of prostatic urethra developing postoperatively from stump of congenital recto-urethral fistula. Am. J. Roentgenol., 106:211, 1969.

Currarino, G., and Fuqua, F.: Cowper's glands in the urethrogram. Am. J. Roentgenol. Rad. Ther. Nucl. Med., 116:838, 1972.

Das, S., and Brosman, S. A.: Duplication of the male urethra. J. Urol., 117:452, 1977.

Devereaux, M. H., and Williams, D. I.: The treatment of urethral stricture in boys. J. Urol., 108:489, 1972.

Dorairajan, T.: Defects of spongy tissue and congenital diverticula of the penile urethra. Aust. N.Z. J. Surg., 32:209, 1963.

Downs, R. A.: Congenital polyps of the prostatic urethra: a review of the literature and report of two cases. Br. J. Urol., 42:76, 1970.

Duckett, J. W.: Current management of posterior urethral valves. Urol. Clin. North Am. 1:471, 1974a.

Duckett, J. W.: Cutaneous vesicostomy in infants and children. Urol. Clin. North Am., 1:484, 1974b.

Duckett, J. W.: The prune belly syndrome. In Kelalis, P. P., King, L. R., and Belman, A. B. (Eds.): Clinical Pediatric Urology. Philadelphia, W. B. Saunders Co., 1976, p. 615.

Edling, N. P.: The radiologic appearance of diverticula of the male cavernous urethra. Acta. Radiol., 40:1, 1953.

Effmann, E. L., Lebowitz, R. L., and Colodny, A. H.: Duplication of the urethra. Radiology, 119:179, 1976.

Egami, K., and Smith, E. D.: A study of the sequelae of posterior urethral valves. J. Urol., 127:84, 1982.

Eklof, O., and Ringertz, H.: Pre- and postoperative urography: findings in posterior urethral valves. Pediatr. Radiol., *4*:43, 1975.

Ericsson, N. O.: Posterior urethral valves. *In* Bergsma, D., and Duckett, J. W. (Eds.): Urinary System Malformations in Children. New York, Alan R. Liss, 1977.

Field, P. L., and Stephens, F. D.: Congenital urethral membranes causing urethral obstruction. J. Urol., *111*:250, 1974.

Firlit, C. F., and King, L. R.: Anterior urethral valves in children. J. Urol., *108*:972, 1972.

Firlit, R. S., Firlit, C. F., and King, L. R.: Obstructing anterior urethral valves in children. J. Urol., *119*:819, 1978.

Firlit, C. F., Smey, P., Cook, W., and King, L. R.: Micturition urodynamic flow studies in children. J. Urol., *119*(2):250, 1978.

Forbes, P. A., Drummond, K. A., and Nogrady, M. B.: Meatotomy in girls with meatal stenosis and urinary tract infection. J. Pediatr., *75*:937, 1969.

Forgaard, D. M., and Ansell, J. S.: Trifurcation of the anterior urethra: a case report. J. Urol., *95*:785, 1966.

Gairdner, D.: The fate of the foreskin: a study of circumcision. Br. Med. J., *2*:1433, 1949.

Gee, W. F., and Ansell, J. S.: Neonatal circumcision: a ten-year overview: with comparison of the Gomco clamp and the plastibell device. Pediatrics, *58*:824, 1976.

Glassberg, K. I., Schneider, M., Haller, J. O., Moll, D., and Waterhouse, K.: Observations on persistently dilated ureter after posterior urethral valve ablation. Urology, *20*:20, 1982.

Graham, J. B., King, L. R., Kroop, K. A., and Uehling, D. T.: The significance of distal urethral narrowing in young girls. J. Urol., *97*:1045, 1967.

Greenfield, S. P., Hensle, T. W., Berdon, W. E., and Geringer, A. M.: Urinary extravasation in the newborn male with posterior urethral valves. J. Pediatr. Surg., *17*:751, 1982.

Gross, R. E., and Bill, A. H., Jr.: Concealed diverticulum of the male urethra as a cause of urinary obstruction. Pediatrics, *1*:44, 1948.

Gross, R. E., and Moore, T. C.: Duplication of the urethra. Arch. Surg., *60*:749, 1950.

Halverstadt, D. B., and Leadbetter, G. W.: Internal urethrotomy and recurrent urinary tract infection in female children. I. Results in the management of infection. J. Urol., *100*:297, 1968.

Harshman, M. W., Cromie, W. J., Wein, A. J., and Duckett, J. W.: Urethral stricture disease in children. J. Urol., *126*:650, 1981.

Hendren, W. H.: A new approach to infants with severe obstructive uropathy: early complete reconstruction. J. Pediatr. Surg., *5*:184, 1970.

Hendren, W. H.: Posterior urethral valves in boys, a broad clinical spectrum. J. Urol., *106*:298, 1971.

Hendren, W. H.: Complications of urethral valve surgery. *In:* Smith, R. B., and Skinner, D. G. (Eds.): Complications of Urologic Surgery. Philadelphia, W. B. Saunders Co., 1976, p. 303.

Hendry, W. F., Stanton, S. L., and Williams, D. I.: Recurrent urinary infections in girls: effects of urethral dilation. Br. J. Urol., *45*:72, 1973.

Henneberry, M. O., and Stephens, F. D.: Renal hypoplasia and dysplasia in infants with posterior urethral valves. J. Urol., *123*:912, 1980.

Hoover, D. L., and Duckett, J. W.: Posterior urethral valves, unilateral reflux and renal dysplasia: a syndrome. J. Urol., *128*:994, 1982.

Immergut, M. A., and Wahman, G. E.: The urethral caliber of female children with recurrent urinary tract infections. J. Urol., *99*:189, 1968.

Immergut, M. A., Jacobson, J. J., Culp, D. A., and Flocks, R. H.: Cutaneous pyelostomy. J. Urol., *101*:276, 1969.

Johnson, C. F., Carlton, C. E., and Powell, N. B.: Duplication of penis. Urology, *4*:722, 1974.

Johnston, J. H.: Temporary cutaneous ureterostomy in the treatment of advanced congenital urinary obstruction. Arch. Dis. Child. *38*:161, 1963.

Johnston, J. H.: Posterior urethral valves: an operative technique using an electric auriscope. J. Pediatr. Surg., *1*:583, 1966.

Johnston, J. H.: Other penile anomalies. *In* Eckstein, H. B., Hohenfellner, R., and Williams, D. I. (Eds.): Surgical Pediatric Urology. Philadelphia, W. B. Saunders Co., 1978.

Johnston, J. H., and Kulatilake, A. E.: Posterior urethral valves: Results in sequela. *In* Johnston, J. H., and Scholtmeijer, R. J., (Eds.): Problems in Pediatric Urology. Amsterdam, Excerpta Medica, 1972, p. 161.

Kaplan, G. W., and Brock, W. A.: Urethral strictures in children. J. Urol., *129*:1200, 1983.

Kaplan, G. W., and King, L. R.: Vesical neck. *In* Kelalis, P. P., King, L. R., and Belman, A. B. (Eds.): Clinical Pediatric Urology. Philadelphia, W. B. Saunders Co., 1976, p. 292.

Kaplan, G. W., Picconi, J. R., and Schuhrke, T. D.: Posterior approach to mullerian duct and seminal vesical cysts. *In:* Transactions of the International Pediatric Urological Seminar. New York, Alan R. Liss, 1977.

Kaplan, G. W., Sammons, T. A., and King, L.: A blind comparison of dilatation, urethrotomy and medication alone in the treatment of urinary tract infection in girls. J. Urol., *109*:917, 1973.

Kelalis, P. P.: Anterior urethra. *In* Kelalis, P. P., King, L. R., and Belman, A. B. (Eds.): Clinical Pediatric Urology. Philadelphia, W. B. Saunders Co., 1976, p. 328.

Kerr, W.: Results of internal urethrotomy in female patients with ureteral stenoses. J. Urol., *102*:449, 1969.

Kjellberg, S. R., Ericsson, N. O., and Rudhe, U.: The Lower Urinary Tract in Childhood. Chicago, Yearbook Medical Publishers, 1957, p. 272.

Krueger, R. P., Hardy, B. E., and Churchill, B. M.: Growth in boys with posterior urethral valves. Primary valve resection vs. upper tract diversion. Urol. Clin. North Am., *7*:265, 1980.

Lich, R., Jr., Maurer, J. E., and Burdon, S.: Retropubic approach to vesical neck pathology in children. Br. J. Urol., *22*:21, 1950.

Litvak, A. S., Morris, J. D., and McRoberts, J. W.: Normal size of the urethral meatus in male children. J. Urol., *115*:736, 1976.

Lome, L. G., Howat, J. M., and Williams, D. I.: The temporarily defunctionalized bladder in children. J. Urol., *108*:469, 1972.

Lyon, R. P.: Distal urethral stenosis. *In* Reviews in Pediatric Urology. New York, American Elsevier Pub. Co., 1974, p. 1.

Lyon, R. P., and Smith, D. R.: Distal urethral stenosis. J. Urol., *89*:414, 1963.

Mackie, G. G., and Stephens, F. D.: Duplex kidneys: a correlation of renal dysplasia with position of the ureteral orifice. J. Urol., *114*:274, 1975.

Mahony, D. T.: Studies on enuresis. I. Incidence of obstructive lesions and pathophysiology of enuresis. J. Urol., *106*:951, 1971.

Mahony, D. T., et al.: Congenital posterior urethral valves in adult males. Urology, *3*:724, 1974.

Maizels, M., Stephens, F. D., King, L. R., and Firlit, C.

F.: Cowper's syringocele: a classification of dilatations of Cowper's gland duct based upon clinical characteristics of eight boys. J. Urol., *129*:111, 1983.

Marion, G.: Surgery of the neck of the bladder. Br. J. Urol., *5*:351, 1933.

McGuire, E. J., and Weiss, R. M.: Secondary bladder neck obstruction in patients with urethral valves: Treatment with phenoxybenzamine. Urology, *5*:756, 1975.

Milliken, L. D., et al.: Renal dysplasia and urethral valves. J. Urol., *108*:960, 1972.

Mitchell, M. E.: Persistent ureteral dilatation following valve resection. Dialogues in Pediatr. Urol., *5*:8, 1982.

Mitchell, M. E., and Garrett, R. A.: Perirenal urinary extravasation associated with urethral valves in infants. J. Urol., *124*:688, 1980.

Monfort, G., et al.: Valves of posterior urethra in boys. Ann. Chir. Inf., *17*:15, 1976.

Morton, H. G.: Meatus size in 1000 circumcised children from two weeks to sixteen years of age. J. Fla. Med. Assoc., *50*:137, 1963.

Mowad, J. J., and Michaels, M. M.: Meatal stenosis associated with vesicoureteral reflux in boys. Management of 25 cases. J. Urol., *3*:100, 1974.

Myers, D. A., and Walker, R. D.: Prevention of urethral strictures in the management of posterior urethral valves. J. Urol., *126*:655, 1981.

Nesbitt, T. E.: Congenital megalourethra. J. Urol., *73*:839, 1955.

Noe, H. N., and Dale, G. A.: Evaluation of children with meatal stenosis. J. Urol., *114*:455, 1975.

Ochsner, M. G., Burns, E., and Henry, H. H.: Incidence of retrograde ejaculation following bladder neck revision as a child. J. Urol., *104*:596, 1970.

Osathanondh, V., and Potter, E. L.: Pathogenesis of polycystic kidneys. Arch. Pathol., *77*:459, 1964.

Parkkulainen, K. V.: Posterior urethral obstruction; valvular or diaphragmatic? *In* Bergsma, D., and Duckett, J. W. (Eds.): Urinary System Malformations in Childhood. New York, Alan R. Liss, 1977.

Perlmutter, A. D.: Temporary urinary diversion in the management of the chronically dilated urinary tract in childhood. *In* Reviews in Pediatric Urology, p. 447. New York, American Elsevier Publishing Co., 1974.

Perlmutter, A. D., and Tank, E. S.: Loop cutaneous ureterostomy in infancy. J. Urol., *99*:559, 1968.

Rabinowitz, R., Barkin, M., Schillinger, J. F., Jeffs, R. D., and Cook, G. T.: Upper tract management when posterior urethral valve ablation is insufficient. J. Urol., *122*:370, 1979.

Remzi, D.: Diphallia. Urology, *1*:462, 1973.

Richardson, D. A., Hajj, S. N., and Herbst, A. L.: Medical treatment of urethral prolapse in children. Obstet. Gynecol., *59*:69, 1982.

Robertson, W. B., and Hayes, J. A.: Congenital diaphragmatic obstruction of the male posterior urethra. Br. J. Urol., *41*:592, 1969.

Rudhe, U., and Ericsson, N. O.: Congenital urethral diverticula. Ann. Radiol., *13*:289, 1970.

Shopfner, C. E.: Roentgen evaluation of distal urethral obstruction. Radiology, *88*:222, 1967.

Shrom, S. H., Cromie, W. J., and Duckett, J. W.: Megalourethra. Urology, *17*:152, 1981.

Smith, D. R.: Critique on the concept of vesical neck obstruction in children. J.A.M.A., *207*:1686, 1969.

Snyder, H. M., Kalichman, M. A., Charney, E., and Duckett, J. W.: Vesicostomy for neurogenic bladder with spina bifida: follow-up. J. Urol., *130*:724, 1983.

Sober, I.: Pelvio-ureterostomy-en-Y. J. Urol., *107*:473, 1972.

Soderdahl, D. W., Brosman, S. A., and Goodwin, W. E.: Penile agenesis. J. Urol., *108*:496, 1972.

Spence, H. M., Murphy, J. J., McGovern J. H., Hendren, W. H., and Pryles, C. V.: Urinary tract infections in infants and children. J. Urol., *91*:23, 1964.

Stephens, F. D.: Congenital malformations of the rectum, anus and genitourinary tract. London, E. & S. Livingston Co., 1963.

Stephens, F. D.: Caeco-ureterocele and concepts on the embryology and aetiology of ureterocele. Aust. N.Z. J. Surg., *40*:239, 1971.

Stephens, F. D.: Urologic aspects of recurrent urinary tract infections in children. J. Pediatr., *80*:725, 1972.

Stephens, F. D.: Congenital intrinsic lesions of the posterior urethra. *In* Congenital Malformations of the Urinary Tract. New York, Praeger Pub., 1983, p. 95.

Tanagho, E. A., Miller, E. R., Lyon, R. P., and Fisher, R.: Spastic striated external sphincter and urinary tract infection in girls. Br. J. Urol., *43*:69, 1971.

Turner-Warwick, R. T., Whiteside, G., Worth, P., Milroy, E., and Bates, P.: A urodynamic view of the clinical problems associated with bladder neck dysfunction. Br. J. Urol., *45*:25, 1973.

Uehling, D. T., and King, L. R.: Limitations in the diagnostic value of the voiding cystourethrogram. J. Pediatr. *69*:744, 1966.

Venable, D. D., and Markland, C.: Urethral prolapse in girls. South. Med. J., *75*:951, 1982.

Vermillion, D. D., Halverstadt, D. B., and Leadbetter, G. W., Jr.: Internal urethrotomy and recurrent urinary tract infection in female children. II. Long-term results in the management of infection. J. Urol., *106*:154, 1971.

Whitaker, R. H.: Methods of assessing obstruction in dilated ureters. Br. J. Urol., *45*:15, 1973a.

Whitaker, R. H.: The ureter in posterior urethral valves. Br. J. Urol., *45*:395, 1973b.

Whitaker, R. H., Keeton, J. E., and Williams, D. I.: Posterior urethral valves: a study of urinary control after operation. J. Urol., *108*:167, 1972.

Williams, D. E., and Bloomberg, S.: Bifid urethra with preanal accessory tract (Y duplication). Br. J. Urol., *47*:877, 1976.

Williams, D. I.: Urology in Childhood. New York, Springer Verlag, 1974, p. 196.

Williams, D. I.: Urethral valves: a hundred cases with hydronephrosis. *In* Bergsma, D., and Duckett, J. W. (Eds.): Urinary System Malformations in Children. New York, Alan R. Liss, 1977.

Williams, D. I., and Retik, A. B.: Congenital valves and diverticula of the anterior urethra. Br. J. Urol., *41*:228, 1969.

Williams, D. I., and Woodard, J. R.: Complications of ectopic ureterocele. J. Urol., *92*:635, 1964.

Williams, D. I., et al.: Urethral valves. Br. J. Urol., *45*:200, 1973.

Wirtshafter, A., Carrion, H. M., Morillo, G., and Pollitano, V. A.: Complete trifurcation of the urethra. J. Urol., *123*:431, 1980.

Woodhouse, C. R. J., and Williams, D. I.: Duplications of the lower urinary tract in children. Br. J. Urol., *51*:481, 1979.

Young, B. W.: The retropubic approach to vesical neck obstruction in children. Surg. Gynecol. Obstet., *96*:150, 1953.

Young, B. W.: Lower Urinary Tract Obstruction in Childhood. Philadelphia, Lea & Febiger, 1972.

Young, B. W., and Goebel, J. L.: Retropubic wedge excision in congenital vesical neck obstruction. Stanford Med. Bull., *12*:106, 1954.

Young, H. H., Frontz, W. A., and Baldwin, J. C.: Congenital obstruction of the posterior urethra. J. Urol., *3*:289, 1919.

CHAPTER 49

Vesicoureteral Reflux, Megaureter, and Ureteral Reimplantation

LOWELL R. KING, M.D.
SELWYN B. LEVITT, M.D.

VESICOURETERAL REFLUX

The recognition of vesicoureteral reflux as an abnormal phenomenon in man, often associated with urinary infection and with both developmental and acquired renal abnormalities, has led to the study of the embryology, anatomy, and physiology of the ureterovesical junction. From a gradual understanding of the causes, consequences, and natural history of vesicoureteral reflux, generally accepted principles of patient management have evolved. The gap has narrowed between the proponents of surgical and "conservative" (i.e., nonoperative) management of patients with reflux. Specific indications for antireflux surgery have been defined, and surgical techniques have been improved to the point at which operative correction, when necessary, is relatively safe and reliable. New renal scars are encountered in only about 3 per cent of patients with uncomplicated reflux, whether they are treated by early surgery or by surveillance until the reflux stops with growth.

Historical Perspective

Semblinow observed reflux of urine stained with methylene blue from the bladder into the ureters of both dogs and rabbits in 1883. Pozzi reported the first case of vesicoureteral reflux in humans in 1893. He noted the appearance of urine from the distal end of a ureter divided during a transabdominal gynecologic procedure. In experiments with human cadavers, Young was unable to make urine flow backward from the bladder into the ureter, irrespective of the pressure used in filling (1898). In 1929, Gruber noted that the structure of the trigone and ureterovesical junction varied in different animal species and that the incidence of vesicoureteral reflux varied directly with the length of the intravesical ureter and the muscular development of the trigone. Kretschmer (1916) and Bumpus (1924) presented early observations on the clinical use of cystography and the occurrence of vesicoureteral reflux.

Partly because reflux is normal in many mammals, its presence in humans was not always considered to be abnormal until Hutch (1958) convincingly demonstrated that acquired periureteral diverticula commonly resulted in reflux, which led to renal damage from hydronephrosis or supraimposed infection. The cystogram came into general use as a clinical tool through the 1950's, and with it the recognition that reflux was not uncommon and had several specific causes.

Anatomy and Function of the Ureter

The ureter is a muscular conduit that contracts in response to the stretch reflex to transport a bolus of urine to the bladder. Distally, it passes through a hiatus in the posterolateral

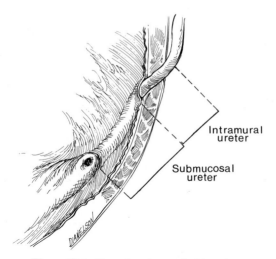

Figure 49–1. Normal ureterovesical junction.

aspect of the bladder wall. The long spiral muscle fibers of the ureter, which transmit peristaltic waves, terminate at this point, and only longitudinal muscle fibers continue in the intravesical ureter, covered by bladder mucosa and buttressed by the underlying detrusor muscle. As the intravesical ureter passes from the hiatus to its orifice, the longitudinal muscle fibers decussate, passing medially to form Mercier's bar and inferiorly to form Bell's muscle, the borders of the superficial trigone. Thus, the

musculature of the ureter and the trigone is in continuity because the ureteral muscular coat passes through the hiatus and fans out on the floor of the bladder to form the superficial trigone (Figs. 49–1 and 49–2).

The adventitia of the juxtavesical ureter is composed of a superficial and a deep periureteral sheath, the former derived from the bladder and the latter derived from the ureter. A plane of cleavage occupied by loose connective tissue, the space of Waldeyer, separates the superficial from the deep periureteral sheath (Fig. 49–3).

When a bolus of urine passes down the ureter, several factors operate to facilitate its passage through the intravesical segment into the bladder. The longitudinal muscle of the intravesical ureter contracts as the bolus presents at the hiatus. This shifts the orifice cranially and laterally toward the hiatus, shortening and widening the intravesical ureter and reducing resistance to the passage of the bolus into the lumen of the bladder.

After the bolus has passed the intravesical ureter, the intrinsic ureteral musculature relaxes, permitting the intravesical ureter to resume its resting configuration beneath the bladder mucosa. The intravesical ureter is a delicate structure. The low pressure normally present in the resting bladder (8 to 15 mm Hg) is sufficient

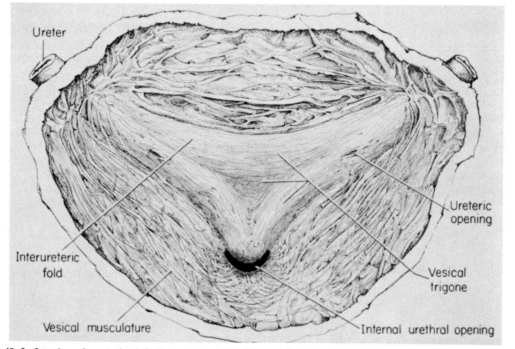

Figure 49–2. Interior of posterior-inferior portion of bladder; vesical trigone, ureteric and urethral apertures. (From Woodburne, R. T.: J. Urol., 92:431, 1964.)

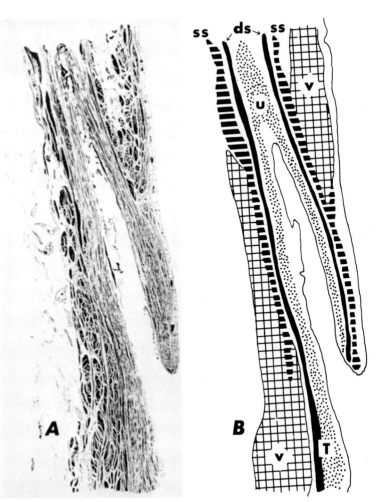

Figure 49–3. Ureterovesical junction in longitudinal section. *A,* Photomicrograph. *B,* Diagrammatic representation. Ureteral muscularis *(u)* is surrounded by superficial *(ss)* and deep *(ds)* periureteral sheaths, which extend in roof of submucosal segment and continue beyond orifice into trigonal muscle *(T).* Relationship of superficial sheath to vesical muscularis *(v)* is clearly seen. Transverse fascicles in superior lip of ureteral orifice belong to superficial and deep sheaths. No true space can be seen separating ureter from bladder. Plane between the two sheaths is occupied by loose connective tissue. Modified trichrome stain, reduced from ×9 (muscle, black; connective tissue, gray). Diagram was drawn by tracing muscular elements of 12 serial sections, including section shown in photomicrograph. (From Elhadaiwi, A.: J. Urol., *107*:224, 1972.)

to passively compress the roof of the intravesical ureter against the underlying detrusor to prevent reflux; peristaltic pressure in the extravesical ureter, between 20 and 35 mm Hg, is sufficient to propel a bolus of ureteral urine rapidly and forcefully into the bladder in an abrupt spurt. Thus, normal compliance and elasticity of the intravesical ureter are crucial, and inflammation of the overlying bladder mucosa may alter the function of the ureterovesical junction significantly.

Critical to the normal absence of reflux in man are the length of the intravesical ureter relative to its diameter and the intrinsic longitudinal muscular coat of the submucosal ureter that inserts onto the superficial trigone (Paquin, 1959) (Fig. 49–4). These factors are reflected in the appearance of the ureteral orifice, described by Lyon et al. (1969) as normally resembling a cone, but sometimes resembling a stadium, horseshoe, or golf hole with increasing tendency toward laterality and reflux (Fig. 49–5).

Ambrose and Nicolson (1962), Stephens and Lenaghan (1962), and others also noted that as the orifice becomes more abnormal in appearance, it usually occupies a more lateral position (ureteral ectopia lateralis), and more of the intravesical ureter is missing. As a result, the more lateral the orifice, the more likely it is that reflux will occur. Such reflux is congenital and often familial and has been termed primary reflux (Garrett et al., 1963).

It is important to realize that reflux is a radiographic sign (typically detected by instilling radiographic contrast material into the bladder), which can be caused by one of several different mechanisms (Table 49–1). For example, lack of an adequate detrusor buttress under the intravesical ureter may result in reflux. If the ureterovesical junction is of marginal competence intrinsically, infection may reduce the compliance of the roof of the intravesical ureter and permit reflux to occur. Although such reflux is often transient or inconsistent, it must be

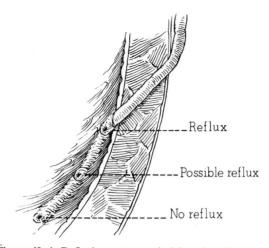

Figure 49–4. Refluxing ureterovesical junction. Same anatomic features as nonrefluxing orifice, except for inadequate length of intravesical submucosal ureter, are shown. Some orifices reflux intermittently with borderline submucosal tunnels. (From Glenn, J. (Ed.): Urologic Surgery. 2nd ed. New York, Harper & Row, 1975.)

understood and recognized as such so that it can be categorized in each patient, for this will have major therapeutic implications, particularly in deciding whether operative correction is likely to be needed.

Incidence and Epidemiology of Reflux

The incidence of reflux in individuals without urologic symptoms is quite low, varying from 0 to 2 per cent in reported series, including premature infants and adults of both sexes (Estes and Brooks, 1970; Gibson, 1949; Leadbetter et al., 1960; Lich et al., 1964; McGovern et al., 1960; Peters et al., 1967; Ransley, 1978). Such studies suggest that the incidence of reflux in healthy children is less than 1 per cent.

When urinary infection is the reason for investigation, reflux has been discovered in 20 to 50 per cent of children (Walker et al., 1977; Shopfner, 1970; Smellie and Normand, 1966. In children with urinary tract infection the prevalence of reflux seems directly proportional to age (Smellie, 1975b; Baker et al., 1966). Infants in particular seem prone to develop reflux in association with infection. With growth, the submucosal ureter elongates and the ratio between the length and diameter of the submucosal tunnel increases (King, 1976; Stephens, 1976; Lenaghan et al., 1976), making noncompliance of the valve mechanism less likely as a cause of reflux.

There is a high prevalence of reflux in

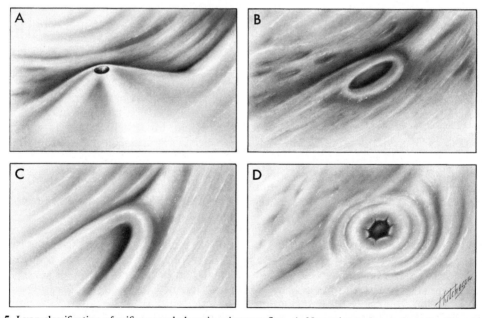

Figure 49–5. Lyon classification of orifice morphology in primary reflux. *A,* Normal or volcano-shaped orifice at cystoscopy by the right-angle lens system. *B,* Stadium orifice. Usually slightly more lateral than the normal orifice, and sometimes associated with reflux. The intravesical ureter, however, is usually well developed, and reflux associated with such orifices will usually stop with growth. *C,* Horseshoe orifice. Part or most of the intravesical ureter is represented by the longitudinal muscle in the ridges above and below the orifice. The proximal submucosal ureter may be well fused but is usually short, and reflux will often persist, at least for several years. *D,* A golf-hole orifice is most lateral in position and lacks any vestige of an intravesical ureter. Associated reflux is quite persistent and usually continues after full growth is achieved. (From Kelalis, P. P., and King, L. R. (Eds.): Clinical Pediatric Urology. Philadelphia, W. B. Saunders Co., 1976.)

TABLE 49–1. CAUSES OF REFLUX

Primary Cause	Mechanisms Resulting in Reflux
Short or absent intravesical ureter (Synonyms: primary reflux; ureteral ectopia lateralis; gaping or golf-hole orifice)	End on opening between ureter and bladder
Absence of adequate detrusor buttress	Congenital paraureteral bladder diverticulum Acquired paraureteral diverticulum (urethral obstruction) Weak and thin detrusor, as in flaccid neurogenic bladder or closed exstrophy
Cystitis-inflammation of the intravesical ureter	Alone, this probably rarely results in reflux, but it operates with any of the factors listed above when the ureterovesical junction is of marginal competence
Ectopic ureter High intravesical pressure Iatrogenic reflux	Mechanisms described in text

siblings of children with known reflux. Dwoskin (1976) found reflux in approximately 30 per cent of siblings. In a review by Jenkins and Noe (1982), 104 siblings of 78 patients with reflux were screened by cystogram without anesthesia. Twenty-four (33 per cent) were found to have reflux. Seventy-three per cent of this group had no history of infection or any abnormal voiding symptoms. Reflux was more likely to occur in the siblings of patients with urographic evidence of renal damage, irrespective of the sex of the patient. Prevalence of both reflux and renal scarring is therefore estimated to be at least ten times greater in siblings of school-aged children with known reflux than in an unselected age-matched population (Lancet editorial, 1978).

A review of 88 families at Christchurch Hospital revealed increased frequency of the genes HLA A9 and B12 in patients with end-stage renal disease due to renal scarring associated with reflux (Bailey and Wallace, 1978). In addition, Torres et al. (1980a), have found HLA B8 and BW15 more frequently in such patients. These genes may become "markers" for reflux. However, the pattern of genetic transmission remains undetermined. Most investigators favor a polygenic or multifactorial mode of inheritance (King, 1976; Lancet editorial, 1982). However, an autosomal dominant or sex-linked mode of inheritance is suggested in some families (Lewy and Belman, 1975). Also of interest from a genetic standpoint is the observation that reflux is perhaps only one tenth as common in black American girls with infection compared with white girls (Askari and Belman, 1981).

It is also apparent that reflux can be intermittent, unilateral, or bilateral. Failure to demonstrate reflux during a single cystogram does not preclude its presence. Conversely, the observation of minor degrees of transient reflux on a single examination is of limited significance.

Diagnosis of Reflux

Reflux can be detected at the time of cystoscopy by filling the bladder with a solution containing methylene blue or indigo carmine and then noting the color of the efflux from each ureteral orifice after the bladder is emptied and refilled with clear sterile water (Amar, 1966). Advanced sonographic techniques can also be used to detect severe reflux, as the ureter will appear more dilated during and immediately after voiding.

Reflux may be suspected from the appearance of the kidneys and ureters on intravenous pyelography. In particular, a dilated lower ureter, a ureter visible for its entire length, ureteral or pelvic striations from redundant mucosa, vascular markings on the ureter, hydronephrosis, calyceal distortion, and renal scarring may be clues to the presence of vesicoureteral reflux or its existence in the past. With the aid of fluoroscopy during voiding after intravenous pyelography, it is often possible to detect vesicoureteral reflux with a high degree of certainty. However, retrograde cystography remains the most sensitive and accurate study to detect or exclude reflux.

CYSTOGRAPHY

Cystography is performed prior to intravenous pyelography in order to avoid confusion about the source of contrast material in the upper tracts. Cystography involves the insertion of a catheter into the bladder after a preliminary radiograph of the abdomen has been obtained; the bladder is filled with a radiopaque solution from a drip chamber approximately 60 to 80 cm above the pubic symphysis. Radiographs are taken in the supine position and the right and left lateral oblique projections. Additional films are exposed during and after voiding. Fluoroscopy and modern cineradiographic equipment facilitate the voiding portion of the study and maximize the amount of information obtainable. In particular, observation of the presence of posterior urethral valves and dynamic changes in the configuration of ureteroceles, bladder diverticula, and ureteral duplications during voiding are critical to proper patient management when these related anomalies are present.

Variations in the technique of cystography are numerous. Delayed films are useful when reflux is intermittent or when the patient is unable to void during the examination. Expression cystography under anesthesia may demonstrate reflux in patients who do not show reflux while awake (Woodard and Filardi, 1976) and vice versa (Vlahakis et al., 1971; Timmons et al., 1977). Timmons found that in 23 of 67 refluxing ureters, reflux was detected only with the patient awake; in five instances, however, reflux was detected only with the child anesthetized. Depending upon the filling pressure and volume, reflux under anesthesia may not be representative of the usual behavior of the ureterovesical junction being studied. Various anesthetic agents may influence bladder tone and capacity (Doyle and Briscoe, 1976). Nevertheless, this technique can be useful in the uncooperative patient.

A distinction is often made between reflux occurring during the filling phase and that seen only during voiding. The implication is that reflux seen only during voiding is occurring at higher intravesical pressures and is therefore less likely to be associated with a relatively severe degree of derangement of the ureterovesical junction than is reflux seen in the filling phase. Because the child is in very abnormal surroundings during cystography, however, this is not necessarily the case. The patient is likely to contract the bladder to resist filling, and usually he or she then can develop a high intravesical pressure—higher than that at which voiding normally occurs if no urethral obstruction is present. Conway and Kruglik (1976), using isotope techniques of cystography in which the entire urinary tract is visualized throughout the examination, found that reflux occurring only during the filling phase is three times as common as reflux occurring only during the voiding phase. Thus, the pressure is higher during the filling phase in many patients. Unless the intravesical pressure is monitored during the cystogram, cystoscopic evaluation of the refluxing ureterovesical junction (to determine orifice position and morphology and to permit estimation of the length of the intravesical ureter) is a

more accurate means to gauge the prognosis for spontaneous cessation of reflux.

Timing of the cystogram in relationship to the presence of infection must be taken into consideration, since round cell infiltration of the intravesical ureter or the overlying mucosa may reduce the compliance of the roof of the ureter and result in transient reflux at normal voiding pressures. There is also some evidence that intravesical pressure is sometimes elevated during acute infections (Van Gool and Tanagho, 1977). Therefore, an infection-free interval of 2 to 4 weeks is recommended before the cystogram is performed. If the clinical situation demands an earlier diagnosis, however, cystography is not harmful and early diagnosis may facilitate therapy. Mild reflux in association with cystitis usually resolves quickly after the infection is eliminated. Reflux of more significant degree will require further evaluation.

RADIONUCLIDE SCANNING

The use of radionuclide scanning techniques in the detection of vesicoureteral reflux is an attractive alternative to conventional cystography (Conway et al., 1972, 1975; Conway and Kruglik, 1976; Winter, 1959). Approximately 1 μC of ^{99m}Tc-pertechnetate is instilled into the bladder through a catheter, and the bladder is then filled slowly with normal saline. The urinary tract is continuously monitored on a persistence scope attachment to the scintillation camera, and images are recorded on Polaroid film at intervals. The special advantage of this technique is that it allows continuous monitoring of the patient with minimal radiation exposure. The limitation of radionuclide cystography is that the resolution of the image does not approach that of roentgenography. Abnormalities of the urethra and bladder, or reflux into the distal ureter only, may not be documented.

Nuclear cystography is especially useful in following patients with known reflux and in checking to be certain that reflux is indeed absent after antireflux surgery (Fig. 49–6). In following patients with reflux, radioactive emissions are counted continuously over various areas of the abdomen, allowing ready calculation of the bladder volume at which reflux begins or ceases, the volume of the reflux, the rate of upper tract drainage (renogram), and the residual urine after voiding. There is real benefit in recording these parameters, because the bladder volume at which reflux begins is significant in predicting when reflux will cease (Fig. 49–7).

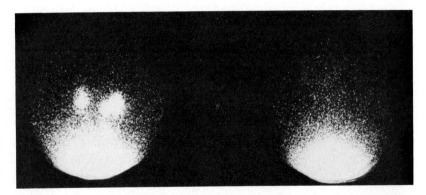

Figure 49–6. Pre- and postoperative nuclear cystograms. Bilateral reflux, evident on the initial study *(left)* is absent 6 months following surgery.

CLASSIFICATION AND GRADING OF REFLUX

Classification of the degree of reflux is as significant clinically as determination of its presence. Reflux as demonstrated by cystography can be readily graded on a scale of increasing severity of 1 to 4 (Dwoskin and Perlmutter, 1973). Grade 1 represents lower ureteral filling only; Grade 2A represents ureteral and pelvicalyceal filling without dilatation; Grade 2B represents pelvicalyceal filling with mild calyceal blunting; Grade 3 represents ureteral and pelvicalyceal filling, calyceal clubbing, and minor to moderate pelvic dilatation without extreme ureteral tortuosity; and Grade 4 represents massive ureteral dilatation and tortuosity. In general, the lower the grade of reflux, the greater the chance of spontaneous cessation (Fig. 49–8).

Several other grading systems have been proposed based on the severity of reflux judged from the cystogram (Rolleston et al., 1975; Heikel and Parkkulainen, 1966). Some have emphasized ureteral caliber as well as the degree of pelvicalyceal dilatation (Howerton and Lich, 1963; Bridge and Roe, 1969; Edelbrook and Mickelson, 1970), whereas other investigators have graded reflux according to bladder pressure (i.e., filling vs. voiding) (Lattimer et al., 1963; Melick et al., 1962; Smellie et al., 1968).

Recently, an international grading system has been proposed that aims to provide a common standard for the assessment of the severity of reflux, thereby allowing for more objective comparison of therapeutic modalities. This international system is based primarily on the appearance of the calyx on the cystogram (Fig. 49–9). Although the degree of dilatation of the ureter usually parallels the degree of dilatation of the pyelocalyceal system, this is not always the case. Also, it should be remembered that in

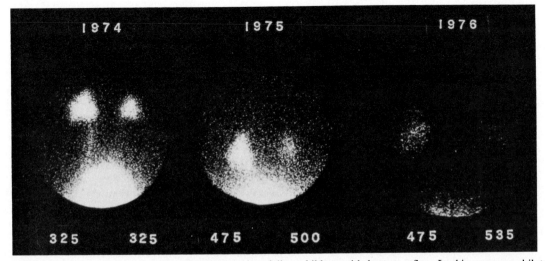

Figure 49–7. Nuclear cystograms are usually employed to follow children with known reflux. In this sequence, bilateral reflux was noted when the bladder had been filled to 325 ml. One year later, reflux did not begin on the right until 475 ml. had been instilled. Mild reflux was noted on the left with 500 ml. in the bladder. The next year, reflux was minimal. Increasing bladder volume before reflux occurs indicates growth of the intravesical ureter, as does a reduced volume of refluxed urine.

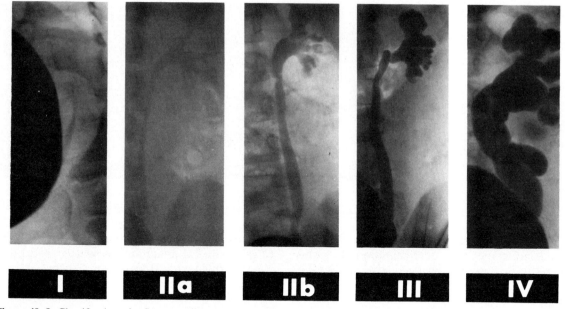

Figure 49–8. Classification of reflux according to the volume of urine seen to reflux on cystogram. Grade I: Lower ureteral filling only. Grade IIa: Ureteral and pelviocalyceal filling, without dilatation. Grade IIb: Ureteral and pelviocalyceal filling with mild calyceal blunting but without clubbing and without dilatation of the pelvis or tortuosity of the ureter. Grade III: Ureteral and pelviocalyceal filling, calyceal clubbing, and minor to moderate pelvic dilatation without tortuosity of the ureter. Grade IV: Massive ureteral dilatation and tortuosity. (From Dwoskin, J. Y., and Perlmutter, A. D.: J. Urol., *109*:888, 1973.)

the awake child the intravesical pressure may be considerably higher than the normal voiding pressure during the cystogram. Reflux may therefore at times be overgraded in systems of this type.

The overall prognostic factors of importance in grading reflux are (1) the degree of hydronephrosis seen on the cystogram; (2) the degree of laterality of the orifice within the bladder; (3) the morphology of the orifice in the Lyon classification (1969); (4) the estimated length of the intravesical ureter; (5) the age of the patient, reflecting potential for growth of the intravesical ureter; and (6) the presence or absence of other factors that may cause or

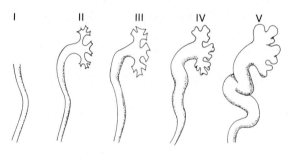

Figure 49–9. Classification of reflux.

contribute to reflux, such as bladder outlet obstruction or neurogenic bladder (Table 49–1).

Any of these factors may be used as guides in deciding whether reflux is likely to persist after full growth has been achieved. Any one factor may at times be misleading, so it is safest to assess all factors in deciding whether a trial of nonoperative therapy is warranted. The exception is mild reflux in an infant or younger child, in whom cystoscopic evaluation is now usually deemed unnecessary.

The cystogram, particularly a single cystogram, may fail to detect primary reflux. The degree of ureterectasis, which influences grading, is subject to variation owing to the bladder pressure at the time of each film and may be quite inconsistent. The degree of orifice laterality is a fairly dependable concept but is difficult to judge at cystoscopy because of the absence of local landmarks. It may be determined in conjunction with an estimation of the length and diameter of the intravesical ureter. These, however, are also subjective measurements, made by inserting a ureteral catheter into the orifice and estimating the length of intravesical ureter elevated by the catheter until it passes through the hiatus (Fig. 49–10). Since a 4:1 or 5:1 ratio of length to width in the intravesical

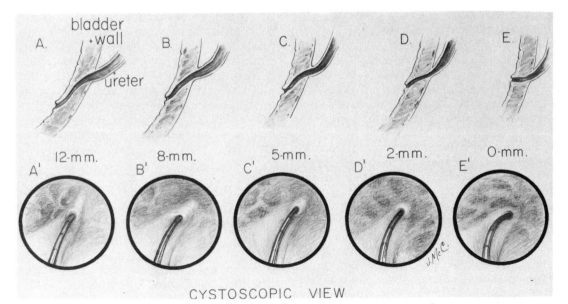

Figure 49–10. The cystoscopic appearance of the ureterovesical junction. A ureteral catheter is used to estimate the length of the submucosal tunnel. The ureter is drawn as normal in diameter to emphasize the appearance of the flap elevated by the catheter. (From Kelalis, P. P., and King, L. R. (Eds.): Clinical Pediatric Urology. Philadelphia, W. B. Saunders Co., 1976.)

ureter is necessary to prevent reflux (Paquin, 1959), diameter must be estimated also.

The morphology of the refluxing orifice is easier to determine, although the appearance of the orifice may change with the degree of bladder filling, and many horseshoe and stadium orifices do not reflux. Age is important in the equation because the more growth potential remains (the younger the child), the more likely it is that defects in the ureterovesical junction will eventually correct themselves. Finally, although small paraureteral diverticula may vanish with time, larger diverticula and ureters entering such diverticula will require surgical correction. Although an obstruction, such as a urethral valve, may be relieved, resulting in cessation of reflux, the presence of chronic cystitis may dictate early antireflux surgery in an attempt (not always successful [Govan et al., 1975]) to protect the kidneys from pyelonephritic scarring and atrophy.

In general, the classification of reflux and the decision to recommend or withhold ureteral reimplantation depend on an assessment of all the foregoing factors. The presence of pyelonephritic scarring (as distinct from a thin renal parenchyma) is used by some as an indication for early surgery. Such kidneys are also likely to exhibit hydronephrosis. Although Stamey (1972) has shed some doubt on the concept that residual urine per se predisposes to chronic infection, most clinicians agree that a severe

degree of reflux, representing residual urine in the upper tracts, predisposes to urinary infections.

Relative indications for early surgery are Grade 4 or Grade 5 reflux (international classification); lateral, golf-hole, or horseshoe orifice; and short (2 to 5 mm) or absent intravesical ureter. Recurrences of infection or progressive renal scarring mandate antireflux surgery.

Factors suggesting that reflux will cease with growth and will not impede renal development or function include Grade 3 reflux or less; orifice in the "B" or "C" position with a stadium or horseshoe configuration; intravesical ureter more than 5 mm in length; relatively young child; and freedom from obstruction or infection. The need for some safe chemotherapeutic agent to keep the urine clear is not viewed as a contraindication to nonoperative management, but those children with a tendency toward asymptomatic reinfection must be followed very carefully. Home urine cultures, such as those done with Uricult tubes, are a great help in this regard.

Primary Reflux

If the normal position of the ureteral orifice on the corner of the trigone is designated as the "A" position, then orifices that are progressively more lateral than normal can be designated as

"B," "C," and "D," in order of their laterality (Lyon et al., 1969; Mackie and Stephens, 1975). The "D" position represents an orifice that opens on the edge of (D_1) or into (D_2) a diverticulum. In general, the more lateral the orifice, the more gaping and abnormal its appearance cystoscopically; the shorter its effective submucosal course, the more prone it is to reflux (Fig. 49–11).

Such lateral ectopia has been explained in two ways: first, as a result of intrinsic weakness in the muscular attachment of the terminal ureter to the trigone (Tanagho, 1976), and second, as a consequence of an abnormality in the location of the ureteral bud on the wolffian duct (Ambrose and Nicolson, 1964; Stephens, 1976). The former explanation is a functional one based on physiologic observations and animal experimentation; the second is a pathoembryologic explanation based on the correlation of clinical and post-mortem observations with the embryology of the ureter.

Both provide a framework for viewing the phenomenon of reflux as a manifestation of a primary abnormality of the ureterovesical junction, caused by a deficiency in the longitudinal muscle of the submucosal ureter. Because the incidence of reflux decreases with age, it is apparent that certain defects that allow reflux to occur in childhood may correct themselves with growth and development. This concept of primary reflux and the knowledge that it may subside spontaneously form the foundation for the nonoperative management of vesicoureteral reflux.

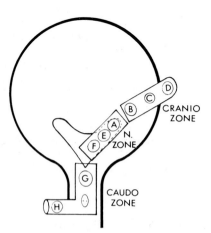

Figure 49–11. Diagram of bladder and urethra, showing three zones of ureteral orifices. *A, E,* and *F,* Normal zone. *B, C,* and *D,* Lateral in cranio zone (*D* in diverticulum). *G* and *H,* Caudo zone with *G* in urethra and *H* in sex ducts. (From Mackie, G. G., and Stephens, F. D.: J. Urol., *114*:274, 1975.)

Further considerations in formulating a program of patient care include whether or not reflux itself poses a threat to renal function, either directly or indirectly. The potential coexistence of reflux with urinary tract infection, lower urinary obstruction, and renal hypoplasia or dysplasia contributes to the complexity of this problem. Each aspect must be reviewed before a rational plan of treatment can be outlined.

Embryology and Association Between Primary Reflux and Abnormal Renal Morphology and Function

The embryology of the urinary tract is described in Chapter 37. Stephens (1976), particularly, and Stephens and associates (1980) have described how an abnormal ureteral bud site may result in reflux (or obstruction) and abnormal development or dysgenesis of the kidney or renal segment drained by the displaced ureteral bud. The association of segmental renal hypoplasia and dysplasia in kidneys with total duplication of the ureters that arise from cranially or caudally ectopic ureteral buds supports the view that the position at which the ureteral bud contacts the metanephric blastema determines the quality of the kidney that results (Fig. 49–12).

Sommer and Stephens (1981) have also examined the role of the position of the orifice associated with dysplasia and renal scarring in children with reflux compared with those with partial ureteral obstruction but no reflux. The groups had comparable degrees of calycectasis. Histologic examination of the kidneys of those with partial obstruction revealed obstructive atrophy but not dysplasia. Only refluxing renal units with abnormal orifice sites contained dysplastic elements. The authors conclude that these findings support the concept of renal parenchymal maldevelopment occurring pari passu with reflux, and they believe that the renal changes seen in patients with reflux are developmental (or secondary to superimposed infection but not to hydrodynamic effects of the reflux).

In this sense, therefore, primary reflux results from the site of the ureteral bud, determined in the fourth week of gestation. Further, the reflux itself probably has little or no effect on the kidney, as faulty induction of the metanephros is ordained when the displaced ureteral bud fails to contact the renal blastema near

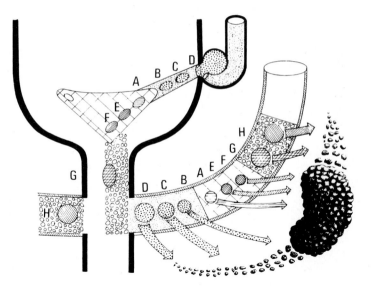

Figure 49–12. Relationship of orifice zones in bladder and urethra and points of origin from wolffian duct is shown, as well as relationship of bud positions on wolffian duct and nephrogenic blastema. (From Mackie, G. G., and Stephens, F. D.: J. Urol., *114*:274, 1975.)

enough to the normal junction site to permit formation of a normal kidney.

These embryologic studies explain the association between reflux and renal anomalies that result in poor renal function at birth or progressive renal deterioration in later life in the absence of any history of urinary infection or obstruction as an obvious cause. Such faulty kidneys may be adequate to support life in childhood and even to sustain nearly normal growth and development for a time, but they remain abnormal and may be unable to grow to meet the load imposed by an ever-increasing body mass. Renal failure is not uncommon in these patients at puberty or when nearly full growth has been achieved. Anemia, hypertension, lethargy, or growth arrest results in the discovery of the problem, and the reflux may then be detected for the first time.

Other factors may operate to produce acquired vesicoureteral reflux or to increase voiding pressure, which then markedly worsens the degree of existing reflux. Sphincter dyssynergia and forceful inappropriate involuntary voiding contractions are two common acquired conditions that may have this effect.

Detrusor-Sphincter Dyssynergia

This condition, also termed the neurogenic/non-neurogenic bladder, clearly seems to be acquired and has not been recognized in infants or very young children. It may result from early and forceful efforts at toilet training; it is also often recognized in children in very adverse family situations. Most commonly, such

children present with inappropriate wetting during the day, but some present only with a history of urinary infections. Upon investigation they are often found to have vesicoureteral reflux, frequently associated with otherwise unexplained bladder trabeculation with or without bladder decompensation and residual urine. The diagnosis is partly one of exclusion of infravesical obstruction and is confirmed by the persistent presence of spontaneous bladder contractions on cystometric studies, failure of one or both sphincters to open during voiding, or both. Sphincter dyssynergia especially is associated with high intravesical pressures, at least during voiding, and if reflux is present, these pressures may be transmitted to the upper tract, causing increased dilatation. If reflux is initially absent, the resultant detrusor hypertrophy and elevated intravesical pressures may result in periureteral diverticula breaking down the normal antireflux mechanism and resulting in reflux, which becomes progressively worse if the condition persists.

Bladder hyperreflexia, instability, and noncompliance are other causes of relatively elevated intravesical pressures. The pressure may rise quite rapidly as the resting bladder begins to fill (Koff and Murtagh, 1983; Glassberg, 1982). If reflux is present, these pressures are transmitted to the kidney, increasing the degree of hydronephrosis.

When antireflux surgery is carried out on children with detrusor-sphincter dyssynergia or hyperreflexia, ureteral reimplantation is often unsuccessful. Surgical correction of reflux should not be attempted until the detrusor dysfunction is properly controlled.

Urinary Tract Infection

Urinary tract infection is the problem most closely associated with vesicoureteral reflux. Reflux is more commonly diagnosed in boys during infancy and in girls during early childhood, peaking at 3 to 7 years of age. Reflux, usually mild in degree, has been noted to occur clinically in association with acute urinary tract infection and to disappear when the urine becomes sterile. Thus, inflammation of the ureterovesical junction can contribute to the occurrence of reflux.

Conversely, severe reflux contributes to the occurrence of urinary infection because it provides a reservoir of residual urine. Thus, although infection contributes to the occurrence of reflux when the ureterovesical junction is marginally competent, it does not play a crucial role in the causation of reflux in the majority of cases, especially in patients with more severe degrees of reflux and when hydronephrosis is present on the intravenous urogram. In other words, it is not uncommon to find the marginal ureterovesical junction refluxing during episodes of acute cystitis, but this is not an important cause of reflux because the kidneys are normal on intravenous pyelograms, ureterectasis is slight, and the reflux abates soon after infection is eliminated.

The incidence of recurrent urinary tract infection in children without reflux or in children in whom reflux has been surgically corrected does not differ greatly from that in children with reflux. However, the incidence of clinical pyelonephritis is greatly reduced by the correction of reflux in children prone to recurrent infection. The danger posed by vesicoureteral reflux is its potential to convert lower urinary tract infection into pyelonephritis with consequent renal damage (Fair and Govan, 1976; Govan et al., 1975).

Infection, superimposed on vesicoureteral reflux, may arrest the normal development of the kidney. Sequential measurements of renal length alone may be used to assess renal growth, but the length of normal kidneys has been shown to be affected by numerous factors (Hernandez et al., 1979). Hypertrophy of the intervening normal renal parenchyma and the predominantly polar distribution of renal scars make interpretation of renal size using length alone inaccurate and somewhat unreliable. Most studies of renal growth in kidneys with reflux suffer from this deficient methodology (Redman et al., 1974).

Claësson et al. (1980, 1981) critically addressed the question of how to best measure renal parenchymal volume. They devised a nomogram to compare observed and expected renal mass derived from linear measurements taken from the urogram. Further work by the same group has produced a technique of computerized planimetry to measure total renal parenchymal area in units of square centimeters. Measurements reflect considerable anatomic detail, as areas of compensatory hypertrophy are indexed and sequential measurements can then be accurately compared.

Renal scans can also be used to estimate the function of the individual kidney. The function can be calculated from the uptake of I-131 hippuran (measuring effective renal plasma flow) or ^{99m}Tc DTPA (technetium-99m-diethylenetriaminepentacetic acid), used to estimate glomerular filtration rate. DMSA (2,3 dimercaptosuccinic acid), a newer cortical imaging agent, provides good anatomic detail when compared with the aforementioned compounds and can reveal small areas of diminished renal function that are not detectable on conventional urography. In addition, DMSA uptake can be used to calculate unilateral renal function. At present, however, no ideal technique for the measurement of renal mass is available.

Given the shortcomings of bipolar renal length measurements, Lyon (1973) and Redman et al. (1974) observed a subnormal rate of renal growth in the presence of reflux without documented urine infection. Kelalis (1971), on the other hand, reported resumption of growth in kidneys with reflux after infection alone had been eliminated.

Longitudinal measurements of bipolar renal length were used by Smellie et al. (1981) to monitor the effects of reflux on the kidney in a series of 76 children with persistent reflux of varying grades. Renal growth was impaired (bipolar length less than half the increment expected for the child's linear growth) in only 5 of 93 kidneys drained by undilated ureters. Of the 18 kidneys drained by a dilated ureter, 6 had growth impairment; however, 5 were already scarred at the time of presentation. The sixth developed new renal scarring. All had episodes of documented infection. The overall relationship between the grade of reflux, the presence of infection, and the rate of renal growth can be summarized as follows: If no infection (or obstruction) is present, normal renal growth can be expected. Renal growth is retarded in about half the refluxing patients with chronic or recurrent episodes of infection. The more severe the reflux, the greater the likelihood of renal growth impairment.

The effect of antireflux surgery on renal growth has been examined by several investigators. McRae et al. (1974) reported accelerated growth after successful surgery. Babcock et al. (1976), considering the effects of unilateral reflux, observed neither radiographic improvement nor a change in the ratio of size in the refluxing kidney compared with the normal contralateral kidney after elimination of reflux. On the other hand, Willscher et al. (1976a), demonstrated normal rates of growth in nonscarred kidneys with severe reflux. However, these kidneys showed accelerated growth after surgical elimination of the reflux. Where renal scarring was present, this accelerated pattern of growth following surgery was seen only in patients with bilateral scarring. Murnaghan (1980) observed significant focal nodular parenchymal hypertrophy in two postpubertal patients following successful antireflux surgery. In addition, somatic growth of prepubertal children with reflux has been observed to accelerate after successful surgical correction (Merrell and Mowad, 1979). However, physical growth alone, particularly during puberty, may account for the increased renal growth rate that has been observed (Claësson et al., 1981).

In 1960, Hodson and Edwards demonstrated the association between reflux and renal scarring. Such renal damage takes three forms on urography: (1) characteristic focal pyelonephritic scarring, in which the contracted parenchyma is seen as a dimple on the outer perimeter of the renal shadow, the clubbed calyx being directly beneath; (2) generalized calyceal dilatation and parenchymal atrophy (Fig. 49–13); and (3) failure of renal growth with the kidney smaller than expected, often associated with either focal scarring or generalized atrophy. *Reflux nephropathy* has been suggested as a preferable term for the scarred kidney associated with reflux. Hypertension, proteinuria, or reduced renal function, or any combination of these, may also be present.

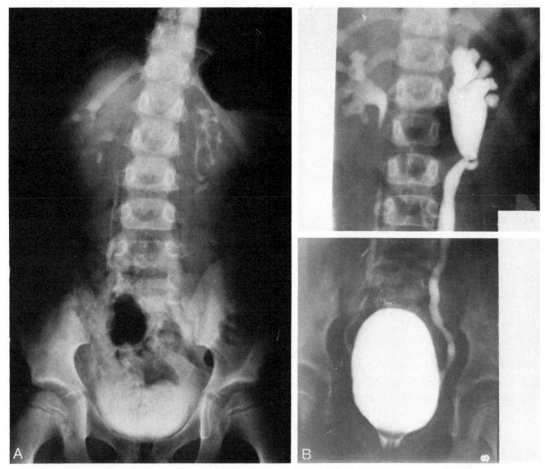

Figure 49–13. *A,* Small atrophic-appearing kidney with clubbed calyces on IVP. This appearance is almost invariably associated with reflux and a history of superimposed infection. *B,* The reflux is demonstrated on cystogram.

Radiographic evidence of scarring is almost always accompanied by reflux. In some instances the scars may be evidence of reflux that has subsequently stopped because of growth of the intravesical ureter. Conversely, between 30 and 60 per cent of children with reflux are found to have renal scarring. The higher figure is derived from data originating in surgical clinics (Williams and Eckstein, 1965), the lower from medical surveys (Smellie and Normand, 1979). It has been suggested that sterile reflux alone may be sufficient to cause renal scarring (Rolleston et al., 1975). Nevertheless, the appearance of fresh scars or the extension of established scars in the absence of obstruction, neuropathic bladder, or sphincter dyssynergia has been documented only in children with urinary infection. Smellie (1975b) reported no new scars in 150 normal or scarred kidneys in children with uncomplicated primary reflux in whom low-dose chemoprophylaxis was successful in maintaining sterile urine. In an additional group of 121 normal or scarred kidneys with reflux, only 2 developed a new scar when the children were maintained on continuous low-dose therapy for a 7- to 15-year follow-up period (Edwards et al., 1977). Both cases were associated with breakthrough infections, and in both there was a moderate to severe degree of reflux.

Lenaghan et al. (1976) used intermittent short courses of antibacterial drugs for the treatment of recurrent infection only in 102 children with reflux. In 76 kidneys that were initially normal, scarring developed in 16 (21 per cent). Of 44 kidneys with established scars, 29 progressed (66 per cent). Filly et al. (1974) observed two new scars in 16 initially normal kidneys with reflux while the children were on "intermittent" therapy. However, scars also developed in 2 of 15 (13 per cent) initially normal kidneys in which reflux was not demonstrated. Cystoscopic examination of these latter children demonstrated poorly muscularized ureteral orifices, suggesting that reflux may have been present at some time in the past. Fifteen of 24 (62 per cent) initially scarred kidneys showed progression of scarring. Intermittent antibacterial therapy does not protect against renal scarring; thus, the need for safe, low-dose, continuous antibacterial therapy seems clear in the follow-up of children with known reflux.

A history of bacteriuria can often be elicited in children with reflux and scarring. The higher the grade of reflux, the more likely is the occurrence of new or progressive scarring associated with recurrent urinary infection (Rolleston et al., 1970). The radiographic appearance of renal scarring develops over a period of at least 8 months (Hodson et al., 1975). It is sometimes difficult to determine whether earlier scars actually progress or simply become more obvious as the surrounding healthy renal parenchyma hypertrophies.

If renal scars occur in conjunction with reflux, they are usually present at the time of the initial intravenous pyelogram. Some investigators believe that scars rarely occur in kidneys beyond infancy and that, when present, they seldom progress even when reflux and infection coexist (Ransley and Risdon, 1981). Older children who have sphincter dyssynergia, bladder instability, or noncompliant bladders are at risk for renal scarring when reflux is also present, however (Koff et al., 1979b); if reflux is present together with unrecognized obstruction, progressive renal damage is the rule.

Experimental Studies

Reflux is virtually always present in the rat and is normal in many rodents. Reflux is also often encountered in rabbits and dogs (Winter, 1959). When absent, it can be induced by incising the trigone (Tanagho et al., 1965b); by crushing a part of the bladder and introducing bacteria, causing chronic cystitis (Schoenberg et al., 1964); or by interfering with the innervation of the trigone as is sometimes seen clinically following lumbar sympathectomy (Tanagho, 1976). Resection of the roof of the submucosal tunnel will also consistently result in reflux. The adage that "reflux, if present, may be demonstrated only intermittently" is probably even more true in animals than in humans (Winter, 1959). Jeffs and Allen (1962) as well as Kaveggia et al. (1966) induced acute pyelonephritis by the introduction of bacteria through a nephrostomy tube and were able to produce reflux without direct manipulation of the normal ureteral vesical junction in puppies and dogs. Contralateral reflux often occurred as well. These investigations suggest that reflux can be caused by pyelonephritis and bacteria in the absence of disease of the bladder or urethra. Boyarsky's demonstration of the toxic effect of bacteria on the ureter, with consequent interference with normal peristalsis, may explain this effect, since normal peristalsis is known to be one of the defense mechanisms that protects against reflux in the human (Boyarsky and Labay, 1972). Grana et al. (1965) found E. coli exotoxins particularly effective in ablating peristalsis.

Experimental work in the pathogenesis of

renal scarring has recently centered on the concept of intrarenal reflux (IRR). This is defined as reflux of urine into the collecting tubules and parenchyma; it provides a readily apparent mechanism whereby urinary microorganisms can gain access to the renal parenchyma and produce renal scarring. Roberts et al. (1982) produced IRR in primates with a bacterial inoculum in order to define the precise mechanism of tubular damage secondary to bacterial infection. Phagocytosis of bacteria by invading neutrophils produces superoxide, an enzyme toxic to renal tubular cells. Administration of superoxide dismutase, an antagonist of superoxide, seemed successful in preventing renal tubular cell damage histologically but did not interfere with phagocytosis. Thus, the work of these investigators suggests that the inflammatory response itself, while eliminating invading bacteria by neutrophil phagocytosis, also produces the irreversible damage that occurs in the renal tissue.

Besides inflammation of the parenchyma due to bacterial infection, other mechanisms have been proposed to explain the pathogenesis of scar formation. Cotran and colleagues (1981) have investigated the role of Tamm-Horsfall protein (THP). This mucoprotein is produced in high concentration by the tubular epithelial cells in the loop of Henle and distal nephron and is a primary constituent of renal tubular casts. Immunofluorescent techniques have demonstrated extratubular THP in the interstitium of kidneys with intrarenal reflux. Extratubular THP, therefore, may serve as a marker of urinary extravasation.

Experimental studies by Ransley and Risdon (1978) and Tamminen and Kaprio (1977) indicate that the areas of renal parenchyma susceptible to intrarenal reflux and subsequent scarring are drained by flat, concave, or compound papillae, which occur predominantly in the polar regions of the human kidney (Fig. 49–14). Among experimental animals, only the pig possesses renal papillary morphology similar to that of man. Thus, this animal has been used to study the mechanism of intrarenal reflux and renal scarring. Studies suggest that in the presence of infected urine, intrarenal reflux results in the development of scarring in less than 4 weeks. However, antimicrobial treatment, introduced after 1 week of urine infection in models that are prone to such scar formation, significantly reduces the extent of the scarring (Ransley and Risdon, 1981).

Hodson et al. (1975), also using the pig model, demonstrated that focal scarring can be

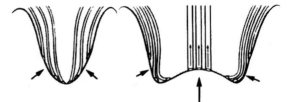

Figure 49–14. Papillary factors in intrarenal reflux. *A,* Convex papilla (nonrefluxing papilla)—crescentic or slitlike openings of collecting ducts opening obliquely onto the papilla. *B,* Concave or flat papilla (refluxing papilla)—round collecting ducts opening at right angles onto flat papilla. (From Ransley, P. G., and Risdon, R. A.: Br. J. Radiol. [Suppl.], *14*:1, 1978.)

produced by sterile reflux but only in the presence of a sustained increase in intravesical pressure produced by incorporating ureteral obstruction into the refluxing model. Ransley and Risdon (1981), using three strains of pigs and sophisticated urodynamic monitoring, found that parenchymal scarring occurred only when there was sufficient bladder outlet obstruction, due to a partially occluding urethral ring, to result in bladder decompensation. They concluded that during the relatively brief interval of high intravesical pressure without bladder decompensation, no lesions were produced, but that once bladder decompensation supervened, scarring was induced. Thus, if these results can be extrapolated to humans, it seems unlikely that sterile reflux results in renal damage in the absence of significant obstruction. This conclusion, in fact, correlates with almost all clinical observations.

Clinical Correlation

In the clinical context, intrarenal reflux has been defined radiographically as the appearance of contrast material in the renal parenchyma during the voiding cystourethrogram. However, visualization of intrarenal reflux may be difficult when the upper tracts are dilated and filled with nonopacified urine that dilutes the contrast. Radiographic detection of intrarenal reflux almost certainly underestimates its true prevalence. Such reflux has been observed in 5 to 15 per cent of neonates and infants with reflux (Rolleston et al., 1974; Rose et al., 1975). Rolleston et al. (1975) reviewed the cystograms of several hundred children with reflux. Intrarenal reflux was detected only in children under the age of 5 years and was seen only in conjunction with moderate or severe degrees of reflux. There was a significant correlation between the presence of intrarenal reflux and the subsequent development of renal scarring in the affected area.

The more frequent detection of intrarenal reflux in neonates and infants with vesicoureteral reflux can be explained by the relatively large size of the collecting ducts, which allows better visualization of contrast in the renal parenchyma. In older children in whom scarring has already occurred, parenchymal fibrosis may prevent intrarenal reflux into the affected segments. Studies of papillary morphology in human kidneys indicate that at least two thirds possess papillae of the type that may permit intrarenal reflux. Controversy exists concerning the clinical significance of intrarenal reflux in predicting the production of renal scars, however, as some infants who exhibit such reflux never develop scars.

The "big bang" theory of Ransley and Risdon (1978) has attempted to reconcile the clinical, radiologic, and pathologic features of intrarenal reflux–related renal scarring in the majority of infants and children in whom the scars are already present on the initial urogram. These investigators suggest that the initial infection in the child with reflux and nonconical papillae results in pyelonephritic scarring of one or both poles. Since all susceptible segments of the kidney are generally affected simultaneously, sequential scar formation with subsequent infections is unusual. However, on occasion, marginally refluxing papillae may be transformed into the refluxing variety, accounting for new scarring with new infections as opposed to progressive contraction of the renal parenchyma following an initial insult.

Despite the very impressive evidence that the combination of moderate to severe vesicoureteral reflux, intrarenal reflux, and bacteriuria may result in pyelonephritic scarring, at least 30 to 40 per cent of patients investigated for renal insufficiency and found to have the radiographic features of reflux nephropathy have no definite history of a urinary infection. Family surveys of index patients with reflux regularly report other individuals with advanced reflux nephropathy who have no history of urinary tract symptomatology or infection. In addition, reflux nephropathy is often detected during the course of diagnostic evaluation for hypertension or proteinuria in the older child or young adult. There are several mechanisms by which reflux nephropathy and end-stage renal disease associated with reflux may be produced, and it seems likely that each predominates in some patients.

From a clinical point of view, there are four possible explanations for renal failure in these patients without a history of infection to account for severe reflux nephropathy: (1) Asymptomatic infections in conjunction with reflux resulted in renal damage; (2) sterile reflux persisting over many years damaged the kidneys permanently; (3) the renal damage occurred when an episode of sphincter dyssynergia or bladder hyperreflexia resulted in elevated voiding pressures, worsening reflux, and initiation of or compounding of parenchymal damage; or (4) renal dysgenesis was present at birth, resulting in a relatively fixed renal mass, with renal failure occurring only when the kidneys were overwhelmed by ever-increasing body mass.

The embryologic studies cited earlier indicate that the last explanation is often the correct one. Children or adults may harbor urinary infections that cause so few symptoms that they are not perceived as infections. Most patients with such infections, however, will admit to some symptoms when closely questioned (urgency, enuresis, episodic incontinence, and the like), and the majority of such patients have no renal impairment. Similarly, functional urodynamic abnormalities that can result in elevated voiding pressure are not silent but are manifested by diurnal enuresis and poor urinary control. Usually, at least a few random urine specimens have been examined in childhood; if these were normal, it is difficult to imagine that intercurrent infections could often produce profound kidney damage without symptoms. Indirect evidence for this statement is derived from monitoring children with known reflux. Renal arrest, failure of the kidney to develop as expected (let alone atrophy), or the onset of renal scarring is unknown in prospective studies in children unless infection has recurred or obstruction was overlooked at the time of the initial evaluation.

On the other hand, even though primary reflux has been reported as an incidental finding in septuagenarians with normal (for age) renal function, the lifelong effect of reflux on renal function in the human is unknown and probably cannot be studied except in retrospect. Since the follow-up of patients with reflux is costly and time-consuming over a very long time span, persistent reflux in the adult should usually be treated by antireflux surgery once the diagnosis has been established (Hawtrey et al., 1983).

In any event, the embryologic study of primary reflux implies that the common clinical association of abnormal renal structure and function with abnormal ureteral orifice position may represent faulty development of the derivatives of the nephrotome rather than progressive pathologic change secondary to hydrostatic effects or intervening infection.

Associated Anomalies

NEUROPATHIC BLADDER

There is an increased incidence of reflux in individuals of any age with congenital or acquired neuropathic bladder. Although there is evidence in animals that interference with either the sympathetic or the parasympathetic innervation of the trigone and distal ureter can predispose to reflux, clinically a combination of factors usually seems to be operative. In the presence of elevated intravesical pressure, trabeculation and paraureteral diverticulum formation associated with functional bladder outlet obstruction can render the ureterovesical junction incompetent. The incomplete bladder emptying commonly associated with neuropathic bladder predisposes the patient to chronic urinary tract infection and the development of bladder calculi. These conditions promote edema and inflammation of the ureterovesical junction and may also alter its function, thus permitting reflux. In myelodysplasia there is also an increased incidence of concomitant urinary tract malformations, including the primary abnormalities of the ureterovesical junction associated with reflux (Hutch, 1962).

Bauer and associates (1984) have recently shown that babies with neurogenic bladder are at very high risk for reflux if sphincter dyssynergia is present on screening urodynamic studies.

Associated Anomalies of the Ureterovesical Junction

URETERAL DUPLICATION

There is also an increased incidence of vesicoureteral reflux in patients with complete duplication of the ureters. Following the Weigert-Meyer rule, the ureter draining the upper pole of the kidney opens into the vesicourethral canal medial and caudal to the ureter draining the lower pole. Although reflux may affect either ureter, it is much more common in the ureter draining the lower pole because of the more lateral orifice of that ureter and its tendency to have only a short (or absent) submucosal tunnel. When the upper pole ureter demonstrates reflux despite its longer submucosal course, the defect often proves to be one of deficient muscularization of the submucosal ureter, or the orifices may be side by side, both lacking sufficient intravesical ureteral length.

Although the presence of duplication does not preclude the spontaneous cessation of reflux, the orifice draining the middle and lower pole calyces is apt to be lateral and to have a golf-hole appearance, and early surgical correction is often elected (King, 1976).

The study of total duplication of the ureters has illuminated the role of the ureteral bud in the differentiation of the kidney to a considerable degree, as noted in Chapter 37.

BLADDER DIVERTICULUM

The other trigonal abnormality that is at times associated with reflux is vesical diverticulum. A diverticulum can be congenital or acquired and can occur anywhere in the bladder. An acquired diverticulum represents herniation of mucosa through an area of relatively deficient muscularization in the bladder wall in the presence of elevated intravesical pressure and bladder outlet obstruction. A congenital diverticulum, which is encountered more commonly in children, is a similar herniation caused by incomplete muscularization in the presence of normal intravesical pressure, in an otherwise normal urinary tract. An acquired diverticulum is associated with gross trabeculation of the bladder and is secondary to anatomic or functional obstruction of the vesicourethral outlet, e.g., urethral valve, sphincter dyssynergia, neurogenic bladder, or similar entities.

The ureteral hiatus represents a potential weak spot in the posterolateral wall of the bladder and is analogous in this respect to the inguinal canal; it is the most common site of both congenital and acquired diverticula. A diverticulum at or near the hiatus predisposes to reflux if it is large enough to impinge upon muscular support of the intravesical ureter. Spontaneous cessation of reflux in the presence of such a diverticulum is unusual, and early surgical correction of both lesions is generally indicated. However, small diverticula and associated reflux have been noted to disappear with growth during childhood (King, 1976; Colodny 1983). Occasionally, a diverticulum may interfere with drainage of the ureter in addition to or instead of predisposing to reflux. Surgical repair is indicated in such instances, unless renal function is so poor in the affected unit that nephroureterectomy, as well as diverticulectomy, becomes the treatment of choice.

Reflux and Renal Function

When reflux is relatively severe in degree and marked ureterectasis is present, the voiding pressure is transmitted more or less directly to the renal pelvis (Ong et al., 1974). It has been suggested that such intermittent elevation of the intrapelvic pressure during voiding acts as a water hammer and in certain instances produces progressive renal damage. Support for the supposition that sterile reflux interferes with intrarenal circulation is derived from animal models in which glomerular and tubular function decreased following the creation of surgical reflux (Helin, 1975).

Although this mechanism may play a role in renal atrophy secondary to bladder outlet obstruction when the intravesical pressures generated during voiding are much higher than normal, any "water hammer" effect has not been observed to cause progressive parenchymal thinning in patients with unobstructed and uninfected bladders who are followed prospectively. Perhaps the pressures generated during voiding by the normal unobstructed bladder are simply not high enough or sustained enough to cause a measurable increase in calyceal dilatation. The retrograde peristaltic wave in the relatively undilated ureter will probably damp such pressure somewhat. An alternative explanation for the calycectasis seen with severe but uncomplicated reflux is that the faulty ureteral bud was able to induce only a thin kidney that is deficient in renal pyramid development and is unable to concentrate the urine to a normal degree (see previous discussion).

Uehling (1971) and Walker et al. (1973) have made use of the diminished concentrating ability seen in children with reflux and hydronephrosis by following such children with overnight concentration tests to assess the severity of the reflux. When medical surveillance is elected as the primary form of treatment in the expectation that reflux may stop with growth, concentrating ability improves as the severity of the reflux diminishes. Failure of the concentrating ability to improve is seen in patients with fixed calycectasis and in those in whom reflux does not decrease with age. If sequential concentration tests for a period of 2 or 3 years demonstrate no improvement, cystoscopic reevaluation is indicated, as the refluxing orifice may not have improved with growth as initially anticipated. Clinically, correction of reflux may result in improved concentrating ability (Uehling and Wear, 1976) and renal growth (Willscher et al., 1976a), but calycectasis is often fixed in patients in whom surgical correction is necessary (Babcock et al., 1976), so some permanent diminution in overall concentrating ability is the rule.

Management

In practice, children who demonstrate vesicoureteral reflux require classification of the type and degree of reflux, as outlined previously, as well as measurement of renal size and cortical thickness and study of the calyceal architecture, abnormalities of which may indicate primary renal malformation or acquired renal damage. The presence of ureteral duplication, bladder diverticula, and other abnormalities of the genitourinary tract and the skeletal, nervous, and gastrointestinal systems are noted. Urinalysis and urine culture and sensitivity tests should be performed. Urinary infection should be treated with specific antibiotic therapy. The medical history should be obtained, with particular attention paid to family history and to bladder and bowel habits.

When reflux is marked in degree, cystoscopy should be done to evaluate the vesicourethral outlet, the appearance of the interior of the bladder, and the architecture and location of the ureteral orifices. The length of the submucosal course of the ureter when the bladder is full is the single most useful guideline in estimating the probability that reflux will subside spontaneously (Fig. 49–15). It normally measures approximately 5 mm at birth, 10 mm by age 10 years, and 13 mm in adulthood (Hutch, 1962). Many studies have shown that in at least 50 to 60 per cent of cases primary reflux will cease spontaneously, particularly if the submucosal tunnel is more than 5 mm at the time of diagnosis. If the submucosal tunnel is between 2 and 5 mm, the probability that reflux will stop is about 33 per cent. If no submucosal tunnel is present, the chances that reflux will subside spontaneously, particularly if the child is older than 2 years of age, is less than 10 per cent (see Fig. 49–9). Conversely, the younger the child at diagnosis, the more likely it is that the intravesical ureter will elongate enough to prevent reflux before full growth is achieved.

Prompt eradication of urinary tract infection is necessary if a trial of nonoperative management is elected. This entails regular examination and culture of the urine at intervals of 8 weeks to exclude asymptomatic reinfection. Home culture kits are useful. The urine should also be tested whenever the child becomes ill.

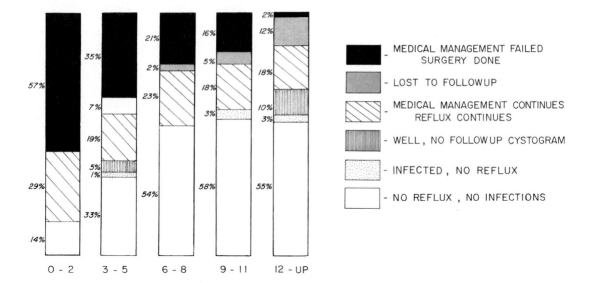

LENGTH OF INTRAMURAL URETER IN MILLIMETERS

Figure 49–15. This graft depicts the relationship between the estimated length of the intravesical ureter at the time of diagnosis and the outcome of a trial of nonoperative management in 247 refluxing units in which the tunnel length was estimated in patients followed 4 to 10 years. There is a nearly linear relationship between original tunnel length and eventual cessation of reflux, indicating the importance of this parameter. (From Kelalis, P. P., and King, L. R. (Eds.): Clinical Pediatric Urology. Philadelphia, W. B. Saunders Co., 1976.)

Recurrence of urinary tract infection despite appropriate specific chemotherapy and long-term prophylactic chemotherapy is a major indication for surgical correction of reflux in children in whom a trial of nonoperative management was elected.

If the child remains healthy, intravenous pyelograms should be obtained at intervals of 1 to 3 years. The development of renal scarring during the period of surveillance is likewise generally an indication for surgery. Cystograms should be obtained at yearly intervals to follow the degree of reflux. The radionuclide cystogram is advantageous in this situation for the reasons outlined earlier. Poor parental cooperation in administering prescribed medication and in keeping follow-up appointments may become a factor in electing early surgical intervention.

It has been suggested that spontaneous resolution of reflux is most likely to occur within the first months or years following diagnosis, but it now seems that the rate at which reflux disappears remains relatively constant throughout childhood, being approximately 20 per cent in each 2-year period (Normand and Smellie, 1979). Reflux was as likely to disappear in children who had recurrent infections as in those without further infection. Puberty is not associated with an increased rate of spontaneous cessation (Edwards et al., 1977).

Even reflux associated with paraureteral diverticula has been observed to undergo spontaneous cessation. Colodny (1983) reported eight children, all with Grade III or IV (international classification) reflux and periureteral diverticula up to 2 cm in diameter, who each experienced cessation of reflux without surgery. In seven of the eight instances the diverticula also disappeared, as judged by follow-up cystogram. However, when the ureter actually enters the diverticulum, associated reflux cannot be expected to resolve spontaneously.

Persistence of reflux into the teenage years is a relative indication for corrective surgery because reflux cannot be expected to stop after growth is completed, and surgery will allow the patient to avoid an indefinite period of surveillance as an adult.

Antireflux surgery in patients with advanced reflux nephropathy remains controversial. Torres et al. (1980b) reported continuing renal deterioration in 11 patients with bilateral reflux and renal scars. Mean creatinine values were greater than 2.75 mg/dl prior to surgery. Progression of renal failure occurred despite successful surgical correction of the reflux. In children with severe bilateral reflux, Burger and Smith (1971) have suggested that proteinuria and a creatinine clearance of less than 25 ml/m² portend progressive renal insufficiency regardless of therapy.

Salvatierra and Tanagho (1977) recommend

antireflux surgery even in children and adolescents with advanced renal insufficiency. While protection of the already compromised renal parenchyma from the risk of offending infection is of obvious benefit, surgical reimplantation has implications in the future management of end-stage renal disease in such patients. In particular, bilateral nephroureterectomy is performed for severe reflux with ureteral dilatation in preparation for a renal transplant because of the risk of recurrent pyelonephritis in such patients receiving immunosuppressive therapy after the transplantation. Although there is no firm evidence that reimplantation will delay progression of end-stage renal failure, the success rate of antireflux surgery is high. A successful procedure may obviate the need for pretransplant bilateral nephroureterectomy, making management during periods of dialysis less complex in terms of fluid balance and anemia (Malek et al., 1983b).

Continued surveillance is necessary after reflux stops spontaneously or after successful antireflux surgery because urinary infections may occur and will require recognition and treatment. Late obstruction of the ureterovesical junction is seen in 0.5 to 1 per cent of patients after successful antireflux surgery (Weiss and Lytton, 1974), so pyelography or sonography should be repeated every 2 to 3 years, even in asymptomatic postoperative patients, until the child is fully grown.

Hypertension

Hypertension is a well-known, long-term complication encountered in children and adults with reflux and renal scarring. A review of 100 children with severe hypertension (diastolic blood pressure greater than 100 mm Hg) revealed 14 with reflux nephropathy, all presenting between the ages of 6 and 15 years (Gill et al., 1976). Pyelonephritic scarring was second in frequency only to chronic glomerulonephritis as the etiology of the high blood pressure. Holland (1979) has reviewed 177 cases of hypertension with scarred atrophic kidneys under various diagnostic terms in 16 series. She suggests that all these terms, in fact, refer to the same pathologic entity, namely reflux nephropathy.

Smellie's long-term study of a large population of children with reflux showed progression of renal damage in the patients who developed hypertension (Smellie and Normand, 1979). The prevalence of high blood pressure in patients

with such scarring is unknown, but hypertension was a significant feature of those developing end-stage renal failure. In Smellie's series, hypertension was detected in 20 per cent of the children with established scars. Six of the 17 hypertensive children had severe hypertension, and eight had some degree of renal insufficiency. However, at least half had normal or near-normal renal function, indicating that the appearance of hypertension is not necessarily related to the development of renal failure but probably associated with vascular lesions within the kidney (Kincaid-Smith, 1975). In favor of such a mechanism is the finding of a high plasma renin activity in two girls with hypertension and reflux nephropathy in whom serum creatinine levels were 0.6 and 1.2 mg/dl, respectively (Siegler, 1976).

Savage et al. (1978) studied 100 normotensive children with reflux nephropathy and found eight with increased plasma renin levels. After 5 years of follow-up, two of the eight children had developed high blood pressure (Dillon, 1982). An additional 51 patients with hypertension at the same center were found on examination to have coarse renal scarring. Almost all those studied had evidence of reflux; 36 had elevated plasma renin activity. Smellie (1975b) has suggested that hypertension associated with reflux and renal scarring is age-related, with increasing risk above age 15 years. Thus, the long-term outcome of patients with renal scarring needs to be accurately defined. Wallace et al. (1981) reported hypertension in 18.5 per cent of children with bilateral renal scars and in 11.3 per cent with unilateral renal scars more than 10 years following surgery for reflux. Stecker et al. (1977) reported hypertension in 3 of 70 children 1 to 19 years after ureteral reimplantation and state that elimination of reflux did not protect against the development of hypertension. No improvement in hypertension occurred in two patients following successful correction of reflux.

In addition to pharmacologic antihypertensive therapy, unilateral nephrectomy has been advocated for relief of hypertension associated with reflux when the affected kidney has very poor function. Dillon (1982) performed 46 renal vein renin studies in 44 hypertensive patients with renal scarring. Ten patients with unilateral scars, in nine of whom the renal vein renin ratio was greater than 1.5, underwent nephrectomy. Eight were cured, and two were improved. Six patients with asymmetric bilateral involvement, with renal vein renin ratios greater than 1.5, also underwent surgery. Five had unilateral nephrectomy, and one had a unilateral nephrectomy with contralateral partial nephrectomy. Three were cured, and three were improved. Of special interest is the observation that approximately half these 44 patients required segmental renal vein renin determinations in order to define the source of their hypertension. Bailey (1979a) described two patients who had unilateral renal scarring and hypertension with renal vein renin ratios of greater than 1.5, yet with low peripheral renin levels. This report confirms the importance of segmental renal vein renin sampling.

Reflux and Pregnancy

Surgical correction of reflux is generally recommended when the reflux persists beyond puberty. An additional rationale is the protection of the sexually active and potentially pregnant woman from pyelonephritic episodes, thereby reducing the risk of maternal renal damage, premature delivery, and increased fetal or perinatal loss. Hutch et al. (1958) demonstrated reflux during pregnancy in 5 of 12 women whose gestation was complicated by pyelonephritis. He also reported a disproportionately high incidence of pyelonephritis during pregnancy among 23 women known to have recurrent bacteriuria and a radiologic diagnosis of chronic pyelonephritis with reflux.

Heidrick et al. (1967) performed 200 cystograms in the last trimester of pregnancy in an unselected population; seven studies revealed reflux (3.5 per cent). An additional 121 women underwent cystography within 30 hours of delivery; two of these also refluxed. Three of these nine women with reflux had developed pyelonephritis earlier in their pregnancy compared with only 4.8 per cent in those without reflux. Thus, it appears that reflux is a significant risk factor predisposing to pyelonephritis during pregnancy.

Williams et al. (1968) evaluated 100 women with asymptomatic coliform bacteriuria during pregnancy. All were treated with a standard course of antibiotic therapy. They were studied radiographically 4 to 6 months post partum. Cystography demonstrated reflux in 21; bacteriuria was again found at the time of the study in 13 of these (62 per cent) compared with only 16 per cent of women without reflux. Ten of the 21 patients with reflux (48 per cent) had renal scarring compared with only 9 per cent of the nonrefluxing group. Two thirds of those with reflux required two or more courses of antibiotics to clear their infection compared with less than one quarter of those without reflux. These data suggest that in pregnant women bacteriuria with reflux is more difficult to eradicate than bacteriuria not complicated by reflux. Moreover, persistent bacteriuria during pregnancy in the face of therapy appears to identify a population of women with a high incidence of reflux nephropathy. Other authors have noted that bacteriuria with reflux in pregnancy tends to persist post partum. Pyelonephritis, which is observed in only 1 to 3 per cent of all pregnancies, occurs in about 30 per cent of pregnant women with otherwise asymptomatic bacteriuria (Whalley and Cunningham, 1977). Although there is a strong suspicion that reflux during pregnancy predisposes to bacteriuria, lack of a longitudinal study in a population of pregnant women with known reflux does not allow a definite conclusion. Since we cannot predict which women will develop bacteriuria during pregnancy, we continue to recommend surgical correction of reflux when it persists beyond puberty.

Clinical Trials of Medical versus Surgical Treatment

Only a randomized prospective clinical trial can determine whether spontaneous cessation of reflux, when it occurs, is preferable to surgery, and which course of therapy has the best potential in terms of renal growth. Moreover, the issue of sterile reflux in conjunction with ureterectasis and its possible eventual deleterious effect on the kidney can be resolved only by such a study. In the only prospective randomized trial yet published, Scott and Stansfeld (1968) compared the results of early surgical correction of reflux with prophylactic antibiotic therapy and observed that the renal growth in children in whom the reflux was surgically cured exceeded that observed in children in whom the reflux was still present. The population sampled was small, however, and the follow-up period was short.

In 1980, an international prospective randomized clinical trial was instituted among a group of major teaching hospitals in the United States and Europe. Because children with moderate to severe reflux present the most difficult management problems, particularly in choice of therapy, this was the group that was selected for study. All patients less than 9 years of age with primary Grade IV (international classification) reflux are accepted into the trial as well as patients with Grade III reflux persisting beyond infancy (the latter in the European branch only). The aims of the study are to compare the effects of successful antireflux surgery performed at the time of diagnosis with effective, continuous, low-dose antibiotic prophylaxis. This therapeutic trial is designed to test whether sterile high-grade reflux is harmful in and of itself, and whether a difference exists between early successful surgery and effective medical management in preventing the possible deleterious effects of reflux on renal growth, creatinine clearance, development of new renal scars, or progression of established scars. In addition, this study will establish the true incidence of recurrent urine infections and hypertension in surgically and medically treated patients.

This prospective approach employs random allocation. Precise criteria are used to select patients, and the standardization of diagnostic, therapeutic, and follow-up procedures should permit an accurate comparison of the two therapeutic modalities. Preliminary results may be available shortly.

Summary

Vesicoureteral reflux is most often a manifestation of a congenital abnormality of the ureterovesical junction. Depending upon the degree of derangement, primary reflux may subside spontaneously during childhood or may persist after full growth has been achieved. However, the presence of reflux places the kidney at risk to deleterious effects from urinary tract infections. Therefore, diligent surveillance for and prevention of urinary tract infection are mandatory in children with reflux; judicious operative intervention is required to correct vesicoureteral reflux in those patients with severe derangement of the ureterovesical junction or intractable recurrent urinary tract infection. The surgical techniques employed are described later in this chapter.

MEGAURETER

Much of the debate surrounding the diagnosis and treatment of "megaureter" stems from confusion in nomenclature, the term meaning a single specific disease to some while carrying a more general connotation to others. Caulk (1923) first used the term to denote the condition of a 32-year-old woman with distal ureterectasis without pyelectasis or calycectasis. The

word itself is simply a combination of *mega*, meaning "big," and ureter. Thus, it may be argued that the term can be applied to any dilated ureter.

Cussen (1967) has established normal measurements of ureteral diameter in infants and children from 30 weeks of gestation to 12 years of age. Any ureter outside these norms, 7 mm at age 12 years, is abnormal and could be considered a megaureter. However, in the clinical setting, megaureter usually denotes more than minimal ureterectasis. The term has been expanded to include dilated ureters with or without pyelocalycectasis, which may or may not be associated with demonstrable obstruction. Debate centers on precise differentiation of the obstructed from the nonobstructed megaureter. The practical reason for differentiating these causes is that obstructed ureters require surgical correction, whereas dilated ureters without reflux or obstruction can generally be successfully managed with a modicum of surveillance only or, at most, antibacterial prophylaxis. In addition, nonobstructed but dilated ureters do not often improve after successful reimplantation but seem prone to surgical complications, which may result in increased hydronephrosis. Recent emphasis on the furosemide (Lasix)–assisted IVP and renogram and the Whitaker test in differentiating the obstructed from the nonobstructed state has advanced our understanding of the causes of ureterectasis.

The purposes of this discussion are to define megaureter in a reasonable way and to establish guidelines for differential diagnosis that are of practical use to the clinician. Emphasis is placed on the classification of megaureter so that the various causes will leap to mind when one is confronted with such a case. The various anatomic causes of obstructed meagureter are described, but once this diagnosis is made, techniques of successful surgical correction become much more important than considerations of etiology, which may remain, in any case, somewhat unclear in individual cases.

All dilated ureters have characteristics in common, especially lack of effective peristalsis caused by inability of the walls of the dilated ureter to coapt. However, lack of peristalsis does not itself result in renal damage or in failure of the kidney to grow. Therefore, to stop the evaluation at the diagnosis of "big ureter" or to advise ureteral tailoring and reimplantation in all such cases is to do the patient a disservice. Furthermore, the congenital nonobstructed megaureter is often associated with megacalycosis, which is calyceal dilatation without obstruction. Thus, the presence of ureteral dilatation with calycectasis is not in itself absolutely indicative of ureterovesical junction (UVJ) obstruction. It is safest to initially consider megaureter a radiographic finding and to train oneself to proceed systematically to exclude reflux or UVJ obstruction as causes.

Classification of Megaureter

All modern attempts to classify megaureter have been in response to the practical need to differentiate the obstructed from the unobstructed variety. Whitaker (1973) and others have pointed out that relatively severe reflux may result in the appearance of megaureter on IVP. More recent classifications have attempted to start with ureterectasis, with or without calycectasis, and include all possible causes. The international classification of Smith et al. (1977) is the most comprehensive (Table 49–2). In this scheme, megaureter may be due to obstruction or reflux, or it may be idiopathic—that is, developmental—and not associated with either reflux or obstruction. Each of these major categories may then be subdivided into a primary and secondary group. Thus, the cause of primary obstructive megaureter is obstruction at or just above the ureterovesical junction. In secondary obstructive megaureter, the ureterectasis is due to intravesical obstruction from valves, prolapsing ureterocele, and the like.

Primary refluxing megaureter is due to a short or absent intravesical ureter, congenital paraureteral diverticulum, or other derangement of the ureterovesical junction. In secondary refluxing megaureter, reflux is present together with another anomaly, such as neuropathic bladder or infravesical obstruction.

In primary nonobstructive, nonrefluxing megaureter there is no juxtavesical obstruction, reflux, bladder anomaly, or outlet obstruction. The ureterectasis is isolated or associated with calycectasis, but upper tract drainage is good by all functional parameters. In children, such systems tend to improve in radiographic appearance with growth, although some ureterectasis usually persists. In secondary nonrefluxing, nonobstructive megaureter the dilatation of the upper tract is due to urinary infection, diabetes insipidus, or other rare causes of very high rates of urine formation.

This is an exhaustive classification. The main advantage is that all patients with ureterectasis can be classified within the system. Glassberg (1977), and others have found its use cumbersome, however, when dealing with what most consider typical megaureter. They argue that in general use the term "megaureter" is not applied to hydroureter caused by overt neuropathic bladder or typical bladder outlet obstruction with bladder trabeculation and residual urine. Megaureter is usually reserved for more mystifying conditions in which the bladder and bladder outlet are normal but the ureter is dilated to some extent (Figs. 49–16 and 49–17).

Dilated ureters of the prune belly syndrome are given a category of their own. However, it must be recognized that in this syndrome the ureterectasis commonly associated may be due to reflux or ureterovesical junction obstruction or may be of the nonobstructive variety and can be categorized according to these characteristics. Glassberg et al. (1982) have also addressed the cause of residual ureterectasis commonly seen after successful resection of urethral valves.

Our own practical classification of megaureter is given in Table 49–3. We tend to agree that the international classification is more complex than necessary and that megaureter means ureteral dilatation in the absence of another overt disease to most urologists. The prune belly and iatrogenic megaureters can be categorized, after evaluation, into one of the four groups, as appropriate diagnostic studies need to be done in nearly every case to rule out obstruction. We added the "reflux with UVJ obstruction" category to call attention to the fact that reflux and obstruction can coexist in a small proportion of patients. In these instances, the reflux is often the most obvious finding, and concomitant obstruction may not be considered unless the possibility of dual lesions is kept in mind. If a

TABLE 49–2. INTERNATIONAL CLASSIFICATION OF MEGAURETER

	Primary	Secondary
Obstructed	Intrinsic ureteral obstruction	To urethral obstruction or extrinsic lesions
Reflux	Reflux is only abnormality	Associated with bladder outlet obstruction or neurogenic bladder
Nonrefluxing, nonobstructed	Idiopathic ureteral dilation	To polyuria (diabetes insipidus) or infection (?)

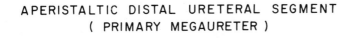

APERISTALTIC DISTAL URETERAL SEGMENT
(PRIMARY MEGAURETER)

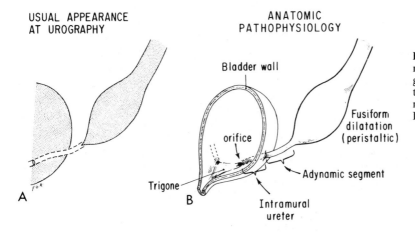

USUAL APPEARANCE
AT UROGRAPHY

ANATOMIC
PATHOPHYSIOLOGY

Bladder wall

Fusiform
dilatation
(peristaltic)

orifice

Adynamic segment

Trigone

Intramural
ureter

A

B

Figure 49–16. Artist's conception of megaureter. Ureteral dilatation begins above the ureterovesical junction, usually a few millimeters or more above the bladder. (Courtesy of Dr. A. P. McLaughlin, III.)

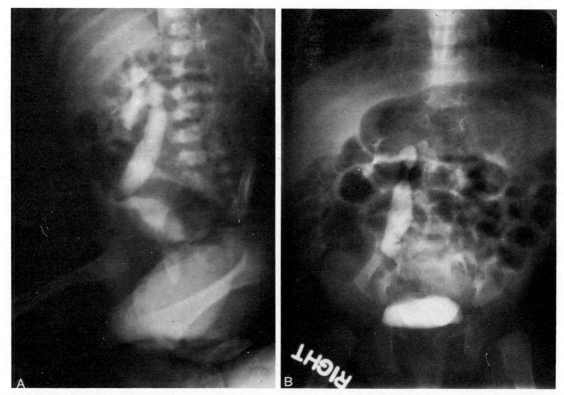

Figure 49–17. Megaureter with calycectasis was diagnosed on fetal ultrasound. *A,* At 1 week of age, an IVP revealed ureteral dilatation but less calycectasis than was suggested by the degree of ureterectasis. There was no reflux. A renogram showed an obstructive curve with prompt drainage after furosemide administration. *B,* Three months later, the calycectasis has resolved.

TABLE 49–3. SIMPLIFIED CLASSIFICATION OF
PRIMARY MEGAURETER*

1. Nonobstructing, nonrefluxing megaureter—without
   obstruction or reflux
2. Obstructive megaureter—due to ureterovesical
   obstruction
3. Refluxing megaureter
4. Megaureter due to ureterovesical obstruction masked
   by reflux

*This simplified system is useful when there is not
intravesical obstruction, reflux, or overt abnormality of the
urinary tract except for hydroureteronephrosis. Megaureter
can then be due to UVJ obstruction or reflux, and category
4 is included to remind the clinician that these lesions can
coexist. Ureterectasis not associated with obstruction or
reflux is also a variety of primary megaureter (category 1).

delayed film is obtained after the cystogram,
poor drainage of one or both upper tracts may
suggest associated UVJ obstruction (Fig.
49–18). This can then be confirmed or excluded
by further evaluation. In a series of over 400
refluxing renal units, Weiss and Lytton (1974)
found concomitant UVJ obstruction in nine.
This can be an important observation, since
proven obstruction generally requires early surgical correction, whereas reflux is often treated
by surveillance, at least for a time.

The reader should employ the system of
megaureter classification that seems most useful.
The main thing to be kept in mind is that
ureterectasis does not always mean obstruction
even when calycectasis is also present. Primary
megaureter is an inherently compound term and
usually includes both primary obstructed megaureter and primary nonobstructive megaureter.

Etiology

NONOBSTRUCTIVE, NONREFLUXING MEGAURETER

The cause of isolated nonobstructed megaureter is not clear. There is no stenosis of the
juxtavesicular ureter, but the ureter is usually
dilated beginning at a point just above the
bladder. The dilatation may involve the entire
ureter or may be segmental. The lowermost
ureter is usually the widest and is bulbous in
appearance, with a sharp cut-off and little tortuosity. Rarely, only the midportion of the
ureter may be dilated. This configuration is
sometimes reminiscent of the dilated ureters
often seen in boys with the prune belly syndrome, so a primary abnormality of the ureteral
musculature is a suspected cause.

REFLUXING MEGAURETER

This term implies that the appearance of
megaureter on IVP, minimally some ureterec-

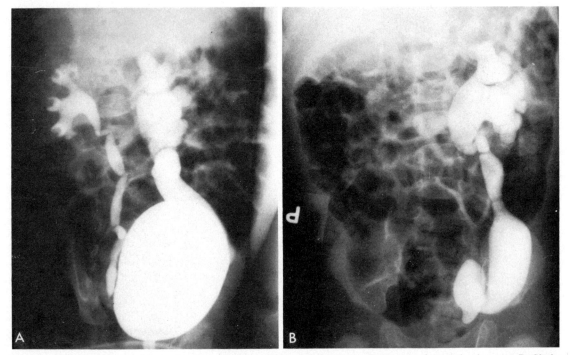

Figure 49–18. *A,* Child with bilateral reflux, dilated collecting system with significant calycectatic changes. *B,* Six-hour
drainage film. Note right side completely empty and sharp cutoff on left at ureterovesical junction. This left side combines
the worst features of two problems—reflux and obstruction.

tasis, is due to reflux. The presence of reflux is usually noted on cystogram. Any of the various causes of reflux maybe responsible. The reflux can be managed according to the etiology, that is, by surveillance or by early operative correction. The choice of therapy in such instances is discussed earlier in this chapter.

OBSTRUCTED MEGAURETER

The juxtavesical ureter may be normal in caliber and yet be the site of functional obstruction, causing proximal ureterectasis, as discussed in Chapter 38. In such instances, the undilated segment does not conduct the peristaltic wave, usually owing to a deficiency in the muscle fibers, which are oriented in spiral fashion. Occasionally, circular muscle bundles are hypertrophied and appear to cause obstruction. The presence of a narrowed juxtavesicular ureteral segment that will not convey the peristaltic wave or dilate enough to permit free passage of urine is the most important cause of primary obstructive megaureter, however. The narrow segment measures from 0.5 to 4 cm in length. Gregoir and Debled (1969) described four his-

tologic types, the majority (60 per cent) exhibiting increased collagenous tissue in the terminal 3 to 4 cm of the ureter. A band of circumferential tissue devoid of muscle in the most distal portion of the narrowed segment is another cause (MacKinnon, 1977). At times a band of thickened muscle is arranged in a nearly circular pattern and seems to be the site of obstruction. It is postulated that such obstruction is initially caused by focal congenital absence of the spiral musculature of the lowermost ureter and that consequent local secondary muscular hypertrophy compounds the problem.

McLaughlin et al. (1973) reviewed the histopathology of 32 typical primary megaureters (obstructed and nonobstructed). Four anatomic varieties could be distinguished. Five ureters were normal histologically in the narrowed portion and contained longitudinal as well as spiral muscle fibers (Fig. 49–19). These patients presumably had nonobstructive megaureter, but physiologic studies to rule out obstruction were not performed, as the furosemide renogram and Whitaker test were not then in use.

The smooth muscle in two specimens was

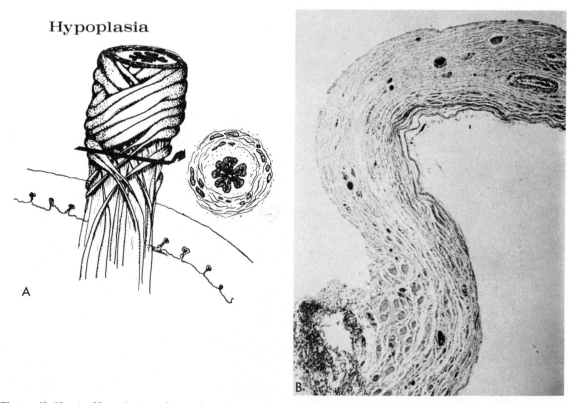

Figure 49–19. *A,* Hypoplasia and atrophy of ureteral muscle as seen in 22 patients in McLaughlin's series. *B,* Photomicrograph from section of ureter. (From McLaughlin, A. P., III, Pfister, R. C., Leadbetter, W. F., et al.: J. Urol., *109*:805, 1973. © 1973, The Williams & Wilkins Company, Baltimore.)

predominantly circular in orientation, while three showed mural fibrosis with little or no musculature.

The fourth and most common type (69 per cent) was characterized by pronounced muscular hypoplasia and atrophy of the muscle fibers, which were separated by sheets of fibrotic tissue (Fig. 49–19). The authors concluded that obstruction had two causes: (1) absence of muscle fibers, which prevents transmission of peristalsis, and (2) fibrotic rigidity of the ureteral wall, which prevents expansion and free passive urine egress.

Tanagho (1973) presented an embryologic explanation of these changes, based on studies in the fetal lamb. He noted that the distal ureter is the last portion to develop its muscular coat and that early muscular differentiation is primarily of the muscle with circular orientation. This observation suggests that arrest late in development results in absence of the longitudinally oriented musculature that conducts the peristaltic wave, and that this, in turn, results in obstruction by the circular muscle fibers, which then often undergo hypertrophy.

When conveying a bolus of urine, each muscular component of a ureteral segment or spindle contracts to force the fluid into the adjacent spindle (Murnaghan, 1957). Obstruction at the terminal ureter causes partial retrograde emptying. Ureteral dilatation is potentially dependent upon the rate of urine flow, in that all ureters become dilated if their volume capacity is exceeded (Hutch and Tanagho, 1965). The retrograde flow of urine from the most distal ureter combined with newly excreted urine produces an excessive load, resulting in dilatation of the normal ureter proximal to the stenotic segment. Vesicoureteral reflux, in quantity, evokes a similar response, and ureterectasis occurs when refluxed bladder urine exceeds the ureter's normal carrying capacity.

Several electron microscopic studies of the lower ureter in nonrefluxing megaureter confirm the variable nature of the lesion (Tokunaka et al., 1982; Hanna and Jeffs, 1975; Pagano and Passerini, 1977). Moreover, pathologic studies of the narrow ureteral segment have not yet been correlated in adequate numbers of patients with the findings on diuretic renogram or Whitaker test to define which lesions are truly obstructive.

Ureterectasis without obstruction must occur by a different mechanism, or obstruction might be present during early development, which results in residual ureterectasis even though the obstruction itself somehow resolves.

At the time of his original description, Caulk (1923) equated megaureter and Hirschsprung's disease, a concept supported by Swenson and Fisher (1955) and Grana and Swenson (1965). Absence of ureteral parasympathetic ganglia, as found in Hirschsprung's disease, has not been noted in children with ureterectasis, however (Gregoir and Debled, 1969; Leibowitz and Bodian, 1963; Notley, 1972).

Radiographic Appearance

In obstructive megaureter the narrow, most distal segment is so close to the bladder wall that this segment is usually obscured by the overlying contrast-filled bladder; it was visualized on the initial IVP in only 3 of 38 megaureters reviewed by Pfister and Hendren (1978). The chances of visualizing the obstructing segment are improved by obtaining oblique views or postvoiding films. Distal ureteral dilatation may be so severe that the bulbous lower ureter prolapses below the proximal portion of the narrowed segment so that the distal dilated portion and the narrow lowermost ureter appear side by side. This has given birth to the term "ureteral valve," which is quite descriptive but sometimes misleading. First, the term "ureteral valve" is too easily confused with "urethral valve" phonetically. More important, the septum or valve between the dilated portion of the ureter and the narrow part is seldom, if ever, the primary cause of the obstruction, which seems clearly to be due to intrinsic stenosis of the most distal segment. The valvelike flap may compound the obstruction but rarely, if ever, occurs without a very narrow, more distal juxtavesical segment, which is the hallmark of obstructed megaureter.

Regardless of the severity of upper ureteral dilatation, active movement of the ureteral wall is seen on cineradiographic studies in almost all cases. Effective peristalsis is absent when the walls of the ureter cannot coapt, and, like ureteral peristalsis generally, this movement is reduced by bacterial exotoxins during some infections. Usually the ureteral movements convey contrast media to the narrowed segment, where most of the bolus simply floods back up the ureter. If the upper ureter is of normal or near-normal caliber, this "refluxed" urine will initiate a wave of retrograde peristalsis. It seems likely that such peristalsis damps the pressure and prevents dilatation of the pelvis. When only the lower ureter is dilated, the pelvis is usually normal in size. When the entire ureter is dilated, some pelvic dilatation is often present also.

Mode of Presentation

Most children with megaureter with or without calycectasis present with urinary infection (which may be cystitis and unrelated to the upper tract anomaly), with hematuria, or with otherwise unexplained abdominal pain. It is not unusual for the dilated ureter to be noted at the time of appendectomy or other abdominal surgery. Uremia, anemia, renal rickets, failure to thrive, or other signs of renal failure are, fortunately, rare presenting complaints. Megaureter is bilateral in about 25 per cent of patients. Children presenting prior to 1 year of age are more apt to have bilateral megaureter than are older patients (Williams and Hulme-Moir, 1970). The incidence in males is 1.5 to 4.8 times greater than in females. The left ureter is involved 1.6 to 4.5 times more often than the right. The incidence of contralateral renal agenesis is about 9 per cent (Table 49–3). The condition is not known to be hereditary, but families with more than one member with megaureter have been described.

Methods for the Differential Diagnosis of Obstructive versus Nonobstructive Megaureter

Since reflux of moderate or severe degree is usually diagnosed without difficulty on cystogram, this discussion will center on differentiating obstructed from nonobstructed megaureter. Many tests are clinically useful in this regard, and these are summarized later. Since the child with megaureter usually presents with urinary tract infection, hematuria, or a flank mass, we assume that a cystogram and IVP are performed and that the x-rays show the ureteral dilatation without reflux or infravesical obstruction as an obvious cause. Renal scans are preferred to excretory urography in the neonate, performed as described further on.

FUROSEMIDE RENOGRAM

The next evaluation can be cystoscopy but is now commonly a renogram using furosemide (Lasix) to stimulate washout of the dilated collecting system if the renogram curve appears obstructive (see also Chapter 7). This test is in wide use, but normal parameters that rule out obstruction have not yet been clearly established. The reason for this difficulty in interpretation is that if the hydronephrosis is very severe, even a relatively well-functioning kidney may not be able to diurese fast enough to clearly demonstrate good drainage after the administration of furosemide. A poorly functioning kidney may not be able to excrete enough urine under any conditions to clear the radioactivity at a "normal" rate. Finally, differences in the degree of hydroureteronephrosis mean that varying degrees of diuresis will dilute the radioactive isotope already excreted by varying amounts, so a spectrum of unobstructed drainage patterns is to be expected. Therefore, the furosemide renogram allows various interpretations, e.g., severely and unequivocally obstructed, unobstructed, and a group in which the diagnosis is not certain. This last group needs further definition. However, some guidelines for the test can be summarized.

The child should have no prior dehydration or enemas. Technetium-labeled DPTA is used to estimate renal blood flow. I-131 labeled hippuran is given, and images of the kidney and ureter are made at 2, 5, 10, 15, 20, 25, and 30 minutes. The counting crystals should be centered over the area where the isotope is pooled, and a catheter should be indwelling to keep the bladder empty. The hippuran renogram is a sensitive test, so the initial renogram curve will usually look obstructed in most cases of megaureter of any etiology. If a catheter is not in place, the child is asked to void, or is catheterized, to determine the effect of bladder emptying on the curve. If the curve continues to appear obstructed, 1 mg of furosemide per kg of body weight is administered. If the amount of radioactivity is reduced by half in less than 10 minutes, the study is normal and UVJ obstruction is not present. When the half-time clearance is 10 to 20 minutes, the study is equivocal and further tests are needed. A half-time clearance of radioactivity requiring longer than 20 minutes is indicative of obstruction unless renal function is very poor or hydronephrosis is extreme, as described earlier.

Some potential pitfalls in the use of the furosemide renogram can be avoided by careful attention to test conditions. Accidental dehydration may minimize the diuresis effect. The technician may accidentally alter the "Y" axis of the renogram curve. The furosemide dose must be standardized and weight-related, as the diuretic effect increases with larger doses. Hippuran, not DTPA, must be used to gauge the furosemide response. Furosemide affects tubular function; hippuran is secreted by the tubules, and hippuran is cleared faster than DPTA. Furosemide administration less than 30 minutes after DTPA administration may result in the collecting system being washed out by "hot," i.e., radioactive, urine, which would produce a false positive test. The child's position during the test should be standardized, as posture may affect drainage of the dilated collecting system. If only the ureter is dilated, the counting crystal should be placed over the area of ureterectasis, not over the kidney.

In spite of these qualifications, the furosemide renogram is a useful test. In fact, Kass et al. (1982) compared it with the more invasive Whitaker test and found the results to be as accurate. Patients with hydroureter without obstruction are then spared more invasive investigations. Also, even though some furosemide renograms are equivocal in some patients with megaureter, such tests are quite reproducible in the same patient when performed in exactly the same manner. Therefore, if the results fall into the equivocal range, a follow-up study done several months after the first may demonstrate improved drainage and thereby exclude obstruction.

OTHER STUDIES

In children who continue to appear to have possible ureteral obstruction, an equivocal or obstructed furosemide renogram is often an indication for further diagnostic studies. These include (1) cystoscopy with ureteral catheterization to see if a "hydronephrotic drip" is present, and (2) measurement of the renal pelvic pressure at which fluid flows into the bladder across the site of possible obstruction (Whitaker test) (Fig. 49-20). It is difficult to make a firm rule as to which of these examinations should be performed first. Many children with megaureter have had previous cystoscopic examinations to rule out urethral obstruction, so a Whitaker test often seems the more pertinent. If cystoscopy has not been done, one may choose to do that first. The anterior urethra is calibrated with bougies and is inspected for an anterior or posterior valve. More than mild bladder trabeculation suggests outflow obstruction. Since the voiding cystogram was normal in these children, the urethra will usually be normal; outlet obstruction, however, may be caused by sphincter dyssynergia, and the hydroureter may be the result of the neurogenic/non-neurogenic bladder syndrome. Urodynamics are then indicated. Attention is next turned to the ureteral orifices. Are they normal, or do their size and position suggest reflux, which is occasionally not detected on cystogram? Is there a small ureterocele? If the orifice is normal, the next step is to pass a 4 or 5 F ureteral catheter, the caliber depending on the size of the child. At least a 4 F is preferred, so that a hydronephrotic drip can be

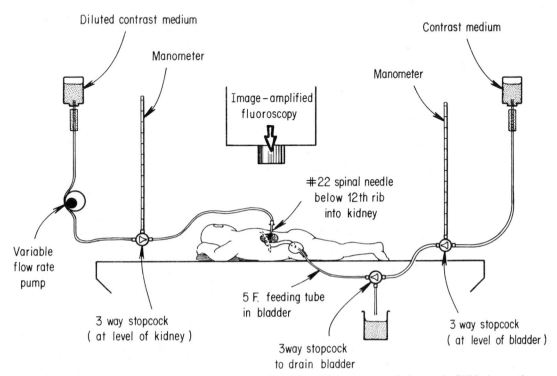

Figure 49-20. Schematic diagram of antegrade pyelography with pressure-perfusion study (Whitaker test).

detected. Occasionally, the ureteral catheter will not pass. This may be due to technical factors, e.g., a difficult angle, or to ureteral meatal stenosis, which is an uncommon cause of ureterectasis but usually susceptible to transurethral or percutaneous meatotomy. Usually, in primary obstructive megaureter the point of obstruction is above the ureteral hiatus, about 5 to 15 mm from the bladder. The ureteral catheter may stop at that point but will usually pass. If a large volume of urine then comes out of the ureteral catheter in a steady drip, a so-called hydronephrotic drip, obstruction is deemed likely to be present.

Contrast material is then introduced, and drainage films are made. The normal rate of drainage from a dilated collecting system in a dehydrated child has not been quantitated, but persistence of contrast in the ureter for 6 hours is usually indicative of obstruction. Conversely, complete drainage within an hour or two is usually most compatible with the diagnosis of nonobstructed, nonrefluxing megaureter. If obstruction is absent, the total volume of the continuous hydronephrotic drip is also apt to be less than one would expect from the size of the dilated collecting system on IVP. These cystoscopic tests to differentiate obstructed from nonobstructed megaureter are all subjective, and yet the results seem fairly accurate. It is hard to conceive that a dilated ureter that produces 20 ml immediately after catheterization and retains contrast for several hours after filling is not an obstructed ureter.

WHITAKER TEST

The other method permitting more complete evaluation of the dilated ureter is measurement of the renal pelvic pressure at which a high volume of fluid, 10 ml per minute, passes the site of possible obstruction. This is a well thought out, physiologic test that has the great advantage of being quantitative. A number, the maximum renal pressure during sustained flow minus the bladder pressure, is produced. The drawbacks are that the test is relatively invasive and usually requires a general anesthetic in children; like the furosemide renogram, it is at times difficult to interpret with certainty. Nonetheless, it has come into wide use to differentiate hydroureteronephrosis due to obstruction from the nonobstructive causes of ureterectasis or calycectasis.

The test requires a nephrostomy or pyelostomy or, most commonly, insertion of long percutaneous needles under fluoroscopic control. Needles of gauge 20 or 22 are usually

employed, although some prefer a larger bore. The needle resistance is subtracted from the renal pressure. An urethral catheter is inserted. A pump capable of delivering a constant flow then perfuses the renal pelvis at a standard rate, 10 ml per minute. Manometers or strain gauges are attached to the perfusion catheter and bladder outflow tubing. Perfusion is maintained until the collecting system is filled and the renal pressure either reaches a plateau or is obviously increasing and is far above the physiologic range, indicating obstruction. Maximum renal relative pressures (renal pelvis pressure minus needle resistance minus bladder pressure) below 15 cm of H_2O are considered to indicate an absence of obstruction. Conversely, higher pressures are regarded as indicative of obstruction, although some cases of marginal elevation may remain equivocal, as discussed later. In typical ureteropelvic junction (UPJ) obstructions, the relative renal pressure may be very elevated during the test; however, most UPJ obstructions are readily diagnosed by the typical appearance of the dilated pelvis and calyces on IVP or ultrasound. Megacalycosis, defined as underdevelopment of the renal pyramids in the absence of obstruction, may occur with ipsilateral nonobstructed megaureter (Von Niederhausern and Tuchschmid, 1971; Talner and Gittes, 1974; Whitaker and Flower, 1981), as noted earlier. In this situation, further evaluation is generally needed, as it is when pyelocalycectasis is combined with typical megaureter. A Whitaker test is usually diagnostic in this situation and will yield relative renal pressures in the normal (usually low normal) or the unequivocally obstructed range. Patients with obstruction are then operated upon, while those without obstruction are followed with an occasional IVP or diuretic renogram to make absolutely certain that the upper tracts do not deteriorate.

When the test is normal, there does not appear to be much risk of misdiagnosis. Witherow and Whitaker (1981) reported on 21 patients, all but 4 of whom were children, evaluated by the Whitaker test in 1973. Patients were divided into four groups. Nine of 11 with elevated pressures who underwent corrective surgery exhibited improved pyelograms or clearances, or both, more than 5 years later. In five children with elevated relative renal pressure, no operation was performed. Four of these patients were boys with valves, in whom the hydroureteronephrosis persisted after valve resection and in whom reimplantation was deferred. In two, the bladder pressures indicated a noncompliant bladder; this elevated pressure was reflected in the kidney, although the relative renal pressure (renal pressure minus bladder pressure) was not elevated. Renal function deteriorated with time in both patients. One of the patients with valves was studied soon after valve resection. The relative renal pressures were elevated. This boy improved. It is surmised that the ureters were obstructed by the hypertrophied detrusor and that as the hypertrophy subsided, the obstruction was relieved.

In seven patients, the pressure-flow study was normal and no operation was performed. After 5 to 9 years, all upper tracts were stable in appearance and function. In four patients, a low relative pressure was found, but operation was performed on clinical grounds. The Whitaker test was introduced in 1973, but its accuracy then was uncertain, so these four patients were treated surgically. Two had bilateral and two had unilateral megaureter. A good surgical result was obtained in each instance. However, after 5 to 8 years, the pyelographic appearance of the kidneys had not changed, except that the tailored lowermost ureter looked less dilated, and renal function was stable. One must conclude that these were patients with nonobstructed megaureter, and that ureteral tailoring and reimplantation could not improve them even though an optimal surgical result was achieved.

The false positive test in the boy with valves, alluded to earlier, is illustrative of problems in interpretation, which are not uncommon. Two groups of children seem particularly prone to misleading or uninterpretable test results. Some are boys with residual hydroureteronephrosis after relief of bladder outlet obstruction; others are children of either sex with persistent or worsened ureterectasis after ureteral reimplantation. The vagaries of the Whitaker test in boys with residual hydronephrosis after valve resection are so great that Glassberg et al. (1982) use the test results to define four different types of megaureter encountered in such patients. They consider relative renal pressures between 15 and 20 cm of H_2O to be inherently equivocal; 3 of 14 renal units studied fell into this marginal category. Only four of the kidneys had low pressures with the bladder both full and empty and were clearly unobstructed. No evaluated patients had unequivocally high relative renal pressures, but in 7 of 14 renal units the test was difficult to interpret. The reason was that renal pressures were normal with the bladder empty but rose quickly into the pathologic range when the bladder began to fill. Thus, strictly speaking, the Whitaker test is normal if done as originally described, with a catheter draining the bladder. However, since some boys with noncompliant bladders after valve ablation develop progressive renal damage, it seems that this observation is important. Also, it seems futile to reimplant such ureters into the bladder with the expectation that drainage will be improved or that the bladder will then somehow function more normally. Glassberg et al. (1982) advise following such patients for at least 6 months. If the upper tracts do not improve and renal pressures remain elevated when the bladder fills, these investigators, and Mitchell (1981), advocate augmentation ileocecocystoplasty to reduce the bladder pressure, using the plicated, reinforced, or intussuscepted ileocecal valve as the antireflux mechanism and moving the ureters into the terminal ileum above the valve. This is also our usual preference, although we think that the success of either operation depends upon removal of the bulk of the noncompliant bladder, retaining only the disc around the urethra or trigone to which the bowel segment is anastomosed. Moreover, we find that only a small proportion of boys with residual hydronephrosis and no reflux after valve resection need further intervention, and that loss of bladder compliance, rather than ureteral obstruction, is the major indication for such surgery.

Other common problems with interpretation of the Whitaker test and results falsely negative for obstruction are seen in children who have persistent or worsening hydronephrosis after ureteral reimplantation. The ureter may be "hooked" as it passes into the vesical hiatus, often around the obliterated umbilical artery, or by the peritoneum. In this situation, the ureter may drain well with the bladder empty. However, as the bladder fills, the entrapped extravesical ureter is immobilized; as the intravesical ureter is shifted laterally, the ureter is angulated at the ureterovesical junction, producing obstruction (Mayo and Ansell, 1980). Such children may also exhibit noncompliant bladders, with renal pressure rising sharply as the bladder begins to fill. Most of these children have normal relative renal pressures with the bladder empty, and most do well over the long term. The bladder seems usually to recover with time, and the child then does well, although interval vesicostomy or intermittent catheterization may be required if ureterectasis increases. Occasionally, specific children will have a completely normal test with a compliant bladder and a low relative renal pressure. In spite of this, hydronephrosis may occasionally increase dramatically, even over only a few months. The reason for this appears to be that, as scar matures, the once unobstructed ureter becomes obstructed, usually at the new hiatus as it passes through the detrusor. This is not a common sequence of events, but it occurs often enough to warn that the Whitaker test must be interpreted with caution in postoperative patients. A negative test does not necessarily mean that obstruction will not occur in the future.

Even with all these provisos, renal pressure-flow measurements have become our most accurate test to differentiate obstructed from non-obstructed megaureter. The test is quite accurate in patients who have not been operated upon and in whom the bladder is compliant. Alternatively, it may be performed intraoperatively to document obstruction, although at that point it is a little late if obstruction is not found. The dilated ureters in the prune belly syndrome may be obstructed or nonobstructed, just as in other types of megaureter, and can be accurately categorized using the Whitaker test.

The only potential problem caused by non-obstructed megaureter is due to stasis caused by the inability of the walls of the ureter to coapt. This loss of effective peristalsis clearly seems not to prevent renal growth, either in children or in animal models, but such ureterectasis occasionally seems to be the predisposing cause of urine infection.

Management of Primary Obstructed Megaureter

HISTORY OF SURGICAL TREATMENT

Caulk treated his initial patient with trans-urethral endoscopic meatotomy in 1923. The patient did well clinically, but, of course, it is not certain whether the surgeon was dealing with an obstructed or nonobstructed megaureter. Lewis and Kimbrough (1952) performed ureteral meatotomy after ureteral dilations and nephroureterolysis failed to result in improvement, but reflux resulted. In 1954, in view of the poor surgical results up to that time, Nesbit and Withycombe concluded that megaureter should not be treated surgically. In retrospect, it seems that ureteral meatotomy was doomed to fail, since the obstruction, when present, is extravesical. In fact, the intravesical ureter is seldom involved, although an occasional child will have severe stenosis at the ureteral meatus without a ureterocele.

The use of a tapered, isolated portion of small bowel to replace the ureter in patients

with extreme hydronephrosis was reported by Swenson et al. (1956). No attempt was made to form an antireflux anastomosis with the bladder. Also in 1956, Lewis and Cletsoway reported using a ureteral nipple similar to that fashioned in a Paquin ureteral reimplantation for reflux. The ureter was not tapered, but the lower, extremely dilated portion was excised. Good surgical results were achieved, and reflux was not demonstrable postoperatively in any of 12 ureters so treated.

Goodwin and associates (1957) also replaced the dilated ureter with isolated ileal segments. Partial extravesical intussusception of the upper ileum into the lower for a distance of 1 to 2 inches was the antireflux mechanism employed. Good long-term results have been achieved. Politano (1972) also successfully used small bowel to replace megaureters. He incorporated a long everted nipple of the distalmost ileal segment through the bladder anastomosis as the antireflux mechanism. All authors have emphasized the need to remove a disc of bladder equal in size to the lumen of the bowel to prevent obstruction when an ileal segment is employed to replace the ureter; the orientation of the bowel loop must always be isoperistaltic. Hirschhorn (1964) and Politano (1972) sought to restore ureteral peristalsis in patients with megaureter by wrapping the dilated ureter with an isolated segment of small bowel from which the mucosa had been removed. The bowel segment must always run the full length of the ureter, preferably from the renal hilum to the bladder, as ureteral dilatation may increase postoperatively above the wrapped segment.

Creevy (1967) was the first to report extensive ureteral tailoring combined with a Politano type of antireflux reimplantation. He clearly defined the radiographic characteristics of the different types of megaureter and felt that ureteral reimplantation was generally indicated when calycectasis was present. Thus, some of his patients probably had nonobstructed megaureter with megacalycosis. Bischoff (1957) advocated tapering of only the lowermost ureter in most instances in order to achieve an antireflux reimplantation.

CURRENT THERAPY

The majority of patients with primary megaureter, particularly those who present as older children or adults, prove to have the nonobstructed variety and do not require surgical intervention. The ureter generally becomes less dilated as the child grows. In a review of their experience with primary megaureter, Williams and Hulme-Moir (1970) presented in detail many cases of children followed for more than 5 years. Those with terminal ureterectasis only always remained stable or improved.

Surgery should be reserved for patients with progressive ureterectasis or extreme generalized hydroureteronephrosis with parenchymal loss, and for those with lesser degrees of dilatation in whom diagnostic tests indicate obstruction.

Another indication for surgery in children with megaureter is recurrent or persistent infection that can be localized to the hydronephrotic system by culturing samples taken from the upper tracts. The urine can be obtained by ureteral catheterization or by percutaneous aspiration. This group may include some with nonobstructed megaureter but severe stasis. As noted earlier, nonobstructed upper tracts seldom improve after surgery in function or appearance, but the infection may be eliminated. It is in this group with persistent infection that the strongest case can be made for tailoring the dilated ureter above the bladder, wrapping the ureter with denuded bowel, or replacing the ureter with a bowel segment to restore peristalsis.

Summary

The diagnosis of primary megaureter is fulfilled under the following conditions:

1. The bladder and bladder outlet appear normal.

2. Ureterectasis begins above a narrow, usually short, distal ureteral segment, which may be difficult to visualize on the IVP. The ureter is dilated for a varying length above, but is usually not as tortuous as one would expect, given the degree of ureterectasis. Calycectasis may or may not be present.

3. Vesicoureteral reflux is absent (except in refluxing megaureter).

4. The ureteral orifice has a normal appearance endoscopically.

Such ureters must then be further studied to differentiate obstructed from nonobstructed megaureter. If intrinsic obstruction is present, a ureteral catheter may not pass through the narrow juxtavesicular ureter. When it does pass, a large volume of urine comes out steadily in a hydronephrotic drip. Contrast instilled for retrograde pyelography will remain in an obstructed system for several hours. The renogram curve on hydrated renal scan has an obstructed pattern that does not change much with the administration of a diuretic. Finally, renal pressures are elevated when the pelvis or upper ureter is perfused with fluid at 10 ml per minute (Whitaker test).

In primary nonobstructive megaureter, a ureteral catheter will pass easily unless technical problems are present. Although some urine may come out in a steady drip, the volume is less than would be expected considering the volume of the system. Similarly, contrast instilled through the catheter tends to drain more quickly, although this is still a function of the volume of the hydroureteronephrosis or ureterectasis. The diuretic renogram may be equivocal, but the Whitaker test will show low relative renal pressures. When marked calycectasis is present with nonobstructed megaureter, this is usually due to megacalycosis. A clue may be that the renal pelvis is usually not as dilated as one would expect with apparent calycectasis of severe degree.

Although the diagnosis of no obstruction can be established with relative certainty, children with nonobstructive megaureter should be followed to be certain that the upper tracts are stable or do improve, as expected, with growth.

The treatment of refluxing megaureter, or the appearance of a typical megaureter on IVP that turns out to be due to reflux, depends on the etiology of the reflux and the chance that the reflux may subside spontaneously. Reflux can occur in conjunction with obstructive megaureter—they are different lesions—and this possibility should be considered when the reflux is severe in grade and the ureter drains poorly.

Megaureter of iatrogenic cause, following prior ureteral reimplantation, or ureterectasis seen in boys with prune belly syndrome can be evaluated and categorized according to whether or not ureteral obstruction is present.

Secondary obstructive megaureter is initially treated by correcting the primary problem. When bladder outlet obstruction is the cause, the hydroureter will usually improve as detrusor hypertrophy regresses. When ureterectasis persists in such circumstances, re-evaluation will permit differentiation of the megaureters into the obstructed or nonobstructed category or detection of a noncompliant bladder. Hydrated, diuretic augmented renograms and the Whitaker test may indicate obstruction until the detrusor hypertrophy has had time—6 months to a year—to subside. However, the results of ureteral reimplantation are usually better when the detrusor is normal. Partly for this reason, such ureterectasis should be given a chance to improve after the outlet obstruction is relieved.

Reimplantation into a noncompliant bladder should be avoided and alternatives, such as bladder augmentation or ileocecal cystoplasty, considered, as discussed in the section on urethral valves.

Neuropathic bladder is another common cause of secondary megaureter. Here again, reflux and obstruction may be combined. When urine is retained in the bladder, the keystone of therapy has become intermittent catheterization on a regular timed basis, although ureteral reimplantation or bladder augmentation may be needed.

Other causes of acquired obstructed megaureter include calculus, granulomatous disease, and the rare ureteral valve or midureteral stricture.

URETERAL REIMPLANTATION

Ureteroneocystostomy

In 1900 Bovee reviewed ureteral surgery and credited Tauffer with performing the first ureteroneocystostomy in 1877. Eighty cases had been reported, most of which were performed after accidental division of the ureter at the time of laparotomy or during surgery for ureteral fistulas following difficult labor or forceps delivery. Bovee mentions several operations for "abnormal congenital ureteral openings" but none for vesicoureteral reflux. Concerning the technique of ureteroneocystectomy, he commented that a transabdominal extraperitoneal approach was appropriate and noted that "an effort has been made to imitate the normal oblique bladder implantation of the ureter to prevent reflux." Ancillary techniques used to correct the difficult clinical situation of inadequate ureteral length that were mentioned in this early article include the psoas hitch, transureteroureterostomy, and inferior nephropexy!

In 1934 Vermooten and Neuswanger described a "submucous" (sic) technique of ureteral reimplantation in dogs that lessened the incidence of vesicoureteral reflux postoperatively compared with direct ureterovesical anastomosis. In 1943, Stevens and Marshall reported ten patients in whom a similar technique had been employed. Dodson (1946) reviewed the techniques of ureteroneocystostomy and mentioned the "advantage of mobilizing or straightening the ureter to lengthen it and lessen the distance that it must traverse to reach the bladder" when the ureter was dilated and tortuous.

Pioneering studies of patients with spinal cord injury after World War II demonstrated that reflux was the most common cause of hydronephrosis and led to progressive renal deterioration in the presence of urinary tract infection. Talbot and Bunts (1949) suggested that ureteral reimplantation to correct vesicoureteral reflux would be beneficial in such cases. In 1952, Hutch reported success in 8 of 11 ureteral reimplantations for vesicoureteral reflux in nine paraplegic patients. Hutch then employed a combined extravesical and intravesical approach to the distal ureter. In 1952, Hutch reported satisfactory results in 11 of 13 ureteral reimplantations in seven children, four of whom had myelodysplasia.

In 1958, Politano and Leadbetter described their technique of intravesical mobilization of the terminal ureter with subsequent reimplantation through a new vesical hiatus and submucosal tunnel. They reported the elimination of reflux in 14 patients requiring a total of 21 ureteral reimplantations. One case of postoperative ureteral obstruction required reoperation. The four patients reported in detail in their series were children who did not have overt neuropathic bladders (Fig. 49–21).

Paquin (1959) summarized the fundamental requirements of a satisfactory antireflux operation. These include a tension-free anastomosis between the ureter and bladder, a submucosal tunnel that is five times as long as the diameter of the ureter, and firm support for the intravesical ureter from the underlying bladder muscle. The ureter should be straightened when necessary to secure proper drainage, but care should be taken to preserve its blood supply. Finally, the terminal 3 to 4 cm of ureter should be tapered if its diameter is greater than 8 to 10 mm in order to restore the proper ratio of length to width in the intramural ureter. Paquin also reported a technique of ureteroneocystostomy that included both extravesical and intravesical dissection to create the new vesical hiatus and submucosal tunnel as well as formation of an everted nipple at the ureterovesical anastomosis (Fig. 49–22). This technique has also remained in general use, except that formation of the intravesical nipple is now generally omitted.

Lich and coworkers (1961) described an extravesical approach to create a submucosal tunnel for the ureter and a new hiatus in the muscular wall of the bladder. This technique does not disturb the continuity of the ureterovesical mucosa, nor does it alter the position of the ureteral orifice (Fig. 49–23). It is employed primarily in situations in which there is little ureterectasis, as the amount of lengthening of

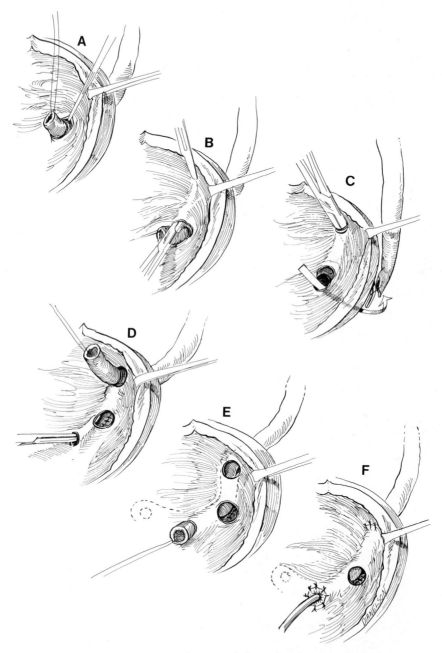

Figure 49–21. Politano-Leadbetter technique of ureteroneocystostomy.

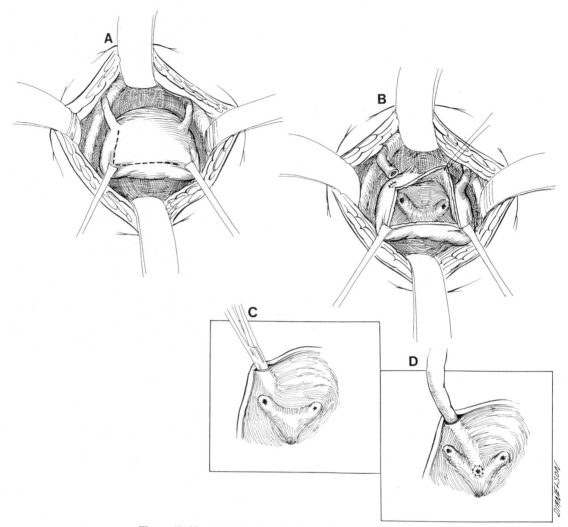

Figure 49–22. *A–D,* Paquin technique of ureteroneocystostomy.

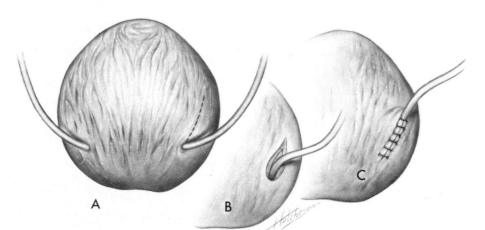

Figure 49–23. Lich's technique of vesicoureteroplasty. (From Kelalis, P. P., and King, L. R. (Eds.): Clinical Pediatric Urology. Philadelphia, W. B. Saunders Co., 1976.)

the intravesical ureter that can be obtained without angulation is limited.

Williams (1961), Hutch (1963), and Glenn and Anderson (1967) all described intravesical ureteral advancement procedures. Each requires mobilization of the ureter from its attachments as it traverses the muscular wall of the bladder, with advancement of its orifice to a new location on the floor of the bladder in order to secure a longer intravesical segment. These procedures are also originally limited to patients in whom the ureter is of relatively normal caliber and in whom there is sufficient room for advancement of the ureter on the floor of the bladder (Fig. 49–24).

Stephens (1977) and Glenn and Anderson (1967) later refined the intravesical advancement technique (Fig. 49–25). After mobilization of the ureter within the deep periureteral sheath, the bladder wall at the superior margin of the vesical hiatus is incised for a distance of 2 to 3 cm; the hiatus is closed inferiorly in order to buttress the intravesical ureter, displace the hiatus superiorly, and gain more length for the submucosal tunnel. The orifice is then advanced to a new location on the floor of the bladder. Utilizing the exposure obtained by initially enlarging the hiatus, a dilated, tortuous ureter can be satisfactorily shortened and tapered from within the bladder prior to reimplantation; this technique is also applicable to the reimplantation of double ureters.

Cohen (1975) modified the advancement technique and obtained additional length for creation of an adequate submucosal tunnel by leading the reimplanted ureter across the midline (Fig. 49–26). The Cohen operation has become very popular because of its versatility. It must be employed when the trigone is tubularized to form a sphincter in incontinence operations, and the results achieved after conventional antireflux surgery have been very good. Perhaps because the original urinary hiatus is usually maintained, there is a very low incidence of obstruction following reimplantation using this technique. One often cited drawback to the

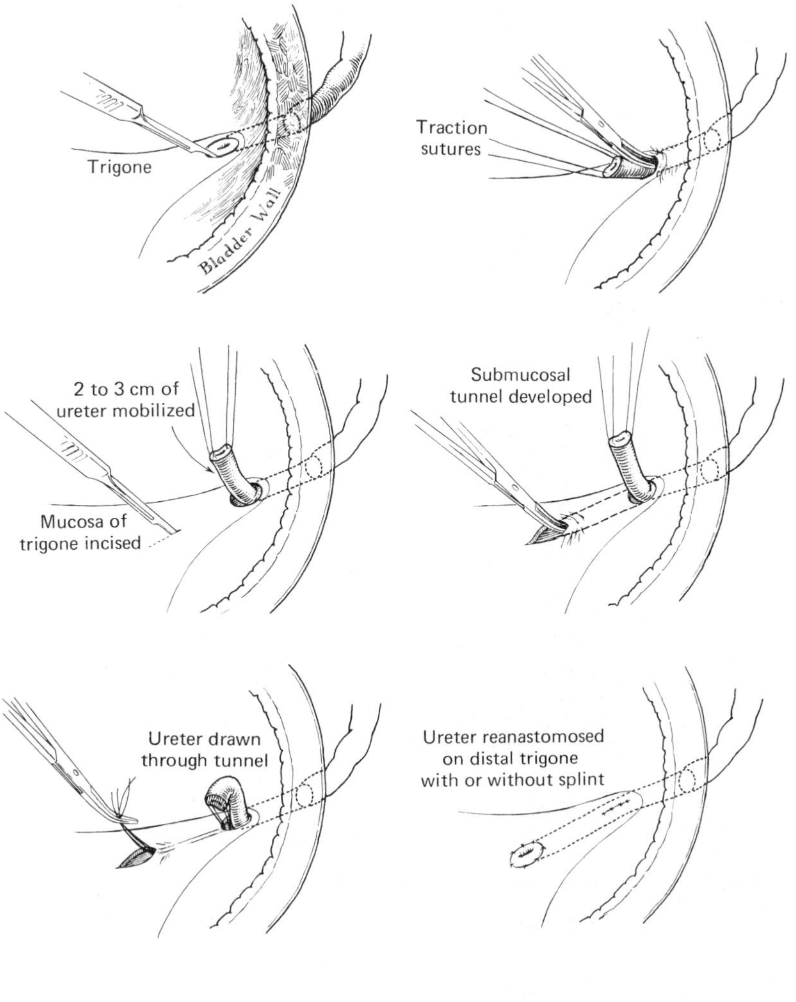

Figure 49–24. Glenn-Anderson distal tunnel ureteral reimplantation. Mobilization of distal tunnel and development of submucosal tunnel distally across trigone obviates some of the potential difficulties of ureteral advancement procedures. (From Glenn, J. F. (Ed.): Urologic Surgery, 2nd ed. New York, Harper & Row, 1975.)

Cohen procedure is that the reimplanted orifices tend to face laterally, as each ureter commonly crosses the midline. Subsequent instrumentation through a cystoscope may be difficult. However, it is possible to fill the bladder and puncture the anterior wall percutaneously with a Cystocath sheath under direct cystoscopic visualization. The sheath of the Cystocath is placed opposite the lateral facing reimplanted orifice, and a ureteral catheter is usually then easily passed percutaneously (Lamesch, 1981). This method of retrograde catheterization following a Cohen reimplant seems very safe. Catheter drainage after bladder puncture is generally unnecessary, as the puncture wound in the bladder usually seals almost immediately. An additional advantage is that adult-sized instruments that will not pass through pediatric cystoscopes can be intro-

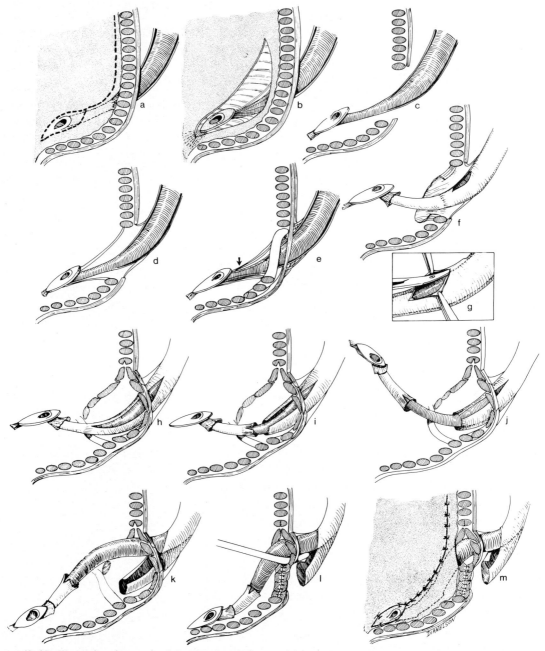

Figure 49–25. Illustration (*a* to *m*) of Stephens' techniques of intravesical mobilization of the ureter within the deep periureteral sheath, displacement of the ureteral hiatus superiorly, and advancement of the ureteral orifice inferomedially in order to lengthen the submucosal ureter.

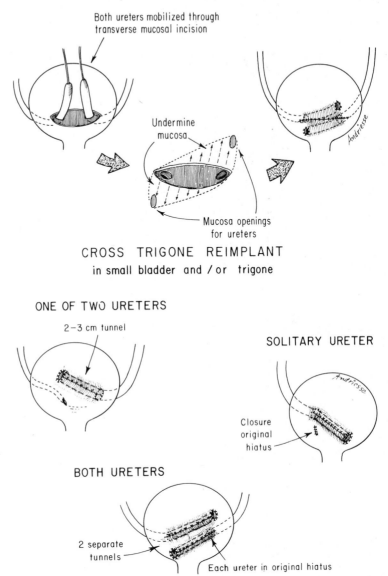

CROSS TRIGONE REIMPLANT

Both ureters mobilized through
transverse mucosal incision

Undermine
mucosa

Mucosa openings
for ureters

CROSS TRIGONE REIMPLANT

in small bladder and / or trigone

ONE OF TWO URETERS

2–3 cm tunnel

SOLITARY URETER

Closure
original
hiatus

BOTH URETERS

2 separate
tunnels

Each ureter in original hiatus

Figure 49–26. Cross trigone reimplantation technique. (From Hendren, W. H.: *In* Smith, R. B., and Skinner, D. G. (Eds.): Complications of Urologic Surgery: Prevention and Management. Philadelphia, W. B. Saunders Co., 1976.)

duced in this way. For instance, a stone basket can often be inserted into such a ureter by percutaneous puncture, whereas the instrument will not pass through a cystoscope that can be employed in boys. Transurethral scissors are also occasionally useful to incise an ischemic stricture of the distalmost ureter following reimplantation.

SURGICAL CORRECTION OF MEGAURETER

The standard surgical therapy for primary obstructive megaureter derives from the work of Politano and Leadbetter (1958), Paquin (1959), Creevy (1967), and Hendren (1968).

Creevy (1967) and Bischoff (1972) advocated tapering only that portion of the wide ureter which would become the new intravesical ureter after reimplantation, but would then permit a reliable type of antireflux anastomosis. Hendren (1968) showed that, with care, more of the lower ureter could be narrowed without devascularizing the most distal portion. The key to success is atraumatic manipulation of the ureter and preservation of the blood vessels that enter the wall of the dilated ureter on its medial aspect (Fig. 49–27). If dilatation of the upper ureter persists or infection ensues, the upper ureter is occasionally narrowed in a similar fashion 6 to

Text continued on page 2075

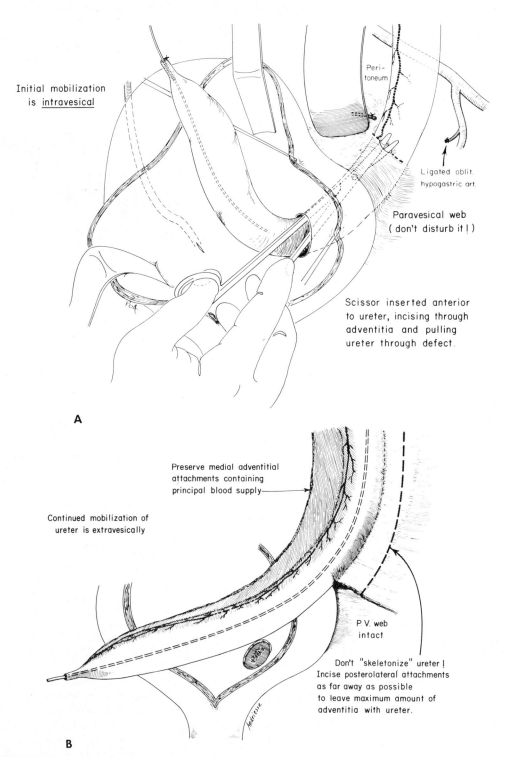

Initial mobilization
is <u>intravesical</u>

Peri-
toneum

Ligated oblit.
hypogastric art.

Paravesical web
(don't disturb it !)

Scissor inserted anterior
to ureter, incising through
adventitia and pulling
ureter through defect.

A

Preserve medial adventitial
attachments containing
principal blood supply

Continued mobilization of
ureter is extravesically

P. V. web
intact

Don't "skeletonize" ureter !
Incise posterolateral attachments
as far away as possible
to leave maximum amount of
adventitia with ureter.

B

Figure 49–27. Hendren's technique of reimplantation of megaureter. *A*, Initial mobilization of ureter from inside bladder. *B*, Continued extravesical mobilization of bladder after dividing obliterated hypogastric ligament. (From Hendren, W. H.: *In* Smith, R. B., and Skinner, D. G. (Eds.): Complications of Urologic Surgery: Prevention and Management. Philadelphia, W. B. Saunders Co., 1976.)

Illustration continued on opposite page

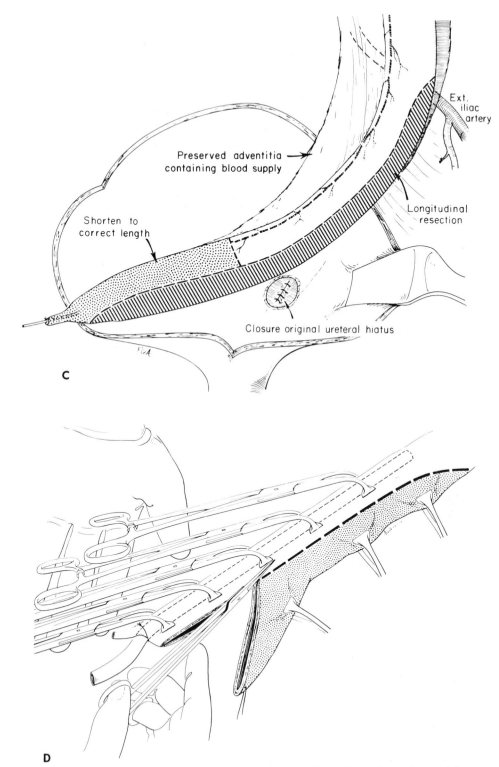

Figure 49–27 *Continued. C,* Planning the amount of resection. *D,* Technique of resection, using special clamps.

Illustration continued on following page

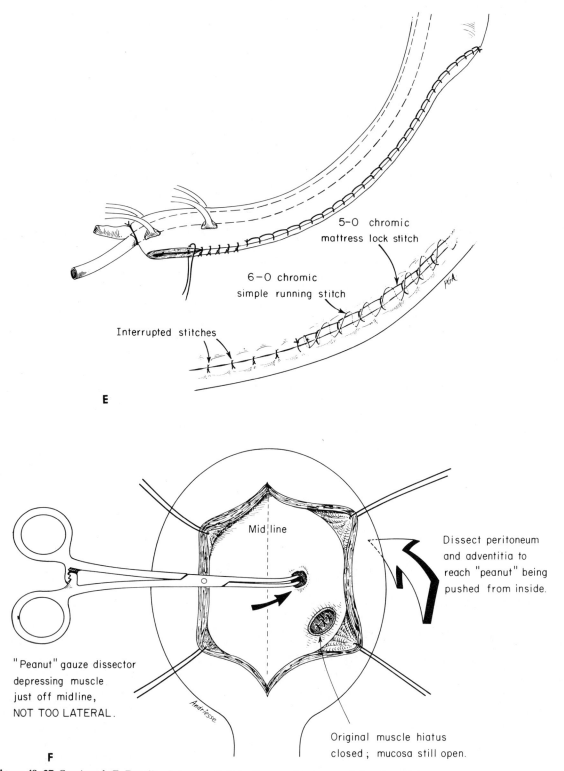

E, Details of closure. **F,** Selecting new hiatus, craniad and medial to original one.

Figure 49–27 *Continued.* E, Details of closure. F, Selecting new hiatus, craniad and medial to original one.

Illustration continued on opposite page

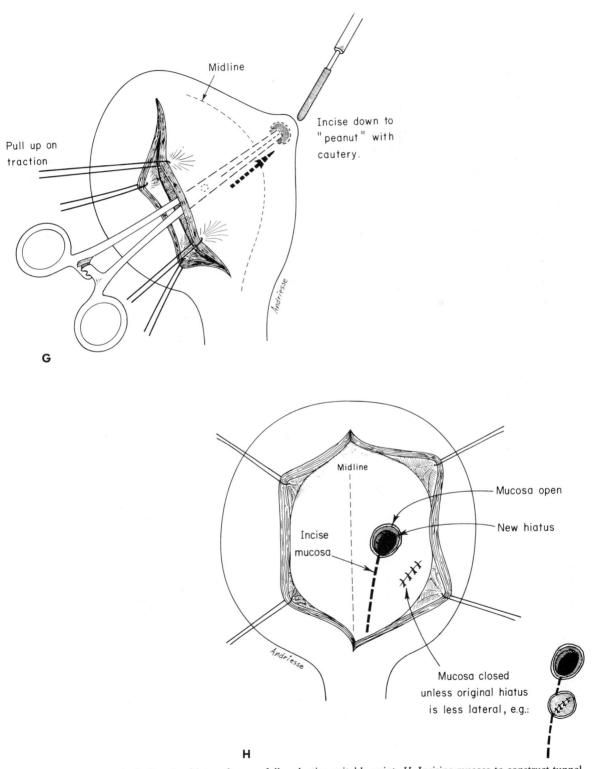

Midline

Incise down to
"peanut" with
cautery.

Pull up on
traction

Andriesse

G

Midline

Mucosa open

New hiatus

Incise
mucosa

Mucosa closed
unless original hiatus
is less lateral, e.g.:

Andriesse

H

Figure 49–27 *Continued.* *G,* Opening hiatus after carefully selecting suitable point. *H,* Incising mucosa to construct tunnel.

Illustration continued on following page

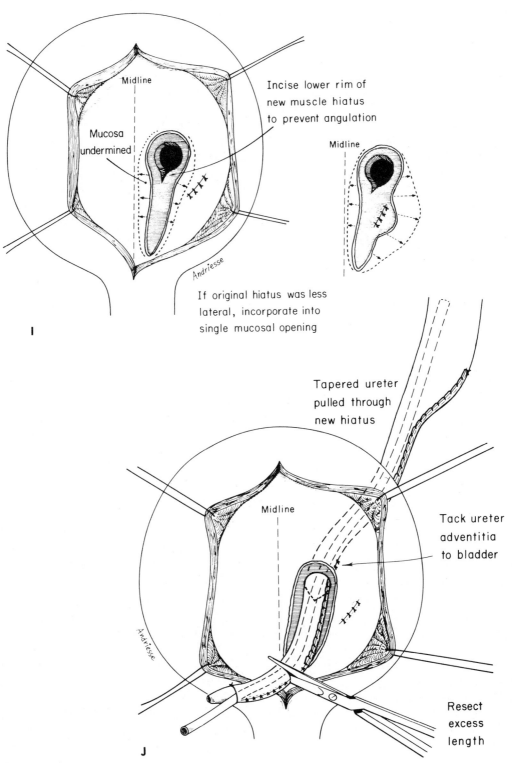

Figure 49–27 *Continued. I,* Elevating mucosal flaps. *J,* Resecting excess length.

Illustration continued on opposite page

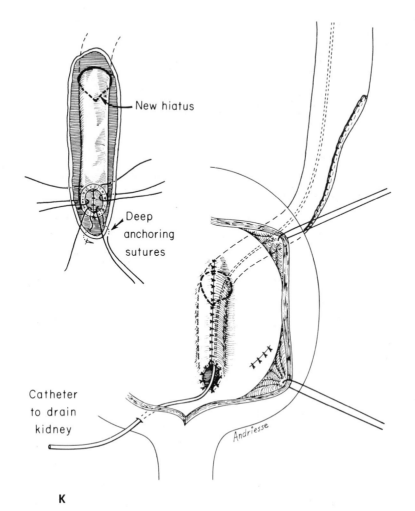

New hiatus

Deep
anchoring
sutures

Catheter
to drain
kidney

Andriesse

K

Figure 49–27 *Continued. K,* Completing repair. Ureteral suture line lies posteriorly.

8 weeks later. Hanna (1979) has devised a technique to permit narrowing the entire length of the ureter in a single operation. In this procedure, the ureteral adventitia with its rich blood supply is preserved intact. Above the bladder, stepwise windows are made in the adventitia to permit exposure of the dilated ureter. A strip of the medial and posterior aspects of the ureter, 12 to 14 cm in width, is left attached to the adventitia. This strip is tubularized with two layers of absorbable suture to narrow the ureter to a uniform caliber of approximately 12 F. Stents are left in place for a week or more after ureteral reimplantation with extravesical tailoring.

The simpler, limited approach has proved to be adequate in most children with obstructed megaureter. If obstruction is relieved and reflux prevented, the dilated ureter above the bladder will narrow and straighten as the child grows.

This means that tailoring long ureteral segments, with an increased risk of distal ureteral ischemia and stenosis even when care is taken to preserve the blood supply, is unnecessary. In practice, we find that tailoring the lowermost 5 cm of ureter, which is to be retained and to serve mainly as the new intravesical ureter after reimplantation, is adequate. This tapered segment, about 12 F in diameter, is reimplanted into the bladder medial to and above the original hiatus so that a 4 cm intravesical course can be achieved, with care taken so that the medial blood supply of the justavesical ureter is not disrupted (Hendren, 1969). Alternatively, a cross-trigone method of implantation can be employed. This also permits a relatively long intravesical course, and Hensley et al. (1982), Ahmed (1980), and Cohen (1975) believe that intravesical tailoring and preservation of the original hiatus reduces the risk of distal ureteral

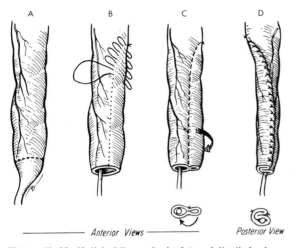

A   B   C   D

——— Anterior Views ———   Posterior View

Figure 49–28. Kalicinski's method of "modeling" the lowermost portion of the dilated ureter to facilitate antireflux ureteral reimplantation. Excessive ureteral length is trimmed away after the lower extravesical ureter is straightened, with care to preserve the major ureteral blood supply. The surgical steps are described in the text. Tailoring only the portion that becomes the new intravesical ureter makes subsequent ischemic stenosis unlikely.

ischemia or obstruction due to angulation outside the bladder.

An alternative to tailoring of the lower ureter to achieve an adequate length to width ratio to prevent reflux has been described by Kalicinski et al. (1977) and evaluated by Starr (1979), Politano (1981), and Ehrlich (1982) (Fig. 49–28). In their view, the risks of devascularization of the distalmost remaining ureter following straightening and tapering of the dilated ureter are best avoided by leaving intact the full circumference of the distal dilated ureter. A 10 or 12 F catheter is passed into the ureter. A running absorbable suture is then used to exclude the excess lateral dilated portion of the ureter from the lumen, the continuity of which is protected by the presence of the catheter. This unused portion of the dilated ureter is then rolled over the lumen and the stent. Interrupted adventitial sutures are used to hold the excluded segment in place. The result of such "modeling" or "folding" results in less ureteral bulk than might be expected, and antireflux anastomosis through a long submucosal tunnel is then readily accomplished. The new orifice is anchored to the detrusor and overlying mucosa with interrupted sutures, as in the more standard techniques. We have not seen obstruction or persistence of reflux in six patients in whom this procedure was employed, and Ehrlich (1982) reports 17 consecutive successes.

Surgical Alternatives

Very good results (99 per cent success) have been obtained with Lich's operation (McDuffie et al., 1977; Gregoir, 1964; Marberger et al., 1978), but it is difficult to quantitate the degree to which the extravesical ureter is compressed, and perhaps compromised, by closing the bladder muscle behind the ureter. Also, this operation is not applicable when the ureter is dilated to more than one or two times its normal diameter. Perhaps for these reasons the procedure is not in very general use.

The procedures in common use today are those of Politano and Leadbetter (1958) and Cohen (1975), and the advancement operations, particularly as modified by Glenn and Anderson (1967) and Stephens (1977), to recess the hiatus and permit a greater increase in the length of the intravesical ureter. The Politano-Leadbetter procedure can be made more versatile by incorporating an extravesical approach to mobilize the distal ureter and to free the posterolateral wall of the bladder in order to create the new vesical hiatus under direct vision. This reduces the risk of kinking the lower ureter, facilitates tapering or modeling what will become the new intravesical ureter when needed, and obviates any risk of perforating the peritoneum or adjacent viscera, since these structures are all then visualized directly (Fig. 49–29).

A ureteral stent is employed postoperatively if tapering of the reimplanted ureter is required. Soft Silastic tubing (No. 8 F) is ideal for this purpose. It can be readily brought through the bladder through a stab wound and connected to dependent drainage. If extensive tapering has been performed, the stent is left in place for 7 to 10 days. Use of a stent, at least on one side, during the first 24 to 72 hours after bilateral reimplantation without tapering is also often beneficial to avoid any risk of oliguria during the period of maximal postoperative edema. The bladder is usually drained by a suprapubic catheter in males and a urethral catheter in females for 5 to 7 days after simple reimplantations, or until all stents are removed after more complicated procedures.

Uncomplicated implantations may not require such a prolonged period of bladder drainage, and Gonzales and associates (1978) have often been able to discharge patients 2 to 4 days after such surgery. Often, however, there is considerable persistence of dysuria when the catheter is removed so soon. Early discharge is most often feasible when a Lich type of reim-

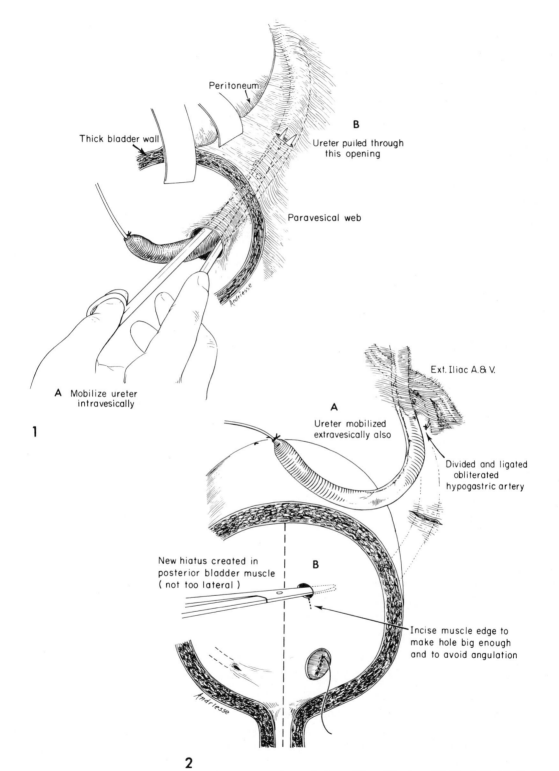

Figure 49–29. Combined intravesical-extravesical reimplantation technique. (From Hendren, W. H.: *In* Smith, R. B., and Skinner, D. G.: Complications of Urologic Surgery: Prevention and Management. Philadelphia, W. B. Saunders Co., 1976.)

Illustration continued on following page

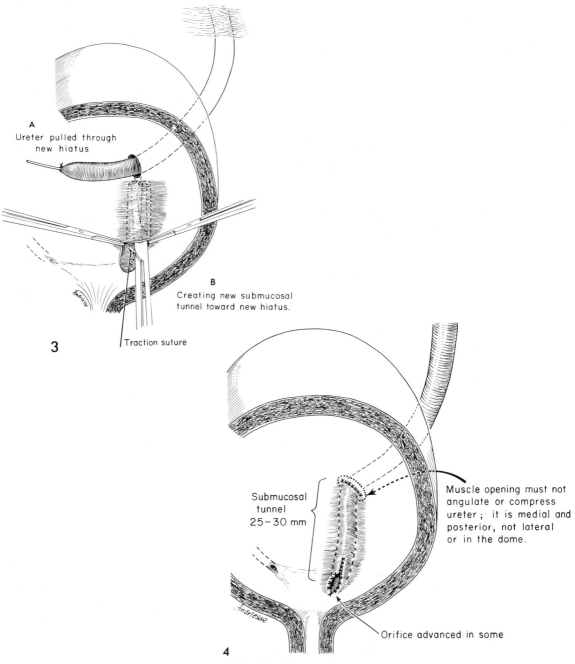

A
Ureter pulled through
new hiatus

B
Creating new submucosal
tunnel toward new hiatus.

3   Traction suture

Submucosal
tunnel
25–30 mm

Muscle opening must not
angulate or compress
ureter; it is medial and
posterior, not lateral
or in the dome.

Orifice advanced in some

4

Figure 49–29 *Continued.*

plantation has been performed, in which the bladder was unopened.

Patients who have had previous antireflux surgery should undergo a combined intravesical-extravesical approach if they require reoperation. It is often convenient to utilize a low midline incision and then open the peritoneum and identify the dilated ureters at the pelvic brim. The lower ureters are then mobilized toward the bladder, and extreme care is taken to preserve the adventitial blood supply and the entire length of ureter that is not involved in stricture or ischemic stenosis. The umbilical arteries are divided if this has not already been done, so that they will not angulate the ureter after reimplantation. If ureteral length is adequate for an antireflux reimplantation without tension, this is carried out using the open Politano-Leadbetter, Cohen, or Paquin technique. The portion of the ureter that will become intravesical is tapered or folded, if necessary, to achieve a 4:1 or 5:1 ratio of length to width. The suture line in the ureter after tapering is oriented against the detrusor and away from the bladder lumen in order to minimize the risk of a fistula between the ureter above the new orifice and the bladder lumen. The ureter is anchored in place with three or four absorbable sutures, generally 4-0 chromic catgut, between the muscle of the trigone and all layers of the ureter on either side of the posterior ureteral suture line that results from tapering. If available, bladder mucosa is drawn over the reimplanted ureter, but if mucosa is friable and has been torn, the intravesical surface of the ureter will quickly epithelialize.

If the ureter will not reach the trigone without tension, there are several alternatives that may be satisfactory. The bladder may be mobilized and drawn over to the ureter by sewing the superolateral aspect of the bladder to the psoas muscle with heavy absorbable sutures, a psoas hitch.

If the contralateral ureter is functioning normally and is neither obstructed nor refluxing, transureteroureterostomy is an attractive alternative, provided that the discrepancy in the diameter of the ureters is not too great. A ureter 1 cm in diameter, or a little more in its collapsed state, may be anastomosed to a ureter of little more than normal caliber with great reliability, and if the recipient ureter is more than twice the normal caliber, anastomosis of a transposed ureter of any size can be accomplished without difficulty. Transureteroureterostomy should not be performed when retroperitoneal inflammation is present. The technique of transureteroureterostomy is described in Chapter 68.

The Boari bladder flap is often an alternative to transureteroureterostomy when a psoas hitch alone will not make up the needed deficiency in ureteral length. This procedure is also described in Chapter 68. The flap is rotated upward toward the mobilized ureter, where a submucosal tunnel is developed in the flap, and the ureter is reimplanted as in the Paquin or Politano-Leadbetter procedure. The flap is then closed in two layers; it encloses the submucosal tunnel and, in effect, provides an extension of the bladder into which a shortened ureter can be implanted without tension in the bladder by an antireflux technique.

When the ureter is extremely dilated, straightening and resection of excessive tortuous redundant ureteral length improve drainage and lessen residual urine in the upper tracts. Tapering or folding of the remaining distal portion of the ureter that becomes the new intravesical segment is necessary to secure an adequate submucosal tunnel to prevent reflux.

As noted, reflux and ureteral obstruction can coexist in megaureter, but antireflux ureteral reimplantation is designed to correct both conditions.

RESULTS

Satisfactory results are obtainable in more than 90 per cent of operations overall for primary vesicoureteral reflux and in over 95 per cent of patients without severe hydronephrosis or infection (Hendren, 1968; Woodard and Keats, 1973). The most frequent complication of ureteroneocystostomy is persistence of reflux in the reimplanted ureter. Failure to correct reflux is more common in those who have had previous ureterovesical surgery and in those with dilated ureters or scarred and noncompliant bladders. The most frequent reasons for continued reflux are (1) failure to position the orifice correctly, placing it too far lateral or too far superior on the mobile portion of the bladder wall, as opposed to securing it on the relatively immobile floor of the bladder; and (2) failure to create an adequate length of submucosal tunnel. The minimal acceptable ratio of tunnel length to ureteral diameter is about 4:1. However, a ratio of 5:1 is ideal.

Reflux is also much more prone to recur when the patient has a noncompliant bladder or untreated sphincter dyssynergia. The good results now being reported after reimplantation into a neuropathic bladder suggest that prompt reinstitution of intermittent catheterization after surgery minimizes the risk of failure.

The other frequent complication is obstruction of the ureter. This may be extrinsic or intrinsic. The former is due to (1) angulation of the ureter proximal to its entry into the bladder, or (2) failure to create a large enough hiatus in the bladder wall, so that the ureter is compressed as it enters the bladder. Stenosis of the reimplanted ureter implies ischemia caused by vascular compromise or tension on the anastomosis. Ureteral meatotomy alone will suffice to correct meatal stenosis at times, but, more often, resection of the narrowed terminal ureter and reimplantation are required after more adequate mobilization of the ureter.

Intravenous pyelography performed during the first 6 weeks after ureteroneocystostomy may demonstrate a mild to moderate increase in hydronephrosis, which generally improves in time as postoperative edema resolves and healing progresses. In postoperative films, one expects no more hydroureteronephrosis than was noted on the preoperative cystogram. This degree of dilatation is probably physiologic and represents "ureteral memory," in that the once dilated ureter will often look dilated on intravenous urogram when presented with a high fluid load (Lebowitz, 1983). However, delayed visualization, particularly if accompanied by febrile urinary tract infection, is an indication for nephrostomy drainage in order to prevent irreversible kidney damage. Percutaneous nephrostomy is often useful in this context.

If the postoperative patient is doing well, intravenous pyelography is deferred until 1 to 2 months after surgery. A nuclear cystogram is performed 3 to 6 months postoperatively. If a cystogram is performed in the immediate postoperative period, reflux is often present owing to edema and inflammation secondary to surgery and incomplete healing. At 3 months, reflux is usually absent, but its occurrence at this time does not mean that it will persist. In 30 per cent of patients with postoperative reflux, such reflux is not present on a second cystogram made 6 to 9 months after surgery. If reflux persists this long, reoperation is generally necessary because healing is then complete, and the scar at the site of reimplantation precludes improvement with further growth.

If the initial intravenous pyelogram is satisfactory and the upper tracts are normal or improved, pyelography is repeated every 2 to 3 years until full growth is achieved, because of the slight risk of late ureteral obstruction due to scar maturation or changing anatomic relationships. Once reflux is demonstrated to be absent on an adequate cystogram, cystography is not repeated unless the child suffers recurrent infections or unless hydronephrosis is detected.

Ideally, urinary tract infection should be eradicated prior to antireflux surgery, and prophylactic chemotherapy should be administered during the immediate postoperative period while catheter drainage is employed. The urine is then recultured after all catheters and drains are removed, and specific antibacterial therapy is started. If the urine is sterile, prophylactic chemotherapy such as nitrofurantoin, sulfa, or nalidixic acid is continued during the first 6 to 8 weeks after hospitalization.

The development of reflux in the contralateral ureter after unilateral ureteroneocystostomy has been noted to occur in as many as 15 to 20 per cent of patients (Warren et al., 1972), and especially in children with neuropathic bladders (Johnston et al., 1976). If the ureteral orifice is normally developed and has an adequate submucosal tunnel, this reflux subsides spontaneously with the resolution of postoperative edema. However, if this ureterovesical junction possessed only borderline competency initially, reflux may not subside and a second operative procedure is occasionally necessary. For this reason, if a nonrefluxing orifice appears gaping and has a short or absent submucosal tunnel, "prophylactic" reimplantation is at times indicated when the contralateral ureter is reimplanted, even though bilateral reflux was not demonstrated on the preoperative cystogram.

Summary

Surgical correction of reflux has become relatively reliable. Modern techniques of ureteral tailoring or "molding" can be incorporated into each of the commonly used methods of ureteral reimplantation to enable a 5:1 ratio of length to width in the intravesical ureter to be achieved. The transverse Cohen method of implantation is quite versatile and is gaining in popularity, especially in the treatment of near-normal or moderately dilated ureters.

References

Vesicouretal Reflux

Allen, T. D.: Vesicoureteral reflux as a manifestation of dysfunctional voiding. In Hodson, C. J., and Kincaid-Smith, P. (Eds.): Reflux Nephropathy. New York, Masson Publishing USA, 1979, pp. 171–180.

Al-Magousy, A., Hanafy, M. H., Saad, S. M., El-Rifaie, M., and Al-Ghorab, J. M.: Early Arabian medicine. Urology, 8:63, 1976.

Amar, A. D.: Calicotubular backflow with vesicoureteral reflux. JAMA, 213:293, 1970.

Amar, A. D.: Cystoscopic demonstration of vesicoureteral reflux: Evaluation in 250 patients. J. Urol., 95:776, 1966.

Ambrose, S. S.: Reflux pyelonephritis in adults secondary to congenital lesions of the ureteral orifice. J. Urol., 102:302, 1969.

Ambrose, S. S., and Nicolson, W. P.: The causes of vesicoureteral reflux in children. J. Urol., 87:688, 1962a.

Ambrose, S. S., and Nicolson, W. P.: Vesicoureteral reflux secondary to anomalies of the ureterovesical junction: Management and results. J. Urol., 87:695, 1962b.

Ambrose, S. S., and Nicolson, W. P.: Ureteral reflux in duplicated ureters. J. Urol., 92:439, 1964.

Ambrose, S. S., Parrott, T. S., Woodard, J. R., and Campbell, W. G., Jr.: Observations on the small kidney associated with vesicoureteral reflux. J. Urol., 123:349, 1980.

Aperia, A., Broberger, O., Ericsson, N. O., and Wikstad, I.: Effect of vesicoureteral reflux on renal function in children with recurrent urinary infection. Kidney Int., 9:418, 1976.

Apperson, J. W., Atkins, H., and Fleming, R.: The value of the isotope cystogram in determining pressure and volume at which ureteral reflux occurs. J. Urol., 89:405, 1963.

Arant, B. S., Jr., Sotelo-Avila, C., and Bernstein, J.: Segmental "hypoplasia" of the kidney (Ask-Upmark). J. Pediatr., 95:931, 1979.

Askari, A., and Belman, A. B.: Vesicoureteral reflux in black girls. J. Pediatr. Nephrol. Urol., *1*:11, 1981.

Ask-Upmark, E.: Uber juvenile maligne nephrosklerose und ihr verhöltnis zu störungen in der nierenen twickling. Acta Pathol. Microbiol. Scand., 7:383, 1929.

Atwell, J. D., Cook, P. L., Strong, L., and Hyde, I.: The inter-relationship between vesicoureteral reflux, trigonal abnormalities and a bifid collection system: A family study. Br. J. Urol., *49*:97, 1977.

Auer, J., and Seager, L. D.: Experimental local bladder edema causing urine reflux into ureter and kidney. J. Exp. Med., *66*:741, 1937.

Babcock, J. R., Keats, G. K., and King, L. R.: Renal changes after uncomplicated antireflux operation. J. Urol., *115*:720, 1976.

Bailey, M., and Wallace, M.: HLA-BIZ as a genetic marker for vesicoureteral reflux? (Letter). Br. Med. J., *1*:48, 1978.

Bailey, R. R.: Reflux nephropathy and hypertension. *In* Hodson, C. J., and Kincaid-Smith, P. (Eds.): Reflux Nephropathy. New York, Masson Publishing USA, 1979*a*, pp. 263–267.

Bailey, R. R.: Sterile reflux: Is it harmless? *In* Hodson, C. J., and Kincaid-Smith, P. (Eds.): Reflux Nephropathy. New York, Masson Publishing USA, 1979*b*, pp. 334–339.

Baker, R., and Barbaris, H. T.: Comparative results of urological evaluation of children with initial and recurrent urinary tract infection. J. Urol., *116*:503, 1976.

Baker, R., Masted, W., Maylath, J., and Shuman, I.: Relation of age, sex, and infection to reflux: Data indicating high spontaneous cure rate in pediatric patients. J. Urol., *95*:26, 1966.

Bakshandah, K., Lynne, C., and Carrion, H.: Vesicoureteral reflux and end-stage renal disease. J. Urol., *116*:557, 1976.

Barrett, D. M., Malek, R. S., and Kelalis, P. P.: Problems and solutions in surgical treatment of 100 consecutive ureteral duplications in children. J. Urol., *114*:126, 1975.

Bauer, S. B., Hallett, M., Khoshoin, S., et al.: Predictive valve of urodynamic evaluation in newborns with myelodysplasia. JAMA, 232:650, 1984.

Bell, C.: Account of the muscles of the ureters and their effects in irritable states of the bladder. Trans. Med. Chir. (Lond.), *3*:171, 1812.

Benjamin, J. A.: The use of X-ray cinematography in urological studies. J. Urol., *81*:227, 1959.

Berger, R. E., Ansell, J. S., Shurtleff, D. B., and Hickman, R. O.: Vesicoureteral reflux in children with uremia. JAMA, 246:56, 1981.

Bialestock, D.: Studies of renal malformations and pyelonephritis in children, with and without associated vesicoureteral reflux and obstruction. Aust. N.Z. J. Surg., *35*:120, 1965.

Bischoff, P. F.: Problems in treatment of vesicorenal reflux. J. Urol., *107*:133, 1972.

Blank, E.: Caliectasis and renal scars in children. J. Urol., *110*:255, 1973.

Blaufox, M. D., Gruskin, A., Sandler, P., Goldman, H., Ogwo, J. E., and Edelmann, C. M., Jr.: Radionuclide scintigraphy for detection of vesicoureteral reflux in children. J. Pediatr., *79*:239, 1971.

Blight, E. M., and O'Shaughnessy, E. J.: Vesicoureteral reflux in children: A prospective study. J. Urol., *102*:44, 1969.

Boyarsky, S., and Labay, P.: Ureteral dynamics. Baltimore, The Williams & Wilkins Co., 1972, p. 354.

Boyarsky, S., Lebay, P., Kirshner, N., and Gerber, C.: Does the ureter have nervous control? J. Urol., 97:627, 1967.

Bredin, H. C., Winchester, P., McGovern, J. H., and Degan, M.: Family study of vesicoureteral reflux. J. Urol., *113*:623, 1975.

Bridge, R. A. C., and Roe, C. W.: The grading of vesicoureteral reflux: A guide to therapy. J. Urol., *101*:831, 1969.

Briggs, E. M., Constantine, C. E., and Govan, D. E.: Dynamics of the upper urinary tract: IV. The relationship of urine flow rate and rate of ureteral peristalsis. Invest. Urol., *10*:56, 1972.

Bumpus, H. C.: Urinary reflux. J. Urol., *12*:341, 1924.

Bunge, R. G.: Delayed cystograms in children. J. Urol., 70:729, 1953.

Bunts, R. C.: Vesicoureteral reflux in paraplegic patients. J. Urol., *79*:747, 1958.

Burger, R. H.: A theory on the nature of the transmission of congenital vesicoureteral reflux. J. Urol., *108*:249, 1972.

Burger, R. H., and Smith, C.: Hereditary and familial vesicoureteral reflux. J. Urol., *106*:845, 1971.

Claësson, I., Jacobsson, B., Jodal, U., and Winberg, J.: Compensatory kidney growth in children with UTI and unilateral renal scarring: an epidemiologic study. Kidney Int., *20*:759, 1981.

Claësson, I., Jacobsson, B., Olsson, T., and Ringertz, H.: Assessment of renal parenchymal thickness in normal children. Acta Radiol. Diagn., *97*:291, 1980.

Colodny, A. H., and Lebowitz, R. L.: The importance of voiding during a cystourethrogram. J. Urol., *111*:838, 1974*a*.

Colodny, A. H., and Lebowitz, R. H.: A plea for grading vesicoureteric reflux (Editorial). Urology, *4*:357, 1974*b*.

Colodny, A. H., et al.: Disappearance of Periureteral Diverticula and Reflux. Presented at Section on Urology, American Academy of Pediatrics. San Francisco, October 1983.

Conway, J. J., and Kruglik, G. D.: Effectiveness of direct and indirect radionucleotide cystography in detecting vesicoureteral reflux. J. Nucl. Med., *17*:81, 1976.

Conway, J. J., Belman, A. B., King, L. R., and Filmer, R. B.: Direct and indirect radionucleotide cystography. J. Urol., *113*:689, 1975.

Conway, J. J., King, L. R., Belman, A. B., and Thorson, T.: Detection of vesicoureteral reflux with radionucleotide cystography. Am. J. Roentgenol. Radium Ther. Nucl. Med., *115*:720, 1972.

Corriere, J. N., Lipshutz, L. I., Judson, F. N., and Murphy, J. J.: Autoradiographic localization of refluxed live and dead *E. coli* and sulfur colloid particles in the rat kidney. Invest. Urol., *6*:364, 1969.

Corriere, J. N., Sanders, T. P., Kuhl, D. E., Schoenberg, H. W., and Murphy, J. J.: Urinary particle dynamics and vesicoureteral reflux in the human. J. Urol., *103*:599, 1970.

Cotran, R. S., and Pennington, J. E.: Urinary tract infection, pyelonephritis, and nephropathy. *In* Brenner, B. M., and Rector, F. C., Jr. (Eds.): The Kidney. Vol. II. 2nd ed. Philadelphia, W. B. Saunders Co., 1981, pp. 1571–1632.

Cunningham, F. G., Morris, G. B., and Mickal, A.: Acute pyelonephritis of pregnancy: a clinical review. Obstet. Gynecol. 42:112, 1973.

Damanski, M.: Vesicoureteric reflux in paraplegia. Br. J. Surg., *52*:168, 1965.

Deture, F. A., and Walker, R. D.: Measurement of the distance from the ureteral orifice to the bladder neck: Additional objective data in the cystoscopy of patients with reflux. J. Urol., *112*:326, 1974.

De Vargas, A., Evans, K., Ransley, P., et al.: A family study of vesicoureteric reflux. J. Med. Genet., *15*:85, 1978.

Dillon, M. J.: Personal communication, 1982.

Doyle, P. T., and Briscoe, C. E.: The effects of drugs and anesthetic agents on the urinary bladder and sphincters. Br. J. Urol., 48:329, 1976.

Duckett, J. W.: Editorial comment. J. Urol., 123:350, 1980.

Duckett, J. W.: Editorial comment. J. Urol., 125:71, 1981.

Duckett, J. W., and Bellinger, M. F.: A plea for standardized grading of vesicoureteral reflux. Eur. Urol., 8:74, 1982.

Dwoskin, J. Y.: Sibling uropathology. J. Urol., 115:726, 1976.

Dwoskin, J. Y., and Perlmutter, A. D.: Vesicoureteral reflux in children: A computerized review. J. Urol., 109:888, 1973.

Edelbrook, H. H., and Mickelson, J. C.: Selection of children for vesicoureteroplasty. J. Urol., 104:342, 1970.

Edwards, D., Nomand, I. C. S., Prescod, N., et al.: Disappearance of reflux during long-term prophylaxis of urinary tract infection in children. Br. Med. J., 2:285, 1977.

Ehrlich, R.: Success of the transvesical advancement technique for VUR. J. Urol., 128:554, 1982a.

Ehrlich, R. M.: Society for Pediatric Urology Newsletter. Dec. 1982b.

Ekman, H., Jacobsson, B., Kock, N. G., et al.: High diuresis: a factor in preventing vesicoureteral reflux. J. Urol., 95:511, 1966.

Elbadawi, A.: Anatomy and function of the ureteral sheath. J. Urol., 107:224, 1972.

Ellis, G. V.: An account of the arrangement of the muscular substance in the urinary and certain of the generative organs. Trans. Med. Chir. (Lond.), 39:327, 1856.

Estes, R. C., and Brooks, R. T.: Vesicoureteral reflux in adults. J. Urol., 103:603, 1970.

Fair, W. R., and Govan, D. E.: Influence of vesicoureteral reflux on the response to treatment of urinary tract infections in female children. Br. J. Urol., 48:111, 1976.

Fairley, K. F.: The effects of a diuresis on vesicoureteric reflux. In Hodson, C. J., and Kincaid-Smith, P. (Eds.): Reflux Nephropathy. New York, Masson Publishing USA, 1979, p. 102.

Filly, R. F., Friedland, G. W., Govan, F., et al.: Development and progression of clubbing and scarring in children with recurrent urinary tract infection. Radiology, 113:145, 1974.

Fisher, J. H., and Darling, D. B.: The course of vesicoureteral reflux associated with urinary tract infection in children. J. Pediatr. Surg., 2:221, 1967.

Friedland, G. W.: The voiding cystourethrogram: an unreliable examination. In Hodson, C. J., and Kincaid-Smith, P. (Eds.): Reflux Nephropathy. New York, Masson Publishing USA, 1979, pp. 93–99.

Fryjordet, A.: Sympathectomy and ureteral reflux. Scand. J. Urol. Nephrol., 2:196, 1968.

Galen: Cited in Polk, H. C., Jr.: Notes on Galenic urology. Urol. Surv., 15:2, 1965.

Garrett, R. A., Rhamy, R. K., and Newman, D.: Management of nonobstructive vesicoureteral reflux. J. Urol., 90:167, 1963.

Geist, R. S., and Antolak, S. J., Jr.: The clinical problems of children with sterile ureteral reflux. J. Urol., 108:343, 1972.

Gibson, H. M.: Ureteral reflux in the normal child. J. Urol., 62:40, 1949.

Gill, D. G., Mendes da Costa, B., Cameron, J. S., Joseph, M. C., Ogg, C. S., and Chantler, C.: Analysis of 100 children with severe and persistent hypertension. Arch. Dis. Child., 51:951, 1976.

Govan, D. E., and Palmer, J. M.: Urinary tract infection in children: the influence of successful antireflux operations in morbidity from infection. Pediatrics, 44:677, 1969.

Govan, D. E., Fair, W. R., Friedland, G. W., and Filly, R. H.: Management of children with urinary tract infections. Urology, 6:273, 1975.

Grana, L., Kidd, J., and Idriss, F.: Effect of chronic urinary tract infection on ureteral peristalsis. J. Urol., 94:652, 1965.

Graves, R. C., and Davidoff, L. M.: Studies on the bladder and ureters with especial reference to regurgitation of the vesical contents. J. Urol., 14:1, 1925.

Gruber, G. M.: A comparative study of the intravesical ureter in man and in experimental animals. J. Urol., 21:567, 1929.

Habib, R., Courtecuisse, V., Ehrensperger, J., et al.: Hypoplasie segmentaire du rein avec hypertension arterielle chez l'enfant. Ann. Pediatr. (Paris), 12:262, 1965.

Harrison, R.: On the possibility and utility of washing out the pelvis of the kidney and the ureters through the bladder. Lancet, 1:463, 1888.

Harrow, B. R.: Ureteral reflux in children. Child. Pediatr., 6:83, 1967.

Hawtrey, C. E., Culp, D. A., Loening, S., et al.: Ureterovesical reflux in an adolescent and adult population. J. Urol., 130:1067, 1983.

Heidrick, W. P., Mattingly, R. F., and Amberg, J. R.: Vesicoureteral reflux in pregnancy. Obstet. Gynecol., 29:571, 1967.

Heikel, P. E., and Parkkulainen, K. V.: Vesico-ureteric reflux in children: A classification and results of conservative treatment. Ann. Radiol., 9:37, 1966.

Helin, I.: Clinical and experimental studies on vesicoureteral reflux. Scand. J. Urol. Nephrol. (Suppl.) 28:1, 1975.

Hernandez, R. J., Poznanski, A. K., Kuhns, L. R., et al.: Factors affecting measurement of renal length. Radiology, 130:653, 1979.

Hicks, C. C., Woodward, J. R., Walton, K. W., et al.: Hypertension as complication of vesicoureteral reflux in children. Urology, 7:587, 1976.

Hinman, F., and Baumann, F. W.: Vesical and ureteral damage from voiding dysfunction in boys without neurologic or obstructive disease. J. Urol., 109:727, 1973.

Hinman, F., and Hutch, J. A.: Atrophic pyelonephritis from ureteral reflux without obstructive signs (reflux pyelonephritis). J. Urol., 87:230, 1962.

Hodson, C. J.: The effects of disturbance of flow on the kidney: J. Infect. Dis., 120:54, 1969.

Hodson, C. J.: The radiological contribution toward the diagnosis of chronic pyelonephritis. Radiology, 88:857, 1967.

Hodson, C. J., and Edwards, D.: Chronic pyelonephritis and vesicoureteric reflux. Clin. Radiol., 11:219, 1960.

Hodson, C. J., Maling, T. M. J., McManaman, P. H., et al.: Pathogenesis of reflux nephropathy. Br. J. Radiol. (Suppl.), 13:1, 1975.

Holland, N.: Reflux nephropathy and hypertension. In Hodson, C. J., and Kincaid-Smith, P. (Eds.): Reflux Nephropathy. New York, Masson Publishing USA, 1979, pp. 257–262.

Howerton, L. W., and Lich, R., Jr.: The cause and correction of ureteral reflux. J. Urol., 89:762, 1963.

Huland, H., and Busch, R.: Chronic pyelonephritis as a cause of end stage renal disease. J. Urol., 127:642, 1982.

Hutch, J. A.: The Ureterovesical Junction. Berkeley, University of California Press, 1958.

Hutch, J. A.: Theory of maturation of the intravesical ureter. J. Urol., 86:534, 1961.

Hutch, J. A.: The role of the ureterovesical junction in the natural history of pyelonephritis. J. Urol., *88*:354, 1962.

Hutch, J. A.: Ureteric advancement operation: anatomy, technique and early results. J. Urol., *89*:180, 1963.

Hutch, J. A., and Tanagho, E. A.: Etiology of nonocclusive ureteral dilatation. J. Urol., *93*:177, 1965.

Iannaccone, G., and Panzironi, P. E.: Ureteral reflux in normal infants. Acta Radiol., *44*:451, 1955.

Ireland, G. W., and Cass, A. S.: The clinical measurement of the intravesical pressure during voiding. Invest. Urol., *2*:303, 1965.

Jakobsen, B. E., Genster, H., Olesen, S., and Nygaard, E.: Vesicoureteral reflux in children. Br. J. Urol., *49*:119, 1977.

Jeffs, R. D., and Allen, M. S.: The relationship between ureterovesical reflux and infection. J. Urol., *88*:691, 1962.

Jenkins, G. R., and Noe, H. N.: Familial vesicoureteral reflux: A prospective study. J. Urol., *128*:774, 1982.

Johnston, J. H.: Vesical diverticula without urinary obstruction in childhood. J. Urol., *84*:535, 1960.

Johnston, J. H.: Vesicoureteral reflux: its anatomical mechanism, causation, effects and treatment in the child. Ann. R. Coll. Surg. Engl., *30*:324, 1962.

Johnston, J. H.: Vesicoureteral reflux with urethral valves. Br. J. Urol., *51*:100, 1979.

Johnston, J. H., and Mix, L. W.: The Ask-Upmark kidney: a form of ascending pyelonephritis? Br. J. Urol., *48*:393, 1976.

Jones, B. W., and Headstream, J. W.: Vesicoureteral reflux in children. J. Urol., *80*:114, 1958.

Kaplan, W. E., Nasrallah, P., and King, L. R.: Reflux in complete duplication in children. J. Urol., *120*:220, 1978.

Kass, E. J., Koff, S. A., and Diokno, A. C.: Fate of vesicoureteral reflux in children with neuropathic bladders managed by intermittent catheterization. J. Urol., *125*:63, 1981.

Kass, J., Majd, M., and Belman, B. A.: The accuracy of the indirect radionuclide cystogram in children. Presented at the urologic section of the 51st American Academy of Pediatrics meetings. October 6, 1982.

Kaveggia, L., King, L. R., Grana, L., and Idriss, F. S.: Pyelonephritis: A cause of vesicoureteral reflux? J. Urol., *95*:158, 1966.

Kelalis, P. P.: Subject review: Proper perspective on vesicoureteric reflux. Mayo Clin. Proc., *46*:807, 1971.

Kincaid-Smith, P.: Glomerular and vascular lesions in chronic atrophic pyelonephritis and reflux nephropathy. Adv. Nephrol., *5*:3, 1975.

King, L. R.: Vesicoureteral reflux: History, etiology and conservative management. *In* Kelalis, P. P., and King, L. R. (Eds.): Clinical Pediatric Urology. Vol. 1. Philadelphia, W. B. Saunders Co., 1976, pp. 342–365.

King, L. R., and Sellards, H. G.: The effects of vesicoureteral reflux on renal growth and development in puppies. Invest. Urol., *9*:95, 1971.

King, L. R., Kazmi, S. O., and Belman, A. B.: Natural history of vesicoureteral reflux. Urol. Clin. North Am., *1*:441, 1974.

King, L. R., Mellens, H. A., and White, H.: Measurement of the intravesical pressure during voiding. Invest. Urol., *2*:303, 1965.

King, L. R., Surian, M. A., Wendel, R. M., and Burden, J. J.: Vesicoureteral reflux: The importance of etiology in management. Trans. Am. Assoc. Genitourin. Surg., *59*:110, 1967.

Koff, S. A., and Murtagh, D. S.: The uninhibited bladder in children: Effect of treatment on recurrence of urinary infection and on vesicoureteral reflux resolution. J. Urol., *120*:1138, 1983.

Koff, S. A., Lapides, J., and Piazza, D. H.: Association of urinary tract infection and reflux with uninhibited bladder contractions and voluntary sphincter obstruction. J. Urol., *122*:373, 1979a.

Koff, S. A., Lapides, J., and Piazza, D. H.: The uninhibited bladder in children: a cause for urinary obstruction, infection and reflux. *In* Hodson, C. J., and Kincaid-Smith, P. (Eds.): Reflux Nephropathy. New York, Masson Publishing USA, 1979b, pp. 161–170.

Kogan, S. J., and Freed, S. W.: Postoperative course of vesicoureteral reflux associated with benign obstructive prostatic disease. J. Urol., *112*:322, 1974.

Kretschmer, H. L.: Cystography, its value and limitations in surgery of the bladder. Surg. Gynecol. Obstet., *23*:709, 1916.

Kunin, C.: Significance of urinary infection in childhood. N.Y. J. Med., *64*:729, 1964.

Kunin, C. M., Deutscher, R., and Paquin, A.: Urinary tract infection in school children. Medicine, *43*:91, 1964.

Lancet editorial, July 1, 1978.

Lancet editorial. Screening for reflux. 2:23, 1978.

Lancet editorial, 2:44, 1982.

Langworthy, O. R., and Kolb, L. C.: Histological changes in the vesical muscle following injury of the peripheral innervation. Anat. Rec., *71*:249, 1938.

Lattimer, J. K., Apperson, J. W., Gleason, D. M., Baker, D., and Fleming, S. S.: The pressure at which reflux occurs: An important indicator of prognosis and treatment. J. Urol., *89*:395, 1963.

Leadbetter, G. W., Danbury, J. H., and Dreyfuss, J. R.: Absence of vesicoureteral reflux in normal adult males. J. Urol., *84*:69, 1960.

Lenaghan, D., Whitaker, J. G., Jensen, F., and Stephens, F. D.: The natural history of reflux and long-term effects of reflux on the kidney. J. Urol., *115*:738, 1976.

Lewy, P. R., and Belman, A. B.: Familial occurrence of non-obstructive, non-infectious vesicoureteral reflux with renal scarring. J. Pediatr., *86*:851, 1975.

Lich, R., Howerton, L. W., Goode, L. S., and Davis, L. A.: The uretero-vesical junction of the newborn. J. Urol., *92*:436, 1964.

Lines, D.: 15th century ureteric reflux. Lancet, *2*:1473, 1982.

Lyon, R. D.: Discussion, Birth Defects: Original Articles Series (New York), *13*:364, 1977.

Lyon, R. P.: Renal arrest. J. Urol., *109*:707, 1973.

Lyon, R. P., Halverstadt, D., Tank, E. S., et al.: Vesicoureteral reflux. *In* Dialogues in Pediatric Urology. Vol. I. New York, Wm. J. Miller Assoc., 1977, pp. 1–8.

Lyon, R. P., Marshall, S., and Tanagho, E. A.: The ureteric orifice: Its configuration and competency. J. Urol., *102*:504, 1969.

Mackie, C. G., and Stephens, F. S.: Duplex kidneys: a correlation of renal dysplasia with position of the ureteral orifice. J. Urol., *114*:274, 1975.

Malek, R. S., Svensson, J., and Torres, V. E.: Vesicoureteral reflux in the adult. I. Factors in pathogenesis. J. Urol., *130*:37, 1983a.

Malek, R. S., Svensson, J., Neves, R. J., and Torres, V. E.: Vesicoureteral reflux in the adult. III. Surgical correction: Risks and benefits. J. Urol., *130*:882, 1983b.

Marshall, F. C.: Excretory urographic changes in children which suggest occurrence of reflux. J. Urol., *87*:681, 1962.

Mattingly, R. F., and Borkowf, H. I.: Clinical implications of ureteral reflux in pregnancy. Clin. Obstet. Gynecol., 21:863, 1978.

Mazze, R. I., Schwartz, F. S., Slocum, H. C., and Barry, K. G.: Renal function during anesthesia and surgery. Anesthesiology, 24:279, 1963.

McAlister, W. H., Schackelford, G. S., and Kissane, L.: The histological effects of 30% Cystokon, Hypaque 25% and Renografin-30 in the bladder. Radiology, 104:563, 1972.

McGovern, J. H., Marshall, V. F., and Paquin, A. J.: Vesicoureteral regurgitation in children. J. Urol., 83:122, 1960.

McRae, C. U., Shannon, F. T., and Utley, W. L. F.: Effect on renal growth of reimplantation of refluxing ureters. Lancet, 1:1310, 1974.

Mebust, W. K., and Foret, J. D.: Vesicoureteral reflux in identical twins. J. Urol., 108:635, 1972.

Melick, W. F., Brodeur, A. E., and Karellos, D. N.: A suggested classification of ureteral reflux and suggested treatment based on cineradiographic findings and simultaneous pressure recordings by means of the strain gauge. J. Urol., 83:35, 1962.

Mendoza, J. M., and Roberts, J. A.: Effects of sterile high pressure vesicoureteral reflux on the monkey. J. Urol., 130:602, 1983.

Merrell, R. W., and Mowad, J. J.: Increased physical growth after successful antireflux operation. J. Urol., 122:523, 1979.

Middleton, G. W., Howards, S. S., and Gillenwater, J. Y.: Sex-linked familial reflux. J. Urol., 114:36, 1975.

Morillo, M. M., Orandi, A., Fernandes, M., and Draper, J. W.: Vesicoureteral reflux in male adults with bladder neck obstruction. J. Urol., 89:389, 1963.

Murnaghan, G. F.: Urologists' correspondence club letter. March 1980.

Neumann, P. Z., deDomenico, I. J., and Nogardy, M. B.: Constipation and urinary tract infection. Pediatrics, 52:241, 1973.

Normand, C., and Smellie, J.: Vesicoureteral reflux: The case for conservative management. In Hodson, C. J., and Kincaid-Smith, P. (Eds.): Reflux Nephropathy. New York, Masson Publishing USA, 1979, pp. 281–286.

Ong, T. H., Ferguson, R. S., and Stephens, F. D.: The pattern of intrapelvic pressure during vesicoureteral reflux in the dog with normal caliber ureter. Invest. Urol., 11:347, 1974.

Paquin, A. J.: Ureterovesical anastomosis: The description and evaluation of a technique. J. Urol., 82:573, 1959.

Pellman, C.: The neurogenic bladder in children with congenital malformation of the spine: A study of 61 patients. J. Urol., 93:472, 1965.

Peters, P. C., Johnson, D. E., and Jackson, J. H.: The incidence of vesicoureteral reflux in the premature child. J. Urol., 97:259, 1967.

Pfister, R. R., Biber, R. J., Rose, J. S., Johnson, M. L., and Parrish, R. G.: Monitoring ureteral reflux with ultrasound. Presented at the Urologic Section of the 51st American Academy of Pediatrics meetings. October 6, 1982.

Politano, V. A.: Ureterovesical junction. J. Urol., 107:239, 1972.

Pollet, J. E., Sharp, P. F., Smith, R. W., Davidson, A. I., and Miller, S. S.: Intravenous radionuclide cystography for the detection of vesicorenal reflux. J. Urol., 125:75, 1981.

Poznanski, E., and Poznanski, A. K.: Psychogenic influences on voiding: observations from voiding cystourethrography. Psychosomatics, 10:339, 1969.

Pozzi, S.: Ureteroverletzung bei laparatomie. Zbl. Gynack., 17:97, 1893.

Prather, G. C.: Vesicoureteral reflux, report of a case cured by operation. J. Urol., 52:437, 1944.

Quinby, W. C.: Observations on the physiology and pathology of the ureter. J. Urol., 7:259, 1922.

Randel, D. R.: Surgical judgement in the management of vesicoureteral reflux. J. Urol., 119:113, 1978.

Ransley, P. G.: Vesicoureteral reflux: Continuing surgical dilemma. Urology, 3:246, 1978.

Ransley, P. G., and Risdon, R. A.: Renal papillae and intra-renal reflux in the pig. Lancet, 2:1114, 1974.

Ransley, P. G., and Risdon, R. A.: Reflux and renal scarring. Br. J. Radiol. (Suppl.), 14:1, 1978.

Ransley, P. G., and Risdon, R. A.: Reflux nephropathy: Effects of antimicrobial therapy on the evolution of the early pyelonephritic scar. Kidney Int., 20:733, 1981.

Redman, J. F., Scriber, L. J., and Bissad, N. K.: Apparent failure of renal growth secondary to vesicoureteral reflux. Urology, 3:704, 1974.

Report of the International Reflux Study Committee: Medical versus surgical treatment of primary vesicoureteral reflux. Pediatrics, 67(3):392, 1981.

Reuterskiold, A. G.: The abnormal ureter in children. Scand. J. Urol. Nephrol., 4:99, 1970.

Roberts, J. A., Roth, J. K., Jr., Domingue, G., Lewis, R. W., Kaack, B., and Baskin, G.: Immunology of pyelonephritis in the primate model. V. Effect of superoxide dismutase. J. Urol., 128:1394, 1982.

Rolleston, G. L., Maling, T. M. J., and Hodson, C. J.: Intrarenal reflux and the scarred kidney. Arch. Dis. Child., 49:531, 1974.

Rolleston, G. L., Shannon, F. J., and Utley, W. L. F.: Relationship of infantile vesicoureteral reflux to renal damage. Br. Med. J., 1:460, 1970.

Rolleston, G. L., Shannon, F. T., and Utley, W. L. F.: Follow up of vesicoureteric reflux in the newborn. Kidney Int., 8:59, 1975.

Rose, J. S., Glassberg, K. I., and Waterhouse, K.: Intrarenal reflux and its relationship to renal scarring. J. Urol., 113:400, 1975.

Ross, J. C.: Some complications of the neurogenic bladder. Br. J. Urol., 33:31, 1961.

Salvatierra, O., and Tanagho, E. A.: Reflux as a cause of end stage kidney disease: Report of 32 cases. J. Urol., 117:441, 1977.

Salvatierra, O., Kountz, S. L., and Belzer, F. O.: Primary vesicoureteral reflux and end stage renal disease. JAMA, 226:1454, 1973.

Sampson, J. A.: Ascending renal infection, with special reference to the reflux of urine from the bladder into the ureters as an etiological factor in its causation and maintenance. Bull. Johns Hopkins Hosp., 14:334, 1903.

Satani, Y.: Histologic study of the ureter. J. Urol., 3:247, 1919.

Savage, D. C. L., Wilson, M. I., Ross, E. M., et al.: Asymptomatic bacteriuria in girl entrants to Dundee Primary School. Br. Med. J., 3:75, 1969.

Savage, J. M., Shah, V., Dillon, M. J., et al.: Renin and blood pressure in children with renal scarring and vesicoureteric reflux. Lancet, 2:441, 1978.

Schmidt, J. D., Hawtry, C. E., and Flocks, R. H.: Vesicoureteral reflux: an inherited lesion. JAMA, 220:821, 1972.

Schoenberg, H. W., Beisswanger, P., Howard, W. J., et al.: Effect of lower urinary tract infection upon ureteral function. J. Urol., 92:107, 1964.

Schulman, C. C., Duarte-Escalante, O., and Boyarsky, S.: The ureterovesical innervation. Br. J. Urol., 44:698, 1972.

Scott, J. E. S.: The role of surgery in the management of vesicoureteric reflux. Kidney Int., 8:73, 1975.

Scott, J. E. S.: The management of ureteric reflux in children. Br. J. Urol., 49:109, 1977.

Scott, J. E. S., and Stansfeld, J. M.: Ureteric reflux and kidney scarring in children. Arch. Dis. Child., 43:468, 1968.

Semblinow, V. I.: Zur Pathologie der duech Bacterien bewinkten ambsteifenden Nephritis. 1883 Dissertation. Cited by Alksne, J.: Folia Urol., 1:338, 1907.

Shopfner, C. E.: Vesicoureteral reflux. Radiology, 95:637, 1970.

Siegler, R. L.: Renin dependent hypertension in children with reflux nephropathy. Urology, 7:474, 1976.

Smellie, J. M.: The disappearance of reflux in children with urinary tract infection during prophylactic chemotherapy. In Proceedings of the 4th International Congress on Nephrology (Stockholm). Vol. 3. Basel, S. Karger, 1969, p. 357.

Smellie, J. M., and Normand, C.: Reflux nephropathy in childhood. In Hodson, C. J., and Kincaid-Smith, P. (Eds.): Reflux Nephropathy. New York, Masson Publishing USA, 1979, pp. 14–20.

Smellie, J. M., and Normand, I. C. S.: Experience of follow-up of children with urinary tract infection. In O'Grady, F., and Brumditte, W. (Eds.): Urinary Tract Infection. London, Oxford University Press, 1968, p. 123.

Smellie, J. M., and Normand, I. C. S.: Bacteriuria, reflux and renal scarring. Arch. Dis. Child., 50:581, 1975.

Smellie, J. M., and Normand, I. C. S.: The clinical features and significance of urinary infection in childhood. Proc. R. Soc. Lond., 59:415, 1966.

Smellie, J. M., Edwards, D., Hunter, N., et al.: Vesicoureteric reflux and renal scarring. Kidney Int., 8:565, 1975a.

Smellie, J., Edwards, D., Hunter, N., Normand, I. C. S., and Prescod, N.: Vesicoureteric reflux and renal scarring. Kidney Int. (Suppl.), 8:65, 1975b.

Smellie, J. M., Edwards, D., Normand, I. C. S., and Prescod, N.: Effect of VUR on renal growth in children with UTI. Arch. Dis. Child., 56:593, 1981.

Smith, A. M.: Comparison of standard and cinecystography for detecting vesicoureteral reflux. J. Urol., 96:49, 1966.

Sommer, J. T., and Douglas, F. D.: Morphogenesis of nephropathy with partial ureteral obstruction and vesicoureteral reflux. J. Urol., 125:67, 1981.

Sommer, J. T., and Stephens, F. D.: Morphogenesis of nephropathy with partial ureteral obstruction and vesicoureteral reflux. J. Urol., 125:67, 1981.

Stamey, T. A.: The question of residual urine. In Stamey, T. A. (Ed.): Urinary Infections. Baltimore, The Williams & Wilkins Co., 1972, pp. 230–231.

Stecker, J. F., Jr., Read, B. P., and Poutasse, E. F.: Pediatric hypertension as a delayed sequela of reflux induced pyelonephritis. J. Urol., 118:644, 1977.

Stephens, F. D.: Correlation of ureteric orifice position with renal morphology. Trans. Am. Assoc. Genitourin. Surg., 1976, p. 53.

Stephens, F. D.: Ureteric configurations and cystoscopy schema. Soc. Pediatr. Urol. Newsletter, Jan. 23, 1980, p. 2.

Stephens, F. S., and Lenaghan, D.: Anatomical basis and dynamics of vesicoureteral reflux. J. Urol., 87:669, 1962.

Stewart, C. M.: Delayed cystograms. J. Urol., 70:588, 1953.

Stickler, G. B., Kelalis, P. P., Burke, E. C., et al.: Primary interstitial nephritis with reflux—A cause of hypertension. Am. J. Dis. Child., 122:144, 1971.

Talbot, H. S., and Bunts, R. C.: Late renal changes in

paraplegia: Hydronephrosis due to vesicoureteral reflux. J. Urol., 61:870, 1949.

Tamminen, T. E., and Kaprio, E. A.: The relation of the shape of renal papillae and of collecting duct openings to intrarenal reflux. Br. J. Urol., 49:345, 1977.

Tanagho, E. A.: Embryologic basis for lower ureteral anomalies: A hypothesis. Urology, 7:451, 1976.

Tanagho, E. A., and Hutch, J. A.: Primary reflux. J. Urol., 93:158, 1965.

Tanagho, E. A., and Puch, R. C. B.: The anatomy and function of the ureterovesical junction. Br. J. Urol., 35:151, 1963.

Tanagho, E. A., Hutch, J. A., Meyers, F. H., et al.: Primary vesico-ureteral reflux: Experimental studies of its etiology. J. Urol., 93:165, 1965.

Timmons, J. W., Watts, F. B., and Perlmutter, A. D.: A comparison of awake and anesthesia cystography. Birth Defects: Original Articles Series (New York), 13:364, 1977.

Tokunaka, S., Koyanagi, T., Matsuno, T., Gotoh, T., and Tsuji, I.: Paraureteral diverticula: Clinical experience with 17 cases with associated renal dysmorphism. J. Urol., 124:791, 1980.

Torbey, K., and Leadbetter, W. F.: Innervation of the bladder and lower ureter: Studies on pelvic nerve section and stimulation in the dog. J. Urol., 90:395, 1963.

Torres, V. E., Moore, S. B., Kurtz, S. B., Offord, K. P., and Kelalis, P. P.: In search of a marker for genetic susceptibility to reflux nephropathy. Clin. Nephrol., 14:217, 1980a.

Torres, V. E., Velosa, J. A., Holley, K. E., Kelalis, P. P., Stickler, G. B., and Kurtz, S. B.: The progression of vesicoureteral nephropathy. Ann. Intern. Med., 92:776, 1980b.

Tremewan, R. N., Bailey, R. R., Little, T. M. J., Peters, T. M., and Tait, J. J.: Diagnosis of gross vesico-ureteric reflux using ultrasonography. Br. J. Urol., 48:431, 1976.

Uehling, D. T.: Effect of vesicoureteral reflux on concentrating ability. J. Urol., 106:947, 1971.

Uehling, D. T., and Wear, J. B., Jr.: Concentrating ability after antireflux operation. J. Urol., 116:83, 1976.

Van Gool, J. D.: Bladder infection and pressure. In Hodson, C. J., and Kincaid-Smith, P. (Eds.): Reflux Neprhopathy. New York, Masson Publishing USA, 1979, pp. 181–189.

Van Gool, J., and Tanagho, E. A.: External sphincter activity and recurrent urinary tract infections in girls. Urology, 10:348, 1977.

Vermillion, C. D., and Heale, W. F.: Position and configuration of the ureteral orifice and its relationship to renal scarring in adults. J. Urol., 109:579, 1973.

Vermooten, V., and Neuswanger, C. H.: Effects on the upper urinary tract in dogs of an incompetent ureterovesical valve. J. Urol., 32:330, 1934.

Vlahakis, E., Hartman, G. W., and Kelalis, D. D.: Comparison of voiding cystourethrography and expression cystourethrography. J. Urol., 106:414, 1971.

Walker, D., Richard, G., and Dobson, D.: Maximum urine concentration: early means of identifying patients with reflux who may require surgery. Urology, 1:343, 1973.

Walker, R. D., Duckett, J., Bartone, F., et al.: Screening school children for urologic disease. Pediatrics, 60:239, 1977.

Wallace, D. M. A., Rothwell, D. L., and Williams, D. I.: The long-term follow-up of surgically treated vesicoureteric reflux. Br. J. Urol., 50:479, 1978.

Warren, M. M., Kelalis, P. P., and Stickler, G. B.: Unilateral ureteroneocystostomy: The fate of the contralateral ureter. J. Urol., 107:466, 1972.

Warshaw, B. L., Edelbrock, H. H., Ettenger, R. B., et al.: Renal transplantation in children with obstructive uropathy. J. Urol., *123*:737, 1980.

Wein, H. A., and Schoenberg, H. W.: A review of 402 girls with recurrent urinary tract infections. J. Urol., *107*:329, 1972.

Weiss, R. M., and Lytton, B.: Vesicoureteral reflux and distal ureteral obstruction. J. Urol., *111*:245, 1974.

Weiss, R. M., Schiff, M., Jr., and Lytton, B.: Late obstruction after ureteroneocystostomy. J. Urol., *106*:144, 1971.

Wesson, M. B.: Anatomical, embryological and physiological studies of the trigone and neck of the bladder. J. Urol., *4*:297, 1920.

Whalley, P. J., and Cunningham, F. G.: Short-term vs. continuous antibiotic therapy for asymptomatic bacteriuria in pregnancy. Obstet. Gynecol., *49*:292, 1977.

White, R. H. R.: Personal communication, 1982.

Williams, D. I.: The ureter, the urologist and the pediatrician. Proc. R. Soc. Lond., *63*:595, 1970.

Williams, D. I.: Obstructive uropathy: The urethra. *In* Williams, D. I. (Ed.): Urology in Childhood. Berlin, Springer-Verlag, 1974, pp. 207–229.

Williams, D. I., and Eckstein, H. B.: Surgical treatment of reflux in children. Br. J. Urol., *37*:12, 1965.

Williams, D. I., Scott, J., and Turner-Warwick, R. T.: Reflux and recurrent infection. Br. J. Urol., *33*:435, 1961.

Williams, G. L., Davies, D. K. L., Evans, K. T., and Williams, J. E.: Vesicoureteral reflux in patients with bacteriuria in pregnancy. Lancet, *2*:1202, 1968.

Willscher, M. K., Bauer, S. B., Zammuto, P. J., and Retik, A. B.: Renal growth and urinary infection following antireflux surgery in infants and children. J. Urol., *115*:722, 1976*a*.

Willscher, M. K., Bauer, S. B., Zammuto, P. J., et al.: Infection of the urinary tract after antireflux surgery. J. Pediatr., *89*:743, 1976*b*.

Winter, C. C.: A new test for vesicoureteral reflux: An external technique using radioisotopes. J. Urol., *81*:105, 1959.

Woodard, J. R., and Filardi, G.: The demonstration of vesicoureteral reflux under anesthesia. J. Urol., *116*:501, 1976.

Woodburne, R. T.: Anatomy of the ureterovesical junction. J. Urol., *92*:431, 1964.

Young, H. H.: Johns Hopkins Hosp. Bull., *9*:100, 1898.

Young, H. H., and Wesson, M. B.: The anatomy and surgery of the trigone. Arch. Surg., *3*:1, 1921.

Zinner, N. R., Foster, E. A., Spaulding, B. H., and Paquin, A. J.: Experimental vesicoureteral reflux: Comparison of three cystographic techniques. J. Urol., *90*:405, 1963.

Megaureter

Albertson, K. W., and Talner, L. B.: Valves of the ureter. Radiology, *103*:91, 1972.

Allen, T. D.: Congenital ureteral strictures. J. Urol., *104*:196, 1970.

Belman, A. B.: Megaureter classification, etiology, and management. Urol. Clin. North Am., *1*:497, 1974.

Bischoff, P. F.: Megaureter. Br. J. Urol., *29*:46, 1957.

Boxer, R. J., Fritsche, P., Skinner, D. F., et al.: Replacement of the ureter by small intestine: clinical application and results of the ileal ureter in 89 patients. J. Urol., *121*:728, 1979.

Caine, M., and Hermann, G.: The return of peristalsis in the anastomosed ureter: A cine-radiographic study. Br. J. Urol., *42*:164, 1970.

Caulk, J. R.: Megaloureter: the importance of the ureterovesical valve. J. Urol., *9*:315, 1923.

Considine, J.: Retrocaval ureter: A review of the literature with a report on two new cases followed for fifteen years and two years, respectively. Br. J. Urol., *38*:412, 1966.

Creevy, C. D.: The atonic distal ureteral segment (ureteral achalasia). J. Urol., *97*:457, 1967.

Cussen, L. J.: Dimensions of normal ureter in infancy and childhood. Invest. Urol., *5*:164, 1967.

Cussen, L. J.: The morphology of congenital dilatation of the ureter: intrinsic ureteral lesions. Aust. N.Z. J. Surg., *41*:185, 1971.

Derrick, F. C.: Management of the large, tortuous, adynamic ureter with reflux. J. Urol., *108*:153, 1972.

Deter, R. L., Hadlock, F. P., Gonzales, E. T., and Wait, R. B.: Prenatal detection of primary megaureter using dynamic image ultrasonography. Obstet. Gynecol., *56*:759, 1980.

Fitzer, P. M.: Congenital ureteral valve. Pediatr. Radiol., *8*:54, 1979.

Flatmark, A. L., Maurseth, K., and Knutrud, O.: Lower ureteric obstruction in children. Br. J. Urol., *42*:431, 1970.

Garrett, W. J., Kossoff, G., and Osborn, R. A.: The diagnosis of fetal hydronephrosis, megaureter and urethral obstruction by ultrasonic echography. Br. J. Obstet. Gynaecol., *82*:115, 1975.

Glassberg, K. I.: Dilated ureter: Classification and approach. Urology, *9*:1, 1977.

Glassberg, K. I., Schneider, M., Haller, D. O., et al.: Observations on persistently dilated ureter after posterior urethral valve ablation. Urology, *20*:20, 1982.

Goodwin, W. E., Burke, D. E., and Muller, W. H.: Retrocaval ureter. Surg. Gynecol. Obstet., *104*:337, 1957.

Gosling, J. A., and Dixon, J. S.: Functional obstruction of the ureter and renal pelvis. A histological and electron microscopic study. Br. J. Urol., *50*:145, 1978.

Grana, L., and Swenson, O.: A new surgical procedure for the treatment of aperistaltic megaloureter. Am. J. Surg., *109*:532, 1965.

Gregoir, W., and Debled, G.: L'etiologie du reflux congenital et du mega-uretere primaire. Urol. Int., *24*:119, 1969.

Hanna, M. K.: Early surgical correction of massive refluxing megaureter in babies by total ureteral reconstruction and reimplantation. Urology, *18*:562, 1981.

Hanna, M. K., and Jeffs, R. D.: Primary obstructive megaureter in children. Urology, *6*:419, 1975.

Heal, M. R.: Primary obstructive megaureter in adults. Br. J. Urol., *45*:490, 1973.

Hensley, T. W., Berdon, W. E., Baker, D. H., and Goldstein, H. R.: The ureteral "J" sign: radiographic demonstration of iatrogenic distal ureteral obstruction after ureteral reimplantation. J. Urol., *127*:766, 1982.

Hirschhorn, R. C.: The ileal sleeve. II. Surgical technique in clinical application. J. Urol., *92*:120, 1964.

Hodgson, N. B., and Thompson, L. W.: Technique of reductive ureteroplasty in the management of megaureter. J. Urol., *113*:118, 1975.

Hurst, A. F., and Gaymer-Jones, J.: A case of megaloureter due to achalasia of the ureterovesical sphincter. Br. J. Urol., *3*:43, 1931.

Hutch, J. A.: Nonobstructive dilatation of the upper urinary tract. J. Urol., *71*:412, 1954.

Hutch, J. A., and Tanagho, E. A.: Etiology of nonocclusive ureteral dilatation. J. Urol., *93*:177, 1965.

Johnston, J. H.: Reconstructive surgery of mega-ureter in childhood. Br. J. Urol., *39*:17, 1967.

Johnston, J. H.: Hydro-ureter and mega-ureter. *In* Williams, D. I. (Ed.): Pediatric Urology. London, Butterworth and Co., 1968, pp. 160–174.

Johnston, J. H., and Farkas, A.: The congenital refluxing megaureter: Experiences with surgical reconstruction. Br. J. Urol., *47*:153, 1975.

King, L. R.: Megaloureter: definition, diagnosis and management (Editorial). J. Urol., *123*:222, 1980.

Koff, S. A., Thrall, J. H., and Keyes, J. W., Jr.: Diuretic radionuclide urography. J. Urol., *122*:451, 1979.

Koff, S. A., Thrall, J. H., and Keyes, J. W., Jr.: Assessment of hydroureteronephrosis in children using diuretic radionuclide urography. J. Urol., *123*:531, 1980.

Leibowitz, S., and Bodian, M.: A study of the vesical ganglia in children and the relationship to the megaureter megacystis syndrome and Hirschsprung's disease. J. Clin. Pathol., *16*:342, 1963.

Lewis, E. L., and Cletsoway, R. W.: Megaloureter. J. Urol., *75*:643, 1956.

Lewis, E. L., and Kimbrough, J. C.: Megaloureter: New concept in treatment. South. Med. J., *45*:171, 1952.

Lockhart, J. L., Singer, A. M., and Glenn, J. F.: Congenital megaureter. J. Urol., *122*:310, 1979.

MacKinnon, K. J.: Primary megaureter. Birth Defects, *13*:15, 1977.

Mayo, M. E., and Ansell, J. S.: The effect of bladder function on the dynamics of the ureterovesical junction. J. Urol., *123*:229, 1980.

McLaughlin, A. P., Pfister, R. C., Leadbetter, W. F., et al.: The pathophysiology of primary megaloureter. J. Urol., *109*:805, 1973.

Mitchell, M. E.: The rate of bladder augmentation in undiversion. J. Pediatr. Surg., *16*:790, 1981.

Mollard, P., and Paillot, J. M.: Primary megaureter (pathogenesis and treatment of 104 patients—131 ureters. Prog. Pediatr. Surg., *5*:113, 1973.

Murnaghan, G. F.: Experimental investigation of the dynamics of the normal and dilated ureter. Br. J. Urol., *29*:403, 1957.

Nesbit, R. M., and Withycombe, J. F.: The problem of primary megaloureter. J. Urol., *72*:162, 1954.

Notley, R. G.: Electron microscopy of the primary obstructive megaureter. Br. J. Urol., *44*:229, 1972.

Pagano, P., and Passerini, G.: Primary obstructed megaureter. Br. J. Urol., *49*:469, 1977.

Passaro, E., and Smith, J. P.: Congenital ureteral valve in children: a case report. J. Urol., *84*:290, 1960.

Pfister, R. C., and Hendren, W. H.: Primary megaureter in children with adults. Clinical and pathophysiologic features of 150 ureters. Urology, *12*:160, 1978.

Pitts, W. R., and Muecke, E. C.: Congenital megaloureter: A review of 80 patients. J. Urol., *111*:468, 1974.

Politano, V. A.: Ureterovesical junction. J. Urol., *107*:239, 1972.

Rabinowitz, R., Barkin, M., Schillinger, J. F., Jeffs, R. D., and Cook, G. T.: Salvaging the iatrogenic megaureter. J. Urol., *121*:330, 1979.

Retik, A. B., McEvoy, J. P., and Bauer, S. B.: Megaureters in children. Urology, *11*:281, 1978.

Skinner, D. G., and Goodwin, W. E.: Indications for the use of intestinal segments in management of nephrocalcinosis. Trans. Am. Assoc. Genitourin. Surg., *66*:158, 1974.

Smith, E. D., et al.: Report of Working Party to Establish an International Nomenclature for the Large Ureter. *In* Bergsma, D., and Duckett, J. W. (Eds.): Birth Defects. Original Articles Series. Vol. 13, No. 5, 1977, pp. 3–8.

Stephens, F. D.: Treatment of megaureters by multiple micturition. Aust. N.Z. J. Surg., *27*:130, 1957.

Swenson, O., and Fisher, J. H.: The relation of megacolon and megaloureter. N. Engl. J. Med., *253*:1147, 1955.

Swenson, O., Fisher, J. H., and Cendron, J.: Megaloureter:

Investigation as to the cause and report on the results of newer forms of treatment. Surgery, *40*:223, 1956.

Talner, L. B., and Gittes, R. F.: Megacalyces: Further observation and differentiation from obstructive renal disease. Am. J. Roentgenol., *121*:473, 1974.

Tanagho, E. A.: Ureteral tailoring. J. Urol., *106*:194, 1971.

Tanagho, E. A.: Intrauterine fetal ureteral obstruction. J. Urol., *109*:196, 1973.

Tatu, W., and Brennan, R. E.: Primary megaureter in a mother and daughter. Urol. Radiol., *3*:185, 1981.

Tokunaka, S., and Koyanagi, T.: Morphologic study of primary nonreflux megaureters with particular emphasis on the role of ureteral sheath and ureteral dysplasia. J. Urol., *128*:399, 1982.

Tokunaka, S., Koyanagi, T., Tsuji, I., and Yamade, T.: Histopathology of the nonrefluxing megaloureter: A clue to its pathogenesis. J. Urol., *17*:238, 1982.

Tscholl, R., Tettamatti, F., and Singg, E.: Ileal substitutes of ureter with reflux-plasty by terminal intussusception of bowel. Urology, *9*:385, 1977.

Turner, R. D., and Goodwin, W. E.: Experiments with intussuscepted ileal valve in ureteral substitution. J. Urol., *81*:526, 1959.

Tveter, K. J., and Goodwin, W. E.: The use of ileum as substitute for the ureter. *In* Resnick, M. I. (Ed.): Current Trends in Urology. Vol. 2. Baltimore, Williams & Wilkins Co., 1982, pp. 1–51.

Uson, A. C., Braham, S. B., Abrams, C. A., et al.: Retrocaval ureter in a child with Turner's syndrome. Am. J. Dis. Child., *119*:267, 1970.

Von Niederhausern, W., and Tuchschmid, D.: Une association mal connue: le mega-uretere congenital primaire et le rein a mega-calices. Ann. Urol., *5*:225, 1971.

Weiss, R. M., and Lytton, B.: Vesicoureteral reflux and distal ureteral obstruction. J. Urol., *111*:245, 1974.

Weiss, R. M., Schiff, M., Jr., and Lytton, B.: Late obstruction after ureteroneocystostomy. J. Urol., *106*:144, 1971.

Whitaker, R. H.: Methods of assessing obstruction in dilated ureter. Br. J. Urol., *45*:15, 1973.

Whitaker, R. H., and Flower, C. D.: Megacalices—how broad a spectrum? Br. J. Urol., *53*:1, 1981.

Williams, D. I., and Hulme-Moir, I.: Primary obstructive megaureter. Br. J. Urol., *42*:140, 1970.

Witherow, R. O., and Whitaker, R. H.: The predictive accuracy of antigrade pressure flow studies in equivocal upper tract obstruction. Br. J. Urol., *53*:496, 1981.

Ureteral Reimplantation

Ahmed, S.: Transverse advancement ureteral reimplantation: pull-through alternative in megaureter. J. Urol., *123*:218, 1980.

Ahmed, S., and Tan, H.: Complications of transverse advancement ureteral reimplantation: Diverticulum formation. J. Urol., *127*:970, 1982.

Bischoff, P.: Betrachtungen zur Genese des Megaureters. Urol. Int., *11*:257, 1961.

Bischoff, P. F.: Problems in treatment of vesicoureteral reflux. J. Urol., *107*:133, 1972.

Bishop, M. C., Askew, A. R., and Smith, J. C.: Reimplantation of the wide ureter. Br. J. Urol., *50*:383, 1978.

Bjordal, R. I., Stake, G., and Knutrud, O.: Surgical treatment of megaureter in the first few months of life. Ann. Chir. Gynaecol. Fenn., *69*:10, 1980.

Bovee, J. W.: A critical survey of ureteral implantation. Ann. Surg., *31*:165, 1900.

Burkowski, A.: Operative treatment of megaureter in adults. Int. Urol. Nephrol., *9*:105, 1977.

Caine, M., and Hermann, G.: The return of peristalsis in the·anastomosed ureter: a cine-radiographic study. Br. J. Urol., 42:164, 1970.

Carlson, H. E.: The intrapsoas transplant of megalo-ureter. J. Urol., 72:172, 1954.

Clark, P., and Hosmame, R. U.: Reimplantation of the ureter. Br. J. Urol., 48:31, 1976.

Cohen, S. J.: Ureterozystoneostome: Eine neue antireflux-technik. Aktuel. Urol., 6:1, 1975.

Creevy, C. D.: The atomic distal ureteral segment (ureteral achalasia). J. Urol., 97:457, 1967.

DeWeerd, J. H., Farsund, T., and Burke, E. C.: Uretero-neocystostomy. J. Urol., 101:520, 1969.

Dodson, A. I.: Some improvements in the technique of ureterocystostomy. J. Urol., 55:225, 1946.

Ehrlich, R. M.: Ureteral folding technique for megaureter surgery. Soc. Pediatr. Urol. Newsletter, May 5, 1982, pp. 56–57.

Filly, R. A., Friedland, G. W., Fair, W. R., and Govan, D. E.: Late ureteric obstruction following ureteral reimplantation for reflux. Urology, 4:540, 1974.

Gearhart, J. P., and Woolfenden, K. A.: The vesicopsoas hitch as an adjunct to megaureter repair in childhood. J. Urol., 127:505, 1982.

Glenn, J. F., and Anderson, E. E.: Distal tunnel ureteral reimplantation. J. Urol., 97:623, 1967.

Gonzales, E. T., Caffarena, E., and Carlton, C. E.: The advantages of short-term vesical drainage after antire-flux operation. J. Urol., 119:817, 1978.

Gregoir, W.: Le traitement chirurgical du reflux vesico-ureteral congenital. Acta Chir. Belg., 63:431, 1964.

Gregoir, W., and Schulman, C. C.: Die extravesikale anti-reflux plastik. Urologie, A16:124, 1977.

Gregoir, W., and Van Regemorter, G.: Le reflux vésico-urétéral congénital. Urol. Int., 18:122, 1964.

Hampel, N., Richter-Levin, D., and Gersh, I.: Extravesical repair of primary vesicoureteral reflux in children. J. Urol., 117:335, 1977.

Hanna, M. K.: New surgical method for one stage total remodeling of massively dilated and tortuous ureter: tapering in situ technique. Urology, 14:453, 1979.

Hendren, W. H.: Ureteral reimplantation in children. J. Pediatr. Surg., 3:649, 1968.

Hendren, W. H.: Operative repair of megaureter in children. J. Urol., 101:491, 1969.

Hendren, W. H.: Complications of megaureter repair in children. J. Urol., 113:238, 1975.

Hendren, W. H.: Tapered bowel segment for ureteral replacement. Urol. Clin. North Am., 5:697, 1978.

Hensley, T. W., Berdon, W. E., Baker, D. H., and Goldstein, H. R.: The ureteral "J" sign: radiographic demonstration of iatrogenic distal ureteral obstruction after ureteral reimplantation. J. Urol., 127:766, 1982.

Hutch, J. A.: Vesicoureteral reflux in the paraplegic: Cause and correction. J. Urol., 68:457, 1952.

Hutch, J. A., Smith, D. R., and Osborne, R.: Review of a series of ureterovesicoplasties. J. Urol., 100:285, 1968.

Jeffs, R. D., Jonas, P., and Schillinger, J. F.: Surgical correction of vesicoureteral reflux in children with neurogenic bladder. J. Urol., 115:449, 1976.

Johnston, J. H., and Heal, M. R.: Reflux in complete duplicated ureters in children: Management and technique. J. Urol., 105:881, 1971.

Johnston, J. H., Shapiro, S. R., and Thomas, G. G.: Anti-reflux surgery in the congenital neuropathic bladder. Br. J. Urol., 48:639, 1976.

Kalicinski, Z. H., Kansy, J., Kotarbinska, B., and Juszt, W.: Surgery of megaureters—modification of Hendren's operation. J. Pediatr. Surg., 12:183, 1977.

Lamesch, A. J.: Retrograde catheterization of the ureter after antirefluxplasty by the Cohen technique of transverse advancement. J. Urol., 125:73, 1981.

Lebowitz, R. L.: Section on Urology. American Academy of Pediatrics Annual Meeting. San Francisco, October 1983.

Lich, R., Howerton, L. W., and Davis, L. A.: Recurrent urosepsis in children. J. Urol., 86:554, 1961.

Marberger, M., Altwein, J. E., Straub, E., Wulff, H. D., and Hohenfellner, R.: The Lich-Gregoir antireflux plasty: experiences with 371 children. J. Urol., 120:216, 1978.

Mayo, M. E., and Ansell, J. S.: The effect of bladder function on the dynamics of the ureterovesical junction. J. Urol., 123:229, 1980.

McDuffie, R. W., Litin, R. B., and Blundon, K. E.: Ureteral reimplantation: Lich method. Urology, 10:19, 1977.

Nanninga, J., King, L. R., Downing, J., et al.: Factors affecting the outcome of 100 ureteral reimplantations done for vesicoureteral reflux. J. Urol., 72:162, 1954.

Paquin, A. J.: Ureterovesical anastomosis: The description and evaluation of a technique. J. Urol., 82:573, 1959.

Paquin, A. J.: Surgery of the ureterovesical junction. In Glenn, J. F., and Boyce, W. H. (Eds.): Urologic Surgery. New York, Harper & Row, 1969, pp. 191–252.

Politano, V.: Poster session, American Urological Association. Boston, 1981.

Politano, V. A., and Leadbetter, W. F.: An operative technique for the correction of vesicoureteral reflux. J. Urol., 79:932, 1958.

So, E. P., Brock, W. A., and Kaplan, G. W.: Ureteral reimplantation without catheters. J. Urol., 125:551, 1981.

Starr, A.: Ureteral plication: A new concept in ureteral tailoring for megaureter. Invest. Urol., 17:153, 1979.

Stephens, F. D.: A new technique of ureteral reimplantation based on anatomical principles. Presented at the meeting of the Society for Pediatric Urology, 1977.

Stevens, A. R., and Marshall, V. F.: Reimplantation of the ureter into the bladder. Surg. Gynecol. Obstet., 77:585, 1943.

Talbot, H. S., and Bunts, R. C.: Late renal changes in paraplegia: Hydronephrosis due to vesicoureteral reflux. J. Urol., 61:810, 1949.

Tocci, P. E., Politano, V. A., Lynne, C. M., and Carrion, H. M.: Unusual complications of transvesical ureteral reimplantation. J. Urol., 115:1731, 1976.

Udall, D. A., Hodges, C. V., Pearse, H. M., et al.: Transureterostomy: Experience in pediatric patient. Urology, 2:401, 1973.

Vermooten, V., and Neuswanger, O. H.: Effects on the upper urinary tract in dogs of an incompetent uretero-vesical valve. J. Urol., 32:330, 1934.

Warren, M. M., Kelalis, P. P., and Stickler, G. B.: Unilateral ureteroneocystostomy: The fate of the contralateral ureter. J. Urol., 107:466, 1972.

Weiss, R. M., Schiff, M., and Lytton, B.: Late obstruction after ureteroneocystostomy. J. Urol., 106:144, 1971.

Whitaker, R. H.: Diagnosis of obstruction in dilated ureters. Ann. R. Coll. Surg., 53:153, 1973.

Williams, D. I., and Eckstein, H. B.: Surgical treatment of reflux in children. Br. J. Urol., 37:13, 1965.

Woodard, J. R., and Keats, G.: Ureteral reimplantation: Paquin's procedure after 12 years. J. Urol., 109:819, 1973.

CHAPTER 50

Ectopic Ureter and Ureterocele

ALAN B. RETIK, M.D.

ECTOPIC URETER

A ureter that opens anywhere except on the trigone of the bladder is considered to be ectopic (Fig. 50–1). In girls, the usual sites for an ectopic orifice are the bladder neck, proximal or distal urethra, vestibule, and vagina. Ectopic orifices have also been reported in the uterus and the cervix. In the male, ectopic ureters usually drain into the prostatic urethra, prostatic utricle, seminal vesicle, vas deferens, or ejaculatory duct. Openings into the rectum occur rarely in both sexes. In the female an ectopic ureteral orifice may be either within or outside the urinary sphincter. Therefore, ectopic ureters in girls are one of the more important causes of urinary incontinence. Because the ureteral orifice during embryonic growth is occasionally incorporated into the structures derived from the müllerian ducts, the ureter may empty into the uterus, vagina, or vestibule. In the male the ureter, even if ectopic, will be proximal to the verumontanum and will not cause urinary incontinence.

Embryologically, an ectopic ureteral orifice results when a ureteral bud or, more often, a second or accessory ureteral bud arises from the mesonephric (wolffian) duct more craniad than is usual and is not incorporated into the trigone but "carried" farther medially and downward into the urethra through the common excretory duct. In general, abnormally located ectopic ureteral orifices within the bladder produce no symptoms. However, should the ureter arise from the mesonephric duct at a still higher level, it will fail completely to become incorporated into the lower urinary tract and will remain confluent with the mesonephric duct in the male

or with its vestiges in the female; this type of ureter will invariably cause symptoms.

The incidence of ectopic ureters has been reported to be higher in females than in males. Because ureteral ectopia usually produces incontinence in females, its discovery at an earlier age is far more likely.

Ectopic Ureter in Girls

Ectopic ureteral orifices in girls are most often associated with renal duplication and may be an important cause of urinary incontinence.

CLINICAL MANIFESTATIONS

Continuous incontinence in a girl with an otherwise normal voiding pattern after toilet training is the classic sign of an ectopic ureteral orifice. Such incontinence will occur if the ectopic orifice is located in the distal urethra, vagina, or vestibule. If the urine drains only when the child assumes the erect position, incontinence may be diurnal when the renal unit drained by the ectopic orifice is dysplastic and poorly functioning. On occasion, incontinence becomes apparent at a later age and may be confused with stress incontinence or incontinence associated with neurogenic bladder dysfunction. A persistent vaginal discharge from an ectopic orifice located in the vagina is another presentation. Most ectopic ureters are associated with urinary tract infection. Ectopic ureters draining into the proximal urethra often reflux, and urge incontinence is common. On occasion, an ectopic ureter may be severely obstructed, causing massive hydronephrosis and hydro-

Female

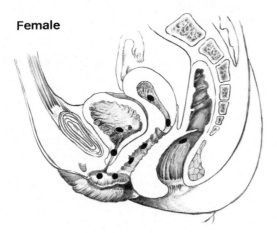

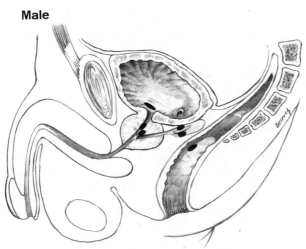

Figure 50–1. Sites of ectopic ureteral orifices in boys and girls.

Male

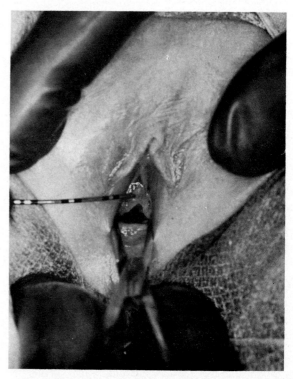

Figure 50–2. Gross photograph of an ectopic ureteral orifice in the urethrovaginal septum. A ureteral catheter is in the orifice.

ureter, and it may present as an abdominal mass (Uson et al., 1972), especially in the neonate.

DIAGNOSIS

In a girl, the diagnosis of an ectopic ureter can sometimes be made by history, and physical examination with direct visualization of the vulva will reveal continuous urinary dribbling or wetness. Often a punctum or orifice is apparent in the urethrovaginal septum (Fig. 50–2). In the absence of neurogenic vesical dysfunction or a urethral sphincter defect, an ectopic ureter is likely.

In most instances the diagnosis of an ectopic ureter is confirmed by excretory urography (Figs. 50–3, 50–4). The usual radiographic feature is a nonvisualizing or poorly visualizing upper pole of a duplex system that may be massively hydronephrotic. The upper pole displaces the lower pole downward and outward, the so-called drooping flower appearance. The calyces of the lower pelvis are fewer in number than in the normal kidney, and the uppermost calyx is usually farther from the upper limit of the renal border than is the lowest calyx from the corresponding lower limit. In addition, this pelvis and the upper portion of its ureter may be farther from the spine than on the contralateral side, and the lower pole ureter may also be scalloped and tortuous secondary to a markedly dilated upper pole ureter wrapped around it. When an ectopic ureter drains a nonvisualizing, diminutive, dysplastic renal unit, the typical radiologic features mentioned above may not be demonstrated. Particular attention should be paid to the contralateral kidney on excretory urography to avoid missing bilateral ureteral ectopia, which classically is stated to occur in about 5 per cent of cases (Mandell et al., 1981) but in one series (Campbell, 1951b) was noted in 25 per cent of cases (Fig. 50–5). In addition, reflux into the lower pole ureter is not uncommon.

Ectopic ureteral orifices may be identified at the time of cystourethroscopy and vaginoscopy. Careful inspection of the vestibule, urethra, and vagina will sometimes reveal the ectopic orifice. I have not found the intravenous injection of indigo carmine to be particularly helpful because of the very poor function of the segment drained by the ectopic center. However, filling the bladder with a dye solution such as methylene blue or indigo carmine is sometimes helpful in detecting the elusive ectopic orifice; if a clear fluid continues to drain into the vulva, one can be certain that an ectopic ureteral orifice is present.

Sometimes the diagnosis must be made by exclusion—i.e., the vestibule is damp, no orifice is found, the excretory urogram shows subtle changes suggesting a tiny dysplastic upper segment of a duplex system, and the patient is cured by surgery!

TREATMENT

The usual treatment for an ectopic ureter associated with a poorly visualizing or nonvisualizing upper pole of a renal duplication is partial nephrectomy and ureterectomy through a standard flank incision (Fig. 50–6). The entire kidney is mobilized, and both ureters are identified. There are usually two or three small arteries with corresponding veins supplying the upper pole; these are divided. Although the renal capsule is often markedly adherent to the scarred upper pole parenchyma, it is usually possible to strip the capsule well back onto the normal lower pole parenchyma. In most instances, it is helpful to place an atraumatic

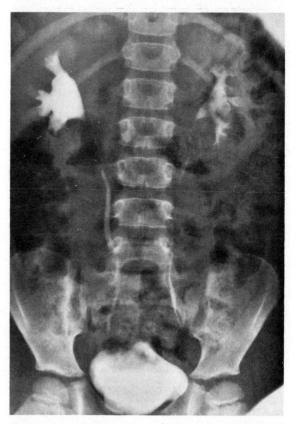

Figure 50–3. Excretory urogram in a 5-year-old girl with urinary incontinence shows a nonvisualizing upper pole on the right side displacing the lower pole downward and outward. Also note the right renal pelvis and upper ureter to be farther from the spine than on the left side.

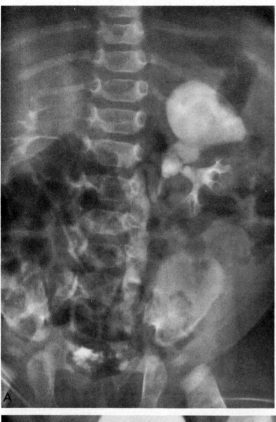

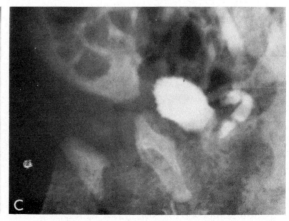

Figure 50–4. *A,* Excretory urogram in a 4-month-old girl with a urinary tract infection reveals a left renal duplication with hydronephrosis and hydroureter of the upper pole system. *B* and *C,* A voiding cystourethrogram demonstrates reflux to the ectopic ureter, whose orifice was located in the proximal urethra.

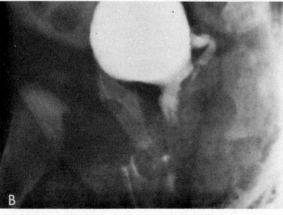

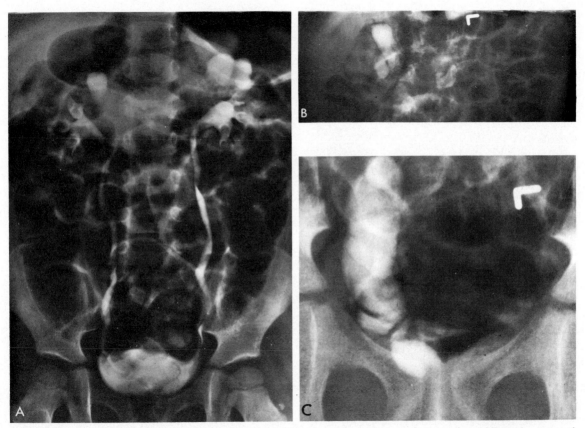

Figure 50–5. *A,* Excretory urogram in a 3-year-old girl with two severe urinary infections shows bilateral upper pole hydronephrosis and hydroureter. *B* and *C,* Voiding cystourethrography demonstrates reflux to the ectopic right upper pole ureter.

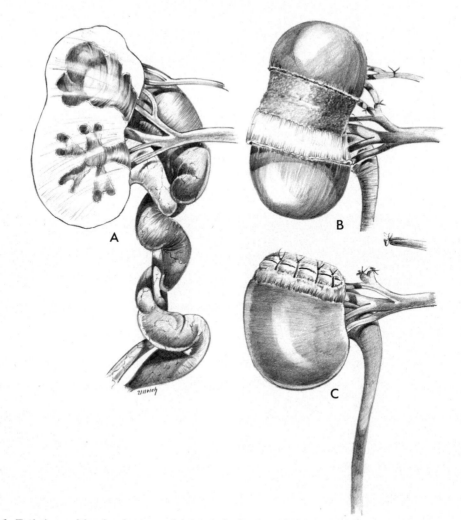

Figure 50–6. Technique of heminephrectomy for renal duplication. *A,* Upper pole ureter is usually very dilated and tortuous and is wrapped around the lower pole ureter. *B,* Two or three arteries usually supply the upper pole. *C,* It is usually possible to obtain a satisfactory capsular closure.

vascular clamp on the main renal artery prior to incising the renal parenchyma. Before the renal circulation is occluded, mannitol is injected intravenously. There is usually a rather clear-cut demarcation between the dysplastic, hydronephrotic upper pole and the lower pole. After the upper pole is removed, the parenchyma is reapproximated with interrupted sutures of 4–0 chromic catgut. The upper pole ureter is then dissected from the lower pole ureter and excised at a level below the iliac vessels. It is important in this dissection not to injure the blood supply of the lower pole ureter or its adventitia. It should not be necessary to mobilize the lower pole ureter from its bed.

Complete distal ureterectomy is not usually necessary unless reflux into the ectopic ureter is present. Rarely will the retained segment cause

symptoms and require subsequent surgical excision (Mandell et al., 1981). If the ectopic ureter refluxes, its distal portion should be excised through a separate suprapubic or groin incision. A Robinson catheter inserted into the distal portion at the time of partial nephrectomy makes the ectopic ureter more readily identifiable through the small second incision. It is usually very difficult to separate the distal 2.5 cm of the upper pole ureter from the lower pole ureter. The ectopic ureter can be completely excised up to this point, and its outer wall is then incised or excised only down to the level of the bladder, where a transfixing suture will obliterate its lumen; care should be taken not to ligate the lumen of the orthotopic ureter (Fig. 50–7).

In a minority of cases when the upper pole

is not markedly hydronephrotic and has decent parenchyma, the upper pole ureter can be anastomosed to the lower pole pelvis. When reflux to the lower pole ureter is significant and when the ectopic ureter is not severely dilated and drains a renal unit worth saving, as demonstrated by renal scanning using the isotope ^{99m}technetium-labeled dimercaptosuccinic acid, common sheath reimplantation may be performed with or without tailoring of the ectopic ureter.

Ectopic Ureter in Boys

Ectopic ureter is not as common in boys and is more often associated with a single renal unit than with renal duplication. Because ec-

topic ureters in boys always drain proximal to the external urinary sphincter, dribbling incontinence is not a presenting feature unless there is an associated abnormality of the sphincter mechanism. In general, the more distant the ectopic orifice is located from the trigone, the more likely the involved kidney is to be dysplastic. The majority of single ectopic ureters in the male open into the prostatic urethra or into the genital tract. The presenting symptoms are those of urinary infection when the orifice drains into the prostatic urethra and those of epididymo-orchitis when drainage involves the genital tract. The ureter may enter the seminal vesicle or ejaculatory duct, but in some instances the ureter and vas deferens join to share a common terminal duct, as in the embryo; reflux of urine into the ureter or vas deferens is

Figure 50–7. Surgical management of the refluxing ureteral stump. *A,* It is difficult to completely separate the distal 2 to 3 cm of the upper pole ureter from the lower pole ureter. The ectopic ureter is excised to this point. *B,* The outer wall of the ectopic ureter is excised to the bladder level. *C,* A transfixing suture obliterates its lumen, with care being taken not to injure the orthotopic ureter.

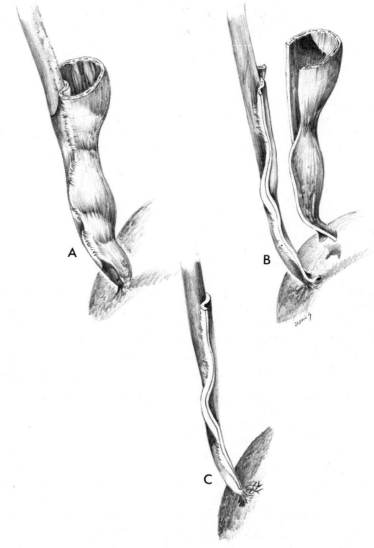

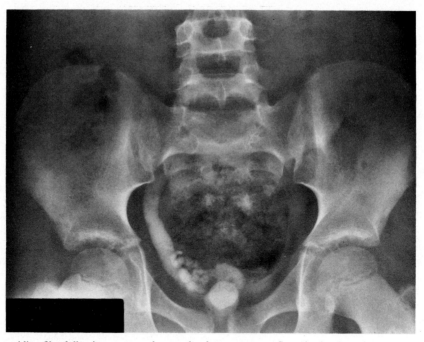

Figure 50–8. Postvoiding film following cystourethrography demonstrates reflux of urine into the ureter and seminal vesicle in a 5-year-old boy with a urinary tract infection.

common during voiding cystourethrography (Fig. 50–8). Excretory urography often reveals a nonvisualizing kidney on the affected side. At cystoscopy, the ectopic orifice is usually just distal to the bladder neck or adjacent to the verumontanum.

As the kidney is generally dysplastic, treatment of an ectopic ureter associated with a single renal system will usually consist of nephrectomy, and, if reflux is present, total ureterectomy. When the ureter enters the genital tract, even if reflux is not present, total ureterectomy, excision of the common duct, and ligation of the vas are necessary to prevent subsequent epididymitis and pyoureter. Treatment of the ectopic ureter associated with renal duplication is the same as that described previously in the female.

The Single System Ectopic Ureter

The single system ectopic ureter is more common in males than in females, as discussed in the previous section. In girls too it is very likely to be associated with a dysplastic, poorly visualizing, or nonvisualizing kidney on excretory urography (Fig. 50–9). Occasionally, an ectopic ureter is associated with an ectopic kidney that may be fused with the contralateral

organ. Uncommonly, a single ectopic ureter in the female opens in or just distal to the bladder neck and drains a relatively normal ureter and kidney. Reflux in this type of situation is common (Fig. 50–10).

The diagnosis of a single ectopic ureter in the female may be difficult, especially if the orifice drains outside of the sphincter mechanism and the associated kidney is nonvisualizing by excretory urography. Diagnostic ultrasound or arteriography may sometimes be helpful in locating the kidney. Rarely, exploratory laparotomy is indicated when the diagnosis cannot be made by the conventional methods.

Treatment depends upon the function of the kidney. In most instances, treatment will consist of nephrectomy or nephroureterectomy. When the ectopic ureter opens just distal to the bladder neck, is refluxing, and is associated with a relatively normal kidney, antireflux surgery is indicated.

BILATERAL SINGLE SYSTEM ECTOPIC URETERS

Bilateral single system ectopic ureters are fortunately rare, as they present a complex therapeutic problem. In this condition, the ureters usually drain into the prostatic urethra in the male and into the distal urethra in the female. Bladder capacity is invariably de-

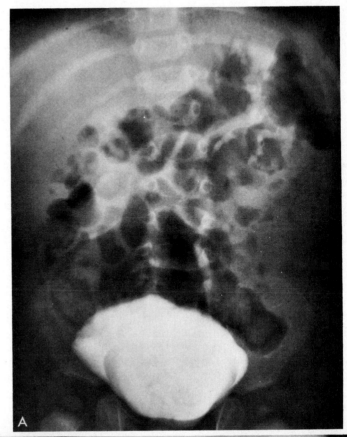

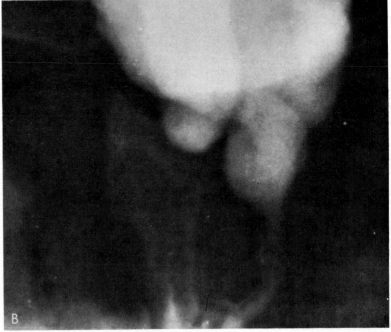

Figure 50–9. *A*, Excretory urogram in a 3-year-old girl reveals a poorly visualizing right kidney. *B*, Voiding cystourethrography demonstrates severe reflux into an ectopic ureter whose orifice was in the proximal urethra.

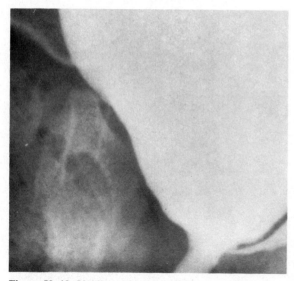

Figure 50–10. Voiding cystogram in a 2-year-old girl shows a refluxing ectopic ureter associated with a single system. The intravenous pyelogram was normal.

creased, reflux is usually present, and, most important, the bladder neck fails to develop. Embryologically, the portion of the urogenital sinus between the orifices of the wolffian duct and the ureter develops the bladder neck musculature. This development does not occur if both ureters remain in the position of the wolffian duct orifice. Because there is no formation of the trigone and base plate, a very wide, poorly defined, incompetent vesical neck results. In rare instances, bilateral single ectopic ureters are associated with agenesis of the bladder and urethra. This condition is usually but not always incompatible with life (Glenn, 1959).

Commonly, the involved kidneys are dysplastic or display varying degrees of hydronephrosis (Fig. 50–11). The ureters are usually dilated, and the bladder has a small capacity, so the child dribbles continuously. In the male, incontinence is not as severe because the external sphincter provides a variable degree of control.

At cystoscopy, the ureteral orifices can be easily identified in the male, usually just distal to the bladder neck. The bladder neck is lax and the bladder is small. In the female, it can be difficult to find both ureteral orifices, which are usually located in the distal urethra but occasionally enter the genital tract.

The abnormality per se is more akin to epispadias, with the basic defect being a short urethra and incompetent bladder neck. However, unlike epispadias, there is also a high incidence of renal and ureteral abnormalities

with this condition as well as a small bladder capacity.

Treatment usually consists of ureteral reimplantation and reconstruction of the bladder neck for continence by one of the tubularization procedures—e.g., the Young-Dees procedure. It is often helpful to employ a vesicourethral suspension at the same time. The success rate is higher in boys than in girls. Bladder capacity in the child who gains satisfactory control will often increase. A colocystoplasty to increase bladder capacity is desirable in selected instances.

Although urinary diversion should rarely be needed for incontinence alone, a few children with incontinence and severe renal dysplasia may require it.

ECTOPIC URETER WITH RENAL TRIPLICATION

This is one of the rarest of all anomalies. The incidence is higher in females. I have seen two cases in young adult females—one had mild incontinence and the other a persistent vaginal discharge.

Like other forms of ureteral ectopy, treatment depends upon the severity of renal involvement and the specifics of each case (Gill, 1952; Gilmore, 1974; Spangler, 1963).

URETEROCELES

Ureterocele is a cystic dilatation of the terminal ureter within the bladder or urethra, or both. In the "simple" or "orthotopic" variety, the ureterocele is located on the trigone at the usual location of the ureteral orifice. In the ectopic type, the ureterocele is located distal to the trigone and may project well into the urethra. The ectopic orifice is located at the bladder neck or in the urethra.

Simple or Orthotopic Ureterocele

Simple or orthotopic ureteroceles are more common in adults. They usually occur as a normally placed ureter on the trigone, associated either with a single collecting system or, very rarely, with the upper pole ureter of a complete duplication. The etiology of simple ureteroceles is debatable, and a complete discussion is beyond the scope of this chapter (see Chapter 38). Although most simple ureteroceles have obstructing pinpoint orifices, nonobstructed ureteroceles do exist.

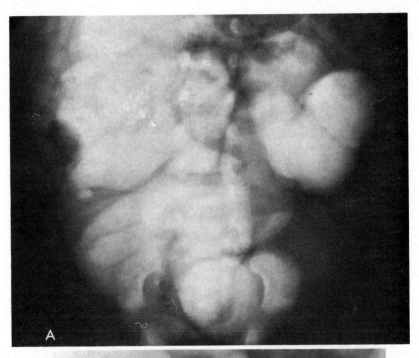

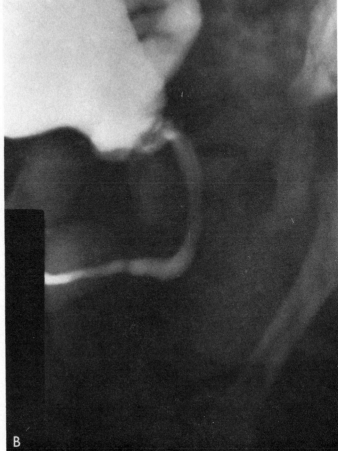

Figure 50–11. *A,* Excretory urogram in a 6-day-old boy shows very severe bilateral hydronephrosis and hydroureter. *B,* A voiding cystourethrogram demonstrates refluxing ectopic ureters draining into the prostatic urethra.

The ureterocele may vary in size from a tiny cystic dilatation of the submucosal ureter to a large balloon that fills the bladder. Histologically, the wall of the ureterocele contains varying degrees of attenuated smooth muscle bundles and fibrous tissue. The ureterocele is covered by vesical mucosa and lined with ureteral mucosa.

Most children present with symptoms of urinary tract infection. Stasis and infection predispose to stone formation in the ureterocele and upper urinary tract. Rarely, large simple ureteroceles will prolapse through the bladder neck, causing urinary obstruction.

Excretory urography often demonstrates the characteristic "cobra-head" deformity, an area of increased density similar to the head of a cobra with a halo or less dense shadow around it. Larger ureteroceles often fail to fill early with contrast material, resulting in a sizable filling defect in the bladder (Fig. 50–12). These findings are associated with varying degrees of hy-dronephrosis and hydroureter. The upper urinary tract changes associated with a simple ureterocele are usually not as severe as those associated with an ectopic ureterocele. Vesicoureteral reflux is rarely seen with a simple ureterocele. At cystoscopy, the ureterocele usually will expand rhythmically with each peristaltic wave of urine that fills it and then shrink as a thin jet of urine drains (usually continuously) through the small orifice.

Transurethral resection of simple ureteroceles, previously recommended as a method of decompression, invariably results in vesicoureteral reflux and infection. Transurethral distal incision of *small* simple ureteroceles, making a tiny slit with a Bugbee electrode, often is therapeutic and leaves the intravesical hood of the ureter intact. Reflux is not the usual result, and if it occurs, a secondary elective ureteral reimplantation can be done when required. However, in most instances, primary excision of the ureterocele and reimplantation of the

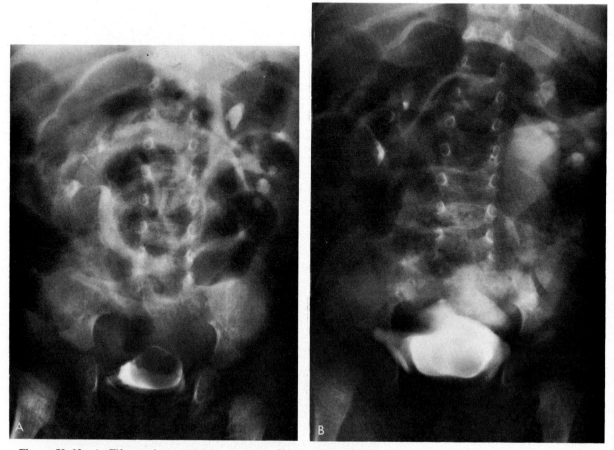

Figure 50–12. *A,* Fifteen-minute excretory urogram film reveals a filling defect in the bladder, which was a simple ureterocele. *B,* Severe left hydronephrosis and hydroureter are seen on a delayed film.

involved ureter by one of the advancement techniques or by the standard Politano-Leadbetter procedure (Politano and Leadbetter, 1958) is the surgical procedure of choice (Fig. 50–13). If the lower ureter is extremely dilated, it may have to be tapered as well. In rare instances, when kidney damage is very severe, nephroureterectomy is indicated.

In the uncommon situation of a simple ureterocele associated with a duplication, treatment depends upon the obstructive effects of the ureterocele and whether or not reflux to the lower pole ureter is present. At times, the ureterocele is associated with minimal dilatation of the upper pole ureter, and surgery may not be indicated (Fig. 50–14). Surgery for obstruction or reflux in this case is similar to that used when there is a single ureter—i.e., excision of the ureterocele and distal portions of both ureters, with common sheath reimplantation of both ureters by advancement or by the Politano-Leadbetter technique.

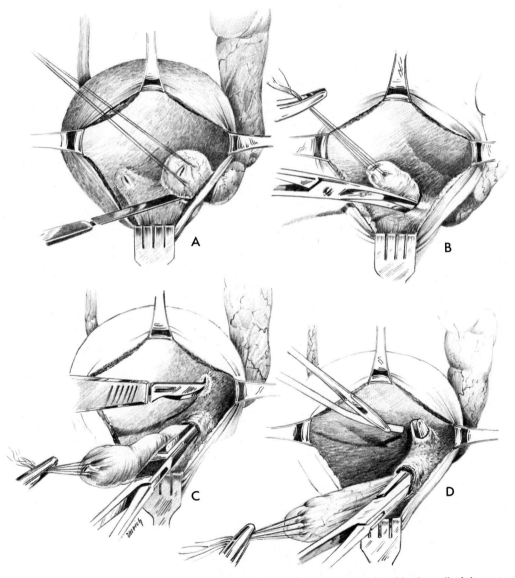

Figure 50–13. Surgical correction of simple ureterocele. *A,* After traction sutures are placed in the wall of the ureterocele, an incision is made with cautery around its circumference. *B,* The ureter is dissected from its intra- and extravesical attachments with scissors. *C,* A right angle clamp is passed outside the bladder, sweeping the peritoneum away. An incision is made on the tip of the clamp approximately 3 cm superior and slightly medial to the original orifice. *D,* The clamp is spread widely to ensure an adequate hiatus and grasps a fine French catheter.

Illustration and legend continued on following page.

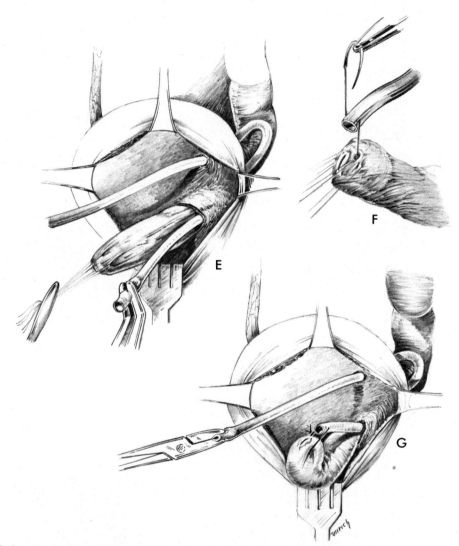

Figure 50–13 *Continued. E* and *F,* The catheter is brought back into the bladder and is sutured to the ureter. *G,* The catheter then guides the ureter through its new entrance into the bladder.

Illustration and legend continued on opposite page.

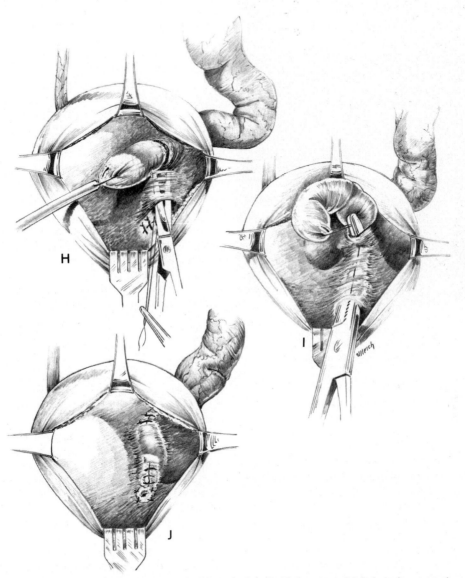

Figure 50–13 *Continued. H,* After the original muscular hiatus is closed with interrupted 4-0 chromic catgut, the surrounding mucosa is mobilized and a submucosal tunnel is made with scissors. *I* and *J,* After the ureter is brought through the tunnel, the redundant ureter is excised and the ureter anastomosed to the bladder with interrupted 4–0 and 5–0 chromic catgut. The mucosa is reapproximated with 5–0 chromic catgut. The very large ureter may be tapered if necessary to achieve the desired result.

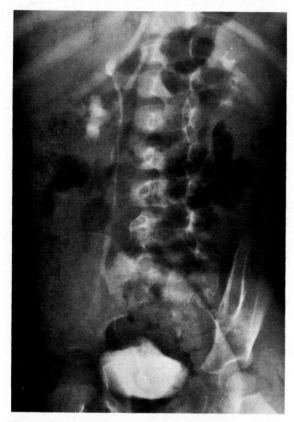

Figure 50–14. Excretory urogram in a 4-year-old girl with two urinary tract infections characterized by irritative symptoms shows the cobra head deformity of a right ureterocele. Note the lack of dilatation of the upper pole ureter.

Ectopic Ureterocele

Ectopic ureterocele is one of the more serious anomalies of the urinary tract in infancy and childhood. It is the most common cause of severe lower urinary tract obstruction in girls. It is far more common in girls than in boys; the reason for this is unknown. Approximately 10 per cent of ectopic ureteroceles are bilateral. There is also an increased incidence of duplication on the contralateral side (Mandell et al., 1980). Rarely, ectopic ureteroceles occur without duplication, usually in males (Johnson and Perlmutter, 1980).

CLASSIFICATION

One classification popularized of late is that of Stephens (1971, 1964, 1963, 1958), who made it to a large extent an anatomic and descriptive one (Figs. 50–15 to 50–17).

A *stenotic ectopic ureterocele* (which occurs in about 40 per cent of cases) is characterized by a small orifice located either at the tip of the cystic dilatation of the ureter or on the superior or inferior surface of the ureterocele.

A *sphincteric ectopic ureterocele* (found in about 40 per cent of cases) terminates within the internal sphincter. The orifice may be normal or large and may open either in the posterior urethra in the male or distal to the external sphincter in the female.

With the *sphincterostenotic ectopic ureterocele* (found in about 5 per cent of cases), the stenotic ureteral orifice is located in the floor of the urethra or beyond.

In the more recently described *cecoureterocele* (rare), the lumen extends distal to the orifice as a long tongue or "cecum" beneath the urethral submucosa, and the orifice communicates with the lumen of the bladder and is large and incompetent.

Other types of ureteroceles that have been described are the *blind ectopic ureterocele* (rare), in which there is atrophy of the portion of ureter extending distal to the ureterocele and there is no orifice, and the *nonobstructed ectopic ureterocele* (rare), in which there is terminal expansion of the ureter, which has a large orifice in the bladder.

A number of theories have evolved to explain the formation of an ectopic ureterocele. In Chwalle's theory, a membrane (Chwalle's membrane) covering the ureteral orifice persists for a prolonged period of time, leading to the formation of a ureterocele (Chwalle, 1927). Ericsson (1954) proposed that there was a failure of reabsorption of a membrane between the wolffian duct and the vesicourethral canal, with the subsequent formation of a caudal opening in this membrane. The ectopic ureteral orifice is buried beneath this membrane. The most popular theory, which can account for all of the various types of ureteroceles including the unobstructed ones, is that of Stephens (1971), who theorizes that there is a failure of expansion of the ureteral orifice rather than temporary occlusion by a membrane.

As in simple ureteroceles, the cystic submucosal dilatation is lined by ureteral mucosa. Similarly, the wall of the ureterocele has varying degrees of markedly attenuated smooth muscle bundles arranged longitudinally, circularly, or in a mixture of the two.

CLINICAL MANIFESTATIONS

The patient often presents during the first few months of life with symptoms of urinary infection or failure to thrive. As mentioned above, ureteroceles in girls may prolapse intermittently through the urethra. Urinary retention

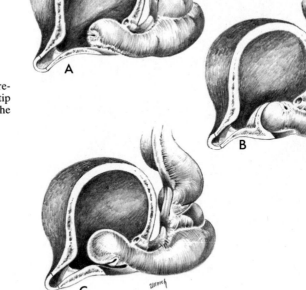

Figure 50–15. *A* to *C*, Stenotic ectopic ureteroceles—orifice may be located at the tip or at the superior or inferior surface of the ureterocele.

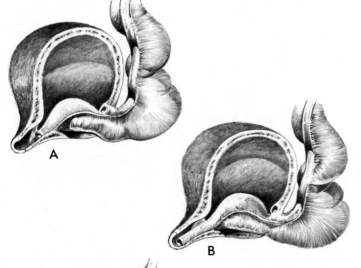

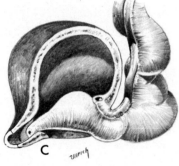

Figure 50–16. *A* and *B*, Sphincteric ectopic ureteroceles. *C*, Sphincterostenotic ectopic ureterocele.

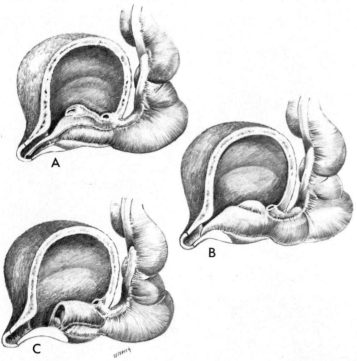

Figure 50–17. *A,* Cecoureterocele—lumen extends distal to the orifice as a long tongue beneath the urethral submucosa. The orifice communicates with the lumen of the bladder and is large and incompetent. *B,* Blind ectopic ureterocele—atrophy of the ureter distal to the ureterocele, which ends blindly. *C,* Nonobstructed ectopic ureterocele—terminal expansion of the ureter, which has a large orifice in the bladder.

is uncommon but occurs when an ectopic ureterocele prolapses through the bladder neck. Some degree of urinary incontinence may occur in a girl with a large intraurethral ectopic ureterocele that has rendered the external urinary sphincter lax and inefficient.

DIAGNOSIS

The renal unit associated with an ectopic ureterocele is commonly dysplastic and has little or no function. The radiologic findings are related to the effect of the ureterocele on the ipsilateral and contralateral ureters and renal units. Large ectopic ureteroceles may obstruct the ipsilateral lower pole ureter and on occasion are large and tense enough to obstruct the contralateral side as well. More often, the ureterocele distorts the ipsilateral lower pole ureteral orifice, effectively shortening the submucosal course of this ureter and producing reflux.

The findings on excretory urography are similar to those described for ectopic ureter, but with ureterocele the upper pole is generally more dilated. Most upper poles are nonvisualizing or show severe hydronephrosis. Characteristically there is a nonopaque filling defect of varying size in the bladder that is usually situated off center and always appears on the bladder outline rather than as a complete circle within the bladder shadow as in a simple ureterocele (Fig. 50–18). The filling defect may

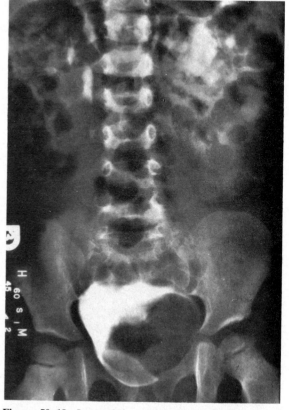

Figure 50–18. Large filling defect in the bladder of an ectopic ureterocele associated with the upper pole of a left renal duplication. A voiding cystogram demonstrated severe reflux to the lower pole.

extend behind or into the prostatic urethra in the male or the entire urethra in the female, thus causing obstruction. Trigonal cysts, which are mentioned in the earlier literature, probably represent subtrigonal extensions of these ureteroceles. The typical filling defect in the bladder associated with an ectopic ureterocele is usually diagnostic. In unusual circumstances, it can be confused with similar defects caused by rhabdomyosarcoma of the bladder or prostate or very severe cystitis cystica.

In addition to outlining the ectopic ureterocele (Fig. 50–19), voiding cystourethrography with diluted contrast medium is important for

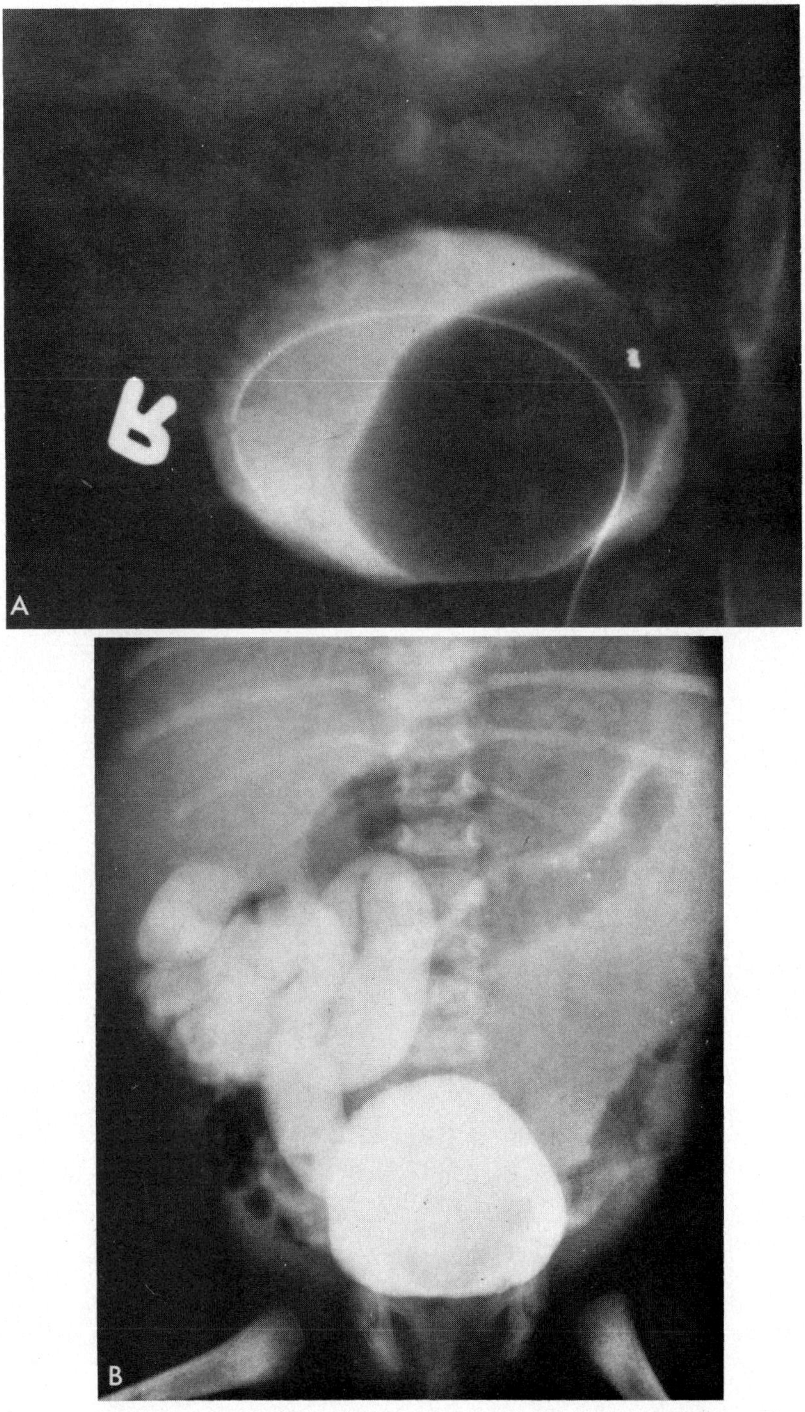

Figure 50–19. *A,* Cystogram outlines a *left* ectopic ureterocele. *B,* Postvoiding film shows reflux to the *right* lower pole. This girl had *bilateral* ectopic ureteroceles, the right being a small subtrigonal one and not demonstrated on the cystogram.

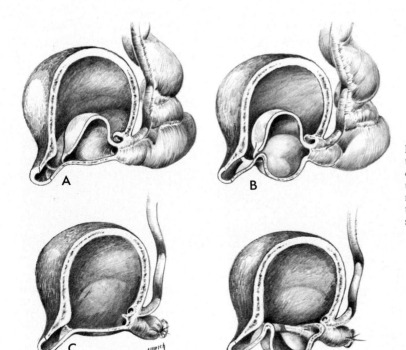

Figure 50–20. *A* and *B,* Ectopic ureterocele with poor backing is displaced outward during voiding. *C* and *D,* If ureterocele is only uncapped, a wide-mouthed diverticulum results, whose distal lip at the bladder neck may be obstructive.

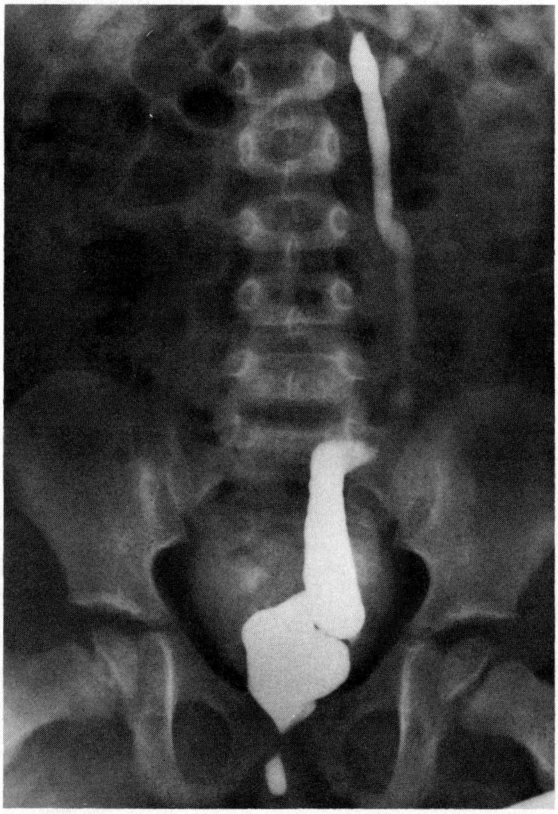

Figure 50–21. Endoscopic injection of a ureterocele outlines the upper pole and the distal extent of the ureterocele.

demonstrating the tension in and compressibility of the ureterocele, the presence of reflux, and the degree of detrusor backing of the ureterocele. The information thus gained has important therapeutic implications. Reflux into the ureterocele is rare but may occur, especially in the cecoureterocele. Reflux into the ipsilateral lower pole ureter, on the other hand, occurs in almost 50 per cent of patients. Ectopic ureteroceles may change in size during voiding, and this to a large extent depends upon their compressibility. Tense ureteroceles will remain the same size during micturition, and the filling defect on the voiding cystogram will not change. However, when the ectopic ureteral orifice is wide and the ureteral contents are at low pressure, the ureterocele is compressed during voiding and its contents either pass into the urethra or empty back into the ureter. In addition, reflux to the lower pole ureter is much more common with a compressible ureterocele than with a tense one. Cystography will also demonstrate whether the detrusor backing is poor or even absent (Fig. 50–20). In the latter situation, filling of the bladder everts the ureterocele, simulating the appearance of a bladder diverticulum.

A ureterocele may be ruptured either spontaneously or following instrumentation. Radiologically, an irregular cavity lying outside the bladder outline with an edge forming a filling defect within the bladder shadow will then be characteristically demonstrated. Here, reflux into the ectopic ureter as well as into the ipsilateral lower pole ureter usually occurs.

Cystourethroscopy can confirm the radiologic findings. It is often very difficult to find the ectopic ureteral orifice, and it may not be clinically important to find it preoperatively by endoscopy. Large ureteroceles will often make visualization difficult and confusing. If the bladder is overfilled at endoscopy, the ureterocele may be effaced and missed; if it everts, the endoscopist may erroneously diagnose a widemouthed diverticulum. It is extremely important to ascertain whether a small ureterocele is present on the contralateral side as well. When the typical radiologic features of a renal duplication are not apparent, it is sometimes helpful to inject the ureterocele with contrast medium through a fine-gauge needle attached to a ureteral catheter to delineate the characteristics of the upper pole kidney and ureter (Fig. 50–21), and this could be important therapeutically (see next section on treatment).

TREATMENT

Ureteroceles have a broad spectrum of presentation, anatomy, and pathophysiology, and thus each child must be treated individually. No single method of surgical repair will suffice for all. Transurethral incision or uncapping of an ectopic ureterocele will almost always lead to reflux into the upper pole collecting system and require one, if not more, additional procedures. Rarely, initial transurethral incision of the ureterocele may be indicated as a temporizing procedure in the extremely ill infant with sepsis who has not responded to intensive intravenous antibiotic therapy. Several nonvisualizing kidneys, after decompression, have been observed to function and have thus been salvaged.

However, the treatment of choice in the majority of children who have an ectopic ureterocele associated with a nonvisualizing or poorly functioning upper renal segment should be upper pole nephrectomy and partial ureterectomy alone. In most cases this is the only procedure necessary both to decompress the ureterocele and to provide adequate drainage of the ipsilateral as well as the contralateral collecting systems and to control infection. I decompress the ureterocele from above with a fine feeding tube at the time of upper pole nephrectomy and partial ureterectomy (as described in the previous section on ectopic ureter). The distal ureteral stump is left open at the time of surgery to avoid pyoureter. During the next several months, the defect caused by the ureterocele usually diminishes, and repeat excretory urography often fails to demonstrate any evidence of the ureterocele (Fig. 50–22).

Kroovand and Perlmutter (1979) advocate total extravesical excision of the ureter to the level of the bladder wall to avoid pyoureter or alternating diverticulum and possible surgical complications from an intravesical procedure in small infants and children with large and distorting ectopic ureteroceles. However, it is our experience that surgery for the retained ureteral stump and ureterocele, per se, is most often not necessary.

Milder degrees of reflux into the ipsilateral and even contralateral ureters usually subside after the ureterocele has been decompressed from above. More severe reflux into the lower pole collecting system, in association with a nonfunctioning upper pole moiety, warrants consideration for repair at the kidney and bladder levels. These severe degrees of reflux are less likely to disappear, especially if the detrusor backing the ureterocele is deficient. In this instance, excision of the ureterocele and ipsilateral lower pole reimplantation (with or without tapering) may be necessary in addition to upper pole nephrectomy. The cross-trigonal technique

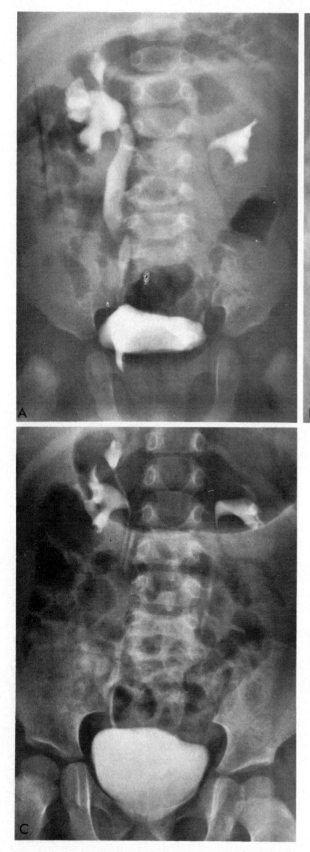

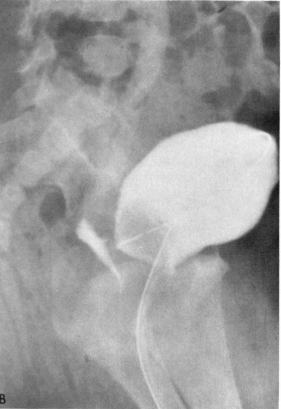

Figure 50–22. *A* Excretory urogram in an 8-month-old female who presented with intermittent prolapse of an ectopic ureterocele. Note the nonvisualizing left upper pole, filling defect in the bladder, and mild dilatation of the right lower pole ureter. *B*, A voiding cystourethrogram revealed reflux to the right lower pole, whose orifice was distorted by the ureterocele. *C*, Excretory urogram 6 months following left upper pole nephrectomy reveals no evidence of the ureterocele and a normal-caliber right lower pole ureter. No reflux was observed on a subsequent voiding cystogram.

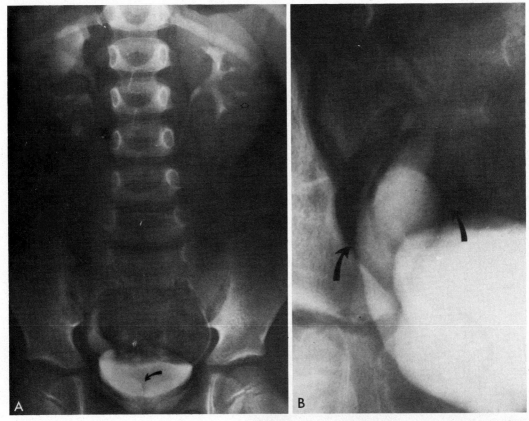

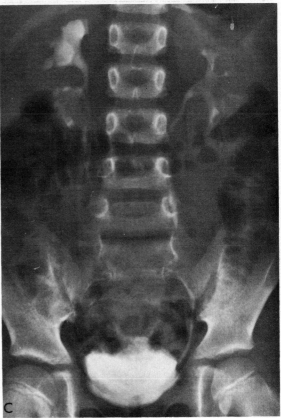

Figure 50–23. *A,* Ectopic ureterocele (dark arrow) associated with a salvageable right upper pole. The right lower pole shows severe pyelonephritis. Light arrow demonstrates a small pyelonephritic scar. *B,* Voiding cystourethrography reveals reflux to both right ureters. In addition, reflux to the left kidney was seen. *C,* Intravenous pyelogram following excision of the ureterocele, right common sheath reimplantation, and left ureteral reimplantation.

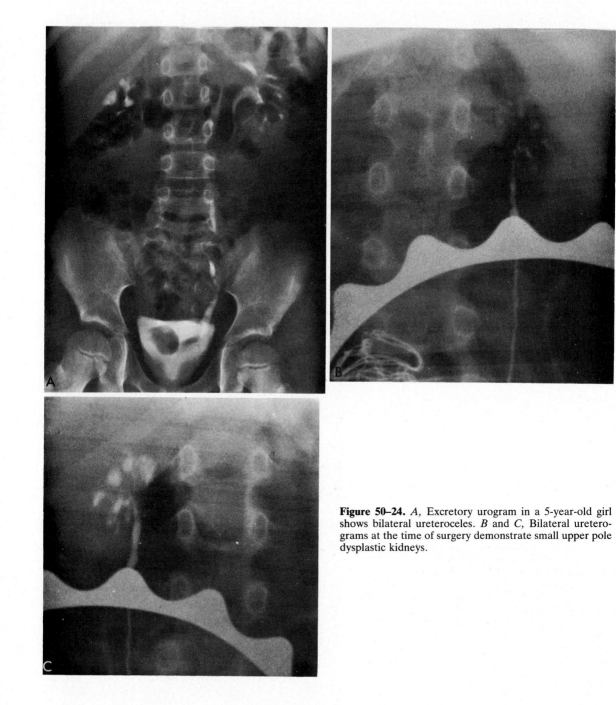

Figure 50–24. *A,* Excretory urogram in a 5-year-old girl shows bilateral ureteroceles. *B* and *C,* Bilateral ureterograms at the time of surgery demonstrate small upper pole dysplastic kidneys.

of ureteral reimplantation is best used in this situation to keep the ureter away from the area of detrusor repair and to prevent postoperative reflux. This entire dissection can often be tedious and time-consuming. The trigonal musculature is reapproximated to reconstitute a strong bladder wall before the reimplantation is completed.

In a few children with massive lower pole ureteral reflux and nonvisualization of both upper and lower renal segments, excision of the ureterocele and complete nephroureterectomy are indicated.

When the upper renal segment demonstrates reasonable function on the basis of an IVP or radionuclide scan, consideration should be given to preserving this portion of the kidney. If the upper pole ureter is not greatly dilated, excision of the ureterocele and common sheath reimplantation should be considered, especially if significant lower pole reflux is present (Fig. 50–23). In the absence of severe lower pole reflux and in the presence of a marked discrepancy between the size of the duplicate ureters, the procedure of choice is ureteroureterostomy or pyeloureterostomy and partial ureterectomy.

In some instances, an ectopic ureterocele drains a tiny, almost atretic ureter attached to a small dysplastic renal segment (Fig. 50–24) (Bauer and Retik, 1978). Ipsilateral lower pole reflux frequently accompanies these findings. In this situation too, excision or uncapping of the ureterocele combined with common sheath reimplantation of both ureters has been employed. In my experience, subsequent heminephrectomy because of infection or hypertension has not been necessary, although the renal unit left behind is dysplastic and nonvisualizing. This approach avoids additional surgery at the kidney level and takes care of the more important problem—i.e., ipsilateral lower pole reflux.

References

Aas, T. N.: Ureterocele: A clinical study of 68 cases in 52 adults. Br. J. Urol., 32:133, 1960.

Abeshouse, B. S.: Ureteral ectopia: Report of a rare case of ectopic ureter opening in the uterus and a review of the literature. Urol. Cutan. Rev., 47:447, 1943.

Ahmed, S.: Ureteral duplication with ectopic ureterocele: Report of a case presenting with peritonitis. J. Urol., 106:287, 1971.

Alfert, H. J., and Gillenwater, J. Y.: Ectopic vas deferens communicating with lower ureter: Embryological considerations. J. Urol., 108:172, 1972.

Amar, A. D.: The management of urinary calculus disease in patients with duplicated ureters. Br. J. Urol., 44:541, 1972.

Amar, A. D.: Lateral ureteral displacement: Sign of nonvisualized duplication. J. Urol., 105:638, 1971a.

Amar, A. D.: Simple ureterocele at the distal end of a blind-ending ureter. J. Urol., 106:423, 1971b.

Amar, A. D.: Ureteropyelostomy for relief of single ureteral obstruction in cases of ureteral duplication. Arch. Surg., 101:379, 1970.

Anhalt, M. A., and Guthrie, T. H.: Management of ectopic ureterocele. J. Urol., 107:856, 1972.

Arey, L. B.: Developmental Anatomy: A Textbook and Laboratory Manual of Embryology. 7th ed. Philadelphia, W. B. Saunders Co., 1974.

Asaad, E. I., Badawi, Z. H., and Gaballah, M. F.: Nature and fate of the ureteric membrane closing the primitive ureterovesical opening. Acta Anat., 92:524, 1975.

Barrett, D. M., Malek, R. S., and Kelalis, P. P.: Problems and solutions in surgical treatment of 100 consecutive ureteral duplications in children. J. Urol., 114:126, 1975.

Bauchard, J.: Un cas de trifidite urétérale bilaterale avec volumineuse hydronephrose. J. Urol. Nephrol. (Paris), 65:476, 1959.

Bauer, S. B., and Retik, A. B.: The nonobstructive ectopic ureterocele. J. Urol., 119:804, 1978.

Beck, A. D.: The effect of intrauterine urinary obstruction upon the development of the fetal kidney. J. Urol., 105:784, 1971.

Belman, A. B., Filmer, R. B., and King, L. R.: Surgical management of duplication of the collecting system. J. Urol., 112:316, 1974.

Bengmark, S., Nilsson, S., and Romanus, R.: Ectopic ureter draining into a seminal megavesicle causing defecation troubles. Report of a case and review of the literature. Acta Chir. Scand., 123:471, 1962.

Berdon, W. E., Levitt, S. B., Baker, D. H., Becker, J. A., and Uson, A. C.: Ectopic ureterocele. Radiol. Clin. North Am., 6:205, 1968.

Boatwright, D. C.: Ureterocele: Surgical treatment. J. Urol., 106:48, 1971.

Boijsen, E.: Angiographic studies of the anatomy of single and multiple renal arteries. Acta Radiol. (Suppl.), 183:1, 1959.

Brannan, W., and Hector, H. H.: Ureteral ectopia: Report of 39 cases. J. Urol., 109:192, 1973.

Burford, C. E., Glen, J. E., and Burford, E. H.: Ureteral ectopia: Review of literature and two case reports. J. Urol., 62:211, 1949.

Campbell, M.: Ureterocele: A study of 94 instances in 80 infants and children. Sur. Gynecol. Obstet., 93:705, 1951a.

Campbell, M. F.: Clinical Pediatric Urology. Philadelphia, W. B. Saunders Co., 1951b.

Campbell, M.: Ureterocele. J. Urol., 45:598, 1941.

Campbell, M.: Ectopic ureteral orifice. Surg. Gynecol. Obstet., 64:22, 1937.

Cendron, J., and Bonhomme, C.: 31 cas d'uretère à abouchement ectopique sous-sphinctérien chez l'enfant du sexe feminin. J. Urol. Nephrol. (Paris), 74:1, 1968a.

Cendron, J., and Bonhomme, C.: Uretère à terminaison ectopique extravésicale chez des sujets de sexe masculin (à propos de 10 cas). J. Urol. Nephrol. (Paris), 74:31, 1968b.

Chidlow, J. H., and Utz, D. C.: Ureteral ectopia in vestibule of vagina with urinary continence. South. Med. J., 63:423, 1970.

Chwalle, R.: The process of formation of cystic dilatations of the vesical end of the ureter and of diverticula at the ureteral ostium. Urol. Cutan. Rev., 31:499, 1927.

Cibert, J., Cibert, J., Gilloz, A., et al.: Triplicite ureterale. J. Urol. Nephrol. (Paris), 71:429, 1965.

Clark, C. W., and Leadbetter, G.: General treatment, mistreatment and complications of ureteroceles. J. Urol., 106:518, 1971.

Constantian, H. M.: Ureteral ectopia, hydrocolpos, and uterus didelphys. JAMA, *197*:54, 1966.

Cox, C. E., and Hutch, J. A.: Bilateral single ectopic ureter: A report of two cases and review of the literature. J. Urol., *95*:493, 1966.

Cukier, J.: Un cas rare d'ectopie urethrale des deux ureteres chez la fille. J. Urol. Nephrol. (Paris), *69*:317, 1963.

Culp, O. S.: Heminephro-ureterectomy: Comparison of one-stage and two-stage operations. J. Urol., *83*:369, 1960.

Cussen, L. J.: The structure of the human ureter in infancy and childhood. Invest. Urol., *5*:179, 1967.

DeWeerd, J. H., and Feeney, D. P.: Bilateral ureteral ectopia with urinary incontinence in a mother and daughter. J. Urol., *98*:335, 1967.

DeWeerd, J. H., and Litin, R. B.: Ectopia of ureteral orifice (vestibular) without incontinence: Report of case. Proc. Staff Meet. Mayo Clin., *33*:81, 1958.

DeWeerd, J. H., Farsund, T., and Burke, E. C.: Ureteroneocystostomy. J. Urol., *101*:520, 1969.

Diaz-Ball, F. L., Finak, A., Moore, C. A., et al.: Pyeloureterostomy and ureteroureterostomy: Alternative procedures to partial nephrectomy for duplication of the ureter with only one pathological segment. J. Urol., *102*:621, 1969.

Dorst, J. B., Cussen, G. H., and Silverman, F. M.: Ureteroceles in children, with emphasis on the frequency of ectopic ureteroceles. Radiology, *74*:88, 1960.

Ellerker, A. G.: The extravesical ectopic ureter. Br. J. Surg., *45*:344, 1957.

Emery, J. G., and Gill, G.: A classification and quantitative histological study of abnormal ureters in children. Br. J. Urol., *46*:69, 1974.

Eneren, M. B.: Absence de la vessie et abouchement direct des deux uretères dans l'urètre postérieur. J. Urol. Nephrol. (Paris), *48*:150, 1939.

Ericsson, N. O.: Ectopic ureterocele in infants and children: A clinical study. Acta Chir. Scand. (Suppl.), *197*:1, 1954.

Friedland, G. W., and Cunningham, J.: The elusive ectopic ureterocele. Am. J. Roentgenol., *116*:792, 1970.

Gibson, T. E.: A new operation of ureteral ectopia: Case report. J. Urol., *77*:414, 1957.

Gill, R. D.: Triplication of the ureter and renal pelvis. J. Urol., *68*:140, 1952.

Gilmore, O. J.: Unilateral triplication of the ureter. Br. J. Urol., *46*:588, 1974.

Glenn, J. F.: Agenesis of the bladder. JAMA, *169*:2016, 1959.

Gordon, H. L.: Ectopic ureter entering the seminal vesicle associated with renal dysplasia. J. Urol., *108*:389, 1972.

Gray, S. W., and Skandalakis, J. E.: Embryology for Surgeons. Philadelphia, W. B. Saunders Co., 1972.

Green, L. F.: Ureteral ectopy in females. Clin. Obstet. Gynecol., *10*:147, 1967.

Greene, L. F., and Ferris, D. O.: Urinary incontinence due to bilateral ectopic ureters. Surg. Gynecol. Obstet., *82*:712, 1946.

Gross, R. E.: The Surgery of Infancy and Childhood. Philadelphia, W. B. Saunders Co., 1953.

Gross, R. E., and Clatworthy, H. W., Jr.: Ureterocele in infancy and childhood. Pediatrics, *5*:68, 1950.

Grossman, H., Winchester, P. H., and Muecke, E. C.: Solitary ectopic ureter. Radiology, *89*:1069, 1967.

Gunther, R. E., Harer, W. B., and Welebir, R.: Ectopic ureter presenting as a tubo-ovarian abscess: Report of a case. Obstet. Gynecol., *25*:259, 1965.

Hamilton, W. J., Boyd, J. D., and Mossman, H. W.: Human Embryology. Baltimore, The Williams & Wilkins Co., 1962.

Hartman, G. W., and Hodson, C. J.: The duplex kidney and related abnormalities. Clin. Radiol., *20*:387, 1969.

Hendren, W. H., and Monfort, G. J.: Surgical correction of ureteroceles in childhood. J. Pediatr. Surg., *6*:235, 1971.

Hutch, J. A., and Chisholm, E. R.: Surgical repair of ureterocele. J. Urol., *96*:445, 1966.

Hutton, I. M., and Green, N. A.: High dose delayed urogram in the detection of the occult ectopic ureter. Br. J. Urol., *46*:289, 1974.

Johnson, D. K., and Perlmutter, A. D.: Single system ectopic ureteroceles with anomalies of the heart, testis and vas deferens. J. Urol., *123*:81, 1980.

Johnston, J. H.: Urinary tract duplication in childhood. Arch. Dis. Child., *36*:180, 1961.

Johnston, J. H., and Davenport, T. J.: The single ectopic ureter. Br. J. Urol., *41*:428, 1969.

Johnston, J. H., and Johnson, L. M.: Experiences with ectopic ureteroceles. Br. J. Urol., *41*:61, 1969.

Katzen, P., and Trachtman, B.: Diagnosis of vaginal ectopic ureter by vaginogram. J. Urol., *72*:808, 1954.

Kelalis, P. P.: Ureterocele. Clin. Obstet. Gynecol., *10*:155, 1967.

Kjellberg, S. E., Ericsson, N. E., and Rudhe, U.: The Lower Urinary Tract in Childhood: Some Correlated Clinical and Roentgenologic Observations. Chicago, Year Book Medical Publishers, 1968.

Kroovand, L. R., and Perlmutter, A. D.: A one-stage surgical approach to ectopic ureterocele. J. Urol., *122*:367, 1979.

Leadbetter, G. W., Jr.: Ectopic ureterocele as a cause of urinary incontinence. J. Urol., *103*:222, 1970.

Leef, G. S., and Leader, S. A.: Ectopic ureter opening into the rectum: A case report. J. Urol., *87*:338, 1962.

Limbert, D. J.: Hypoplastic right kidney with ectopic nonduplicated ureter. Urology, *6*:354, 1975.

Livaditis, A., Maurseth, K., and Skog, P. A.: Unilateral triplication of the ureter and renal pelvis: Report of a case. Acta Chir. Scand., *127*:181, 1964.

Lundin, E., and Riggs, W.: Upper urinary tract duplication associated with ectopic ureterocele in childhood and infancy. Acta Radiol. (Diagn.), *7*:13, 1968.

MacKelvie, A. A.: Triplicate ureter: Case report. Br. J. Urol., *27*:124, 1955.

Mackie, G. G., and Stephens, F. D.: Duplex kidneys: A correlation of renal dysplasia with position of the ureteral orifice. J. Urol., *114*:274, 1975.

Mackie, G. G., Awang, H., and Stephen, F. D.: The ureteric orifice: The embryologic key to radiologic status of duplex kidneys. J. Pediatr. Surg., *10*:473, 1975.

Malek, R. S., Kelalis, P. P., Burke, E. C., et al.: Simple and ectopic ureterocele in infancy and childhood. Surg. Gynecol. Obstet., *134*:611, 1972.

Malek, R. S., Kelalis, P. P., Stickler, G. B., et al.: Observations on ureteral ectopy in children. J. Urol., *107*:308, 1972.

Mandell, J., Bauer, S. B., Colodny, A. H., Lebowitz, R. L., and Retik, A. B.: Ureteral ectopia in infants and children. J. Urol., *126*:219, 1981.

Mandell, J., Colodny, A. H., Lebowitz, R. L., Bauer, S. B., and Retik, A. B.: Ureteroceles in infants and children. J. Urol., *123*:921, 1980.

McCall, I. W., Atkinson, D. O., and Moule, N. J.: Multiple ureteral diverticula associated with bilateral ureteroceles. Br. J. Urol., *47*:538, 1975.

McGovern, J. G., and Marshall, V. F.: Reimplantation of ureters into the bladders of children. J. Urol., *99*:572, 1968.

McKay, R. W., and Baird, H. H.: Bilateral single ureteral

ectopia terminating in the urethra. J. Urol., *63*:1013, 1950.

Mertz, H. O., Hendricks, J. W., and Garrett, R. A.: Cystic ureterovesical protrusion: Report of four cases in children and two in adults. Trans. Am. Assoc. Genitourin. Surg., *40*:180, 1948.

Michelson, L.: Congenital anomalies of the ductus deferens and epididymis. J. Urol., *61*:384, 1949.

Mogg, R. A.: The single ectopic ureter. Br. J. Urol., *46*:3, 1974.

Mogg, R. A.: Some observations on the ectopic ureter and ureterocele. J. Urol., *97*:1003, 1967.

Musselman, B. C., and Barry, J.: Varying degrees of ureteral ectopia and duplication in five siblings. J. Urol., *110*:476, 1973.

Nash, A. G., and Knight, M.: Ureterocele calculi, Br. J. Urol., *45*:404, 1973.

Paquin, A. J., Jr.: Considerations for the management of some complex problems for ureterovesical anastomosis. Surg. Gynecol. Obstet., *118*:75, 1964.

Parsons, C. A., and Malpass, C. P.: Demonstration of simple ureterocele prolapsing into the urethra of an adult male. Br. J. Surg., *60*:501, 1973.

Pearson, H. H.: Results of pyeloureterostomy for bifid ureters (abstract). Br. J. Urol., *40*:483, 1968.

Perkins, P. J., Kroovand, R. L., and Evans, A. T.: Ureteral triplication. Radiology, *108*:533, 1973.

Perrin, E. V., Persky, L., Tucker, A., et al.: Renal duplication and dysplasia. Urology, *4*:660, 1974.

Politano, V. A., and Leadbetter, W. F.: An operative technique for the correction of vesicoureteral reflux. J. Urol., *79*:932, 1958.

Prewett, J. H., Jr., and Lebowitz, R. L.: The single ectopic ureter. Am. J. Roentgenol., *127*:941, 1976.

Riba, L. W., Schmidlapp, C. J., and Bosworth, N. L.: Ectopic ureter draining into the seminal vesicle. J. Urol., *56*:332, 1946.

Redman, J. F.: Unsuspected duplex ureters. Urology, *5*:196, 1975.

Royle, M. G., and Goodwin, W. E.: The management of ureteroceles. J. Urol., *106*:42, 1971.

Sandegard, E.: The treatment of ureteral ectopia. Acta Chir. Scand., *115*:149, 1958.

Schnitzer, B.: Ectopic ureteral opening into seminal vesicle. A report of four cases. J. Urol., *93*:576, 1965.

Scott, R.: Triplication of the ureter. Br. J. Urol., *42*:150, 1970.

Seitzman, D. M., and Patton, J. F.: Ureteral ectopia: Combined ureteral and vas deferens anomaly. J. Urol., *84*:604, 1960.

Shappley, N., and Keeton, J.: Unusual presentation of cecoureterocele. Urology, *6*:605, 1975.

Shaw, R. E.: Ureterocele. Br. J. Surg., *60*:337, 1973.

Sherwood, T., and Stevenson, J. J.: Ureteroceles in disguise. Br. J. Radiol., *42*:899, 1969.

Simms, M. H., and Higgins, P. M.: Diagnosis of the occult ectopic ureter in a duplex kidney. J. Urol., *114*:697, 1975.

Spangler, E. B.: Complete triplication of the ureter. Radiology, *80*:795, 1963.

Srivastava, H. C.: Bilateral termination of the ureter in the uterine tube. Indian J. Med. Sci., *22*:37, 1968.

Stephens, D.: Caecoureterocele and concepts on the embryology and aetiology of ureteroceles. Aust. N. Z. J. Surg., *40*:239, 1971.

Stephens, F. D.: Intramural ureter and ureterocele. Postgrad. Med. J., *40*:179, 1964.

Stephens, F. D.: Congenital Malformations of the Rectum, Anus and Genitourinary Tract. Edinburgh, E. and S. Livingstone, 1963.

Stephens, F. D.: Ureterocele in infants and children. Aust. N. Z. J. Surg., *27*:288, 1958.

Subbiah, N., and Stephens, D.: Stenotic ureterocele. Aust. N. Z. J. Surg., *41*:257, 1972.

Swenson, O., and Ratner, I. A.: Pyeloureterostomy for treatment of symptomatic ureteral duplications in children. J. Urol., *88*:184, 1962.

Tanagho, E. A.: Ureteroceles: Embryogenesis, pathogenesis and management. Urology, *18*:13, 1979.

Tanagho, E. A.: Embryologic basis for lower ureteral anomalies: A hypothesis. Urology, *7*:451, 1976.

Tanagho, E. A.: Anatomy and management of ureteroceles. J. Urol., *107*:729, 1972.

Tanagho, E. A.: Surgically induced partial urinary obstruction in the fetal lamb. III. Ureteral obstruction. Invest. Urol., *10*:34, 1972.

Thompson, G. J., and Greene, L. F.: Ureterocele: A clinical study and a report of thirty-seven cases. J. Urol., *47*:800, 1942.

Thompson, G. J., and Kelalis, P. P.: Ureterocele: Clinical appraisal of 176 cases. J. Urol., *91*:488, 1964.

Timothy, R. P., Decter, A., and Perlmutter, A.: Ureteral duplication: Clinical findings and therapy in 46 children. J. Urol., *105*:445, 1971.

Uson, A. C., and Schulman, C. C.: Ectopic ureter emptying into the rectum: Report of a case. J. Urol., *108*:156, 1950.

Uson, A. C., Lattimer, J. K., and Melicow, M. M.: Ureteroceles in infants and children. A report based on 44 cases. Pediatrics, *27*:971, 1961.

Uson, A. C., Womack, C. E., and Berdon, W. E.: Giant ectopic ureter presenting as an abdominal mass in a newborn infant. J. Pediatr., *80*:473, 1972.

Vanhoutte, J. J.: Ureteral ectopia into a wolffian duct remnant (Gartner's ducts or cysts) presenting as a urethral diverticulum in two girls. Am. J. Roentgenol. Radium Ther. Nucl. Med., *110*:540, 1970.

Weiss, J. M., and Dykhuizen, R. F.: An anomalous vaginal insertion into the bladder: A case report. J. Urol., *98*:610, 1967.

Weiss, R. M., and Spackman, T. J.: Everting ectopic ureteroceles. J. Urol., *111*:538, 1974.

Wigglshoff, C. C., and Kiefer, J. H.: Ureteral ectopia: Diagnostic difficulties. J. Urol., *96*:671, 1966.

Williams, D. I.: Paediatric Urology. London, Butterworth & Co. Ltd., 1968.

Williams, D. I.: Ectopic ureterocele. Proc. R. Soc. Med., *51*:783, 1958.

Williams, D. I.: The ectopic ureter: Diagnostic problems. Br. J. Urol., *26*:253, 1954.

Williams, D. I., and Lightwood, R. G.: Bilateral single ectopic ureters. Br. J. Urol., *44*:267, 1972.

Williams, D. I., and Lillie, J. G.: The functional radiology of ectopic ureterocele. Br. J. Urol., *44*:417, 1972.

Williams, D. I., and Royle, M.: Ectopic ureter in the male child. Br. J. Urol., *41*:421, 1969.

Williams, D. I., and Woodard, J. R.: Problems in the management of ectopic ureteroceles. J. Urol. *92*:635, 1964.

Willmarth, C. L.: Ectopic ureteral orifice within a urethral diverticulum: Report of a case. J. Urol., *59*:47, 1948.

Wines, R. D., and O'Flynn, J. D.: Transurethral treatment of ureteroceles. Br. J. Urol., *44*:207, 1972.

Woodruff, S. R.: Complete unilateral triplication of the ureter and renal pelvis. J. Urol., *46*:376, 1941.

Zielinski, J.: Avoidance of vesicoureteral reflux after transurethral ureteral meatotomy for ureterocele. J. Urol., *88*:386, 1962.

CHAPTER 51

Temporary Urinary Diversion in Infants and Young Children

ALAN B. RETIK, M.D.
ALAN D. PERLMUTTER, M.D.

In recent years, considerable emphasis has been placed on reconstructive surgery of the urinary tract, especially in the pediatric age group (Hendren, 1970, 1972, 1974). Urinary diversion is now less frequently mentioned as a method of management for many conditions in which it had previously been used. However, situations remain for which diversion of urine is indicated on a temporary basis, and there are even occasions when the urinary tract must be diverted permanently. In this chapter, a variety of temporary diversionary procedures will be discussed that seem appropriate to infants and children. Permanent urinary diversion and undiversion are discussed in other chapters.

The management of the severely decompensated upper urinary tract in the infant or child still evokes considerable controversy. Because of recent advances in the medical management of the critically ill infant, improved pediatric anesthesia, and more experience in the surgical techniques of remodeling ureters, primary reconstruction of the disordered urinary tract has been advocated and is being performed successfully in a number of centers. However, temporary urinary diversion in the infant with severe hydronephrosis and hydroureter should still be carefully considered and may be desirable in specific patients, primarily in the severely ill neonate with sepsis and uremia.

This chapter will describe the various types of intubated and nonintubated forms of temporary urinary diversion used in infants and children and will discuss the indications, merits, and disadvantages of each. In general, intubated diversions in the pediatric age group should be used infrequently and for short periods of time because of the hazards and complications of indwelling catheters in children. Therefore, we feel that any form of intubation during childhood, and especially during infancy, obligates the surgeon to develop a plan of management and rehabilitation that includes a specific limitation on the planned duration of tube drainage.

INTUBATED PROCEDURES FOR URINARY DIVERSION

Urethral Catheter

A urethral catheter is the simplest form of intubated diversion. It should be employed for only short periods of time, especially in the infant or young child. We use this catheter primarily in the infant who has lower urinary tract obstruction with azotemia in order to allow renal function to improve and stabilize prior to definitive surgery. It is safest to use a soft No. 5 or No. 8 F. infant feeding tube taped to the penile shaft. In the older child, a balloon catheter can be used, but the retention balloon may increase vesical irritability and spasm. Although successful long-term management of children with urinary tract obstruction by indwelling urethral catheter has been reported (Conger and Toub, 1960), the catheter is often uncomfortable and poorly tolerated. As complications of long-term catheter drainage include urinary tract infections, calculi, urethritis, and stricture formation, we emphasize that the period of drainage should generally be a matter of days rather than weeks.

Percutaneous Cystostomy

This procedure has been used with increasing frequency following the advent of reliable disposable kits. For all practical purposes, trocar or percutaneous cystostomy should replace the formal suprapubic cystostomy as a method of short-term tube diversion. It is particularly useful as a method of diversion for hypospadias repairs, in infants with large, distended bladders (in preference to a urethral catheter), and in children with urethral stricture or severe urethral inflammatory disease.

Either a straight or a balloon type catheter may be used, preferably of Silastic or plastic. It is important that the bladder be distended at the time of cystotomy. If a straight catheter is used, it is advisable not to thread too much catheter into the bladder to avoid severe bladder spasm from trigonal irritation.

Suprapubic Cystostomy

This procedure is now used infrequently in children and has been largely replaced by trocar or percutaneous cystostomy. It is now most useful for short-term diversion in the previously operated bladder. Suprapubic cystostomy is contraindicated for infants and children with severe hydronephrosis and hydroureter with poor ureteral emptying. After open cystostomy, the bladder will often contract down on the foreign body and actually cause increasing ureterovesical obstruction (Raper, 1953). This procedure also has inherent problems of urinary tract infection and stone formation if used for more than a few weeks.

After open cystostomy, prolonged intubation may result in contracture and fibrosis of the anterior bladder wall and mobilized anterior perivesical tissues, especially in infancy. This can be compounded by chronic infection. Cystostomy also may be useful, of course, for short-term drainage in association with definitive corrective intravesical procedures.

TECHNIQUE OF SUPRAPUBIC CYSTOSTOMY
(Fig. 51–1)

Through a small transverse incision two fingerbreadths above the symphysis pubis (or higher when the bladder is tense), the anterior rectus fascia is divided transversely. The fascia is then undermined superiorly and inferiorly, and the rectus muscle is divided or retracted in the midline, exposing the bladder. Because the bladder rises well out of the pelvis in children and because tissue layers are thin, a minimal incision is required. The peritoneum is reflected superiorly, and the bladder is opened between stay sutures. The appropriate-sized catheter is then placed in the *dome*. We usually employ a Malecot catheter. The bladder is then closed in layers, using chromic catgut. The catheter is brought out through a stab wound superior to the skin incision or directly through the skin incision, if the incision is small and the tip of the tube remains well above the trigone. The muscle and fascial layers are closed with interrupted and running chromic catgut, and the subcutaneous tissues are reapproximated with fine plain catgut. After the skin is closed, the suprapubic catheter is sewn in place and secured with tape.

Percutaneous Nephrostomy

Percutaneous nephrostomy was introduced in 1955 by Goodwin et al. and has been used with increasing frequency (Fowler et al., 1975; Ogg et al., 1969). In the pediatric age group, it is most often employed in place of a formal nephrostomy to promote immediate drainage of an acutely obstructed kidney. We also employ this technique to drain a kidney with marginal function, in an effort to determine whether reconstructive surgery rather than nephrectomy will be indicated. Percutaneous nephrostomy also allows antegrade pyelography as well as physiologic testing of intraluminal pressures, including perfusion study, i.e., the Whitaker test (Whitaker, 1973), to determine pressure-flow relationships across ureteropelvic and ureterovesical junctions that are questionably obstructed.

In our experience, percutaneous nephrostomy has largely replaced open nephrostomy, and the tubes used may be left in for several months.

TECHNIQUES OF PERCUTANEOUS NEPHROSTOMY

There are a number of techniques for percutaneous nephrostomy. In general, the procedure can be done under local anesthesia in the x-ray department, using fluoroscopy as a guide or employing ultrasonography to localize the position and size of the renal pelvis.

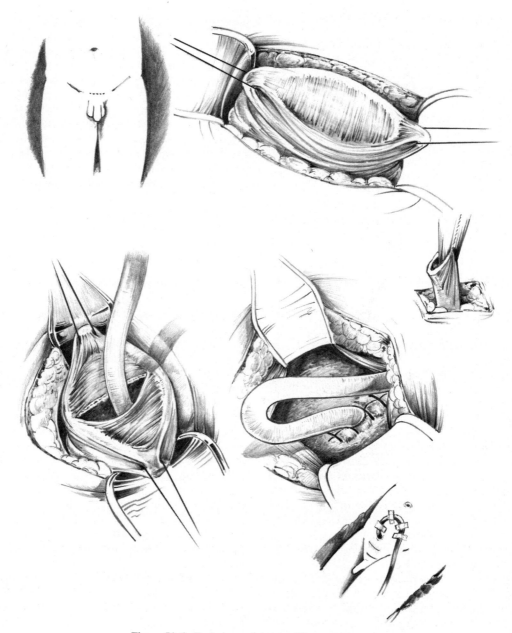

Figure 51–1. Technique of suprapubic cystostomy.

For a giant hydronephrosis, the disposable No. 8 F trocar cystostomy kit is suitable. However, the long length of the trocar blade (1 cm) projecting beyond the sheath makes it dangerous for use in a moderate hydronephrosis, as the far wall is easily punctured and other viscera injured.

Alternative approaches include use of a short-bevel, thin-bore, 13-gauge needle through which a Silastic tube or plastic feeding tube will pass; use of an 18-gauge cardiac needle with a Teflon sheath; or use of angiographic wire and tubing. With the various techniques, it is often possible to coil some extra catheter in the renal pelvis (except for the Teflon, which is too stiff).

Open Nephrostomy

Open nephrostomy placement is useful on rare occasions and for short periods of time when tubeless diversion is contraindicated for technical reasons or when renal biopsy is indicated in questionably salvageable kidneys. It is difficult to keep the tube in place for longer than 2 to 3 weeks in an infant. The tube is readily dislodged and oftentimes may be difficult to replace. Leakage around the tube may be bothersome, and chronic bacilluria usually occurs eventually and is difficult to eradicate. Other complications of nephrostomy have included calculus formation and obstruction at the ureteropelvic junction. Although in the past some authors have treated infants and children with advanced hydronephrosis and hydroureter from posterior urethral valves by initial open nephrostomy drainage, we have avoided this approach. We prefer other forms of management, such as those presented in Chapter 48, or those utilizing tubeless forms of diversion on the rare occasions when this is necessary. Experiences with nephrostomy diversion in children are reported in several series (McGovern, 1972; Parker and Perlmutter, 1969; Rattner et al., 1963; Rickham, 1962; Waldbaum and Marshall, 1970; Williams and Eckstein, 1965; Wosnitzer and Lattimer, 1960).

TECHNIQUE OF OPEN NEPHROSTOMY
(Fig. 51–2)

With the patient in the lateral decubitus position, a standard flank incision is made. The kidney is partially mobilized, exposing the renal pelvis. A short radial pyelotomy incision is made, and a right angle or Kelly clamp is passed into a dilated lower calyx until it can be felt on the lateral border of the kidney. The clamp is then incised upon, and a heavy silk suture or tape is grasped by the clamp and withdrawn into the pelvis (King and Belman, 1972). The suture is tied to the beveled end of a Malecot catheter and is then used to guide the catheter through the nephrotomy. A flexible catheter guide can be used to flatten and narrow the retainer on the catheter. In this manner, a smaller opening is made in the kidney, resulting in less renal damage and better hemostasis. The pyelotomy incision is then reapproximated with fine chromic catgut. The nephrostomy tube and a small Penrose drain are brought out through the wound or through a separate stab wound, and the wound is closed in layers with catgut. When the collecting system is very large and the parenchyma is thin, the tube can be placed directly into the collecting system without the need to mobilize and open the pelvis.

Loop Nephrostomy

This procedure (Fig. 51–3) is most applicable for very long-term diversion. It was initially advocated by Comarr (1966) for use in patients with spinal cord injuries. Loop nephrostomy has little or no use in children. Upper and lower pole nephrotomies are usually made to provide a gentle curve and to avoid kinking. It is preferable to use Silastic tubing with three or four large holes in the portion of tubing that lies within the renal pelvis. Both limbs of the tubing are then attached to a Y-connector (Binder et al., 1971; Bissada et al., 1973; Weyrauch and Rous, 1967).

Ureterostomy In Situ

Diversion of the unmobilized ureter has rarely been employed in children. We have used this procedure on occasion to divert the acutely obstructed ureter following reimplantation. When the obstruction is sudden and severe, the collecting system may dilate only minimally, making percutaneous nephrostomy hazardous and open nephrostomy difficult. Ureterostomy in situ is a rapid and simple procedure and can be performed bilaterally, if needed, with the child in the supine position (Pokorny et al., 1976).

Ureterostomy in situ has also been advocated in adults with distal ureteral obstruction, usually secondary to tumor. The dilated ureter is exposed from the retroperitoneal approach through a small incision above the anterior

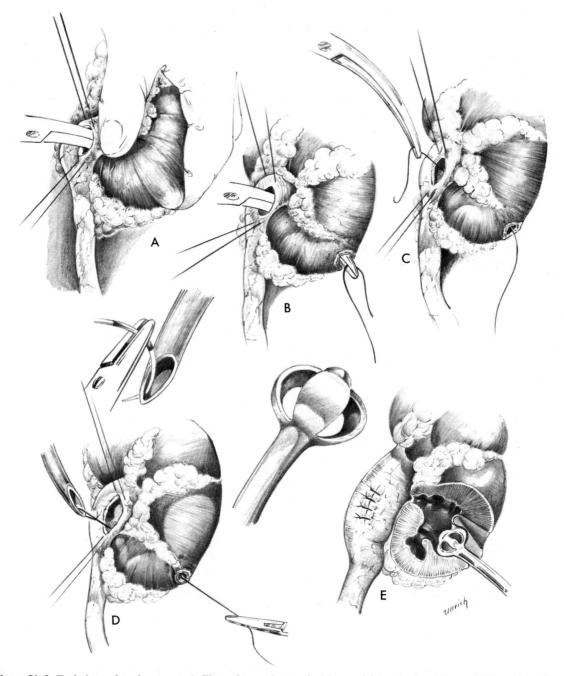

Figure 51–2. Technique of nephrostomy. *A,* Through a pyelotomy incision, a right angle clamp is passed through a dilated lower calyx. *B,* The clamp is then incised upon and a heavy silk suture is *(C)* grasped and drawn into the pelvis. *D,* The suture is tied to the beveled end of a Malecot catheter and *(E)* used to guide the catheter through the nephrotomy.

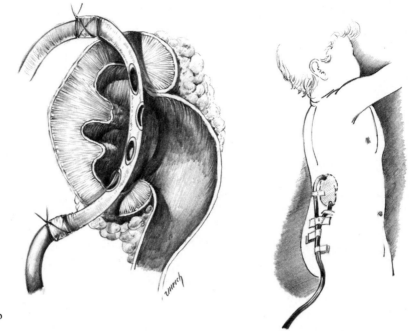

Figure 51–3. Technique of loop
nephrostomy.

superior iliac spine. A segment of ureter is
identified, and a fine Silastic or plastic catheter
is threaded into the pelvis through a small
ureterotomy. The catheter is sutured in place to
the ureter with chromic catgut and is brought
out through a distal stab wound and secured at
the skin level. Once a tract forms, the catheter
may be changed at regular intervals (Walsh,
1974). It is best to use an open-ended catheter
so that a small-caliber ureteral catheter or flexible wire can be inserted as a guide for tube
change.

NONINTUBATED PROCEDURES
FOR URINARY DIVERSION

Temporary tubeless methods of urinary diversion are particularly applicable to infants and
young children who are in diapers. Nonintubated diversions provide maximal decompression of the urinary tract, allowing for optimal
renal function, renal growth, and the unhurried
reassessment of the entire urinary tract, both
radiologically and physiologically, at any later
date. Stomal care and symptomatic urinary tract
infections have, in general, not been problems.
Appliances are not needed in these diaper-aged
infants, and the peristomal skin rarely becomes
inflamed. Diapers have to be changed somewhat
more frequently than ordinarily and have to be
worn at a suitably higher level with renal pelvis
or high ureteral diversions.

Cutaneous Vesicostomy

Blocksom (1957) and Lapides et al. (1960)
popularized tubeless drainage of the bladder.
We regard vesicostomy as a temporary tubeless
method of diversion to be considered in the
infant with chronic bladder distention, especially
when the cause is uncertain. This procedure is
ideally suited to the male infant with neurogenic
bladder dysfunction who has significant hydronephrosis and hydroureter with a large bladder
that fails to empty completely. It is also suitable
for the premature neonate with posterior urethral valves and an extremely narrow urethra in
whom transurethral fulguration of the valves
would not be feasible. We would emphasize that
this diversion is temporary and that when the
true status of bladder function, renal function,
and growth of the child is ascertained, some
type of reconstructive surgery or permanent
diversion may be necessary or desirable. Obviously, this procedure is inappropriate for a
baby with supravesical obstruction. Vesicostomy
is also a reasonable alternative to an upper
urinary tract diversion if ureteral emptying improves after a brief period of drainage by use
of an indwelling urethral catheter.

Vesicostomy has also been advocated as a permanent method of urinary diversion. However, complications over a long period of time have made many urologists unwilling to use this technique. These complications include poor vesical emptying with a significant residual urine, chronic bacilluria, calculus formation, and difficulty in fitting a stomal appliance to the suprapubic region (Ireland and Geist, 1970). A number of authors have reported their experiences with vesicostomy in children (Beland and Weiss, 1965; Bell et al., 1968; Belman and King, 1973; Carlson, 1960; Duckett, 1974; Karafin and Kendall, 1966; Mandell et al., 1981).

TECHNIQUE OF VESICOSTOMY (Fig. 51–4)

We perform a modified Blocksom procedure by making a 2-cm transverse incision halfway between the symphysis pubis and the umbilicus. A transverse incision is made in the rectus fascia; a small triangle of rectus fascia can be excised. The rectus muscles are then divided for 2 cm in the midline, exposing the bladder. With the aid of traction sutures, the bladder is mobilized superiorly, and the peritoneum is peeled off the dome. The dome is then mobilized well out into the incision. Next, the wall of the bladder is sutured to the fascia with the interrupted chromic catgut, and the bladder dome is incised. The edges of the bladder are then sutured to the skin with interrupted chromic catgut or Dexon. To avoid prolapse, it is important to exteriorize the dome rather than the anterior wall of the bladder. Principal complications of this technique have been prolapse and stomal stenosis; revision of the stoma is sometimes necessary.

Vesicostomy may be technically difficult in patients with a very small, thick-walled bladder. Perlmutter has also used a very small 1.5 to 2.0 cm diameter U-flap based inferiorly, midway between the umbilicus and symphysis pubis in neonates, to the bladder dome and has not had to use a counter-incision.

CLOSURE OF VESICOSTOMY

Closure of vesicostomy is simple and is usually performed following definitive treatment of the condition causing urinary retention (e.g., fulguration of posterior urethral valves) or in conjunction with a program of intermittent catheterization in the child with neurogenic bladder dysfunction. The metaplastic mucosa is excised, and the bladder is closed in layers, as are the fascia and skin. The bladder should be drained with a urethral catheter or a suprapubic tube for approximately 1 week.

RESULTS OF VESICOSTOMY

In the series by Mandell et al. (1981), cutaneous vesicostomy was performed on ten infants with severe bilateral dilatation of the upper urinary tract. The etiology of the upper urinary tract dilatation was neurogenic bladder dysfunction secondary to myelodysplasia in eight, and severe vesicoureteral reflux and urinary sepsis in two. The vesicostomy resulted in marked improvement in the drainage and appearance of the upper urinary tract in each child (Fig. 51–5). When other methods of managing the underlying lower urinary tract dysfunction were deemed more appropriate, the vesicostomy was closed. Cutaneous vesicostomy proved to be an effective, simple, and easily reversible means of treating selected infants with lower urinary tract dysfunction.

The Lapides Technique of Vesicostomy (Fig. 51–6)

Lapides in 1960 described a technique for the creation of a vesicocutaneous fistula that has been used in patients with spinal cord injuries and that has also been used in older children. After the bladder is filled, a transverse incision is made two fingerbreadths above the symphysis pubis. The anterior rectus sheath is incised transversely and mobilized superiorly to the umbilicus. A skin flap measuring 3.25 cm wide by 2.25 cm long is outlined on the abdominal wall. The skin flap is then freed from the underlying rectus sheath, and an opening is made in the rectus fascia immediately underneath the skin flap by excising a portion of the anterior rectus sheath. It is important not to make this opening too large to avoid herniation of the bowel or bladder.

The bladder flap, approximately 4 × 4 cm, is then created, with the bladder distended to a volume of 300 ml. The base of the flap is cephalad and in the region of the bladder dome and is made 2 to 3 cm wider than the apex. The bladder flap is then sutured to the skin flap with interrupted fine nonabsorbable sutures. The remainder of the defect in the bladder is closed with interrupted absorbable sutures. This procedure is considerably more extensive than those described earlier; it is particularly suited for the older or obese patient. We feel it is contraindicated in infants, in contrast to the simpler Blocksom procedure.

Immediate complications with the Lapides procedure have included fistula formation and

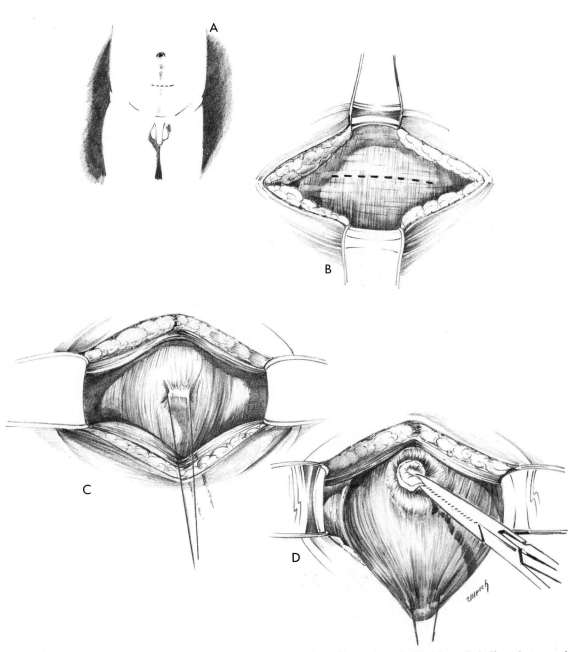

Figure 51–4. Blocksom technique of cutaneous vesicostomy. *A,* A small transverse incision is made halfway between the symphysis pubis and umbilicus. *B,* The rectus fascia is incised transversely, and the rectus muscles are divided in the midline, exposing the bladder. *C* and *D,* The bladder is mobilized superiorly with the aid of traction sutures and the peritoneum peeled off the dome, which is mobilized into the incision.

Illustration and legend continued on following page.

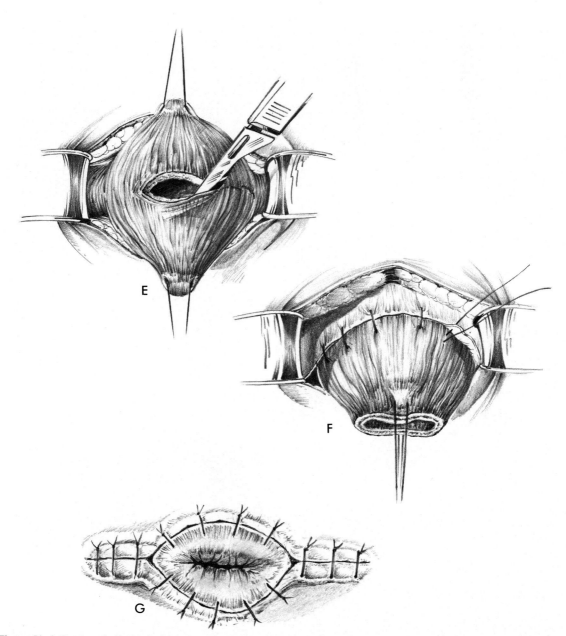

Figure 51–4 *Continued. E,* An incision is made in the dome of the bladder. *F,* The bladder wall is sutured to the fascia with interrupted chromic catgut. *G,* The edges of the bladder are sutured to the skin with interrupted chromic catgut or Dexon.

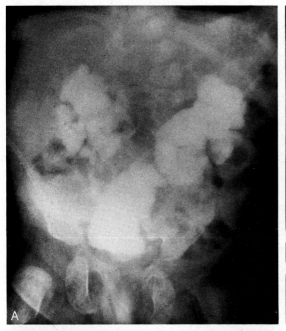

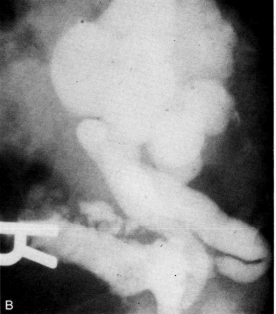

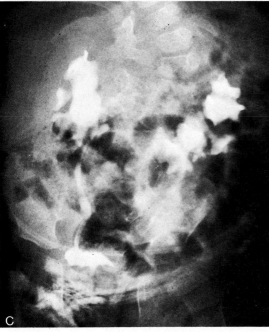

Figure 51–5. *A*, Preoperative IVP in a 3-month-old girl with lumbosacral myelomeningocele shows marked bilateral hydronephrosis. *B,* Preoperative voiding cysto-urethrogram demonstrates bilateral severe vesicoureteral reflux. *C,* IVP following cutaneous vesicostomy shows decompression of the upper urinary tracts. (From Mandell, J., et al.: J. Urol., *126*:92, 1981. Used by permission.)

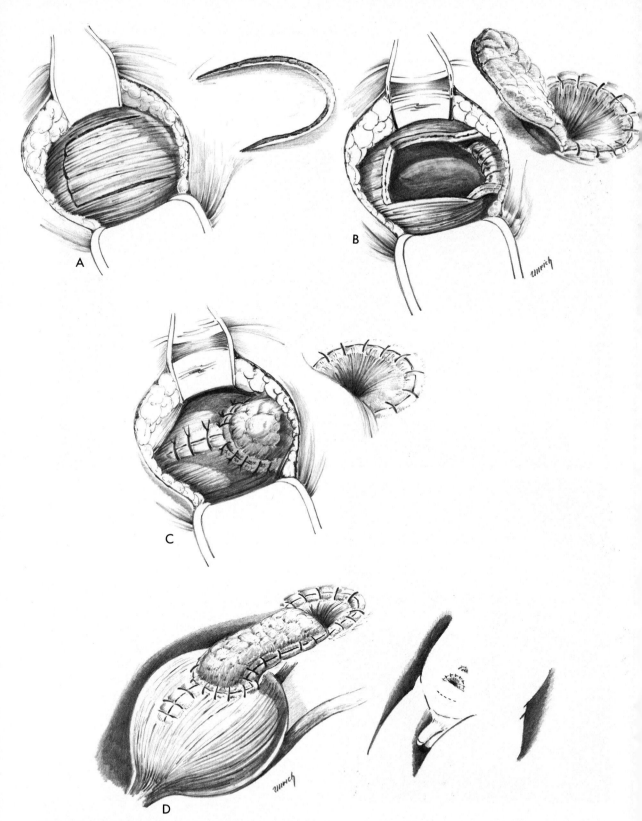

Figure 51–6. Lapides' technique of cutaneous vesicostomy. After the bladder is filled, a transverse incision is made two fingerbreadths above the symphysis pubis. The anterior rectus sheath is incised transversely and mobilized to the umbilicus. *A,* The skin flap, measuring 3.25 cm wide by 2.25 cm long, is outlined on the abdominal wall. The flap is then mobilized, and an opening is made in the rectus fascia immediately underneath the flap. With the bladder distended to a volume of approximately 300 ml, a bladder flap measuring 4 × 4 cm is created. *B,* The bladder flap is sutured to the skin flap with interrupted, fine, nonabsorbable sutures. *C,* The remainder of the defect in the bladder is closed with interrupted absorbable sutures. *D,* The complete vesicostomy.

sloughs of the bladder or skin flap. However, these have not been common. Delayed complications have included calculus formation, severe stomatitis, increased residual urine, chronic bacilluria, and difficulty in wearing a suitable urinary collecting device.

Loop Cutaneous Ureterostomy

Loop cutaneous ureterostomy is the creation of a cutaneous stoma along the lateral wall of a dilated and elongated ureter, maintaining ureteral continuity. Several authors (Fein et al., 1969; Rickham, 1962; Williams and Eckstein, 1965; Williams and Rabinovitch, 1967) have employed this procedure as the initial treatment in patients in the pediatric age group with massively dilated urinary tracts. Johnston (1963) further popularized this technique in a series of ten children whose ureterostomies were subsequently closed. A number of other series of temporary loop cutaneous ureterostomy with subsequent urinary tract reconstruction have been reported (Brueziere and Beurton, 1969, 1970; Ellis et al., 1966; Felderhof et al., 1968;

Leadbetter, 1972; Leape and Holder, 1970; Lome and Williams, 1972; Maloney and Smith, 1970; Perlmutter, 1974; Perlmutter and Patil, 1972; Perlmutter and Tank, 1968; Retik and Ontell, 1977). The majority of these authors have felt that a carefully performed loop cutaneous ureterostomy is well tolerated, that it causes minimal stomal complications, and that in most of the cases the urinary tract can be successfully reconstructed.

Loop cutaneous ureterostomy is ideally suited to the infant with severe upper urinary tract dilatation who is also septic or uremic (Fig. 51–7). It quickly provides excellent upper urinary tract drainage with minimal morbidity. This procedure is appropriate only for the dilated, tortuous ureter that can easily be mobilized to the level of the skin with minimal dissection and without tension.

TECHNIQUE OF LOOP CUTANEOUS URETEROSTOMY (Fig. 51–8)

With the infant in the lateral decubitus position, a posterolateral oblique skin incision is made in the upper flank or midflank region. The muscles are divided, and the retroperito-

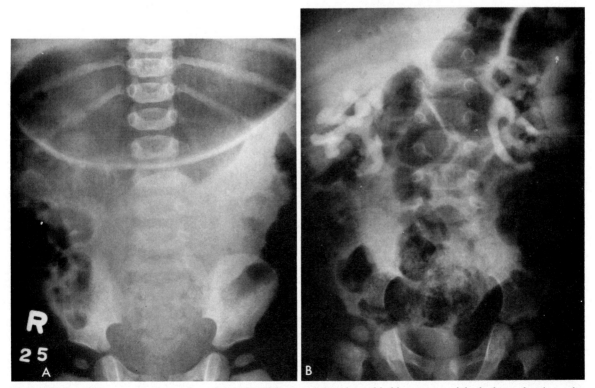

Figure 51–7. *A,* Excretory urogram in a 4-month-old boy reveals a large bladder, severe right hydronephrosis, and a poorly visualizing left kidney. The serum creatinine value was 3.4, and the patient was febrile. A voiding cystourethrogram demonstrated posterior urethral valves. *B,* Excretory urogram 3 weeks following bilateral loop cutaneous ureterostomies shows satisfactory decompression.

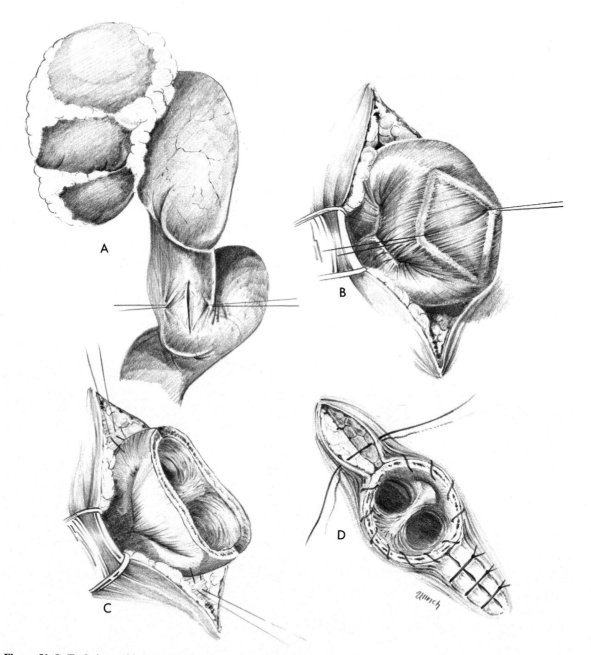

Figure 51–8. Technique of loop cutaneous ureterostomy. *A* and *B,* After the upper ureter is mobilized to reach the skin without tension, a 1- to 1.5-cm incision is made along the lateral aspect of the ureter. *C,* The ureteral adventitia is sutured to the external oblique fascia anteriorly and posteriorly with fine chromic catgut. To avoid obstruction, muscle and fascia are not sutured between the limbs of the ureter. They are reapproximated on both sides of the exteriorized ureter, which is then *(D)* sutured flush at the skin level with interrupted fine Dexon or nylon.

neum is entered. If the muscle layers are split, postoperative shifting of the layers may create obstruction. The upper ureter is mobilized minimally, with care taken not to injure the blood supply. It is helpful at this time to lyse any bands from the proximal ureteral limb to the ureteropelvic junction to make absolutely certain that areas of relative obstruction are not present and are not created by the procedure. Enough ureter is mobilized to reach the skin without tension. Usually a loop of redundant ureter is readily available for this.

Between fine stay sutures, a 1 to 1.5 cm incision is made along the lateral aspect of the ureter, and a fine infant feeding tube is passed proximally to ensure that there is no angulation. Fine chromic catgut is used to suture the ureteral adventitia to the external oblique fascias, anteriorly and posteriorly. Muscle and fascia are not sutured between the limbs of the ureter, as this may cause obstruction and as stomal hernias have not been a problem. The various muscle and fascial layers are then reapproximated on both sides of the exteriorized ureter, which is

then sutured flush at the skin level with interrupted fine Dexon or nylon. The ureter is not intubated. These stomas are relatively easy to care for. Large diapers are used and require frequent changing.

CLOSURE OF LOOP CUTANEOUS URETEROSTOMY (Fig. 51–9)

Although continuity of the ureter can be restored by simple stomal closure (Perlmutter, 1974; Raney and Zimskind, 1972), most authors prefer to resect the limbs of the ureterostomy and reanastomose the ureter, as the excised segment may be adynamic. We prefer to close loop cutaneous ureterostomies at least 4 months after any surgery on the lower ureter, although some authors have done both procedures simultaneously (Dwoskin, 1974).

A circumferential incision is made around the stoma, the proximal and distal ureteral limbs are mobilized, and the stoma and redundant ureter are excised obliquely. The ureteral edges are then spatulated, and the ureter is anastomosed with a continuous fine chromic catgut

Figure 51–9. Closure of loop ureterostomy. A circumferential incision is made around the stoma, the proximal and distal ureteral limbs are mobilized, and the stoma and redundant ureter are excised obliquely. After the ureteral edges are spatulated, the ureter is anastomosed with a continuous fine chromic catgut suture.

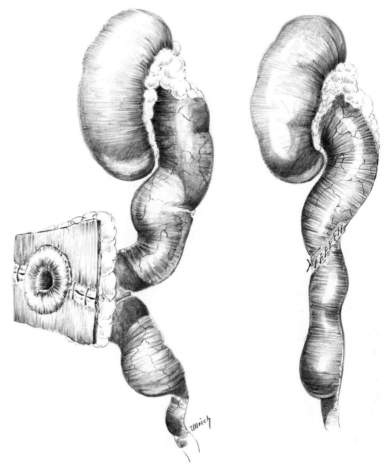

suture. When the ureter is dilated, reduction ureteroplasty is part of the repair, with care taken to preserve the segmental blood supply. In some cases the anastomosis can be made between the renal pelvis and the distal limb if the excised segment is very proximal. It is safest to divert the urine for 7 to 10 days, using a nephrostomy tube or a fine infant nasogastric tube emerging through a stab ureterotomy distal to the anastomosis.

Y-Ureterostomy

Y- or side-limb ureterostomy is a modification of loop cutaneous ureterostomy and is used under the same circumstances. This procedure, popularized by Sober in 1972, permits ureteral shortening reconstruction at the time of diversion and also allows some urine to drain to the bladder, thus preventing bladder contracture (Sober, 1973). This is a more extensive procedure than loop cutaneous ureterostomy; it

should not be attempted if the infant is critically ill.

TECHNIQUE OF Y-URETEROSTOMY
(Fig. 51–10)

The approach to this operation is similar to that for loop cutaneous ureterostomy. A proximal end ureterostomy is established, and the upper ureter is anastomosed to the renal pelvis, at which time it may be shortened and tailored. Postoperatively, most of the urine drains out to the skin, although some drains into the bladder.

Closure of the Y-ureterostomy is relatively simple and involves excising the segment of ureter draining to the skin up to the level of the renal pelvis.

End Cutaneous Ureterostomy

End cutaneous ureterostomy should be performed only on a markedly dilated ureter and is useful as a temporary diversion in two specific

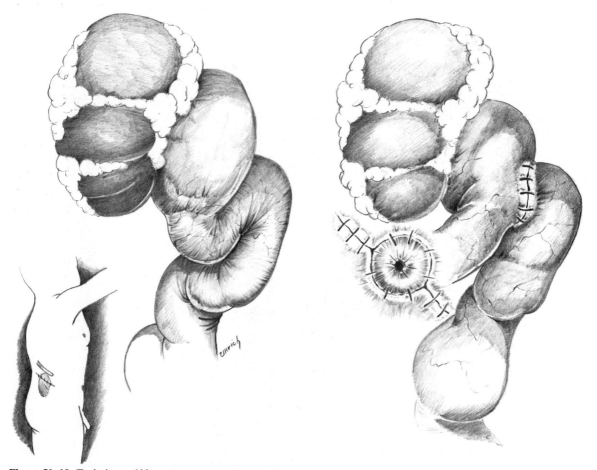

Figure 51–10. Technique of Y-ureterostomy. After a proximal end ureterostomy is established, the transected distal ureter is anastomosed to the renal pelvis.

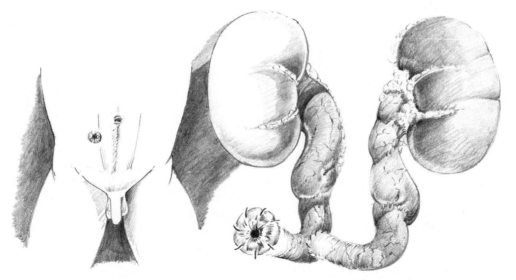

Figure 51–11. Technique of single stoma end cutaneous ureterostomy with transureteroureterostomy.

instances. The first is to divert the upper pole ureter that is associated with an ectopic ureterocele at the time of excision of the ureterocele and reconstruction of the trigone. This procedure allows an interval of time to elapse before deciding upon the definitive procedure to the upper pole, i.e., anastomosis of the upper pole ureter to the lower pole pelvis or partial nephrectomy. The other indication for end cutaneous ureterostomy is that of temporary drainage for a child with severe uremia who requires supravesical diversion and who will be a candidate for renal transplantation. However, some physicians have also employed terminal ureterostomy as a temporary diversion, with the option of later ureteroneocystostomy.

Bilateral end cutaneous ureterostomy is occasionally used for permanent diversion in children or adults with massively dilated ureters (Eckstein, 1963; Feminella and Lattimer, 1971; Flinn et al., 1971; Rickham, 1962; Swenson and Smyth, 1959; Wasserman and Garrett, 1965; Williams and Eckstein, 1965; Williams and Rabinovitch, 1967). Stomal obstruction can result from a compromised blood supply, especially when the dissection is extensive or the ureter is not very dilated (Blanchard et al., 1966; Lome and Williams, 1972; Rinker and Blanchard, 1966).

TECHNIQUE OF END CUTANEOUS URETEROSTOMY (Figs. 51–11 and 51–12)

When this procedure is used to divert the upper pole ureter that is associated with an ectopic ureterocele, the stoma may be placed through the lower transverse incision and should be everted slightly. In the other situations just mentioned, both ureters are isolated in the retroperitoneum through a low transverse incision, freed proximally, and straightened. A single stoma may be made in either lower quadrant or in the midline below the umbilicus. If the stoma is to be in the midline, a button of abdominal wall is excised, and the ureters are brought out through the opening in a gentle curve. It is important to avoid angulation. The redundant ureters are excised, and the ureters are spatulated medially and anastomosed together to form a single stoma. They are then sutured to the skin with Dexon or fine nylon. We usually create a nipple of approximately 0.5 cm. An alternative technique (Fig. 51–13) proposed by Lapides (1962) consists of a transverse skin incision with formation of superior and inferior skin flaps, spatulation of both ureters, and anastomosis of the two skin flaps between the ureters to prevent stricture. If the stoma is to be in the right lower quadrant, the left ureter may be tunneled retroperitoneally and sutured to the right ureter at the skin level or sutured in the retroperitoneum, creating a transureteroureterostomy (Flinn et al., 1971; Halpern et al., 1973; Udall et al., 1973; Weiss et al., 1966). Terminal ureterostomies, in general, should be intubated for 5 to 7 days to promote satisfactory drainage.

Cutaneous Pyelostomy

The indications for cutaneous pyelostomy are similar to those for loop cutaneous ureterostomy (Immergut et al., 1969; Schmidt et al., 1973). However, the renal pelvis must be quite

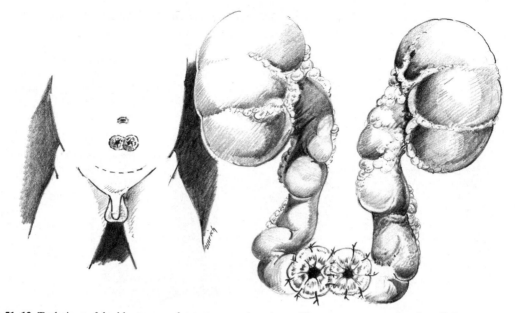

Figure 51–12. Technique of double stoma end cutaneous ureterostomy. The ureters are spatulated medially and anastomosed together to form a single stoma. A nipple of approximately 0.5 cm is created.

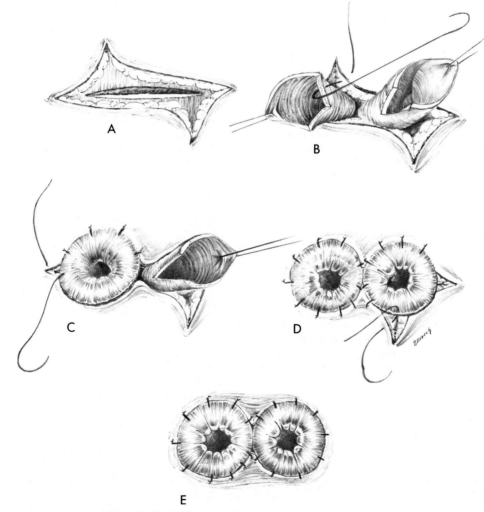

Figure 51–13. Technique of butterfly cutaneous ureterostomy.

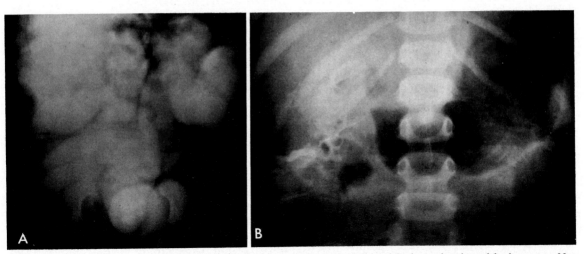

Figure 51–14. *A,* Excretory urogram in a 5-day-old boy reveals severe bilateral hydronephrosis and hydroureter. Note large renal pelves. He had ectopic ureters draining into the prostatic urethra. *B,* Following bilateral cutaneous pyelostomies, an excretory urogram shows excellent drainage.

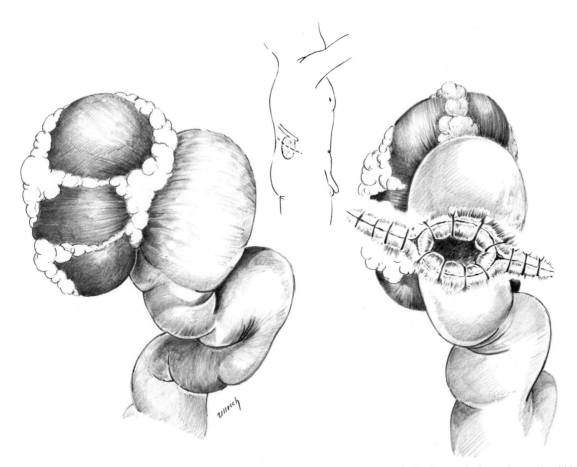

Figure 51–15. Technique of cutaneous pyelostomy. The renal pelvis should be exteriorized posteriorly, and care should be taken not to distort or angulate the ureteropelvic junction.

large to consider this procedure (Fig. 51–14); otherwise mobilization could distort and obstruct the ureteropelvic junction, thus compromising the later closure. Cutaneous pyelostomy also has been advocated as a diagnostic procedure in neonates with giant hydronephrosis from severe ureteropelvic obstruction prior to deciding whether pyeloplasty or nephrectomy is indicated. However, percutaneous nephrostomy (see page 2117) might better serve this purpose, unless the definitive surgery is to be postponed.

TECHNIQUE OF CUTANEOUS PYELOSTOMY
(Fig. 51–15)

The incision and approach are the same as for loop cutaneous ureterostomy. Alternatively, a posterior vertical lumbotomy will easily expose the large pelvis. The retroperitoneum is entered, and the renal pelvis is mobilized sufficiently to exteriorize it. It is important to exteriorize the renal pelvis posteriorly and not to angulate or distort the ureteropelvic junction.

Closure of the cutaneous pyelostomy involves freeing up the pelvis and closing it with a running fine chromic catgut stitch. Again, care must be taken not to disturb the ureteropelvic junction.

Summary of Nonintubated Procedures

Most of the described nonintubated procedures for temporary urinary diversion are technically easy, rapid forms of diversion that can be lifesaving for the neonate with severe hydronephrosis and hydroureter, sepsis, and uremia. They have a low morbidity rate, allow for an indefinite period of growth and development of the child, and provide opportunities for periodic assessment of renal, ureteral, and bladder function. They permit reconstruction to be performed electively when the child is in good health. Unlike intubated diversions, there is no urgency in completing the repair. The problems that have been encountered with these various forms of diversion have usually resulted from inappropriate patient selection and less than meticulous dissection.

Of particular significance is the enhanced growth potential of younger boys with posterior urethral valves and impaired renal function treated by initial, temporary diversion of the upper urinary tract. This is in comparison with the growth potential of boys undergoing treatment by primary valve resection (Krueger et al., 1980). In those boys under 1 year of age who were treated by supravesical diversion, follow-up height and weight percentiles were more nearly normal than those of boys treated with primary valve resection. This was particularly apparent in those who were younger than 1 month of age at the time of presentation. In addition, in both the immediate postoperative and the follow-up periods, renal function was better in the younger patients treated by upper tract diversion.

In our series of patients, failure of antireflux surgery, resulting in persistent reflux or ureterovesical obstruction, was rarely a problem, even with a defunctionalized distal ureter. Also, contrary to the experience of Lome et al. (1972) and Tanagho (1974), in our own series we have not found a defunctionalized bladder that has never contained a suprapubic tube incapable of re-expansion (Schmaelze et al., 1969), even after 2 to 3 years. However, a small bladder capacity in a patient with a chronically infected bladder is still a possibility and may be a problem. Careful preservation of ureteral blood supply during ureteral reconstruction and reimplantation is critical, and cycling of the bladder with saline to simulate normal urinary filling and voiding over a period of 5 to 10 days in the early postoperative period may be helpful. When reflux is mild, urinary tract continuity can be restored before reimplantation is considered. Often such reflux will cease spontaneously after the ureters and bladder resume normal function (Teele et al., 1976).

Bacilluria, present in many of the infants with tubeless forms of diversion, generally has not led to symptomatic infections or progressive renal damage. It is important to treat infection vigorously, of course, during periods of reconstructive surgery.

Other tubeless diversions such as sigmoid conduits and ileal or ileocecal conduits, formerly considered to be permanent, sometimes are reconnected to the urinary tract or intact bowel, and in that sense can also be temporary. These are discussed in another chapter.

References

Beland, G. A., and Weiss, R. M.: Cutaneous vesicostomy in children. J. Urol., 94:128, 1965.

Bell, T. E., Hoodin, A. O., and Evans, A. T.: Tubeless cystostomy in children. J. Urol., 100:459, 1968.

Belman, A. B., and King, L. R.: Vesicostomy: Useful means of reversible urinary diversion in selected infants. Urology; 1:208, 1973.

Binder, C., Gonick, P., and Ciavarra, V.: Experience with Silastic U-tube nephrostomy. J. Urol., 106:499, 1971.

Bissada, N. K., Cole, A. T., and Fried, F. A.: Renal

diversion with silicone circle catheters. Urology, 2:238, 1973.

Blanchard, T. W., Rinker, J. R., and McLendon, R. L.: Cutaneous ureterostomy following blockage of the ureteral vasculature: An experimental study. J. Urol., 96:39, 1966.

Blocksom, B. H., Jr.: Bladder pouch for prolonged tubeless cystotomy. J. Urol., 78:398, 1957.

Brueziere, J., and Beurton, D.: Traitement des megaurétéres de l'enfant et du nourrison par l'urétérostomie cutanée. Ire partie. Ann. d'Urol., 3:189, 1969.

Brueziere, J., and Beurton, D.: Traitement des mégaurétéres de l'enfant et du nourrisson par l'urétérostomie cutanée. 2e partie. Ann. d'Urol., 4:41, 1970.

Carlson, H. E.: Tubeless cystotomy in childhood. J. Urol., 83:669, 1960.

Comarr, A. E.: Experience with the U-tube for renal drainage among patients with spinal cord injury. J. Urol., 95:741, 1966.

Conger, K. B., and Toub, L.: Obstruction of the bladder neck in the male infant and child: Present concepts of diagnostic methods and management, and a report of 14 cases. J. Pediatr., 57:855, 1960.

Duckett, J. W., Jr.: Cutaneous vesicostomy in childhood. The Blocksom technique. Urol. Clin. North Am., 1:485, 1974.

Dwoskin, J. Y.: Management of the massively dilated urinary tract in infants by temporary diversion and single-stage reconstruction. Urol. Clin. North Am., 1:515, 1974.

Eckstein, H. B.: Cutaneous ureterostomy. Proc. R. Soc. Med., 56:749, 1963.

Ellis, D. G., Fonkalsrud, E. W., and Smith, J. P.: Congenital posterior urethral valves. J. Urol., 95:549, 1966.

Fein, R. L., Young, J. G., and Van Buskirk, K. E.: The case for loop ureterostomy in the infant with advanced lower urinary tract obstruction. J. Urol., 101:513, 1969.

Felderhof, J., Van Essen, A. G., and Oosterhof, P. G.: Bilaterale lus-ureterostomie bij jonge kinderen als tijdelijke maatregel bij ernstige obstructie van de urinewegen. Ned. Tidjscher. Geneeskd., 112:1947, 1968.

Feminella, J. G., Jr., and Lattimer, J. K.: A retrospective analysis of 70 cases of cutaneous ureterostomy. J. Urol., 106:538, 1971.

Flinn, R. A., King, L. R., McDonald, J. H., et al.: Cutaneous ureterostomy: An alternative urinary diversion. J. Urol., 105:358, 1971.

Fowler, J. E., Meares, E. M., and Goldin, A. R.: Percutaneous nephrostomy: Techniques, indications and results. Urology, 6:428, 1975.

Francis, D. R., and Bucy, J. G.: Inside-out kidney: An unusual complication of cutaneous pyelostomy. J. Urol., 112:514, 1974.

Goodwin, W. E., Casey, W. C., and Woolf, W.: Percutaneous trocar (needle) nephrostomy in hydronephrosis. JAMA, 157:891, 1955.

Halpern, G. N., King, L. R., and Belman, A. B.: Transureteroureterostomy in children. J. Urol., 109:504, 1973.

Hendren, W. H.: Urinary tract refunctionalization after prior diversion in children. Ann. Surg., 180:494, 1974.

Hendren, W. H.: Restoration of function in the severely decompensated ureter. In Johnston, J. H., and Scholtmeijer, R. J. (Eds.): Problems in Paediatric Urology, p. 1. Amsterdam, Excerpta Medica, 1972.

Hendren, W. H.: A new approach to infants with severe obstructive uropathy: Early complete reconstruction. J. Pediatr. Surg., 5:184, 1970.

Immergut, M. A., Jacobson, J. J., Culp, D. A., and Flocks, R. H.: Cutaneous pyelostomy. J. Urol., 101:276, 1969.

Ireland, G. W., and Geist, R. W.: Difficulties with vesicostomies in 15 children with meningomyelocele. J. Urol., 103:341, 1970.

Johnston, J. H.: Temporary cutaneous ureterostomy in the management of advanced congenital urinary obstruction. Arch. Dis. Child., 38:161, 1963.

Karafin, L., and Kendall, A. R.: Vesicostomy in the management of neurogenic bladder disease secondary to meningomyelocele in children. J. Urol., 96:723, 1966.

King, L. R., and Belman, A. B.: A technique for nephrostomy in the absence of caliectasis. J. Urol., 108:518, 1972.

Krueger, R. P., Hardy, B. E., and Churchill, B. M.: Growth in boys with posterior urethral valves. Urol. Clin. North Am., 7:265, 1980.

Lapides, J.: Butterfly cutaneous ureterostomy. J. Urol., 88:735, 1962.

Lapides, J., Ajemian, E. P., and Lichtwardt, J. R.: Cutaneous vesicostomy. J. Urol., 84:609, 1960.

Leadbetter, G. W.: Skin ureterostomy with subsequent ureteral reconstruction. J. Urol., 107:462, 1972.

Leape, L. L., and Holder, T. M.: Temporary tubeless urinary diversion in children. J. Pediatr. Surg., 5:288, 1970.

Lome, L. G., and Williams, D. I.: Urinary reconstruction following temporary cutaneous ureterostomy diversion in children. J. Urol., 108:162, 1972.

Lome, L. G., Howat, J. M., and Williams, D. I.: The temporarily defunctionalized bladder in children. J. Urol., 107:469, 1972.

Lytton, B., and Weiss, R. M.: Cutaneous vesicostomy for temporary urinary diversion in infants. J. Urol., 105:888, 1971.

Maloney, J. D., and Smith, J. P.: Temporary cutaneous loop ureterostomy. J. Urol., 103:790, 1970.

Mandell, J., Bauer, S. B., Colodny, A. H., and Retik, A. B.: Cutaneous vesicostomy in infancy. J. Urol., 126:92, 1981.

McGovern, J. H.: Urinary diversion by nephrostomy. In Scott, R., Jr. (Ed.): Current Controversies in Urologic Management. Philadelphia, W. B. Saunders Co., 1972.

Ogg, C. S., Saxton, H. M., and Cameron, J. S.: Percutaneous needle nephrostomy. Br. Med. J., 4:657, 1969.

Parker, R. M., and Perlmutter, A. D.: Upper urinary tract obstruction in infants. J. Urol., 102:355, 1969.

Perlmutter, A. D.: Temporary urinary diversion in the management of the chronically dilated urinary tract in childhood. In Johnston, J. H., and Goodwin, W. E. (Eds.): Reviews in Paediatric Urology. Amsterdam, Excerpta Medica, 1974.

Perlmutter, A. D., and Patil, J.: Loop cutaneous ureterostomy in infants and young children: Late results in 32 cases. J. Urol., 107:655, 1972.

Perlmutter, A. D., and Tank, E. S.: Loop cutaneous ureterostomy in infancy. J. Urol., 99:559, 1968.

Pokorny, M., Pontes, J. E., and Pierce, J. M., Jr.: Ureterostomy in situ. Urology, 8:447, 1976.

Raney, A. M., and Zimskind, P. D.: Replacement of loop cutaneous ureterostomy without excision of ureteral segment: An experimental study. J. Urol., 107:39, 1972.

Raper, F. P.: The recognition and treatment of congenital urethral valves. Br. J. Urol., 25:136, 1953.

Rattner, W. H., Meyer, R., and Bernstein, J.: Congenital abnormalities of the urinary system. IV. Valvular obstruction of the posterior urethra. J. Pediatr., 63:84, 1963.

Retik, A. B., and Ontell, R.: Temporary urinary diversion in infants and children. In Libertino, J. A., and Zinman, L. (Eds.): Reconstructive Urological Surgery, p. 135. Baltimore, The Williams and Wilkins Co., 1977.

Rickham, P. P.: Advanced lower urinary obstruction in childhood. Arch. Dis. Child., *37*:122, 1962.

Rinker, J. R., and Blanchard, T. W.: Improvement of the circulation of the ureter prior to cutaneous ureterostomy: A clinical study. J. Urol., *96*:44, 1966.

Schmaelze, J. F., Cass, A. S., and Hinman, F., Jr.: Effect of disease and restoration of function on vesical capacity. J. Urol., *101*:700, 1969.

Schmidt, J. D., Hawtrey, C. E., Culp, D. A., et al.: Experience with cutaneous pyelostomy diversion. J. Urol., *109*:990, 1973.

Sober, I.: Pelvioureterostomy-en-Y. J. Urol., *107*:473, 1973.

Swenson, O., and Smyth, B. T.: Aperistaltic megaloureter: Treatment by bilateral cutaneous ureterostomy using a new technique; preliminary communication. J. Urol., *82*:62, 1959.

Tanagho, E. A.: Congenitally obstructed bladders: Fate after prolonged defunctionalization. J. Urol., *111*:102, 1974.

Teele, R. L., Lebowitz, R. L., and Colodny, A. H.: Reflux into the unused ureter. J. Urol., *115*:310, 1976.

Udall, D. A., Hodges, C. V., Pearse, H. M., et al.: Transureteroureterostomy: A neglected procedure. J. Urol., *109*:817, 1973.

Waldbaum, R. S., and Marshall, V. F.: Posterior urethral valves: Evaluation and surgical management. J. Urol., *103*:801, 1970.

Walsh, A.: Personal communication, 1974.

Wasserman, D. H., and Garrett, R. A.: Cutaneous ureterostomy: Indications in children. J. Urol., *94*:380, 1965.

Weiss, R. M., Beland, J. A., and Lattimer, J. K.: Transureteroureterostomy and cutaneous ureterostomy as a form of urinary diversion in children. J. Urol., *96*:155, 1966.

Weyrauch, H. M., and Rous, S. N.: U-tube nephrostomy. J. Urol., *97*:225, 1967.

Whitaker, R. H.: Methods of assessing obstruction in dilated ureters. Br. J. Urol., *45*:15, 1973.

Williams, D. I., and Eckstein, H. B.: Obstructive valves in the posterior urethra. J. Urol., *93*:236, 1965.

Williams, D. I., and Rabinovitch, H. H.: Cutaneous ureterostomy for the grossly dilated ureter of childhood. Br. J. Urol., *39*:696, 1967.

Wosnitzer, M., and Lattimer, J. K.: Comparison of permanent nephrostomy and permanent cutaneous ureterostomy. J. Urol., *83*:553, 1960.

CHAPTER 52

Urinary Undiversion: Refunctionalization of the Previously Diverted Urinary Tract

W. HARDY HENDREN, M.D.

INTRODUCTION

In the past 30 years many infants and children with various types of urologic malformations have been managed by using various methods of urinary diversion. The majority of these children would be treated today by different means. For example, in the 1950's children with meningomyelocele and neurogenic bladder were often managed by indwelling urethral or suprapubic catheters. Such long-term catheter drainage created many difficulties with recurrent infection, contracture of the bladder, progressive hydronephrosis, and stone formation. In 1950, Dr. Eugene M. Bricker introduced the ileal loop urinary diversion for bladder substitution after pelvic evisceration (Bricker, 1950). This was a major step forward in the management of patients with cancer and also of children with neurogenic bladder and various obstructive uropathies. Today the majority of children with neurogenic bladder are managed by intermittent catheterization or various reconstructive operations, depending on the state of continence, whether there is vesicoureteral reflux, the size of the bladder, and a number of other factors.

In 1950, surgical correction of vesicoureteral reflux did not exist, nor was operative correction of megaureter in the surgeon's armamentarium. Therefore, many children with those problems were treated by urinary diversions such as vesicostomy, end ureterostomy, loop ureterostomy, and nephrostomy. Many infant males with severe dilatation of the upper tracts from urethral valves were treated by temporary loop ureterostomy diversion (Johnston, 1963; Perlmutter and Patil, 1972). Today they are treated by primary endoscopic resection of the urethral valves using modern fiberoptic pediatric endoscopes, followed by reconstructive surgery for severely deformed urinary tracts if needed (Hendren, 1971; 1974).

Improved techniques for repairing deranged urinary tracts has led to re-evaluation of many patients diverted in former years. This chapter will discuss techniques that have been found useful in undiverting 140 patients in the past 15 years, as noted in Figure 52–1. The most common type of urinary diversion was an ileal loop, which was present in almost half of the patients. One quarter of the patients had only one kidney. In three quarters of the patients the diversion had been considered a permanent one, with no anticipation of subsequent reconstruction.

Figure 52–2 shows the age of the patients and Figure 52–3 shows the duration of their urinary diversions. Experience has shown that many years of disuse does not preclude successful rehabilitation of the lower urinary tract. Indeed, 46 of the patients had lived with a urinary diversion between 10 and 20 years.

GENERAL CONSIDERATIONS

When evaluating an individual patient for possible refunctionalization of the previously

URINARY UNDIVERSION
1969 – 1984   140 CASES

60	ILEAL LOOP (12 pyelo-ileal)	**107**	permanent diversions
4	COLON CONDUIT	**33**	temporary diversions
33	LOOP URETEROSTOMY OR PYELOSTOMY	**46**	females
17	END URETEROSTOMY	**94**	males
19	CYSTOSTOMY		
7	NEPHROSTOMY	**35**	patients had one kidney

9 personal diversions;   131 had been diverted elsewhere

Figure 52–1. Undiversion case data.

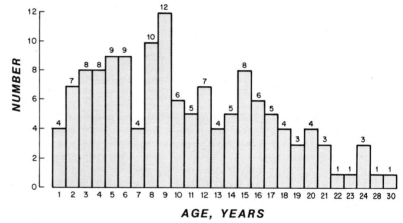

Figure 52–2. Age in 140 undiversion patients.

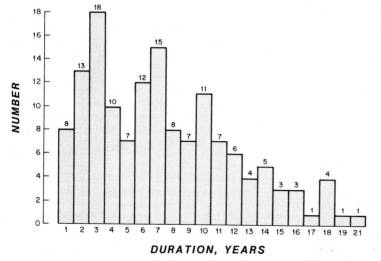

Figure 52–3. Duration of diversion in 140 undiversion patients.

diverted urinary tract, there are a number of factors that must be weighed. Each case differs from the others one may have treated. It is important to examine why the patient's urinary tract was diverted in the first place. The most common causes we have encountered include severe obstructive uropathy from urethral valves, prune belly syndrome, failed ureteral reimplantation, failed repair of megaureter, urinary incontinence, stricture of the urethra, and myelodysplasia with neurogenic bladder. If incontinence was the reason for diversion in the first place, obviously undiversion will also require an incontinence correction. This may mean creating more outlet resistance or increasing the size and compliance of the bladder, or both. Increasing outlet resistence may require narrowing the bladder neck or constructing a distal urethra in females, or both procedures. Bladder augmentation can be done with a patch of sigmoid or small bowel or with an ileocecal segment. Thus the surgeon who undertakes undiversions must have a wide range of technical options.

RENAL FUNCTION

Many diverted patients have reduced renal function. About one third of those patients on whom I have performed reconstruction had such severe upper tract damage at the outset that one could predict that transplantation would likely be necessary in the future. Ten patients have had renal transplantation to date; in none of them did upper tract deterioration occur as a result of undiversion. It is common to see a steady rise in serum creatinine as these children grow, especially at adolescence when the body mass increases to a size greater than poor kidneys can support. In patients with borderline renal function, undiversion has invariably improved the quality of life between the time of reconstruction and the time when dialysis or transplantation, or both, were needed. Many diverted patients have chronic bacilluria. In most it proved possible to maintain a sterile urinary tract after undiversion. When transplantation is necessary, it is much better done into a functioning lower urinary tract instead of into a urinary diversion that imposes many additional possible complications.

If bowel is used in the urinary tract one should anticipate solute resorption through the bowel surface. These patients must be followed closely. All patients with diminished renal function are managed collaboratively with a nephrol-

ogist. This is of great help in maintaining metabolic hemostasis when there is declining renal function. It has provided a smooth transition to dialysis and transplantation for those patients who have reached that stage.

PSYCHOLOGIC FACTORS

A patient with a long-term urinary diversion has grown accustomed to it as a way of life. If undiversion should require temporary or permanent intermittent self-catheterization postoperatively, such as in patients with neurogenic bladder, the patient must be fully prepared. It is essential that he be willing to cooperate if undiversion is to be successful.

ANESTHESIA

Undiversion operations are long and complicated. Seldom do they last less than 5 to 6 hours. The most difficult one I have encountered lasted 20 hours. That child had undergone 13 prior operations. Her undiversion required repair of ureters, bladder neck, urethra, and vagina, and simultaneous repositioning of a previously pulled-through rectum. Obviously, expert anesthesia management is mandatory. There should be constant monitoring of the patient's acid-base balance, blood gases, and replacement of blood and fluids. These patients cannot withstand inadequate fluid replacement for it can cause renal tubular necrosis. Fluid replacement for ordinary intra-abdominal pediatric surgical operations is in the range of 5 ml per kg per hr. In our experience these patients generally require four to five times that volume, that is, 20 to 25 ml per kg per hr, to maintain a satisfactory urinary output intraoperatively. These amounts are scaled down appropriately for older adult patients. Wide retroperitoneal dissection and exposure of the intestines creates enormous fluid losses and "third spacing." If only parameters of blood pressure and hematocrit are followed to estimate fluid requirements, replacement will fall behind. Some patients with renal failure and inability to concentrate the urine have an obligatory high output. Those patients are not put on an ordinary "NPO after midnight regime"; they are maintained on intravenous fluid therapy from the time oral intake is stopped.

Nitrous oxide should be avoided in these long cases. It diffuses into the gut, and creates distention, which makes intraoperative exposure and later wound closure significantly more difficult.

ASSESSMENT OF BLADDER FUNCTION

Urodynamic evaluation of the lower urinary tract is an important tool in modern day urology. Nevertheless, it has not been the keystone for predicting how well a long-defunctionalized bladder will function when urine flow is re-established. Cystography will demonstrate bladder size and sensation as well as the presence of diverticula, urethral valves, and reflux into ureteral stumps. Cystoscopy can provide additional information. Usually the long diverted bladder is small and has a smooth lining, which bleeds readily when filled with irrigating solution under pressure. It is important not to overfill the bladder, which can cause it to rupture, a complication we have encountered on four occasions when attempting to stretch a bladder preoperatively under anesthesia.

The most helpful test we have used is intermittently filling the bladder with saline and observing sensation, size, continence, and ability to void (Kogan et al., 1976). As shown in Figure 52–4, a small Silastic catheter is introduced during cystoscopy. The patient is taught to fill the bladder with saline to test continence and ability to empty, and to see whether the bladder will stretch. Some bladder capacities will increase rapidly in just a week or two from a very small initial capacity of only 2 or 3 ounces, to a normal or near-normal capacity. Others may not. This may signify the need for augmentation during undiversion. The length of time spent doing "bladder cycling" may vary from a few days to several months, depending on the

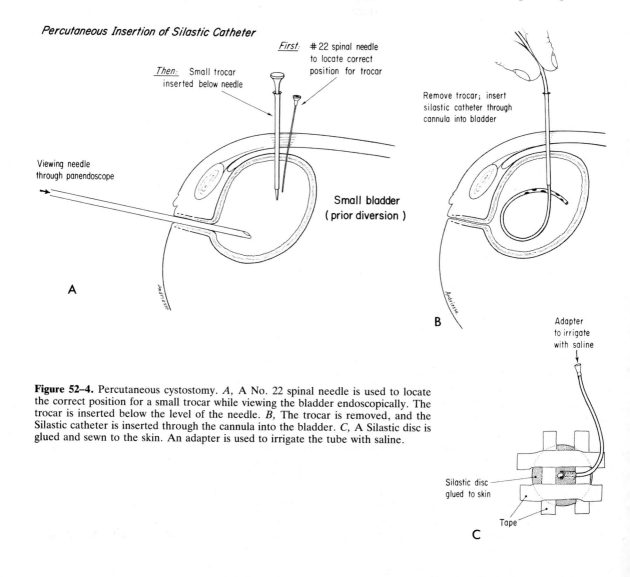

Figure 52–4. Percutaneous cystostomy. *A*, A No. 22 spinal needle is used to locate the correct position for a small trocar while viewing the bladder endoscopically. The trocar is inserted below the level of the needle. *B*, The trocar is removed, and the Silastic catheter is inserted through the cannula into the bladder. *C*, A Silastic disc is glued and sewn to the skin. An adapter is used to irrigate the tube with saline.

findings, the degree of cooperation of the patient, and other factors. Optimally the patient should fill the bladder by rapid drip from a reservoir bottle about 3 to 4 feet above the level of the bladder. This is done as many times during the day as possible. The irrigating fluid is tap water to which 2 teaspoons of salt per quart are added, and it is boiled to sterilize it. To this solution a few milliliters of 0.5 per cent neomycin solution are added to reduce the likelihood of contamination and infection. Occasionally the irrigating catheter will pass through the bladder neck into the urethra so that irrigation will not fill the bladder. It can be pulled back an appropriate distance to remedy the problem. Alternatively, the Stamey Malecot percutaneous catheter can be used. However, the contracting bladder may pull away from the catheter, allowing the irrigating fluid to enter the prevesical space.

When urethral valves are encountered at cystoscopy in a patient whose bladder is diverted, they can be destroyed by fulguration if bladder cycling is to commence immediately. Conversely, urethral valves should never be fulgurated in a "dry urethra" that will remain dry postoperatively. In several cases, we have seen that lead to impermeable strictures, creating a need for an additional reconstructive operation.

SURGICAL PRINCIPLES IN UNDIVERSION OPERATIONS

The bowel is cleansed preoperatively, especially when use of a bowel segment is contemplated. For this we rely on clear fluids by mouth for 2 or 3 days and cleansing saline enemas. Preoperative and intraoperative antibiotic administration is guided by culture with antibiotic sensitivities of the urine.

Wide transabdominal exposure is essential (Hendren, 1978). Although some patients will have had previous urologic surgery through a transverse lower abdominal incision, a long midline incision is preferred, usually from the pubis to the xiphoid sternum. This will give access to all levels of the urinary tract. A large ring retractor is desirable. To expose the kidneys and ureters, the right and left colon are mobilized and reflected medially. When the ureter is mobilized, all of its periureteral tissue should be kept with it, skeletonizing the other structures in the retroperitoneum—not the ureter (Fig. 52–5). The gonadal vessels should be maintained with the ureter for collateral blood supply. We have done this many times without loss of testis or ovary. Similarly the kidney can be mobilized and moved downward and medially to facilitate getting sufficient length for a foreshortened ureter, whether it is to be joined to the bladder or to the contralateral renal pelvis or ureter.

Psoas hitch is a most helpful adjunct (Fig. 52–6). It can compensate for some shortness of the ureter, which must be implanted without tension. It can also allow a super-long tunnel to be obtained, which is necessary if reflux is to be prevented when reimplanting a bowel segment or a slightly dilated and scarred ureter. To obtain a tunnel length:ureter diameter ratio of 5:1 may mandate having a tunnel 5 to 10 cm long. Fixation to the psoas muscle will allow

Figure 52–5. Technique for mobilizing kidney and ureter to gain additional length by wide dissection of structures, while preserving periureteral tissue for blood supply, including gonadal vessels.

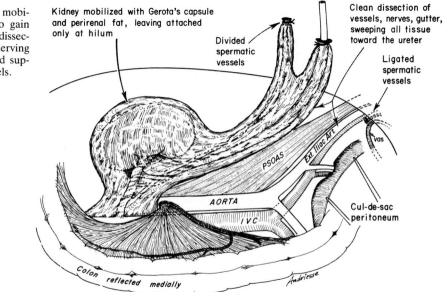

Kidney mobilized with Gerota's capsule and perirenal fat, leaving attached only at hilum

Divided spermatic vessels

Clean dissection of vessels, nerves, gutter, sweeping all tissue toward the ureter

Ligated spermatic vessels

PSOAS

Ext Iliac Art

vas

AORTA

IVC

Cul-de-sac peritoneum

Colon reflected medially

Andriesse

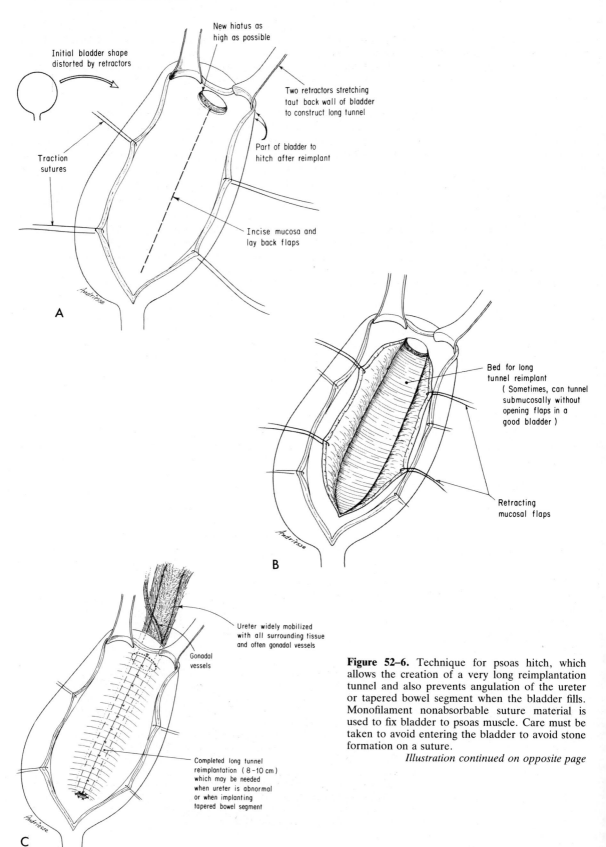

New hiatus as
high as possible

Initial bladder shape
distorted by retractors

Two retractors stretching
taut back wall of bladder
to construct long tunnel

Part of bladder to
hitch after reimplant

Traction
sutures

Incise mucosa and
lay back flaps

A

Bed for long
tunnel reimplant
(Sometimes, can tunnel
submucosally without
opening flaps in a
good bladder)

Retracting
mucosal flaps

B

Ureter widely mobilized
with all surrounding tissue
and often gonadal vessels

Gonadal
vessels

Completed long tunnel
reimplantation (8-10 cm)
which may be needed
when ureter is abnormal
or when implanting
tapered bowel segment

C

Figure 52–6. Technique for psoas hitch, which allows the creation of a very long reimplantation tunnel and also prevents angulation of the ureter or tapered bowel segment when the bladder fills. Monofilament nonabsorbable suture material is used to fix bladder to psoas muscle. Care must be taken to avoid entering the bladder to avoid stone formation on a suture.

Illustration continued on opposite page

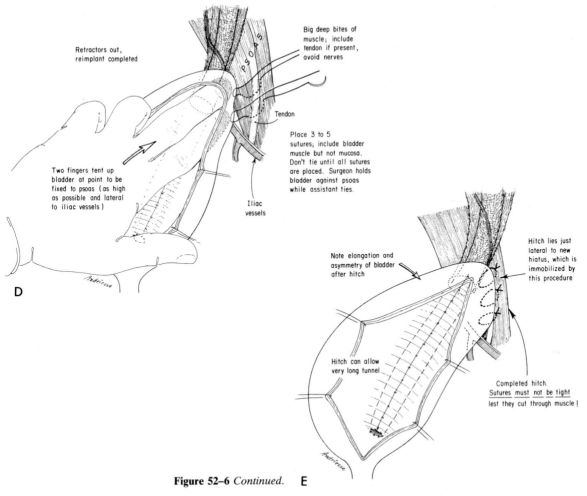

Figure 52–6 *Continued.* **E**

that. It will also fix the ureteral hiatus so that when the bladder fills there will be no angulation and obstruction of the ureter.

Transureteroureterostomy or transuretero-pyelostomy is another extremely useful adjunct in these cases (Fig. 52–7) (Hendren and Hensle, 1980; Hodges et al., 1963). Rarely is it feasible to join two ureters to the bladder. Most often the better ureter has been implanted, draining the other across into it. This must be done without tension. It is important to avoid angulation of a ureter beneath a mesenteric vessel, especially the inferior mesenteric artery.

A cardinal principle in reconstructing these cases is to lay out all of the anatomic structures at the operating table, listing the various options one might pursue and choosing the one that has the greatest likelihood of success. Failure is much more likely when the surgeon attempts to get by with a minimal procedure, with the aim of avoiding a large one. Conversely, most extensive procedures will succeed if they are well conceived and skillfully executed. These patients can not tolerate a major complication

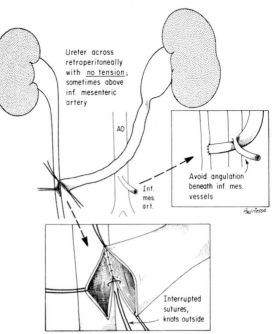

Figure 52–7. Technique for transureteroureterostomy.

such as leakage from an anastomosis under tension, ureteral obstruction, or devascularization of a part of the urinary tract.

There has been no major early postoperative complication in the 140 patients who have undergone undiversion since 1969. There were three late deaths. The first died at age 28 years, 11 years after undiversion, from sepsis during hemodialysis. He had the prune belly syndrome with a solitary kidney. His total creatinine clearance when first seen at age 17 years was only 20 per cent of normal. The second death occurred in a 13-year-old girl 4 years after undiversion during an intravenous pyelogram (IVP) examination elsewhere. An anaphylactic reaction occurred, resulting in her death. The third patient was a 23-year-old woman who died of acute myelocytic leukemia, after having done well for 16 months after undiversion of an ileal loop that had been present for 18 years.

SELECTED CASES

The following cases, and others that have been described previously, will illustrate some of the technical details to be encountered in undiversion surgery (Hendren, 1973; 1974; 1976; 1979). Since the ileal loop is the most common type of previous diversion extant, it will be emphasized. The same principals apply, however, when undiverting patients with long-standing diversion by vesicostomy, end ureter-

ostomy, loop ureterostomy, pyelostomy, or nephrostomy.

The principal options available in reconstruction of the urinary tract in a patient with an ileal loop diversion are shown in Figure 52–8. To this can be added autotransplantation, which will be indicated only rarely. Whenever the bowel loop can be discarded, using one or both ureters to drain the upper tracts into the bladder, that is preferred. Often it is not possible, however.

CASE 1 (Figs. 52–9 and 52–10)

An 11-year-old boy was referred in 1974 with an ileal loop done at age 3 years. His original pathologic condition was urethral valves with hydronephrosis, infection, and stones. Prior surgery included suprapubic cystoscopy at age 3 months, bilateral pyelolithotomies at age 2 years, urinary diversion at age 3 years, and later a second left pyelolithotomy. The ileal loop was tapered and reimplanted with a long tunnel to prevent reflux. The patient is now 21 years of age, more than 10 years after undiversion. He is well, free from urinary infection or stones, and has normal renal function by creatinine clearance determination. Originally a scrawny youngster, with a bag on his abdomen and chronic urinary infection, he is now a robust adult (6 feet 2 inches tall and weighing 170 pounds).

Comment. In tapering an ileal loop that is to serve as a substitute ureter, several important

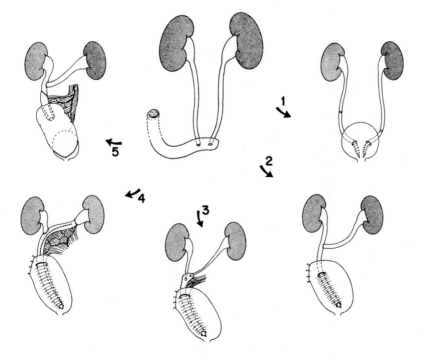

Figure 52–8. Principal options available for undiversion of an ileal loop.

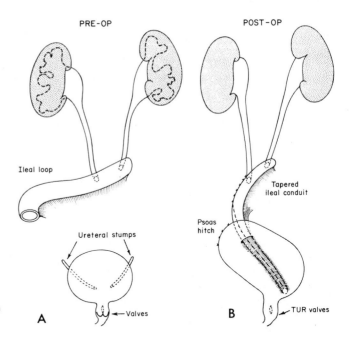

Figure 52–9. Case 1 before *(A)* and after *(B)* reconstruction.

points must be respected. First, mobilizing the ileal loop down from the abdominal wall should be done with great care, because it may be necessary to use the full length of the bowel segment. In dissecting free the intra-abdominal part of the loop, catheters through the loop and up the ureters can prove helpful. This dissection can be facilitated by gently distending the system with saline, with a ligature occluding the end of the loop around the catheters. It is often nec-

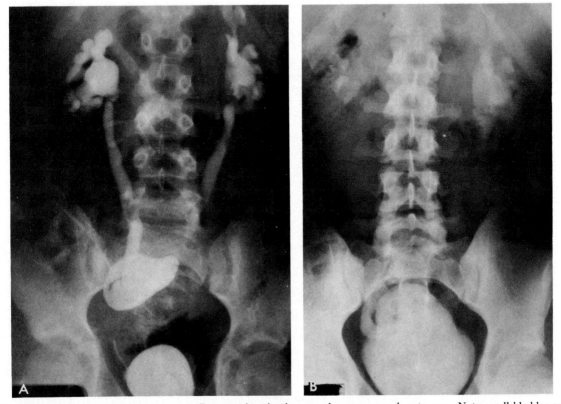

Figure 52–10. Case 1 roentgenograms. *A,* Preoperative simultaneous loopogram and cystogram. Note small bladder and short, unusable ureteral stumps. *B,* Intravenous pyelogram (IVP) 6 years after undiversion. Note normal size of bladder.

essary to incise the mesentery to straighten the loop, taking care not to devascularize the bowel. The strip of bowel to be removed on its anti-mesenteric border should be marked with a skin pencil to ensure accuracy, resecting not more than one third of the circumference of the bowel. A two-layer inverting closure with catgut sutures will use several additional millimeters of bowel circumference. The first layer is a running, inverting suture. The second layer is interrupted sutures. It is important to create a nonrefluxing anastomosis of the tapered bowel to the bladder. Since the bowel loop, even when tapered, will be 1 to 1.5 cm in diameter, the tunnel must be very long (5 to 10 cm). Obviously, this will be possible only in a favorable bladder of good size. It is fruitless to attempt reimplantation of a tapered small bowel segment into a small, scarred, contracted bladder. The optimal method for making a long tunnel is shown in Fig. 52–6. Mucosal flaps are dissected sharply to prepare a bed for the tapered bowel. The tapered bowel is tacked to the muscle of the back wall of the bladder, with its suture line lying posteriorly, not adjacent, to the mucosa to be closed over it in order to avert fistula formation. Psoas hitch is essential to immobilize the hiatus through which the tapered bowel segment enters the bladder wall. This will prevent angulation when the bladder fills. In tapering 28 ileal loops and reimplanting them into the bladder, 19 attempts were completely successful, as was true in this patient. Nine patients required reoperation because of reflux. In six patients it was possible to make a longer tunnel, which stopped the reflux. These were basically good bladders, in which a longer tunnel could be made. Three were poor bladders, indicating that it had been an error in judgment to attempt implantation of a tapered loop in the first place. Ileocecal cystoplasty solved the problem in these small, noncompliant bladders. Avoiding the pitfalls learned from experience, which have been mentioned previously, should lead to a high success rate when implantation of a tapered bowel segment is necessary.

Patients with intestine in the urinary tract will notice mucus in their urine. Occasionally a blob of mucus will temporarily obstruct the urethra in a male during micturition. The amount of mucus, and the patient's awareness of it, seem to diminish in time. Late stricture is a well-known complication of ileal loop urinary diversions. We have encountered late stricture of a tapered bowel segment in three cases as well as in two other cases that were referred with untapered bowel serving as ureter (Hendren and McLorie, 1983). This underscores the need to maintain long-term, continuing surveillance of all patients with bowel in the urinary tract, especially when it has been used as a substitute ureter.

CASE 2 (Figs. 52–11 and 52–12)

A 15-year-old boy with the prune belly syndrome was referred in 1973 for possible undiversion. Bilateral nephrostomies had been done at birth. Later an ileal loop was done but it had never drained. The left ureter was obstructed by the left colic artery; the right kidney was blocked by ureteropelvic junction obstruc-

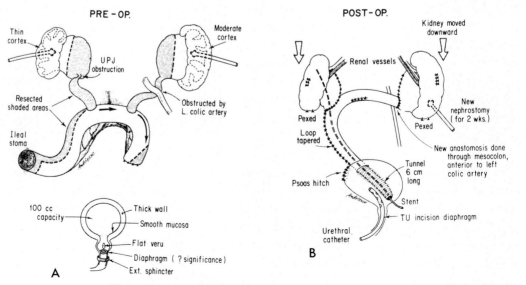

Figure 52–11. Case 2 before *(A)* and after *(B)* reconstruction.

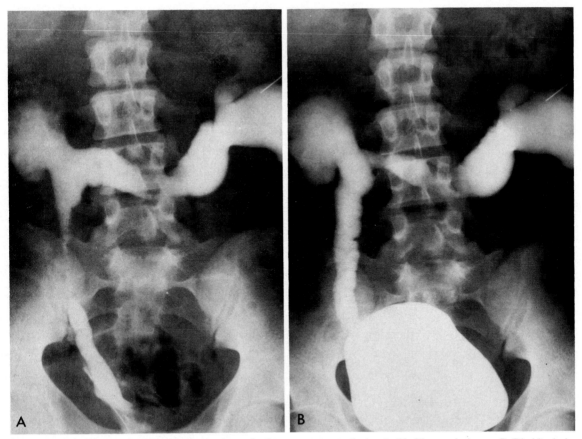

Figure 52–12. Case 2 antegrade perfusion pyelography 8 years postoperatively. *A,* Bladder on drainage. *B,* Bladder being allowed to fill during the study. Note needle in left kidney.

tion. An extensive reconstruction was performed, converting the conduit to a pyeloileal conduit to correct obstruction of both ureters. It was then tapered and implanted with a long tunnel to prevent reflux. It is now more than 10 years after reconstruction, and at age 25 years, the patient is of normal stature, is free from urinary infection, and has stable, though diminished, urinary function. A college graduate, he is an investment counselor and leads an essentially normal life. Renal transplantation may be necessary some day. That should not pose any special problems, because he is free from infection and has a refunctionalized lower urinary tract.

Comment. There were 12 patients with pyeloileal conduits among the 61 patients with ileal loops for undiversion. It is well recognized that patients with pyeloileal loops have the greatest degree of long-term deterioration when the loop drains into a bag on the abdominal wall. Thus these patients in particular can benefit from getting rid of their bags and diverting their drainage into the bladder, provided it is done in a manner that averts reflux.

CASE 3 (Figs. 52–13 and 52–14)

A 14-year-old boy was referred in 1982 with an ileal loop performed 8 years previously after failed ureteral reimplantation surgery. Hydrostatic stretching preoperatively increased the bladder size from about 50 ml to 250 ml. The boy was able to retain saline instilled into the bladder, and he could void it at will. At operation, both previously reimplanted lower ureters were too short to be useful. The strictured ileal loop also was unusable. Because the two kidneys and upper ureters were nearly normal, and this was a favorable bladder in which reimplantation of a ureter should be straightforward, autotransplantation of the right kidney was elected, draining the left one by transureteropyelostomy. The patient convalesced uneventfully following this lengthy operation. His lifestyle has been normal in the 2 years since reconstructive surgery. He is free of urinary infection and has normal renal function. He has been advised to avoid contact sports and other activities that would increase the likelihood of injury to the relatively unprotected kidney in his right lower quadrant.

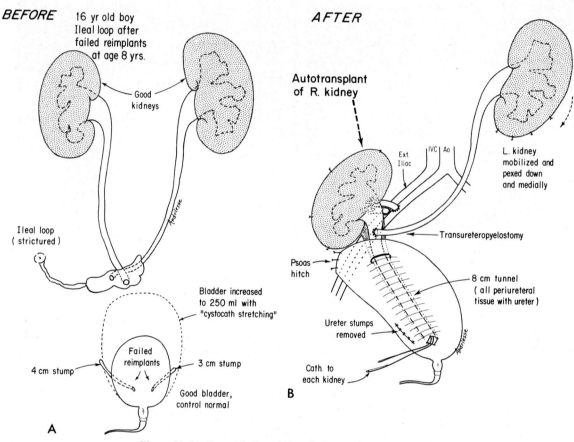

Figure 52–13. Case 3 before *(A)* and after *(B)* reconstruction.

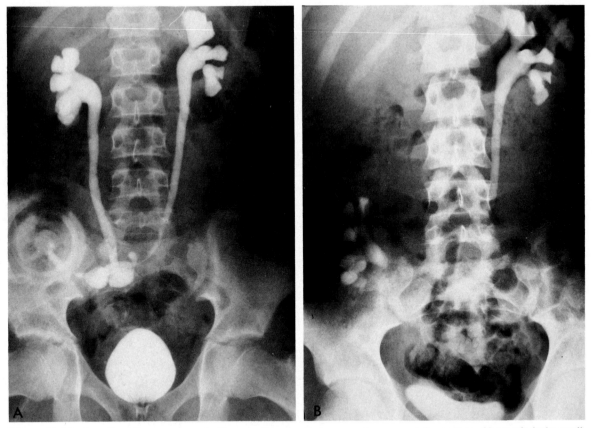

Figure 52–14. Case 3 roentgenograms. *A,* Preoperative simultaneous cystogram and loopogram. Note relatively small bladder and severely strictured ileal loop. *B,* IVP 1 year postoperatively. Note autotransplanted right kidney in right lower quadrant.

Comment. Autotransplantation is an option that can be considered in selected cases. I have felt it was justified in only two patients to date. Both had strictured ileal loops, raising the possibility that they might stricture a bowel segment to be used as a ureter. Both had basically two good kidneys, lending a margin of safety in case the transplanted kidney should sustain a serious complication (though that is a fairly low risk). In the majority of cases undiverted, another option was more appealing. This case, like most, could have been reconstructed by several different methods. It is vital to consider all possible methods in each case. Generally the best choice will be clear when all factors are taken into account, that is, renal function, length of the ureters, state of the bladder, and so on.

CASE 4 (Figs. 52–15 and 52–16)

A 15-year-old girl was referred in 1982 with an ileal loop that had been present for 10 years. The underlying problem was a neurogenic bladder secondary to sacral agenesis. YV plasty had been performed to the bladder neck at age 2

years for an inability to empty the bladder. Ileal loop was elected later because she was incontinent. Hydrostatic "cycling" of the bladder for 3 months showed that there was a small capacity and complete incontinence. From that it could be predicted that undiversion would require increasing outlet resistence as well as augmenting the bladder to provide a low-pressure reservoir of good size. The patient's neurologic deficit showed that she must be prepared to perform intermittent self-catheterization. In the 2 years since her reconstructive surgery this young woman has led a normal lifestyle. She is continent; she empties her bladder every 4 hours. There is no urinary infection. Postoperative urodynamic testing showed urethral resistence of 85 cm of water in a 3.5-cm-long urethra. The bladder held 400 ml. There was no reflux. When the bladder was filled to capacity, spontaneous cecal contractions were noted, but they did not generate pressures high enough to cause wetting.

Comment. Patients with neurogenic bladder create some of the most difficult decisions regarding undiversion. This is especially true

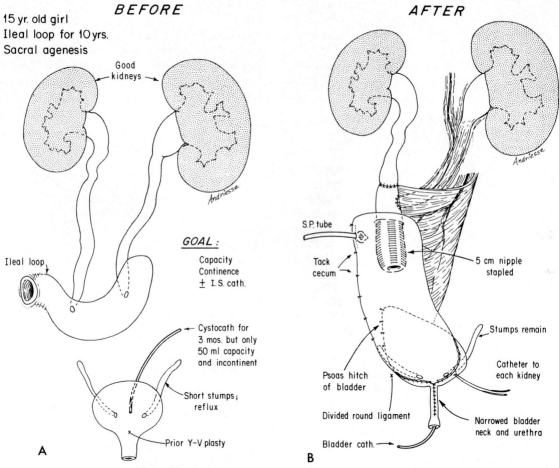

15 yr. old girl
Ileal loop for 10 yrs.
Sacral agenesis

BEFORE

AFTER

Good
kidneys

Ileal loop

GOAL :

Capacity
Continence
± I.S. cath.

Cystocath for
3 mos. but only
50 ml capacity
and incontinent

Short stumps;
reflux

Prior Y-V plasty

A

S.P. tube

Tack
cecum

5 cm nipple
stapled

Stumps remain

Psoas hitch
of bladder

Catheter to
each kidney

Divided round ligament

Narrowed bladder
neck and urethra

Bladder cath.

B

Figure 52–15. Case 4 before *(A)* and after *(B)* reconstruction.

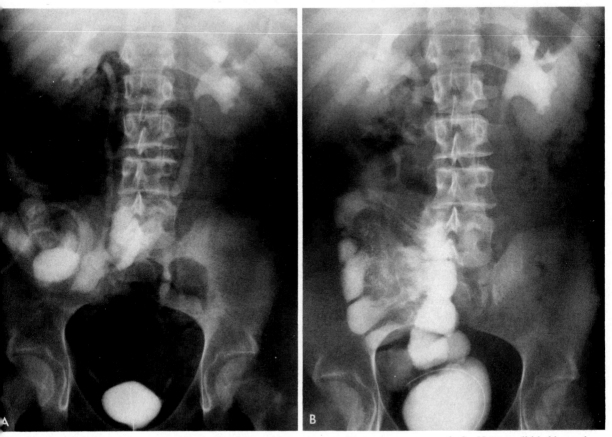

Figure 52–16. Case 4 roentgenograms. *A,* Simultaneous loopogram and cystogram preoperatively. Note small bladder and sacral agenesis. *B,* IVP 9 months postoperatively. Note cecal augmentation of small bladder and filling defect in the cecum, which is intussuscepted terminal ileum. Note staples in nipple.

when there is a prior urinary diversion that is functioning well—that is, without hydronephrosis, infection, stones, or other complications requiring reoperation. An extensive revamping of the urinary tract as in this procedure, which lasted 11 hours, could be a great risk to life if there were a technical misadventure. In a patient with good ureters and a suitable bladder, re-establishment of ureteral continuity or ureteral reimplantation into the bladder would be preferred; augmentation can be done with cecum, a patch of sigmoid, or a patch of small bowel. When joining a ureter to the bladder cannot be done, however, cecal augmentation can be used, preventing reflux with a nipple of terminal ileum.

Special mention should be made concerning prevention of reflux in ileocecal preparations. We have used several methods that work well when tested at the operating table and on early postoperative cystogram examination, but they tend to break down in time. These methods include wrapping the adjacent cecum around the terminal ileum, similar to gastroesophageal

fundoplication for reflux; removing the mesentery from the terminal ileum and creating an intussuscepted nipple 4 to 5 cm long; scarifying the seromuscular layer of the nipple to make its walls adhere; placing multiple sutures through the walls of the nipple to promote their adherence; and even placing four rows of staples longitudinally in the nipple. Although these nipples seem to do well in an isolated ileocecal conduit that is draining to the skin surface, in some cases the same preparation can become reduced when placed on the bladder, which intermittently distends it. It can then reflux. The technique I have used for the past year consists of creating a nipple and placing three rows of staples to maintain it. An incision is then made for the full length of an unstapled side of the nipple, transecting the ileocecal valve and then incising along the adjacent wall of the cecum, which will become the back wall of the augmented bladder. Two parallel running sutures are started at the base of the nipple, sewing it to the adjacent incision in the cecal wall. This technique appears to have maintained the integrity of those nipples created in the past year. It has also been used with success to repair some broken-down nipples that refluxed. The use of staples raises the possibility of stone formation. In my experience most staples become covered by mucosa. In three cases, however, small stones were seen clinging to staples at followup cystoscopy. The staples and stones were easily plucked out using alligator forceps through a cystoscope.

Artificial sphincters are being used today in some centers to create continence in patients like this. It is my opinion, however, that increasing outlet resistence and resorting to intermittent catheterization may prove safer and more satisfactory in the long run for most patients. There is still a substantial long-term failure rate with prosthetic devices. Narrowing the bladder neck does not "burn any bridges." If sphincter technology advances in the future to a point at which there is no failure rate from erosion (which I think is unlikely) or mechanical malfunction (which may well be possible), it would be relatively easy to open the previously narrowed bladder neck by endoscopic resection, to create incontinence, subsequently implanting an artificial sphincter.

CASE 5 (Figs. 52–17 and 52–18)

An 11-year-old girl was referred in 1978 with bilateral end ureterostomies, which she had since age 16 months. Her problem had started at age 3 months with reflux, which was treated by YV plasty to the bladder neck and ureteral reimplants. These failed, as did subsequent re-operation on both ureters, and so ureterostomy was performed. The bladder was small despite 3 weeks of hydrostatic stretching. However, it was possible to obtain one good ureteral reimplantation, draining the second side by transureteroureterostomy. Her bladder capacity was small initially, but it soon increased. Six years postoperatively, the patient is age 16 years and is leading the normal life of a teenage girl. She is continent even while doing competitive roller skating and is free from urinary infection.

Comment. It would be ideal to get two ureters reimplanted into the bladder in every case, but we have found this is usually impossible in undiversion cases. Also we have found that is not feasible in many patients requiring repeat ureteral reimplantation. Reimplanting the better ureter with a long tunnel and psoas hitch, relying on transureteroureterostomy for the second side, has proved to be a very satis-

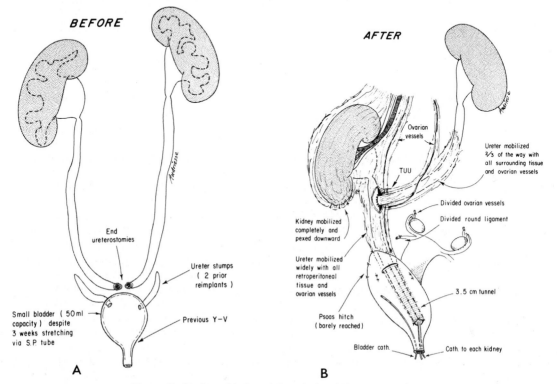

Figure 52–17. Case 5 before *(A)* and after *(B)* reconstruction.

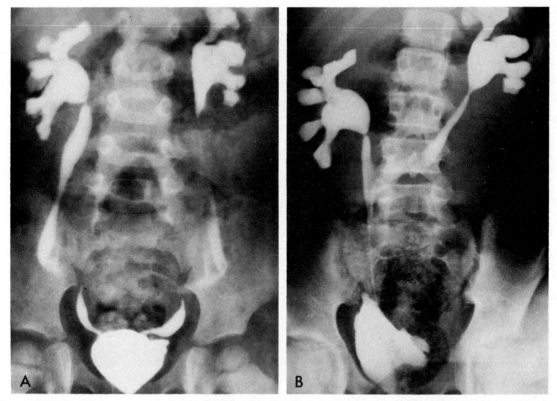

Figure 52–18. Case 5 roentgenograms. *(A),* Preoperative simultaneous cystogram and bilateral ureterograms. The short, previously reimplanted ureteral stumps were not usable. *B,* Retrograde pyelogram 1 year postoperatively (patient was allergic to IVP contrast medium).

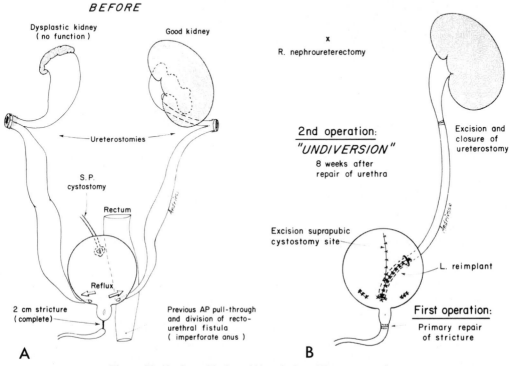

Figure 52–19. Case 6 before *(A)* and after *(B)* reconstruction.

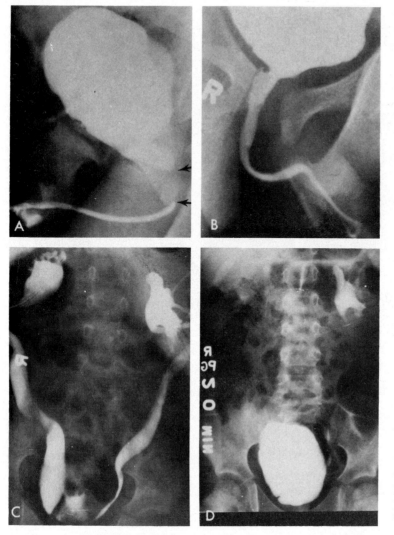

Figure 52–20. Case 6 roentgenograms. *A,* Preoperative cystourethrogram showing long stricture (arrows). *B,* Cystourethrogram after repair of stricture by excision and anastomosis. *C,* Preoperative ureterograms via the bilateral cutaneous loopureterostomies; right kidney was nonfunctional. *D,* IVP 1 year after undiversion. Note normal bladder and normal left ureter.

factory option (Hendren, 1980a). Although she has satisfactory control now, during the first year the small size of her bladder, together with less than normal outlet resistence from the prior YV plasty, caused some frequency and stress incontinence. Today, reconstruction of a similar case might include narrowing the bladder neck and augmentation with a patch of ileum. Despite the serious problems encountered in early infancy, this patient's total urinary function is within the range of normal.

CASE 6 (Figs. 52–19 and 52–20)

A 3-year-old boy was referred in 1977 with bilateral loop cutaneous ureterostomies, suprapubic cystostomy, and complete stricture of the membranous urethra. Imperforate anus had been treated by colostomy when he was a newborn. Subsequent urinary tract evaluation at 6

months disclosed urethral valves and hydronephrosis. Cutaneous vesicostomy was performed, but the bladder prolapsed, causing increasing hydronephrosis. Bilateral skin ureterostomies were performed. Later the valves were resected, and a rectal pull-through was done. The vesicostomy was closed and converted into a suprapubic cystostomy. Pyocystis was treated by antibiotic irrigations. Ileal loop urinary diversion was recommended but was declined by the parents, who then sought further advice.

Hydrostatic testing of the bladder showed good function despite previous diversion and pyocystis. At the first operation the urethral stricture was resected and continuity was reestablished by primary anastomosis. Eight weeks later undiversion was accomplished. This included removing the nonfunctional right kidney, closing the left ureterostomy, reimplanting the left ureter, and excising the suprapubic cystostomy site. Today, at age 10 years, 7 years following reconstruction, the patient is a happy, well-adjusted, normal boy. His renal function is normal.

Comment. This case illustrates several points. First, cutaneous vesicostomy was a simple procedure to perform, but it set the stage for a series of major complications. It failed to drain the bladder adequately (because of prolapse), following which ureterostomies were performed. It would have been better to resect the valves in the first place, probably followed by left ureteral reimplantation and right nephroureterectomy. Second, it is probable that complete stricture of the membranous urethra was caused by endoscopic resection of valves when there was a "dry urethra," that is, supravesical diversion of the urine. Rectal pull-through with division of the rectourethral fistula may also have contributed to that complication,

however. Ileal loop diversion was suggested elsewhere as being the best alternative, since reconstruction would be difficult and might be fraught with some uncertainties. It has been my experience, however, that many more bad results come from trying to get by with a lesser procedure, as compared with doing a major reconstructive operation that is well planned and skillfully performed. In performing reconstructive surgery in patients who have undergone loop ureterostomy, I have found that it is usually best to do the entire reconstruction at one procedure—that is, repair the obstructive problem and close the ureterostomies simultaneously (Hendren, 1978*b*).

CASE 7 (Figs. 52–21 and 52–22)

A 7-year-old girl was referred in 1978 with a nonfunctional bladder, obstructed ureterosigmoidostomies with infection and hydrone-

Figure 52–21. Case 7 before *(A)* and after *(B)* reconstructive operations.

Illustration continued on following page

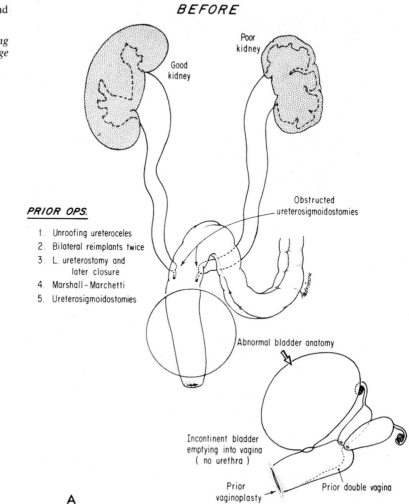

BEFORE

Good kidney

Poor kidney

PRIOR OPS.

1. Unroofing ureteroceles
2. Bilateral reimplants twice
3. L. ureterostomy and later closure
4. Marshall-Marchetti
5. Ureterosigmoidostomies

Obstructed ureterosigmoidostomies

Abnormal bladder anatomy

Incontinent bladder emptying into vagina (no urethra)

Prior vaginoplasty

Prior double vagina

A

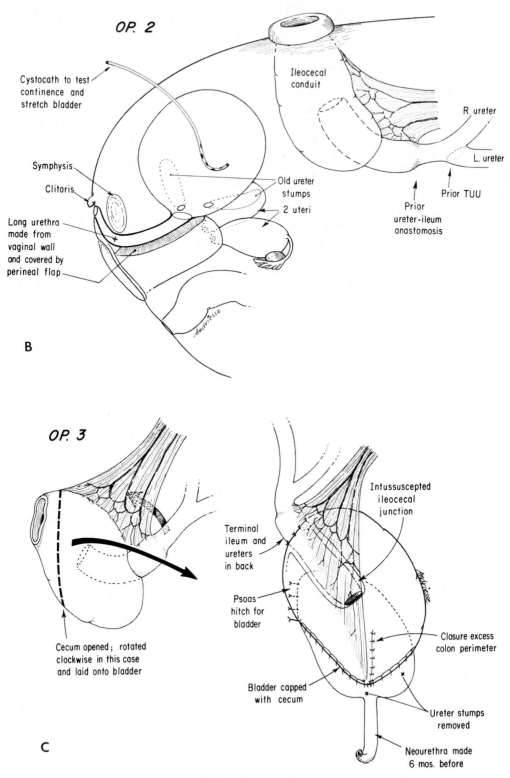

OP. 2

Cystocath to test continence and stretch bladder

Ileocecal conduit

R. ureter

L. ureter

Prior TUU

Prior ureter-ileum anastomosis

Old ureter stumps

2 uteri

Symphysis

Clitoris

Long urethra made from vaginal wall and covered by perineal flap

Andriesse

B

OP. 3

Intussuscepted ileocecal junction

Terminal ileum and ureters in back

Psoas hitch for bladder

Closure excess colon perimeter

Cecum opened; rotated clockwise in this case and laid onto bladder

Bladder capped with cecum

Ureter stumps removed

Neourethra made 6 mos. before

C

Figure 52–21 *Continued.*

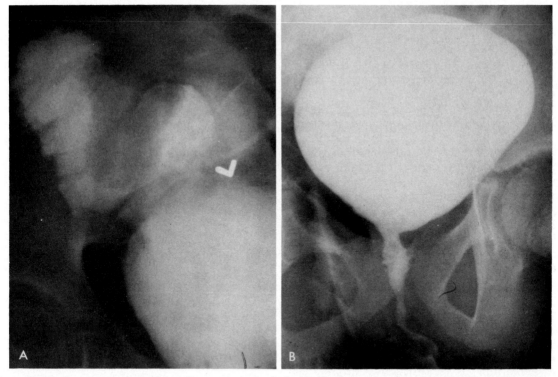

Figure 52–22. Case 7 cystourethrograms 2 years postoperatively. *A,* Cecal augmentation of bladder. Note filling defect in cecum, which is the terminal ileum intussuscepted as a nipple to prevent reflux. Today, the nipple is held with three rows of staples and is also sewn to adjacent back wall of cecum. *B,* Bladder and distal urethra fashioned from a tube of anterior vaginal wall and introitus, covered by a pedicle flap from buttocks. The patient has normal bladder volume. She can void without difficulty, and she is completely continent.

phrosis, and rectal incontinence of stool and urine. Multiple previous operations had been performed. They included vaginoplasty, unroofing of ureteroceles, two ureteral reimplantations, left ureterostomy and later closure, and Marshall-Marchetti suspension of the bladder neck. An ileocecal conduit was fashioned first to deal with the problem of recurrent pyelonephritis. This stopped the problem of recurrent pyelonephritis and got the patient socially continent and free from the malodorous problem of combined urinary and fecal incontinence, which prevented her from attending school. A urethra was constructed 6 months later by tubularizing the anterior wall of the vagina and the introitus (Hendren, 1980b and c; 1982). This neourethra extended from the high opening of the bladder near the cervix out to the clitoris. Later, testing the bladder through suprapubic instillation of saline showed satisfactory function—that is, the ability to hold water and void it at will. The bladder capacity was small. Six months later the ileocecal conduit was taken down and added on to the bladder. Now age 13 years, 4 years following undiversion, this child is doing well. She is continent, free of infection, and has stable renal function.

Comment. Several points are illustrated by this case: (1) Most pediatric urologic malformations can be solved if the proper operation is performed in the first place. Unroofing ureteroceles has little place in modern reconstructive urology. It will uniformly create reflux. (2) Reoperation for failed ureteral reimplants is a difficult undertaking. Often, reimplanting both ureters for a second time will not work, whereas reimplanting one ureter with the adjunct of psoas hitch and draining the other by transureteroureterostomy will solve the problem. (3) Marshall-Marchetti suspension of the bladder neck would not be expected to improve incontinence in a patient lacking resistence from congenital absence of the urethra. That can be best dealt with by creating a urethra using the vaginal wall and a flap from the adjacent buttocks. (4) Ureterosigmoidostomy is certain to fail when the ureters are dilated and scarred from previous surgery. These factors will usually allow colo-ureteral reflux, which will result in pyelonephritis, stones, and eventual upper tract deterioration. (5) The ileocecal preparation can provide a good way to achieve nonrefluxing urinary diversion, when that is needed, as well as providing a means for augmenting the bladder and preventing vesicoureteral reflux when ureteral reimplantation is not possible.

CONCLUSION

Urinary diversion by ileal conduit in children is not the panacea that it once appeared to be in the 1950's and 1960's. Because they have reflux, upper tract deterioration is common (Hendren and Radopoulos, 1983; Middleton and Hendren, 1976; Pitts and Muecke, 1979; Retik et al., 1967). Further, it leaves much to be desired in lifestyle. Many of these problems are best treated today by other means, which include reconstructive surgery for various obstructive uropathies and incontinence, and intermittent catheterization for selected patients with myelodysplasia. In the relatively few patients who will still require urinary diversion, we firmly believe that it is best to use a nonrefluxing colon segment or ileocolic segment (Althausen et al., 1982; Richie and Skinner, 1975; Richie et al., 1974; Skinner et al., 1975; Zinman and Libertino, 1975).

There are many patients who had previous urinary diversions by ileal loop and other methods who deserve re-evaluation for possible undiversion. Success requires knowledge of a wide armamentarium in reconstructive urology as well as meticulous attention to all technical details.

Poor renal function is not a contraindication to undiversion, in my opinion. Indeed, patients with marginal function whose urinary tracts are reconstructed are better candidates for ultimate transplantation. All patients with decreased renal function are followed in close collaboration with the nephrology service to optimize their dietary and metabolic management.

The quality of life, control of infection, and preservation of renal function is better in patients who have a functioning urinary tract, when compared with those who are living with various types of urinary diversion.

References

Althausen, A. F., Hagen-Cook, K., and Hendren, W. H.: Non-refluxing colon conduit: Experience with 70 cases. J. Urol., *120*:35, 1982.

Bricker, E. M.: Bladder substitution after pelvic evisceration. Surg. Clin. North Am., *30*:1511, 1950.

Hendren, W. H.: Posterior urethral valves in boys: A broad clinical spectrum. J. Urol., *106*:298, 1971.

Hendren, W. H.: Reconstruction of previously diverted urinary tracts in children. J. Pediatr. Surg., *8*:135, 1973.

Hendren, W. H.: Urethral Valves: Diagnosis and Endoscopic Resection. Eaton Film Library, 1974*a*.

Hendren, W. H.: Urinary tract refunctionalization after prior diversion in children. Ann. Surg., *180*:494, 1974*b*.

Hendren, W. H.: Non-refluxing colon conduit for temporary or permanent urinary diversion in children. J. Pediatr. Surg., *10*:381, 1975.

Hendren, W. H.: Urinary diversion and undiversion in children. Surg. Clin. North Am., *56*:425, 1976.

Hendren, W. H.: Urinary tract undiversion. *In*, Ravitch, M. M., Welch, K. J., Benson, C. D. et al. (Eds.): Pediatric Surgery, 3rd ed. Chicago, Year Book Medical Publishers Inc., p. 1275, 1979.

Hendren, W. H.: Some alternatives to urinary diversion in children. J. Urol., *119*:652, 1978*a*.

Hendren, W. H.: Complications of ureterostomy. J. Urol., *120*:269, 1978*b*.

Hendren, W. H.: Reoperative ureteral reimplantation: Management of the difficult case. J. Pediatr. Surg., *15*:770, 1980*a*.

Hendren, W. H.: Construction of female urethra from vaginal wall and a perineal flap. J. Urol., *123*:657, 1980*b*.

Hendren, W. H.: Reconstructive problems of the vagina and the female urethra. Clin. Plast. Surg., *7*:207, 1980*c*.

Hendren, W. H.: Further experience in reconstructive surgery for cloacal anomalies. J. Pediatr. Surg., *17*:695, 1982.

Hendren, W. H., and Hensle, T. W.: Transureteroureterostomy: Experience with 75 cases. J. Urol., *123*:826, 1980.

Hendren, W. H., and McLorie, G. A.: Late stricture of intestinal ureter. J. Urol., *129*:584, 1983.

Hendren, W. H., and Radopoulos, D.: Complications of ileal loop and colon conduit urinary diversion. Urol. Clin. North Am., *10*:451, 1983.

Hodges, C. V., Moore, R. J., Lehman, T. H., and Behnam, A. M: Clinical experiences with transureteroureterostomy. J. Urol., *90*:552, 1963.

Johnston, J. H.: Temporary cutaneous ureterostomy in the management of advanced congenital urinary obstruction. Arch. Dis. Child., *38*:161, 1963.

Kogan, S. J., Kim, K., and Levitt, S. B.: Preoperative evaluation of bladder function prior to renal transplantation or urinary tract reconstruction in children: Description of a method. J. Pediatr. Surg., *11*:1007, 1976.

Middleton, A. W., Jr., and Hendren, W. H.: Ileal conduits in children at the Massachusetts General Hospital from 1955 to 1970. J. Urol., *115*:591, 1976.

Perlmutter, A. D., and Patil, J.: Loop cutaneous ureterostomy in infants and young children: Late results in 32 cases. J. Urol., *107*:655, 1972.

Pitts, W. R., Jr., and Muecke, E. C.: A 20 year experience with ileal conduits: The fate of the kidneys. J. Urol., *122*:154, 1979.

Retik, A. B., Perlmutter, A. D., and Gross, R. E.: Cutaneous ureteroileostomy in children. N. Engl. J. Med., *277*:217, 1967.

Richie, J. P., and Skinner, D. G.: Urinary diversion: The physiological rationale for non-refluxing colonic conduits. Br. J. Urol., *47*:269, 1975.

Richie, J. P., Skinner, D. G., and Waisman, J.: The effect of reflux on the development of pyelonephritis in urinary diversion: An experimental study. J. Surg. Res., *16*:256, 1974.

Skinner, D. G., Gottesman, J. E., and Richie, J. P.: The isolated sigmoid segment: Its value in temporary urinary diversion and reconstruction. J. Urol., *113*:614, 1975.

Zinman, L., and Libertino, J. A.: Ileocecal conduit for temporary and permanent diversion. J. Urol., *113*:317, 1975.

CHAPTER 53

Prune-Belly Syndrome

JOHN R. WOODARD, M.D.
TIMOTHY S. TRULOCK, M.D.

Prune-belly syndrome is the most common term for congenital absence, deficiency, or hypoplasia of the abdominal musculature accompanied by a large hypotonic bladder, dilated and tortuous ureters, and bilateral cryptorchidism (Osler, 1901). Because of the abdominal musculature–urinary tract–testicular involvement, the term "triad syndrome" (Stephens, 1963) is often used but is unsatisfactory, since it gives no indication of the nature of the disorder and since there are more than three characteristic anomalies. Another popular eponym is Eagle-Barrett syndrome. The syndrome occurs primarily in boys and is rare, with the incidence reported to be approximately 1 in 35,000 to 50,000 live births (Garlinger and Ott, 1974). Despite its rarity, the syndrome holds great interest for the urologist.

Historically, infants born with the full-blown syndrome have carried a poor prognosis for long-term survival, with a high percentage dying from urinary sepsis or renal failure, or both (Barnhouse, 1972; Burke et al., 1969; Lattimer, 1958; McGovern and Marshall, 1959). Although the prognosis has certainly improved in recent years, we have witnessed a controversy between those who believe that more aggressive surgical reconstruction of the urinary tract might improve a lot of these unfortunate infants (Hendren, 1972; Jeffs et al., 1977; Randolph et al., 1981a; Woodard and Parrott, 1978a) and those who advocate limited, if any, surgical intervention (Duckett, 1980; Woodhouse et al., 1979).

Although in rare instances a girl is affected by the absence of abdominal muscles, it is exceptional to find the characteristic urinary tract anomaly in the female at the same time. The fully developed syndrome occurs almost exclusively in males. A great many questions remain to be answered concerning etiology, pathogenesis, proper management of the uropathy (both upper and lower tract), and proper management of cryptorchidism.

Infants with prune-belly syndrome may be born after entirely normal pregnancies, but oligohydramnios is more the rule and is responsible for some of the associated and complicating conditions, especially those of the pulmonary and skeletal variety. Although the availability of diagnostic fetal ultrasound makes it possible for a presumptive diagnosis of prune-belly syndrome to be made in utero, it appears unlikely that a fetal diagnosis will have much impact upon clinical management. The appearance of the neonate is characteristic (Fig. 53–1) and now well known to neonatologists and pediatricians. The abdominal wall is thin and lax. Because of the sparsity of subcutaneous tissue it tends to crease and wrinkle like a wizened prune.

The cause of the prune-belly syndrome remains unknown. It has been suggested that both the abdominal wall defect and the intra-abdominal cryptorchidism are secondary to distension of the urinary tract. Obstruction in the posterior urethra is a possible cause of this distension and would explain the predominance of male patients. This theory suggests that testicular descent is blocked by a distended bladder and that the abdominal wall defect is secondary to the urinary tract distension. Another commonly quoted theory is that a primary mesodermal error might account for both the abdominal wall defect and the genitourinary abnormalities, since both arise from the paraxial, intermediate, and lateral plate mesoderm (Smith, 1970). More recently, a number of investigators (Monie and Monie, 1979; Moer-

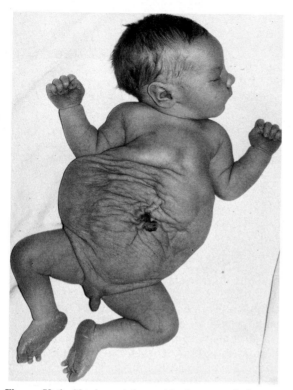

Figure 53–1. Newborn infant with the prune-belly syndrome, showing the characteristic appearance of the abdominal wall, the empty scrotum, and the talipes equinovarus.

man et al., 1984) have suggested that prostatic dysgenesis and fetal ascites are key factors in the causation of the syndrome, with the fetal ascites causing the abdominal wall defect. Although ascites is rarely present in patients with prune-belly syndrome, it is speculated that ascites is transient, with reabsorption toward the end of gestation. It has also been recently suggested that it is caused by a complex chromosomal mutation (Riccardi and Grum, 1977).

PATHOPHYSIOLOGY

Abdominal Wall Defect

Despite the fact that most affected infants have similar appearances, the abdominal wall defect may be quite variable. It is often asymmetric and patchy in distribution. Characteristically, the abdominal muscles are absent in the lower and medial parts of the abdominal wall, though the upper rectus muscles and outer oblique muscles are developed. Some (Welch and Kearney, 1974) claim that the muscles are present but hypoplastic, whereas others (Afifi et al., 1972) find the deficiency to range from

slight hypoplasia to complete absence of muscles. Secondary atrophy interspersed with some muscles that are hypertrophied (Mininburg et al., 1973) has also been reported.

The flanks often bulge markedly, with the thorax demonstrating a secondary flaring at the costal margins. This poor support for the lower chest wall interferes with an effective cough mechanism and contributes to a greater vulnerability to respiratory infections. These children also have difficulty in sitting up from the supine position. Although the wrinkled appearance is typical of the abdominal wall in the infant, the older child tends to take on a pot-bellied appearance (Fig. 53–2).

Surprisingly, the defective abdominal wall has caused little difficulty for operating surgeons. Wound healing proceeds satisfactorily despite the absence of layers for suturing. Wound dehiscence and other wound complications have been rare.

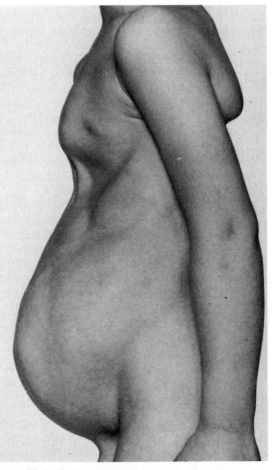

Figure 53–2. Older child with the prune-belly syndrome, showing the absence of wrinkling, the "potbelly" appearance, and the consequent deformity of the lower ribs.

Kidney

Although the kidneys may be normal, renal dysplasia and hydronephrosis are the two renal abnormalities typically associated with the syndrome. Often the prognosis is actually determined by the degree of dysplasia, which seems to be more severe in those patients having urethral stenosis, megalourethra, or imperforate anus (Potter, 1972). The spectrum may vary widely from marked dysplasia to a totally normal histologic appearance, and the findings are often asymmetric. For example, a completely dysplastic, multicystic kidney may be present on one side with normal renal histologic characteristics on the other.

Most patients with prune-belly syndrome will have some degree of hydronephrosis, which may vary from mild to severe and does not appear related to the degree of abdominal wall deficiency. The degree of hydronephrosis is often less than anticipated from the degree of dilatation of the ureter. It is also common to find the renal parenchyma to be thicker and of better quality than might be expected from the degree of distortion in the drainage system. Although these findings have prognostic importance, they also suggest that the mechanism for the hydronephrosis might differ from that of other obstructive uropathies.

The infundibula are often long and narrow, whereas the renal pelvis may vary from small to large. Occasional patients might also have ureteropelvic junction obstructions, and this possibility must not be overlooked in deciding upon a plan of management for the patient. The function in these hydronephrotic kidneys is often surprisingly good, and it appears to be infection rather than obstruction per se that leads to their deterioration.

Ureter

The ureters are characterized by varying degrees of tortuosity and dilatation. Although the tortuosity and dilatation are segmental in distribution, the lower end of the ureter tends to be the most severely affected, with the upper ureter in many patients being actually surprisingly small in caliber (Fig. 53–3). Fluoroscopic studies may reveal poor ureteral peristalsis, but function does seem to improve after surgical straightening and tapering or, in some patients, simply after growth and elongation have occurred. Histologically, the ureteral wall demonstrates fibrosis and a scarcity of muscle bundles (Palmer and Tesluk, 1974). Some have also found a decrease in nerve plexuses (Ehrlich and Brown, 1977). The ureterovesical junction is markedly abnormal in most patients, and vesicoureteral reflux is present in most but not all

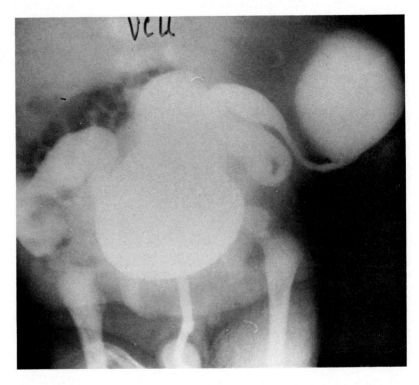

Figure 53–3. Cystogram showing massive bilateral vesicoureteral reflux. Note the marked difference in caliber of the left upper ureter as compared with the lower ureter.

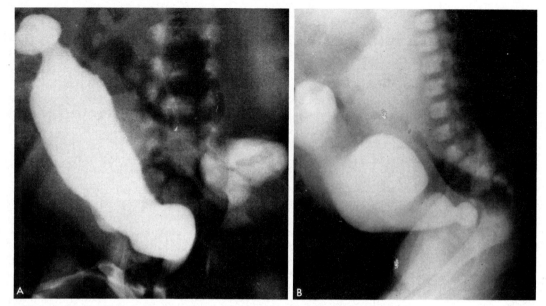

Figure 53–4. *A* and *B*, Voiding cystograms in two patients, showing the pseudodiverticulum configuration of the dome of the bladder. Note the wide, triangular prostatic urethra in both cystograms and the small utricular diverticulum in *B*.

of these ureters. The difference in functional and morphologic quality of the upper and lower ureters is an important consideration in planning corrective surgery, and it may explain some of the failures seen when the distal ureter was used in reconstructive procedures.

Bladder and Urachus

The prune-belly bladder is typically very large and irregular in outline and has a thick

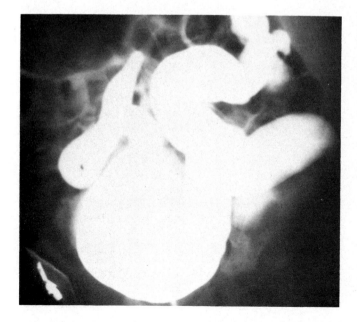

wall. This does not represent true bladder wall hypertrophy, however, and actual trabeculation is unusual. The apex of the bladder is attached to the abdominal wall at the umbilicus. Often, the dome of the bladder will bulge to resemble a pseudodiverticulum (Fig. 53–4). The trigone is very large—at times enormous—with the ureteral orifices posteriorly placed and quite wide apart. Vesicoureteral reflux is commonly present (Fig. 53–5) though, surprisingly, is not demonstrable in some patients. The bladder neck tends to be wide, relaxed, and ill-defined. In

Figure 53–5. Cystogram in a boy with prune-belly syndrome, showing massive bilateral reflux. The upper ureter has an abrupt upper termination without any filling of the renal pelvis, an appearance that is characteristic of the multicystic kidney.

many patients, voiding pressures and urine flow rates are normal, and some are capable of emptying their bladders completely. Others, however, will have significant postvoid residual urine because of unbalanced voiding mechanisms (Snyder et al., 1976). Interestingly, some investigators have reported improved voiding patterns with increasing age (Lee, 1977), whereas others (Williams, 1979) have seen the residual urine increase in age in some patients.

The urachus may be patent. This is likely with urethral atresia but may also occur in some patients without definite urethral obstruction.

Prostate

Below the wide bladder neck, the prostatic urethra has a dilated and somewhat triangular configuration (Fig. 53–6). It tapers to a relatively narrow point in the membranous portion of the urethra at the urogenital diaphragm. On the voiding cystourethrogram, this may produce a configuration that resembles a posterior urethral valve. The coincidental occurrence of a true urethral valve in a patient with prune-belly syndrome must be quite rare. In most cases there is no clear-cut obstruction at this point, even though some obstructive element, occurring perhaps in utero, must be postulated. In a few cases there is complete atresia of the membranous area of the urethra, with consequent

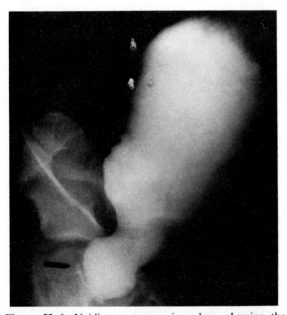

Figure 53–6. Voiding cystogram in a boy, showing the abrupt narrowing of urethra and apex of the wide, triangular prostatic portion. Note the utricular diverticulum (arrow).

destruction of the upper tract. A tubular diverticulum commonly arises from the level of the verumontanum. It is assumed to be of utricular origin (Kroovand et al., 1982). During voiding urethrography, reflux of contrast material into the ejaculatory ducts is also occasionally seen.

Histologic studies of autopsy specimens have revealed a lack of development of the epithelial elements of the prostate gland (Deklerk and Scott, 1978; Moermann et al., 1984). This prostatic hypoplasia or dysgenesis may be a factor in etiology (Monie and Monie, 1979), and it appears to explain the configuration of the prostatic urethra as seen on radiologic studies.

There is little information regarding ejaculation or sexual function in men with prune-belly syndrome, but no cases of fertility can be documented. Recent data suggests that erection and orgasm are normal, but that retrograde ejaculation is common (Woodhouse and Snyder, 1984).

Urethra

The anterior urethra and the penis are normal in most patients with prune-belly syndrome. However, it is well known that congenital megalourethra is occasionally associated with the syndorme (Sellers et al., 1976). In one reported series (Kroovand et al., 1982) this association has been rather prominent, and other anomalies of the penis, including dorsal chordee, ventral cordee, hypospadias, and absence of the corporal bodies were noted.

Testis

Bilateral cryptorchidism is characteristic of the syndrome and, in most patients, both testes lie intra-abdominally, usually overlying the ureter at the pelvic brim near the sacroiliac level. The etiology of this particular cryptorchidism is not known, but it is reasonable to speculate that it might be different from cryptorchidism seen in otherwise normal children. It has been suggested that the failure of descent is the result of the absence of abdominal muscles, absence of the gubernaculum, or an intrinsic abnormality of the testis itself (Nunn and Stevens, 1961; Williams and Burkholder, 1967). Although some observers have noted the testicular histologic appearance to be normal for the age of the patient when the testis is biopsied (Nunn and Stevens, 1961) more recent observations

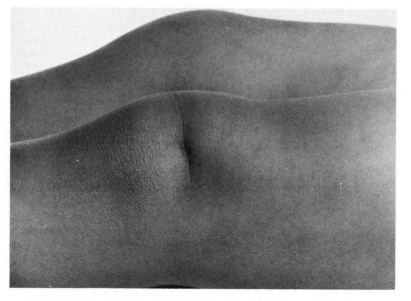

Figure 53–7. The dimple on the outer aspect of the knee characteristic of the prune-belly syndrome.

suggest an absence of spermatogonia in these patients (Uehling, 1982, Hadziselimovic, 1984). Others (Woodhouse and Snyder, 1984) report some patients with spermatogenesis. It has been speculated by some that the neoplastic potential of these testes was not the same as for other intra-abdominal testes. This may not be the case, however, since there are now several reports of neoplasms developing in such testes (Woodhouse et al., 1979; Duckett, 1980). The short spermatic vessels make orchiopexy a difficult operation to perform in these patients.

Limb Deformities

Various orthopedic anomalies of the limbs are commonly associated with and are probably the direct result of fetal compression secondary to oligohydramnios. The most frequent and most benign finding is a dimple on the outer aspect of the knee or elbow (Fig. 53–7) at which point the skin is adherent to the underlying joint structures. It is of no great clinical significance. However, more severe limb deficiencies have been reported in as many as 3 per cent of the patients (Carey et al., 1982). Since there are no reported cases of upper extremity deficiency with this syndrome, the lower limb abnormalities are thought to be due to compression of the iliac vessels from a markedly distended bladder (Ralis and Forbes, 1971). Club feet and, less commonly, congenital hip dislocation are other orthopedic anomalies found with some fre-

quency (Tuck and Smith, 1978). More than half of the patients reported since 1958 have had some musculoskeletal deformity and, as survival improves, the orthopedic surgeon will undoubtedly play a greater role in the future management of these patients.

Gastrointestinal Anomalies

Most individuals with this syndrome have intestinal malrotation secondary to a universal mesentary with an unattached cecum (Silverman and Huang, 1950). Much less frequent is imperforate anus, which is more likely to occur in association with urethral atresia and renal dysplasia (Morgan et al., 1978). Gasroschisis and Hirschsprung disease have also been reported in these patients (Willert et al., 1978; Cawthern et al., 1979). Constipation also appears to be a problem that is secondary to the deficiency of the abdominal musculature, and it may lead to an acquired megacolon. Splenic torsion has also been reported (Heydenrych and DuToit, 1978).

Heart Abnormalities

Ventricular septal defect, atrial septal defect, and tetrology of Fallot occur with increased frequency in this population. It has been estimated that the incidence of heart abnormalities is approximately 10 per cent (Adebonojo, 1973).

CLINICAL PRESENTATION AND NATURAL HISTORY

Prenatal Diagnosis

With the increased use of diagnostic ultrasound to monitor the fetus during pregnancy, there have been several reports of prenatal diagnosis of the prune-belly syndrome (Bovicelli et al., 1980; Christopher et al., 1982; Shih et al., 1982; Smythe, 1981). The sonographic findings include markedly dilated ureters, enlarged bladder, and a flaccid-appearing abdominal wall. Fetal ascites has also been detected (Monie and Monie, 1979). The diagnosis seems to be most readily made at about the 30th week of gestation but can be detected as early as 20 weeks (Okulski, 1977). At present, the role of fetal intervention for the prune-belly syndrome is undefined.

Neonate

Although all cases should be recognized by the pediatrician on routine postnatal examination, there is a considerable variablility in the severity of the disorder and in the urgency with which urologic advice is sought. This is obviously a syndrome with a spectrum, and patients can be placed in groups according to severity. The classification shown in Table 53–1 is simple and clinically useful.

Category I includes those neonates with severe pulmonary difficulty or marked renal dysplasia, either of which precludes survival beyond the first days of life. In some of these infants, there will be a patent urachus and complete urethral obstruction. They are not subject to successful treatment. The more severely affected babies in this category might be stillborn. Because of severe oligohydramnios, others may have some of the features described in cases of renal agenesis, such as Potter facies. The serum creatinine level is normal at birth but rises steadily thereafter. If these babies do not die quickly from pulmonary hypoplasia, they succumb only slightly later from renal failure. Drainage procedures will result in a very scanty flow of dilute urine. In a few of these cases, when there appears to be a possible chance for survival, a simple drainage procedure such as vesicostomy may be justified.

Patients in Category II have the potential to survive the neonatal period. They have the typical, full-blown uropathy with diffuse dilatation of the urinary tract and hydronephrosis. Renal dysplasia may exist, but it is unilateral or less severe than in those patients in Category I. Most of these infants are able to void urine from the bladder and often do so with apparent ease. Others suffer a general failure to thrive, with enormous abdominal distension. It should be emphasized that all such infants should be transferred to expert units before any instrumentation is permitted.

Included in Category III are those infants with definite but relatively mild or incomplete features of the syndrome. Some uropathy is present, but the renal parenchyma is apparently of high quality, and urinary stasis is generally less marked. There is general agreement that patients in Category III may require little if any urologic reconstructive surgery. However, they may later show signs of progressive upper tract deterioration, particularly if they are prone to urinary infection. They will also be candidates for treatment of their cryptorchidism. It is evident that all surviving patients in any of these categories require long-term surveillance and supervision.

Pulmonary Aspects

Infants born with prune-belly syndrome are subject to a variety of pulmonary complications. Alford categorized his patients into two major groups.

The first group included those with pulmonary hypoplasia (Fig. 53–8) secondary to oligohydramnios. The hypoplasia is thought to result from external uterine pressure on the fetal thorax, causing an arrest in the growth of the lung. Pneumomediastinum or pneumothorax are common occurrences in patients with hy-

TABLE 1. The Spectrum of the Prune Belly Syndrome

Distinguishing Characteristics	Category Classification
Oligohydramnios, pulmonary hypoplasia, or pneumothorax. May have urethral obstruction or patent urachus and club foot.	I
Typical external features and uropathy of the full blown syndrome but no immediate problem with survival. May have mild or unilateral renal dysplasia. May or may not develop urosepsis or gradual azotemia.	II
External features may be mild or incomplete. Uropathy is less severe and renal function stable.	III

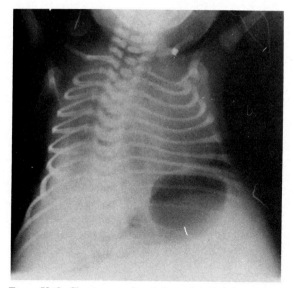

Figure 53–8. Chest x-ray of an infant who died shortly after birth from pulmonary hypoplasia.

poplastic lungs. Neonates in this category commonly die from respiratory failure, but if the patient does survive the neonatal period, the lungs will grow and eventually attain adequate capacity. As the patient becomes older, he still may have respiratory problems secondary to the deficiency of accessory respiratory muscles in the abdominal wall.

Alford's second category includes those patients who are prone to lobar atelectasis and pneumonia. Since the abdominal muscles are important in powerful expiration, patients with prune-belly syndrome have a decreased ability to cough effectively, thus making them more vulnerable to complications during periods of excess mucus production. A number of anesthetic complications have been reported (Hannington-Kiff, 1970; Karamanian et al., 1974). Sedatives and analgesics must be used judiciously so that respiratory depression may be avoided. Apnea monitors play an important role in the neonatal surveillance of these patients.

Adult Presentation

The diagnosis of the prune-belly syndrome is usually made in the neonatal period and almost always during early infancy. However, an occasional, rare patient will escape diagnosis until adulthood. Such patients have been known to present with hypertension and renal insufficiency (Lee, 1977), and others have been seen in middle life with renal insufficiency but no hypertension (Asplund and Laska, 1975). One

would expect such a patient to have renal insufficiency, though not all patients who have presented as adults have had diminished kidney function. Texter and Koontz (1980) reported a 33-year-old man with prune-belly syndrome who presented with decreased libido but had normal renal function.

There is, in fact, a paucity of literature concerning adults with the prune-belly syndrome. Patients have been reported who seem to do well with little if any treatment during their younger years only to succumb to urinary sepsis as adults (Culp and Flocks, 1954).

Female Syndrome

Of all patients properly labeled as having prune-belly syndrome only approximately 3 per cent are genetic females. When higher percentages are quoted, the criteria for diagnosis appear less strict. Affected females appear to have no urethral abnormality. The defect involves the abdominal wall, bladder, and upper urinary tract (Rabinowitz and Schillinger, 1977). Actually, fewer than 20 cases of the female syndrome have been reported, and the principles of management are essentially the same as for male patients. Many of the females have had incomplete forms of the syndrome with normal upper urinary tracts. The syndrome has also been reported in a patient with the Turner (XO karotype) syndrome (Lubinsky et al., 1980).

Incomplete Syndrome

Although it is exceptionally rare to encounter a normal urinary tract in association with the characteristic abdominal wall defect, the converse is not unusual. Some patients with a normal or relatively normal abdominal wall will exhibit many or all of the internal urologic features, usually in a less severe form. This may include dysplastic or dysmorphic kidneys; dilated, tortuous ureters; a large-capacity bladder; and the typical configuration of the bladder neck and prostatic urethra. It is important to avoid labeling those cases with only localized abnormality as incomplete prune-belly syndrome.

GENETIC ASPECTS

The genetic basis of the prune-belly syndrome is still the subject of controversy and speculation. Some suspect that a single gene defect might be responsible (Garlinger and Ott, 1974), whereas others propose that it might result from different genes producing identical results (Riccardi and Grum, 1977). The latter theory proposed that the anomaly might represent a superficial X-linkage mimicry. There is, in fact, other evidence to support a sex-linked inheritance (Adenyokunnu et al., 1975; Lockhart et al., 1979; Adenyokunnu and Familusi, 1982; Woodard, 1978), and the occurrence of prune-belly syndrome in siblings has now been reported several times. In counseling parents of infants with prune-belly syndrome, it is important to make them aware of a possibility of a recurrence in a subsequent sibling, though the degree of risk is, at present, unknown.

Of great interest is the association between twinning and the prune-belly syndrome. Among all pregnancies, the incidence of twinning is about 1 in 80, whereas the incidence of twinning among patients with prune-belly syndrome is about 1 in 23, or four times greater than normal (Ives, 1974). All reported pairs of twins are discordant for the syndrome. The possibility of a normal monozygotic twin must be kept in mind if a kidney donor should be needed for a patient with prune-belly syndrome who develops chroic renal failure.

The karyotype is normal in most prune-belly patients. Only a few cases of chromosomal abnormalities have been reported, including one with a minute additional chromosome (Halbrecht et al., 1972). There have also been reports of two siblings with the syndrome who had mosaicism (Harley et al., 1972) and others in association with the Turner syndrome (Lubinsky et al., 1980).

TREATMENT

Theoretically, at least, treatment might now begin with in utero intervention following a fetal diagnosis by ultrasound. However, at this time there is no evidence that the potential for renal or pulmonary function can be altered by such a procedure. Perhaps further laboratory and clinical investigation will open new horizons in this area. At present, treatment of the infant with prune-belly syndrome begins with his initial neonatal evaluation.

Initial Diagnostic Evaluation

The syndrome is now well known and, because of the typical external features, the diagnosis of prune-belly syndrome **and** the presence of prune-belly uropathy **are** seldom in doubt. Although the urologist is usually notified immediately, the affected neonate rarely represents a true urologic emergency. The most urgent matters are actually those concerned with cardiopulmonary function. Pulmonary hypoplasia, pneumomediastinum, pneumothorax, and heart abnormalities, which are perhaps less evident from external inspection, may demand immediate attention. These matters must not be overlooked by the overzealous urologist. It should be noted whether a patent urachus is present and whether the infant can void. An orthopedic examination should also be done initially.

Early urologic assessment of each patient is necessary in order to individualize treatment (Jeffs et al., 1977). However, some compromises must be made because of the risks inherent in those diagnostic procedures requiring instrumentation of the urinary tract. Clearly, an x-ray examination of the chest, evaluation of pulmonary and heart function, and serial blood studies to estimate the level of renal function are first-priority procedures. An abdominal ultrasound examination will provide considerable useful information and will avoid the disadvantage of either instrumentation or additional x-ray exposure. Since urinary infection may occur even in the absence of instrumentation, urine cultures must be done.

If the baby is stable and the serum creatinine level remains normal, one may wait for several days before obtaining a renal scan or an excretory urogram (intravenous pyelogram [IVP]). However, these studies should be done, and the remainder of the diagnostic evaluation must then be tailored to one's attitude toward definitive management. If the pyelographic findings and renal functional parameters are such that early reconstruction to correct obstruction or reflux, or both, might be considered, a voiding cystourethrogram may be indicated. Any instrumentation of the urinary tract in these patients, however, may result in bacterial contamination that might be exceedingly difficult to eradicate, so care must be taken to insert the catheter under sterile conditions.

By following the serum creatinine levels, urine cultures, pyelographic and sonographic findings, it is possible to formulate a reasonable plan of clinical management. Evidence of infection or deteriorating renal function is usually an indication for surgical intervention. In the absence of such complications, one should monitor the respiratory function closely for 2 to 4 months, at which time a more thorough urologic evaluation might be appropriate. Many different approaches have been advocated for the management of prune-belly uropathy, each with its rationale and each with its own proponents. All methods have the same ultimate aim of maintaining renal function and preventing urinary infection.

Vesicoureteral Dysfunction

In the typical patient, the bladder is large, thick-walled, and flabby, and it tends to empty slowly and incompletely. Usually, but not always, there is vesicoureteral reflux. The ureter is long, redundant, irregularly dilated, and tortuous. There is usually some degree of hydronephrosis. Considerable controversy has arisen concerning the proper management of this aspect of the syndrome.

Nonoperative Treatment. Although successful results are possible with aggressive reconstructive operations, many investigators (Burke et al., 1969; Duckett, 1976; Rogers and Ostrow, 1973; Williams and Burkholder, 1967) contend that extensive reconstructive operations may fail to improve the ultimate fate of these patients. As a result, a "hands-off" attitude has been adopted by many. Despite the rather gross urographic abnormalities, many newborns seem to do quite well (Fig. 53–9). Woodhouse et al. (1979) reviewed a series of prune-belly patients who had been managed conservatively. Nine of eleven of those patients followed from infancy had remained well, except for a few urinary tract infections, for periods up to 24 years. They were said to have normal voiding patterns and normal renal function. Certainly, those patients in Category III are candidates for this type of management. Unfortunately, in the more severe Category II patient, long-term follow-up data are necessary to evaluate the results of either medical management or extensive surgical reconstruction, and such data are not yet available. Many patients with prune-belly syndrome have ultimately required renal transplantation, and others have seemed to do well for years only to succumb to urologic complications later (Culp and Flocks, 1954).

Temporary Diversion. When urinary infection becomes a problem, or it appears that renal function is deteriorating, a urinary drainage procedure must be considered. There are advantages in selecting a tubeless type of diversion, and the simplest of these is *cutaneous*

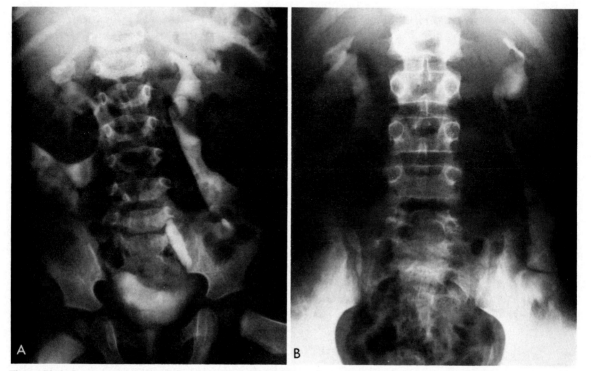

Figure 53–9. Intravenous urograms in a boy with prune-belly syndrome. *A,* At age 2 years, showing classic appearance of tortuous, dilated ureters with relatively well-preserved kidneys. *B,* At age 19 years, showing improvement in ureteric dilatation without surgical treatment and no deterioration in renal function.

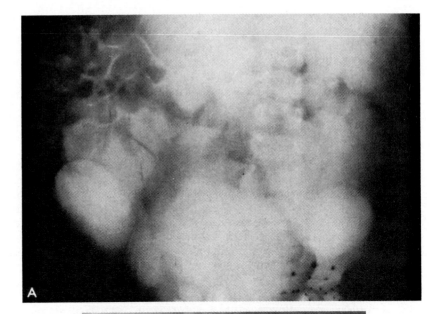

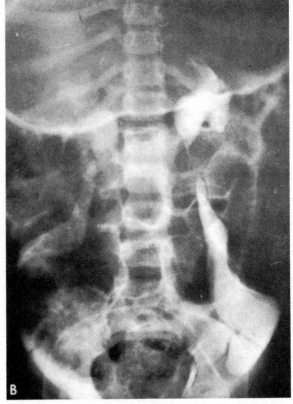

Figure 53–10. Vesicostomy drainage. *A,* Intravenous pyelogram in an 18-month-old boy with prune-belly syndrome. *B,* Intravenous pyelogram 10 years later with cutaneous vesicostomy alone.

vesicostomy (Duckett, 1976). Vesicostomy provides expedient and effective bladder drainage and is easily tolerated by most of these patients (Fig. 53–10). It is performed through a small transverse incision midway between the umbilicus and the pubic symphysis. A small ellipse of skin in rectus fascia is excised, and the dome of the bladder is mobilized and delivered into the incision, at which point it is sutured to the rectus fascia and the skin, and a small bladder stroma is fashioned. The urine is allowed to drain freely into the diaper using no collection device or tubes. Subsequent closure of the vesicostomy is also simple. Vesicostomy is useful either as a primary temporary drainage procedure or as a preliminary drainage procedure prior to a more extensive reconstruction at some later date. It might be argued that in some instances it fails to provide optimal drainage to the upper urinary tract in some patients with markedly redundant and tortuous ureters, in which case one might wonder whether a more proximal drainage procedure would be superior. In addition, there is the occasional patient in whom obstruction exists at the ureteropelvic junction.

High Loop Cutaneous Ureterostomy or Pyelostomy. This procedure has been advocated for those patients having urosepsis or progressive deterioration of renal function (Williams and Parker, 1974). Although not as simple as vesicostomy, it is still an expedient procedure and has the advantage of providing good proximal drainage to each kidney while permitting inspection and biopsy of the kidney at the time of operation. By allowing for a subsequent differential evaluation of kidney function, it may also aid in the planning of subsequent reconstructive operations. Its main disadvantage is that it may hinder an eventual reconstructive procedure by damaging the upper ureter, which is an important consideration in these patients, since it may be the only portion of ureter that is near normal in caliber and function. Although this procedure may have some merit in a few selected cases, its popularity has, with good reason, decreased in recent years.

Extensive Ureteral Reconstruction. The role of extensive surgical remodeling of the urinary tract in patients with prune-belly syndrome is understandably controversial, because some patients appear to do well without major reconstruction and others seem to have been harmed by successful surgical attempts. There is little question, however, that the urinary tract in patients with prune-belly syndrome is characterized by stasis and that this stasis predisposes to bacteriuria, which leads to deterioration of renal function as well as to troublesome clinical symptoms. Therefore, it is likely that many surgeons will continue their efforts at remodeling these distorted urinary tracts. Success in these surgical reconstructions depends to a great extent upon the use of the upper few centimeters of ureter, which are usually less dilated, less tortuous, and of better morphologic appearance than the distal ureter. Meticulous surgical technique with adherence to established principles of ureteral tailoring and reimplantation surgery is required (Fig. 53–11). Unfortunately, both the bladder and the ureter, by the very nature of this bizarre uropathy, are difficult

structures with which to work. Despite these inherent difficulties, in experienced hands a reasonably high degree of success is possible with this extensive reconstructive surgery, both in the neonate as a primary procedure (Figs. 53–12 and 53–13) and in the older infant or child (Fig. 53–14) as a staged procedure (Woodard and Parrott, 1978a).

Vesicourethral Dysfunction

There is little question that poor bladder emptying, with resulting recurrent and chronic urinary tract infection, leads to upper tract deterioration in many of these patients. The large bladder capacity, abnormal bladder wall, and relative narrowing of the membranous urethra may all play some role. Although some efforts have been made to delineate this problem urodynamically (Snyder et al., 1976), such data is still sparse. Efforts have been made toward improving detrusor function and reducing outflow resistance, however.

Reduction Cystoplasty. As has already been noted, the bladders in most of these patients are large and tend to bulge in pseudodiverticulum-like fashion at the dome. Fluoroscopic studies indicate that the dilated dome portion of the bladder may hinder micturition (Perlmutter, 1976). Reduction cystoplasty is a useful procedure in treating such a large, poorly functioning bladder and can be employed alone or as part of a major upper urinary tract reconstructive procedure (Fig. 53–11B and D). The technique involves generous resection of the bladder dome with a significant reduction in bladder capacity. This appears to improve bladder function by creating a more spherical detrusor. Plication of the bladder dome has also proved successful in some instances (Williams and Parker, 1974), and Hanna (1982) has reported improvement in detrusor function by "remodeling" the bladder.

Internal Urethrotomy. Although prune-belly uropathy is compatible with normal voiding dynamics, pressure flow studies in some patients will demonstrate an unbalanced voiding mechanism, and the condition of these patients may be improved by internal urethrotomy (Snyder et al., 1976; Woodhouse et al., 1979; Cukier, 1977). This procedure may be useful for those children who develop difficulty in voiding or who develop increased residual urine. A child with residual urine, a dilated posterior urethra, reflux, or ureteral dilation might be considered a suitable candidate. Internal urethrotomy ap-

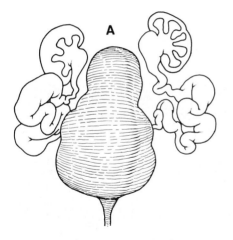

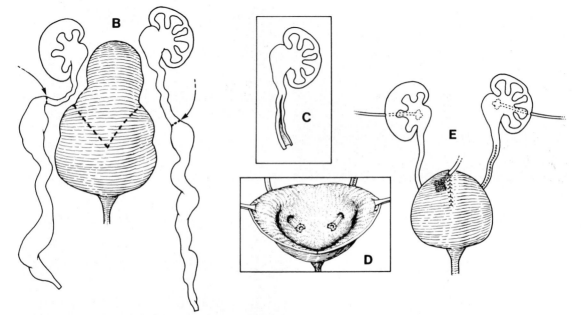

Figure 53–11. Artist's drawings showing surgical technique used for extensive reconstruction of "prune-belly uropathy." The operation is performed transperitoneally. No attempt is made to straighten the lower ureter, since only the upper portion is needed for re-establishing continuity. The ureter may or may not require tapering. Dome of bladder is excised (dotted line) in most patients. Ureteral stents (not shown) are employed, and nephrostomy tubes are frequently used.

pears to be an easy method of improving bladder emptying in these circumstances. Unfortunately, it might also be an easy method of producing urinary incontinence, though its advocates suggest this may be temporary (Williams, 1979). Incontinence would seem to be less of a risk in the unbalanced voiding situation that exists in some of these patients. However, it would perhaps be wise to limit its use to those patients in whom urodynamic evaluation confirms this imbalance. Clearly, urethrotomy has some role to play in the management of many patients with prune-belly uropathy. It may be performed with the Otis urethrotome or visually, using an en-

doscope. Williams (1979) advocates making one or two cuts anteriorly or anterolaterally to size 24 or 30 French followed by a period of catheter drainage. A visual urethrotomy would seem preferable to the Otis procedure and should be made through the narrowed area in the urethra, which is typically at the end of the prostatic portion. Since the bladder neck appears wide in these individuals, a cut in that area does not appear warranted. In some patients, urethrotomy alone produces noticeable improvement in the radiographic appearance of the upper urinary tract (Fig. 53–15).

Megaurethra. In the rare child in whom

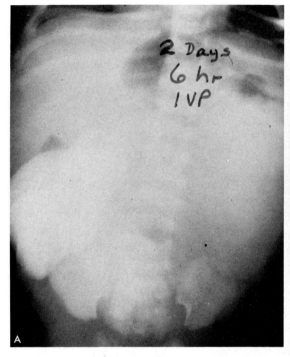

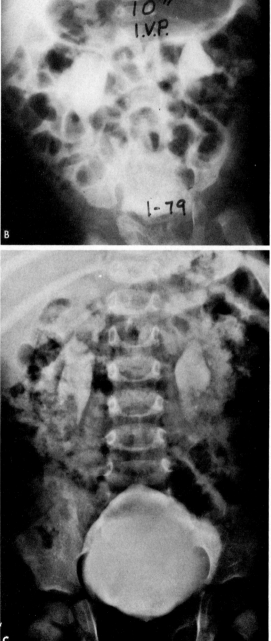

Figure 53–12. Result of neonatal reconstruction. *A,* IVP in a 2-day-old infant prior to primary neonatal reconstruction. *B,* IVP 2 months later. *C,* IVP 3 years later.

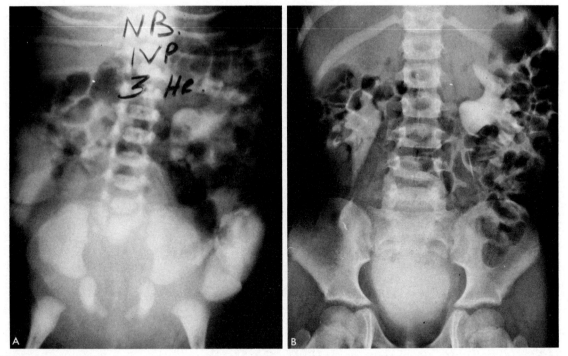

Figure 53–13. Results of neonatal reconstruction. *A,* IVP during first week of life, just prior to reconstruction. *B,* Ten years later after a single primary reconstructive procedure.

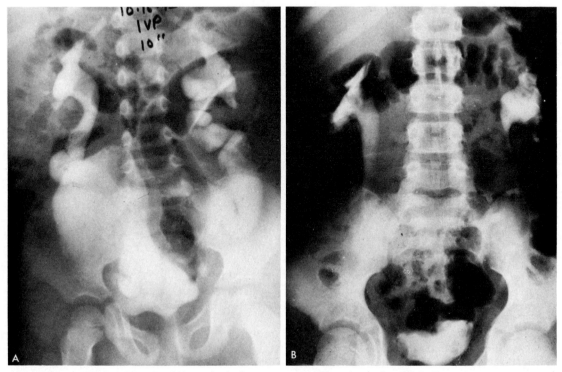

Figure 53–14. *A,* IVP in a 2½-year-old boy who had worn a suprapubic catheter since birth. Extensive reconstruction was done. *B,* The pyelographic result seen 7 years later.

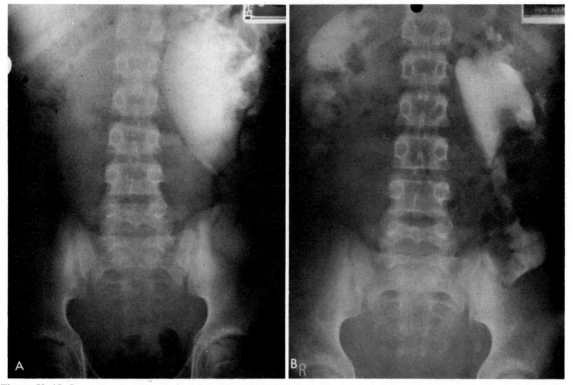

Figure 53–15. Intravenous urograms in a boy 12 years old with prune-belly syndrome. *A,* At presentation with residual urine of 2 L. *E,* Following Otis urethrotomy.

the anterior urethra is grossly dilated, surgery is required to reduce it to a normal caliber. Usually only the penile urethra is involved, the meatus and the glanular portion being normal. In such cases, a circumferential incision around the coronal sulcus with stripping back of the penile skin provides the best approach. The redundant wall of the urethra is then excised, and the lumen is reconstituted over a catheter. The penile skin is then drawn forward and sutured. In more severe examples it may be necessary to cut back from the meatus, excising both redundant skin and urethra, with reconstruction based on the methods of hypospadias repair.

Cryptorchidism

Fertility potential in patients with prune-belly syndrome is, at best, doubtful. Whether the wide bladder neck will allow for normal ejaculation and whether germ cells are present in the testicles of many of these patients has been questioned (Uehling, 1982; Hadziselimovic, 1984; Woodhouse and Snyder, 1984). Nonetheless, these testes have good hormonal function and orchiopexy is attempted in most of these patients. Rarely, if ever, is the standard surgical technique for orchiopexy successful in these circumstances. Staged procedures of the classic type have also been less than satisfactory. At present, three alternatives are available for the management of cryptorchidism in these patients.

Transabdominal Neonatal Orchiopexy. In the neonate, and perhaps in patients up to several months of age, transabdominal complete mobilization of the spermatic cord almost always allows the testis to be positioned in the dependent portion of the scrotum without tension and without dividing the vascular portion of the spermatic cord (Fig. 53–16) (Woodard and Parrott, 1978b). This procedure is particularly applicable in those infants who undergo extensive ureteral reconstructive procedures during the neonatal period, since it can be done simultaneously. In those patients who do not require reconstructive surgery, one might wait 3 or 4 months to ensure stability of the upper urinary tract as well as stability of the cardiopulmonary status before performing the operation.

Fowler-Stephens (Long Loop Vas) Technique. The Fowler-Stephens technique for per-

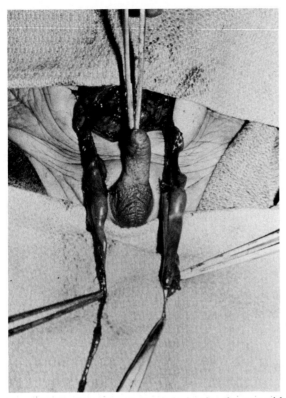

Figure 53–16. Operative photograph showing the ease with which the testes reach the scrotum following neonatal transabdominal mobilization of the spermatic cords.

forming orchiopexy in patients with intra-abdominal testes has become part of the standard urologic armamentarium (Fowler and Stephens, 1963). The operation involves division of the spermatic vessels above the level of the internal ring with preservation of the anastomotic connections between the vessels of the vas deferens and the distal spermatic vessels. A layer of peritoneum should be left over the vas to preserve these collaterals. In patients with prune-belly syndrome, the success rate has been reported as approximately 75 per cent (Gibbons et al., 1979). This procedure, therefore, represents a reasonable approach to the intra-abdominal testis in the patient with prune-belly syndrome and allows for greater flexibility in the timing of the procedure.

Microvascular Autotransplantation. With increased experience in microvascular surgery, autotransplantation of the abdominal testis to the scrotum with anastomosis of the spermatic vessels to the inferior epigastric vessels has become a feasible procedure. This technique has now been applied successfully in many patients of various ages with prune-belly syndrome

(MacMahon et al., 1976; Wacksman et al., 1980).

Although there is no evidence of offspring from fathers with prune-belly syndrome, there does appear to be good androgenic function in these testes and it is likely that orchiopexy will continue to be part of the treatment for these individuals. The recent reports of tumors arising in these cryptorchid testes add some additional importance to the treatment of this aspect of the syndrome.

Abdominal Wall Defect

The most obvious external feature of the prune-belly syndrome is the abdominal wall defect itself. Although it clearly offers a cosmetic disadvantage to the patient, the role this deficiency might play in either pulmonary or bladder function has been difficult to document with any accuracy. Consequently, there has been some controversy regarding the need for surgical procedures to improve the abdominal wall. Enthusiasm for such procedures seems to wax and wane, and many patients are treated simply with abdominal supports or corset devices.

Abdominal Wall Reconstruction. Electromyographic studies have demonstrated that the major functioning or recoverable muscle exists in the lateral and upper section of the abdomen and that there is usually little or no useful muscle present in the lower, more central portion. Based on this information, the technique of abdominal wall plication involving excision of a transverse elliptical portion of the lower abdominal wall, as described by Randolph et al. (1981a), has produced good results and is a procedure worthy of consideration, at least in selected patients (Duckett, 1980). It provides the patient with a waist and allows for wearing normal trousers when this might not otherwise be possible. However, Randolph reports satisfactory results after the first procedure in only about half of his patients, with some requiring repeat operation. The procedure involves removing the full thickness of the abdominal wall in such a way as to spare potentially functioning musculature and corresponding motor nerves (Fig. 53–17).

External Support Devices. The parents of most children with prune-belly syndrome, if left to their own devices, will provide their children with some type of corset or external support device. When properly designed, such a corset will provide the child a fairly normal appearing

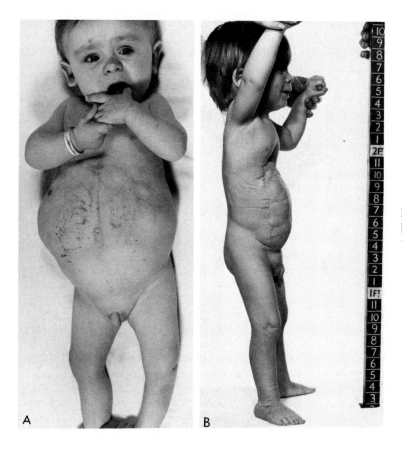

Figure 53–17. Unilateral abdominal wall plication for prune-belly syndrome. *A,* Infant 9 months. *B,* At 2 years.

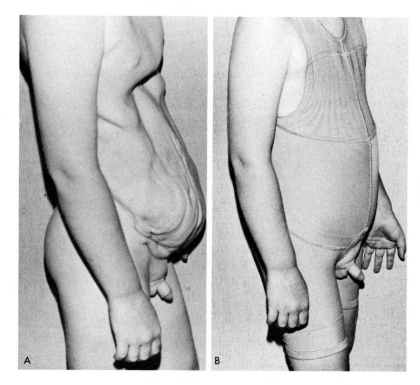

Figure 53–18. Photograph of a 4-year-old boy without *(A)* and with *(B)* his elasticized corset.

physique while clothed (Fig. 53–18). The corsets can be worn with ease and comfort and are relatively inexpensive. Since the abdominal wall deformity in some patients seems to improve slightly with age, external support devices may have an advantage over major surgical abdominal wall plication procedures in many patients.

Outlook

The considerable improvements in the medical, surgical, and urodynamic management of patients born with the prune-belly syndrome will certainly result in a prognosis far better than that previously reported, both for survival and for the quality of life. The syndrome is clearly a spectrum disorder. Some patients may benefit from major urologic reconstruction, but many will require little if any such surgery. All of the patients require careful evaluation and individualized management and since their urodynamics may change with age, long-term surveillance and periodic reappraisal are necessary.

References

Adebonojo, F. O.: Dysplasia of the abdominal musculature with multiple congenital anomalies; prune-belly or triad syndrome. J. Natl. Med. Assoc., 65:327, 1973.

Adenyokunnu, A. A., and Familusi, J. B.: Prune belly syndrome in two siblings and a first cousin. Am. J. Dis. Child., 136:23, 1982.

Adenyokunnu, A. A., Adeniyi, T. M., Kolawole, T. M. et al.: Prune-belly syndrome: A study of ten cases in Nigerian children with common and uncommon manifestations. E. Afr. Med. J., 52:438, 1975.

Afifi, A.K., Rebeiz, J. M., Andonian, S. J. et al.: The myopathy of the prune-belly syndrome. Neurol. Sci., 15:153, 1972.

Asplund, J., and Laska, J.: Prune-belly syndrome at the age of 37. Scand. J. Urol. Nephrol., 9:297, 1975.

Barnhouse, D. H.: Prune-belly syndrome. Br. J. Urol., 44:356, 1972.

Bovicelli, L., Rizzo, N., Orsini, L. F. et al.: Prenatal diagnosis of the prune-belly syndrome. Clin. Genet., 18:79, 1980.

Burke, E. C., Shin, M. H., Kelalis, P. P.: Prune-belly syndrome. Am. J. Dis. Child., 117:668, 1969.

Carey, J. C., Eggert, L., Curry, C. J. R.: Lower limb deficiency and the urethral obstruction sequence. Birth Defects, 18:19, 1982.

Cawthern, T. H., Bottene, C. A., and Grant, D.: Prune-belly syndrome associated with Hirschsprung's disease. Am. J. Dis. Child., 133:652, 1979.

Christopher, C. R., Spinelli, A., and Severt, D.: Ultrasonic diagnosis of prune-belly syndrome. Obstet. Gynecol., 59:391, 1982.

Cukier, J.: Resection of the urethra in the prune-belly syndrome. Birth Defects, 13:95, 1977.

Culp, D. A., and Flocks, R. H.: Congenital absence of abdominal musculature. J. Iowa State Med. Soc., 44:155, 1954.

Deklerk, D. P., and Scott, W. W.: Prostatic maldevelopment in prune-belly syndrome: A defect in prostatic stromal-epithelial interaction. J. Urol., 120:241, 1978.

Duckett, J. W., Jr.: The prune-belly syndrome. In Kelalis, P. P., King, L. R., and Belman, A. B. (Eds.): Clinical Pediatric Urology. Philadelphia, W. B. Saunders Co., 1976, p. 615.

Duckett, J. W.: The prune-belly syndrome. In Holder, T. M., and Ashcroft, K. W. (Eds.): The Surgery of Infants and Children. Philadelphia, W. B. Saunders Co., 1980, pp. 802–815.

Ehrlich, R. M., and Brown, W. J.: Ultrastructural anatomic observations of the ureter in the prune-belly syndrome. Birth Defects, 13:101, 1977.

Fowler, R., Jr., and Stephens, F. D.: The role of testicular vascular anatomy in the salvage of high undescended testes. In Stephen, F. D. (Ed.): Congenital Malformations of the Rectum, Anus, and Genitourinary Tract. Baltimore, The Williams & Wilkins Co., 1963.

Garlinger, P., and Ott, J.: Prune-belly syndrome—possible genetic implications. Birth Defects, 10:173, 1974.

Gibbons, M. D., Cromie, W. J., and Duckett, J. W., Jr.: Management of the abdominal undescended testis. J. Urol., 122:76, 1979.

Hadziselimovic, F.: Personal communication, July 1984.

Halbrecht, I., Komlos, L., and Shabtal, F.: Prune-belly syndrome with chromosomal fragment. Am. J. Dis. Child., 123:518, 1972.

Hanna, M. D.: New concept in bladder remodeling. Urology, 19:6, 1982.

Hannington-Kiff, J. G.: Prune-belly syndrome and general anesthesia. Br. J. Anaesthesiol., 42:649, 1970.

Harley, L. M., Chen, Y., and Rattner, W. H.: Prune-belly syndrome. J. Urol., 108:174, 1972.

Hendren, W. H.: Restoration of function in the severely decompensated ureter. In Johnston, J. H., and Scholtmeijer, R. J. (Eds.): Problems in Paediatric Urology. Amsterdam, Excerpta Medica, 1972, pp. 1–56.

Heydenrych, J., and DuToit, P. E.: Torsion of the spleen and associated prune-belly syndrome—case report and review of the literature. S. Afr. Med. J., 53:637, 1978.

Ives, E. J.: The abdominal muscle deficiency triad syndrome—experience with ten cases. Birth Defects, 10:127, 1974.

Jeffs, R. D., Comisarow, R. H., and Hanna, M. K.: The early assessment for individualized treatment in the prune-belly syndrome. Birth Defects, 13:97, 1977.

Karamanian, A., Kravath, R., Nagashima, H. et al.: Anesthetic management of prune-belly syndrome. Br. J. Anaesthesiol., 46:897, 1974.

King, C. R., and Prescott, G.: Pathogenesis of the prune-belly anomaly. J. Pediatr., 93:273, 1978.

Kroovand, R. L., Al-Ansari, R. M., and Perlmutter, A. D.: Urethral and genital malformations in prune-belly syndrome. J. Urol., 127:94, 1982.

Lattimer, J. K.: Congenital deficiency of the abdominal musculature and associated genitourinary abnormalities: A report of 22 cases. J. Urol., 79:343, 1958.

Lee, M. L.: Prune-belly syndrome in a 54 year old man. JAMA, 237:2216, 1977.

Lockhart, J. L., Reeve, H. R., Bredael, J. J. et al.: Siblings with prune-belly syndrome and associated pulmonic stenosis, mental retardation and deafness. Urology, 14:140, 1979.

Lubinsky, M., Koyle, K., and Trunca, C.: The association of prune-belly with Turner's syndrome. Am. J. Dis. Child., 134:1171, 1980.

MacMahon, R. A., O'Brien, M. C., and Cussen, L. J.: The use of microsurgery in the treatment of the undescended testis. J. Pediatr. Surg., 11:521, 1976.

Martin, D. C., and Salibian, A.: Orchiopexy utilizing microvascular surgical techniques. J. Urol., *123*:263, 1980.

McGovern, J. H., and Marshall, V. F.: Congenital deficiency of the abdominal musculature and obstructive uropathy. Surg. Gynecol. Obstet., *108*:289, 1959.

Mininberg, D. T., Montoya, F., Okada, K. et al.: Subcellular muscle studies in the prune-belly syndrome. J. Urol., *109*:524, 1973.

Moerman, P., Fryns, J., Goddeeris, P., and Lauweryns, J. M.: Pathogenesis of the prune-belly syndrome: A functional urethral obstruction caused by prostatic hypoplasia. Pediatrics, *73*:470, 1984.

Monie, I. W., and Monie, B. J.: Prune-belly syndrome and fetal ascites. Teratology, *19*:111, 1979.

Morgan, C. L., Jr., Grossman, H., and Novak, R.: Imperforate anus and colon calcification in association with the prune-belly syndrome. Pediatr. Radiol., *7*:19, 1978.

Nunn, I. N., and Stephens, F. D.: The triad syndrome: A composite anomaly of the abdominal wall, urinary system and testes. J. Urol., *86*:782, 1961.

Okulski, T. A.: The prenatal diagnosis of lower urinary tract obstruction using B scan ultrasound: A case report. J. Clin. Ultrasound, *5*:268, 1977.

Osler, W.: Congenital absence of the abdominal musculature, with distended and hypertrophied urinary bladder. Bull. Johns Hopkins Hosp., *12*:331, 1901.

Palmer, J. M., and Tesluk, H.: Ureteral pathology in the prune-belly syndrome. J. Urol., *111*:701, 1974.

Perlmutter, A. D.: Reduction cystoplasty in prune-belly syndrome. J. Urol., *116*:456, 1976.

Potter, E. L.: Abnormal development of the kidney. *In* Potter, E. L. (Ed.): Normal and Abnormal Development of the Kidney. Chicago, Year Book Medical Publishers, 1972, pp. 154–220.

Rabinowitz, R., and Schillinger, J. F.: Prune-belly syndrome in the female subject. J. Urol., *118*:454, 1977.

Ralis, Z., and Forbes, M.: Intrauterine atrophy and gangrene of the lower extremity of the fetus caused by megacystis due to urethral atresia. J. Pathol., *104*:31, 1971.

Randolph, J., Cavett, C., and Eng, G.: Abdominal wall reconstruction in the prune-belly syndrome. J. Pediatr. Surg., *16*:960, 1981*a*.

Randolph, J., Cavett, C., and Eng, G.: Surgical correction and rehabilitation for children with "prune-belly" syndrome. Ann. Surg., *193*:757, 1981*b*.

Riccardi, V. M., and Grum, C. M.: The prune-belly anomaly: Heterogeneity and superficial X-linkage mimicry. J. Med. Genet., *14*:266, 1977.

Rogers, L. W., and Ostrow, P. T.: The prune-belly syndrome: Report of 20 cases and description of a lethal variant. J. Pediatr., *83*:786, 1973.

Sellers, B. B., McNeil, R., Smith, R. V. et al.: Congenital megalourethra asssociated with prune-belly syndrome. J. Urol., *16*:814, 1976.

Shih, W., Greenbaum, L. D., and Baro, C.: In utero sonogram in prune-belly syndrome. Urology, *20*:102, 1982.

Silverman, F. M., and Huang, N.: Congenital absence of the abdominal muscle associated with malformation of the genitourinary and alimentary tracts: Report of cases and review of literature. Am. J. Dis. Child., *80*:9, 1950.

Smith, D. W.: Recognizable Patterns of Human Malformation. Philadelphia, W. B. Saunders Co., 1970, p. 5.

Smythe, A. R.: Ultrasonic detection of fetal ascites and bladder dilation with resulting prune-belly. J. Pediatr., *98*:978, 1981.

Snyder, H. M., Harrison, N. W., Whitfield, H. N. et al.: Urodynamics in the prune-belly syndrome. Br. J. Urol., *48*:663, 1976.

Stephens, F. D.: Congenital malformations of the rectum, anus and genito-urinary tracts. London and Edinburgh, Livingstone, 1963, pp. 149, 186, 187.

Texter, J. H., and Koontz, W. W.: Prune-belly syndrome seen in the adult. Soc. Pediatr. Urol. Newsletter, Feb. 6, 1980.

Tuck, B. A., and Smith, T. K.: Prune-belly syndrome: A report of 12 cases and review of the literature. J. Bone Joint. Surg., *60*:109, 1978.

Uehling, D. T.: Testicular histology in triad syndrome. Soc. Pediatr. Urol. Newsletter, Dec. 30, 1982.

Wacksman, J., Dinner, M., and Staffon, R. A.: Technique of testicular autotransplantation using a microvascular anastomosis. Surg. Gynecol. Obstet., *150*:399, 1980.

Welch, K. J., and Kearney, G. P.: Abdominal musculature deficiency syndrome: prune-belly. J. Urol., *111*:693, 1974.

Willert, C., Cohen, H., Yu, Y. T. et al.: Association of prune-belly syndrome and gastroschisis. Am. J. Dis. Child., *132*:526, 1978.

Williams, D. I.: Prune-belly syndrome. *In* Harrison, J. H., Gittes, R. F., Perlmutter, A. D. et al. (Eds.): Campbell's Urology, 4th ed. Philadelphia, W. B. Saunders Co., 1979, pp. 1743–1755.

Williams, D. I., and Burkholder, G. V.: The prune-belly syndrome. J. Urol., *98*:244, 1967.

Williams, D. I., and Parker, R. M.: The role of surgery in the prune-belly syndrome. *In* Johnston, J. H., and Goodwin, W. F. (Eds.): Reviews of Pediatric Urology. Amsterdam, Excerpta Medica, 1974, pp. 315–331.

Woodard, J. R.: The prune-belly syndrome. Urol. Clin. North Am., *5*:73, 1978.

Woodard, J. R., and Parrott, T. S.: Reconstruction of the urinary tract in prune-belly uropathy. J. Urol., *119*:824, 1978*a*.

Woodard, J. R., and Parrott, T. S.: Orchiopexy in prune-belly syndrome. Br. J. Urol., *50*:348, 1978*b*.

Woodhouse, C. R. J., Kellett, M. J., and Williams, D. I.: Minimal surgical interference in prune-belly syndrome. Br. J. Urol., *51*:475, 1979.

Woodhouse, C. R. J., and Snyder, H. M.: Testicular and sexual function in adults with prune-belly syndrome. Submitted for publication, 1984.

CHAPTER 54

Enuresis

STEPHEN A. KOFF, M.D.

Enuresis (from the Greek *enourein,* to void urine) has been defined as an involuntary discharge of urine. The term is often used alone, imprecisely, to describe wetting that occurs only at night during sleep. It is more accurate, however, to refer to nighttime wetting as nocturnal enuresis and to distinguish it from daytime wetting, which is called diurnal enuresis. Since incontinence is normal in young children, the age at which enuresis becomes inappropriate depends on the statistics of developing urinary control, the pattern of wetting, and the sex of the child. Approximately 15 per cent of normal children still wet at night at age 5 years. Nocturnal enuresis occurring after the age of 5 or by the time the child enters grade school is generally considered a cause for concern. With a spontaneous resolution rate of about 15 per cent per year, 99 per cent of children are dry by the age of 15 years (Forsythe and Redmond, 1974). In contrast, diurnal enuresis that persists much after toilet training may be a problem. A larger proportion of girls than boys are dry both day and night by the age of 2 years, and nocturnal enuresis is 50 per cent more common in boys than in girls.

Over 80 per cent of enuretics wet only at night. The remainder have variable and varying patterns of nocturnal and diurnal incontinence. Most nocturnal enuretics have never been dry and are termed primary enuretics. However, the development of urinary control is not always final, and approximately 25 per cent of children who attain initial nighttime dryness by age 12 will relapse and wet for a period averaging 2.5 years. These children are termed secondary enuretics, and in many, emotional stress that occurred during a vulnerable period in their development may be recognized. Children who develop initial daytime dryness by age 12 are less prone to relapse, but at least 10 per cent will redevelop daytime wetting for periods averaging 1.2 years (Oppel et al., 1968).

THE DEVELOPMENTAL BIOLOGY OF URINARY CONTROL

In the infant, micturition occurs spontaneously as a spinal cord reflex. When increasing amounts of urine distend the bladder and sufficiently stimulate the afferent limb of the reflex arc, the detrusor contracts. Even at this young age, the periurethral striated muscles that compose the voluntary (external) urinary sphincter are fully integrated into the voiding reflex so that as the bladder fills, the urinary sphincter constricts progressively to prevent incontinence. During micturition, the striated muscle sphincter relaxes reflexly to allow low-pressure bladder emptying.

The young infant sleeps nearly 60 per cent of the day, and approximately 40 per cent of voidings occur during sleep. In the first year of life, the number of voidings per day remains fairly constant at about 20. Thereafter, during the first 3 years of life, the frequency of urinations per day decreases to about 11, while the mean voided volume increases nearly 4 fold (Goellner et al., 1981). This progressive reduction in bladder responsiveness has been presumed to be due to the unconscious inhibition of the micturition reflex (Yeates, 1973). It appears that these changes in voided volume and frequency of voidings may instead reflect changes in the volume of fluid intake and alterations in the size of the infant's bladder. Daily urine volume correlates closely with oral intake and, when expressed as a percentage of intake, does not change appreciably during the first 3 years of life. Similarly, when mean voided volumes are expressed per unit of body weight, voiding size changes little with age. However, the volume of urine produced per unit of body weight per day decreases and bladder capacity increases during this period (Goellner et al., 1981; Koff, 1983). It thus appears that the reduction in voiding frequency observed during the first 3 years of life is due primarily to a growth-related increase in bladder capacity that is proportionately greater than is the increase in urine volume produced.

As a child matures, the success of toilet training and the development of an adult-type of urinary control depend on the outcome of at least three separate events in the development of bladder form and bladder-sphincter function (Nash, 1949). First, the capacity of the bladder must increase to permit it to function as an adequate reservoir. The capacity of the newborn's bladder is approximately 1 to 2 ounces. Each year until nearly age 12, the bladder enlarges by about 1 ounce per year. As a consequence, bladder capacity in childhood can be accurately estimated and expressed by the formula: bladder capacity (in ounces) equals age plus 2 (in years) (Koff, 1983). Second, voluntary control over the periurethral striated muscle sphincter must occur to permit the decisive initiation and termination of micturition. As with other acquired striated muscle skills, sphincter control fits into an orderly scheme of developmental landmarks, and usually is complete by the age of 3 years. Third, direct volitional control over the spinal micturition reflex must develop in order for the child to initiate or inhibit detrusor contraction voluntarily. This last phase in the development of urinary control is the most complex, but once accomplished, the ability to void or inhibit voiding voluntarily at any degree of bladder filling sets the child apart from all other mammals (except the canine). Although voluntary control over the bladder smooth muscle is somewhat perplexing from a physiologic standpoint, its occurrence has been well documented (Lapides et al., 1957; Muellner, 1960).

Eventually, by the age of 4 years, most children will have developed an adult pattern of urinary control and will be continent day and night. This adult pattern is characterized by the absence of spontaneous uncontrolled infant-type or so-called uninhibited bladder contractions. Urodynamic studies have confirmed that even at bladder capacity, when the desire to void is strongest, the detrusor will not contract unless voluntarily initiated (Diokno et al., 1974). During bladder filling, the striated muscles of the urinary sphincter will be reflexly activated, and their constriction will become maximal at bladder capacity. This is a guarding reflex that prevents urinary incontinence. However, when detrusor contraction is voluntarily initiated, simultaneous reflex relaxation of the striated muscle sphincter will afford low-pressure bladder emptying.

The development of urinary control thus fits into an orderly scheme of overall bowel and bladder control that follows a typical sequence of development: (1) control of bowel function at night; (2) control of bowel function by day; (3) control of bladder function by day; and finally, after a lag of several months or more, (4) control of bladder function by night. However, this sequence of achieving urinary control is malleable and can be overridden by external forces. Consequently, there is a marked individual variability in the age of achieving nighttime urinary control (Stein and Susser, 1967).

ETIOLOGY

A variety of theories have been proposed to explain enuresis. These include developmental delay, sleep abnormalities, genetic factors, stress and psychologic factors, as well as organic urinary tract disease. Since enuresis is, in fact, a symptom rather than a true disease state, it is likely that no single hypothesis will explain all cases and that in each individual instance multiple factors may be operative. However, the vast majority of nocturnal enuretics do not suffer from obvious or treatable psychiatric disease, neurologic abnormalities, or urologic disturbances. As a result, causal analysis is often frustratingly difficult and unrewarding.

Urodynamic Factors

The single most important urodynamic observation in children with enuresis is that they have a reduced bladder capacity compared with normals (Hallman, 1950; Muellner, 1960; Starfield, 1967; Esperanca and Gerrard, 1969a.) The magnitude of this reduction is often in excess of 50 per cent of bladder capacity. Measurements of bladder capacity in enuretics under anesthesia indicate that total bladder capacity is not actually reduced and that the disturbance causing a reduction in capacity is functional rather than anatomic (Troup and Hodgson, 1971). This finding is supported by the results of intravenous anticholinergic therapy for enuresis, which effects an increase in functional bladder capacity of 25 to 600 per cent (Johnstone, 1972).

In addition to small functional bladder capacity, a number of enuretics have diurnal symptoms of frequency, urgency, and incontinence, which suggests the presence of uninhibited bladder contractions. These contractions represent involuntary and insuppressible detrusor activity, which may occur in children who have failed to gain complete voluntary control over the micturition reflex (Lapides and Diokno, 1970; Koff et al., 1979). Although they represent the normal mechanism for infant micturition, the precise cause for persistence of these contractions after toilet training is unknown. They are believed to represent either a delay in central nervous system maturation or a developmental regression (Nash, 1949).

In childhood enuresis, uninhibited contractions have been documented in over 50 per cent of unselected patients (Linderholm, 1966; Pompeius, 1971). Recent studies suggest, however, that this incidence may be underestimated, because when cystometry is performed in only the supine position, it may fail to identify correctly up to two thirds of children with uninhibited contractions. When provocative tests aimed at eliciting uninhibited contractions are performed, such as sitting or standing cystometry or micturition stop testing, a much higher incidence (78–84 per cent) of uninhibited bladder activity is discovered (Giles et al., 1978; Mahony et al., 1981). These findings suggest that uninhibited bladder contractions may be much more common in enuresis than is generally appreciated. However, reliance on symptoms to predict which child will have this problem may be misleading because nearly a third of children with uninhibited contractions have no incontinence at all; conversely, 20 per cent of children with daytime symptoms will have normal cystometric studies (Koff and Murtagh, 1983).

Urodynamic studies performed during sleep or under anesthesia confirm the presence of bladder hyperactivity in a number of enuretics and indicate that the sleep cystometrogram in these enuretics differs from that of controls. Whereas deep anesthesia will depress bladder contractility, bladder contractions can be recorded in over 90 per cent of susceptible children under light anesthesia although the threshold volume at which the contraction occurs may be different from when awake (Grossman et al.,

1977). Sleep cystometrograms recorded from enuretics show spontaneous bladder contractions that are more frequent and of greater amplitude than those of controls. Intravesical pressure during contractions may reach 50 cm of water or higher. These contractions may occur spontaneously, or be secondary either to internal stimuli associated with autonomic changes and alterations in the electroencephalogram (EEG) or to external stimuli such as loud noise. A typical enuretic wetting episode is associated with a series of high-pressure bladder contractions culminating in micturition. Enuretics who happen not to wet during sleep studies will still display the same bladder hyperactivity, but pressures will be lower and frequency less than those preceding an enuretic event. In contrast, normal, nonenuretic individuals will display few, if any, low-pressure bladder contractions during sleep cystometrography (Gastaut and Broughton, 1965; Broughton, 1968).

In summary, these findings suggest that bladder contractions that produce nocturnal enuresis are potentially inhibitable even during sleep and that the ability to suppress bladder hyperactivity while awake and asleep is essential for the successful development of day and nighttime urinary control. Although uninhibited contractions appear to be much more common and more intimately associated with the pathophysiology of nocturnal enuresis than has been generally appreciated, there does not appear to be a direct causal relationship between uninhibited bladder contractions and nighttime wetting for most enuretics. Rather, one may hypothesize that the presence and the awareness of uninhibited contractions that continue through and persist after the developmental stages of toilet training significantly delay and interfere with the learning of behavioral skills required for the acquisition of nocturnal urinary control.

Developmental Delay

In a sense, nocturnal and diurnal enuresis represent an arrest in development, since both occur normally in young children. Consequently, the hypothesis that enuresis represents a developmental delay or maturational lag in central nervous system development is both attractive and well supported by a number of diverse clinical observations.

The aforementioned urodynamic abnormalities of bladder capacity and activity, which occur so commonly in enuresis, tend to improve with time and to resolve spontaneously. Children displaying these abnormalities do not manifest obvious neuropathy, and neurologic disease is rarely identified. It is most likely that these phenomena are a biologic expression of neurophysiologic immaturity rather than a manifestation of an occult organic disease.

A developmental cause for enuresis is also supported by the observation that a number of nonorganic disturbances, such as social factors and stress, can modify the attainment of urinary control and influence the timing and duration of enuresis. Bedwetting is more common in lower socioeconomic groups and occurs twice as often among unskilled workers compared with professionals (Essen and Peckham, 1976). In families undergoing stress, the likelihood for enuresis occurring is increased 3 fold (Miller et al., 1960). MacKeith (1968) has pointed out that the second to the fourth year is a particularly sensitive period in the development of nocturnal bladder control, and is a time when a high proportion of the population develops enuresis. Consequently, children with a significant anxiety-producing episode in this period have a much increased chance for developing enuresis. Young and Morgan (1973) have suggested further that the difference between primary and secondary enuresis is simply related to the timing of stressful events, with primary enuresis resulting from stress during the sensitive period and secondary enuresis being due to stresses occurring after the sensitive developmental period. Although these stressful episodes are typically transient, they may prevent the child from developing nocturnal urinary control at the appropriate point in time and allow the child to pass into a later developmental stage where spontaneous control is less likely to occur. The negative effect of stress on maturation of urinary control is further evidenced by the increased prevalence of enuresis in children from deprived environments, from broken homes, and with a background of temporary institutional habitation. In considering the effect of stress on urinary control, one must recognize that another potential form of stress facing the young child is insuppressible uninhibited bladder activity, which renders the child incontinent during this critical developmental period of toilet training. The occurrence of daytime incontinence at this time may be sufficiently disturbing to further delay the acquisition of nocturnal urinary control.

Critics of developmental delay argue that this hypothesis is not anatomically correct or physiologically valid, and point out that the occurrence of a single dry day and night in an enuretic child is proof that the neurologic pathways are intact and operative (Apley and MacKeith, 1968; MacKeith, 1972). They suggest, instead, that both primary and secondary enuresis are entirely stress-related phenomena, recognizing that in secondary enuresis these stressful events are usually much more obvious. However, to counter these views, it is apparent that despite the fact that neuroanatomic pathways are intact, their successful integration and the acquisition of behavioral skills necessary for nighttime urinary control may be adversely affected by developmental immaturity. This is reflected in the tendency for encopresis to occur more commonly (10–25 per cent) in enuretics and supports the generally apparent clinical observation that children who are retarded in one aspect of sphincter control tend to be retarded in another. In addition, a significantly higher proportion of bedwetting is observed in children who are also delayed in walking and in talking. These findings all suggest that achieving dryness is a sequential part of the child's general development and that when the overall rate of maturation is delayed, the delay appears in most of the individual aspects of development (Stein and Susser, 1967).

Sleep Factors

Objective evaluation of the relationship between sleep and enuresis required the development of sleep laboratories capable of monitoring all night the physiologic variables during sleep. Such studies demonstrated that sleep is not simply the progressive and passive slowing of body and brain processes. Normal sleep begins with so-called nonrapid eye movement (NREM) sleep, which is divisible into four progressively deep sleep stages (Stages 1–4), each characterized by specific electroencephalographic (EEG) changes. In addition, a particularly light stage of sleep is recognized and characterized by bursts of conjugate rapid eye movements (REM). REM sleep is associated with increased autonomic activity, generalized muscle atonia, and dreaming. Normal sleep structure is composed of cycles of NREM sleep, REM sleep, and occasional awakenings. In older children and adults these cycles last about 1 to 1.5 hours, and the percentage of time spent in REM sleep increases as the cycles progress (Rechtschaffen and Kales, 1968).

Historically, enuresis has been considered

a disorder of sleep and more precisely a consequence of deep sleep, recognizing that some enuretics appear to be deep sleepers (Broughton, 1968; Lowy, 1970; Anders and Weinstein, 1972; Kales and Kales, 1974). Early sleep studies supported this view by demonstrating that enuresis occurred during deep sleep and that adult enuretics were often very deep sleepers who required amphetamines to lighten their sleep (Strom-Olsen, 1950). However, the observation that enuretics are often deep sleepers may be biased and partially invalidated by the fact that parents do not regularly attempt to arouse their nonenuretic children from sleep (Hallgren, 1957; Boyd, 1960; McKendry et al., 1968; Graham, 1973). When children are aroused from deep Stage 4 sleep, they may be hard to awaken and appear confused and disoriented. It has been suggested that the degree of "sleep drunkenness" may be more deeply observed in enuretics, and this finding might account in part for the perception that enuretics sleep more soundly than do normals (Lowy, 1970).

Although depth of sleep may be a factor for some enuretic children, recently accumulated evidence has suggested that previously hypothesized relationships between enuresis and sleep may be erroneous. Controlled sleep research studies indicate that children with enuresis sleep no more soundly than do normals and that a proportion of enuretics actually wet during very light sleep or while awake (Ritvo et al., 1969). Findings such as these encouraged the notion that enuresis was a disorder of arousal, implying that enuresis might correlate better with a transition from one level of sleep to another than with an inability to awaken from deep sleep (Broughton, 1968). Two large sleep studies have demonstrated that neither of these hypotheses—deep sleep or arousal—is an accurate description of enuretic sleep structure. Enuretics were observed to sleep no more deeply than age-matched controls, and enuretic events were associated neither with deep sleep nor with a transition between sleep stages or arousal signs. Instead, enuretic episodes were noted throughout the night on a random basis and occurred in each stage of sleep in proportion to the actual amount of time spent in that stage (Kales et al., 1977; Mikkelson et al., 1980). These findings indicate that enuretic sleep patterns are not appreciably different from the sleep patterns of normal children, and that most enuretics do not wet as a consequence of sleeping too deeply.

Genetic Factors

It is an old but valid observation that enuresis tends to run in families. In multiple series, over a third of fathers and a fifth of mothers of enuretics have an enuretic history themselves (Frary, 1935; Hallgren, 1957). Bakwin (1971, 1973) showed further that when both parents had enuresis, 77 per cent of children were enuretic, whereas when one parent was enuretic, 44 per cent of children developed wetting. These figures contrast with a 15 per cent incidence of enuresis in children from nonenuretic parents. Studies in twins indicate as well that when one twin has enuresis the other is predisposed to develop wetting (Bakwin, 1971).

Organic Urinary Tract Disease

Children with enuresis, particularly girls, are predisposed to develop urinary tract infections (Dodge et al., 1970). However, many of these children will have diurnal symptoms due to uninhibited bladder contractions. The mechanism for their infection is voluntary constriction of the urinary sphincter muscles in an attempt to maintain continence during the uninhibited bladder contraction. This produces obstruction with high intravesical pressures of a degree comparable to an anatomic urinary tract obstruction. Not all children will have both day and night wetting, but characteristically their symptoms will persist after the infection is eradicated and they will continue to display a small functional bladder capacity. In contrast to girls, boys with enuresis seem less prone to develop urinary tract infections even if they have associated uninhibited bladder activity (Lapides and Diokno, 1970; Koff et al., 1979; Koff and Murtagh, 1983).

Excluding uninhibited bladder activity, most children with nocturnal enuresis do not have an organic urinary tract cause for their wetting; the incidence of organic disease is less than 10 per cent and probably closer to 1 per cent (Hallgren, 1957; Forsythe and Redmond, 1974; McKendry and Stewart, 1974). However, prior to a decade ago, diseases that nowadays would be classified as normal variants or minor abnormalities were regularly invoked as common causes for enuresis, and many children underwent some type of surgical procedure (Fisher and Forsythe, 1954; Mahony, 1971; Arnold and Ginsberg, 1973). It is now generally appreciated that these minor disorders, such as meatal stenosis, do not cause enuresis, and in only a small percentage of children will relief of symptoms follow an operation such as meatotomy (Kunin et al., 1970). In contrast to pure nocturnal enuresis, Cutler et al. (1978) found an increased incidence of organic abnormalities in children with diurnal symptoms, although not all series have substantiated this finding (Redman and Seibert, 1979).

Psychologic Factors

The occurrence of emotional disturbances in enuretic children is probably slightly higher than in the general population, but most enuretics do not suffer from significant psychologic disease (Werry, 1967). From a psychodynamic viewpoint, if enuresis were the somatic expression of an emotional disorder, its elimination might prove undesirable and result either in a worsening of the psychopathologic disturbance or in the development of substitute symptoms (Young and Morgan, 1973). Such a hypothesis is insupportable by clinical observation and most therapists find precisely the opposite, that childhood adjustment tends to improve rather than worsen after successful treatment of enuresis (Baker, 1969). Bindelglas and Dee (1978) recently reported on the fate of enuretics who had been successfully treated with imipramine 10 years earlier. They convincingly put to rest the notion that enuresis was a symptom of severe psychopathologic disturbance by demonstrating that treatment of enuresis did not produce psychologic decomposition, inhibition of learning, or, in fact, any negative effect on adolescent health, growth, or development. In most instances, enuresis should be considered a disturbance unrelated to psychopathologic abnormality, and its symptomatic treatment is therefore perfectly justifiable.

In some instances, enuresis and a psychopathologic disorder may coexist, although disturbed children are not particularly prone to enuresis. Occasionally, emotional disturbance may actually be due to or exacerbated by enuresis because wetting places an additional burden on the child suffering from multiple difficulties (Young and Morgan, 1973).

Miscellaneous Factors

Although there is no objective evidence relating allergy to enuresis for most patients, in a small number of selected individuals such an association may exist. Zaleski et al. (1972) have shown that food allergy may cause bladder hyperactivity and a reduced functional bladder capacity. Both of these were observed to improve convincingly after elimination of the offending dietary allergen. However, no differences were observed in the level of immunoglobulins often associated with allergenic phenomena (IgE) in enuretics as compared with controls (Kaplan, 1973).

Enuretics have a higher incidence of EEG abnormalities compared with normal children (Campbell et al., 1966; Kajtor et al., 1967; Fermaglich, 1969). This finding has been alternately interpreted as demonstrating mild degrees of cerebral dysfunction in these children or, more probable, as providing evidence for delayed functional maturation of the central nervous system, since many of these described abnormalities were nonspecific and minor.

Sudden onset enuresis and urinary frequency in little girls may be due to *Enterobius vermicularis* (pinworm) infestation without perineal itching. Diagnosis is made by recovery of characteristic eggs in feces, from perianal skin, or from under fingernails. Immediate and dramatic relief of symptoms will follow appropriate anthelmintic therapy (Sachdev and Howards, 1975).

EVALUATION

The enuretic child and family seek medical attention to find cause or cure. Unfortunately, it is often difficult to pinpoint the etiologic factor and to eliminate the symptoms. Out of frustration, the physician may be tempted to perform overly invasive diagnostic testing or to attach pathologic significance to minor anatomic variations and to treat them aggressively. Such an approach is unwarranted for childhood enuresis and is unjustifiable.

Most children with enuresis do not have an organic lesion and those who do are readily detected by routine evaluation. A careful history, physical examination, and urinalysis with culture are needed for all children with bedwetting and are all that is needed for the child with purely nocturnal enuresis. Routine radiographic studies, such as intravenous pyelography or voiding cystourethrography, are not indicated for enuretics who have a normal physical examination, a negative urine, and no obvious neuropathy. This is a view supported by the American Academy of Pediatrics (1980). Likewise, endoscopic evaluation is unwarranted, and urologists must resist the compulsion to inspect and manipulate the lower urinary tracts of children with enuresis simply because they are referred for evaluation. In the vast majority of enuretics, the diagnostic yield from cystourethroscopy is nil, as is the prospect for influencing symptoms by altering urethral caliber or by fulgurating prominent urethral folds.

The nature and extent of the history, physical examination, and urinary examination are important because they will permit wetting pattern recognition, which allows segregation of patients into useful diagnostic and therapeutic categories. Specific features in the voiding history should include the age and success of toilet training, the pattern of urinary incontinence (such as day, night, urgency), maneuvers that are used to stay dry (such as squatting), and the results of prior therapeutic trials. It is often helpful to interview the patient and family privately to assess their perceptions of the problem, to measure the child's maturity and motivation for cure, and to establish rapport. In addition to routine physical examination, neurologic examination is required. Careful palpation and inspection of the lumbosacral spine will reveal hairy patches, lipomata, tracts, or bony irregularities, which suggest occult spinal dysraphism. After a check for rectal sphincter tone and perineal sensation, assessment of the sensory, motor, and reflex functions of the lower extremities is needed to exclude neuropathy. Examination for abnormalities of gait and bony alterations in the lower extremities, such as deformed feet, may reveal evidence of occult neurologic disease. In addition, a complete urinalysis requires a check for proteinuria and for fixed low specific gravity in addition to microscopic examination and urine culture.

The aforementioned evaluation will separate children with only nocturnal enuresis and no infection, who require no additional diagnostic studies, from those with urinary infection or overt neuropathy, who require full urologic investigation. It will also identify those children without infection who either have both daytime and nighttime incontinence or display a variety of dysfunctional voiding symptoms, which may suggest more complicated micturitional disturbances. The majority of these children ultimately prove not to have an underlying anatomic urinary tract abnormality, but instead display urodynamic disturbances such as uninhibited bladder activity. In this group of patients, urinary tract anatomy should be screened and this can be accomplished noninvasively and satisfactorily with an ultrasound examination of the kidneys, ureters, and bladder before and after voiding. This study will effectively exclude even mild degrees of hydroureteronephrosis and will assess the completeness of bladder emptying. Any positive findings can be pursued with conventional urologic studies. When ultrasonography is normal, consideration should be given to an empirical therapeutic trial of pharmacologic agents such as anticholinergic drugs aimed at the suspected urodynamic disturbance. This approach is generally satisfactory provided that the patient continues to be followed closely. If symptoms of wetting persist, complete urodynamic studies are indicated to exclude neuropathy and to identify treatable voiding disturbances.

TREATMENT

A variety of different programs have been used in the treatment of enuresis. They range from home remedies and nonspecific measures, such as decreasing fluids and awakening the child during the night, to sophisticated medical regimens. Because almost all children will eventually outgrow enuresis on their own, it has been genuinely difficult objectively to evaluate even seemingly well controlled treatment programs in order to determine which are effective. This difficulty is compounded by the fact that the yearly spontaneous remission rate is approximately 15 per cent and that the placebo improvement effect may be as high as 68 per cent (Forsythe and Redmond, 1974; Mishra et al., 1980). Despite this analytical handicap, reproducibly proven and effective therapy does exist for enuresis and has evolved along two main lines, pharmacologic therapy and modification of behavior.

Before initiating therapy, the physician must realize, once the parents are reassured that organic causes are excluded, that not all families will desire medical treatment or will accept any risks, inconveniences, or responsibility; some may lack the motivation and intelligence needed to execute and sustain a behavior-oriented therapy. Surprisingly, although most parents generally feel that children should be dry at a much younger age than do physicians, only 63 per cent of parents believe that medical therapy is appropriate treatment for enuresis as opposed to 87 per cent of physicians. Likewise, the vast majority of parents (93 per cent) do not consider drugs a good form of treatment for bedwetting (Haque et al., 1981). It is necessary in developing a treatment plan for the physician to recognize that wide differences exist between parental and physician attitudes and perceptions toward enuresis. For most nocturnal enuretics, therapy should be discouraged before the age of 5 or 6 years. However, for children with significant day and night symptoms, pharmacotherapy may be required at an even younger age (see following).

Pharmacotherapy

AUTONOMIC AGENTS

Effective pharmacologic therapy exists for enuresis, but not in the form of sedatives, stimulants, or sympathomimetic agents (Blackwell and Currah, 1973). Overall, anticholinergic drug therapy has been disappointing. Its effectiveness has been in the range of 5 to 40 per cent, and in some series therapy was unappreciably different from placebo (Leys, 1956; Harrison and Albino, 1970; Kunin et al., 1970; Rapoport et al., 1980). Although anticholinergic drugs have been shown to increase the functional capacity of the bladder in enuretic children, clinical improvement does not follow in about one half of cases (Johnstone, 1972). However, because these agents are very useful in eliminating uninhibited contractions, they may be effective for subgroups of enuretics with this urodynamic disturbance. Indeed, Kass et al. (1979) found anticholinergic therapy to be very effective (87.5 per cent) in treating enuretic patients with symptoms of bladder hyperactivity, such as urgency, frequency, and day and night incontinence, and highly effective (90.6 per cent) in those with proven uninhibited bladder contractions. The success rate was much less (50 per cent) in patients with pure nocturnal enuresis and was only 11 per cent in those with normal cystometrograms. It is apparent that by tailoring pharmacotherapy to clinical symptoms or urodynamic findings that indicate urodynamic disturbances, the results of anticholinergic therapy for enuresis can be improved.

AGENTS AFFECTING URINARY OUTPUT

Reduction of urine output at night is theoretically attractive for treating bedwetting. However, simply limiting fluids or using diuretics during the daytime to produce relative dehydration at night has not been particularly effective (Scott and Morrison, 1980). In contrast, manipulation of antidiuretic hormone levels (ADH, vasopressin) offers a prospect for treatment. Measurements of urinary ADH demonstrate a reversal of the normal diurnal rhythm in some nocturnal enuretics who have lower excretion levels at night (Puri, 1980). Until recently, however, any preparation containing natural vasopressin was not useful for enuresis control because the drug effect was too short or was associated with unpleasant smooth muscle side effects. With the development of desmopressin (DDAVP), an analog of vasopressin, wide potential application for treating enuresis became available. This drug can be given intranasally, has no pressor or smooth muscle activity in the effective dose range, and the effect lasts 7 to 10 hours. In double-blind studies, DDAVP was shown to be an effective treatment in enuresis. By producing a state of antidiuresis early in the night, a 60 per cent reduction in wetting was achieved with up to a 50 per cent cure rate. The dose ranged between 10 and 40 μg and responses were dose-dependent. Best results occurred in older children and no change was noted in morning urine osmolarites. Unfortunately, after treatment most children resumed wetting (Dimson, 1977; Tuvemo, 1978; Birkasova et al., 1978; Puri, 1980; Aladjem et al., 1982).

IMIPRAMINE

Imipramine, typical of a class of tricyclic antidepressants, is probably the most effective and most widely studied of all antienuretic agents. Since its effect on enuresis was first observed in 1960 (MacLean), it has proved to be significantly effective in large numbers of well controlled clinical studies. Overall, enuresis can be cured in over 50 per cent of children and will be improved in another 15 to 20 per cent. However, discontinuation of medication will cause up to 60 per cent of patients to relapse (Hagglund and Parkkulainen, 1965; Poussaint et al., 1966; Kardash et al., 1968; Miller et al., 1968; Milner and Hills, 1968; Shaffer et al., 1968; Esperanca and Gerrard, 1969b; Liederman et al., 1969; Harrison and Albino, 1970; Kunin et al., 1970; Martin, 1971; Blackwell and Currah, 1973). While imipramine (Tofranil) is the most widely used agent, other drugs in this class, such as nortriptyline (Aventyl), amitriptyline (Elavil), and desipramine (Pertofrane), have similar effects.

Imipramine possesses several pharmacologic actions on the central and peripheral nervous system that could be responsible for its effect in enuresis, although its precise mechanism of action remains unknown. Its peripheral effects include: (1) weak anticholinergic activity that is $1/157$ as active as atropine on bladder smooth muscle (Sigg, 1959) but that is ineffective in abolishing uninhibited detrusor contractions (Diokno et al., 1972); (2) direct in vitro antispasmodic activity on bladder smooth muscle that is inapparent at clinically effective antienuretic doses (Labay and Boyarsky, 1973; Stephenson, 1979); and (3) a complex effect on sympathetic input to the bladder, which prevents norepinephrine action on alpha receptors and enhances its effect on beta receptors by inhibiting norepinephrine reuptake (Labay and Boyarsky, 1973; Stephenson, 1979). Combined, these peripheral actions of imipramine produce significant increase in bladder capacity. It has been observed that successful clinical improvement in enuresis correlates with an average 34 per cent increase in bladder functional capacity (Hagglund, 1965), while those children who have no change in bladder capacity are generally not cured (Esperanca and Gerrard, 1969b).

Imipramine effects on the central nervous system include its antidepressant activity and its action on sleep. It is unlikely that antienuretic effect is related to antidepressant activity because the time course of action in enuresis is immediate, whereas the effect on depression requires higher dosage and is often delayed for a period of time (Rapoport et al., 1980). Imipramine significantly alters sleep patterns by decreasing the time spent in REM sleep and increasing the time spent in light non-REM sleep. This REM sleep suppression occurs primarily during the first two thirds of the night, and as a result there are less enuretic events in this period of sleep and more during the last third. In sleep studies, imipramine can be shown to reduce the total number of wetting episodes, but it does not appreciably alter the time at which wetting occurs. Incontinence seems to occur in each sleep stage roughly in proportion to the time spent in that stage (Ritvo et al., 1969; Kales et al., 1977; Rapoport et al., 1980). Compared with placebo, no more frequent night wakenings occur during imipramine therapy and the occurrence of wakenings does not correlate with clinical response. This indicates that imipramine does not work by converting enuresis to nocturia and further supports the observation that its effect on sleep stage is independent of its effect on enuresis (Kales et al., 1977; Rapoport et al., 1980).

Clinical response to imipramine has been shown to correlate with plasma levels, and this has provided a better understanding of drug action and a more rational approach to therapy (Jorgensen et al., 1980; Rapoport et al., 1980). Imipramine is generally prescribed as a single dose of 25 mg for children between 5 and 8 years of age and 50 mg for older children. On a weight basis, the usual recommended dosage is 0.9 to 1.5 mg per kg per day (Maxwell and Seldrup, 1971). Unfortunately, this dosage results in an optimal therapeutic plasma concentration in only 30 per cent of patients (Jorgensen et al., 1980). This finding may explain the variability in clinical effect noted in early reports. An increase of 3- to 5-fold in dose would be required to achieve a therapeutic level in all patients, but this cannot be justified because nearly toxic levels would result for a significant number of patients (Stephenson, 1979). However, even high plasma levels will not ensure a response in all instances, since true nonresponders can be identified as well as patients who have developed a tolerance to the antienuretic effect of the drug.

Imipramine is generally given once per day and usually shortly before bedtime. The exact time of administration does not appear critical, although some children who wet very early at night may benefit from late afternoon administration (Alderton, 1970). A 2-week trial is generally adequate to assess drug responsiveness. Thereafter, adjustments in the dosage and time can be made if necessary. It is not entirely clear how long a satisfactorily responding child should be kept on drug therapy. Since the long-term effects of tricyclic therapy in children are unknown, continued medication is difficult to justify except in instances where the child is extremely distressed or when all other therapies have been exhausted and are unsuccessful. When the decision is made to stop medication, it may be advisable to wean the drug rather than to discontinue therapy abruptly, since some studies have shown a reduced tendency for a relapse using this withdrawal technique (Martin, 1971).

Imipramine drug therapy has two potentially hazardous consequences. The first is a manifestation of drug toxicity. Side effects, although infrequent, include personality changes, adverse effects on sleep and appetite, gastrointestinal symptoms, and nervousness (Shaffer et al., 1968; Kardash et al., 1968). Because of the low ratio between beneficial effect and toxic effect, toxic overdose is a potential hazard. At greatest risk are the younger siblings of enuretics who unwarily ingest the medication in large amounts. Poisoning is characterized by severe myocardial depression and electrocardiographic changes that are not observed at therapeutic levels (Fouron and Chicoine, 1971; Koehl and Wenzel, 1971; Martin, 1973; Rohner and Sanford, 1975). Should a toxic reaction occur, careful attention must be given to specific therapeutic protocols aimed at drug effect reversal (Green and Cromie, 1981).

The second effect of imipramine that is potentially problematic is its ability to improve wetting symptoms not only in cases of enuresis but also when the incontinence is due to an organic abnormality such as neuropathy (Epstein and DeQuevedo, 1964; Cole and Fried, 1972). As a result, the use of imipramine as a therapeutic test to distinguish organic from nonorganic incontinence is not advisable.

Behavioral Modification

Modification of behavior to control enuresis has met with varying success. While generalized supportive measures designed to improve self-confidence and provide encouragement are unpredictably effective, certain specific approaches, when determinedly applied to a motivated child, may produce favorable results. Techniques that have been used include bladder training, responsibility reinforcement, and classical conditioning therapy. Often a successful treatment program for enuresis combines aspects of each specific technique that may be used in conjunction with pharmacotherapy.

BLADDER TRAINING

Bladder training or so-called retention control training (Kimmel and Kimmel, 1970) was developed as specific therapy for the reduced functional bladder capacity that characterizes most enuretics. Since an increase in the functional capacity of the bladder correlates positively with reduced bedwetting, the rationale for this treatment is well founded and the initial results were promising. The goal of therapy is to increase progressively the time interval between voiding so that the bladder capacity is effectively enlarged. Positive reinforcement is provided as the child goes for longer intervals and demonstrates larger recorded urine volumes. With retention control therapy, mean bladder capacity can be increased sizably in enuretic subjects compared with controls (approximately 35 per cent). However, as a cure for enuresis, this method has not met clinical expectations, because the frequency of bedwetting does not appear to decrease significantly in many children so treated. Although enlargement in bladder capacity generally accompanies cure of enuresis, treatments aimed only at bladder capacity, such as retention control therapy and anticholinergic therapy, are not effective for most nocturnal wetters (Doleys, 1977; Harris and Purohit, 1977).

RESPONSIBILITY REINFORCEMENT

Behavioral modification techniques are successful in treating enuresis, but they require a motivated child, conscientious parents, and rapport between the physician and family. The components of a successful responsibility reinforcement program include motivation, reward, response shaping, and reinforcement. The program aims to motivate the child to assume both the responsibility for wetting and the credit for dryness. The child keeps a progress record or "gold star" chart, and by trying to determine what factors are responsible for wetting, attempts to reduce enuresis and to keep totally dry. Progressively longer dry intervals and dry nights are rewarded by stars or an equivalent. The consequence of these stepwise rewards for changes in behavior results, in a generalized molding of responses and progressive attainment of continence.

The results of a responsibility reinforcement program may be difficult to evaluate on a controlled basis because better results are observed when the child takes an active role in therapy compared with a passive role. For selected children, improvement may be more rapid and the relapse rate lower than with other types of programs (Marshall et al., 1973).

CONDITIONING THERAPY

The urinary alarm was popularized by Mowrer and Mowrer in 1938 for the treatment of enuresis. It consists of a battery-operated detector upon which the child sleeps. The detector is activated by urine and the child is awakened by a bell, turns off the alarm, and then gets up and completes voiding in the toilet. The success of the urinary alarm method has been explained by classical conditioning theory. If the alarm that awakens the child and initiates inhibition of micturition is repeatedly followed by the onset of normal voiding, then ultimately those factors causing the reflex micturition at night, such as bladder distention, would produce the same inhibition response as the alarm and awaken the child before enuresis occurs (Doleys, 1977). Although not all investigators agree with the precise mechanism of effect (Lovibond, 1963), conditioning therapy using an alarm appears to be the most statistically effective available therapy for enuresis.

The single most important cause for failure of the alarm has been lack of parental understanding and cooperation. This can be prevented by proper instruction and supervision. However, before embarking on this program, parents and child must be motivated and well selected, and recognize that the period of therapy is long, often lasting approximately 4 months. In addition, there must be no delay between the alarm sounding and the child getting up to void. As a result, parents may have to awaken their child at variable times throughout the night, and this no doubt leads to the high dropout rate observed with conditioning therapy. Once enuresis has been converted to nocturia or cured completely, relapse can be prevented in many instances by using overlearning techniques. These involve forcing fluids prior to bedtime to promote bladder overdistention in order to provide a stronger conditioning stimulus. The likelihood for relapse can also be reduced by having the alarm sound intermittently on some nights but not others.

In controlled studies, the urine alarm is superior to drug therapy, with a cure rate of 60 to 100 per cent. Although over 25 per cent of patients may relapse, in many instances this is preventable and retreatment will effect a cure in a significant proportion (Forsythe and Redmond, 1970; Young and Morgan, 1973; Doleys, 1977). Conditioning therapy is effective under a variety of circumstances; age and intelligence are not factors in achieving dryness, nor is the amount of incontinence.

Even when used as described, the urine alarm is not entirely free of complications. So-called buzzer ulcers have occurred when parts of the body soaked in urine remained in prolonged contact with the passage of a current through the wet pad. Weak batteries producing a continued low-voltage current insufficient to activate the alarm have been implicated and should be avoided (Greaves, 1969; Neal and Coote, 1969). Advances in electronics have made this complication less likely and have enabled production of futuristic "wrist radio" type alarms, which are both appealing and safe for children and reasonably inexpensive.

Miscellaneous Therapy

In addition to the aforementioned programs, numerous other treatments have been used for enuresis. Hypnotherapy and psychotherapy are highly effective for selected patients who have a stressful emotional cause for their wetting or in whom enuresis accompanies psychologic disturbance. However, for most enuretics who have no significant psychopathologic disorder, these approaches would be inappropriate and inefficient (Fraser, 1972).

Certain children will show a marked improvement following recognition and elimination of dietary ingredients that enhance enuresis. The approach to diagnosis is similar to that used to identify food allergens, which involves serial elimination of foods such as chocolate, dairy products, and red-dye containing substances (Esperanca and Gerrard, 1969b). Of course, foods and drinks that contain caffeine may enhance enuresis by producing a diuresis that overwhelms the small functional capacity bladder and should be omitted.

ADULT ENURESIS

Enuresis occurring in adults is seen in two contexts: persistent primary enuresis, which occurs in over 1 per cent of the population (Levine, 1943; Miller et al., 1973), and adult onset enuresis. Unlike the situation in children, a high proportion (over 70 per cent) of adults with persistent primary enuresis will display overt urodynamic abnormalities, generally in the form of uninhibited bladder activity (Torrens and Collins, 1975; Whiteside and Arnold, 1975). These abnormalities are not due to a neuropathic process, and once identified may persist for many years as fixed urodynamic disturbances. Although symptoms from uninhibited bladder dysfunction usually depend on the frequency of detrusor contraction and on the opposing forcefulness of sphincteric constriction, the presence of diurnal symptoms and urge incontinence are often useful predictors of which patient has uninhibited bladder activity and may be a guide to empirical pharmacologic therapy (Hindmarsh and Byrne, 1980). In the absence of overt neuropathy, urinary infection, or obstructive symptoms, the incidence of organic disease does not appear to be appreciably greater for adults with persistent nocturnal enuresis than for children (Torrens and Collins, 1975). Even though the presence of diurnal symptoms may increase the likelihood of urodynamic disturbance in these patients, it is not clear that such symptoms increase the possibility of organic disease. Consequently, it is a matter of clinical judgment in each individual case to determine the need for and the extent of investigation in excess of the evaluation required for childhood enuresis. Once a diagnosis of primary enuresis has been established, treatment may follow the general guidelines described for children.

Acquired or adult onset enuresis is not generally a solitary symptom, but occurs more commonly in association with generalized bladder hyperactivity and with other disturbances of micturition and continence. Even in the absence of urinary infection, patients usually require a thorough anatomic evaluation as well as a careful neurologic and urodynamic study, recognizing that occult neurologic dysfunction and anatomic disease can masquerade as a disturbance of genitourinary tract function and present as adult onset enuresis.

SUMMARY

The physician evaluating and treating enuresis must keep in perspective its medical significance and recognize that for the vast majority of patients the condition is medically benign and subject to a high spontaneous cure rate. Because an organic cause for enuresis is rare, and such patients can usually be readily diagnosed by a systematic history, physical examination, and urinalysis, the evaluation of most enuretics can be accomplished in the office at the first visit. The so-called urologic workup consisting of an intravenous pyelogram, voiding cystogram, and cystoscopy has no place in the routine evaluation of childhood enuretics. Such studies should be considered only after less invasive tests, such as ultrasonography, incriminate structural disease.

For certain enuretics, no therapy is necessary, since none will be successful; all involved must wait frustratingly until spontaneous cure occurs. Assessment of the motivation of the family and particularly the child is important in determining whether therapy more than reassurance alone is actually being sought and in deciding which treatment is likely to succeed. The most statistically effective therapy for enuresis includes conditioning therapy with either the urine alarm or behavior-oriented techniques. These can only be effective provided they are properly supervised and continued sufficiently long in highly receptive and motivated individuals. Considering the potential and unknown risks of long-term pharmacotherapy, drugs such as imipramine probably should be reserved for failures of other therapy or when short-term dry periods are essential.

References

Aladjem, M., Wohl, R., Boichis, H., et al.: Desmopressin in nocturnal enuresis. Arch. Dis. Child., 57:137, 1982.

Alderton, H. R.: Imipramine in childhood enuresis: Further studies on the relationship of time of administration to effect. Can. Med. Assoc. J., 102:1179, 1970.

American Academy of Pediatrics, Committee on Radiology: Excretory urography for evaluation of enuresis. Pediatrics, 65:644, 1980.

Anders, T. F., and Weinstein, P.: Sleep and its disorders in infants: A review. Pediatrics, 50:312, 1972.

Apley, J., and MacKeith, R.: The Child and His Symptoms. 2nd ed. Philadelphia, F. A. Davis Co., 1968.

Arnold, S. J., and Ginsberg, A.: Enuresis, incidence and pertinence of genitourinary disease in healthy enuretic children. Urology, 2:437, 1973.

Baker, B. L.: Symptom treatment and symptom substitution in enuresis. J. Abnorm. Psychol., 74:42, 1969.

Bakwin, H.: Enuresis in twins. Am. J. Dis. Child., 121:222, 1971.

Bakwin, H.: The genetics of enuresis. In Kolvin, I. MacKeith, R. C., and Meadow, S. R. (Eds.): Bladder Control and Enuresis. London, W. Heinemann Medical Books Ltd., 1973, pp. 73–77.

Bindelglas, P. M., and Dee, G.: Enuresis treatment with imipramine hydrochloride: A 10-year follow-up study. Am. J. Psychiatry, 135:12, 1978.

Birkasova, M., Birkas, O., Flynn, M. J., et al.: Desmopressin in the management of nocturnal enuresis in children: A double blind study. Pediatrics, 62:970, 1978.

Blackwell, B., and Currah, J.: The psychopharmacology of nocturnal enuresis. In Kolvin, I., MacKeith, R. C., and Meadow, S. R. (Eds.): Bladder Control and Enuresis. London, W. Heinemann Medical Books Ltd., 1973, pp. 231–257.

Boyd, M. M.: The depth of sleep in enuretic school children and nonenuretic controls. J. Psychosom. Res., 4:274, 1960.

Broughton, R. J.: Sleep disorders: Disorders of arousal? Science, 159:1070, 1968.

Campbell, E. W., Jr., and Young, J. D., Jr.: Enuresis and its relationship to electroencephalographic disturbances. J. Urol., 96:947, 1966.

Cole, A. T., and Fried, F. A.: Favorable experiences with imipramine in the treatment of neurogenic bladder. J. Urol., 107:44, 1972.

Cutler, C., Middleton, A. W., and Nixon, G. W.: Radiographic findings in children surveyed for enuresis. Urology, 11:480, 1978.

Dimson, S. B.: Desmopressin as treatment for enuresis. Lancet, 1:1260, 1977.

Diokno, A. C., Hyndman, C. W., Hardy, D. A., and Lapides, J.: Comparison of action of imipramine (Tofranil) and propantheline (Probanthine) on detrusor contractions. J. Urol., 107:42, 1972.

Diokno, A. C., Koff, S. A., and Bender, L.: Periurethral striated muscle activity in neurogenic bladder dysfunction. J. Urol. 112:743, 1974.

Dodge, W. F., West, E. F., Bridgforth, E. B., and Travis, L. B.: Nocturnal enuresis in 6 to 10 year-old children. Correlation with bacteriuria, proteinuria and dysuria. Am. J. Dis. Child., 120:32, 1970.

Doleys, D. M.: Behavioral treatments for nocturnal enuresis in children: A review of the recent literature. Psychol. Bull. 1:30, 1977.

Epstein, S. J., and DeQuevedo, A.: The control of enuresis with imipramine in the presence of organic bladder disease. Am. J. Psychiatry, 120:908, 1964.

Esperanca, M., and Gerrard, J. W.: Nocturnal enuresis: Studies in bladder function in normal children and enuretics. Can. Med. Assoc. J., 101:324, 1969a.

Esperanca, M., and Gerrard, J. W.: Nocturnal enuresis. Comparison of the effect of imipramine and dietary restriction on bladder capacity. Can. Med. Assoc. J., *101*:721, 1969b.

Essen, J., and Peckham, C.: Nocturnal enuresis in childhood. Dev. Med. Child Neurol., *18*:577, 1976.

Fermaglich, J. L.: Electroencephalographic study of enuretics. Am. J. Dis. Child., *118*:473, 1969.

Fisher, O. D., and Forsythe, W. I.: Micturating cystourethrography in the investigation of enuresis. Arch. Dis. Child., *29*:460, 1954.

Forsythe, W. I., and Redmond, A.: Enuresis and the electric alarm. Study of 200 cases. Br. Med. J., *1*:211, 1970.

Forsythe, W. I., and Redmond, A.: Enuresis and spontaneous cure rate. Study of 1129 enuretics. Arch. Dis. Child., *49*:259, 1974.

Fouron, J., and Chicoine, R.: ECG changes in fatal imipramine (Tofranil) intoxication. Pediatrics, *48*:777, 1971.

Frary, L. G.: Enuresis: A genetic study. Am. J. Dis. Child., *49*:553, 1935.

Fraser, M. S.: Nocturnal enuresis. Practitioner, *208*:203, 1972.

Gastaut, H., and Broughton, R.: A clinical and polygraphic study of episodic phenomena during sleep. *In* Wortis, J. (Ed.): Recent Advances in Biological Psychiatry. New York, Plenum Press, 1965, pp. 197–221.

Giles, G. R., Light, K., and Van Blerk, P. J. P.: Cystometrogram studies in enuretic children. S. Afr. J. Surg., *16*:33, 1978.

Goellner, M. H., Ziegler, E. E., and Fomon, S. J.: Urination during the first three years of life. Nephron, *28*:174, 1981.

Graham, P.: Depth of sleep and enuresis: A critical review. *In* Kolvin, I., MacKeith, R. C., and Meadow, S. R. (Eds.): Bladder Control and Enuresis. London, W. Heinemann Medical Books Ltd., 1973, pp. 78–83.

Greaves, M. W.: Hazards of enuresis alarms. Arch. Dis. Child., *44*:285, 1969.

Green, A. S., and Cromie, W. J.: Treatment of imipramine overdose in children. Urology, *18*:314, 1981.

Grossman, H. B., Koff, S. A., and Diokno, A. C.: Cystometry in children. J. Urol., *117*:646, 1977.

Hagglund, T. B.: Enuretic children treated with fluid restriction or forced drinking. A clinical and cystometric study. Ann. Paediatr. Fenn., *11*:84, 1965.

Hagglund, T. B., and Parkkulainen, K. V.: Enuretic children treated with imipramine (Tofranil). Ann. Paediatr. Fenn., *11*:53, 1965.

Hallgren, B.: Enuresis. A clinical and genetic study. Acta Psychiatr. Neurol. Scand. [Suppl.], *114*:1, 1957.

Hallman, N.: On the ability of enuretic children to hold urine. Acta Paediatr., *39*:87, 1950.

Haque, M., Ellerstein, N. S., Gundy, J. H., et al.: Parental perceptions in enuresis, a collaborative study. Am. J. Dis. Child., *135*:809, 1981.

Harris, L. S., and Purohit, A. P.: Bladder training and enuresis: A controlled trial. Behav. Res. Ther., *15*:485, 1977.

Harrison, J. S., and Albino, V. J.: An investigation into the effects of imipramine hydrochloride on the incidence of enuresis in institutionalized children. S. Afr. Med. J., *44*:253, 1970.

Hindmarsh, J. R., and Byrne, P. O.: Adult enuresis—a symptomatic and urodynamic assessment. Br. J. Urol., *52*:88, 1980.

Johnstone, J. M. S.: Cystometry and evaluation of anticholinergic drugs in enuretic children. J. Pediatr. Surg., 7:18, 1972.

Jorgensen, O. S., Lober, M., Christiansen, J., et al.: Plasma concentration and clinical effect in imipramine treatment of childhood enuresis. Clin. Pharmacokinetics, 5:386, 1980.

Kajtor, F., Ovary, I., and Zsadanyi, O.: Nocturnal enuresis: Electroencephalographic and cystometric examinations. Acta Med. Acad. Sci. Hung., *23*:153, 1967.

Kales, A., and Kales, J. D.: Sleep disorders. Recent findings in the diagnosis and treatment of disturbed sleep. N. Engl. J. Med., *290*:487, 1974.

Kales, A., Kales, J. D., Jacobson, A., Humphrey, F. J., and Soldatos, C. R.: Effect of imipramine on enuretic frequency and sleep stages. Pediatrics, *60*:431, 1977.

Kaplan, G.: Serum IgE and allergy in enuresis. Presented at Section on Urology, American Academy of Pediatrics, Oct. 22, 1973.

Kardash, S., Hillman, E. S., and Werry, J.: Efficacy of imipramine in childhood enuresis: A double blind control study with placebo. Can. Med. Assoc. J., *99*:263, 1968.

Kass, E. J., Diokno, A. C., and Montealegre, A.: Enuresis: Principles of management and result of treatment. J. Urol., *121*:794, 1979.

Kimmel, H. D., and Kimmel, E. C.: An instrumental conditioning method for the treatment of enuresis. J. Behav. Ther. Exp. Psychiatry, *1*:121, 1970.

Koehl, G. W., and Wenzel, J. E.: Severe postural hypotension due to imipramine therapy. Pediatrics, *47*:71, 1971.

Koff, S. A.: Estimating bladder capacity in children. Urology, *21*:248, 1983.

Koff, S. A., and Murtagh, D. S.: The uninhibited bladder in children: Effect of treatment on recurrence of urinary infection and on vesicoureteral reflux resolution. J. Urol. *130*:1138, 1983.

Koff, S. A., Lapides, J., and Piazza, D. H.: The uninhibited bladder in children: A cause for urinary tract infection, obstruction and reflux. *In* Hodson, J., and Kincaid-Smith, P. (Eds.): Reflux Nephropathy. New York, Masson Publishing, 1979.

Kunin, S. A., Limbert, D. J., Platzker, A. C. G., and McGinley, J.: The efficacy of imipramine in the management of enuresis. J. Urol., *104*:612, 1970.

Labay, P., and Boyarsky, S.: The action of imipramine on the bladder musculature. J. Urol., *109*:385, 1973.

Lapides, J., and Diokno, A. C.: Persistence of the infant bladder as a cause of urinary infection in girls. J. Urol., *103*:243, 1970.

Lapides, J., Sweet, R. B., and Lewis, L. W.: Role of striated muscle in urination. J. Urol. 77:247, 1957.

Levine, A.: Enuresis in the Navy. Am. J. Psychiatry, *100*:320, 1943.

Leys, D.: Value of propantheline bromide in treatment of enuresis. Br. Med. J., *1*:549, 1956.

Liederman, P. C., Wasserman, D. H., and Liederman, V. R.: Desipramine in the treatment of enuresis. J. Urol., *101*:314, 1969.

Linderholm, B. E.: The cystometric findings in enuresis. J. Urol., *96*:718, 1966.

Lovibond, S. H.: The mechanism of conditioning treatment of enuresis. Behav. Res. Ther., *1*:17, 1963.

Lowy, F. H.: Recent sleep and dream research: Clinical implications. Can. Med. Assoc. J., *102*:1069, 1970.

MacKeith, R. C.: A frequent factor in the origins of primary nocturnal enuresis: Anxiety in the third year of life. Dev. Med. Child Neurol., *10*:465, 1968.

MacKeith, R. C.: Is maturation delay a frequent factor in the origins of primary nocturnal enuresis? Dev. Med. Child Neurol., *14*:217, 1972.

MacLean, R. E. G.: Imipramine hydrochloride (Tofranil) and enuresis. Am. J. Psychiatry, *117*:551, 1960.

Mahony, D. T.: Studies of enuresis. I. Incidence of obstructive lesions and pathophysiology of enuresis. J. Urol., *106*:951, 1971.

Mahony, D. T., Laferte, R. O., and Blais, D. J.: Studies on enuresis. IX. Evidence of a mild form of compensated detrusor hyperreflexia in enuretic children. J. Urol., *126*:520, 1981.

Marshall, S., Marshall, H. H., and Lyon, R. P.: Enuresis: An analysis of various therapeutic approaches. Pediatrics, *52*:813, 1973.

Martin, G. I.: Imipramine pamoate in the treatment of childhood enuresis. A double-blind study. Am. J. Dis. Child., *122*:42, 1971.

Martin, G. I.: ECG monitoring of enuretic children given imipramine. JAMA, *244*:902, 1973.

Maxwell, C., and Seldrup, J.: Imipramine in the treatment of childhood enuresis. Practitioner, *207*:809, 1971.

McKendry, J. B. J., and Stewart, D. A.: Enuresis. Pediatr. Clin. North Am., *21*:1019, 1974.

McKendry, J. B. J., Williams, H. A. L., and Broughton, C.: Enuresis—a study of untreated patients. Appl. Ther., *10*:815, 1968.

Mikkelsen, E. J., Rapoport, J. L., Nee, L., et al.: Childhood enuresis. I. Sleep patterns and psychopathology. Arch. Gen. Psychiatry, *37*:1139, 1980.

Miller, F. J. W., Court, S. D. M., Walton, N. G., and Knox, E. G.: Growing-up in Newcastle upon Tyne. London, Oxford University Press, 1960.

Miller, F. J. W., Knox, E. G., and Brandon, S.: Children who wet the bed. *In* Kolvin, I., MacKeith, R. C., and Meadow, S. R. (Eds.): Bladder Control and Enuresis. London, W. Heinemann Medical Books Ltd., 1973, pp. 47–52.

Miller, P. R., Champelli, J. W., and Dinello, F. A.: Imipramine in the treatment of enuretic school children. Am. J. Dis. Child., *115*:17, 1968.

Milner, G., and Hills, N. F.: A double-blind assessment of antidepressants in the treatment of 212 enuretic patients. Med. J. Aust., *1*:943, 1968.

Mishra, P. C., Agarwal, V. K., and Rahman, H.: Therapeutic trial of amytriptiline in the treatment of nocturnal enuresis—a controlled study. Indian Pediatr., *17*:279, 1980.

Mowrer, O. H., and Mowrer, W. M.: Enuresis—a method for its study and treatment. Am. J. Orthopsychiatry, *8*:436, 1938.

Muellner, S. R.: Development of urinary control in children. JAMA, *172*:1256, 1960.

Nash, D. F. E.: The development of micturition control with special reference to enuresis. Ann. R. Coll. Surg. Engl., *5*:318, 1949.

Neal, B. W., and Coote, M. A.: Hazards of enuresis alarms. Arch. Dis. Child., *44*:651, 1969.

Oppel, W. C., Harper, P. A., and Rider, R. V.: The age of attaining bladder control. Pediatrics, *42*:614, 1968.

Pompeius, R.: Cystometry in pediatric enuresis. Scand. J. Urol., *5*:222, 1971.

Poussaint, A. F., Ditman, K. S., and Greenfield, R.: Amitriptyline in childhood enuresis. Clin. Pharmacol. Ther., *7*:21, 1966.

Puri, V. N.: Urinary levels of antidiuretic hormone in nocturnal enuresis. Indian Pediatr., *17*:675, 1980.

Rapoport, J. L., Mikkelsen, E. J., Zavodil, A., et al.: Childhood enuresis. II. Arch. Gen. Psychiatry, *37*:1146, 1980.

Rechtschaffen, A., and Kales, A. (Eds.): A Manual of Standardized Terminology, Techniques and Scoring System for Sleep Stages of Human Subjects. Los Angeles, Brain Information Service/Brain Research Institute, UCLA, 1968, pp. 1–12.

Redman, J. F., and Seibert, J. J.: The uroradiographic evaluation of the enuretic child. J. Urol., *122*:799, 1979.

Ritvo, E. R., Ornitz, E. M., Gottlieb, F., Poussaint, A. F., Maron, B. J., Ditman, K. S., and Blinn, K. A.: Arousal and non-arousal enuretic events. Am. J. Psychiatry, *126*:115, 1969.

Rohner, T. J., and Sanford, E. J.: Imipramine toxicity. J. Urol., *114*:402, 1975.

Sachdev, Y. V., and Howards, S. S.: Enterobius vermicularis infestation and secondary enuresis. J. Urol., *113*:143, 1975.

Scott, R., and Morrison, L. H.: Diuretic treatment of enuresis: Preliminary communication. J. R. Coll. Surg. Edinb., *25*:470, 1980.

Shaffer, D., Costello, A. J., and Hill, I. D.: Control of enuresis with imipramine. Arch. Dis. Child., *43*:665, 1968.

Sigg, E. B.: Pharmacological studies with Tofranil. Can. Psychiatr. Assoc. J., *4*:75, 1959.

Starfield, B.: Functional bladder capacity in enuretic and non-enuretic children. J. Pediatr., *5*:777, 1967.

Stein, Z. M., and Susser, M. W.: Social factors in the development of sphincter control. Dev. Med. Child Neurol., *9*:692, 1967.

Stephenson, J. D.: Physiological and pharmacological basis for the chemotherapy of imipramine. Psychol. Med. *9*:249, 1979.

Strom-Olsen, R.: Enuresis in adults and abnormality of sleep. Lancet, *2*:133, 1950.

Torrens, M. J., and Collins, C. D.: The urodynamic assessment of adult enuresis. Br. J. Urol., *47*:433, 1975.

Troup, C. W., and Hodgson, N. B.: Nocturnal functional bladder capacity in enuretic children. J. Urol., *129*:132, 1971.

Tuvemo, T.: DDAVP in childhood nocturnal enuresis. Acta Pediatr. Scand., *67*:753, 1978.

Werry, J. S.: Enuresis—a psychosomatic entity? Can. Med. Assoc. J., *97*:319, 1967.

Whiteside, C. G., and Arnold, E. P.: Persistent primary enuresis: A urodynamic assessment. Br. Med. J., *1*:364, 1975.

Yeates, W. K.: Bladder function in normal micturition. *In* Kolvin, I., MacKeith, R. C., and Meadow, S. R. (Eds.): Bladder Control and Enuresis. London, W. Heinemann Medical Books Ltd., 1973, pp. 28–36.

Young, G. C., and Morgan, R. T. T.: Conditioning technics and enuresis. Med. J. Aust., *2*:329, 1973.

Zaleski, A., Shokeir, M. K., and Gerrard, J. W.: Enuresis: Familial incidence and relationship to allergic disorders. Can. Med. Assoc. J., *106*:30, 1972.

CHAPTER 55

Myelomeningocele

R. LAWRENCE KROOVAND, M.D.

Myelomeningocele has been recognized in skeletons that were found in northeastern Morocco and were estimated to be almost 12,000 years old. The earliest recorded medical description of myelomeningocele was by ancient Greek and Arabian physicians, who felt that the vertebral defect was caused by the tumor (i.e., herniated neural tissue). Professor Nicolai Tulp of Amsterdam first employed the term *spina bifida* in 1552. Although many other terms have been used to describe the defect, spina bifida remains the most useful because it describes the separation of the vertebral bodies in the midline. Morgagni reported the association of lower limb deformities, hydrocephalus, and spina bifida in 1761, and later, in the nineteenth century, Cleland in 1883, Chiari in 1891 and 1896, and Arnold in 1894 described in detail the brain stem anomalies responsible for the hydrocephalus (Frank and Fixsen, 1980) that is commonly associated with myelomeningocele.

Although the first accurate medical description of myelomeningocele occurred more than a century ago, it has been only during the past decade that a more thorough understanding of variations in the disease and a more aggressive approach to the physical, psychologic, and educational deficits that are commonly encountered in these children have led to significant advances in treatment. This chapter will review the multifaceted problems associated with myelomeningocele and will provide a rational approach for the management of these children.

NOMENCLATURE—DEFINITION OF TERMS

There are two major types of spina bifida: *spina bifida cystica (aperta)* and *spina bifida occulta*. Spina bifida occulta, a normal variant, represents an incomplete fusion of the neural arches in the midline. Spina bifida occulta occurs in 5 per cent of the normal population, usually at the L5 to S1 level, and it is virtually never associated with spinal cord abnormality. Spina bifida cystica (aperta) describes the cystic protrusion of the spinal cord or its coverings, or both, through a congenital defect in the posterior neural arches. There are two distinct, different types of spina bifida cystica: *myelomeningocele* and *meningocele*.

Myelomeningocele composes 90 per cent of spina bifida cystica cases and is potentially the most serious because there is usually paralysis at the level of the lesion and below. There is a wide defect in the posterior neural arches caused by defective fusion of one to several of the posterior vertebral arches. The neural spines are absent, and the everted pedicles and laminae are well away from the midline. The meninges and neural tissues protrude through the bony defect (Fig. 55–1). More extensive bony defects can be described as rachischisis (myeloschisis) (Fig. 55–2). Most myelomeningoceles are lumbar or lumbosacral (Table 55–1).

Meningocele is less common than myelomeningocele, accounting for approximately 5 per cent of spina bifida cystica cases. Meningoceles usually occur in the cervical spine and contain a herniated sac covered by meninges but no neural elements. Paralysis and neurologic defects are less common than with myelomeningocele.

Lipomeningocele is an infrequent but important variant of spina bifida cystica in which a lipomatous tumor is embedded within the lumbar spinal cord and often replaces the overlying dura. A soft mass may be palpable overlying the lumbar spine, or a characteristic lesion

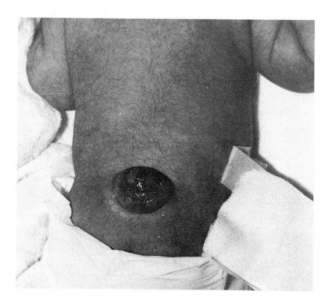

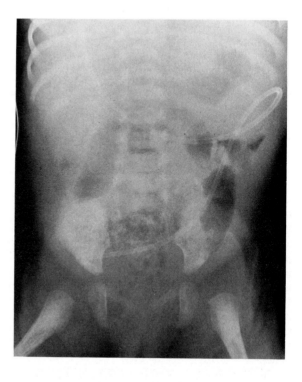

Figure 55–1. A newborn infant with an intact myelo-meningocele.

Figure 55–2. Plain film of the abdomen demonstrating the absence of the posterior lamellae and widening of the interpedicular distance of the vertebrae in a patient with myelomeningocele. Such extensive defects may be described as a rachischisis. Note the presence of the ventriculoperitoneal shunt.

TABLE 55–1. Spinal Level of Myelomeningocele

Location	Incidence
Cervical—high thoracic	2%
Low thoracid	5%
Lumbar	26%
Lumbosacral	47%
Sacral	20%

(tufts of hair, nevi, or a dermal sinus tract or dimple) may be evident overlying the skin in the sacral area (Fig. 55–3). Lipomeningocele causes little if any early impairment but may produce progressive neurologic deficit as the child grows resulting from compression and stretching of nerve roots (Till, 1969).

PATHOGENESIS OF SPINA BIFIDA CYSTICA

Developmentally, the primary failure of neural tube closure that leads to myelomeningocele occurs early during embryogenesis, usually by the twenty-sixth gestational day. Most authorities agree that the lesion begins with a failure of the embryonic neural plate to close in its caudal part, and that from this initial error the changes in the surrounding tissue follow—for example, failure of neural arch fusion.

The occurrence of myelodysplasia may be influenced by a number of poorly understood genetic and environmental factors, including geographic location, socioeconomic status, and dietary intake or deficiency (Laurence, 1969; Naggan and MacMahon, 1967; Renwick, 1972; Yen and MacMahon, 1968). Despite numerous etiologic theories suggested by subprimate teratologic research, no single hypothesis has been widely accepted or rigorously proved. Clusters of cases occur, with a higher incidence among the poor and among those living in wet, temperate climates. Even within the small area of the United Kingdom, there are marked differences in the occurrence rates of spina bifida. Rogers and Weatherhall (1976) reported regional variations in the occurrence of neural tube defects in Wales, with the incidence of spina bifida in the mining valleys being almost twice that in the coastal plain around Cardiff. Seasonal variations were noted by Guthkelch (1962); babies born between December and May have a higher incidence for myelomeningocele than those born between June and November. Carter (1974) found the situation to be reversed in the Southern Hemisphere.

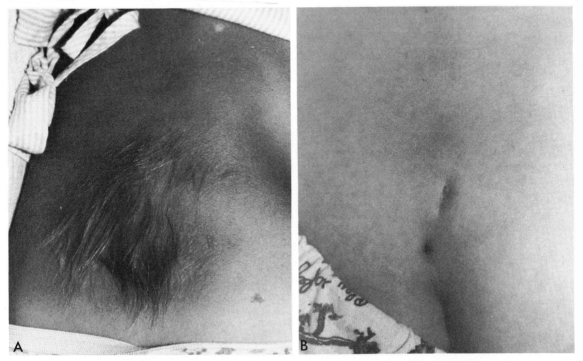

Figure 55–3. *A,* An extensive hairy nevus overlying the lumbosacral spine in a child with a lipomeningocele. *B,* Sinus tract overlying the lumbosacral spine in a child with a lipomeningocele.

Although a genetic component appears to influence the occurrence of spina bifida, more than 90 per cent of all pregnancies that produce neural tube defects occur in families without a history of previously affected members (Haddow and Macri, 1979; Laurence and David, 1965; Laurence, 1969). A first-born child is at greater risk than are subsequent children, and girls are more commonly affected than boys (1.0:0.7) (Nevin et al., 1981). The condition occurs twice as often in mothers past 35 years of age and in parents with a history of pilonidal cyst or scoliosis (Renwick, 1972; Tavafoghi et al., 1978). Ethnic differences, an increased recurrence risk after the birth of an affected child, and a 63 per cent chance that siblings of an affected child will have a similar defect also appear to support a genetic hypothesis. A population with a high incidence tends to take the higher incidence with it on migration (Naggan and MacMahon, 1967). The risk is also greater in the offspring of mixed marriages in which the mother, but not the father, is from a higher-risk population (but not vice versa) (Leck, 1971).

Poor maternal nutrition, particularly folic acid deficiency, has been identified as an environmental factor related to the occurrence of neural tube defects (Laurence, 1982). Smithells provided preconception folic acid supplementation for women who had previously given birth to one or more infants with neural tube defects and found that the women receiving folic acid supplements produced fewer infants with neural tube defects during subsequent pregnancies when compared with a similar control group that was not provided with folic acid dietary supplementation (James, 1981; Smithells et al., 1980). It has been suggested that potato blight was an etiologic factor accounting for the increased incidence of myelomeningocele in the British Isles; however, this theory has not been confirmed. There are most certainly other environmental factors involved, but they are as yet unidentified (Renwick, 1972).

INCIDENCE OF SPINA BIFIDA CYSTICA

The risk of a pregnancy resulting in myelomeningocele is much less than for most other genetic disorders. The incidence of myelodysplasia is highest in the British Isles and lowest in Bogota, Colombia, and in patients from Jewish and black ethnic backgrounds (Alter, 1962; Haddow and Macri, 1979) (Table 55–2).

TABLE 55–2. INTERNATIONAL INCIDENCE OF SPINA BIFIDA CYSTICA PER 1000 LIVE BIRTHS

Country	Incidence
British Isles	2.5
Canada	1.44
United States	0.82
Sweden and Finland	0.45
Australia	0.59
Colombia (Bogota)	0.1

The risk for a second or subsequent pregnancy producing a child with myelomeningocele is increased, as reflected in Table 55–3 (McLaughlin and Shurtleff, 1979; Smithells et al., 1968).

In the United States, the risk for recurrence of myelomeningocele in a family with one previously affected child is approximately 5 per cent and the risk with two previously affected children is 10 to 15 per cent (Table 55–3). The risk appears to be greatest for monozygotic twins (20 per cent); dizygotic twins have a 6 per cent risk. Over the past several decades there appears to have been an annual 3 to 8 per cent decline in the occurrence of myelomeningocele in the United States, occurring from north to south and from east to west (Stein et al., 1969). The rate among stillborn infants has decreased more rapidly than the rate among live-born infants, and the incidence also appears to be declining more rapidly in females than in males. Data from England reflect a larger average annual decline (10.6 per cent). It must be noted, however, that the rates of occurrence for neural tube defects historically have been labile and could increase again at any time (Windham and Edmonds, 1982).

ANTENATAL DIAGNOSIS

Accurate prenatal diagnosis of open neural tube defects first became possible in 1972, when

TABLE 55—3. FAMILIAL RISK OF MYELODYSPLASIA IN THE UNITED STATES PER 1000 LIVE BIRTHS

Relationship	Incidence
General population	0.7–1.0
Mother with one previously affected child	40 to 50
Mother with two previously affected children	100
Patient with myelodysplasia	40
Mother greater than 35 years of age	3
Sister of mother with an affected child	10
Sister of father with an affected child	3
Brother of parent with an affected child	2

Brock discovered higher levels of alpha fetoprotein (AFP) in the amniotic fluid and serum of women bearing fetuses with open neural tube defects than in women bearing normal fetuses (Brock et al., 1973; Crandall, 1981). High-resolution ultrasonography and fetoscopy may also diagnose neural tube defects antenatally, but these methods have not been as accurate as AFP determinations.

AFP is a glycoprotein that is produced by the yolk sac and fetal liver, reaching the amniotic fluid via fetal urine and also through the fetal skin prior to keratinization (about 20 weeks of gestation). An open neural tube defect permits additional AFP to enter the amniotic fluid (Milunsky and Alpert, 1974). The concentration of AFP in maternal serum and amniotic fluid varies during pregnancy; however, it appears that the best time to detect an open neural tube defect by measurement of maternal serum AFP is between 16 and 18 weeks of gestation (Haddow and Macri, 1979); by measurement of amniotic fluid AFP, the best time is between 16 and 17 weeks of gestation. Results can be available in less than a week. Although it not diagnostic of an open tube defect, an elevated maternal serum AFP level greater than 2.5 times normal indicates a high risk for a neural tube defect, but unfortunately it does not indicate its severity (Chamberlain, 1978; Crandall, 1981). An elevated maternal serum AFP measurement should be followed by an amniocentesis to measure amniotic fluid AFP levels. If these studies are also positive, a second maternal serum AFP measurement should be done prior to considering termination of the pregnancy. After appropriate counseling, some families may elect to terminate the pregnancy and try again for a healthy child, whereas others will decline intervention and will require special arrangements for infant care after delivery (Laurence and David, 1965).

AFP determinations are highly sensitive and specific (there is a false positive rate of less than 0.1 per cent). False positive AFP test results occur from contamination of the specimen by fetal blood; from incorrect gestational dates; or in the presence of omphalocele, the Turner syndrome in conjunction with a cystic hygroma, congenital nephrosis, anal atresia, esophageal atresia, threatened abortion, fetal distress, fetal death, erythroblastosis, maternal liver disease, multiple pregnancy, or severe Rh isoimmunization (Milunsky, 1977). The major cause for a false negative result is a closed (skin-covered) neural tube defect. Unfortunately, closed defects represent 5 to 10 per cent of neural tube defects. Obtaining maternal urine rather than fetal amniotic fluid during the amniocentesis may also produce a false negative result, but this can be avoided by performing ultrasonography at the time of amniocentesis.

ASSOCIATED ANOMALIES

It is often the case that a child with one congenital anomaly has others. Spina bifida cystica is no exception; up to one third of affected infants have additional anomalies.

Cryptorchidism is more common in boys with spina bifida cystica than in the general population. Kropp and Voeller (1981) reported 23 boys with myelomeningocele, 6 of whom (25.1 per cent) had an undescended testicle, whereas the incidence in the general population is about 0.8 per cent. The reason is uncertain.

Roberts (1961), in an autopsy study, found that 18 per cent of infants with myelomeningocele had anomalies of the urinary tract, exclusive of hydronephrosis, that might be related to a neurogenic bladder. Fusion anomalies (horseshoe kidney) were the most common, with cystic disease (dysplasia) next; renal agenesis was not rare. Forbes (1972) encountered renal dysplasia in 12 per cent of spina bifida patients at autopsy compared with 0 per cent in a control autopsy series. Exstrophy and cloacal exstrophy occur more frequently in association with myelomeningocele than in the general population (Fig. 55–4).

Approximately 80 per cent of neonates with spina bifida cystica have a normal intravenous pyelogram (IVP) at birth. Deterioration of the upper urinary tract or bladder, or both, can be anticipated in up to 50 per cent of them by age 5 years (Smith, 1965), although it is hoped that modern management techniques will lessen the frequency of upper urinary tract deterioration (Fig. 55–5). Gaum and colleagues (1982) reported that 55 of 68 neonates with spina bifida cystica (80.9 per cent) had normal IVP's. Of the 13 neonates with abnormal IVP's, 7 had bilateral hydronephrosis, 3 had ureterectasis, 1 had pyelectasis, 1 had renal dysplasia, and 1 had a horseshoe kidney. Of those with a normal IVP, 17 (30.9 per cent) had a normal voiding cystourethrogram (no trabeculation or vesicoureteral reflux demonstrated), and the remaining 38 (69.1 per cent) had an abnormal study. Twelve of the 13 patients with an abnormal IVP also had an abnormal VCUG (voiding cystoure-

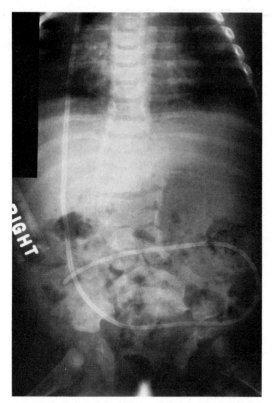

Figure 55–4. A newborn with an extensive vertebral bony defect (rachischisis) and exstrophy of the urinary bladder. (Note widely separated pubic rami.)

throgram) demonstrating bladder trabeculation or vesicoureteral reflux, or both. Other authors (Harlo et al., 1965; Chapman et al., 1969; Thomas and Hopkins, 1971), in reviewing a total of 279 neonates with spina bifida cystica, reported similar findings, with normal IVP's in 81 per cent and abnormal cystograms in up to 80 per cent, including vesicoureteral reflux in 10 to 16.5 per cent. In all reported series, there was little correlation between the level of the spinal lesion and the uroradiographic findings.

Children with myelomeningocele may have, in addition to the obvious spinal defect, other abnormalities of the central nervous system. One quarter of these children have significant hydrocephalus at birth or may develop hydrocephalus after closure of the defect; one third have mild hydrocephalus that may arrest spontaneously in infancy. The deformity responsible for the hydrocephalus is the Cleland-Arnold-Chiari malformation, in which there is herniation of the brain stem and cerebellar vermis through the foramen magnum (Bell et al., 1980). Examination of the cranial nerves may reveal optic nerve palsy, poor gag and swallowing

reflexes, and a croupy, hoarse cry, which is the result of ninth and tenth nerve palsies. Hand-eye coordination and visual perception abnormalities are common in children with myelomeningocele and may be related to lower intellectual achievement in these children (Soare and Raimondi, 1977; Tew and Laurence, 1975).

Orthopedic anomalies occur frequently in infants with myelomeningocele. The more common ones include equinovarus and calcaneovalgus deformity of the feet, hip dysplasia or dislocation, hip flexion and adductor contractures, genu recurvatum (knee flexion contractures), tibial torsion, and kyphos. Early detection and correction of orthopedic anomalies are necessary to prevent progressive deformity and to maximize rehabilitation, because these deformities tend to worsen with persistent muscle imbalance, mild asymmetric spasticity, and increasing age (Bahnson, 1982). Specific management of the orthopedic problems common in children with myelomeningocele is discussed later in this section.

MANAGEMENT OF THE INFANT WITH SPINA BIFIDA CYSTICA

Prior to the 1950's, surgical treatment of spina bifida cystica was uncommon. The management of paraplegia was daunting, and there was no adequate drainage procedure for hydrocephalus. Most infants born with myelomeningocele died in infancy. Failure to treat did not mean that all infants with myelomeningocele died, however. Ten per cent of 381 patients not treated or minimally treated, as described by Laurence and Tew in 1967, were alive from 6 to 12 years after birth; approximately 70 per cent of these survivors were severely handicapped. During the 1950's, advances in the treatment of paraplegia and the development of the various shunting procedures for management of hydrocephalus led to a wave of enthusiasm for emergent and intensive treatment of most neonates with spina bifida cystica, employing early closure of the spinal lesion and cerebrospinal fluid shunting when necessary (Knolson and Spitz, 1952; Sharrard et al., 1963).

In 1971, Lorber analyzed the results of treatment of 524 unselected patients with myelomeningocele; many, in spite of early closure of the spinal lesion and central nervous system shunting, survived with severe disability. Lorber concluded that a better quality of life for survivors would have resulted if a process of selection

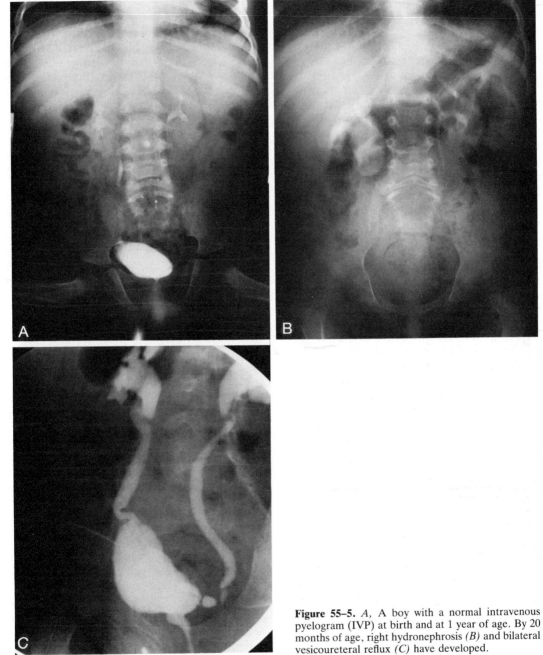

Figure 55–5. *A,* A boy with a normal intravenous pyelogram (IVP) at birth and at 1 year of age. By 20 months of age, right hydronephrosis *(B)* and bilateral vesicoureteral reflux *(C)* have developed.

had been performed at birth (Lorber, 1971) and proposed the following set of adverse physical findings that, if present at birth, are usually associated with a poor prognosis: (1) thoracolumbar lesion, (2) severe paraplegia, (3) grossly enlarged head with occipital circumference that is at least 2 cm above the ninetieth percentile, (4) frankly evident kyphosis or scoliosis, or (5) other gross congenital anomalies or birth injuries.

At about the same time, Smith and Smith outlined a selection program for infants with spina bifida cystica developed at the Royal Children's Hospital in Melbourne, Australia, deferring spinal closure for infants with high-level lesions. If the child survived, despite the withholding of early closure, the infant was reassessed, and active treatment was instituted (Smith and Smith, 1973).

Infants with any one or a combination of

Lorber's criteria for nontreatment receive no active treatment but only supportive nursery care. The intention is that those who are not treated will die. Of the initial series of 37 infants evaluated using his criteria, all 25 not treated died within 9 months (Lorber, 1973). In 1981, Lorber added 83 additional infants to his series (Lorber and Salfield, 1981). Of the total series of 120 infants (1971 and 1981 reports), 71 were not treated and 90 per cent died within 6 months. In another series, 24 of 33 infants evaluated by Gross et al. (1983) and selected for nontreatment received only supportive care; none of the 24 survived beyond 6 months of age. In contrast, Feetham et al. (1979) reported that 70 per cent of 31 neonates initially selected for nontreatment survived to 18 months of age.

In 1965, Shurtleff and colleagues (1975) began selection of patients for nontreatment based on an early assessment of potential cerebral function and intellectual prognosis. Thirty-six infants born after 1965 were selected for nontreatment on the basis of intellectual prognosis; 10 per cent of this group survived into the second year of life. Shurtleff compared this group with a study of 52 children with myelomeningocele initially managed prior to implementing the intellectual prognosis criteria for nontreatment in 1965. Thirty per cent of this pre-1965 group survived to the second decade. Both Lorber's and Shurtleff's groups demonstrate that some infants will survive despite a dismal initial prognosis and that reassessment of a nontreatment decision may be necessary.

Although selection criteria for nontreatment and survival statistics differ, the application of selection policies depends on the philosophy of the physicians involved, the attitudes and religious beliefs of the parents, the social conditions of the family, and the local medicolegal climate (Stark, 1975; Shurtleff et al., 1975; Stark and Drummond, 1974; Parkin, 1975). Unfortunately, the crucial decision to begin active treatment must be made within the first 24 hours after birth. Because of the many problems associated with myelomeningocele, a team approach is mandatory for contemporary management of the infant with myelomeningocele. Such a team should consist of pediatrician, urologist, neurosurgeon, orthopedic surgeon, and experienced clinical staff (nurse, social worker, psychologist, orthotist) who can rapidly and thoroughly evaluate the infant and appropriately educate and counsel the family so that they can give informed consent for treatment or nontreatment (Sharrard, 1969).

Early management should be directed to minimizing complications that might occur before a thorough diagnostic evaluation is completed. The neonate should be transferred to a center specializing in the management of myelomeningocele and placed in an Isolette or covered incubator to allow observation and temperature stabilization. To minimize injury and the risk of infection, the exposed neural elements should be covered immediately with a nonadherent sterile dressing and kept moist with sterile saline. The neonate should undergo a general examination, with special note taken of the nature of the spinal lesion, the level and degree of any paraplegia, lower limb deformities, anal tone, head size, signs of hydrocephalus, and the presence of other gross anomalies. There is often great variability in neurologic involvement as compared with the vertebral level of the spinal lesion. Therefore, a careful assessment is necessary to define the exact nature of the neurologic deficit.

If the decision has been made to refrain from active treatment ("nontreatment"), the guidelines laid out by Lorber should be followed. The infant is kept in a crib, and no incubator is used. A clean dressing is placed over the spinal lesion, no antibiotics are given, and the neonate is fed only by bottle—no tube or intravenous feeding is given. Sedation is not offered unless the neonate is excessively restless, when chloral hydrate may be administered. If the neonate survives, once the lesion has epithelialized, the chances of early death as a result of central nervous system infection will be markedly reduced, and the decision for nontreatment (not to treat actively) should be revised. Frequently, hydrocephalus will be established at this stage; however, in some instances the hydrocephalus will not progress because the persistent spinal lesion allows for decompression. If hydrocephalus has progressed, ventricular shunting should be considered. The delay in treatment does not inevitably worsen the long-term prognosis; these children by definition are the most severely handicapped; therefore, most would have been paraplegic and incontinent and would probably have required central nervous system shunting even if they were treated in the neonatal period.

Neurosurgical Management

Once the decision to treat the neonate actively has been made, the spinal lesion is usually closed within 24 hours of birth (Sharrard, 1969). Antibiotics, such as gentamicin and penicillin, should be administered preoperatively. An obviously purulent lesion is best left open until infection is controlled. Careful observation of the neonate for urinary retention should be made following back closure, with appropriate management instituted if it is present.

If progress following spinal closure is smooth, the next decision is whether and when to treat the hydrocephalus that may be present at birth or that is likely to supervene after closure of the spinal lesion in at least 80 per cent of infants. No consensus exists as to precise timing for cerebrospinal fluid shunting; however, postclosure hydrocephalus is usually evident within the first several weeks postoperatively. Computerized tomography (CT) scanning or ultrasonography, or both, through the open fontanelle will establish the severity of ventricular enlargement and may aid in the decision-making. Long-term follow-up is required to detect shunt malfunction, progression of hydrocephalus, or neurologic deterioration. Shunt infection, although infrequent, remains a significant problem because of its potential to produce cerebritis and subsequent mental impairment. Shunt infection, especially after ventriculovenous shunts, may produce anemia, splenomegaly, or glomerulonephritis with microhematuria (shunt nephritis).

As the child grows, the lumbosacral cord segments may be stretched by scarring of the neural elements to overlying tissue or by congenital attachments to the sacrum of abnormal structures such as a filum terminalis, fibrous bands, or scarred nerve roots. Such spinal cord tethering (tethered cord) may present with progressive motor or sensory deficit in the legs, pes cavus, changing bowel or bladder function, scoliosis, or leg or back pain (Fedun, 1982).

Urologic Evaluation and Management

The aim of urologic care for the infant or child with spina bifida cystica is to preserve renal function and, when possible, to attain socially appropriate urinary continence. A urologic investigation should be done at the first convenient opportunity during the initial hospital admission and should include at least a urinalysis and urine culture, blood urea nitrogen (BUN) and creatinine determinations, and an excretory urogram. Renal ultrasonography may be done early in the neonatal period and an IVP may be obtained after renal function is more mature, prior to discharge from the hospital. We do not routinely perform voiding cystourethrography because with a normal IVP, including the absence of any ureteral fullness, any reflux present will be minimal and of little consequence when the urine remains sterile. Radionuclide studies may be substituted for standard uroradiography. In approximately 80 per cent of neonates with myelomeningocele, the excretory urogram will be normal. For the infant with an abnormal excretory urogram, a voiding cystourethrogram should be done because up to 16 per cent of these neonates will demonstrate significant vesicoureteral reflux (Fig. 55–6).

The reliability and usefulness of urodynamic evaluation in the neonate and infant have not been well established. Bauer et al. (1984) performed urodynamic evaluations in 36 neonates with myelomeningocele and identified a population of neonates at risk for rapid deterioration of the upper urinary tract. Half of the 36 neonates urodynamically investigated demonstrated detrusor sphincter dyssynergia; 72 per cent of this group developed decompensation of the upper urinary tract by 2 years of age, indicating that the observation of dyssynergia in the neonate was highly predictive for subsequent

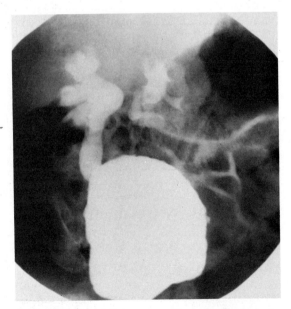

Figure 55–6. A voiding cystourethrogram demonstrating bilateral vesicoureteral reflux in a newborn infant with myelomeningocele.

deterioration of the upper urinary tract. In those children with sphincter activity but initially without dyssynergia (22 per cent of the 36 neonates), none deteriorated unless dyssynergia developed. Therefore, on the basis of Bauer's data, it might be helpful to add a urodynamic evaluation to the initial neonatal evaluations and as part of routine follow-up. If the initial excretory urogram is abnormal or the urodynamic study reveals dyssynergia of the detrusor and external urinary sphincter, or both of these conditions occur, a voiding cystourethrogram should be done. Subsequent follow-up evaluations would then be dictated by urodynamic findings. Employing the data of Bauer and associates (1984) on detrusor sphincter dyssynergia, long-term follow-up might be modified, as discussed further on.

Routine circumcision should be avoided in the incontinent infant boy with myelomeningocele because the prepuce protects the neurologically insensitive glans penis from dermatitis and ulceration or trauma from continually wet diapers (Klauber, 1979).

For the newborn with myelomeningocele and a normal upper urinary tract, manual suprapubic expression (the Credé maneuver) may be used initially to produce bladder emptying, provided that the bladder is easily emptied and the amount of residual urine is negligible. In this group of children with normal upper urinary tracts, the Credé maneuver is done with the infant in a prone position, and the first two fingers of each hand are used while the thumbs remain in the back. Pressure is exerted downward toward the rectum starting at the dome of the bladder; no pressure should be placed on the spinal defect. The Credé maneuver may be continued indefinitely; however, as the child grows older it frequently becomes difficult because of local discomfort or abdominal muscle resistance, and it is often no longer successful in emptying the bladder; furthermore, the Credé maneuver does not produce meaningful urinary continence in older children. At this time, urinary evacuation must be provided by other means.

In those infants with bladder outflow obstruction, urinary infection, upper urinary tract changes, or vesicoureteral reflux, the Credé maneuver is unwise, and clean intermittent catheterization should be started or a cutaneous vesicostomy should be done (Fig. 55–7). Overdilation of the female urethra or Y-V-plasty of the bladder neck are not consistently effective in improving bladder emptying and may destroy the continence mechanism, limiting the effectiveness of clean intermittent catheterization.

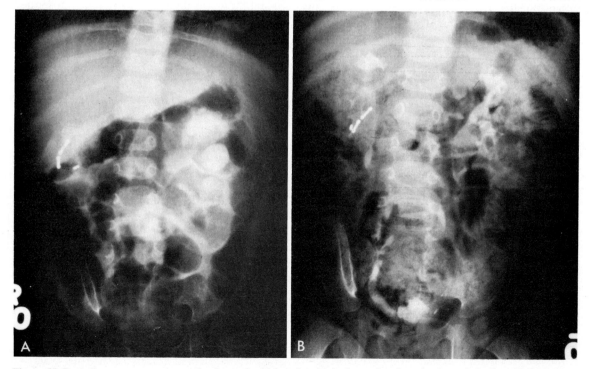

Figure 55–7. *A,* Intravenous urogram of a 6-month-old female with hydronephrosis and urinary infection. *B,* Intravenous urogram of the same patient 3 months after cutaneous vesicostomy.

These procedures, therefore, are no longer recommended.

Follow-up in the infant with a normal upper urinary tract and no urinary infection or vesicoureteral reflux includes a urinalysis and culture and sensitivity tests, if indicated, at intervals of 3 to 6 months. A renal ultrasound, IVP, or radionuclide renal scan should be done at 6 months and 1 year of age, and yearly thereafter until 5 years of age, when such studies should be done biannually. The place for urodynamic evaluation during follow-up has been discussed previously.

For babies with detrusor sphincter dyssynergia (at high risk for upper urinary deterioration), a renal ultrasound (or excretory urogram or nuclide study), a urodynamic study, and voiding cystourethrogram can be repeated at intervals of 6 months for the first 2 years of life and yearly thereafter, if stable, until 5 years of age. If the pressures associated with filling or emptying of the bladder are elevated or if the volume of residual urine begins to increase, anticholinergic medication and clean intermittent catheterization should be instituted or a cutaneous vesicostomy should be done.

Babies with synergic activity are followed at yearly intervals with renal ultrasonography (or excretory urogram) and a urodynamic study to detect the development of dyssynergia. Those with complete denervation of the external urethral sphincter (lowest-risk group) require only a yearly ultrasound study or excretory urogram. If hydronephrosis or a distended bladder is found or if urinary infection develops, a voiding cystourethrogram and urodynamic studies should be performed.

When infection is detected, it should be treated aggressively, and, once under control, a voiding cystourethrogram should be done to assess whether vesicoureteral reflux has developed. Approximately 6 per cent of children with myelomeningocele will demonstrate vesicoureteral reflux after infection (Culp et al., 1970).

With vesicoureteral reflux, a persistently distended bladder, or deterioration of the upper urinary system (whether during the neonatal period or later in life), close surveillance is necessary to detect recurrent urinary infection or urinary retention, or both. Regular decompression of the bladder is necessary. Indwelling catheters (urethral or suprapubic) are unsatisfactory for long-term management because they may contribute to infection and calculus formation and may contribute to upper tract deterioration and promote bladder fibrosis. Intermittent catheterization should suffice in most instances, but it is often not appropriate because of parental inhibitions and the technical difficulties in catheterizing small infants, especially in the home situation. In this case, a cutaneous vesicostomy provides a simple and readily reversible method for decompressing the urinary bladder without introducing a foreign body (see Fig. 55–6). The technique described by Blocksom (1957) and popularized by Duckett (1974) brings the urachal portion of the dome of the bladder to the lower abdominal skin as a small vesicocutaneous fistula without skin flaps, providing satisfactory temporary urinary diversion to manage the deteriorating upper urinary tract in the infant or young child. Infection is usually controlled with prophylactic antibacterial medications, and the upper urinary tract generally will decompress or stabilize postoperatively. Management of the wet stoma associated with the vesicostomy has not proved to be a burden to parents caring for these infants. Diapers may be used for collection. Diaper dermatitis occasionally is a problem because of continuous wetness but may be minimized by meticulous hygiene and the use of barrier ointments such as Desitin or 1 per cent hydrocortisone (Cohen et al., 1978; Duckett, 1974).

Complications after cutaneous vesicostomy are uncommon but include stomal stenosis, squamous metaplasia, bladder prolapse requiring revision (occurring in up to 25 per cent of patients), chronic bacilluria, and calculi, especially on hair-bearing surfaces after puberty (Cohen et al., 1978).

INTERMITTENT CATHETERIZATION

Sterile intermittent catheterization was first described by Guttmann and Frankel in 1966 as a method for managing urinary tract infection in patients with spinal cord injury. In 1972, Lapides demonstrated that a clean, unsterile technique was acceptable for intermittent catheterization (Lapides et al., 1972; Lapides, 1974). Emphasizing the frequency rather than the sterility of the technique, Lapides found that a significant number of patients with neurogenic bladders remained free of infection. Over time, clean intermittent catheterization has proved a safe and well-accepted technique for the management of urinary infection and urinary incontinence while often permitting the stabilization or improvement of changes in the upper urinary tract (Diokno et al., 1976; Lyon et al., 1975; Plunkett and Braren, 1979; Kass et al., 1979) (Fig. 55–8). Older girls who dislike clean intermittent catheterization in spite of its effectiveness in keeping them dry are a notable exception

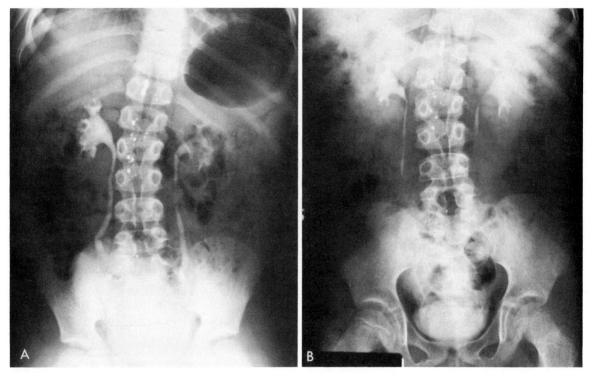

Figure 55–8. *A,* Intravenous urogram of a 7-year-old girl, demonstrating bilateral early hydronephrosis. *B,* Intravenous urogram of the same patient 5 months after instituting intermittent catheterization.

to the wide acceptance of the technique, as are older boys, especially those with normal urethral sensation.

Despite an early optimism concerning clean intermittent catheterization for the management of urinary infection and urinary incontinence and for stabilizing or improving the morphologic characteristics of the upper urinary tract, not all children on clean intermittent catheterization are free of infection and continent. Nor do all upper urinary tracts stabilize or improve.

Contemporary data reflecting the incidence of bacteriuria are quite divergent, with some reports of up to 65 per cent of those managed on clean intermittent catheterization having persistently sterile urine (Plunkett and Braren, 1979; Light and Van Blerk, 1977; Drago et al., 1977; Lapides et al., 1974; Lapides et al., 1976), whereas others report more dismal results. Ehrlich and Brem (1982) report persistently sterile urine in only 16 per cent of children who perform clean intermittent catheterization. Asymptomatic bacteriuria is more common in girls than in boys, but febrile urinary infections are unusual in either sex in the absence of vesicoureteral reflux. Although the current literature generally supports a 50 to 60 per cent occurrence of asymptomatic bacteriuria in children on clean

intermittent catheterization, few authors have commented on the long-term significance of such asymptomatic bacteriuria (Kass et al., 1981). Lapides et al. (1974), noting chronic or recurrent bacteriuria in 35 per cent of their patients who performed clean intermittent catheterization, felt that in this context it was not significant. With a proper program of clean intermittent catheterization, overdistention of the bladder was avoided, and emptying was frequent and complete enough to negate the adverse effect of the bacteriuria. Obviously, such bacteriuria is of concern in children with vesicoureteral reflux and increased intravesical pressures, which may predispose to upper urinary tract deterioration. Some authors note that antibacterial prophylaxis in patients on clean intermittent catheterization does not appear to be helpful and may lead to selection of resistant organisms on subsequent cultures (Drago et al., 1977).

UPPER TRACT CHANGES

Upper tract changes respond to intermittent catheterization with stabilization or improvement in most children (see Fig. 55–8). Enrile and associates (1980) demonstrated stabilization of upper urinary dilation in 46 per cent of 39 patients (10 boys and 29 girls) and improvement in 38 per cent; clean intermittent catheterization failed to stabilize or halt progression of upper urinary deterioration in 16 per cent of patients with abnormal IVP's demonstrating hydroureter or hydronephrosis. Those children who did not respond to intermittent catheterization had vesicoureteral reflux and outlet obstruction secondary to bladder hypertonicity that was poorly managed with anticholinergic medications. Perez-Marreno et al. (1982) recorded similar results in 15 children with upper urinary abnormalities who were managed by intermittent catheterization. Ehrlich and Brem (1982) reported on one child on clean intermittent catheterization who developed hydronephrosis after a previously normal IVP, indicating that clean intermittent catheterization is not completely safe for all children and that children on clean intermittent catheterization require close observation. Ideally, urodynamic studies should be done prior to starting clean intermittent catheterization to determine precisely the pathophysiology of the incontinence (Bauer et al., 1977). This will identify those children requiring adjunctive neuropharmacologic treatment and perhaps also those with detrusor sphincter dyssynergia who appear to require more careful observation (Mandel et al., 1980).

CONTINENCE

Untreated, 95 per cent of children with myelomeningocele will have urine incontinence (Lorber, 1981; Winemiller and Lehman, 1973). Early reports suggested that 50 to 60 per cent of those performing clean intermittent catheterization became socially continent (Katzen, 1981). However, in reviewing more recent series, it is apparent that the results reported are at least partially governed by preselection of patients for clean intermittent catheterization (Altshuler et al., 1977) and the use of adjunctive neuropharmacology. Further, such data may be biased favorably because of inaccurate patient reporting.

Enrile and Crooks (1980) and Drago et al. (1977) determined that only 76 of 375 children (20 per cent) in their clinics with myelodysplasia were suitable candidates for intermittent catheterization. The indications for selection are not clearly defined but appear to be related to intelligence, mobility, manual dexterity, and motivation. Of these 76 children, only 30 (39 per cent) became socially dry, 13 (17 per cent) were improved (less wet), and 31 (41 per cent) were unaltered. None of these children was treated with clean intermittent catheterization

and adjunctive neuropharmacology simultaneously. Using neuropharmacology to increase functional bladder capacity or bladder outlet resistance, or both, Hilwa and Perlmutter (1978) achieved continence in 16 of 19 girls and 8 of 9 boys who were not continent performing intermittent catheterization alone. Similar results were obtained by Mulcahy et al. (1977) in 21 of 25 children (84 per cent) who were managed with intermittent catheterization and adjunctive neuropharmacology.

As already stated, urinary incontinence is present in up to 95 per cent of children with myelomeningocele (Lorber, 1981; Winemiller and Lehman, 1973). Early management of bladder emptying employing the Credé maneuver, intermittent catheterization, or cutaneous vesicostomy has been discussed previously. External collecting devices and penile clamps are generally unsatisfactory for managing urinary incontinence and are not universally applicable for both sexes.

As school age approaches, it is desirable to have achieved urinary and fecal continence for both psychologic and social reasons. Excessive constipation or fecal soiling, or both, may adversely affect attempts at achieving urinary continence. The damp, soiled child who has a foul smell is unwelcome at school and becomes a personal and social nuisance. Prior to starting a program to promote urinary continence, one must determine whether the child's bladder is one that fails to store urine or one that does not empty well. In some children, the clinical history, physical findings, and appearance of the bladder and bladder outlet on intravenous urography or cystography may be adequate for evaluation. However, uroradiographic and urodynamic studies permit classification of the abnormal lower urinary tract as a "failure to store" because of hypertonicity, inadequate outlet resistance, or inadequate bladder capacity, or as a "failure to empty" because of increased outlet resistance or poor bladder contractility. At times, both hypertonicity and increased outlet resistance may be present and, if untreated, may predispose to upper tract deterioration.

For the child who is unable to empty the bladder, the alternatives include clean intermittent catheterization, overdilation of the infant female urethra, internal urethrotomy, Y-V-plasty of the bladder neck, external sphincterotomy, and electrical stimulation of the detrusor muscle. Shochat and Perlmutter (1972) and Johnston (1968) used overdilation of the urethra to manage urinary outlet obstruction in female infants with myelomeningocele, but this treatment antedates the popularization of intermittent catheterization. Over time, both overdilation of the urethra and internal urethrotomy may interfere with the continence that is desirable for an effective intermittent catheterization program and consequently are no longer recommended for such purpose.

Similarly, Y-V-plasty or transurethral resection of the bladder neck were popular in the past to improve bladder emptying and may be beneficial in selected patients whose urodynamic evaluation demonstrates sufficient bladder capacity and external sphincter resistance to store and evacuate urine (Navarro et al., 1978). However, these procedures most often have led to intractable incontinence. Likewise, external sphincterotomy may be done in selected children to reduce outflow resistance and improve bladder emptying. A more balanced detrusor external sphincter function has been achieved in some patients, with improved urinary continence and more complete bladder emptying. However, because of the difficulties of obtaining a balanced bladder and the risks of incontinence, any of these techniques should be avoided unless it is part of a planned procedure to be followed by implantation of an artificial sphincter (Kaplan and King, 1970; Koontz and Smith, 1977).

Electrical stimulation of the detrusor muscle or pelvic plexus to produce a sustained detrusor contraction has been a disappointing and unreliable method for promoting bladder emptying in children with myelomeningocele (Cooper, 1968; Wheatley et al., 1982; Halverstadt, 1971). Direct stimulation of the spinal cord to promote bladder emptying is still investigational (Jonas et al., 1975).

Approximately one third of bladders associated with myelomeningocele will not store urine adequately because of severe uninhibited bladder contractions, inadequate bladder capacity, or inadequate outlet resistance. In this situation, a complete uroradiographic and urodynamic assessment of the lower urinary tract is essential for understanding the pathophysiology of the incontinence and directing the most appropriate plan of management. Neuropharmacologic agents may be successful in some cases to control uninhibited bladder contractions or to improve bladder outlet resistance.

Any program to promote storage of urine must be coordinated with a program to provide regular and complete emptying, using clean intermittent catheterization or the Credé or Valsalva maneuvers. The Valsalva and Credé maneuvers are infrequently effective in totally emptying the bladder in these children. The role of intermittent catheterization with and without adjunctive neuropharmacologic agents to produce urinary continence in children with neurogenic bladders has been discussed previously (Hilwa and Perlmutter, 1978; Kass et al., 1979).

For some children with reduced bladder capacity secondary to uninhibited detrusor contractions who are unresponsive to neuropharmacology, bilateral pudendal neurectomy may improve bladder capacity (Mullholland et al., 1974; Stark, 1969). The success of the procedure can usually be predicted by preoperative nerve blocks combined with pre- and postblock urodynamic studies. Similarly, selective sacral rhizotomy has been successful in controlling incontinence in some girls with hypertonic bladders and urinary incontinence when other, less involved methods have failed or were contraindicated (Manfredi and Leal, 1968). Bilateral pudendal neurectomy may produce erectile impotence in boys and penile or clitoral anesthesia (if the patient had preoperative sensation) and therefore should only be done unilaterally.

Bladder augmentation using the isolated ileocecal segment or sigmoid colon offers an alternative method for salvaging the small-capacity, noncompliant bladder or for modifying intractable hyperreflexia and hypertonicity. Perlmutter and Kroovand (1983) presented a series of bladder augmentations in 15 children, 9 of whom had neurogenic bladders and intractable hyperreflexia or hypertonicity. Satisfactory bladder capacity was achieved in all nine patients and urinary continence was achieved in seven of the nine children, five of them requiring an artificial sphincter (Fig. 55–9). The long-term results and consequences of bladder augmentation are as yet unknown and will require careful follow-up.

Chronic electrical stimulation of the pelvic floor musculature via an anal plug or implanted electrodes has had only limited success in achieving urinary continence and is no longer widely employed (Caldwell et al., 1969; Godec and Cass, 1978).

Unfortunately, in some children the degree of bladder neck and pelvic floor dysfunction is such that the child remains incontinent despite appropriate attempts to manage the incontinence. For these children, the artificial urinary sphincter offers a universally applicable method for achieving and maintaining social urinary continence combined with preservation of renal function and normal urinary flow. Early results of the use of the artificial urinary sphincter in children were not encouraging; however, after

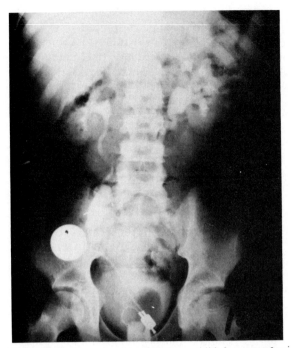

Figure 55–9. Postoperative IVP in a child 2 years after bladder augmentation and placement of a Scott artificial urinary sphincter.

several device modifications, current results are very acceptable. Kroovand has implanted the artificial sphincter in 44 incontinent children with neurogenic bladders.

Over a follow-up period of 1 year to 7 years, 38 of the 44 children are continent for at least 3 hours during the day and are dry at night; 4 children have occasional stress urinary incontinence. Eight of these children empty their bladders completely; 5 void but require supplemental intermittent catheterization to drain postvoid residual urine; and 29 utilize clean intermittent catheterization exclusively. None of the children has required revision of the device because of somatic growth. Most postimplantation complications involve device malfunction or noncompliance. Erosion of the device into the urinary tract or perforation requiring device removal are relatively uncommon in children (Kroovand, 1983). The experiences of other authors (Gonzalez and Sheldon, 1982; Light et al., 1983) also support the current optimism concerning the artificial urinary sphincter in children with neurogenic bladders.

URINARY DIVERSION

Until recently, supravesical cutaneous urinary diversion, ordinarily achieved by ileal conduit, has been considered by many the most satisfactory method of urinary management for the child with myelodysplasia. The majority of patients undergoing ileal conduit urinary diversion initially demonstrated either stabilization or improvement of renal morphology. However, in long-term follow-up of 10 years or more, many series report recurring episodes of pyelonephritis or progressive renal deterioration, or both, in many patients (Wainsten et al., 1972; Kass et al., 1979; Dretler, 1973; Glenn et al., 1968; Bellman, 1972; Hendren, 1978; Merrill and Conway, 1974).

In 1975, the first reports of long-term complications of ileal conduit urinary diversion appeared in the urologic literature. Schwartz and Jeffs (1975) reported a 50 per cent incidence of pyelonephritic deterioration in 41 patients with ileal conduits who were followed for 2 to 16 years. Soon thereafter, Shapiro et al. (1975) showed that one fourth of the renal units in 86 surviving children with ileal conduit urinary diversion had evidence of upper urinary deterioration in follow-ups of 10 to 16 years. Only 13.2 per cent of this same series had no late complications. Kyker and associates (1977) reported 26 children (52 renal units) who had undergone ileal conduit urinary diversion. Sixty per cent of the renal units were normal at the time of the diversion, but 13 per cent subsequently deteriorated. Of the 21 (40 per cent) renal units that were abnormal at the time of the diversion, 14 per cent deteriorated further, 67 per cent remained stable, and 19 per cent improved after urinary diversion. Similar reports by other authors cite upper urinary deterioration and progressive pyelonephritic scarring in up to 56 per cent of renal units after cutaneous diversion (Smith, 1972a,b; Shapiro et al., 1975; Middleton and Hendren, 1976; Schwartz and Jeffs, 1975; Smith et al., 1979; Schmidt et al., 1973). Other long-term complications after ileal conduit urinary diversion include stomal stenosis, conduit elongation, conduit stenosis, stomal prolapse, and parastomal hernia.

For salvage of the deteriorating ileal conduit, Reiner and Jeffs (1979) described a technique of ileal intussusception in ileal conduits to prevent reflux of infected urine from the appliance into the conduit and then into the upper urinary tract in the hope of preventing further upper urinary tract deterioration. Although this technique is unlikely to supplant the current use of colon conduits as a preferred structure into which to fashion antirefluxing ureteral anastomoses, it nevertheless appears to be useful for those ileal conduits in need of revision.

The high frequency of upper urinary tract deterioration and other complications after ileal conduit urinary diversion prompted a search for alternatives to ileal conduit cutaneous diversion. Recent advances in the understanding of the neurophysiology of bladder function, clean intermittent catheterization, and the use of the artificial sphincter have reduced the indications for urinary diversion. Unfortunately, there will still be a few children for whom cutaneous urinary diversion offers the only method to manage urinary incontinence and urinary infection. For these children, a nonrefluxing colon conduit employing either the sigmoid colon or the ileocecal segment may ultimately prove of importance not only for urinary diversion but also, more importantly, for preservation of the upper urinary tract. The use of the large intestine for cutaneous urinary diversion permits a technically easier antirefluxing ureterocolonic anastomosis and creation of a large abdominal wall stoma that is less prone to stomal stenosis. Surgical complications after colon conduit urinary diversion appear significantly lower than those described after ileal conduit urinary diversion (Altwein et al., 1977). However, in a recent study, Hill and Ransley (1983) reported 47 children followed for 2 to 21 years after colonic conduit diversion with an overall complication rate of 81 per cent, including upper tract deterioration in 36 per cent and stomal stenosis in 34 per cent. Therefore, the nonrefluxing colon conduit in children with myelomeningocele will have to pass the test of time before any authoritative statement can be made concerning the long-term effectiveness of this procedure. To maximize the potential benefit from colon conduit urinary diversion, it probably should be done before the onset of pyelonephritis and deteriorating upper tracts. This is in contrast to most series reporting ileal conduits in which the urinary diversion was often done after the onset of upper tract deterioration (Shapiro et al., 1975; Mogg, 1967; Altwein et al., 1977; Kelalis, 1974; Ritchie et al., 1974).

Cutaneous vesicostomy can also serve as a form of permanent urinary diversion. Because of chronic residual urine and bacteriuria, there is concern about maintaining a vesicostomy for a prolonged time, especially in the presence of reflux (Blocksom, 1957). In addition, because of difficulties with appliance fit, a vesicostomy is not always well tolerated after early childhood. Therefore, with an established vesicostomy, it is generally necessary to reassess the indications for it later in childhood and to choose between definitive urinary reconstruction or another form of permanent diversion.

Any child with a urinary diversion should have lifelong follow-up. A limited IVP 4 to 6 weeks after diversion will rule out urinary obstruction. Renal functional parameters and serum electrolyte levels should be assessed several times yearly. An IVP, radionuclide study, or ultrasonogram should be repeated annually for 2 or 3 years and then at least once every 2 years thereafter. The substitution of radionuclide scans or ultrasonography for IVP reduces or avoids radiation exposure and may be appropriate for long-term postdiversion follow-up.

Although there have been no consistent recommendations for management of the defunctionalized bladder after urinary diversion (Lome et al., 1972), reports of pyocystis and delayed development of malignancy indicate a need for systematic follow-up, including studies such as periodic bladder irrigations for cytology, cystography, and endoscopy (Garvin et al., 1972).

URINARY UNDIVERSION

During the past decade, urinary undiversion and the re-establishment of continuity of the previously diverted urinary tract has become an increasingly acceptable mode of therapy. The enthusiasm for urinary undiversion has in part stemmed from dissatisfaction with the long-term results after ileal conduit urinary diversion, from the changing indications for cutaneous diversion, and from the realization that some patients, particularly teenagers, cannot psychologically tolerate cutaneous urinary diversion. The decision to remove a satisfactorily functioning urinary conduit must not be taken lightly. Strict criteria for the selection of patients to undergo undiversion are necessary to ensure a successful outcome with minimal morbidity, especially in children with neurogenic bladder dysfunction, who pose special problems with undiversion because of associated skeletal and neurologic problems. Urinary undiversion is discussed in greater detail elsewhere.

Clinically, the results after urinary undiversion in children with spina bifida cystica have been encouraging. In 1979, Borden and associates compiled a series of 25 selected patients with neurogenic bladder dysfunction who had undergone urinary undiversion. Seventeen of the 25 (68 per cent) had excellent results, and eight (32 per cent) had less than optimal results because of incontinence, increasing hydronephrosis, or declining renal function. Bauer et al. (1980) performed undiversion in 15 children with myelodysplasia and ileal conduits. A successful outcome was achieved in 66 per cent (two void spontaneously, six require clean intermittent catheterization, and two have had artificial urinary sphincters). Poor results occurred in four children (27 per cent) because of poor urinary control. These four children are awaiting secondary operations to establish urinary continence. A failure, requiring rediversion, occurred in one child. The most recent reports on urinary undiversion in children with myelodysplasia by Kass and Koff (1983), Light and associates (1983), and Menon and associates (1983) cite a 5-year follow-up on a total of 24 patients. All patients did well in terms of stability of the upper urinary tract and renal function after undiversion and all are continent, using either clean intermittent catheterization or the artificial urinary sphincter. Again, careful follow-up is necessary to correctly assess the long-term consequences of urinary undiversion.

For children with a cutaneous urinary diversion and a small or noncompliant bladder, severe hyperreflexia, or urinary incontinence after urinary undiversion, bladder augmentation using an intestinal segment has proved successful in producing a lower-pressure bladder with increased capacity, thus improving urinary capacity and continence and stabilizing the upper urinary system (Perlmutter and Kroovand, 1983). For those who remain incontinent after bladder augmentation, later placement of a Scott sphincter usually establishes urinary continence (Kroovand, 1983).

Orthopedic Follow-Up

The ultimate goal for orthopedic care is a stable posture and the promotion of ambulation, when possible. An ambulatory status is important because it maximizes independence and prevents deformity, thus improving the child's self-esteem (Hoffer et al., 1973). In infancy, orthopedic abnormalities should be treated as early as possible, because they tend to worsen with persistent muscle imbalance and muscle spasticity. Early, careful casting and splinting, combined with physical therapy, permit easier correction of orthopedic abnormalities. The management of hip subluxation and hip dislocation must be individualized, depending on the functional capabilities of the child. Soft tissue contractures may require surgical release to preserve functional motion of the hips and knees, balancing existing muscle forces to ensure maximum ambulatory achievement that is compatible with the level of the lesion. Most required operative procedures should be completed in as few steps as possible by the time the child is a few years of age.

FRACTURES

Pathologic fractures are a frequent problem in children with myelomeningocele, especially involving the osteoporotic bones of the lower extremities in more severely paralyzed patients who have undergone prolonged immobilization in casts. Fractures are insidious in their presentation, often resembling cellulitis. They heal slowly and infrequently require surgical stabilization.

SCOLIOSIS

The incidence of structural spinal problems in children with myelodysplasia is high. Kyphosis, scoliosis, or lordosis may occur individually or concurrently and may progress with growth, affecting as many as 60 to 80 per cent of patients with high-level lesions, 5 to 15 per cent of those with lumbar lesions, and 5 per cent of those with sacral lesions. Combinations of these conditions are frequently associated with and are compounded by structural vertebral anomalies such as hemivertebrae, failure of segmentation, and unilateral bars. Both kyphosis and scoliosis may convert the marginally ambulatory patient into a wheelchair patient. A kyphotic defect (a severe posterior angulation of the vertebral column) is best treated at birth during the initial spinal operation, since later procedures involve osteotomy or excision of vertebrae and are formidable. Initially, scoliosis management should be conservative (nonoperative). Bracing and physical therapy should be tried in all patients, but they are generally unsuccessful in paraplegics. Curves of more than 20 degrees are initially managed with a brace program, which may delay surgery. Scoliosis of more than 40 degrees tends to be progressive and is best treated operatively. The timing and type of operative correction remain controversial.

AMBULATION

Children with myelomeningocele may demonstrate varying degrees of partial or complete paralysis in either lower extremity. For those children who cannot walk, functional wheelchair mobility, including independent transfer, should remain the goal unless there is severe upper extremity involvement or marked obesity occurs. Children with myelomeningocele can be divided into four general categories related to their motor level.

Thoracic level patients (L1 and higher) are generally paralyzed from the waist down and in childhood are able to walk with the aid of knee-ankle-foot orthoses (bilateral long leg braces with pelvic support). However, as they grow, walking requires increased effort, and for that reason these children usually cease functional ambulation in the preteens and elect for a wheelchair ambulatory existence. Some will continue to walk mainly during physical therapy sessions and are therefore classified as *"therapy ambulators."* Such therapeutic ambulation promotes weight control, balance, lower extremity bone and soft tissue development, and upper extremity strength. It also improves pulmonary function. Thoracic-level children often require stabilization of the kyphotic or scoliotic spine in order to provide maximum sitting height and balance and to distribute the weight evenly over the perineum. A plantigrade foot is desirable for transfer and cosmetic reasons.

Upper lumbar level (L2–L3) myelomeningocele patients walk with the assistance of knee-ankle-foot orthoses or bilateral long leg braces. They require less energy for ambulation than do those with a thoracic level lesion; however, the majority elect wheelchair ambulation as their primary means of transportation by the time they are teenagers. In the absence of complications, continued ambulation should be encouraged, because ambulation aids in weight control, promotes strength and balance, and improves cardiopulmonary reserve. Children with upper lumbar level lesions are usually classified as *"household ambulators,"* though some may become "community ambulators."

The *lower lumbar level* (L4–L5) patients have active quadriceps muscles and are able to walk in ankle-foot orthoses or bilateral short leg braces. The majority of these children are *"community ambulators"* and will remain so throughout life with the aid of short leg braces. Many require multiple orthopedic procedures to correct foot deformities, maintain equal weight distribution, avoid decubiti, and improve balance.

For practical purposes, the *sacral level* myelomeningocele patients are normal, with the exception of some numbness of the soles of their feet. Most ambulate without braces or crutches; observation for and treatment of scoliosis are mandatory (Sharrard, 1969; Menelaus, 1976).

Pediatric Follow-Up

Because of expertise in well-child care (preventive medicine) and knowledge of motor, cognitive, and psychologic development, the pediatrician specializing in the handicapped child, is the key member and coordinator of the myelomeningocele management team. The pediatrician not only directs the general pediatric care but also provides genetic counseling both for the parents of the infant or child and eventually for the affected adolescent or young adult.

Intellectual development is often below normal in children with myelomeningocele. Soare and Raimondi (1977) studied 173 children with myelomeningocele, 133 of whom developed hydrocephalus, and noted that 63 per cent of those with hydrocephalus had IQs greater than 80, whereas 87 per cent of those without hydrocephalus had IQs greater than 80. When compared with 80 normal siblings, those with hydrocephalus were significantly less intelligent, whereas those without hydrocephalus were not. Soare and Raimondi (1977) also noted that most children with myelomeningocele, with or without hydrocephalus, had visual-perceptual deficits and fine motor disabilities that impaired learning and required special educational attention. Children with hydrocephalus often appear brighter than testing indicates and have misleading vocabulary and social abilities. These children may even learn to read clearly but have difficulty with comprehension. It may be necessary for the pediatrician to meet with school personnel prior to schooling to outline the child's special educational and medical needs.

Obesity is common, is difficult to prevent, and has a detrimental effect on ambulation, often being severe enough to necessitate permanent use of a wheelchair. Careful attention to diet and exercise and maintenance of the proper height:weight ratio are important. Maceration and pressure decubitus ulcers are common in children with myelomeningocele.

Maceration decubiti, the result of stool soiling and wetness, are easily managed by improved perineal hygiene, exposure, and avoidance of occlusive clothing. Pressure decubiti arise from subcutaneous tissue breakdown around bony prominences and become secondarily infected. They are difficult to manage. The use of neurosensory island skin flaps to treat or prevent decubitus ulcers is generally unsuccessful. A ring cushion, foam pillow, silicone or gel pad, or lamb's wool blanket may aid in distributing pressure around bony prominences. Maintenance of proper pelvic alignment, symmetry of weight bearing, a low weight:height ratio, preservation of mobility, and proper perineal hygiene also contribute to prevention of pressure decubiti.

BOWEL MANAGEMENT

Of all accidents that might trouble a child, fecal incontinence is the most annoying and most damaging to self-esteem. In addition, inadequate rectal emptying may inhibit attempts to achieve urinary continence or make it difficult to treat urinary infections. A colostomy should rarely be needed to achieve fecal continence, since this merely substitutes an abdominal stoma for a perineal one.

Normal anorectal function depends on an adequate appreciation of rectal fullness, satisfactory peristalsis, and properly balanced tone and function of the anal sphincter mechanisms. Anorectal manometry measuring rectal sensation to fullness and anal sphincter tone in myelomeningocele patients has demonstrated that fecal incontinence in the child with a neurogenic bowel is due to weak or absent contracture of the external anal sphincter when the rectum is distended. Internal sphincter tone is generally spared from paralysis (Meunier et al., 1976; White et al., 1972). These studies suggest that the management of neurogenic rectal incontinence is best achieved by encouraging regular evacuation of the fecal reservoir to avoid elevated rectal pressures and thus prevent reflex relaxation of the internal sphincter and inadvertent defecation (Engel et al., 1974). We also occasionally encounter children with fecal incontinence due to a hypertonic colon and rectum are especially difficult management problems.

In the myelomeningocele patient, bowel regulation should start early, generally in the newborn period, and not as an afterthought as the child is preparing for school. Avoiding constipating foods and encouraging foods that increase bulk aid in development of bowel control. Regular stool evacuation and scheduled toileting aid in colonic transit and should be encouraged. In infancy and early childhood, bowel emptying may be achieved with glycerin suppositories and manual expression. As the child grows, regular stool evacuation is desirable and is aided by bulk laxatives. Daily suppositories or disposable enemas may be used, followed by scheduled toileting and encouraging the child to strain or use abdominal expression. The child may also be taught to employ the Valsalva maneuver by grunting or blowing up a balloon. Daily rectal washouts are useful but are time-consuming and may be hazardous in inexpert hands. Toileting after meals increases the chance of a more complete evacuation by taking advantage of the gastrocolic reflex, and the sitting position increases intra-abdominal pressure. Initially, 3 to 5 minutes after each meal suffices with gradual increases in time to 15 to 20 minutes as the child's tolerance allows (Engel et al., 1974).

Employing these principles, White and associates (1972) managed 29 children with a program of daily evacuations to empty the anorectal area and avoid overfilling the rectum, relying on the resting tone of the internal sphincter to maintain fecal continence. Seventeen of the 29 (55 per cent) were clean, 2 (6 per cent) had occasional soiling, and 10 (32 per cent) had frequent staining. Twelve of the 29 (41 per cent) learned regular bowel habits, while 17 required assistance in evacuation.

Using manometric data on rectal tone and sensation, Engel and associates (1974) added biofeedback training to an unsuccessful bowel management program and achieved fecal continence in seven patients with myelomeningocele. Whitehead and associates (1981) taught eight children with myelodysplasia to voluntarily contract the anal sphincter or nearby gluteal muscles in response to rectal distention and to maintain these contractions for a sustained duration. Six of these eight children had been persistently incontinent of feces even though they were already using enemas or suppositories. Five achieved excellent fecal continence and two were able to discontinue enemas and suppositories after attaining fecal continence. A sixth child was continent 80 per cent of the time. Two children did not benefit from the biofeedback regimen (Whitehead et al., 1981). In a similar study, Wald (1981) achieved excellent fecal control in four of eight myelomeningocele patients.

SEXUALITY

Questions and concerns about later sexual function may occur early in the child's life; however, few data exist concerning the sexuality and sexual function of the patient with myelomeningocele. There are few recorded observations relating anal tone, bulbocavernous reflex, glans sensitivity, analgesia or anesthesia, and the presence or absence of reflex erection in infancy or childhood to later erotic sensation or gratification in either sex. Unfortunately, most information concerning sexuality and actual sexual activity in neurologically impaired patients is derived from traumatic paraplegics and may not be applicable to those with myelodysplasia.

The issue of sexuality should have been addressed early in infancy; however, most parents are unaware of their child's potential for sexual function, marriage, and parenthood. Traditionally, most of these children are sheltered and have few social contacts. Nevertheless, adolescent myelomeningocele patients have normal concerns about the opposite sex and the possibility of sexual function, marriage, and procreation. Because of a disproportionate emotional immaturity and lack of experience, sexual interest may not be fully developed or may appear later than in normal children. Many feel disqualified from marriage and parenthood because of their disabilities (Passo, 1978; Shurtleff and Sousa, 1977). Only 18 of 63 myelodysplastic teenagers interviewed by Dorner (1977) reported a relationship with the opposite sex, as contrasted with 80 per cent of this same group who expressed an interest in the opposite sex but were unwilling or unable to fulfill their interests.

The mean age for developing secondary sexual characteristics and the onset of menses tends to be earlier in girls with myelomeningocele and is commonly early in most girls with hydrocephalus (Passo, 1978; McLaughlin and Shurtleff, 1979). The girls are most concerned with their capacity to conceive and expect erotic pleasure to come from kissing and cuddling. Despite a frequently observed lack of genital sensation, most women with myelomeningocele have the potential for relatively normal sexual intercourse and pregnancy; however, when pelvic deformity is present, a cesarean section is usually necessary. Any renal impairment may place the pregnancy in a high-risk category. Up to 89 per cent of girls older than 25 years of age report sexual activity (McLaughlin and Shurtleff, 1979).

Boys with myelomeningocele experience more difficulties. Boys are most concerned about their capacity for sexual intercourse and their ability to derive pleasure from it (Passo, 1978; Dorner, 1977). Secondary sexual characteristics develop normally; however, heterosexual activity is delayed and appears closely related to mobility. The capacity for erection, sexual intercourse, and ejaculation is variable but is usually impaired. Many experience spontaneous erections during infancy; however, whether these observations are predictive of later erectile potency is unknown. Partial or complete glandular anesthesia is common; again, the influence on sexual function is uncertain. Masturbation is reported in fewer than one third of boys, although as many as 39 per cent of those over 25 years of age have claimed sexual activity. For those with erectile failure, penile implants are now available. Although

fathering is possible, it is much less likely than is fertility in the female (McLaughlin and Shurtleff, 1979).

Only two reports cite pregnancy related to a parent with myelodysplasia. In 1973, Carter and Evans reported 215 patients with myelomeningocele who had produced 104 children. Fourteen of the 100 males had 35 children, and 38 of the 115 females had 69 children. One man had a child with spina bifida cystica, and one woman had a child with anencephaly. In a later study, Laurence and Beresford (1975) provided long-term follow-up on 51 adults (28 men and 23 females) with myelodysplasia. Eleven men and 11 women were married, with 18 of the married couples producing 39 pregnancies. There were 32 live-born normal children (19 boys, 13 girls), 1 girl with spina bifida who is surviving and another who died as a neonate, and 5 stillborns (3 of which were anencephalic). There were also four known miscarriages and one termination, on psychiatric grounds, of a normal pregnancy. Of the two childless women, one avoided pregnancy because of her disability; the other had an anencephalic birth and miscarriages. Two males were childless. These data should not be interpreted overly optimistically, because all of these adults were born before the era of early spinal closure or of aggressive management of hydrocephalus, and they therefore represent less severely handicapped patients. Since children with more severe defects are now surviving, it is unlikely that these children will be capable of leading such normal lives.

SACRAL AGENESIS

Sacral agenesis (Fig. 55–10) occurs in 0.09 to 0.43 per cent of pregnancies (Schanz and Bundens, 1956) and is frequently associated with other orthopedic anomalies, imperforate anus, and urologic and neurologic malformations. In general, the absence of three or fewer sacral segments does not interfere with normal voiding; however, more extensive sacral defects, especially those involving the second to fourth nerve roots, may produce a neuropathic bladder and fecal incontinence with similar implications for management and complications as for myelodysplasia (Williams and Nixon, 1957). Although saddle anesthesia may be extensive, there is often no obvious neurologic deficit or external evidence of sacral agenesis; related signs and symptoms are often subtle and diagnosis is often delayed (White and Trowbridge,

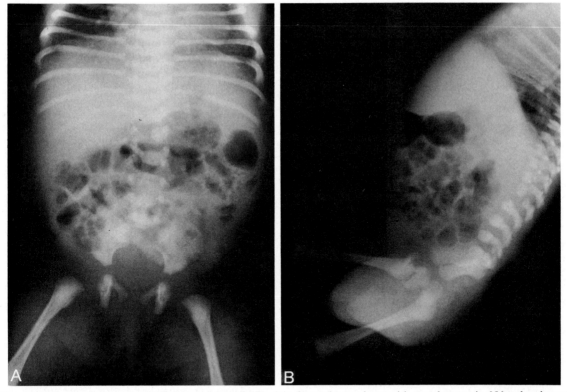

Figure 55–10. Anteroposterior (AP) *(A)* and lateral *(B)* plain films of a newborn with sacral agenesis. Note the absence of the sacrum and coccyx.

1976; Braren and Jones, 1979). When diagnosed, sacral agenesis should be investigated and managed in a manner similar to the management of the infant or child with myelodysplasia.

References

Alter, M.: Anencephalus, hydrocephalus and spina bifida. Arch. Neurol., 7:411, 1962.

Altshuler, A., Meyer, J., and Butz, M. K. J.: Even children can learn to do clean self-catheterization. Am. J. Nurs., 97:101, 1977.

Altwein, J. E., Jonas, U., and Hohenfellner, R.: Long-term follow-up of children with colon conduit urinary diversion and ureterosigmoidostomy. J. Urol., 118:832, 1977.

Bahnson, D. H.: Myelomeningocele and its problems. Pediatr. Ann., 11:528, 1982.

Bauer, S. B., Colodny, A. H., Hallet, M., Khoshbin, S., and Retik, A. B.: Urinary undiversion in myelodysplasia: Criteria for selection and predictive value of urodynamic evaluation. J. Urol., 124:89, 1980.

Bauer, S. B., Hallett, N., Koshbin, S., Lebowitz, R. L., Winston, K. R., Gibson, S., Colodny, A. H., and Retik, A. B.: Predictive value of urodynamic evaluation of newborns with myelodysplasia. JAMA, 252:650, 1984.

Bauer, S. B., Labib, K. B., Dieppa, R. A., and Retik, A.

B.: Urodynamic evaluation of boy with myelodysplasia and incontinence. Urology, 10:354, 1977.

Bell, J. E., Gordon, A., and Maloney, A. F. J.: The association of hydrocephalus and Arnold-Chiari malformation in the fetus. Neuropathy Appl. Neurobiol., 6:29, 1980.

Bellman, A. B.: Penicillin therapy for metaplasia of the ileal conduit stoma. J. Urol., 107:141, 1972.

Blocksom, B. H., Jr.: Bladder pouch for prolonged tubeless cystostomy. J. Urol., 78:398, 1957.

Borden, T. A., McGuire, E. J., Woodside, J. R., et al.: Urinary undiversion in patients with myelodysplasia and neurogenic bladder dysfunction. Urology, 18:223, 1981.

Braren, V., and Jones, W. B.: Sacral agenesis: diagnosis, treatment and follow-up of urologic complications. J. Urol., 121:543, 1979.

Brock, D. J. H., Bolton, A. E., and Monaghan, A. M.: Prenatal diagnosis of anencephaly through maternal serum AFP measurement. Lancet 2:385, 1973.

Caldwell, K. P. S., Martin, M. R., Flack, F. C., and James, E. D.: An alternative method of dealing with incontinence in children with neurogenic bladders. Arch. Dis. Child., 44:625, 1969.

Carter, C. O.: Clues to the aetiology of neural tube malformations. Dev. Med. Child Neurol., (Suppl) 16(32):3, 1974.

Carter, C. O., and Evans, K.: Children of adult survivors with spina bifida cystica. Lancet, 2:924, 1973.

Cass, A. S.: Urinary complications in myelomeningocele patients. J. Urol., 115:102, 1976.

Chamberlain, J.: Human benefits and costs of a national

screening program for neural tube defects. Lancet, 2:1293, 1978.

Chapman, W. H., Shurtleff, D. B., Eckert, D. W., and Ansel, J. S.: A prospective study of the urinary tract from birth in patients with myelomeningocele. J. Urol., 102:363, 1969.

Cohen, J. S., Harback, L. B., and Kaplan, G. S.: Cutaneous vesicostomy for temporary urinary diversion in infants with neurogenic bladder dysfunction. J. Urol., 119:120, 1978.

Cooper, D. G. W.: Bladder studies in children with neurogenic incontinence. With comments on the place of pelvic floor stimulation. Br. J. Urol., 40:157, 1968.

Crandall, B. F.: Alphafetoprotein: The diagnosis of neural tube defects. Pediatr. Ann., 10:38, 1981.

Culp, D. A., Bekhrad, A., and Flocks, R. H.: Urologic management of the myelomeningocele patient. JAMA, 213:753, 1970.

Diokno, A. C., Kass, E. J., and Lapides, J.: A new approach to myelodysplasia. J. Urol., 116:771, 1976.

Dorner, S.: Sexual interest and activity in adolescents with spina bifida. J. Child Psychol. Psychiatry, 18:229, 1977.

Drago, J. R., Wellner, L., Sanford, B. J., et al.: The role of intermittent catheterization in the management of children with myelomeningocele. J. Urol., 118:92, 1977.

Dretler, S. P.: Pathogenesis of urinary tract calculi occurring after ileal conduit diversion: I. Clinical study. II. Conduit study. III. Prevention. J. Urol., 109:204, 1973.

Duckett, J. W., Jr.: Cutaneous vesicostomy in childhood. The Blocksom technique. Urol. Clin. North Am., 1:485, 1974.

Ehrlich, O., and Brem, A. S.: A prospective comparison of urinary tract infections in patients treated either with clean intermittent catheterization or urinary diversion. Pediatrics, 70:655, 1982.

Engel, B. T., Nikoomanesh, P., and Shuster, M. M.: Operant conditioning of retrosphincteric responses in the treatment of fecal incontinence. N. Engl. J. Med., 290:646, 1974.

Enrile, B. G., and Crooks, J. K.: Clean intermittent catheterization for home management in children with myelomeningocele. Clin. Pediatr., 19:743, 1980.

Fedun, P. C.: Tethered cord syndrome. J. Neurosurg. Nurs., 14:114, 1982.

Feetham, S., Tweed, J., and Perrin, J. S.: Practical problems in selection of spina bifida infants for treatment in the USA. Z. Kinderchir., 28:301, 1979.

Forbes, N.: Renal dysplasia in infants with neural spinal dysraphism. J. Pathol., 107:13, 1972.

Frank, J. D., and Fixsen, J. A.: Spina bifida. Br. J. Hosp. Med., 24(5)422, 1980.

Garvin, D. D., Weber, C. H., Jr., and Olsky, M. S.: Carcinoma in the defunctionalized bladder: Report of a case and a review of the literature. J. Urol., 117:669, 1972.

Gaum, L. D., Wese, F. X., Alton, D. J., Hardy, B. E., and Churchill, B. M.: Radiologic investigation of the urinary tract in the neonate with myelomeningocele. J. Urol., 127:510, 1982.

Glenn, J. F., Small, M. P., and Boyarsky, S.: Complications of ileal segment urinary diversion in children. Urol. Int., 23:97, 1968.

Godec, C. J., and Cass, A. S.: Electrical stimulation for incontinence in myelomeningocele. J. Urol., 120:729, 1978.

Gonzalez, R., and Sheldon, C. A.: Artificial sphincters in children with neurogenic bladders: Long-term results. J. Urol., 128:1270, 1982.

Gross, R. H., Cox, A., Tatyrek, R., Pollay, M., and Barnes, W. A.: Early management and decision making for treatment of myelomeningocele. Pediatrics, 72:450, 1983.

Guthkelch, A. N.: Studies in spina bifida cystica III. Seasonal variations in the frequency of spina bifida births. Br. J. Prevent. Soc. Med., 16:159, 1962.

Guttmann, L., and Frankel, H.: Value of intermittent self-catheterization in early management of traumatic paraplegia and tetraplegia. Paraplegia, 4:63, 1966.

Haddow, J. E., and Macri, J. N.: Prenatal screening for neural tube defects. JAMA, 242:515, 1979.

Halverstadt, D. B.: Electrical stimulation of the bladder: Three years later. J. Urol., 106:673, 1971.

Harlo, S. E., Merrill, R. E., Lee, E. N., Turman, A. E., and Trapp, J. D.: Clinical evaluation of the urinary tract in patients with myelomeningocele. J. Urol., 93:411, 1965.

Hendren, W. H.: Some alternatives to urinary diversion in children. J. Urol., 119:652, 1978.

Hill, J. T., and Ransley, P. G.: The colonic conduit: a better method of urinary diversion? Br. J. Urol., 55:629, 1983.

Hilwa, N., and Perlmutter, A. D.: Adjunctive drug therapy for intermittent catheterization and self-catheterization. J. Urol., 119:551, 1978.

Hoffer, M. M., Feiwell, E., Perry, R., et al.: Functional ambulation in patients with myelomeningocele. J. Bone Joint Surg., 55A:157, 1973.

James, W. H.: Recurrence rates for neural tube defects and vitamin supplementation. J. Med. Genet., 18:249, 1981.

Johnston, J. H.: The neurogenic bladder in the newborn infant. Paraplegia, 6:157, 1968.

Jonas, V., Jones, L. W., and Tanagho, E. A.: Spinal end stimulation versus detrusor stimulation. Invest. Urol., 13:171, 1975.

Kaplan, G. S., and King, L. R.: Results of Y-V vesico-urethroplasty in children. Surg. Gynecol. Obstet., 130:1059, 1970.

Kass, E. J., and Koff, S. A.: Bladder augmentation in the pediatric neuropathic bladder. J. Urol., 129:552, 1983.

Kass, E. J., Koff, S. A., Diokno, A. C., and Lapides, J.: The significance of bacilluria in children on long-term intermittent catheterization. J. Urol., 126:223, 1981.

Kass, E. J., McHugh, T., and Diokno, A. C.: Intermittent catheterization in children less than six years old. J. Urol., 121:792, 1979.

Katzen, M.: The total care of spina bifida cystica. Surg. Ann., 13:325, 1981.

Kelalis, P. P.: Urinary diversion in children by sigmoid conduit: its advantages and limitations. J. Urol., 112:666, 1974.

Klauber, G. T., Chairman: Action Committee on Myelodysplasia, Section of Urology, American Academy of Pediatrics. Current approaches to evaluation and management of children with myelodysplasia. Pediatrics, 63:663, 1979.

Knolson, F. E., and Spitz, E. B.: Treatment of hydrocephalus by direct shunt to jugular vein. Surg. Forum, 2:399, 1952.

Kogan, S. J., and Levitt, S. B.: Bladder evaluation in pediatric patients before undiversion in previously diverted urinary tracts. J. Urol., 118:443, 1977.

Koontz, W. W., Jr., and Smith, M. J. V.: Transurethral external sphincterotomy in boys with myelodysplasia. J. Urol., 117:500, 1977.

Kroovand, R. L.: The artificial sphincter for urinary continence. Dev. Med. Child Neurol., 25:520, 1983.

Kropp, K. A., and Voeller, K. K. S.: Cryptorchism in myelomeningocele. J. Pediatr. 99:110, 1981.

Kyker, J., Gregory, J. G., Shah, J., and Schoenberg, H. W.: Comparison of intermittent catheterization and supravesical diversion in children with myelomeningocele. J. Urol., 118:90, 1977.

Lapides, J.: Neurogenic bladder: Principles of treatment. Urol. Clin. North Am., 1:81, 1974.

Lapides, J., Diokno, A. C., Gould, F. R., et al.: Further observations on self-catheterization. J. Urol., 116:169, 1976.

Lapides, J., Diokno, A. C., Lowe, B. S., et al.: Follow-up on unsterile intermittent self-catheterization. J. Urol., 111:184, 1974.

Lapides, J., Diokno, A. C., Silber, S. J., and Lowe, B. S.: Clean intermittent self-catheterization in the treatment of urinary tract disease. J. Urol., 107:458, 1972.

Laurence, K. M.: The recurrence risk of spina bifida cystica and anencephaly. Dev. Med. Child Neurol., (Suppl) 11(20):23, 1969.

Laurence, K. M.: Neural tube defects: a two-pronged approach to primary prevention. Pediatrics, 70:648, 1982.

Laurence, K. M., and Beresford, A.: Continence, friends, marriage and children in fifty-one adults with spina bifida. Dev. Med. Child Neurol., (Suppl) 17(35):123, 1975.

Laurence, K. M., and David, P. A.: The incidence of major central nervous system malformations in South Wales: Investigation of the possible etiology. Proceedings of the fifth international conference on neuropathology: Excerpta Medica International Congress Series, 100:740, 1965.

Laurence, K. M., and Tew, B. S.: Follow-up of 65 survivors from 425 cases of spina bifida born in South Wales between 1956 and 1962. Dev. Med. Child Neurol., (Suppl) 13:1, 1967.

Leck, I.: The etiology of human malformations: insights from epidemiology. Teratology, 5:303, 1971.

Light, J. K., Flores, F. N., and Scott, F. B.: Use of the AS792 artificial sphincter following urinary undiversion. J. Urol., 129:548, 1983.

Light, J. K., and Van Blerk, J. P. J.: Intermittent catheterization in congenital neurogenic bladder: A preliminary report. Br. J. Urol., 45:523, 1977.

Lome, L. G., Howat, J. M., and Williams, D. I.: The temporarily defunctionalized bladder in children. J. Urol., 108:162, 1972.

Lorber, J.: Results of treatment of myelomeningocele: an analysis of 524 unselected cases with special reference to possible selection for treatment. Dev. Med. Child Neurol., 13:279, 1971.

Lorber, J.: Early results of selection treatment in spina bifida cystica. Br. Med. J., 4:201, 1973.

Lorber, J., and Salfield, S. A. W.: Results of selective treatment of spina bifida cystica. Arch. Dis. Child, 56:822, 1981.

Lyon, R. P., Scott, M. P., and Marshall, S.: Intermittent catheterization rather than urinary diversion in children with myelomeningocele. J. Urol., 113:409, 1975.

Mandel, J., Lebowitz, R. L., Hallett, M., Koshbin, S., and Bauer, S. B.: Urethral narrowing in the region of the external sphincter: radiologic-urodynamic correlations in boys with myelodysplasia. AJR, 134:731, 1980.

Manfredi, R. A., and Leal, J. F.: Selective sacral rhizotomy for dysplastic bladder syndrome in patients with spinal cord injuries. J. Urol., 100:17, 1968.

McLaughlin, J., and Shurtleff, D. B.: Management of the newborn with myelodysplasia. Clin. Pediatr., 18:463, 1979.

Menelaus, M. B.: Orthopaedic management of children with myelomeningocele: A plea for realistic goals. Dev. Med. Child Neurol., (Suppl) 37:3, 1976.

Menon, M., Elder, J., Manley, C. B., and Jeffs, R. D.: Undiverting the ileal conduit. J. Urol., 129:998, 1983.

Merrill, D. C., and Conway, C. J.: Clinical experience with the Mentor bladder stimulator. 1. Patients with upper motor neuron lesions. J. Urol., 112:52, 1974.

Meunier, P., Molar, P., and Dedeaujeum, J.: Manometric studies of anorectal disorders in infancy and childhood: An investigation of physiopathology of incontinence and defecation. Br. J. Surg., 63:402, 1976.

Middleton, A. W., Jr., and Hendren, W. H.: Ileal conduits in children at the Massachusetts General Hospital from 1955 to 1970. J. Urol., 115:591, 1976.

Milunsky, A.: Prenatal detection of neural tube defects: False positive results. Pediatrics 59:782, 1977.

Milunsky, A., and Alpert, E.: The value of alphafetoprotein in the prenatal diagnosis of neural tube defects. J. Pediatr., 84:889, 1974.

Mogg, R. A.: Urinary diversion using the colon conduit. Br. J. Urol., 39:687, 1967.

Mulcahy, J. J., James, H. E., and McRoberts, J. W.: Oxybutynin chloride combined with intermittent catheterization in the treatment of myelomeningocele patients. J. Urol., 118:95, 1977.

Mullholland, G. S., Yalla, S. V., Raezer, D. M., et al.: Primary external urethral sphincter hyperkinesia in a boy. Urology, 4:577, 1974.

Naggan, A. L., and MacMahon, B.: Ethnic differences in the prevalence of anencephaly and spina bifida in Boston, Massachusetts. N. Engl. J. Med., 227:1119, 1967.

Navarro, M. D., Madduri, M. D., Iglesias, J. J., and Seebode, J. J.: Transurethral resection of the bladder neck in neurogenic bladder secondary to myelomeningocele. J. Med. Soc. N. J., 75:52, 1978.

Nevin, N. C., Johnston, W. P., and Merrett, J. D.: Influence of social class on the risk of recurrence of anencephalus and spina bifida. Dev. Med. Child Neurol., 23:155, 1981.

Parkin, J. M.: Ethics of selective treatment of spina bifida, report by a working party. Lancet 1:85, 1975.

Passo, S.: Parents' perception, attitudes and needs regarding sex education for the child with myelomeningocele. Res. Nurs. Health, 1:53, 1978.

Perez-Marreno, R., Dimlock, W., Churchill, B. M., and Hardy, B. E.: Clean intermittent catheterization in myelomeningocele children less than three years old. J. Urol., 128:779, 1982.

Perlmutter, A. D., and Kroovand, R. L.: Use of bowel for bladder augmentation in children. Presented to the American Association of Genitourinary Surgeons Annual Meeting, May 1983. Greenbriar, West Virginia.

Plunkett, J. M., and Braren, V.: Clean intermittent catheterization of children. J. Urol., 121:469, 1979.

Reiner, W. G., and Jeffs, R. D.: Ileal intussusception as an antireflux mechanism in urinary diversion for myelomeningocele. J. Urol., 121:212, 1979.

Renwick, J. H.: Potato babies. Lancet, 2:336, 1972.

Ritchie, J. P., Skinner, D. G., and Waisman, J.: The effect of reflux on the development of pyelonephritis and urinary diversion: an experimental study. J. Surg. Res., 16:256, 1974.

Roberts, J. B. M.: Congenital anomalies of the urinary tract and their association with spina bifida. Br. J. Urol., 33:309, 1961.

Rogers, S. C., and Weatherhall, J. A. C.: Anencephalus, spina bifida and congenital hydrocephalus: England and Wales 1964–72. Studies on medical and population subjects No. 32. Office of Population Censuses and Survey. HMSO. London, 1976.

Schanz, A. R., Jr., and Bundens, W. D.: Congenital malformations of the spine: an analysis of roentgenograms of 700 children. Bull. Hosp. Joint Dis., 17:110, 1956.

Schmidt, J. D., Hawtrey, C. E., Flocks, R. H., and Culp, D. A.: Complications, results and problems of ileal conduit diversions. J. Urol., 109:210, 1973.

Schwartz, G. R., and Jeffs, R. D.: Ileal conduit urinary diversion in children: Computer analysis of follow-up from two to sixteen years. J. Urol., 114:285, 1975.

Shapiro, S. R., Lebowitz, R., and Colodny, A. H.: Fate of 90 children with ileal conduit urinary diversion a decade later: Analysis and complications, pyelography, renal function and bacteriology. J. Urol., 114:289, 1975.

Sharrard, W. J. W.: Newer orthopaedic aspects of myelomeningocele. In Wilkinson, A. W. (Ed.): Recent Advances in Pediatric Surgery. London, Churchill Livingstone, 1969, p. 71.

Sharrard, W. J. W., Zachary, R. B., Lorber, J., and Bruce, A. M.: A controlled trial of immediate and delayed closure of spina bifida cystica. Arch. Dis. of Child., 38:18, 1963.

Shochat, S. J., and Perlmutter, A. D.: Myelodysplasia with severe neonatal hydronephrosis: the value of urethral dilation. J. Urol., 107:146, 1972.

Shurtleff, D. B., and Sousa, J. C.: The adolescent with myelodysplasia: development, achievement, sex and deterioration. Del. Med. J., 49:631, 1977.

Shurtleff, D. B., Hayden, T. W., Lower, J. D., and Kronmal, R. A.: Myelodysplasia: Decision for death or disability. N. Engl. J. Med., 291:1005, 1975.

Smith, E. D.: Spina bifida and the Total Care of Spinal Myelomeningocele. Springfield, Ill., Charles C Thomas, 1965.

Smith, E. D.: Follow-up studies on 105 ileal conduits in children. J. Pediatr. Surg., 7:1, 1972a.

Smith, E. D.: Urinary prognosis in spina bifida. J. Urol., 108:815, 1972b.

Smith, G. K., and Smith, E. D.: Selection for treatment in spina bifida cystica. Br. J. Med. 4:189, 1973.

Smith, H. P., Russell, J. M., Boyce, W. H., and Alexander, E., Jr.: Results of urinary diversion in patients with myelomeningocele. J. Neurosurg., 50:773, 1979.

Smithells, R. W., D'Arcy, E. E., and McAllister, E. F.: Outcome of pregnancies before and after birth of infants with nervous system malformations. Dev. Med Child. Neurol., (Suppl) 10(15):6, 1968.

Smithells, R. W., Sheppard, S., Schorah, C. J., et al.: Possible prevention of neural tube defects by preconceptional vitamin supplementation. Lancet, 1:339, 1980.

Soare, P. L., and Raimondi, A. J.: Intellectual and perceptual motor characteristics of treated myelomeningocele children. Am. J. Dis. Child., 131:199, 1977.

Stark, G. D.: Myelomeningocele: The changing approach to treatment. In Wilkinson, A. W. (Ed.): Recent Advances in Pediatric Surgery. London, Churchill Livingstone, 1975, p. 73.

Stark, G. D., and Drummond, M.: Results of selective early operation in myelomeningocele. Arch. Dis. Child., 48:676, 1974.

Stark, J.: Pudendal neurectomy in management of neurogenic bladder in myelomeningocele. Arch. Dis. Child., 44:698, 1969.

Stein, S. C., Feldman, J. G., Friedlander, M., and Klein, R. J.: Is myelomeningocele a disappearing disease? Pediatrics, 65:511, 1969.

Tavafoghi, V., Gandehi, A., Hembrick, G. W., et al.: Cutaneous signs of spina dysraphism. Arch. Dermatol., 114:573, 1978.

Tew, B. J., and Laurence, K. M.: The effects of hydrocephalus on intelligence, visual perception and school attainments. Dev. Med. Child Neurol., (Suppl) 17(35):129, 1975.

Thomas, M., and Hopkins, J. N.: A study of the renal tract from birth in children with myelomeningocele. Dev. Med. Child Neurol., (Suppl)25(13):96, 1971.

Till, K.: Spinal dysraphism: A study of congenital malformations of the lower back. J. Joint Bone Surg., (B) 51B:415, 1969.

Wainsten, M., Richard, D. E., Nulsen, S., and Persky, L.: Fever in the child with myelomeningocele and ileal diversion. Am. J. Surg., 124:317, 1972.

Wald, A.: Use of biofeedback in treatment of fecal incontinence in patients with myelomeningocele. Pediatrics, 68:45, 1981.

Wheatley, J. K., Woodard, J. R., and Parrott, T. S.: Electronic bladder stimulation in the management of children with myelomeningocele. J. Urol., 127:283, 1982.

White, J. J., Suzuki, H., El Shafie, M., Kumar, M., et al.: A physiologic rationale for management of neurologic rectal incontinence in children. Pediatrics, 49:888, 1972.

White, R. I., and Trowbridge, E. T.: Sacral agenesis. An analysis of 22 cases. Urology, 8:521, 1976.

Whitehead, W. E., Parker, L. H., Masek, B. J., et al.: Biofeedback treatment of fecal incontinence in patients with myelomeningocele. Dev. Med. Child Neurol., 23:313, 1981.

Williams, D. I., and Nixon, H. H.: Agenesis of the sacrum. Surg. Gynecol. Obstet., 103:84, 1957.

Windham, G. C., and Edmonds, L. D.: Current trends in the incidence of neural tube defects. Pediatrics, 70:333, 1982.

Winemiller, J. H., Lehman, T. H.: An eight-year-old urologic experience in the multidisciplinary approach of the care of the myelomeningocele patient. J. Urol., 110:138, 1973.

Yen, S., and MacMahon, B.: Genetics of anencephaly and spina bifida. Lancet, 2:623, 1968.

CHAPTER 56

Neonatal and Perinatal Emergencies

JOHN R. WOODARD, M.D.

INTRODUCTION

Neonate is the term generally applied to the newborn infant during his or her first and most critical month of life (Behrman, 1973). While approximately two thirds of all infant deaths occur during the first year of life, most are during the neonatal period, with the first day of life being the most hazardous. Between 10 and 15 per cent of all neonatal deaths are attributable to gross congenital malformations (Schaffer and Avery, 1977). In a series of 543 autopsies performed on neonates and stillborn infants, 264 different urologic abnormalities were discovered in 91 infants or fetuses. That is, 17 per cent had one or more urologic abnormalities (Woodard and Lasky, unpublished data). In the same institution, the incidence of recognizable urologic abnormalities in surviving neonates was 0.8 per cent, with hypospadias and cryptorchidism being the most common findings.

The urgency of diagnosis and treatment in infants with congenital abnormalities depends upon the risk associated with that abnormality. A disorder that produces the most marked abnormality of form may not be as urgent a problem as one that produces a major abnormality of function (Keay and Morgan, 1974). That is, the least easily recognizable urologic abnormality may be the one that requires the most urgent attention. A *neonatal urologic emergency* is any genitourinary condition during the first month of life that jeopardizes the gonads, the kidneys, or the life of the infant, should there be a delay in either diagnosis or treatment. Therefore, it is crucial that urologists involved in the care of newborn infants be alert to the clues of underlying genitourinary anomalies or diseases in the neonate and be acutely aware of those conditions requiring immediate attention. Since the pathophysiology and management of many of these conditions are dealt with extensively elsewhere in this text, this chapter will emphasize early detection and initial management.

CLUES TO THE PRESENCE OF UROLOGIC DISORDERS

During Pregnancy. A family history or past history in the mother of previous *fetal wastage* should alert one to an increased likelihood of malformation, as should a family history of *chromosomal abnormalities*, such as translocation. Although severe obstructive uropathy, the prune-belly syndrome, or renal agenesis might be signaled by the presence of *oligohydramnios*, neonatal ovarian cysts are said to be more common in pregnancies characterized by *polyhydramnios*. A pregnancy complicated by *bleeding*, especially in the first trimester, is more likely to produce a baby with congenital malformation(s). *Illnesses* in the mother during the pregnancy, particularly rubella and diabetes, are known to be associated with abnormalities in the baby, as are certain *drugs* administered during the period of gestation. Intrauterine growth retardation should further alert one to the possibility of an anomaly. As the *age of the prospective mother* passes 35 years, perinatal mortality more than doubles (Behrman, 1973; Keay and Morgan, 1974; Schaffer and Avery, 1977; Vulliamy, 1972).

During Labor and Delivery. If the mother is given *magnesium sulfate* for toxemia during labor, the neonate may have neuromuscular blockade with both generalized hypotonia and bladder distention (Cockburn and Drillien, 1974). Asphyxia from a *traumatic delivery* can result not only in renal cortical or tubular necrosis but also in inappropriate antidiuretic hormone (ADH) secretion, leading to generalized edema. Congenital malformations are almost twice as likely to occur in babies born by *breech delivery* (Schaffer and Avery, 1977).

Approximately 0.9 per cent of all babies are born with a *single umbilical artery,* and there is an ongoing controversy regarding its urologic significance. The mortality rate in infants born with single umbilical arteries is almost four times that of newborns in general, and of those infants who die, approximately 28 per cent have genitourinary malformations. However, of babies born with malformations but not with single umbilical arteries, the incidence of genitourinary abnormalities almost equals the same 28 per cent. From the information currently available, it still appears that surviving infants with a history of single umbilical artery are suspect of having a urologic malformation and should be so investigated (Altshuler et al., 1975; Bryan and Kohler, 1975; Feingold et al., 1964; Froehlich and Fujikura, 1973; Gellis, 1975; Lemtis and Klemme, 1971).

From External Features of the Neonate. Despite the foregoing discussion, most clues are derived from actual examination of the newborn baby. *Potter's facies,* characterized by large, low-set, and flabby ears and widely spaced eyes, is now well known as a sign of renal agenesis (Fig. 56–1) (Potter, 1946). These facies might also occur in some infants with the prune-belly syndrome and with bilateral multicystic kidneys (Williams, 1974). Abnormalities of the external ear alone may signal the presence of a uropathy. Many syndromes in which urologic defects are a major feature are also characterized by *widely spaced nipples. Deficiency of the abdominal musculature* is a reliable indication of prune-belly uropathy (Fig. 56–2) and cryptorchidism. *Renal enlargements* are usually easily detectable during the initial examination of the newborn, and *abnormalities of the genitalia and anus* should also be obvious. Subtle clues such as a *sacral dermal sinus* may indicate either a spinal abnormality or the presence of a teratoma. Although this list could be expanded, Smith (1976) states that if as many as three minor abnormalities are present, there is a 90 per cent likelihood of a major abnormality.

SIGNS AND SYMPTOMS OF GENITOURINARY EMERGENCIES IN NEONATES

Abdominal Mass

An abdominal mass is by far the most common sign or symptom ultimately leading to urologic surgery in the newborn infant (Parrott and Woodard, 1976). With approximately one half of the neonatal abdominal masses arising in the kidney, one should not assume that a mass presenting anteriorly cannot arise from the retroperitoneal area. Table 56–1 is a composite inventory derived from three published series reporting on abdominal masses and shows the relative frequency of various entities that are likely to present in the neonate as an abdominal mass (Longino and Martin, 1958; Raffensperger and Abousleiman, 1968; Wedge et al., 1971). It

TABLE 56–1. FREQUENCY OF CAUSES OF NEONATAL ABDOMINAL MASSES IN 115 PATIENTS*

Site and Cause	No. of Patients
KIDNEY	
Hydronephrosis	33
Multicystic kidney	35
Polycystic kidney	2
Renal vein thrombosis	3
Solid tumors	2
RETROPERITONEUM	
Neuroblastoma	7
Teratoma	2
Hemangioma	1
BLADDER	
Urethral valves	1
FEMALE GENITAL TRACT	
Hydrocolpos	7
Ovarian cyst	5
GASTROINTESTINAL TRACT	
Duplications	5
Giant cystic meconium peritonitis	2
Mesenteric cyst	1
Volvulus of ileum	1
Teratoma of stomach	1
Leiomyoma of colon	1
HEPATIC OR BILIARY TRACT	
Hemangioma of liver	2
Solitary cyst of liver	1
Hepatoma	1
Distended gallbladder	1
Choledochal cyst	1

*Data from Longino, L. A., and Martin, L. W.: Pediatrics, *21*:596, 1958; Raffensperger, J., and Abousleiman, A.: Surgery, *63*:514, 1968; Wedge, J. J., et al.: J. Urol., *106*:770, 1971.

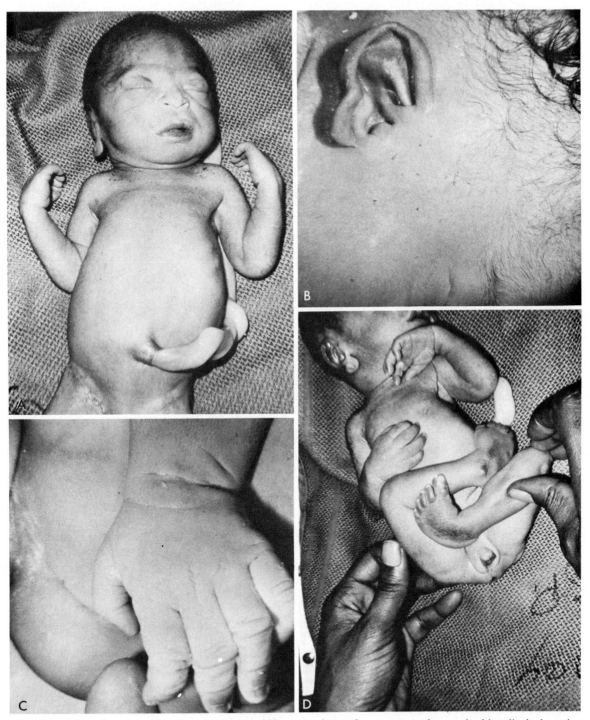

Figure 56–1. This newborn with bilateral multicystic kidneys was born of a pregnancy characterized by oligohydramnios, and he died from pulmonary hypoplasia. He illustrates the features of Potter's syndrome: *(A)* flattened face, "beaked" nose, apparent hypertelorism, skin fold below the eye, and micrognathia; *(B)* low-set, abnormally shaped ears with large lobes; *(C)* abnormally large hands with flabby digits; and *(D)* bowed legs with clubbed feet.

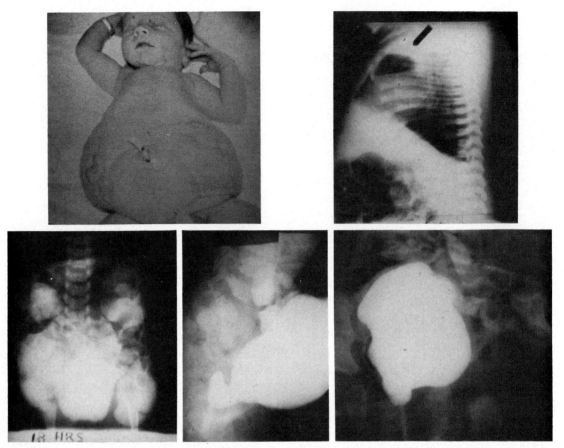

Figure 56–2. Infant with congenital hypoplasia of the abdominal musculature demonstrating the typical features of "prune-belly uropathy" and pneumomediastinum.

is noteworthy that disorders of the kidney accounted for well over 50 per cent of these abdominal masses, with hydronephrosis and multicystic kidney being approximately equal in frequency. Of all masses recorded, 83 per cent originated in the kidney, retroperitoneal area, or female genital tract. Only 17 per cent were related to the liver or the gastrointestinal tract. Consequently, it is obvious that diagnostic evaluations should seldom begin with barium studies of the gastrointestinal tract (Longino and Martin, 1958; Raffensperger and Abousleiman, 1968; Wedge et al., 1971).

The most important aspect in managing the neonate with an abdominal mass is an accurate diagnosis, and Table 56–1 lists most of the diagnostic possibilities. The evaluation of such a mass should proceed in a logical and systematic fashion, beginning with careful abdominal palpation that will usually provide important information. The size, contour, location, and mobility of the mass help to determine its site of origin. For example, a mass in the epigas-

trium that moves with respiration is likely to be hepatic, omental, or gastric in origin. When masses are bilateral, they are more often of renal origin, with hydronephrosis and polycystic kidneys (Fig. 56–3) being the more likely lesions. A smooth lower midline abdominal mass could represent a distended bladder, but in the female patient, it might be of uterine or ovarian origin (Figs. 56–4 and 56–5).

Following abdominal palpation, the simplest and often most useful diagnostic tool is transillumination. This examination should be carried out in a completely darkened room with a powerful light source, such as a fiberoptic system. It is more useful in white than in black infants, and many cystic lesions will clearly transilluminate, as will some hydronephrotic kidneys. Transillumination is particularly useful in distinguishing the solid from the cystic or fluid-filled lesion.

Clearly, radiographic examination of the abdomen in neonates with abdominal masses is the most definitive diagnostic modality. Plain

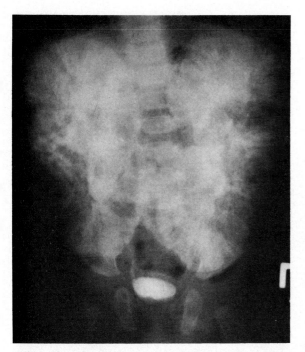

Figure 56–3. Excretory urogram (4 hours after contrast injection) in a neonate having bilateral abdominal masses. The film illustrates the "sunburst" appearance typical of infantile polycystic kidney disease.

films of the abdomen will usually confirm the presence of a mass and help in localizing it by showing displacement of the abdominal viscera with shifting of the intestinal gas pattern. These films should be made in the anteroposterior and lateral projections, with erect films sometimes proving helpful. Penetration should be sufficient to allow the detection of subtle calcifications that might be present in patients with meconium peritonitis, neuroblastoma, or teratoma.

The initial plain radiograph should be followed by excretory urography. Some physicians suggest that in the young neonate the examination can be done through the patent umbilical artery, if a cannula can be easily inserted. This might allow an aortogram to precede the intravenous pyelogram (Lebowitz and Griscom, 1977). Otherwise, the contrast medium is injected in the routine fashion. Infants tolerate up to 4 ml/kg of contrast material, and satisfactory visualization of the urinary tract can usually be obtained. The immature neonatal nephron excretes slowly and concentrates poorly. It requires a high dose of contrast material and delayed filming (Fig. 56–6) for maximum information. The quality of the excretory urogram is usually better by the third week of life (Martin et al., 1975).

If opacification is inadequate by excretory urography, a renal scan will often yield complementary information. However, it is generally agreed that the *intravenous pyelogram (IVP) is the single most important diagnostic tool* in the evaluation of neonatal abdominal masses. This is obvious when the lesion is of renal origin, but it is also true for other retroperitoneal lesions as well as for lesions arising from the female genital tract. Again, oblique and lateral views are important, and delayed filming (up to 24 hours following injection) is helpful in making a diagnosis of hydronephrosis (Fig. 56–6). The total body opacification that results from high-dose contrast injection in the neonate is often useful when evaluating abdominal masses from any source (Martin et al., 1972).

At this point, if the lesion appears to be intraperitoneal, barium studies of the gastrointestinal tract may prove helpful. Additional means of evaluating abdominal masses include angiography, either inferior venacavography or arteriography, and ultrasonography. Angiographic studies are likely to be useful in evaluating renal or other retroperitoneal solid masses and suspected renal vein thromboses. Use of ultrasonic evaluation of the abdomen in neonates is increasing. It is a safe, noninvasive, informative technique that complements intravenous urography and involves minimal discomfort to the patient without further radiation exposure (Teele, 1977). Abdominal arteriography can be done in neonates, particularly when umbilical artery catheterization is used (Emmanouilides and Rein, 1964). While computerized axial tomography is occasionally indicated, abdominal ultrasonography is generally more useful in evaluating neonatal abdominal masses.

Most neonatal abdominal masses will require surgical intervention, either for therapeutic reasons or to finalize the diagnosis.

Hematuria

It is an axiom in urologic practice that either microscopic or gross hematuria must be fully evaluated in all patients. In the newborn this becomes an emergency. Gross hematuria in the newborn is rare, as evidenced by only 35 neonatal admissions to the Children's Memorial Hospital in Chicago for that reason between 1950 and 1967 (Emanuel and Aronson, 1974). Table 56–2 lists the narrow spectrum of causes of gross hematuria found in those 35 neonates. In the 11 undiagnosed cases the possibilities

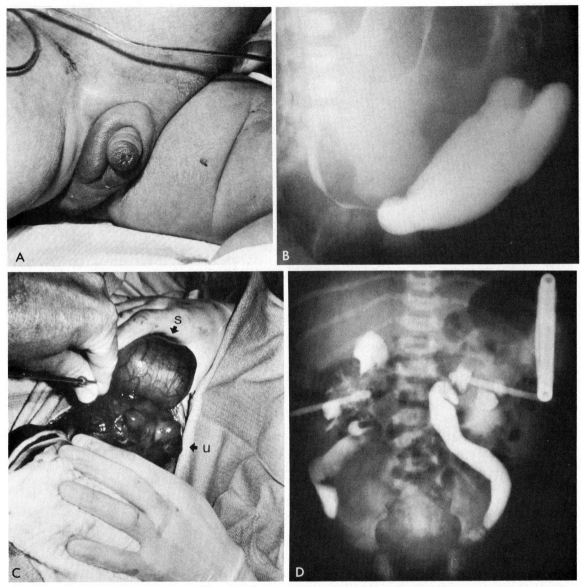

Figure 56–4. This female neonate with imperforate anus had a midline lower abdominal mass found to be hydrometrocolpos. *A,* The external genitalia appear ambiguous. *B,* The mass displaces the ureter posterolaterally and the bladder anteriorly. *C,* At operation the distended uterus(u) is seen adjacent to the sigmoid(s). *D,* Postoperative antegrade pyelograms show lower ureteral obstruction persisting despite catheter drainage of the uterus. The baby died of sepsis.

TABLE 56–2. Findings in 35 Neonates
Hospitalized for Hematuria*

Cause	No. of Patients
Renal vein thrombosis	7
Obstructive uropathy	7
Polycystic kidney disease	6
Sponge kidney	3
Wilms' tumor	1
Undiagnosed	11

*From Emanuel, B., and Aronson, N.: Am. J. Dis. Child., *128*:204, 1974.

included neonatal glomerulonephritis, hemorrhagic disease of the newborn, traumatic delivery, intravascular coagulation, and renal necrosis.

In the author's experience the neonate is vulnerable to three lethal conditions in which hematuria is likely to be a prominent sign or symptom (Table 56–3). These require immediate recognition and prompt and appropriate therapy if survival is to be expected. The management of these three entities will be discussed individually later in this chapter.

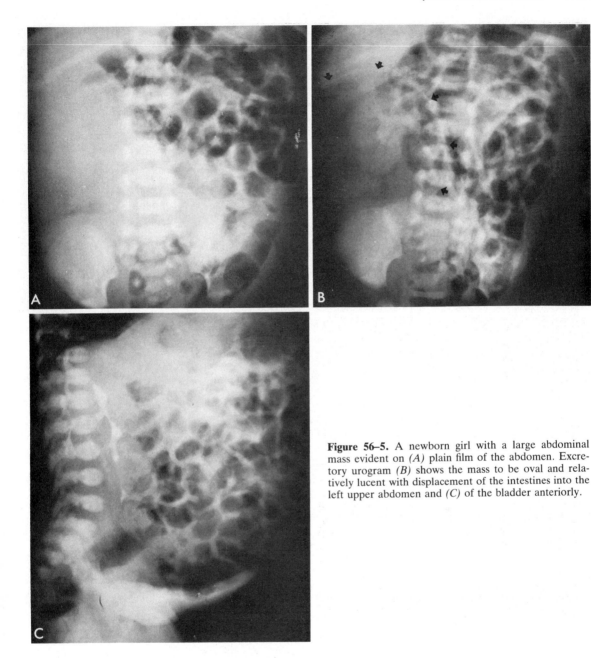

Figure 56–5. A newborn girl with a large abdominal mass evident on *(A)* plain film of the abdomen. Excretory urogram *(B)* shows the mass to be oval and relatively lucent with displacement of the intestines into the left upper abdomen and *(C)* of the bladder anteriorly.

Not to be discussed here are a variety of birth traumas such as rupture of a distended bladder or hydronephrotic kidney during a difficult or traumatic delivery. In these circumstances hemoperitoneum may be more prominent than hematuria (Cywes, 1967; Ravitch and Schell, 1961).

Hypertension

Although hypertension in other age groups is a true emergency only occasionally, systemic hypertension in the neonate always requires an immediate explanation and usually necessitates treatment. Such treatment may be urgently needed to combat congestive heart failure.

TABLE 56–3. EMERGENCY CONDITIONS PRESENTING
IN THE NEONATE AS HEMATURIA

Renal artery thrombosis
Renal vein thrombosis
Renal cortical necrosis

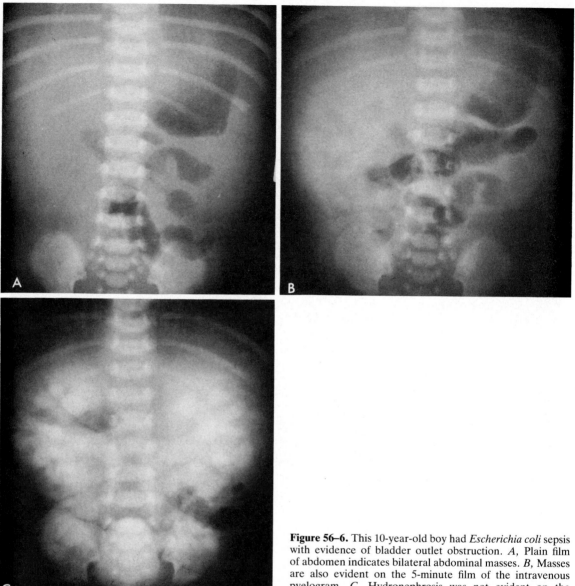

Figure 56–6. This 10-year-old boy had *Escherichia coli* sepsis with evidence of bladder outlet obstruction. *A,* Plain film of abdomen indicates bilateral abdominal masses. *B,* Masses are also evident on the 5-minute film of the intravenous pyelogram. *C,* Hydronephrosis was not evident on the pyelogram until 3 hours later.

The average normal blood pressure for a full-term newborn infant is 72 mm Hg systolic and 47 mm Hg diastolic in the resting state. This pressure may be increased by 20 mm Hg, both systolic and diastolic, if the infant is crying (Moss et al., 1963). The method for determining blood pressure has improved considerably with the use of the Doppler reflected ultrasound technique. The blood pressure in the legs should be within 20 mm Hg of the pressure in the arms, whether by the flush or by the Doppler technique (Lees, 1973).

The major cause of hypertension in the neonate has been said to be coarctation of the aorta. Nephrogenic causes are second in frequency (Lees, 1973). Among the nephrogenic causes of hypertension, perhaps the most important is that resulting from renal artery thrombosis. This phenomenon may produce severe hypertension, rapidly leading to congestive heart failure (Woodard et al., 1967). In a recent report of hypertension in ten infants under the age of 3 months, eight cases had a renal origin with seven having thrombosis of either the renal artery or the abdominal aorta. Hypertension is also known to occur in infants with hydronephrosis secondary to vesicoureteral reflux or to obstruction and is possibly aggravated by infection or surgical procedures (Munoz et al., 1977; Plummer et al., 1975).

Hypertension has also been associated with the adrenogenital syndrome, in which an enzymatic block results in excessive excretion of mineralocorticoids. A deficiency of 11-hydroxylase causes accumulation of desoxycorticosterone (DOC), a potent mineralocorticoid, as well as of 11-deoxycortisol. The 17-alpha hydroxylase defect also results in hypertension. However, the hypertension in these forms of adrenogenital syndrome is inconsistent, and it is not certain whether this occurs during the neonatal period (Avery, 1975; Eberlein and Bongiovanni, 1956). Other rare causes of hypertension in the neonate include pheochromocytoma, Cushing's disease, primary hyperaldosteronism, and neuroblastoma.

Abnormal Micturition

The presence of oliguria, anuria, or a poor urinary stream in the neonate may be an indication of a urologic emergency. Micturition will have occurred in two thirds of all neonates within 12 hours of birth and in at least 90 per cent of newborns during the first 24 hours (Table 56–4) (Sherry and Kramer, 1955). Failure of micturition to occur during the first 24 hours should arouse concern. Approximately 10 ml of urine is excreted during the first day, with the urine volume increasing to about 200 ml by the twelfth day (Sherry and Kramer, 1955).

Delayed micturition in a neonate with a palpably distended bladder should alert one to the possible presence of lower urinary tract obstruction, such as posterior urethral valves. A weak urinary stream, with or without a distended bladder, was the presenting sign or symptom in 15 per cent of the neonates requiring major urologic surgery in the author's experience (Woodard and Parrott, 1976). One must also remember that *neuropathic bladders* may be distended in the neonatal period and that when the neurologic defect is subtle, the palpable bladder may be the initial sign of this defect.

TABLE 56–4. Time of Passage of Urine
in 500 Neonates

Time (Hours)	Per Cent
0–12	67.6
12–24	92.4
24–48	99.4
over 48	0.6

The infant with anuria and Potter's facies is likely to have renal agenesis, while oliguria and hematuria may signal a vascular catastrophe such as renal vein thrombosis, renal artery thrombosis, or renal cortical necrosis.

However, there are less ominous reasons for delayed voiding and bladder distention, such as *magnesium sulfate* administered to the mother for toxemia during delivery. This may produce neuromuscular blockade in the infant with generalized hypotonia and may result in severe, though transient, bladder atony.

Scrotal Mass

Any firm enlargement of the testis in the neonate must be considered a possible torsion of the spermatic cord until proved otherwise. Although fewer than 75 cases have been found in the literature (Treadwell et al., 1976), such torsion undoubtedly occurs with a much greater frequency. Unlike the older children, in whom torsion of the cord occurs intravaginally in a "bell clapper" situation, prenatal and neonatal torsion almost always occurs extravaginally, occasionally even intra-abdominally (Campbell and Schneider, 1976; Heydenrych, 1974; Watson, 1974).

In addition to torsion of the spermatic cord, the differential diagnosis of a testicular or scrotal mass in the older child includes epididymitis, incarcerated inguinal hernia, torsion of the appendix testis or epididymis, orchitis, and testicular tumor. These various conditions may also occur in the neonate, although they are considerably less common at this age (Gierup et al., 1975; Qvist, 1955). However, hemorrhage into the testicle resulting from birth trauma might be found in the neonate. Further, testicular tumors also occur in the neonate. In fact, approximately one fourth of all pediatric testicular teratomas occur at or shortly after birth (Giebink and Ruymann, 1974). There have been several instances of acute nonspecific epididymitis reported in neonates as well as reports of incarcerated inguinal hernia. (Gierup et al., 1975; Qvist, 1955).

Spermatic cord torsion in the neonate may occur in an intra-abdominal testis and present as an abdominal mass or hemoperitoneum (Campbell and Schneider, 1976; Heydenrych, 1974).

The management of scrotal masses in the neonate, barring some major mitigating circumstance, is immediate surgical exploration.

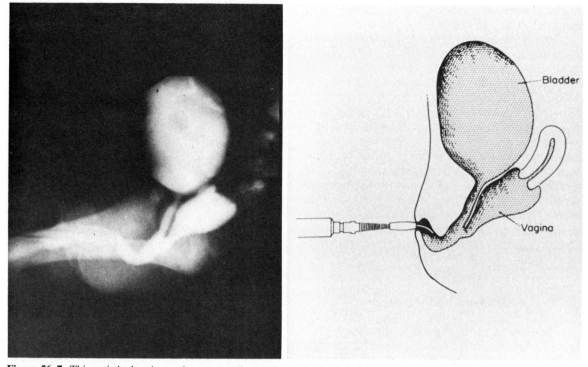

Figure 56–7. This artist's drawing and corresponding radiograph of a female neonate with congenital adrenal hyperplasia illustrate the simple radiographic technique for examining infants with urogenital sinus and cloacal anomalies.

Ambiguous Genitalia

The embryology, pathophysiology, and management of abnormalities of the genitalia are dealt with in other sections of this text. However, infants born with ambiguous genitalia constitute at least a "social emergency" and require urgent evaluation.

The most common cause of sexual ambiguity is congenital adrenal hyperplasia. If unrecognized, the salt-losing variety of this disorder carries a high mortality rate. Therefore, such infants should first be evaluated for congenital adrenal hyperplasia and monitored with appropriate blood and urine studies. Second, the actual sex of the infant and plan of management must be determined as soon as reasonably possible in order to minimize trauma to the parents and problems in dealing with relatives and with the community. A diagnosis should not be forthcoming and corrective surgery should not be performed until the evaluation is completed. The diagnostic evaluation should include serum electrolyte determinations, blood and urine steroid studies, x-ray examination of the urogenital sinus (Fig. 56–7), cystoscopy and vaginoscopy, x-ray studies to determine bone age, buccal mucosal smear for Barr body and Y

body studies, and karyotype. Diagnostic laparotomy with gonadal biopsies is also indicated in some instances. Data obtained from any or all of these studies plus evaluation of the potential of the external organs allow for a diagnosis and a proposed therapeutic plan.

It is increasingly evident that individuals considered at birth to have hypospadias should be more thoroughly evaluated in order to avoid erroneous assignment or delay complications (Aarskog, 1971).

Ascites

Ascites is the abnormal accumulation of fluid within the peritoneal cavity. An infant with ascites has a bulging abdomen in which radiographic examination demonstrates gas-filled loops of bowel floating in a densely opaque background (Fig. 56–8). This disorder is relatively rare in neonates, in whom the various forms include chylous ascites, ascites caused by syphilis, hepatobiliary obstruction with bile ascites, ascites due to meconium peritonitis, and urinary ascites. Ascites might also occur with the nephrotic syndrome, when the fluid is an exudate having a protein content usually less than 500 mg/dl (Spitzer et al., 1973).

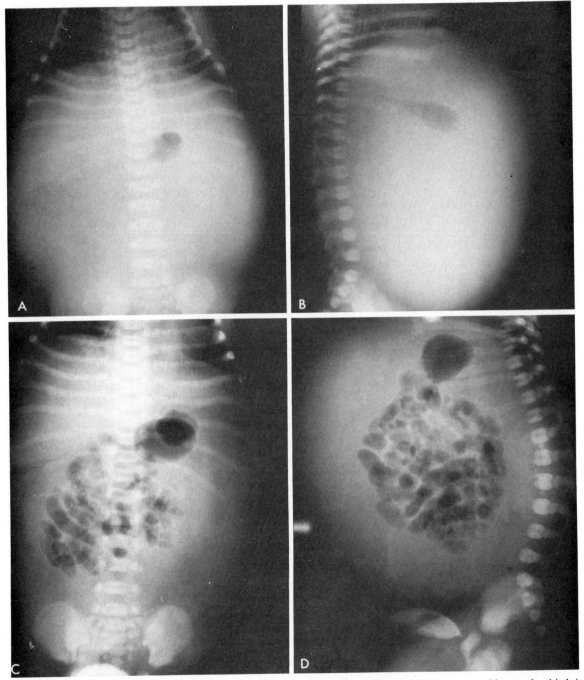

Figure 56–8. Plain films (*A* and *B*) made at birth and intravenous pyelograms (*C* and *D*) made several hours after birth in a female infant born with severe ascites. These films show the typical appearance of ascites with intestines "floating" toward the center of the abdomen. This child did not have an obstructive uropathy, and her ascites subsided.

Urine is the fluid most commonly found in neonatal ascites (Moncada et al., 1973), and obstructive uropathy is the usual underlying cause (Garrett and Franken, 1969; Krane and Retik, 1974; Mann et al., 1974; Moncada et al., 1973; Parker, 1974; Scott, 1976; Williams and Eckstein, 1965). This is a lethal condition with a mortality rate of approximately 45 per cent. It occurs seven times more often in male infants, with the common primary obstructive lesion being posterior urethral valves. The second most common cause of urinary ascites is hydronephrosis from congenital ureteropelvic junction obstruction. In lesser numbers, ascites has been reported to occur as a result of urethral stricture, urethral atresia, bladder neck obstruction, ectopic ureterocele, neurogenic bladder, hydrocolpos, and sacrococcygeal teratoma.

The urine may enter the peritoneal cavity either by transudation through the retroperitoneum or by direct communication between the retroperitoneum and the peritoneal cavity. Although transudation through the intact urinary tract was originally thought to be responsible for most cases of ascites, later reports emphasized rupture of the urinary tract directly into the peritoneal cavity as the cause. This perhaps occurs most frequently from the calyceal fornices, producing perirenal and eventually peritoneal urinary collection. The site of rupture has been found in many instances.

The true incidence of urinary ascites in association with posterior urethral valves is rather difficult to determine, since Garrett and Franken (1969) reported ascites in one third of their infants with valves while Williams and Eckstein (1965) found only one example among 104 patients.

After ascites is suspected from the physical examination and after radiographic studies have distinguished it from intestinal obstruction, a paracentesis will yield a urine-colored fluid that may have an elevated creatinine and urea content. However, since absorption of urine from the peritoneal cavity is rapid, equilibration of the creatinine and urea contents of the peritoneal fluid and the plasma occurs promptly. This raises the blood urea and creatinine content to a level disproportionate to the level of renal function. It may also reduce the urea content in the ascitic fluid to a level lower than expected.

Because of the high reported mortality rate, it is essential that urinary ascites be detected promptly, evaluated properly, and treated expeditiously. In addition to those studies already listed, a voiding cystourethrogram and an intravenous pyelogram are essential to the evaluation.

Treatment begins with immediate correction of fluid and electrolyte imbalance, keeping the patient under close observation for respiratory distress. Paracentesis may be necessary to combat respiratory embarrassment. Prompt and appropriate urinary drainage is then indicated. Although prompt upper urinary tract diversion or drainage has improved the previously poor record of survival, some have suggested that the surgical approach be the simplest appropriate to the problem and that lower urinary tract drainage via bladder catheter may be satisfactory in some instances. However, when suprapubic cystostomy alone was used as the drainage procedure, there was a two-thirds mortality rate, suggesting that more proximal drainage has contributed to the improved survival (Garrett and Franken, 1969; Krane and Retik, 1974; Mann et al., 1974; Moncada et al., 1973; Parker, 1974; Scott, 1976; Weller and Miller, 1973; Williams and Eckstein, 1965).

After suitable correction of fluid and electrolyte problems and satisfactory drainage of the urinary tract, the infant is allowed to recover and stabilize before definitive treatment of the primary obstructive disorder is begun.

Other Signs and Symptoms of Genitourinary Emergencies

Individuals born with *cloacal exstrophy,* the most extreme variation of the exstrophy-epispadias complex, present an early problem in management. They are apt to have multiple system involvement in addition to a markedly shortened intestinal tract, resulting in poor potential for survival. In addition, there is reason to think that all such infants should be assigned as female at the outset (Marshall and Muecke, 1962; Tank and Lindenauer, 1970).

Infants born with *classic exstrophy* of the bladder, however, are usually not acutely ill and present no immediate problem. If functional closure is anticipated, however, Ansell (1971) suggests that these babies might best be operated upon during the first or second day of life when the bony pelvis can be brought together anteriorly without iliac osteotomy. Therefore, under these circumstances the baby with classic bladder exstrophy would require immediate urologic attention.

Congenital *absence of the abdominal musculature* is readily apparent in the newborn. It signals the typical prune-belly uropathy (see Fig. 56–2). Such infants require immediate evaluation and close monitoring. While some will have pulmonary hypoplasia and/or extreme degrees of renal dysplasia that makes survival impossible, others will have no problems whatsoever. Between these two extremes are the majority of infants, who may have some pulmonary difficulties resulting from either pneumomediastinum or pneumothorax and severe urinary stasis, making them vulnerable to bacteriuria with the possibility of increasing azotemia. Immediate drainage or reconstructive procedures in these instances may greatly alter the eventual prognosis (Williams and Parker, 1974; Woodard, 1978).

It is common knowledge that a male infant with *imperforate anus* is likely to have a fistula connecting the distal gastrointestinal tract with the prostatic urethra or bladder and that a female infant with imperforate anus is likely to have a rectovaginal fistula. It is becoming increasingly apparent, however, that infants with imperforate anus are likely to have other major internal genitourinary abnormalities (Belman and King, 1972; Hall et al., 1970; Parrott and Woodard, unpublished data; Puckner et al., 1975; Singh et al., 1974; Williams, 1974). At our institution, among the last 40 neonates evaluated because of imperforate anus there were 21 urogenital abnormalities exclusive of rectourinary fistulae. These included ten instances of vesicoureteral reflux and/or hydronephrosis and three of fused or ectopic kidneys (Parrott and Woodard, unpublished data).

Other studies indicate that between 25 and 50 per cent of all infants with imperforate anus will have associated urogenital abnormalities other than fistulae. Renal agenesis is frequently reported. It is obvious that all patients with imperforate anus should have a voiding cystourethrogram and an excretory urogram as a part of their initial evaluation.

Persistent cloaca warrants special consideration because of the extent and severity of both the primary and the associated abnormalities. The "cloacogram," in addition to endoscopic examination, is helpful in delineating the abnormal anatomy. A much higher incidence of genital and urinary abnormalities is reported in patients with persistent cloaca than in those with the other forms of imperforate anus (Parrott and Woodard, unpublished data). Such infants are prone to having hydrometrocolpos (Cheney et al., 1974; Raffensperger and Ramenofsky, 1973), the treatment of which will be discussed later in this chapter. Various degrees of vaginal and uterine duplication are also common.

SPECIFIC DISORDERS REQUIRING PROMPT UROLOGIC MANAGEMENT

Hydronephrosis

The evaluation and management of hydronephrosis are dealt with extensively elsewhere in this text. It is, nonetheless, the most common cause of a neonatal abdominal mass and one of the most common abnormalities in the neonate requiring surgical correction. Therefore, it will be discussed at some length in this section.

Neonatal hydronephrosis usually presents as a palpable abdominal mass for which the differential diagnosis has already been discussed. The most common causative lesion is obstruction at the ureteropelvic junction (commonly referred to as congenital hydronephrosis). It is perhaps slightly more common in male infants, occurring bilaterally in 20 to 30 per cent of newborns with the condition. When hydronephrosis occurs bilaterally, one must take care to ensure that bladder outlet obstruction does not exist. Primary obstruction at the ureterovesical junction (see Fig. 56–9) is less likely to be recognized in the neonate. Polycystic kidneys and renal tumors are the lesions most commonly confused with hydronephrosis.

Diagnosis. Transillumination is a simple and often helpful means of making a diagnosis. Ultrasonography has also proved helpful. The excretory urogram, however, is the most useful diagnostic study, especially in conjunction with a large dose of contrast material and delayed films. Retrograde studies are often necessary to confirm the normality of the ureter below the level of apparent obstruction. Voiding cystourethrography should be done to evaluate the lower urinary tract and is very important in ruling out associated reflux.

Treatment. Once the evaluation is complete, treatment should be diligently directed toward preservation of renal substance. Pyeloplasty and other reconstructive procedures in the newborn can be very successful, and the kidney should be preserved in the presence of even a thin rim of recognizable renal parenchyma (Fig. 56–9).

It has been shown that even severe degrees of hydronephrosis and hydroureter in the neonate can result from sepsis and that complete

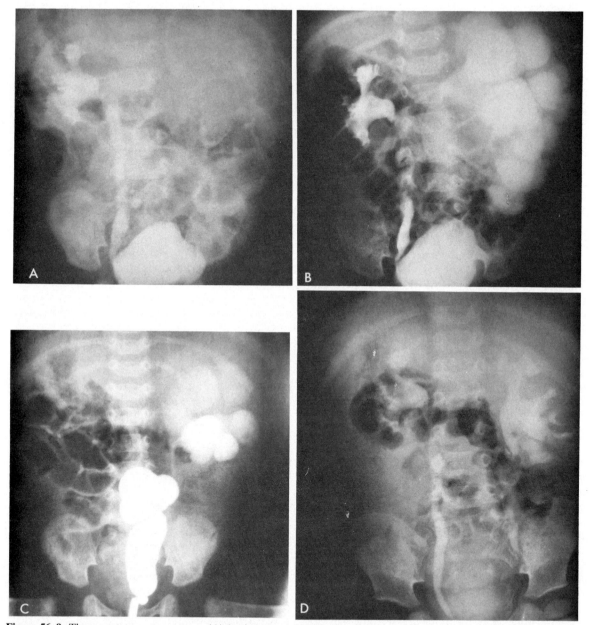

Figure 56–9. These excretory urograms at *(A)* 1 minute and *(B)* 2 hours in an infant with a left flank mass show massive left hydronephrosis with extremely thin renal parenchyma. Retrograde pyelogram *(C)* localizes the obstruction at the ureterovesical junction. An intravenous pyelogram *(D)* 2 years after tailoring and reimplanting the left ureter demonstrates the remarkable recovery potential of the neonatal obstructed kidney.

reversal may occur with proper antibiotic treatment (Alton, 1977; Lebowitz and Griscom, 1977; Uson et al., 1968). This possibility must be borne in mind when evaluating an infant with hydronephrosis and urinary sepsis (Pais and Retik, 1975).

Multicystic Kidney

Multicystic kidney is one of the two most common causes of neonatal abdominal masses. The importance of this disorder perhaps lies in its frequency (Longino and Martin, 1958; Parrott and Woodard, 1976; Raffensperger and Abousleiman, 1968; Wedge et al., 1971). It represents an extreme form of dysplasia that is associated with atresia of the ureter and is classified as Potter Type II (Potter, 1972). On histologic examination there is renal dysplasia with reduction in the number of nephrons and no normal renal parenchyma. In most instances multicystic kidney is a unilateral phenomenon, although bilateral cases have been reported in association with Potter's facies (Williams, 1974). The cysts are relatively few in number, large and heterogeneous in size, and loosely bound together.

Diagnosis. The patient usually presents with a palpable mass that is often noted to be lobulated and is functionless on excretory urography. Retrograde studies, when done, demonstrate ureteral atresia. Although ultrasonography is quite useful in making this diagnosis (Sanders, 1975), excretory urography is important to ensure normality of the contralateral kidney.

Treatment. Most multicystic kidneys are operated upon and removed during the neonatal period, although this does not appear to be an urgent matter. Operation is perhaps more important diagnostically than therapeutically, since late complications from this lesion are poorly documented.

Renal Vein Thrombosis

Although uncommon, renal vein thrombosis is the cause of approximately 20 per cent of the cases of gross hematuria occurring in the first month of life and also is a prominent cause of renal enlargement (Emanuel and Aronson, 1974; Longino and Martin, 1958; Parrott and Woodard, 1976; Raffensperger and Abousleiman, 1968; Wedge et al., 1971). It is considered

to carry a grave prognosis. Of renal vein thromboses in the pediatric age group, approximately 40 per cent have occurred during the first 2 weeks of life, with the majority occurring in the first 2 months. The arterial pressure in the neonate is uniformly low and is reflected in low venous pressure. The nature of renal circulation, with a double capillary network, results in considerable slowing of the blood stream in the renal vein. This sluggish renal perfusion in the normally polycythemic neonate, when combined with trauma, dehydration, infection, vascular endothelial damage, or the dehydrating effects of a diabetic mother, creates an ideal situation for renal vein thrombosis to occur at this stage of the baby's existence. (Belman et al., 1970; McFarland, 1965; Verhagen et al., 1965).

Primary renal vein thrombosis occurs suddenly in a previously healthy neonate, whereas *secondary renal vein thrombosis* results from a known cause, such as diarrhea with dehydration. The latter disorder carries a poorer prognosis (McFarland, 1965). The site of origin of the thrombotic process is variable. However, in unilateral renal vein thrombosis the thrombus usually originates peripherally in the small intrarenal branches of the renal vein. In bilateral renal vein thrombosis the thrombus is primarily in the vena cava and the main renal veins. It is unlikely that unilateral renal vein thrombosis will ever progress to become bilateral (Belman et al., 1970; Lowry et al., 1970; McFarland, 1965; Seeler et al., 1970; Thompson et al., 1974; Verhagen et al., 1965).

The clinical features of renal vein thrombosis are listed in Table 56–5. The typical clinical picture is that of a firm enlarging kidney accompanied by hematuria and proteinuria in a sick infant, although occasionally the constitutional disturbance is mild. Gross *hematuria* is a consistent finding and is due to hemorrhagic renal infarction. *Anemia* may occur secondary to hemolysis, hematuria, or the trapping of erythrocytes in the thrombotic process, and blood transfusion is occasionally necessary. Also,

TABLE 56–5. CLINICAL FEATURES OF RENAL VEIN THROMBOSIS

Renal enlargement
Hematuria
Thrombocytopenia
Anemia
Azotemia
Nonfunction on intravenous pyelogram
Proteinuria
"Shock-sepsis"

thrombocytopenia secondary to trapping of platelets within the thrombotic process is a remarkably consistent finding. However, it has generally not resulted in bleeding problems from other sites or during operation. Thrombocytopenia is such a consistent feature of this disorder that when this finding is absent, one suspects the renal vein thrombosis to have occurred some time earlier and to be in the resolving stage. The *renal enlargement* is readily apparent, smooth, and firm. Initially the mass enlarges but can be felt to diminish as the process resolves. Although *proteinuria* occurs in neonatal renal vein thrombosis, it is not as prominent a feature as it is in the adult type of thrombosis, in which it may be massive. *Shock* or sepsis is variable and may be due in part to the predisposing factors as well as to the infarction itself. The septic picture can be confusing until the renal mass is detected. *Azotemia* is usually present, even in unilateral thromboses (Belman et al., 1970; McFarland, 1965).

Diagnosis. Included in the diagnostic evaluation are blood studies appropriate for detecting and monitoring the anemia, thrombocytopenia, and azotemia. Excretory urography demonstrates "nonfunction" of the involved kidney(s). Retrograde pyelograms are rarely indicated unless obstructive uropathy must be ruled out. Inferior venacavography is an essential part of the evaluation of suspected bilateral renal vein thrombosis and may be the best method of distinguishing it from early renal cortical necrosis. Blood and urine cultures should be obtained. Renal arteriography is not a definitive study in this disorder and usually merely confirms the renal enlargement by demonstrating widening of the intrarenal vessels. Since excretory urograms in the neonate are often difficult to evaluate, radionuclide scan may be helpful in confirming "nonfunction" initially and in following recovery subsequently. If the diagnosis is still in doubt, surgical exploration with renal biopsy is occasionally necessary (Belman et al., 1970).

Treatment. The treatment of renal vein thrombosis should begin with hydration and correction of any electrolyte imbalance. Antibiotics are also recommended. Beyond that, treatment becomes somewhat controversial. After Campbell and Matthews (1942) reported two successful results of unilateral renal vein thrombosis treated by nephrectomy, this became the standard approach. It is now evident that the reasons for immediate nephrectomy are tenuous and that spontaneous recovery from

renal vein thrombosis in the neonatal kidney is possible and does occur. Surgical thrombectomy may possibly enhance that recovery potential (Thompson et al., 1974). The fate of the involved kidney may depend upon the degree and the speed of venous occlusion. The chief indication for early nephrectomy in the treatment of unilateral renal vein thrombosis is infection.

Although heparin is recommended by some, there are no controlled studies confirming its usefulness. Heparin was advocated because of its activity against thrombin formation and platelet aggregation and its success in treating disseminated intravascular clotting. When heparin is used, the dose schedule starts with 1 mg/kg every 4 hours to keep the clotting time in the range of 20 to 30 minutes. Treatment with heparin should last for 1 to 2 weeks (Belman et al., 1970; Seeler et al., 1970).

The initial medical management for bilateral renal vein thrombosis is the same as for unilateral thrombosis. However, most of the few reported survivals have resulted from an aggressive surgical approach. Once venacavography has demonstrated thrombosis of the vena cava and main renal veins (Fig. 56–10), consideration must be given to an early surgical thrombectomy. At operation, both kidneys should be preserved, whether or not good "back bleeding" is achieved after extraction of thrombi. Vigorous postoperative care, which may include peritoneal dialysis is required.

Following renal vein thrombosis, the involved kidney may recover completely or may show evidence of damage. The result may be nonfunction with complete fibrosis, partial fibrosis with diminished function, renal hypertension, nephrotic syndrome, or chronic renal infection. Chronic renal tubular dysfunction may occur (Stark and Geiger, 1973). If sufficiently severe, these late complications may necessitate delayed nephrectomy.

Massive Adrenal Hemorrhage

The occurrence of small hemorrhages into the adrenal gland of the neonate is surprisingly frequent, being found in between 1 and 2 per cent of those undergoing autopsy examination (Black and Williams, 1973; DeSa and Nicholls, 1972). Massive adrenal hemorrhage, however, is an entirely different entity. It is an uncommon occurrence that carries a high mortality rate. Before 1965 only three cases were reported in which the diagnosis was made prior to death

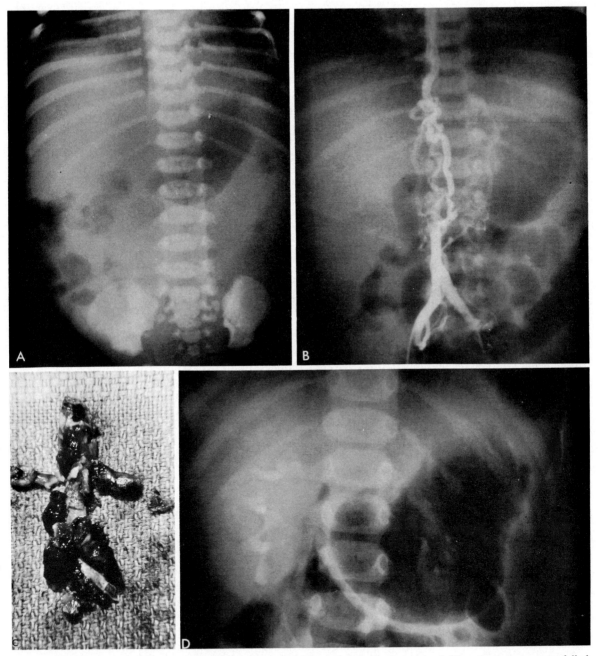

Figure 56–10. This 1-day-old infant had gross hematuria and bilateral abdominal masses. *A*, The excretory urogram failed to show any excretion at 4 hours. *B*, An inferior venacavogram demonstrated caval obstruction at the level of the renal veins with collateral venous return via the azygous system. *C*, At operation the thrombus was extracted from the cava and both renal veins, with subsequent renal vein "back bleeding." Three years later the child was normotensive with normal blood urea nitrogen and creatinine values. *D*, An intravenous pyelogram shows bilateral renal function but a small left kidney.

(Sober and Hirsch, 1965). Until 1970 only 13 cases had been accurately diagnosed and successfully treated during the neonatal period (Eklof et al., 1975). Improved neonatal care has, it appears, led to the discovery of an increasing number of adrenal hematomas during the first week of life (Eklof et al., 1975; Glenn, 1962). Yet, uniform diagnostic and therapeutic guidelines are lacking, and indications for conservative versus surgical management are vague.

The traumatic events of childbirth—prolonged labor, difficult or traumatic delivery, and possible resuscitative efforts—appear to be the leading etiologic factors. These events tend to produce prolonged abdominal compression that renders the neonate susceptible to massive adrenal hemorrhage, especially when coupled with, or in any combination with, hypoprothrombinemia, increased vascular fragility, and disseminated thromboembolic lesions with possible thrombocytopenia.

Diagnosis. The diagnosis of massive adrenal hemorrhage may be difficult. It must be distinguished from renal vein thrombosis, hydronephrosis in the upper pole of a duplicated collecting system, and other causes of renal or adrenal masses. Adrenal hemorrhage might be particularly difficult to distinguish preoperatively from hemorrhage within a neuroblastoma.

The clinical features of massive adrenal hemorrhage include the presence of a mass in one or both flanks; signs of blood loss, such as anemia, paleness, shock, or lethargy; jaundice; and urinary infection or sepsis. Azotemia may be present. Whereas gross hematuria usually occurs with renal vein thrombosis, microscopic hematuria is likely in adrenal hemorrhage.

Opacification is usually present on the excretory urogram (Fig. 56–11), although the mass displaces the pyelogram downward with outward rotation. Calcifications occur late in the course, or following recovery, and may persist indefinitely (Eklof et al., 1975). The diagnostic study of most importance is probably the excretory urogram. During the total body opacification stage, the area of hemorrhage appears lucent. Retrograde pyelograms might be indicated in cases in which renal function is severely impaired. Arteriography (Fig. 56–11) should outline the lesion nicely but is not indicated routinely. Ultrasonography is highly important in making the diagnosis and in following resolution of the hematoma.

Treatment. Because of the high mortality rate of massive adrenal hemorrhage, one must be most thoughtful and deliberate in planning the management of such an infant. Some physicians advocate conservative management with careful monitoring and replacement of fluids, electrolytes, and steroids as indicated. Blood transfusion may play an important part in such management, as may antibiotics (Black and Williams, 1973). However, the majority of reported survivors appear to have been treated surgically (Eklof et al., 1975; Glenn, 1962; Gross et al., 1967). The likelihood is considerable that massive adrenal hemorrhage will produce rupture of the adrenal gland with massive bleeding into the retroperitoneal or peritoneal cavity, resulting in vascular collapse and shock. Therefore, the case for aggressive surgical management appears to be a strong one. The difficulty in distinguishing adrenal hemorrhage from hemorrhage into an adrenal neuroblastoma may also be a strong indication for surgical intervention (Sober and Hirsch, 1965). The operation for massive adrenal hemorrhage in the neonate is directed toward evacuation of the hematoma with ligation of the vessels. Adrenalectomy may be necessary, and nephrectomy has occasionally resulted. However, one should strive to preserve renal tissue as well as adrenal tissue when feasible (Gross et al., 1967).

Although the neonatal adrenal gland produces minimal amounts of steroids during the first week of life, most urologists advocate the use of steroids in managing this condition, particularly if the hemorrhage is bilateral or if shock develops in infants with unilateral disease. Steroids should also be given if the patient is subjected to an anesthetic or operative procedure.

Renal Tumors

The most common renal tumor in childhood is nephroblastoma (Wilms' tumor) (see also Chapter 57). Although Wilms' tumors have been reported to occur in the fetus and neonate (Hartenstein, 1949), it is now apparent that most solid renal tumors in the neonate are not true Wilms' tumors. Rather, they have different morphologic and clinical characteristics (Fig. 56–12) (Richmond and Dougall, 1970; Waisman and Cooper, 1970; Wigger, 1969). It is important that these predominantly mesenchymal tumors be recognized as an entity separate from Wilms' tumor in order to avoid the hazards of overtreatment. Although the benign nature of this tumor is now widely known, a single designation has not been generally accepted. It is

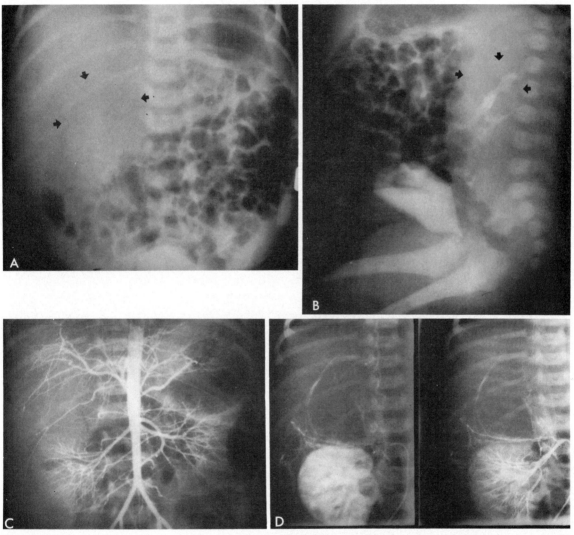

Figure 56–11. *A* and *B,* Excretory urograms in an infant with massive adrenal hemorrhage, showing a mass above the right kidney. Aortogram *(C)* and selective renal arteriograms *(D)* confirm that the mass is of adrenal origin with an avascular center.

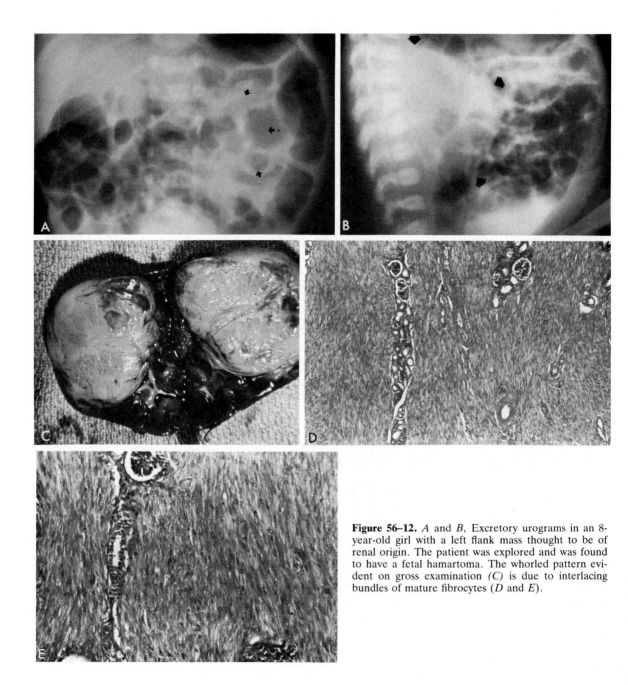

Figure 56–12. *A* and *B,* Excretory urograms in an 8-year-old girl with a left flank mass thought to be of renal origin. The patient was explored and was found to have a fetal hamartoma. The whorled pattern evident on gross examination *(C)* is due to interlacing bundles of mature fibrocytes *(D* and *E).*

best known as either fetal hamartoma or mesoblastic nephroma.

Diagnosis. The presentation is usually that of an incidentally discovered mass, with pyelographic features of a renal mass lesion. Typically, the cut surface of the tumor has a whorled pattern, with interlacing bundles of mature fibrocytes seen microscopically.

Treatment. The patients are generally cured by surgical removal of the tumor; metastases are not reported. Further treatment with irradiation and/or chemotherapy is contraindicated, since the few reported fatalities have resulted from the treatment rather than from the disease (Richmond and Dougall, 1970; Waisman and Cooper, 1970; Wigger, 1969).

Renal Cortical Necrosis

Symmetric renal cortical necrosis may occur early in the neonatal period as the result of hypoxia, dehydration, sepsis, or blood loss or may be caused by birth trauma or intrauterine distress of sufficient severity and duration to lead to renal ischemia (Reisman and Pathole, 1966). The clinical features include pallor, flaccidity, and cyanosis. In the acute stage the kidneys are enlarged and thrombocytopenia, anemia, azotemia, and hematuria may be present. Accordingly, renal cortical necrosis may be easily confused with bilateral renal vein thrombosis.

Diagnosis. Although renal biopsy may be necessary to finally confirm the diagnosis of renal cortical necrosis, inferior venacavography is useful in distinguishing it from bilateral renal vein thrombosis.

Treatment. Renal cortical necrosis generally is fatal. The treatment is supportive and includes management for renal failure (Bernstein and Meyer, 1961; Reisman and Pathole, 1966).

Renal Artery Thrombosis

Until recently there were few reports of renal artery thrombosis (Fig. 56–13) in newborns, and most of those were reports based on autopsy statistics (Waisman and Cooper, 1970). Congenital heart disease and sepsis were considered possible etiologic factors, although it was felt that thrombosis of the ductus arteriosus was the source of embolism in most cases. There has been an increase in the number of reported cases of renal artery thrombosis in neonates (Bauer et al., 1975; Ford et al., 1974; Plummer et al., 1975). The increase is apparently due to the growing use of umbilical artery catheterization for diagnostic and therapeutic management in neonates. This is a procedure with specific indications for use, and renal artery thrombosis is now a well-documented complication. In fact, in a report of ten young infants with hypertension, five had renal artery thrombosis and two had thrombosis of the abdominal aorta. Eight of these ten infants had histories of umbilical artery catheterization (Plummer et al., 1975).

The clinical features of renal artery thrombosis in the neonate include hematuria, proteinuria, azotemia, hypertension frequently leading to congestive heart failure, and nonopacification of the involved kidney on excretory urography (Table 56–6). Although there are only a few reported survivors, most of those have been treated by removal of the involved kidney (Woodard et al., 1967). It is likely that with an increased awareness of this condition in the neonate and an earlier diagnosis, more of these infants will be saved.

Because of the importance of making an accurate diagnosis promptly, one should consider renal artery thrombosis in any infant having unexplained hematuria, hypertension, or congestive heart failure. With the increased use of umbilical artery catheterization this entity is destined for an increased incidence.

Renal Agenesis

Unilateral renal agenesis occurs approximately once per 1000 births. It is more common in boys, occurs more often on the left side, and is not likely to be noted clinically in the neonate (Kissane, 1977). Bilateral renal agenesis occurs approximately one third as often and is the most ominous urologic malformation. It is readily identified at birth by the features termed Potter's facies (see Fig. 56–1), which include wide-set eyes, "parrot beak" nose, receding chin, and

TABLE 56–6. CLINICAL FEATURES OF RENAL ARTERY THROMBOSIS

Hematuria
Proteinuria
Azotemia
Hypertension
Congestive heart failure
Nonfunction on intravenous pyelogram

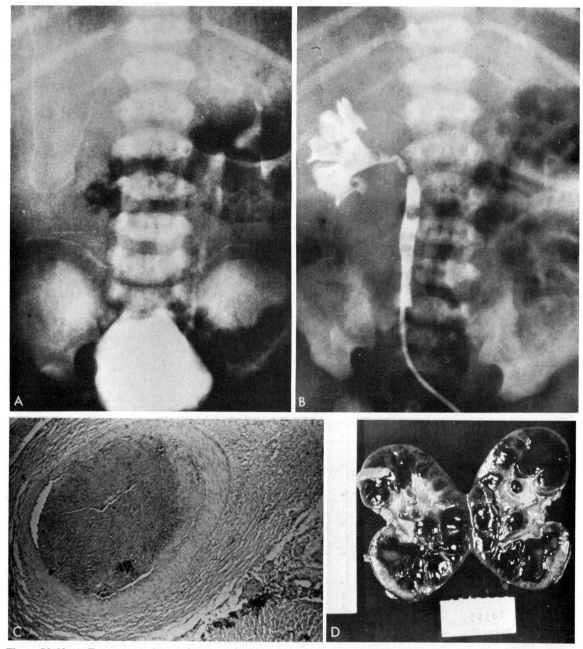

Figure 56–13. *A,* Excretory pyelogram in a 1-week-old boy with hematuria and hypertension showing no contrast excretion from the right kidney. *B,* On retrograde study the kidney is not obstructed. *C,* Operation revealed an organizing thrombus completely occluding the main renal artery, and there was diffuse hemorrhagic medullary necrosis of the kidney *(D)*. The infant was cured by nephrectomy. (From Woodard, J. R., Patterson, J. H., and Brinsfield, D.: Am. J. Dis. Child., *114*:191, 1967.)

large, low-set, flabby ears. Severe oligohydramnios is the rule and results in amnion nodosum and pulmonary hypoplasia. Paradoxically, death is rarely due to uremia but rather to the result of pulmonary hypoplasia. Other major malformations may coexist, and heroic therapeutic measures are inappropriate (Cockburn and Drillien, 1974; Potter, 1946).

Hydrometrocolpos

Although rare, hydrometrocolpos is an important abdominal mass occurring in the neonate. It is produced by fluid distention of the vagina and uterus. The circumstances necessary for its development are vaginal obstruction and excessive secretion of the cervical glands in response to circulating maternal estrogen. It is less common than the hematocolpos that occurs at menarche. Although imperforate hymen can produce the vaginal obstruction, vaginal atresia is more common and has been shown to be inherited as a simple autosomal recessive disorder (McKusick et al., 1964).

Diagnosis. Hydrometrocolpos produces a mass that is large, firm, and midline in position, and arises from the pelvis (see Fig. 56–14). On rectal examination or on plain lateral radiograph of the abdomen it is easily seen to be anterior to the rectum and posterior to the bladder. Since it commonly produces ureteral obstruction with hydronephrosis, an excretory urogram is an essential part of the evaluation. Intestinal or vascular obstruction might also result from the mass. When hydrometrocolpos is secondary to imperforate hymen, the diagnosis is easily made from external examination. However, in the more frequently encountered vaginal atresia, a vaginal examination might be confusing. As is so often true, an accurate diagnosis depends upon an awareness of the condition by the examiner. In one series of 49 cases, only half were diagnosed correctly, a third were operated upon with an inadequate diagnosis, and half of those were subjected to hysterectomy (Cook and Marshall, 1964).

The knowledge that hydrometrocolpos is likely to occur in female infants with imperforate anus or cloacal anomalies is essential, since rectal palpation is not possible in these instances and the external genitalia may have an ambiguous appearance (see Fig. 56–4) (Parrott and Woodard, 1976).

Treatment. The treatment of hydrometrocolpos should be aggressive (Ramenofsky and Raffensperger, 1971). Whereas imperforate hymen can usually be managed by simple incision, the more common vaginal atresia requires a major surgical correction. The distended uterus is opened through a lower abdominal incision. Incision of the obstructing vaginal septum by a combined vaginal and abdominal approach with indwelling catheter drainage of the uterus has been used in the past, but this form of treatment has been followed by an excessive number of deaths from sepsis and is considered inadequate (Ramenofsky and Raffensperger, 1971). Accordingly, the vaginal pull-through operation (Fig. 56–14) as described by Snyder (1966) is recommended. This procedure adequately separates the genital and urinary tracts.

In general, the obstructive uropathy can be expected to resolve following satisfactory drainage of the uterus. Occasionally, however, surgical intervention will be necessary, either for persistent urinary obstruction or for the occurrence of urinary sepsis.

Ovarian Cysts

In the female infant one must consider ovarian cyst as a possible cause of an abdominal mass (Wedge et al., 1971). Most cysts are follicular in type and are usually quite large. Malignant ovarian tumors during the first year of life, and especially during the neonatal period, are rare. The cause of ovarian cysts in the neonate is not known, but placental and maternal hormones probably play an important role in the etiology (Marshall, 1965). Some physicians have noted that polyhydramnios is present before neonatal ovarian cysts are subsequently discovered, and diabetes in the mother may be an underlying contributing factor (Bowen et al., 1974).

Diagnosis. Clinically, the ovarian cyst usually presents as an abdominal mass in the lower abdomen but occasionally occupies the entire abdomen and resembles ascites. When smaller, it is usually mobile. Radiographically, it is noted to be relatively central in position, with intestinal shadows displaced laterally or circumferentially (see Fig. 56–5). An ovarian cyst must be distinguished from the various other types of abdominal masses.

Sudden and severe complications caused by this cyst are common, so that a delay in diagnosis and treatment is unwarranted and may jeopardize the patient. The major complication is torsion or rupture, producing an acute abdo-

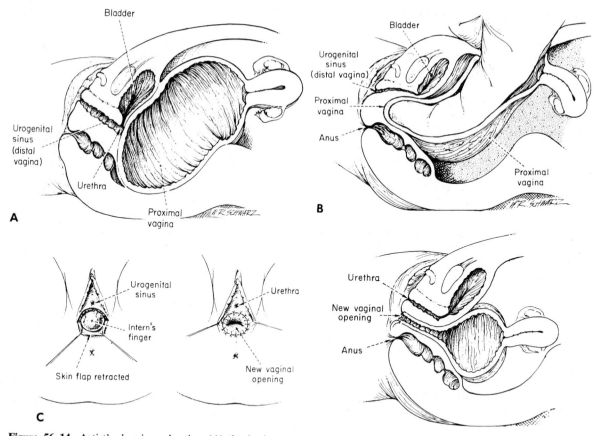

Figure 56–14. Artist's drawings showing *(A)* the basic anatomy of hydrometrocolpos and *(B, C, D)* the pull-through operation. The abdomen is opened through a transverse incision. The anterior vaginal wall is opened, and its contents are evacuated and cultured. With a finger in the vagina *(B)* an incision is made behind the urogenital sinus in the perineum, raising an inverted U flap of skin *(C)*. The incision is deepened to meet the posterior wall of the vagina, which is being pushed down by the finger. When the back wall of the vagina is completely mobilized through the perineum, it is opened and sutured to the perineal skin behind the urogenital sinus *(C and D)*. (From Ramenofsky, M. I., and Raffensperger, J. G.: J. Pediatr. Surg., 6:381, 1971.)

men (Longino and Martin, 1955). Rupture of an ovarian cyst may cause hemoperitoneum.

Treatment. Many times treatment has consisted of removal of the cyst along with the ovary and, in some instances, the fallopian tube. Some cysts are so large that no ovarian tissue is recognizable. In the majority, however, it would appear that a more conservative approach would be possible, such as aspiration of the cysts with resection of the cyst wall and preservation of whatever functional ovarian tissue is present at the base. This would be especially important in bilateral cases (Aamed, 1971).

Torsion of the Spermatic Cord

Torsion of the spermatic cord resulting in testicular infarction can occur at any age and constitutes one of the true urologic emergencies.

Animal studies indicate that complete occlusion to the spermatic circulation results in some damage to the spermatogenic cells after 2 hours, severe damage after 4 hours, and complete loss after 6 hours (Smith, 1955). The Leydig cells are severely damaged after 8 hours and completely lost after 10 hours. Immediate surgical intervention is, therefore, necessary if one is to salvage a functional testis. As already stated, neonatal torsion is typically of the extravaginal type (Frederick et al., 1967).

Some consider neonatal torsion to be related to birth trauma (Lattimer et al., 1962); however, it is also known to occur in utero (Peterson, 1961). Accordingly, some instances of neonatal torsion will result in nonsalvageable testes.

Diagnosis. The physical findings are rather typical, with induration and enlargement of the scrotal contents. Anatomic detail may be obscured, and the testicular mass may be several times normal size with a hard consistency and some overlying ecchymosis. These findings, although suggestive of birth trauma, may reflect failure of the infarction and extravasation to be contained by the tunic. The right and left testes are affected with equal frequency, and a number of bilateral cases have been reported (Atallah et al., 1975; Auldist and Ferguson, 1975; Frederick et al., 1967; Papadatos and Monsouris, 1967).

Treatment. The treatment is immediate surgical intervention, barring some contraindication to operation. Manipulative reduction has no place in the management, and inguinal exploration is preferable to the trans-scrotal route. This is particularly true because incarcerated inguinal hernia is sometimes difficult to distinguish preoperatively. Surgical exploration should not be tantamount to orchiectomy. The treatment of choice should be surgical exploration with detorsion of the spermatic cord and biopsy of the involved testis followed by orchiopexy. Even if the gonad appears nonviable, it may retain some hormonal function. However, if the infant is toxic and the organ is clearly necrotic, orchiectomy should be carried out.

Some question remains regarding management of the contralateral testis in patients with unilateral neonatal torsion. There are now enough instances of bilateral involvement to warrant contralateral orchiopexy, which is the standard procedure in older children with intravaginal torsion.

References

Aamed, S.: Neonatal and childhood ovarian cysts. J. Pediatr. Surg., 6:702, 1971.

Aarskog, D.: Intersex conditions masquerading as simple hypospadias. Birth Defects, 7:122, 1971.

Alton, D. J.: Pelviureteric obstruction in childhood. Radiol. Clin. North Am., 15:61, 1977.

Altshuler, G., Tsang, R. C., and Ermocilla, R.: Single umbilical artery. Am. J. Dis. Child., 129:697, 1975.

Ansell, J. S.: Primary closure of exstrophy in the newborn. Northwest Med., 70:842, 1971.

Atallah, M. W., Ippolito, J. J., and Rubin, B. W.: Intrauterine bilateral torsion of the spermatic cord. J. Urol., 116:128, 1975.

Auldist, A. W., and Ferguson, R. F.: Torsion of the testicle in the newborn. Aust. N.Z. J. Surg., 45:14, 1975.

Avery, G. B.: Endocrine disorders. In Moshang, T., and Bongiovanni, A. M. (Eds.): Neonatology, pp. 945–971. Philadelphia, J. B. Lippincott Co., 1975.

Bauer, S. B., Feldman, S. M., Gellis, S. S., and Retik, A. B.: Neonatal hypertension: A complication of umbilical artery catheterization. N. Engl. J. Med., 293:1032, 1975.

Behrman, R. E.: The higher risk infant. In Behrman, R. E. (Ed.): Neonatology, pp. 1–49. St. Louis, C. V. Mosby Co., 1973.

Belman, A. B., and King, L. R.: Urinary tract abnormalities associated with imperforate anus. J. Urol., 108:823, 1972.

Belman, A. B., Susmano, D. F., Burden, J. J., and Kaplan, G.: Non-operative treatment of unilateral renal vein thrombosis in the newborn. JAMA, 211:1165, 1970.

Bernstein, J., and Meyer, R.: Congenital abnormalities of the urinary system. II. Renal cortical and medullary necrosis. J. Pediatr., 59:657, 1961.

Black, J., and Williams, D. I.: Natural history of adrenal hemorrhage in the newborn. Arch. Dis. Child., 48:183, 1973.

Bowen, R., Dehner, L. P., and Ternberg, J. L.: Bilateral ovarian cysts in the newborn. Am. J. Dis. Child., 128:731, 1974.

Bryan, E. M., and Kohler, H. G.: The missing umbilical artery: II. Pediatric follow-up. Arch. Dis. Child., 50:714, 1975.

Campbell, J. R., and Schneider, C. P.: Intrauterine torsion of an intraabdominal testis. Pediatrics, 57:262, 1976.

Campbell, M. F., and Matthews, W. F.: Renal thrombosis in infancy. J. Pediatr., 20:604, 1942.

Cheney, G. K., Fisher, J. H., O'Hare, K. H., Retik, A. B., and Darling, D. B.: Anomaly of the persistent cloaca in female infants. Am. J. Roentgenol., 120:413, 1974.

Cockburn, F., and Drillien, C. M.: Pharmacology. In Cockburn, F., and Drillien, C. M. (Eds.): Neonatal Medicine, pp. 752–787. Oxford, Blackwell Scientific Publishers, 1974.

Cook, G. T., and Marshall, V. F.: Hydrocolpos causing urinary obstruction. J. Urol., 92:127, 1964.

Cywes, S.: Haemoperitoneum in the newborn. S. Afr. Med. J., 41:1063, 1967.

DeSa, D. J., and Nicholls, S.: Haemorrhagic necrosis of the adrenal gland in perinatal infants: a clinical pathological study. J. Pathol., 106:133, 1972.

Eberlein, W. R., and Bongiovanni, A. M.: Plasma and urinary corticosteroids in hypertensive forms of congenital adrenal hyperplasia. J. Biol. Chem., 223:85, 1956.

Eklof, O., Grotte, G., Garulf, H., Lohr, G., and Ringerts, H.: Perinatal hemorrhagic necrosis of the adrenal gland. Pediatr. Radiol., 4:31, 1975.

Emanuel, B., and Aronson, N.: Neonatal hematuria. Am. J. Dis. Child., 128:204, 1974.

Emmanouilides, G. C., and Rein, B. I.: Abdominal aortography via umbilical artery in newborn infants. Radiology, 82:447, 1964.

Feingold, M., Fine, R. M., and Ingall, D.: Intravenous pyelography in infants with single umbilical artery. N. Engl. J. Med., 270:1178, 1964.

Ford, K. T., Teplick, S. K., and Clark, R. E.: Renal artery embolism causing neonatal hypertension. Radiology, 113:169, 1974.

Frederick, P. L., Dusha, N., and Eralkis, A. J.: Simultaneous bilateral torsion of the testis in a newborn infant. Arch. Surg., 94:299, 1967.

Froehlich, L. A., and Fujikura, T.: Follow-up of infants with single umbilical artery. Pediatrics, 52:6, 1973.

Garrett, R. A., and Franken, E. A., Jr.: Neonatal ascites: perirenal extravasation and bladder outlet obstruction. J. Urol., 102:627, 1969.

Gellis, S. S.: Editorial comment. In Gellis, S. S. (Ed.): Yearbook of Pediatrics, p. 42. Chicago, Yearbook Medical Publishers, Inc., 1975.

Giebink, G. S., and Ruymann, F. B.: Testicular tumors in childhood. Am. J. Dis. Child., 127:433, 1974.

Gierup, J., Hedenberg, C., and Osterman, A.: Acute non-specific epididymitis in boys. Scand. J. Urol. Nephrol., 9:5, 1975.

Glenn, J. F.: Neonatal adrenal hemorrhage. J. Urol., 87:639, 1962.

Griscom, N. T., Colodny, A. H., Rosenberg, H. K., Fliegel, C. P., and Hardy, B. E.: Diagnostic aspects of neonatal ascites: Report of 27 cases. Am. J. Roentgenol., 128:961, 1977.

Gross, M., Kottmeier, P. K., and Waterhouse, J.: Diagnosis and treatment of neonatal hemorrhage. J. Pediatr. Surg., 2:308, 1967.

Gross, R. E.: Arterial embolism and thrombosis in infancy. Am. J. Dis. Child., 70:61, 1945.

Hall, J. W., Tank, E. S., and Lapides, J.: Urogenital anomalies and complications associated with imperforate anus. J. Urol., 103:810, 1970.

Hartenstein, H.: Wilms' tumor in a newborn infant. J. Pediatr., 35:381, 1949.

Heydenrych, J. J.: Haemoperitoneum and associated torsion of the testicle in the newborn. S. Afr. Med. J., 48:2221, 1974.

Hilson, D.: Malformation of ears as a sign of malformation of the genitourinary tract. Br. Med. J. 2:785, 1957.

Keay, A. J., and Morgan, D. M.: Congenital anomalies. In Keay, A. J., and Morgan, D. M. (Eds.): Craig's Care of the Newly Born Infant, pp. 191–262. Edinburgh, Churchill Livingston, 1974.

Kissane, J. M.: Congenital malformations. In Stepinstall, R. H. (Ed.): Pathology of the Kidney, pp. 69–120. Boston, Little, Brown & Co., 1977.

Krane, R. J. and Retik, A. B.: Neonatal perirenal urinary extravasation. J. Urol., 111:96, 1974.

Lattimer, J. K., Uson, A. C., and Melicow, M. M.: Urologic emergencies in newborn infants. Pediatrics, 29:310, 1962.

Lebowitz, R. L., and Griscom, N. T.: Neonatal hydronephrosis: 146 cases. Radiol. Clin. North Am., 15:49, 1977.

Lees, M. H.: Diseases of the cardiovascular system. In Behrman, R. E. (Ed.): Neonatology, pp. 241–344. St. Louis, C. V. Mosby Co., 1973.

Lemtis, H. G., and Klemme, G.: Is there any correlation between aplasia of one umbilical artery and other congenital malformations? In Proceedings of the Second European Congress of Perinatal Medicine, pp. 308–309. Basel, S. Karger, 1971.

Longino, L. A., and Martin, L. W.: Abdominal masses in the newborn infant. Pediatrics, 21:596, 1958.

Longino, L. A., and Martin, L. W.: Torsion of the spermatic cord in the newborn infant. N. Engl. J. Med., 253:695, 1955.

Lowry, M. F., Mann, J. R., Abrams, L. D., and Chance, G. W.: Thrombectomy for renal venous thrombosis in infant of diabetic mother. Br. Med. J., 3:687, 1970.

McFarland, J. B.: Renal venous thrombosis in children. Q. J. Med., 34:269, 1965.

McKusick, V. A., Bauer, R. L., Koop, C. E., and Scott, R. B.: Hydrometrocolpos as a simply inherited malformation. JAMA, 189:813, 1964.

Mann, C. M., Leape, L. L., and Holden, T. M.: Neonatal urinary ascites: a report of two cases of unusual etiology and a review of the literature. J. Urol., 111:124, 1974.

Marshall, J. R.: Ovarian enlargements in the first year of life: a review of 45 cases. Ann. Surg., 161:372, 1965.

Marshall, V. F., and Muecke, E. C.: Variations in exstrophy of the bladder. J. Urol., 88:766, 1962.

Martin, D. J., Gilday, D. L., and Reilly, B. J.: Evaluation of the urinary tract in the neonatal period. Radiol. Clin. North Am., 13:359, 1975.

Martin, D. J., Griscom, N. T., and Newhauser, E. B. D.: A further look at the total body opacification effect. Br. J. Radiol., 45:185, 1972.

Moncada, R., Cooper, R. A., Reynes, C. J., and Greene, R.: Neonatal urine ascites associated with urinary outlets obstruction: another survivor. Br. J. Radiol., 46:1005, 1973.

Moss, A. J., Duffie, E. R., Jr., and Emmanouilides, G.: Blood pressure and vasomotor reflexes in the newborn infant. Pediatrics, 32:175, 1963.

Mullin, E. M., and Paulson, D.: Renal cystic disease. Urology, 8:5, 1976.

Munoz, A. I., Baralt, J. F. P., and Melendez, M. T.: Arterial hypertension in infants with hydronephrosis. Am. J. Dis. Child., 131:38, 1977.

Ornoy, A., Benaday, S., Kohen-Raz, R., and Russell, A.: Association between maternal bleeding during gestation and congenital anomalies in the offspring. Am. J. Obstet. Gynecol., 124:474, 1976.

Pais, V. M., and Retik, A. B.: Reversible hydronephrosis in the neonate with urinary sepsis. N. Engl. J. Med., 192:465, 1975.

Papadatos, C., and Monsouris, C.: Bilateral testicular torsion in the newborn. J. Pediatr., 71:249, 1967.

Parker, R. M.: Neonatal urinary ascites. Urology, 3:589, 1974.

Parrott, T. S., and Woodard, J. R.: Urologic surgery in the neonate. J. Urol., 116:506, 1976.

Parrott, T. S., and Woodard, J. R.: Unpublished data.

Peterson, C. G.: Testicular torsion and infarction in the newborn. J. Urol., 85:65, 1961.

Plummer, L. B., Mendosa, S. A., and Kaplan, G. W.: Hypertension in infancy: The case for aggressive management. J. Urol., 113:555, 1975.

Potter, E. L.: Normal and Abnormal Developments of the Kidney, pp. 1–305. Chicago, Yearbook Medical Publishers, 1972.

Potter, E. L.: Bilateral renal agenesis. J. Pediatr., 29:68, 1946.

Puckner, P. J., Santulli, T. B., and Lattimer, J. K.: Urological problems associated with imperforate anus. Urology, 6:205, 1975.

Qvist, O.: Swelling of the scrotum in infants and children and non-specific epididymitis. Acta Chir. Scand., 110:418, 1955.

Raffensperger, J., and Abousleiman, A.: Abdominal masses in children under one year of age. Surgery, 63:514, 1968.

Raffensperger, J. G., and Ramenofsky, M. L.: The management of a cloaca. J. Pediatr. Surg., 8:647, 1973.

Ramenofsky, M. L., and Raffensperger, J. G.: An abdomino-perineal vaginal pull-through for definitive treatment of hydrometrocolpos. J. Pediatr. Surg., 6:381, 1971.

Ravitch, L., and Schell, N. B.: Rupture of the kidney in the newborn infant. N.Y. State J. Med., 61:2823, 1961.

Reisman, L. E., and Pathole, A.: Bilateral renal cortical necrosis in the newborn. Am. J. Dis. Child., 111:541, 1966.

Richmond, H., and Dougall, A. J.: Neonatal renal tumors. J. Pediatr. Surg., 5:413, 1970.

Rouquette, C., Etienne, C., and Goujard, J.: Bleeding in the first trimester of pregnancy and congenital defects. In Proceedings of the Second European Congress of Perinatal Medicine, pp. 300–301. Basel, S. Karger, 1971.

Sanders, R. C.: The place of diagnostic ultrasound in the examination of kidneys not seen on excretory urography. J. Urol., 114:813, 1975.

Schaffer, A. J., and Avery, M. E.: Introduction. In Schaffer, A. J., and Avery, M. E. (Eds.): Diseases of the Newborn, pp. 1–13. Philadelphia, W. B. Saunders Co., 1977.

Scott, T. W.: Urinary ascites secondary to posterior urethral valves. J. Urol., 116:87, 1976.

Seeler, R. A., Kapadia, P., and Moncado, R.: Non-surgical management of thrombosis of bilateral renal veins and inferior vena cava in a newborn infant. Clin. Pediatr., 9:543, 1970.

Sherry, S. N., and Kramer, I.: The time of passage of first stool and first urine by the newborn infant. J. Pediatr., 46:158, 1955.

Singh, M. P., Haddadin, A., Zachary, R. B., and Pilling, D. W.: Renal tract disease in imperforate anus. J. Pediatr. Surg., 9:197, 1974.

Smith, D. W.: Introduction. In Smith, D. W. (Ed.): Recognizable Patterns of Human Malformation, pp. 1–5. Philadelphia, W. B. Saunders Co., 1976.

Smith, G. I.: Cellular changes from graded testicular ischemia. J. Urol., 73:355, 1955.

Snyder, W. H., Jr.: Some unusual forms of imperforate anus in female infants. Am. J. Surg., 111:319, 1966.

Sober, I., and Hirsch, M.: Unilateral massive adrenal hemorrhage in the newborn infant. J. Urol., 93:430, 1965.

Spitzer, A., Bernstein, J., and Edelman, C. M., Jr.: Diseases of the kidney and urinary tract. In Behrman, R. E. (Ed.): Neonatology, pp. 485–513. St. Louis, C. V. Mosby Co., 1973.

Stark, H., and Geiger, R.: Renal tubular dysfunction following vascular accidents to the kidney in the newborn period. J. Pediatr., 83:933, 1973.

Sutton, T. J., Leblanc, A., Gauthier, N., and Hassan, M.: Radiological manifestations of neonatal renal vein thrombosis on follow-up examination. Radiology, 122:435, 1977.

Tank, E. S., and Lindenauer, S. M.: Principles of management of exstrophy of the cloaca. Am. J. Surg., 119:95, 1970.

Teele, R. L.: Ultrasonography of the genitourinary tract in children. Radiol. Clin. North Am., 15:109, 1977.

Thompson, I. M., Schneider, R., and Lababidi, Z.: Thrombectomy for renal vein thrombosis. J. Urol., 113:396, 1974.

Treadwell, T. A., Andrassy, R. J., and Ratner, I. A.: Spermatic cord torsion in the newborn. Tex. Med., 72:43, 1976.

Uson, A. C., Cox, L. A., and Lattimer, J. K.: Hydronephrosis in infants and children. JAMA, 205:323, 1968.

Verhagen, A. D., Hamilton, J. P., and Genel, M.: Renal vein thrombosis in infants. Arch. Dis. Child., 40:214, 1965.

Vulliamy, D. G.: Congenital anomalies and deformities with some genetic disorders. In Vulliamy, D. G. (Ed.): The Newborn Child, pp. 142–180. Baltimore, Williams & Wilkins Co., 1972.

Waisman, J., and Cooper, P. H.: Renal neoplasms of the newborn. J. Pediatr. Surg., 5:407, 1970.

Watson, R. A.: Torsion of the spermatic cord in the neonate. Urology, 5:439, 1974.

Wedge, J. J., Grosfeld, J. L., and Smith, J. P.: Abdominal masses in the newborn: 63 cases. J. Urol., 106:770, 1971.

Weller, M. H., and Miller, K.: Unusual aspects of urine ascites. Radiology, 109:665, 1973.

Wiener, E. S., and Kiesewetter, S. W.: Urological abnormalities associated with imperforate anus. J. Pediatr. Surg., 8:151, 1973.

Wigger, H. J.: Fetal hamartoma of the kidney. Am. J. Clin. Pathol., 51:323, 1969.

Williams, D. I.: Renal anomalies. In Williams, D. I. (Ed.): Urology in Childhood, pp. 70–80. New York, Springer-Verlag, 1974.

Williams, D. I., and Eckstein, H. R.: Obstructive valves in the posterior urethra. J. Urol., 92:236, 1965.

Williams, D. I., and Parker, R. M.: The role of surgery in the prune belly syndrome. In Johnston, H., and Goodwin, W. E. (Eds.): Reviews in Pediatric Urology, pp. 315–331. Amsterdam, Excerpta Medica, 1974.

Woodard, J. R.: The prune belly syndrome. Urol. Clin. North Am., 5:75, 1978.

Woodard, J. R., and Lasky, R.: Unpublished data.

Woodard, J. R., and Parrott, T. S.: Urologic surgery in the neonate. J. Urol., 116:506, 1976.

Woodard, J. R., Patterson, J. H., and Brinsfield, D.: Renal artery thrombosis in newborn infants. Am. J. Dis. Child., 114:191, 1967.

CHAPTER 57

Pediatric Oncology

HOWARD McC. SNYDER, III, M.D.
GIULIO J. D'ANGIO, M.D.
AUDREY E. EVANS, M.D.
R. BEVERLY RANEY, M.D.

WILMS' TUMOR AND OTHER RENAL TUMORS OF CHILDHOOD

History

Rance in 1814 apparently was the first to describe it, but Max Wilms in 1899 better characterized the tumor that has become associated with his name. Other more descriptive terms, including mixed tumor of the kidney, embryoma of the kidney, and nephroblastoma, are commonly used.

These neoplasms often grow to massive size before becoming clinically evident, so that into the twentieth century only rare efforts were made to excise them, and most children died. By the 1930's, better surgical techniques, especially improvements in anesthesia, and better understanding of pediatric surgical care led to lowering of the operative mortality rates; survival rates of up to 25 per cent were achieved by the fourth decade (Gross and Neuhauser, 1950).

The multimodal approach to the management of pediatric solid tumors originated with Wilms' tumor, when it was learned that this lesion was responsive to radiation therapy. With this addition, survivals rose to the 50 per cent range, where they remained until the advent of chemotherapy.

In the 1940's, the introduction of aminopterin for the treatment of leukemia opened the era of chemotherapy for pediatric cancers, and Sidney Farber and coworkers at the Boston Children's Hospital in 1956 reported actinomycin D to be effective for Wilms' tumor. This marked the first successful treatment of a pediatric solid neoplasm by chemotherapy. By 1966, Farber could report a survival rate of 81 per cent for children with Wilms' tumor treated by surgery, radiotherapy, and chemotherapy with actinomycin D at the Boston Children's Hospital as compared with a 40 per cent survival rate for children treated by surgery and radiotherapy alone. Wolff et al. (1968) reported that multiple courses of chemotherapy were more effective than a single course.

At about the same time, the vinca alkaloids were found to be effective oncolytic agents. The successful use of vincristine as a single agent in the treatment of Wilms' tumor was reported (Sutow and Sullivan, 1965; Sullivan et al., 1967). It was also shown to be effective in patients who had previously been treated with actinomycin D (Sutow et al., 1963). Subsequently, high-dose cyclophosphamide (Finklestein et al., 1969) and Adriamycin (Wang et al., 1971) were demonstrated to be useful in the treatment of Wilms' tumor.

Modern therapy for Wilms' tumor owes much to the cooperative studies carried out in many centers to compare different modes of treatment. The intergroup National Wilms' Tumor Study (NWTS) in the United States and trials conducted by the International Society of Pediatric Oncology and the United Kingdom Medical Research Council helped guide the development of current treatment, as will be discussed further on.

Incidence

Wilms' tumor is the most common malignant neoplasm of the urinary tract in children and is responsible for 8 per cent of all childhood solid tumors. It makes up more than 80 per cent of genitourinary cancers below the age of 15 years (Young et al., 1978). There are approximately 7 new cases per 1 million children per year in the United States, for a total of about 350 new cases a year. In about 75 per cent of cases, the diagnosis is made between the ages of 1 and 5 years. Ninety per cent are seen before age 7 years, with a peak incidence between ages 3 and 4 years. The male to female ratio is almost equal (0.97/1.0). Occasionally, the tumor occurs in adults (Olsen and Bischoff, 1970). Familial cases are rare (1 per cent).

Etiology and Embryology

Wilms' tumor is believed to be the result of an abnormal proliferation of metanephric blastema without normal differentiation into tubules and glomeruli. The median age incidence of 3 1/2 years makes it unlikely that Wilms' tumor is a truly congenital neoplasm. Recent evidence (Machin, 1980; Bove and McAdams, 1976) suggests that the lesions of the nephroblastomatosis complex may function as a carrier state, bringing blastemal tissue to a point at which a subsequent change leads to the development of clinical Wilms' tumor. This is in accord with the two-hit theory of oncogenesis of Knudson and Strong (1972).

The etiology of Wilms' tumor is probably heterogeneous, as has been pointed out in a review by Belasco (1982). There is a genetic component (McBride, 1979). An 11-p deletion, especially when seen with aniridia (Riccardi et al., 1978), has been associated. Trisomies 8 and 18, 45X Turner's syndrome, and pseudohermaphroditism with an XX/XY mosaicism have been found with Wilms' tumor, as has BC translocation (Giangiacomo et al., 1975). In spite of these associations, in a review of 1926 cases, Cochran and Froggatt (1967) found that familial-genetic factors could be found in only about 1 per cent. The association of pseudohermaphroditism, nephron disorders, and Wilms' tumor raises the question of an embryologic event occurring before the differentiation of renal and genital structures, and therefore affecting both (Drash et al., 1970). Teratogens in animal models have also produced Wilms' tumor as well as other neoplasms.

Associated Anomalies

About 15 per cent of children with Wilms' tumor have other congenital abnormalities (Pendergrass, 1976; Miller et al., 1964; Miller, 1968). *Aniridia* was found in 1.1 per cent of the children in the first National Wilms' Tumor Study. While the occurrence of aniridia in the general population is 1 in 50,000, it is present in about 1 in 70 patients with Wilms' tumor. It is the sporadic form of aniridia rather than the familial one that is associated with Wilms' tumor. The full syndrome, in addition to the tumor and congenital eye lesions, includes presentation generally before 3 years of age, genitourinary anomalies, deformities of the external ear, mental retardation, and, less frequently, facial or skull dysmorphism, inguinal and umbilical hernias, and hypotonia (Haicken and Miller, 1971).

Hemihypertrophy, characterized by an asymmetry of the body, has been found in 2.9 per cent of cases of Wilms' tumor, not necessarily lateralized to the side of the tumor. It may even become evident after the Wilms' tumor has appeared (Janik and Seeler, 1976). The incidence of hemihypertrophy in the general populations is 1 in 14,300, whereas in Wilms' tumor it is found in 1 in 32 patients. An increased incidence of other cancers is associated with hemihypertrophy, e.g., embryonal carcinomas, especially adrenocortical carcinoma and hepatoblastomas. These patients also often manifest multiple pigmented nevi, hemangiomas, and genitourinary anomalies (Meadows and Jarrett, 1978).

The *Beckwith-Wiedemann syndrome* (Fig. 57–1) consists of visceromegaly involving the adrenal cortex, kidney, liver, pancreas, and gonads. Additionally, omphalocele, hemihypertrophy, microcephaly, mental retardation, and macroglossia may be found. Approximately one in ten children with this syndrome develops a neoplasm (Sotelo-Avila et al., 1980). The malignancies affect the liver, adrenal cortex, and kidney, the same organs that are at risk in children with hemihypertrophy. It is possible that many cases listed as hemihypertrophy represent incomplete forms of the Beckwith-Wiedemann syndrome.

Musculoskeletal anomalies have been found in 2.9 per cent of Wilms' tumor patients, who demonstrate a 7.9 per cent incidence of hamartomas, including hemangiomas, multiple nevi, and café-au-lait spots. There is a 30-fold increase in neurofibromatosis with Wilms' tumor (Stay and Vawter, 1977).

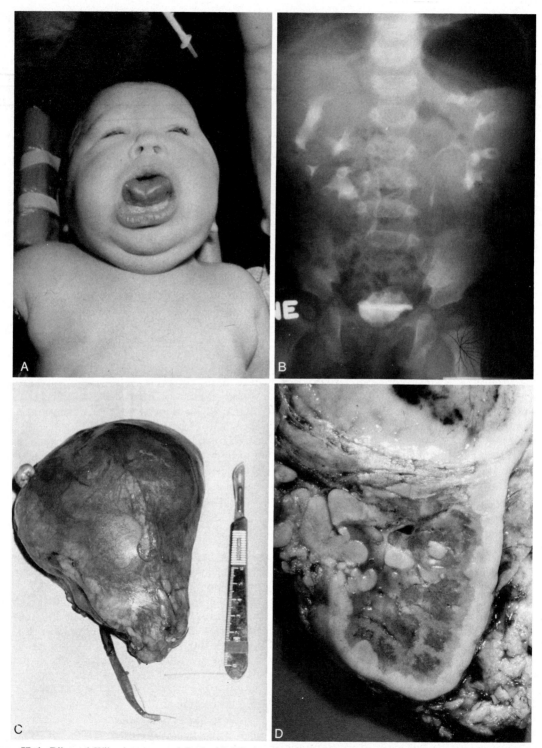

Figure 57–1. Bilateral Wilms' tumor and Beckwith-Wiedemann syndrome. *A,* Associated macroglossia. *B,* Intravenous pyelogram showing calyceal distortion in both kidneys. *C,* Right kidney with large upper pole Wilms' tumor. *D,* Cut specimen showing Wilms' tumor and inferior rim of nephroblastomatosis and Wilms' tumorlets.

Genitourinary anomalies are found in 4.4 per cent of cases. Most often seen is renal hypoplasia, ectopia, fusions, duplications, cystic disease, hypospadias, cryptorchidism, and pseudohermaphroditism. As mentioned before, this may suggest that the primary event in the genesis of this tumor occurs before the differentiation of renal and genital structure has taken place and accordingly affects both.

A number of associated *second malignant neoplasms* have been reported in long-term survivors of Wilms' tumor. These have included brain tumors, sarcomas, adenocarcinomas, and leukemias. Most of the sarcomas (generally osteogenic) and carcinomas have been found within previous fields of radiation therapy. Such tumors may be induced by prior treatment or may result from a genetic predisposition to the second tumor. Perhaps others are a result of a combination of these factors.

Pathology

GROSS FEATURES

Classic Wilms' tumor is a sharply demarcated and usually encapsulated solitary tumor occurring in any part of the kidney (Fig. 57–2). The cut tumor bulges with a fleshy tan surface. Necrosis is frequent. This may lead to hemorrhage or to the appearance of cyst formation. True cysts are seen occasionally. The tumor distorts the calyceal anatomy, accounting for the typical radiographic picture. Uncommonly, the tumor grows into the renal pelvis, where it may lead to hematuria or obstruction. Renal venous invasion occurs in 20 per cent of cases (Fig. 57–3). While lymph node metastases often appear to be present at surgery, histologic examination frequently proves this to be a false impression, making gross assessment of nodal involvement unreliable (Martin et al., 1979). It may be possible, however, to distinguish Wilms' tumor from some other renal tumors on gross examination. Congenital mesoblastic nephroma, on examination of the cut surface, has a typical interlacing pattern that is similar to a uterine fibroid (Fig. 57–4). If multiple small lesions are present, this suggests the diagnosis of nephroblastomatosis with or without Wilms' tumor.

Rarely, extrarenal Wilms' tumors have been found (Aterman et al., 1979), such as in the retroperitoneum and inguinal regions, or as part of complex teratomas. Other sites include the posterior mediastinum, posterior pelvis, and sacrococcygeal area (McCauley et al., 1979).

MICROSCOPIC FEATURES

It is difficult to describe a "typical" Wilms' tumor, as the neoplasm can exhibit a wide spectrum of the structures of the metanephros and mesoderm from which it takes its origin. The tumor is triphasic. The most diagnostic feature is a swirl of "nephrogenic" cells having a tubuloglomerular pattern against a background of "stromagenic" cells (Fig. 57–5). These are undifferentiated and generally compact but may have a myxoid appearance. The stromal component may occasionally differentiate into striated muscle (frequent), cartilage or fat (rare), or bone (very rare). The epithelial component of Wilms' tumor can be well differentiated with characteristic mature tubules, or it may be very primitive.

Experience with the pathologic examination of large numbers of specimens has suggested histologic characteristics that tend to be associated with a favorable or an ominous prognosis. Chatten (1976) recognized that epithelial predominance may indicate a better prognosis (Lawler et al., 1977). Although data from the Medical Research Council Nephroblastoma Trial have supported this concept, the National Wilms' Tumor Study has not (Beckwith and Palmer, 1978). The reason may be that overall survival for Wilms' tumor is now so high (approaching 90 per cent) that it may be impossible to separate histologic features that confer a particularly favorable prognosis. While the poor outlook predicted for those with tumors having unfavorable histologic features may be confirmed by the clinical course, it may be that especially favorable histologic variants cannot be recognized because the overall success with the tumor prevents singling out these cases.

Unfavorable Histologic Types. One of the first important pathologic correlations to come from the National Wilms' Tumor Study was the recognition of three particularly unfavorable histologic types. Although these three categories made up only about 10 per cent of the cases studied, they accounted for at least 60 per cent of the deaths.

Anaplasia is strictly defined as a threefold variation in nuclear size with hyperchromatism and abnormal mitotic figures. These features may be found in any of the various elements of a Wilms' tumor. When anaplasia is diffuse rather than focal, the prognosis is more unfavorable. It has an increased incidence in older children.

The second unfavorable category is the *rhabdoid* tumor (Fig. 57–6). Histologically, the

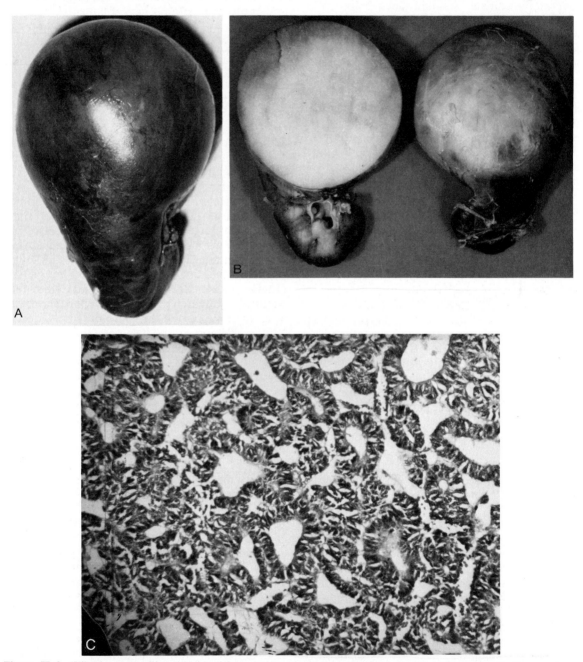

Figure 57–2. Wilms' tumor with epithelial differentiation. *A*, Kidney with large upper pole tumor. *B*, Cut specimen showing well-encapsulated tumor. *C*, Histology (320 ×): Well-differentiated Wilms' tumor with epithelial component forming tubules (favorable histology).

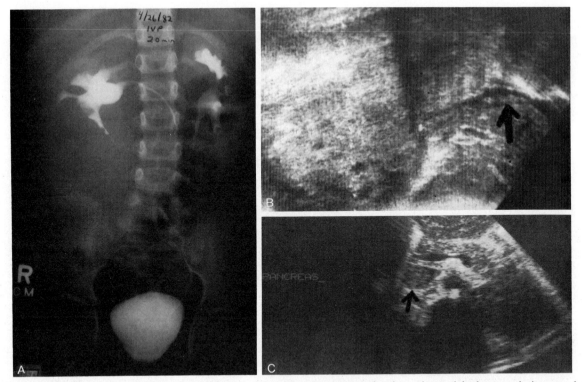

Figure 57–3. Wilms' tumor with caval invasion. *A,* Intravenous pyelogram showing a large right lower pole intrarenal tumor displacing the collecting system upward. Note course of ureter coursing over tumor. Abdominal ultrasound study showing tumor (arrow) in inferior cava on sagittal *(B)* and transverse *(C)* views.

cells are uniform and large with large nuclei and very prominent nucleoli. The cystoplasm contains eosinophilic inclusions, which by electron microscopy can be shown to be fibrils. These large cells are suggestive of rhabdomyoblasts and gave the tumor its name, but neither light nor electron microscopy actually confirms the presence of muscle. Indeed, if striated muscle can be identified, as may be seen in conventional Wilms' tumor, it excludes the diagnosis of a rhabdoid tumor and the outlook is not bad. In fact, this neoplasm may not be a form of Wilms' tumor at all. It is now considered by many to be a distinct sarcoma of childhood, not of metanephric origin. It tends to metastasize to the brain and to have a high association with independent primary central nervous system tumors (Palmer and Beckwith, 1981).

The third unfavorable variant has been referred to as *clear cell sarcoma* of the kidney and seems to be the same as the "bone metastasizing renal tumor of childhood" described by Marsden and Lawler (1980). Histologically, these tumors are characterized by a spindle cell pattern with a vasocentric arrangement. The nucleoli are not prominent, and the cytoplasm is scanty with variably eosinophilic characteristics. As tubules may be seen in the primary lesion but are not seen in metastatic sites, this may indicate that tubules are merely being trapped by the tumor. The tumor characteristically metastasizes to bone (Morgan and Kidd, 1978) and is frequent in males. Opinion is building to classify this tumor as a distinct entity rather than as a variant of Wilms' tumor (Carcassonne et al., 1981). Some ultrastructural studies have suggested that the tumor may be derived from blastemal cells (Novak et al., 1980). It is possible that clear cell sarcoma reflects a malignant phase of the normally benign congenital mesoblastic nephroma.

Favorable Histologic Types. There are several other renal lesions found in children that have a characteristic morphology and tend to have a relatively benign course. Their exact relationship to classic Wilms' tumor continues to be debated, but perhaps they are best considered as variants rather than as distinct pathologic entities (Ganick et al., 1981).

MULTILOCULAR CYSTS (MLC). The characteristic aspect of MLC is its gross appearance. Typically, the lesion is round and smooth on its

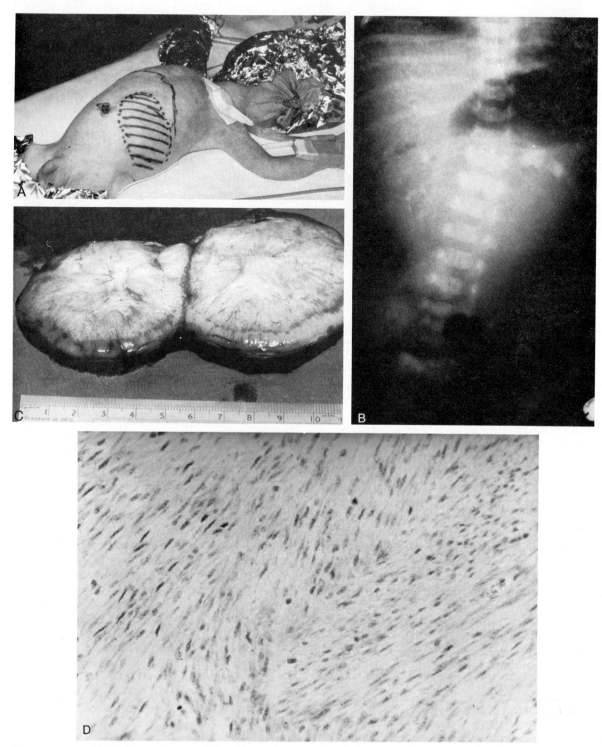

Figure 57–4. Congenital mesoblastic nephroma. *A,* Newborn infant who presented with a left flank mass (outlined). *B,* Intravenous pyelogram showing large left lower pole renal tumor displacing collecting system superiorly. *C,* Gross specimen: characteristic dense pale tumor composed of interlacing bundles grossly resembling a leiomyoma. *D,* Histology: tumor composed of sheets of uniform spindle-shaped cells with no capsule.

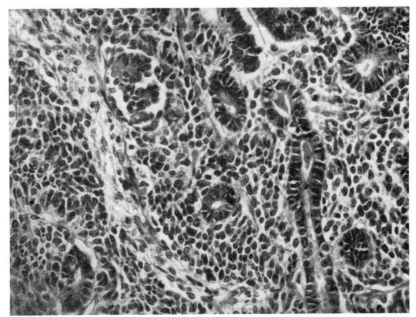

Figure 57–5. Wilms' tumor pathology: Classic triphasic histology showing swirls of primitive renal blastema and tubules against a background of undifferentiated stroma.

external border. It consists of a localized cluster of cysts within the kidney and is almost always unilateral. There are two peaks in the age incidence of MLC (Coleman, 1980; Banner et al., 1981). The first peak occurs in the pediatric age group and is characterized by the presence of blastema in the septa of the cyst. While this may have the potential for eventually developing into a classic Wilms' tumor (Fig. 57–7), the MLC itself has a benign course. Local excision constitutes adequate treatment. The second peak incidence occurs in the adult, and the tumor is seen more commonly in females than in males. Histologically, there is more mature fibrous tissue in the wall. Again, this is a benign tumor. Unfortunately, not all cystic localized lesions of the kidney fall into such a straightforward classification (Cho et al., 1979).

CONGENITAL MESOBLASTIC NEPHROMA (CMN). This is a renal tumor typically presenting in early infancy before the age peak for classic Wilms' tumor (Howell et al., 1982).

Figure 57–6. Rhabdoid Wilms' tumor: unfavorable histology. Uniform cells with large nuclei and prominent nucleoli. The cytoplasm contains eosinophilic inclusions, which by electron microscopy can be shown to be fibrils.

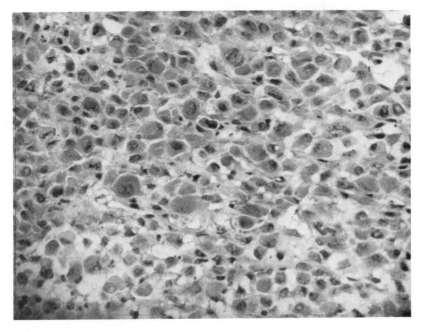

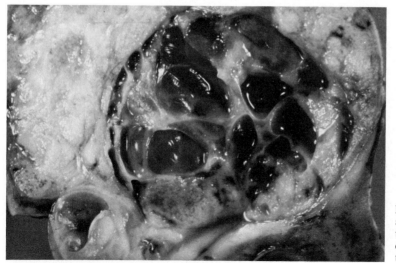

Figure 57–7. Wilms' tumor containing a multilocular cyst that demonstrates a typical characteristic series of adjacent cysts with an overall round configuration.

There is a frequent association with polyhydramnios (Blank et al., 1978). A male predominance has been noted. Grossly, this lesion is a massive, firm tumor, which on cut surface demonstrates interlacing bundles of whitish tissue grossly resembling a leiomyoma. (Fig. 57–4). Microscopically, the tumor consists of sheets of spindle-shaped uniform cells (Bolande, 1973, 1974); ultramicroscopically, the cells appear to be fibroblasts or myofibroblasts (Wockel et al., 1979). The margin of the tumor tends to infiltrate locally rather than having the pseudocapsule of classic Wilms' tumor. There may be cartilaginous tissue at the tumor margin, a characteristic suggesting dysplasia.

When completely excised, classic CMN has a uniformly benign course (Snyder et al., 1981). More morbidity has resulted from the treatment of small infants with radiation therapy and chemotherapy, in the belief that this was a true Wilms' tumor, than from the tumor itself. Wigger (1969) has argued that this is a hamartoma and not a form of Wilms' tumor.

Occasionally, a "cellular variant" of CMN is seen. This tumor has a higher mitotic index and more of a sarcomatous appearance. The distinction between this variant and clear cell sarcoma of the kidney may be difficult. Indeed, the age and sex incidence, spindle morphology, prominent vascularity, and trapping of mature renal elements may suggest that clear cell sarcoma is the malignant counterpart of the normally benign classic CMN (Hartman et al., 1981).

RHABDOMYOSARCOMA TUMOR. This is a rare but favorable Wilms' tumor variant characterized by the presence of fetal striated muscle. It should not be confused with the unfavorable rhabdoid tumor, which does not contain muscle (Harms et al., 1980).

It can be seen that when any high grade of differentiation can be recognized in pediatric renal tumors, it tends to impart a better prognosis to the various lesions that are collectively termed nephroblastoma.

NEPHROBLASTOMATOSIS COMPLEX AND RELATION TO WILMS' TUMOR

In 1976, Bove and McAdams made a major contribution to our understanding of Wilms' tumor by their description of the nephroblastomatosis complex (NBC) of lesions. The possible role of NBC as a precursor to Wilms' tumor has been well summarized in a series of three articles by Machin (1980). Microscopically, nephroblastomatosis is defined by the presence of primitive metanephric elements beyond the thirty-sixth week of gestation, when nephrogenesis normally ceases. Usually, persistent nests of metanephric blastema are recognized in the nephrogenic zones of the kidney (subcapsular and column of Bertin). Grossly, the lesions vary from abnormal clefts on the surface of the kidney to patches of discoloration to frank multicentric tumors. The rarest form of NBC is the diffuse *superficial infantile* form (Hou and Holman, 1961). Affected children present with massive nephromegaly and die shortly after birth, as no functioning renal tissue is present. Histologic examination reveals that the entire kidney has been replaced by nephroblastomatosis. The more common form of NBC is the *multifocal juvenile* one. When the lesions are microscopic only, they are referred to as *nodular renal blastema* (NRB) (Fig. 57–8), but when they are grossly visible, they are termed *metanephric hamartomas* and may exhibit sclerotic characteristics or be glomerulocystic or papillary. *Wilms' tumorlets* show the typical triphasic histology of classic Wilms' tumor but are usually well differentiated and are defined as being less than 3.5 cm and greater than 1 cm in diameter.

One hundred per cent of patients with bilateral Wilms' tumor can be shown microscopically to exhibit some component of nephroblastomatosis. Classic solitary Wilms' tumors on careful microscopic examination are found to have elements of NBC in about 40 per cent of cases, and an even higher incidence is anticipated as more systematic searches for the lesions in large Wilms' tumors are performed.

Certain aspects of the lesions of the nephroblastomatosis complex suggest they may be precursors of Wilms' tumor (Bove and Mc-Adams, 1976; Machin, 1980; Shanklin and Sotelo-Avila, 1969). The peak age incidence of

Wilms' tumor at 3 years suggests that it is not a truly congenital tumor. It has been speculated that lesions of the nephroblastomatosis complex may represent the first "hit" in a two-step process leading to Wilms' tumor (Knudson and Strong, 1972). Nephroblastomatosis is discovered in approximately 1 in every 300 autopsies in infants. When cases associated with lethal anomalies are subtracted, one is left with an incidence of 1 in 10,000, approximately the incidence of Wilms' tumor. It may be that after the first mutagenic event producing an NBC lesion, the likelihood of a second "hit" is near 100 per cent, accounting for these figures. This would be in contradistinction to neuroblastoma in situ, which is found in 1 in 200 neonatal autopsies but only rarely goes on to produce clinical neuroblastoma.

The therapeutic implications of discovering nephroblastomatosis continue to be debated. As it is likely that NBC, while itself benign, will eventually be followed by the development of a frank Wilms' tumor, chemotherapy appears reasonable. Lesions of the complex do respond to the same chemotherapy as for conventional Wilms' tumor, at least in some cases. The optimal program is as yet undefined. It is also important to single out patients with NBC in one kidney for particularly careful follow-up. Bilateral Wilms' tumors frequently develop in such circumstances, and patients with metachronous bilateral tumors have a worse prognosis.

Wilms' Tumor Presentation

An abdominal mass or increasing abdominal girth is the most frequent presenting sign leading to the diagnosis of Wilms' tumor. It is seen in over three quarters of cases. Usually, the child is well, without a history of worrisome symptoms. About one third of patients present with abdominal pain. This may range from vague, poorly localized discomfort to acute flank pain reflecting hemorrhage into the tumor. A history of acute onset of pain with fever, abdominal mass, anemia, and hypertension suggests Wilms' tumor with sudden subcapsular hemorrhage (Ramsey et al., 1977). Rarely, a child may present with the signs of an acute abdomen secondary to intraperitoneal rupture of the tumor (Thompson et al., 1973). While gross hematuria is uncommon, microscopic blood may be found in up to 25 per cent of cases. A history of minor renal trauma is often elicited.

On physical examination, a firm, nonten-

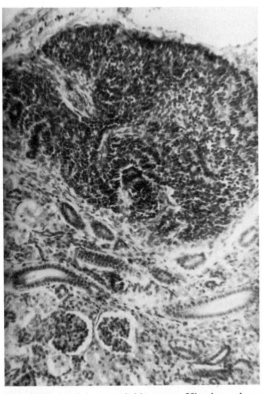

Figure 57–8. Nodular renal blastema. Histology demonstrates microscopic nodules of metanephric blastema in infant beyond 36 weeks of gestation. The lesion is subcapsular here but may also be found in the columns of Bertin.

der, smooth, unilateral abdominal mass is most common. Very large tumors may cross the midline, but most do not. This is in contradistinction to neuroblastoma, which often presents with a more nodular, irregular tumor growing across the midline. The child with neuroblastoma also usually looks sick.

Hypertension may be found in Wilms' tumor patients if the blood pressure is carefully checked—a practice not common in the past. The incidence has been reported to range from 25 per cent to 63 per cent. Hypertension may result from compression of normal renal tissue (renal ischemia) or from the direct production of renin by the tumor itself (Ganguly et al., 1973; Marosvari et al., 1972).

Rare cases of Wilms' tumor associated with polycythemia secondary to erythropoietin production by the tumor have been reported (Shalet et al., 1967). Occasionally, a patient with Wilms' tumor is found to have an associated nephrotic syndrome, leading to the term "Wilms' nephritis." This may be a chance association, since neither problem is rare; however, it has been proposed that both conditions may result from a common embryologic renal misadventure and that the relationship thus may not be due to chance alone (Drash et al., 1970).

Even more rare presentations of Wilms' tumor have included varicocele, hernia, enlarged testis, congestive failure from propagation of tumor into the heart or because of intrarenal AV fistula, hypoglycemia, Cushing's syndrome, hydrocephalus from a brain metastasis, and acute renal failure (Sanyal et al., 1976). Occasionally, pulmonary metastases may lead to an initial presentation with cough, pleural effusion, or pleural pain.

DIFFERENTIAL DIAGNOSIS

The differential diagnosis for Wilms' tumor is the same as that for any abdominal mass (Table 57–1).

Renal tumors can usually be separated from nonrenal ones by a combination of intravenous pyelography and ultrasonography. Neuroblastoma may present diagnostic problems even after these two tests, particularly if the tumor arises intrarenally (Shende et al., 1979), but a bone marrow aspiration positive for neuroblastoma cells or an elevation of the urinary catecholamine levels is conclusive. The diagnosis of the other malignant tumors is usually not difficult once the origin of the abdominal mass is identified correctly. Most of the benign abdominal masses can be separated from Wilms' tumor by intravenous pyelography or ultrasonography,

TABLE 57–1. DIFFERENTIAL DIAGNOSIS OF WILMS' TUMOR

Malignant Tumors
Renal: Renal cell carcinoma
Neuroblastoma
Rhabdomyosarcoma
Hepatoblastoma
Lymphoma, lymphosarcoma
Benign Abdominal Masses
Renal: Renal abscess, multicystic dysplastic kidney, hydronephrosis, polycystic kidney, congenital mesoblastic nephroma
Mesenteric cysts
Choledochal cysts
Intestinal duplication cysts
Splenomegaly

or both. An intrarenal abscess may be confusing if signs of sepsis are not prominent (Simonowitz and Reyes, 1976). Splenomegaly is occasionally confused for a left-sided Wilms' tumor. Age is of importance in the differential diagnosis; in the newborn period, a renal mass is most likely to be ureteropelvic junction obstruction or a multicystic dysplastic kidney. Infantile polycystic disease usually presents with bilateral nephromegaly. The rare congenital mesoblastic nephroma, found early in life, requires histopathologic examination for accurate diagnosis. It is of interest that in the first National Wilms' Tumor Study (NWTS), 5 per cent of the patients were misdiagnosed preoperatively (Ehrlich et al., 1979). The most common diagnostic errors were neuroblastoma or renal cystic disease.

DIAGNOSTIC IMAGING

In spite of the recent enormous advances in radiology, the conventional intravenous pyelogram continues to be the mainstay of the diagnosis of Wilms' tumor. The characteristic radiographic appearance is of deformation and distortion of the calyceal morphology by an intrarenal mass (Figs. 57–1B and 57–3A). There may be radiolucent areas produced by hemorrhage or necrosis in the tumor. The initial plain film of the abdomen should be examined carefully. Calcification is rarely present but, when found, has a characteristic peripheral "eggshell" pattern resulting from old hemorrhage. If there is a stippled pattern, the diagnosis of neuroblastoma is probable. The intravenous pyelogram also permits an assessment of the kidney opposite the side of the clinical mass. It is important to make certain that a contralateral renal anomaly is not present before removing the tumor. About 10 per cent of Wilms' tumors are bilateral.

Nonvisualization of the affected kidney on the intravenous pyelogram occurs in about 10 per cent of cases. This may suggest renal vein invasion by the tumor or massive parenchymal replacement by tumor. It is in the evaluation of a nonvisualizing kidney that ultrasound is particularly valuable.

Modern real-time ultrasonography has eliminated much of the diagnostic doubt that occasionally surrounded renal masses in the past. Renal agenesis, hydronephrosis, and multicystic kidneys can be rapidly separated from Wilms' tumor, which has a characteristic echogenic pattern separate from that of a number of other infiltrative renal diseases (Hunig and Kinser, 1973). Ultrasound also permits an assessment of the renal vein and inferior vena cava for intraluminal tumor (Green et al., 1979) (Fig. 57–3*B* and *C*). Retroperitoneal nodes and possible liver metastases can be ascertained. By observing movement of the tumor in relation to the liver during breathing, it may be possible to determine if there is direct involvement of the liver. Assessment of the contralateral kidney may detect small tumors missed by intravenous pyelography and may show a pattern suggestive of nephroblastomatosis. This is of importance in directing attention to specific areas of the opposite kidney for biopsy. In the great majority of cases, ultrasonography and intravenous pyelography will establish the diagnosis and extent of the disease accurately and will obviate the need for other time-consuming and costly examinations, e.g., retrograde pyelography, angiography, or computerized tomography. Other studies thus are undertaken only infrequently in the evaluation of children with Wilms' tumor.

Arteriography, which carries a significant morbidity in childhood, is recommended by the NWTS only in the following circumstances: (1) the mass is not clearly intrarenal; (2) the mass is so small that it cannot be assessed by other modalities; (3) tumors are suspected to be bilateral, especially if heminephrectomy is being considered; and (4) nonvisualization of the kidney is present, and adequate assessment cannot be made by other means. In practice, angiography is rarely needed. Inferior venacavography to evaluate renal vein or caval involvement is subject to false positive studies from blood shunting—the result of the Valsalva effect during crying. The opaque column is forced into the paravertebral plexus of veins, suggesting inferior vena caval obstruction. Ultrasound is the more reliable study.

Computerized tomography can provide precise anatomic delineation of renal and retroperitoneal anatomy, but it requires a general anesthetic in the small child and is usually not necessary in Wilms' tumor. The study may have a greater role in the evaluation of neuroblastoma. As a rule, renal scans are needed only in the evaluation of a possible renal pseudotumor. In this situation, a 99m Tc DMSA or glucoheptonate renal scan is useful (Katz and Landau, 1979). A renal pseudotumor exhibits normal function, whereas a Wilms' tumor is cold.

A retrograde ureteropyelogram is rarely needed today. It is indicated in the presence of hematuria, especially when the kidney does not visualize by intravenous pyelography. Ureteral metastases from calyceal invasion (Stevens and Eckstein, 1976) and direct ureteral invasion by Wilms' tumor have occasionally been reported and are important to diagnose in order to permit an en bloc resection.

Evaluation for metastatic disease in children with Wilms' tumor routinely involves careful imaging of the chest because the lungs are the most frequent sites of metastases. Our practice at the Children's Hospital of Philadelphia is to obtain chest x-ray films in frontal, lateral, and both oblique views. Tomography is useful to evaluate any suspicious areas. Other imaging studies are generally not carried out until pathologic studies have been done. If a rhabdoid tumor is found, imaging of the brain by radionuclear scan or computerized tomography is indicated because of the high incidence of CNS involvement with either metastases or second, independent brain tumors. The finding of a clear cell sarcoma should lead to a skeletal survey or radionuclide bone scan because of the high incidence of bony metastases with this tumor. Roentgenography is said to be more sensitive than bone scans in these cases.

LABORATORY STUDIES

Standard laboratory evaluations of a child with a retroperitoneal mass include a complete blood count and urinalysis. To help rule out neuroblastoma in questionable cases, the LaBrosse spot test for urinary catecholamines is useful (Evans et al., 1971). Bone marrow aspiration and biopsy usually are not carried out unless the diagnosis of neuroblastoma is suspected; Wilms' tumor rarely infiltrates the marrow in the absence of bone metastases, if then. A BUN and serum creatinine, as well as liver enzymes, are usually drawn preoperatively to provide baseline comparisons. Although formal creatinine clearances are seldom needed prior to surgery, they may be useful to assess renal function following treatment. GFR calculations by nuclear medicine studies can provide similar follow-up information.

SURGICAL TREATMENT

Until the introduction of radiotherapy, increased survival in Wilms' tumor in this century correlated with improved surgical and anesthetic techniques; the hallmark of success with Wilms' tumor continues to be the complete removal of the tumor. Although surgery is no longer regarded as the emergency it once was, surgical exploration of the abdomen should be undertaken as soon as the child can be completely evaluated diagnostically and his condition stabilized appropriately for surgery.

We usually position the child with rolls beneath the back to hyperextend the back, with the involved side elevated approximately 30 degrees. A very generous incision is made from below the tip of the twelfth rib on the involved side to the lateral margin of the opposite rectus muscle. This generally affords excellent exposure; today we rarely find it necessary to resort to the thoracoabdominal approach. The extent of the tumor is first evaluated. The liver should be inspected and palpated as well as the para-aortic and hilar lymph nodes and cava. Although node assessment can be frustratingly inaccurate at surgery, the presence of large node masses is certainly an indication for biopsy.

Exploration of the contralateral kidney should be carried out prior to efforts to remove the tumor. The colon is reflected and Gerota's capsule entered, with mobilization of the uninvolved kidney adequate to permit a careful palpation and visual study of its entire surface. The presence of nephroblastomatosis may be suggested by an abnormal-looking cleft or discoloration on the surface of the kidney. Biopsy should be done on any suspicious lesion.

The resectability of the tumor must then be determined . It is not unusual for Wilms' tumor to invade through the renal capsule and be adherent to or invade adjacent organs or structures, such as the adrenal, duodenum, liver, pancreas, spleen, diaphragm, colon, or muscles of the abdominal wall. Although it may be appropriate to do a limited resection of these involved organs in order to permit primary extirpation of the tumor, a heroic initial undertaking is not justified. Pretreatment with chemotherapy, with or without radiation therapy, will shrink the size of a tumor (see further on) and generally render it capable of removal.

The approach to the tumor begins with the reflection of the colon on the involved side. If the mesocolon appears to be adherent, it may

be left with the tumor, as the bowel will generally be adequately vascularized through the marginal vessel (Williams and Martin, 1982). When approaching a large left-sided tumor, it may be useful to reflect the cecum and the base of the mesentery to permit exposure of the infrarenal vena cava. This quickly may permit exposure of the left renal vein and artery, which can be thus ligated from a right-sided approach (Todani et al., 1976). We usually begin the tumor mobilization by establishing a plane of dissection inferiorly against the posterior abdominal wall and along the great vessels medially. The ureter is divided early below the level of the iliac vessels along with the gonadal vessels. The advantage of establishing these planes of dissection is that they are as far away from the tumor as possible, thus helping to avoid rupture of the tumor. The dissection along the great vessels leads to the early identification of the renal vessels. It is in keeping with the basic principles of cancer surgery always to try to ligate the renal artery and vein prior to mobilization of the tumor in order to avoid hematogenous spread. With renal tumors, division of the renal artery prior to division of the vein has been advocated in order to avoid venous engorgement of the tumor. Although we do try to adhere to that principle, we have not hesitated to divide the renal vein first when exposure of the artery was difficult. We have not noted that this has materially affected the tumor or the difficulty of the operation.

Major efforts should be made to avoid tumor rupture and spill of viable cells into the peritoneal cavity. This has been shown to be associated with an increased incidence of abdominal relapse (Pochedly, 1971; Cassady et al., 1973). Occasionally, there will be a limited rupture that can be contained by the judicious use of surgical sponges or suction. Keeping the tumor from diffusely spilling may avoid the need for total abdominal irradiation.

The adrenal gland is taken with the tumor if it involves the upper pole. However, the adrenal may be spared when the upper pole of a kidney is normal.

It is important to establish by careful palpation whether the renal vein and cava contain tumor, as renal vein ligation when a tumor thrombus is present may lead to the separation of a tumor embolus (Shurin et al., 1982). Engorgement of retroperitoneal venous collaterals indicates obstruction of the renal vein. Surgical management requires cross-clamping the cava above the neoplastic plug and opening the renal vein and cava if necessary to extract the thrombus. The tumor is usually free and may be extracted with surprising ease. Pretreatment with chemotherapy or radiation therapy has been reported to lead to dense adherence of the tumor to the vein wall, making subsequent surgical removal more difficult (DeLorimier, 1976). If a right-sided mass has grown into the wall of the cava, the vessel can be resected up to the level of the hepatic veins. The left kidney has adequate venous collaterals through gonadal and adrenal veins to survive caval resection (Duckett et al., 1973). For tumor that extends into the atrium, it may be necessary to place the child on cardiopulmonary bypass in order to extract the thrombus (Murphy et al., 1973). The use of preoperative embolization of Wilms' tumor to facilitate removal has been reported (Danis et al., 1979); however, we have not found this necessary.

Although some have advocated a formal radical lymph node dissection for Wilms' tumor (Martin and Reyes, 1969), no better survival has been achieved by radical dissection when the nodes were positive (Jereb et al., 1980). With Wilms' tumor, there are often enlarged hilar or para-aortic nodes that are reactive and do not contain tumor. Nonetheless, they should always be biopsied and the site of large masses of matted nodes marked with metal clips. The presence of positive nodes has important prognostic implications. When tumor excision has been incomplete, it is advisable to use a limited number of metal clips to mark the extent of tumor. This assists the radiation therapist in designing treatment. Use of many clips is inadvisable because they interfere with computerized tomography of the area postoperatively, should it become necessary.

When a tumor seems unresectable, consideration should be given to pretreatment with chemotherapy or radiation therapy, or both, with a subsequent surgical attempt at tumor removal. This approach to pretreatment has become popular in Europe. Radiation therapy as well as chemotherapy with actinomycin D and vincristine has been shown to produce good preoperative shrinkage of tumors (Bracken et al., 1982; Waggert and Koop, 1970; Lemerle et al., 1976, 1983). The NWTS has shown that in the United States, the preoperative diagnostic error is on the order of 5 per cent. Because of both this and concerns that treatment might change the pathologic findings, making it more difficult to ascertain the need for subsequent treatment, pretreatment before surgical exploration of a tumor has not been popular (D'Angio, 1983). There is no evidence that pretreat-

ment with radiotherapy (Lemerle et al., 1976) or chemotherapy (D'Angio et al., 1976a; Lemerle et al., 1983) influences long-term survival. However, the incidence of surgical rupture of the tumor has been shown by the International Society of Pediatric Oncology (SIOP) to be decreased by preoperative radiation or chemotherapy (Lemerle et al., 1976, 1983). SIOP data have also shown that actinomycin D and vincristine given preoperatively produce results at least as good as those of preoperative radiotherapy (Lemerle et al., 1983).

Staging. There have been a number of different staging systems advocated for Wilms' tumor, notably that of Garcia as modified by others (Cassady et al., 1973). The clinicopathologic grouping system used by the NWTS has been the one most widely adopted (Table 57–2).

One problem that emerged from NWTS-1

TABLE 57–2. NATIONAL WILMS' TUMOR STUDY GROUPING SYSTEM

Group	Features
I	*Tumor limited to kidney and completely excised* Surface of renal capsule is intact. Tumor was not ruptured before or during removal. There is no residual tumor apparent beyond margins of resection.
II	*Tumor extends beyond kidney but is completely excised* There is local extension of tumor, that is, penetration beyond pseudocapsule into pararenal soft tissues, or para-aortic lymph node involvement. Renal vessel outside kidney substance is infiltrated or contains tumor thrombus. There is no residual tumor apparent beyond margins of resection.
III	*Residual nonhematogenous tumor confined to abdomen* Any of the following may occur: a. Tumor has ruptured before or during surgery, or biopsy has been performed. b. Implants are found on peritoneal surfaces. c. Lymph nodes are involved beyond abdominal para-aortic chains. d. Tumor is not completely resectable because of local infiltration into vital structures.
IV	*Hematogenous metastases* Deposits are beyond Group III, affecting lung, liver, bone, and brain.
V	*Bilateral renal involvement either initially or subsequently*

From D'Angio, G. J., Evans, A. E., Breslow, N., et al.: Cancer *47*:2302, 1981.

and NWTS-2 was the inadequate discrimination between Groups II and III. In NWTS-2, the 2-year relapse-free survival rates for patients in Groups II and III were 80 per cent and 72 per cent, respectively, with survival rates of 86 per cent and 84 per cent, respectively. It had been previously noted that lymph node involvement was associated with a poor prognosis (Jereb and Eklund, 1973). The grouping method was therefore modified, notably by assigning all patients with positive lymph nodes to Stage III (see further on). When analyses based on NWTS-2 experience were performed, it was found that the relapse-free survival rates of NWTS-2 patients became 85 per cent and 69 per cent for Stages II and III, respectively; survival rates were 94 per cent and 79 per cent, respectively. This better discrimination between these two forms of localized but extensive disease promises to be useful in NWTS-3 (Farewell et al., 1981). The differences between the grouping method and the staging system used in the third National Wilms' Tumor Study are presented in Table 57–3.

Results and Conclusions from National Wilms' Tumor Studies 1 and 2. The results of these studies are summarized in Table 57–4.

TABLE 57–3. NATIONAL WILMS' TUMOR STUDY 3 STAGING: DIFFERENCES FROM GROUPING SYSTEM*

Stage	Features
I	Same as Group I
II	Same as Group II except: a. Biopsy or local spillage of tumor may have occurred. b. Lymph nodes may not be involved.
III	Same as Group III except: a. Lymph nodes at any level are involved. b. There has been massive tumor spillage (local spills or positive biopsy specimens do not qualify).
IV	Same as Group IV
V	Bilateral renal involvement at diagnosis

*Staging criteria are the same for tumors of favorable or unfavorable histologic pattern. Both staging and histologic type should be specified for all patients.

NWTS-1 (running from 1969 to 1974) showed that routine radiotherapy was not needed after surgery in children under 2 years of age with Group I tumors as long as they received actinomycin D for 15 months postop-

TABLE 57–4. RESULTS OF NATIONAL WILMS' TUMOR STUDY 1 AND 2:
Outcome by Randomized Groups and Regimens

Group and Regimen*	No.	% 4-Year RFS†	% 4-Year Survival
NWTS-1			
I < 2 yrs old			
A (RT)	38	89 P = 0.85	94 P = 0.46
B (no RT)	41	88	90
I ≥ 2 yrs old			
A (RT)	42	76 P = 0.06	38 P = 0.015
B (no RT)	42	57	81
II/III			
A (AMD)	63	56	71
B (VCR)	44	57 P = 0.01	71 P = 0.01
C (AMD + VCR)	63	79	84

	% 3-Year No.	RFS	Survival
NWTS-2			
I E (short)	106	96 P = 0.21	97 P = 0.15
F (long)	109	90	91
II/III/IV C	159	65 P = 0.0006	74 P = 0.06
D (C + ADR)	155	79	84

*Regimen IA = Postoperative actinomycin D (AMD) for 15 months plus irradiation (RT)
     IB = Postoperative AMD for 15 months without RT
     IE = Postoperative AMD + vincristine (VCR) for 6 months without RT
     IF = Postoperative AMD + VCR for 15 months without RT
II/III/(IV) A = Postoperative RT + AMD for 15 months
     B = Postoperative RT + VCR for 15 months
     C = Postoperative RT + AMD + VCR for 15 months
     D = Postoperative RT + AMD + VCR + Adriamycin for 15 months
†RFS = Relapse-free survival.
From D'Angio, G. J., et al.: *In* Frontiers of Radiation Therapy and Oncology. Vol. 16. Basel, S. Karger, 1982.

eratively. Over 2 years of age, there was a significantly worse survival, largely because of recurrent intra-abdominal disease. NWTS-1 also demonstrated that chemotherapy with vincristine and actinomycin D together was more effective than either drug given alone. This study also demonstrated that preoperative vincristine conferred no additional advantage to patients with Group IV disease, all of whom were treated after surgery with radiation therapy, actinomycin D, and vincristine. Delays of more than 10 days in initiating radiation therapy appeared to be deleterious. No additional benefit could be shown from giving doses of radiation therapy of more than 1000 rad. Whole abdominal irradiation conferred no additional benefit when compared with localized radiation therapy for children who had a tumor biopsy or who had localized tumor spillage at surgery (D'Angio et al., 1976a, 1978, 1980).

The second NWTS (begun in 1974), evolved from observations made in the first study. Group I patients received no radiation therapy but were randomized to either 6 or 15 months of double-agent chemotherapy with actinomycin D and vincristine. The longer course of treatment was found to convey no statistically significant benefit (D'Angio et al., 1981). At 2 years, survival was 95 per cent, with no suggestion that age was important in the results. Patients with Groups II, III, and IV disease received, in addition to radiation therapy, actinomycin D and vincristine for 15 months, and half were randomized to receive doxorubicin (Adriamycin). Three-drug chemotherapy was demonstrated to be significantly better than the two-drug regimen.

A number of factors that were at one time thought to be important have been proved to be of less significance. NWTS-1 found that Group I children under 2 years of age and those with tumors less than 250 gm in weight had a better prognosis. Subsequent treatment improvements have shown that excellent survival expectancy is the rule regardless of tumor size or age for these children (see further on). NWTS-1 also showed that extension of tumor into the renal vein and cava does not have an adverse prognosis as long as the tumor is completely removed. Direct extension of tumor beyond the kidney likewise does not adversely affect the prognosis as long as it is completely removed. Biopsy of the tumor or localized operative spill does not upgrade the tumor from Stage II unless it is massive. The result is that in most of these cases, postoperative radiation therapy, when needed, can be safely limited to the flank. Overall survival today in Wilms' tumor is summarized from NWTS-2 in Table 57–5.

Prognostic Factors. As Wilms' tumor has been more intensively studied, the major prognostic factors have devolved into three areas. *Histology* is the most important. Patients with unfavorable histology make up only 10 to 15 per cent of all Wilms' tumors; however, they account for more than half of all deaths. In NWTS-2, there was a 90 per cent survival at 2 years for those with favorable histology versus a 54 per cent survival for those with unfavorable histology (D'Angio et al., 1981).

The second unfavorable prognostic determinant is the presence of *hematogenous metastases,* whether they involve the lung (as is most common), liver, bone, or brain. This is the stage of Wilms' tumor with the worst prognosis and at which the most intensive chemotherapeutic attack is being addressed by NWTS-3 (see further on).

The third negative prognostic factor is the presence of *lymph node involvement.* In NWTS-2, there was an 82 per cent overall survival for those with negative nodes versus a 54 per cent survival for those with positive nodes (D'Angio et al., 1981). Any patient with lymph node involvement is now placed in Stage III for the third National Wilms' Tumor Study.

The data presented in Table 57–4 helped design the protocol for the third National Wilms' Tumor Study (Fig. 57–9).

The intent of NWTS-3 is to reduce treatment for children who have a good prognosis. A reduced course of treatment for Stage I patients with favorable histology is being tried by randomizing chemotherapy with actinomycin D and vincristine between 10 weeks and 6 months. Stages II and III patients are being randomized between intensive actinomycin D and vincristine, and those two drugs plus doxorubicin, in an effort to see whether the cardio-

TABLE 57–5. SURVIVAL IN WILMS' TUMOR

Characteristic	2-Year Survival (Per Cent)
Group I	95
Group II	90
Group III	84
Group IV	54
Positive nodes	54
Negative nodes	82
Unfavorable histology	54
Favorable histology	90

From D'Angio, G. J., Evans, A. E., Breslow, N., et al.: Cancer, *47*:2302, 1981.

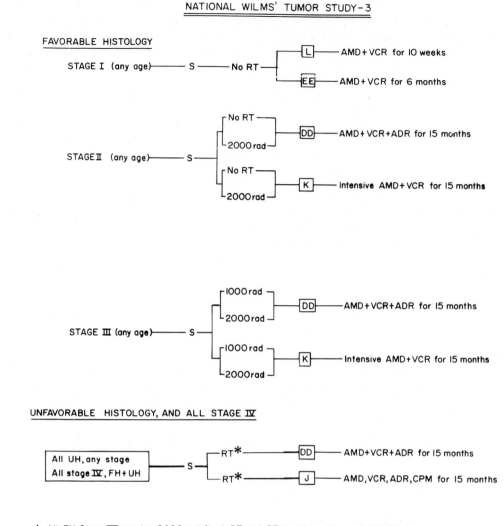

NATIONAL WILMS' TUMOR STUDY-3

FAVORABLE HISTOLOGY

STAGE I (any age)——— S ——— No RT ——— [L] ——— AMD + VCR for 10 weeks
                                        [EE] ——— AMD + VCR for 6 months

STAGE II (any age)——— S ——— No RT
                            2000 rad ——— [DD] ——— AMD + VCR + ADR for 15 months
                            No RT
                            2000 rad ——— [K] ——— Intensive AMD + VCR for 15 months

STAGE III (any age)——— S ——— 1000 rad
                             2000 rad ——— [DD] ——— AMD + VCR + ADR for 15 months
                             1000 rad
                             2000 rad ——— [K] ——— Intensive AMD + VCR for 15 months

UNFAVORABLE HISTOLOGY, AND ALL STAGE IV

All UH, any stage
All stage IV, FH + UH ——— S ——— RT* ——— [DD] ——— AMD + VCR + ADR for 15 months
                                RT* ——— [J] ——— AMD, VCR, ADR, CPM for 15 months

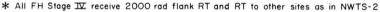

* All FH Stage IV receive 2000 rad flank RT and RT to other sites as in NWTS-2

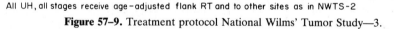

All UH, all stages receive age–adjusted flank RT and to other sites as in NWTS-2

Figure 57–9. Treatment protocol National Wilms' Tumor Study—3.

toxic drug (doxorubicin) can be safely eliminated from their program. Radiotherapy is being studied with relation to Stage II disease to see whether it is possible to eliminate its use. In Stage III disease, children are being randomized to lower-dose or high-dose radiotherapy. Patients with an unfavorable prognosis (that is, any stage with an unfavorable histology and all Stage IV cases) are being randomized into a more intensive chemotherapeutic program.

Preliminary results indicate that patients with Stages II and III tumors of favorable histology do not benefit from the addition of doxorubicin to actinomycin D and vincristine. Also, the patients with Stage II tumors who received

no radiotherapy fared no worse than those receiving 2000 rad. These results, if they continue to hold up, may permit the future simplification of treatment of tumors of favorable histology. Unfortunately, the more intensive chemotherapy protocol of NWTS-3 does not appear to be improving the prognosis for Stage IV tumors or those with unfavorable histology (D'Angio et al., 1984).

X-RAY THERAPY—GENERAL PRINCIPLES

Radiation therapy generally is begun 1 to 3 days after surgery. Two thousand rad is delivered to the flank of all children with tumors of unfavorable histology because they have been shown to be at high risk for abdominal relapse (D'Angio et al., 1978). No children with Stage I tumors of favorable histology are irradiated. The role of radiation therapy after surgery for Stages II and III patients treated with combination chemotherapy is being questioned at present (see earlier). Until the final result of NWTS-3 is available, it appears advisable in Stages II and III patients to continue to give 2000 rad to the tumor bed, except in babies under 1 year of age, in whom the dose is 1000 rad. This helps to protect against infradiaphragmatic relapses, which have been shown to be associated with poor outcomes (Sutow et al., 1982). Whole-abdomen irradiation (2000 rad) is recommended for Stage III tumors with abdominal dissemination. The opposite kidney should be shielded at 1500 rad because radiation nephrotoxicity is a risk when doses exceeding 1500 rad are given. Supplemental doses of 500 to 1000 rad are delivered to regions of residual bulky disease, including portions of the liver, if necessary. Portals similar to those described are used for tumors with unfavorable histology, but higher doses (1200 to 4000 rad) are given, modulated according to age. This is because it has been recognized that growth deformities are more pronounced in the smaller child with the same dose of radiation therapy (Neuhauser et al., 1952).

CHEMOTHERAPY—GENERAL PRINCIPLES

Chemotherapy is usually commenced after surgery once bowel function has been regained. The administration of prolonged courses of chemotherapy in small children has been greatly facilitated by the advent of Broviak central venous lines, which can be placed and maintained for long periods. The doses and schedule followed for the most commonly utilized four drugs are outlined in Table 57–6.

TABLE 57–6. CHEMOTHERAPY FOR WILMS' TUMOR

Actinomycin
    15 μg/kg/day × 5 consecutive days; repeat at 6 weeks, at 3 months, and thereafter at 12- to 13-week intervals
Vincristine
    1.5 mg/m² weekly for 8 to 10 weeks initially; thereafter, at beginning of each course of actinomycin D and 1 week later
Doxorubicin
    20 mg/m²/day × 3 days every 12 weeks; alternate doxorubicin and actinomycin D
Cyclophosphamide
    10 mg/kg/day for 3 consecutive days; thereafter, every 6 weeks

Blood counts should be carefully monitored; it is appropriate to withhold radiation therapy as well as chemotherapy when the total neutrophil count is less than 1000/ml³ and the platelet count less than 75,000/ml³. The recommendation of the National Wilms' Tumor Study is to reduce the dose of all drugs to one-half standard for a child less than 13 months of age because of increased toxicity in this age group.

Inanition may be encountered in children receiving combination chemotherapy, especially when wide-field radiation therapy is also employed. Hyperalimentation via an enteral feeding tube or intravenously may permit the completion of a successful course of chemotherapy in this situation (Donaldson et al., 1982).

Cyclophosphamide should be administered with copious hydration, as this drug has an associated significant incidence of chemical cystitis, which can lead to fibrosis of the bladder wall. This side effect is due to the irritative nature of a breakdown product of cyclophosphamide—acrolein—which has no oncolytic activity. This by-product is chemically bound by Mesna, a drug that has been in use in Europe but is not yet available in the United States. Its use intravenously in combination with cyclophosphamide administration should reduce this complication (Ehrlich et al., 1984).

Doxorubicin is cardiotoxic and has occasionally resulted in the death of a Wilms' tumor patient. Careful monitoring by EKG is important if this drug is used.

TREATMENT OF METASTATIC AND RECURRENT TUMOR

The lungs are the most common location for hematogenous metastases of Wilms' tumor. If pulmonary metastases are present, both lungs should be irradiated regardless of the number or location of the metastases. A dose of 1200 rad is appropriate. The second most common site is the liver. It should be stressed that liver scans may show focal defects secondary to irradiation that can be misinterpreted as metastases. Regenerating liver can produce identical confusion. Thus, it is wise to have tissue confirmation before irradiating the liver. Three thousand rad to liver metastases is delivered over 3 to 4 weeks. If a significant hepatic resection for metastatic disease is undertaken, it must be kept in mind that radiation therapy and chemotherapy begun during the period of liver regeneration can abort the process and lead to severe chronic hepatic impairment (Filler et al., 1969). A large hepatic resection as part of the initial tumor resection may thus not be advisable because it would delay the initiation of postoperative chemotherapy and radiation therapy. It may be wiser to consider hepatic resection if liver involvement does not respond to initial treatment with radiation and chemotherapy (Jenkin, 1976). There are documented cases of patients with both pulmonary and hepatic metastases who have achieved long-term cure by judicious combinations of radiation therapy, chemotherapy, and selective surgery (Smith et al., 1974; Wedemeyer et al., 1968; White and Krivit, 1962).

Wilms' tumor can metastasize to such unlikely sites as the salivary gland and tonsil (Movassaghi et al., 1974), but those instances are rare. It is well to recall that the sarcomatous clear cell tumor tends to metastasize to bone and the rhabdoid lesion tends to metastasize to the brain. Involvement of those organs by a tumor of favorable histology is uncommon. An occasional patient with cerebral metastases will survive after radiation therapy and chemotherapy with or without surgical removal of the tumor (Mohammad et al., 1977; Traggis et al., 1975).

Chemotherapy for metastatic or locally recurrent Wilms' tumor depends on the drugs used before that event. Doxorubicin is the mainstay for children who have received only actinomycin D and vincristine, and it is added to those two drugs. No well-established regimen can be recommended for those who relapse after therapy with actinomycin D, vincristine, and doxorubicin. The addition of cyclophosphamide plus actinomycin D and vincristine was used by Ortega et al. (1980) to retrieve patients who developed metastatic disease while receiving vincristine and actinomycin D. Their regimen used vincristine more intensively than shown in Table 57–6. The United Kingdom Medical Research Council has shown that aggressive use of vincristine is more effective than the usual doses and schedule. Contrariwise, NWTS-3 has not demonstrated any major gain in cases of either favorable or unfavorable histology when cyclophosphamide was added to actinomycin D and vincristine. Those wishing to use these three drugs for children in relapse should therefore follow the specific recommendations of Ortega et al. (1980). DTIC (dimethyltriazeno-imidazole-carboxamide) (Cangir et al., 1976) and cis-platinum (Baum and Gaynon, 1981) may also be useful.

Complications of Chemotherapy and Radiation Therapy. There may be considerable acute and chronic morbidity, and indeed mortality, from the treatment of Wilms' tumor (Mathe and Oldham, 1974; Jaffe et al., 1980). The problem is compounded by the ability of actinomycin D and doxorubicin to potentiate the toxicity of radiotherapy. The infant is at particular risk (Siegel and Moran, 1981). Li et al. (1975) reported on 14 deaths occurring among 140 patients with Wilms' tumor who survived 36 months after diagnosis. Nine died as a result of treatment-associated problems without evidence of any residual cancer. In the second National Wilms' Tumor Study, 2 per cent of the children treated died of causes directly attributable to complications of therapy (D'Angio et al., 1981).

Acute hematologic toxicity due to the effects of chemotherapy on bone marrow is very common and well known and will not be discussed further. Acute gastrointestinal toxicity from chemotherapy, in the form of nausea, vomiting, and diarrhea, is common in the postoperative period, especially in patients who are young or who require total abdominal irradiation. A syndrome of delayed radiation enteritis may appear within a couple of months of completion of radiotherapy. Symptoms include the secondary onset of vomiting and diarrhea with a distended abdomen. It has been reported by Donaldson et al. (1975) that a diet free of lactose, gluten, and bovine protein along with limited dietary fat and residue may be able to improve the malabsorption that is produced by radiation enteritis. Over a longer course, intestinal obstruction may result from intussusception, fibrosis, or postoperative adhesions (Kuffer et al., 1968).

Hepatic toxicity may be acute or long-term, or both. This occurs especially in children with right-sided tumors in whom the radiation field includes a portion of the right lobe of the liver, or when the liver is irradiated as part of total abdominal irradiation. In the first National Wilms' Tumor Study, liver dysfunction was noted in 6 per cent of irradiated children. Initially, there may be a transient hepatic enlargement, abnormalities in liver functions, and a thrombocytopenia with hypoproteinemia and ascites (Jayabose and Lanzkowsky, 1976; McVeagh and Ekert, 1975; Samuels et al., 1971). Selective thrombocytopenia may be a particularly prominent aspect of hepatotoxicity. It is probably the result of platelet entrapment either from radiation-induced hyperemia with hepatic congestion and secondary portal hypertension or from a consumption coagulopathy in the congested liver (Tefft, 1977). Symptoms of liver toxicity may reappear during subsequent treatment with actinomycin D (Tefft et al., 1971) or doxorubicin.

Late orthopedic complications are distressingly frequent, with up to 30 per cent of irradiated children sustaining clinically appreciable sequelae (Katzman et al., 1969; Riseborough et al., 1976). Orthopedic changes are most severe when children under the age of 2 years are treated with high-dose radiation therapy (Neuhauser et al., 1952). Vertebral hypoplasia and scoliosis are produced by the direct effect of radiation therapy. Care is taken at present to treat the entire width of the vertebral bodies in an effort to minimize scoliosis. Even when spinal irradiation is evenly administered, soft tissue fibrosis in an asymmetric fashion may produce tethering, with resulting scoliosis. The lower doses and high-energy beams now being used can be expected to produce less bony damage (Heaston et al., 1979).

Renal problems may also follow radiation of the kidney. Acute changes occur beginning 1 to 2 months after completion of radiotherapy. Potentiating chemotherapeutic agents make the kidney more susceptible (Tefft, 1977). Acutely, the patient may demonstrate microscopic hematuria, azotemia, and edema. It is also possible for chronic nephritis to develop without acute changes having been manifested. Long-term follow-up has indicated that normal renal function usually results after unilateral nephrectomy and combination chemotherapy/radiotherapy if the opposite kidney is not irradiated beyond a dose of 1200 rad (Mitus et al., 1969).

Pulmonary complications are related to the amount of lung treated, the concomitant chemotherapy used, and complicating factors such as infection (Wara et al., 1973). An acute interstitial radiation pneumonitis may begin 1 to 3 months after radiotherapy. There may be no symptoms or a mild cough and fever. Generally, symptoms resolve in less than a month. The long-term effects of pulmonary radiation therapy in children may be an eventual decrease in both lung and chest wall size (Wohl et al., 1975). Fortunately, today these problems are less common than they once were (Littman et al., 1976).

Myocardial damage may occur with the use of doxorubicin, with or without thoracic radiotherapy. The clinical picture is that of congestive heart failure with cardiomegaly, and it is not reversible. Fortunately, this is rare with the doses employed in the NWTS.

The *ovary* is unfortunately quite sensitive to the effects of radiation therapy, and following whole abdomen radiation, ovarian failure may be noted in the postpubertal period (Scott, 1981). This usually presents with poor development of secondary sexual characteristics and primary amenorrhea. FSH and LH levels are elevated. Hormonal replacement therapy may be required. Of those women with preserved fertility, abdominal orthovoltage radiotherapy may predispose to low birth weight infants (Green, 1982). The scatter dose of radiation therapy to the testis may be sufficient to produce oligospermia (Shalet and Beardwell, 1979). Drugs, especially cyclophosphamide, also may contribute to these effects on the ovary and testis (Shalet, 1982).

There have been numerous reports of *secondary neoplasms* occurring in patients treated previously for Wilms' tumor. The exostosis is the most common of the benign tumors. Malignant neoplasms include soft tissue sarcomas, bone tumors (especially osteosarcomas), hepatomas, thyroid carcinomas, and leukemias (Li et al., 1975). Colon cancer also has been reported (Opitz, 1980). Most of these secondary malignancies have developed in fields of prior radiation therapy. The cumulative probability of a second cancer in a long-term survivor of Wilms' tumor treated with radiotherapy has been calculated to be 17 per cent over 5 to 25 years, with a peak incidence at 15 to 19 years after initial diagnosis (Li et al., 1975). Mike and her colleagues (1982) found a lower incidence (3 per cent) among 20-year survivors of Wilms' tumor. It is of interest that the risk of developing a secondary neoplasm may be decreased in patients who received actinomycin D in addition to radiation therapy (D'Angio et al., 1976b). Lifelong surveillance nonetheless is important for those cured of Wilms' tumor.

BILATERAL WILMS' TUMOR

A review of all patients from the National Wilms' Tumor Study entered between 1969 and 1980 by Breslow and Beckwith (1982) reported an incidence of 4.2 per cent with synchronous, and 1.6 per cent with metachronous, bilateral Wilms' tumor. The reviews of bilateral Wilms' tumor undertaken by Bond at the Hospital for Sick Children at Great Ormond Street (1975 *a* and *b*) revealed some interesting epidemiologic characteristics of bilateral, synchronous Wilms' tumors (Table 57–7).

The fact that these tumors can always be demonstrated to exhibit features of nephroblastomatosis may indicate, as Bond has suggested, a major genetic role in the etiology of this

TABLE 57–7. BILATERAL WILMS' TUMOR

	Unilateral	Bilateral
Distribution	Unifocal (usual)	Multifocal (nephroblastomatosis)
Patient age (average)	42 months	15 months
Maternal age (average)	28 years	34 years
Associated anomalies	4%	45%
Inheritance	Sporadic	? Dominant

tumor. When metachronous, the tumors can be separated by as much as 10 years. These are believed to be separate primary tumors rather than the result of metastatic spread, a belief supported by the fact that although metastases from Wilms' tumor usually are first seen in the lung, in patients with bilateral renal involvement, pulmonary metastases are seldom seen at diagnosis (D'Angio et al., 1976a).

Bilateral tumors usually exhibit favorable histologic features. When synchronous, the tumors have an excellent prognosis with an 87 per cent survival rate, as opposed to a 40 per cent survival rate when the tumors arise metachronously (Jones, 1982; Malcolm et al., 1980).

There has been no uniform treatment scheme for patients with synchronous bilateral Wilms' tumors. Of the 30 patients reviewed by Bishop et al. (1977), 26 (87 per cent) survived in spite of the fact that only 25 per cent had complete excision of all tumor at one or more operations. All were treated with chemotherapy and most with radiation therapy.

Surgical approaches have varied, but, in general, the most involved side was excised with marking of the contralateral tumor after biopsy. A second-look operation was then carried out after chemotherapy or radiation therapy, or both. Altman et al. (1977) have employed bench surgery successfully. Bilateral nephrectomy and renal transplantation may also be used. The results, however, have not been as good as those in patients treated conservatively with limited surgery and combination radiation and chemotherapy (DeLorimier et al., 1971). If transplantation is contemplated, some advocate a waiting period of as long as 2 years to be certain that no metastatic disease is present (Penn, 1979). The continued advances being made in the chemotherapy realm make it difficult to justify such an aggressive surgical posture. Rather, we would support Bishop and his colleagues (1977), who recommend bilateral biopsies followed by chemotherapy with actinomycin D plus vincristine. Radiation therapy or doxorubicin can be added if prompt shrinkage does not occur. Re-exploration is performed when the bulk of disease has been significantly reduced. We have seen quite massive tumors shrink to sizes treatable by partial nephrectomy with this approach. The goal is to preserve as much functional parenchyma as possible without compromising the survival expectancy (Wasiljew et al., 1982).

The Future

The history of the treatment of Wilms' tumor has been one of the success stories of pediatric oncology, and the future offers hope for further advances. From the surgeon's standpoint, the experience with partial nephrectomy in bilateral Wilms' tumor is beginning to suggest that total nephrectomy may not be required in children with unilateral disease either. The goal of the third National Wilms' Tumor Study is to minimize chemotherapy and radiation therapy for patients who have a favorable prognosis. This may enable us to reduce the morbidity produced by these treatment modalities even further. Conversely, patients with a poor prognosis are being treated more intensively with new chemotherapy regimens in an effort to salvage more of these difficult cases. Because nodal disease carries an ominous prognosis and is difficult to ascertain at operation by nodal palpation, studies are under way to determine if a systematic node dissection for Wilms' tumor will result in better staging, and thus treatment, of patients. Most important, epidemiologic studies are in progress seeking to determine possible environmental and genetic causes of Wilms' tumor. One would hope that prevention of at least some of these cases may some day be achieved.

OTHER RENAL TUMORS OF CHILDHOOD

Primary renal neoplasms of childhood other than Wilms' tumor are rare; *renal cell carcinoma* is the most common of them. Although it is the most frequent malignant tumor of the kidney in adults, it constitutes less than 7 per cent of all renal tumors in those under 21 years of age. Most children with renal cell carcinoma are 5 years of age or older at diagnosis, but cases in the first year of life have been reported (Castellanos et al., 1974). The signs and symptoms are the same as in the adult: hematuria, abdominal or flank pain, an abdominal mass, or nonspecific symptoms such as weight loss, anorexia, and fever. Intravenous pyelography reveals calyceal deformation resembling Wilms' tumor, but calcifications are more common. The metastatic spread of renal cell carcinoma is to regional lymph nodes, bones, lungs, and liver. Renal vascular invasion or the absence of a pseudocapsule around the tumor is an ominous anatomic feature (Dehner et al., 1970).

Most renal cell carcinomas in children appear to be sporadic cases, as in the adult, but some families with an increased incidence have been reported. The tumor, in one family with ten involved members, appeared to be passed as an autosomal dominant trait with a characteristic chromosomal translocation (Cohen et al., 1979). An increased incidence of renal cell carcinoma has also been reported in patients with von Hippel–Lindau disease and polycystic kidney disease (Kantor, 1977). Reviews of renal cell carcinoma in childhood by Raney et al. (1983), Castellanos et al. (1974), and Dehner et al. (1970) reveal an overall survival rate of about 50 per cent. The outlook seems best in children under 11 years of age and in those with Stage I lesions. All six children under 11 years of age and all five with Stage I lesions survived in the series reported by Raney et al. (1983). Radiation therapy, chemotherapy, and hormonal therapy did little, if anything, to improve survival over that produced by nephrectomy alone. At present, the most effective treatment appears to be a radical nephrectomy with regional lymph node dissection.

In 1980, Chatten et al. reported two male infants with what was termed *ossifying tumor of the infantile kidney*. The infants presented with hematuria and were found to have small calcified renal masses that appeared to be calculi. At histologic examination, there were dense cores of bone surrounded by a periphery of undifferentiated cells firmly adherent to the renal parenchyma. The authors postulate that these tumors were derived from urothelium rather than from metanephric blastema, and that this tumor was a separate benign pediatric renal tumor distinct from Wilms' tumor.

There are additional very rare primary intrarenal tumors in children, including neuroblastoma, rhabdomyosarcoma, leiomyosarcoma, fibroma, hemangiopericytoma, cholesteatoma, lymphangioma, and hamartoma. The diagnosis of these tumors is rarely made prior to histologic examination. The renal *angiomyolipoma* is a form of hamartoma usually seen in adulthood but rarely occurring in childhood (Bennington and Beckwith, 1975). This tumor is very common in patients with tuberous sclerosis and may be bilateral. Diagnostic and therapeutic measures are similar to those used in adults. Although more commonly found in the pararenal retroperitoneal space, *teratomas* may rarely present as an intrarenal tumor.

By far the most common *secondary tumor* seen in the kidney is involvement produced by non-Hodgkin's lymphoma or leukemia. Tumor involvement is generally diffuse. Unlike the other non-Wilms' renal tumors discussed, treatment consists of radiation therapy or chemotherapy, or both.

Although rare, both benign and malignant tumors of the renal pelvis and ureter have been reported. Ureteral lesions are most commonly benign fibrous polyps located in the upper third of the ureter. Symptoms usually consist of intermittent pain from obstruction. Treatment is by local excision with a ureteroureterostomy or ureteropyelostomy (Colgan et al., 1973). Very rarely, a transitional epithelial cancer of the renal pelvis will be seen in infancy or childhood (Koyanagi et al., 1975).

NEUROBLASTOMA

History

In 1864 Virchow was the first to characterize neuroblastoma, which he labeled a glioma. Marchand in 1891 commented on the histologic similarities between neuroblastoma and developing sympathetic ganglia. Herxheimer (1914), using a specific neural silver stain, showed that fibrils in neuroblastoma shared staining characteristics with nervous tissue. This contributed to establishing the tissue of origin of this tumor.

The biochemical aspects of neuroblastoma began to be understood as Mason et al. (1957) reported the presence of pressor amines in the urine of a child with neuroblastoma. Subsequently, we have come to recognize elevated levels of norepinephrine and its precursors and metabolites in the urine of patients with this tumor.

Another landmark in our understanding of neuroblastoma came in 1927 when Cushing and Wolbach reported for the first time a transformation of neuroblastoma into benign ganglioneuroma. Everson and Cole (1966) noted that this generally occurred in infants under the age of 6 months. That spontaneous regression of neuroblastoma may be more common than is clinically evident was suggested by Beckwith and Perrin (1963), who noted microscopic clusters of neuroblastoma cells in the adrenal glands of a number of infants under 3 months of age who had died of other causes. These foci of tumor cells they called neuroblastoma in situ. They estimated neuroblastoma in situ to occur about 40 times more frequently than the number of cases of neuroblastoma clinically diagnosed. Under normal circumstances, recession appeared usually to be complete after 3 months of age.

Etiology

Although the cause of neuroblastoma, as for most other carcinomas, is unknown, it arises from cells of the neural crest that form the sympathetic ganglia and adrenal medulla. Bolande (1979) has termed this tumor a type of neurocristopathy. Other neurocristopathies include pheochromocytoma, paraganglioma, medullary carcinoma of the thyroid, carcinoid, melanoma, neurocutaneous melanosis, neurofibromatosis, and multiple endocrine neoplasia. Sympathetic nervous system tumors can apparently differentiate along two lines: the pheochromocytoma line and the sympathoblastoma line. It is this latter line that forms neuroblastoma, ganglioneuroblastoma, and ganglioneuroma.

There appears to be a genetic influence in this tumor. Knudson and Strong (1972) have suggested that approximately 20 per cent of cases arise in children predisposed to the tumor by a dominant transmittable mutation. Knudson and Meadows (1976) have suggested that familial cases result from a prezygotic mutation and the nonfamilial ones from a postzygotic somatic mutation. Rare families having more than one member affected with this tumor have been described (Chatten and Vorhees, 1967; Arenson et al., 1976).

Incidence

Neuroblastoma is the most common malignant tumor of infancy and, after brain tumors, the most common malignant solid tumor of childhood (Young and Miller, 1975). Neuroblastoma accounts for 6 to 8 per cent of all childhood malignancies. In the United States, the incidence is 9.6 per million in white children and 7.0 per million in black children per year. There is a slight male predominance of 1.1:1 (Miller et al., 1968). It should be remembered that the actual incidence is much higher than reported because of the proclivity for spontaneous regression of neuroblastoma in situ.

Although neuroblastoma may occur throughout childhood and occasionally in adulthood, the tumor usually develops early in life. Fifty per cent of the cases occur in children under the age of 2 years, and over 75 per cent of cases have been encountered by the fourth year of life (Peterson et al., 1969; Fortner et al., 1968). This is a younger age of distribution than that of Wilms' tumor. Unlike Wilms' tumor, neuroblastoma has a low incidence of associated congenital anomalies. One exception is an increased incidence of brain and skull defects, approaching 2 per cent in children with neuroblastoma (Miller et al., 1968). There also is an association with neurofibromatosis and Hirschsprung's disease (Hope et al., 1965; Knudson and Amromin, 1966).

Pathology

Neuroblastoma. On gross examination, small tumors usually are well encapsulated and firm. On cut surface, the tumor is fairly soft and lobulated, with a grayish-to-pink color. The tumor has a tendency to break through its pseudocapsule and infiltrate surrounding tissues. When it does, it generally is found to be friable and very soft, with hemorrhage and necrosis. Cystic areas may be present.

Histologically, neuroblastoma is one of the small round cell tumors of childhood. There is a similarity by light microscopy between neuroblasts, lymphocytes, and the cells of lymphomas, embryonal myosarcomas, and Ewing's sarcomas. When the tumor cells can be seen to form themselves into rosettes and neurofibrils are evident, the degree of differentiation is quite good and the tumor is recognizable as a neuroblastoma. Unfortunately, these signs are often absent. Ewing's sarcoma and rhabdomyosarcoma usually contain glycogen, which can be seen by PAS staining. Neuroblastoma lacks glycogen. Neuroblastoma cells may be recognized by the use of a rapid fluorescence assay for intracellular catecholamines or tissue culture assay for neurite outgrowth (Reynolds et al., 1981). Neuron-specific enolase staining of tumor has also been reported by Odelstad et al. (1982) to be fairly specific for neuroblastoma. This test is useful to separate neuroblastoma from poorly differentiated Wilms' tumor. The importance of this is the different responses of these neoplasms to chemotherapy.

The ultrastructure of neuroblastoma is

quite distinctive and reflects the neural crest derivation of neuroblasts. Characteristic peripheral dendritic processes that contain longitudinally oriented microtubules are seen. Small spherical membrane-coated granules with electron dense cores representing cytoplasmic accumulations of catecholamines are seen. The larger number of granules seen in some tumors reflects a higher degree of differentiation and has been reported by Romansky et al. (1978) to be a favorable prognostic factor. Conventional microscopy, occasionally supplemented by electron microscopy, usually enables a bone marrow aspirate to be diagnosed as neuroblastoma, avoiding the need for an open biopsy in a child with disseminated disease.

Efforts have been made to correlate the histologic grade of a tumor with its biologic behavior. It has been suggested that the presence of abundant cytoplasm and cystoplasmic processes, vesicular nuclei, mature ganglion cells, and rosette formation suggests better differentiation of the tumor and carries a more favorable prognosis (Makinen, 1972). Beckwith and Martin (1968) suggested that if at least 5 per cent of the cellular elements demonstrated eosinophilic cytoplasm, nerve processes, or large nuclei, the prognosis would be more favorable. By these criteria, tumors were graded from 1 to 4, with 4 being most undifferentiated. Unfortunately, histologic grading has not measured up to expectations because of the many exceptions that have been found and the high incidence of tumors with poor differentiation (Koop and Schnaufer, 1975).

Recently, a grading system devised by Shimada, which includes the number of mitotic cells per high-power field among other characteristics, has proved to have significant prognostic value in patients with local and regional neuroblastoma (Littman et al., 1984).

Ganglioneuroma. At the other end of the spectrum of neuroblastoma lies its benign counterpart, the ganglioneuroma. By definition, these tumors do not metastasize, but they can become quite large, with projections that envelop adjacent structures and occasionally extend through intervertebral foramina to produce neurologic symptoms through cord compression. On cut surface, they tend to be firmer and better encapsulated than neuroblastoma. Histologically, they are composed of large mature ganglion cells with abundant cytoplasm and a large nucleus. They are scattered through a collagen-rich background with bundles of neurofibrils.

Ganglioneuroblastoma. This tumor is intermediate between neuroblastoma and ganglioneuroma. Histologically, there are grades of ganglioneuroblastoma exhibiting the full spectrum from benign ganglioneuroma to malignant neuroblastoma. Attempts have been made to correlate prognosis with the degree of differentiation (Makinen, 1972). Unfortunately, most have reported a poor correlation between the histology of ganglioneuroblastomas and prognosis (Adam and Hochholzer, 1981). About 20 per cent of ganglioneuroblastomas metastasize in the form of neuroblastoma. Indeed, there is no firm correlation between the degree of differentiation of the primary tumor and the degree of differentiation found in metastatic lesions.

Location, Presentation, and Differential Diagnosis

Because neuroblastomas and their more benign variants may occur anywhere along the sympathetic chain from the head to the pelvis, their presentation and differential diagnosis will vary with the site of tumor origin (Fig. 57–10). Over half of neuroblastomas have their origin

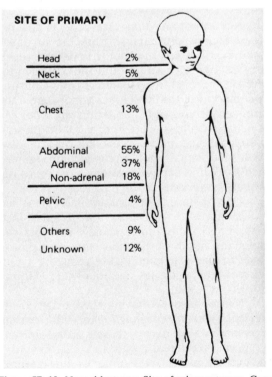

Figure 57–10. Neuroblastoma: Site of primary tumor. Composite data from the literature. (From Williams, T. E., and Donaldson, M. H.: Neuroblastoma. In Sutow, W. W., Vietti, T. J., and Fernback, D. J. (Eds.): Clinical Pediatric Oncology. St. Louis, The C. V. Mosby Co., 1973, p. 388. Used by permission.)

in the abdomen, and two thirds of these arise in the adrenal. When a tumor originates in the adrenal, there is less likelihood of metastases than from nonadrenal abdominal paravertebral sites. A mass is the most common presenting symptom. It is characteristically an irregular, firm, nontender, fixed mass, often extending beyond the midline. This is in contrast to Wilms' tumor, which usually presents with a smooth flank mass not crossing the midline.

Neuroblastoma that arises from an *abdominal paravertebral sympathetic ganglion* has a higher likelihood of growing through an intervertebral foramen to form a dumbbell-shaped tumor compressing the spinal cord (Akwari et al., 1978; Traggis et al., 1977). In about 40 per cent of these cases, the intraspinal component will be asymptomatic. Paravertebral tumors should always be evaluated for possible intraspinal extension. Prompt recognition may prevent permanent neurologic sequelae. Early neurosurgical intervention is warranted, as patients with these dumbbell neuroblastomas generally have an excellent prognosis. It is interesting that these tumors may be more mature or even completely benign within the spinal canal and less mature in their abdominal extension. They must be differentiated from primary intraspinal tumors.

Neuroblastoma may also arise in the *presacral* region, presumably from the organs of Zukerkandl. Here the tumor may lead to urinary frequency or retention from extrinsic pressure on the bladder (Hepler, 1976). Constipation may also result. These tumors are quite rare, constituting only approximately 4 per cent of neuroblastomas. The differential diagnosis of abdominal and pelvic neuroblastoma involves other abdominal and retroperitoneal tumors such as Wilms' tumor, teratomas, or more rare primary neoplasms in the pancreas or liver.

One of the rarest primary sites for a neuroblastoma is the *olfactory bulb* (esthesioneuroblastoma). This tumor usually presents with unilateral nasal obstruction and epistaxis. It tends to be seen later in life than the typical neuroblastoma arising in other sites (Homzie and Elkon, 1980).

Neuroblastomas having their origin in the *cervical sympathetic ganglion* account for approximately 5 per cent of these tumors. Horner's syndrome may result, with a sinking inward of the eyeball, ptosis of the upper eyelid, elevation of the lower eyelid, pupillary constriction, narrowing of the palpebral fissure, and anhidrosis. Because the sympathetic nervous system is involved with the development of pigmentation in

the iris, neuroblastoma affecting the ophthalmic sympathetic nerves can lead to heterochromia iridis, an unequal color between the two irises. Both syndromes may occur together (Jaffe et al., 1975). Hoarseness may indicate compression of the recurrent laryngeal nerve by tumor. Cervical neuroblastoma may present as a neck mass and must be differentiated from branchial cleft cysts, benign adenopathy, lymphoma, leukemia, and other malignant tumors found in the neck.

Thoracic neuroblastoma, accounting for 13 per cent of all neuroblastomas, may become massive before becoming clinically evident. It is often discovered by radiographs taken for the diagnosis of an unrelated disease. There may be cough, dyspnea, or pulmonary infection from tracheal or bronchial compression. The superior vena cava may be compressed. Weakness of an upper extremity may indicate brachial plexus involvement. There may be pain in the neck, back, abdomen, or pelvis caused by a dumbbell extension of the tumor to produce spinal cord compression. In the posterior mediastinum, neuroblastoma must be differentiated from teratomas, esophageal duplications, and bronchogenic cysts.

In its early stages, neuroblastoma is usually a silent tumor. *Metastatic* dissemination of the tumor may occur early and does not appear to be related to the size of the primary lesion. Up to 70 per cent of patients have metastatic disease at the time of diagnosis (Gross et al., 1959). In the young, metastases tend to go to the liver; in older children, bony metastases are more common. Unexplained fever, general malaise, anorexia, weight loss, irritability, bone pain, and pallor secondary to anemia are all common manifestations of widespread disease. Occasionally, such symptoms may be noted without evidence of dissemination. The high incidence of disseminated disease with neuroblastoma accounts for the more frequent presentation of a generally unwell child, this is in contradistinction to the child with Wilms' tumor, who is usually robust.

The liver suffers the brunt of metastatic dissemination, especially in the infant (Fig. 57–11A). The tumor may present as a rapidly growing hepatic neoplasm that may embarrass respiration (Bond, 1976). Primary hepatoblastoma must be ruled out.

Often, the first symptoms from neuroblastoma reflect *bony involvement*. The skull and long bones are most commonly involved. Metastatic disease usually occurs in the diaphysis and may be bilaterally symmetric. By x-ray, metastases appear as lytic defects with an irreg-

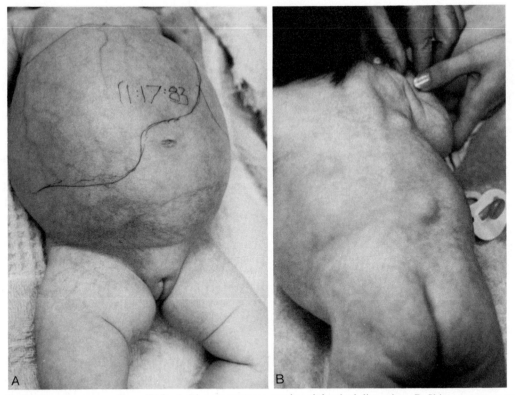

Figure 57–11. Neuroblastoma: Stage IV-S. *A,* Liver metastases causing abdominal distention. *B,* Skin metastases on back.

ular margin and some periosteal reaction. Symptoms may include local bone pain or a limp. Metastatic bone lesions must be differentiated from primary bone tumors, lymphoreticular malignancies, and infectious processes.

Over 50 per cent of children with neuroblastoma have *bone marrow involvement,* even in the absence of x-ray evidence of change in the bone (Finklestein et al., 1970). Bone marrow replacement with depletion of one or more cell lines in the peripheral blood may lead to the incorrect diagnosis of aplastic anemia or other diseases that may cause thrombocytopenia or anemia (Quinn and Altman, 1979). Neuroblastoma cells in the bone marrow can usually be distinguished from leukemic infiltration because neuroblastoma appears in small clusters and may exhibit rosettes and neurofibrils. Electron microscopy, as mentioned earlier, may occasionally be useful in distinguishing neuroblastoma from other malignancies that invade the bone marrow.

Subcutaneous nodules (Fig. 57–11*B*) are also a common metastatic pattern for neuroblastoma. They often have a bluish color and have been likened to blueberry muffins. Such subcutaneous nodules have been reported in up

to one third of neonates with neuroblastoma (Schneider et al., 1965). These skin lesions may become erythematous for several minutes after palpation and then blanch, presumably as a result of vasoconstriction secondary to catecholamine release from the tumor cells. When present, this reaction may be a diagnostic sign of neuroblastoma (Hawthorne et al., 1970). These nodules must be differentiated from leukemic infiltrates of the skin.

Periorbital metastatic disease is also common in children with neuroblastoma (Fig. 57–12). Retrobulbar soft tissue involvement may cause periorbital edema and proptosis. Periorbital ecchymoses may give a "raccoonlike" appearance to the child. Ecchymosis typically occurs in the upper eyelid. This is in contradistinction to lower eyelid ecchymosis, which is more commonly seen with trauma.

Certain organs including the heart, lungs, brain, and spinal cord, are rarely the site of metastases. Pulmonary metastases are occasionally seen in very advanced disease secondary to extensive lymphatic spread or direct growth through the diaphragm.

Occasionally, children are seen whose symptoms are produced by the *biochemical ac-*

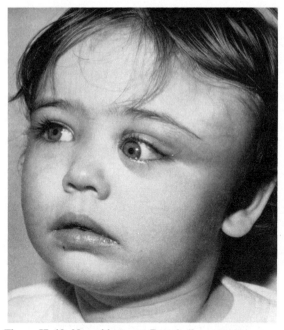

Figure 57–12. Neuroblastoma: Retrobulbar metastases producing proptosis.

tivity of the tumor. As neural crest tumors, neuroblastomas usually secrete *catecholamines.* Occasional children are seen with paroxysmal attacks of sweating, pallor, headaches, hypertension, palpatations, and flushing. Voute et al. (1970) have even reported six mothers who had these symptoms in the eighth and ninth months of pregnancy and were subsequently delivered of infants diagnosed as having neuroblastoma during the first few months of life. The mother's symptoms presumably were caused by fetal catecholamines entering the maternal circulation. When symptoms of catecholamine release are prominent, neuroblastoma may simulate pheochromocytoma.

Children have also presented with persistent, intractable, watery diarrhea and hypokalemia. This has now been found to be due to tumor secretion of an enterohormone known as *vasoactive intestinal peptide* (VIP) (Mitchell et al., 1976; El Shafie et al., 1983). It has now been demonstrated that a variety of other tumors besides neuroblastoma secrete VIP, including pancreatic tumors and bronchogenic carcinoma. Pearse (1978) has suggested that these tumors have a common ancestor cell in the neural crest. The tumors share cytochemical characteristics. The most important is the ability to absorb amines from the environment and convert them into hormones or hormone-like products. This ability is referred to as APUD (amine precursor uptake and decarboxylation), and these tumors are thus termed apudomas.

One of the most interesting systemic manifestations of neuroblastoma is *acute myoclonic encephalopathy.* This is seen in approximately 2 per cent of children with neuroblastoma. The syndrome consists of rapid multidirectional eye movements (opsoclonus), myoclonus, and truncal ataxia in the absence of increased intracranial pressure (Senelick et al., 1973). Although it was initially felt that the encephalopathy was caused by a toxic neurologic effect of circulating catecholamine catabolites, at least one child has been reported who developed this neurologic symptom 7 months after removal of a primary tumor and return to normal of previously elevated levels of urinary catecholamines (Delalieux et al., 1975). An alternative explanation may be the existence of an autoimmune factor—perhaps an antibody directed against a neuroblastoma antigen that is cross-reacting with a common antigen in the cells of the cerebellum, resulting in damage (Bray et al., 1969). Tumors associated with this syndrome are often located in the thorax, are well differentiated, and are associated with a good prognosis (Altman and Baehner, 1976).

On rare occasions, a neonate presents with a rare syndrome that may mimic *erythroblastosis.* Massive metastasis to the liver and bone marrow may produce jaundice, anemia, and hepatosplenomegaly. This syndrome may mimic hemolytic disease in the newborn. Two patients with congenital neuroblastoma metastatic to the liver and placenta who were thought to have hydrops fetalis have been reported by Anders et al. (1973).

From the foregoing descriptions of the multiple possible sites and presentation of neuroblastoma, it should be readily evident why this tumor has been referred to as the great mimicker. A prepared mind is a requisite for making a proper diagnosis in many of these enigmatic cases (Jaffe, 1976).

Diagnostic Evaluation

Hematologic Studies. The complete blood count (CBC) is usually normal in a child with neuroblastoma until the disease becomes disseminated. With dissemination, anemia may be present owing to bone marrow involvement by tumor or hemorrhage into the tumor. Rarely, thrombocytopenia may be seen because of bone marrow involvement or platelet trapping in the tumor. Liver involvement may cause a bleeding diathesis through disseminated intravascular coagulopathy. The erythrocyte sedimentation rate is usually raised in the child with systemic disease.

Bone marrow aspiration is indicated in every suspected case of neuroblastoma. As many as 70 per cent of bone marrow aspirates in patients with neuroblastoma have been reported to be positive (Finklestein et al., 1970). While it is not unusual to find tumor cells in the bone marrow aspirate with no evidence of skeletal metastases, occasionally a patient may demonstrate widespread bony metastases with no cells in the marrow. As discussed earlier under pathologic aspects of the tumor, neuroblastoma will frequently form pseudorosettes in the bone marrow. This helps to separate neuroblastoma in the marrow from such other processes as leukemia and metastatic carcinomas such as lymphosarcoma, retinoblastoma, Ewing's sarcoma, and other small round cell tumors that have a proclivity to metastasize to bone. In the child with disseminated disease, careful evaluation of the bone marrow may obviate the need for an open biopsy of the tumor.

Catecholamine Excretion. Since the first report of urinary catecholamine excretion in neuroblastoma was made by Mason et al. in 1957, much attention has been given to the biochemical products of this tumor. The two major metabolites of catecholamine production by neuroblastoma are vanillylmandelic acid (VMA) and homovanillic acid (HVA). Williams and Greer (1963) have reported 95 per cent of patients with neuroblastoma to have an elevated urinary excretion of VMA or HVA, or both. Occasional patients with no elevation of catecholamine excretion are seen (Voorhees, 1971). Tumors in these individuals are most commonly found in the thorax and probably have arisen from dorsal spinal nerve roots and ganglia that are nonsecretors of catecholamines. There is no correlation between the pattern of catecholamine excretion and the age of patients, symptomatology, or histologic pattern.

As hypertension is not common in neuroblastoma, it is interesting to speculate why elevated catecholamine production does not lead to clinical symptoms in most cases. It may be that norepinephrine is catabolized within the tumor and thus does not become systemically active (LaBrosse and Karon, 1962). Also, it is possible that the initial enzyme in catecholamine synthesis, tyrosine hydrolase (TH), is subject to normal feedback inhibition by norepinephrine, dopamine and dopa (Imashuku et al., 1971).

This may help to explain why high levels of serum norepinephrine and hypertension are uncommon in neuroblastoma. This is in contrast to pheochromocytoma, in which there are excessive amounts of TH present because of lack of normal feedback inhibition.

Although quantitative determination of all catecholamines and their metabolites in a 24-hour urine collection is clearly the most accurate method of biochemical diagnosis of neuroblastoma, the collection of 24-hour urine specimens in infants and small children is difficult. This led Gitlow et al. (1970) to propose the simultaneous assay of VMA and/or HVA and creatinine in a single spot urine specimen. The upper limits of normal have been found to be 20 µg/mg of creatinine for VMA and 40 µg/mg of creatinine for HVA. While this is a very accurate diagnostic approach, it is also quite cumbersome. In 1968, LaBrosse developed a filter paper spot test for VMA in the urine. This test has approximately 75 per cent positivity when used in the diagnosis and follow-up of patients with neuroblastoma (Evans et al., 1971a). There is, however, general agreement that VMA screening tests, although useful, lack total reliability and that confirmation by specific quantitative assays is important (Johnsonbaugh and Cahill, 1975).

As will be discussed later, urinary levels of catecholamines are of importance in following neuroblastoma. The persistence, reappearance, or development of elevated urinary catecholamines during or after therapy suggests a poor prognosis (De Gutierrez Moyano et al., 1971). LaBrosse et al. (1976) reported that when initially elevated urinary metabolites returned to normal, 80 to 82 per cent of patients survived. Urinary excretion remained elevated in 4 to 5 per cent of survivors but in 90 to 95 per cent of those who died.

Cystathionine and carcinoembryonic antigen have also been described to be elevated in patients with neuroblastoma. The lack of specificity of these products for neuroblastoma, however, has limited the clinical usefulness of urinary assays.

Imaging. Appropriate roentgenographic and nuclear medicine diagnostic studies are useful to localize the site of primary disease as well as to define the presence and extent of metastatic spread. For abdominal tumors, an *intravenous pyelogram* should be routinely carried out. With a suprarenal neuroblastoma, the kidney is characteristically displaced inferiorly and laterally with maintenance of a normal calyceal pattern (Figs. 57–13 and 57–14). This is in

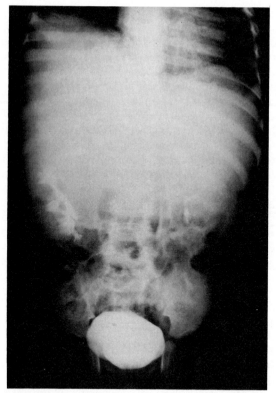

Figure 57–13. Neuroblastoma: Intravenous pyelogram showing inferior and lateral displacement of right kidney by adrenal neuroblastoma.

contrast to an intrarenal Wilms' tumor, which distorts the calyceal pattern. Very rarely, intrarenal neuroblastoma will closely mimic Wilms' tumor (Gibbons and Duckett, 1979). An abdominal paravertebral neuroblastoma may displace the ureter laterally. Occasionally, there will be delayed visualization or nonvisualization of the kidney if ureteral obstruction is present. Calcification in a characteristically speckled pattern can be seen in 50 per cent of patients by plain films (Fig. 57–14). Computerized axial tomography can pick up calcification in an additional 30 per cent. This speckled pattern contrasts with the less frequent calcification seen with Wilms' tumor, which tends to be curvilinear.

Ultrasonography may be very useful in determining the exact location of an intra-abdominal primary tumor. The ability of ultrasound to evaluate the retroperitoneum may give evidence of direct spread or nodal involvement. The cava is well visualized by ultrasound and is often anteriorly displaced. Complete obstruction or tumor invasion of the cava is rare. The liver can be examined, making a liver scan usually unnecessary. *Computerized axial tomography* adds little to the information that can be gained from the IVP and abdominal ultrasound and is rarely justified.

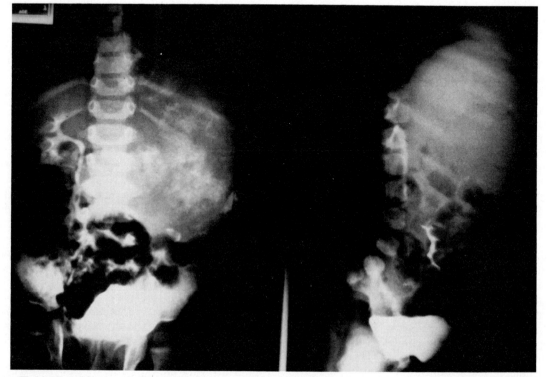

Figure 57–14. Neuroblastoma: Left suprarenal tumor with characteristic speckled calcification. Intravenous pyelogram (PA and lateral) shows inferior and lateral displacement of kidney.

A *chest x-ray* should be routinely carried out. Careful examination of the posterior mediastinum in patients with abdominal tumors is important, as extension can take place through the diaphragm. Thoracic neuroblastomas are second in frequency to abdominal tumors. Usually the tumor is in the posterior mediastinum. Both sides of the thorax are affected equally, and calcification is seen in about half the cases. Oblique views as well as anterior and posterior ones are important to detect dumbbell tumors with invasion of the neural foramina. The posterior portion of the ribs may be separated and the ribs themselves narrowed by erosion.

As metastatic involvement of the skeleton is so common, a *skeletal survey* should be routinely included in the evaluation of a patient with neuroblastoma. Bony metastases occur most commonly in the skull and in the diaphyses of the distal tubular bones, the femur and humerus. Metastatic spread is rare distal to the elbow and knee. Metastases may also be seen in the ribs, scapula, vertebral bodies, or pelvis. The distribution of metastases is often both bilateral and symmetric but rarely involves epiphyses. The lesions are usually lytic and irregular with periosteal reaction. Occasionally, a pathologic fracture occurs. The degree of involvement varies from barely perceptible to massive. A radionuclear *bone scan* may be useful in detecting disease not seen by radiographic bone survey (D'Angio et al., 1969).

Arteriography and venography are not generally required in the evaluation of patients with neuroblastoma.

Staging

Accurate staging of patients with neuroblastoma is of critical importance both for the information this provides regarding prognosis and for the determination of the extent of treatment to be employed. Although in the 1960's a number of staging systems for neuroblastoma were proposed, the one advocated by Evans et al. (1971) is in widest clinical use today (Table 57–8).

For tumors that arise in midline structures such as the sympathetic tissue at the origin of the inferior mesenteric artery (organs of Zuckerkandl), extension beyond the capsule and involvement of lymph nodes on the same side is considered Stage II disease. Bilateral extension of any type is considered Stage III.

Stage IV-S (Fig. 57–11) is a unique form of disseminated disease that occurs most com-

TABLE 57–8. STAGING OF NEUROBLASTOMA

Stage 0	Neuroblastoma in situ
Stage I	Tumors confined to the organ or structure of origin
Stage II	Tumors extending in continuity beyond the organ or structure of origin but not crossing the midline. The regional lymph nodes on the ipsilateral side may be involved.
Stage III	Tumors extending in continuity beyond the midline. Regional lymph nodes may be involved bilaterally.
Stage IV	Distant metastases involving bones, bone marrow, brain, skin, liver, lung, soft tissues, or distant lymph node groups.*
Stage IV-S	Patients who would otherwise be Stage I or II but who have remote spread of tumor confined to one or more of the following sites: liver, skin, or bone marrow (without roentgenographic evidence of bone metastases on complete skeletal survey).†

*These patients usually have elevated ferritin levels and E-rosette inhibitory factor, which helps to distinguish these patients from those who are Stage IV-S.

†Inclusion of bone marrow disease in this stage may not be justifiable. If the marrow is extensively involved, the prognosis is probably poor.

monly in infancy. In contradistinction to Stage IV neuroblastoma, which has an approximate 5 per cent survival rate, Stage IV-S has a survival rate in the order of 80 per cent (D'Angio et al., 1971). These children usually appear to have robust good health and lack the malaise, weight loss, fever, and anemia that are often seen with typical Stage IV disseminated disease. Disease in children with IV-S neuroblastoma is limited to the liver, skin, or bone marrow. There is no x-ray evidence of bony metastases. Although local tumor growth may rarely cause serious problems, generally the tumor regresses spontaneously without treatment, and these infants have an excellent prognosis.

The Evans classification continues to be the most widely used one because of its clinical applicability. As will be discussed, other factors are critical to the prognosis of neuroblastoma, but a staging system incorporating them would become so unwieldy as to be impractical.

Prognostic Factors and Survival

A number of variables determine the prognosis for neuroblastoma. In general, survival for 2 years with no evidence of disease is equivalent to cure (Gross et al., 1959; DeLorimier et al.,

1969). Occasional later deaths have been reported, and chemotherapy may have prolonged somewhat the lives of some children with disease without influencing overall survival.

The *stage of disease* is an important prognostic factor and appears to be independent of age at diagnosis or site of the tumor (Coldman et al., 1980). When the disease is localized (Stages I and II), survival rates of 80 per cent can be expected. Disseminated disease of the IV-S type also has a similar survival rate. In contrast, Stage III disease has a survival of approximately 37 per cent and Stage IV, 5 to 7 per cent (Breslow and McCann, 1971; Grosfeld, 1983).

In neuroblastoma, survival is inversely correlated with *age at diagnosis* (Sutow, 1958). In the review of Breslow and McCann (1971), children under 1 year of age had a survival rate of 74 per cent. Between 12 and 23 months, survival was 26 per cent, and in those over 2 years of age it was only 12 per cent. Spontaneous remission of neuroblastoma appears to be most likely in children under 6 months of age. Interestingly, there are now accumulating data that may indicate that survival expectancy improves for children who present over the age of 6 years (Evans, 1980; Sather et al., 1981). Nonetheless, only approximately one child in four with neuroblastoma in this age group will survive.

The *site of origin* is also a factor of prognostic significance. Coldman et al. (1980) have reported that nonadrenal abdominal tumors have a greater likelihood of survival than adrenal primary tumors. This appears to be independent of age and stage. Mediastinal neuroblastoma, even when there is node involvement, Horner's syndrome, bony erosion, or cord compression, also has an improved prognosis (Filler et al., 1972). This may be due to the fact that tumors above the diaphragm usually are less disseminated at presentation (Evans et al., 1976). Five-year actuarial survival rates for posterior mediastinal tumors have been reported to be as high as 88 per cent (Adam and Hochholzer, 1981). Neuroblastoma that originates in the neck or pelvis also has an improved prognosis, perhaps because these tumors become symptomatic early in their course and are diagnosed before dissemination occurs.

Beckwith and Martin (1968) developed a *histopathologic grading* for neuroblastoma and attempted to correlate the degree of histologic differentiation with survival. Their data suggested a direct correlation between degree of histologic differentiation and survival. With well- or moderately differentiated tumors, 30 per cent of patients survived 2 years, in contrast to only 9 per cent of those with poorly differentiated tumors. In the minds of many pathologists, this classification is difficult to apply clinically because of the degree of variability in histologic criteria, sampling errors, and difficulty in quantifying the mixed cell populations.

Laug et al. (1978) correlated the prognosis of children with neuroblastoma with the urinary *VMA/HVA ratio*. Although the absolute amounts of these two compounds do not influence the prognosis, a higher level of VMA compared with HVA appears to indicate a better outcome. Thus, the higher the VMA/HVA ratio, the better the prognosis. LaBrosse et al. (1976) pointed out that the periodic study of urinary VMA and HVA during the course of treatment is of prognostic value. If urinary catecholamines remain elevated, the prognosis is grim, with less than 10 per cent survival. It has also been noted that the presence of vanillactic acid, a dopa metabolite, adversely influences the prognosis. It has been found that neuroblastoma excretes elevated levels of a serum protein, *ferritin*, which can be detected in the serum (Hann et al., 1979). Neuroblastoma patients, like others with malignant disease, may have reduced *E-rosette formation* by T-lymphocytes (Fuks et al., 1976). It has been speculated that ferritin may be responsible for this. That these factors are of prognostic significance is suggested by the report of Hann et al. (1981) that the majority of children with Stage IV disease have elevated serum ferritin levels but those with IV-S disease do not. E-rosette inhibition was seen frequently in Stage IV but seldom in Stage IV-S patients. Thus, elevated serum ferritin and the presence of E-rosette inhibition appear to be unfavorable prognostic factors.

Treatment of Localized Disease—Stages I, II, and III

In any discussion of the management of neuroblastoma, it must be emphasized that this remains one of the most frustrating pediatric malignancies to treat. In spite of extensive efforts to improve outcome, little has changed in the prognosis of these children over the past 20 years. The recommendations made here reflect the current state of knowledge, which, it is hoped, will be improved in the future.

Surgery. In the treatment of well-localized disease, surgery continues to be the primary mode of treatment. Complete surgical removal often may be accomplished in Stages I and II disease but may not be possible once the midline has been crossed in Stage III disease, when the aorta and inferior vena cava are frequently involved. In general, although total excision is the goal, en bloc removal of major organs in continuity with the tumor is not justified. An exception to this is the adjacent kidney for adrenal tumors. In clinical practice, tumors tend either to be well enough localized to permit excision or to be so extensive that even heroic operations would be impossible.

A second important role for the surgeon is to stage the neoplasm. It must be determined if the tumor infiltrates across the midline or involves contralateral lymph nodes. Biopsy of lymph nodes with a benign appearance is warranted because occult tumor may be found. This is a staging maneuver, and there is no evidence that radical node dissection is of value. Accurate staging is essential because, with the good prognosis for Stage II disease, therapy can be limited.

Second-look surgical procedures have a role with Stage III, and occasionally Stage II, inoperable tumors. Through chemotherapy and radiation therapy, it may be possible to produce adequate tumor shrinkage to permit a secondary complete removal. The timing of a second-look procedure is critical. Too early exploration is likely to find the tumor highly vascular and friable. An appropriate delay allows maturation and encapsulation of the tumor with the establishment of better tissue planes for dissection (Smith et al., 1980). Ideally, the appropriate time for secondary surgery is after a favorable tumor response to treatment but before the responsiveness of the tumor is lost. The secondary operation should be more aggressive in an effort to completely remove the tumor, because chemotherapy may be limited in its ability to produce effective suppression of the tumor unless the primary lesion is completely removed. Grosfeld et al. (1977) have reported survivors with Stage IV disease converted to complete responders by removal of the primary tumor at a secondary operation. Operations that "debulk" but do not completely remove the tumor, however, have not been shown to produce improved long-term survival (Sitarz et al., 1983).

Radiotherapy. While neuroblastoma is regarded as a generally radiosensitive tumor, the exact role of radiation therapy continues to be defined. In Stage I or II tumors, even if there is minimal residual disease after surgery, radiation therapy does not appear to improve the outcome (Evans et al., 1984). In Stage III disease, when gross residual tumor remains following surgery, irradiation does appear to be of significant benefit and to improve survival (Koop and Schnaufer, 1975). Usually, 1500 to 2500 rad, administered at 150 to 200 rad daily, is sufficient to control local disease.

Chemotherapy. Neuroblastoma in Stages I and II has an 80 per cent survival rate, and there is no evidence that chemotherapy improves this (Evans et al., 1984). Stage III disease, however, has a 50 per cent recurrence rate. Accordingly, the Children's Cancer Study Group has been exploring the effects of vincristine, cyclophosphamide and dacarbazine (DTIC) for 2 years with local radiotherapy and delayed surgery for these patients. The value of this treatment has yet to be demonstrated.

Treatment of Disseminated Disease—Stage IV

Surgery. There does not, at present, appear to be a role for the surgeon in the primary treatment of Stage IV neuroblastoma. Although for a period there was enthusiasm for an "assault" on the tumor in the belief that this might affect the outcome, this has unfortunately not resulted in any improvement in the dismal prognosis for this stage of neuroblastoma. Indeed, the results of the Children's Cancer Study Group (CCSG) suggest that initial surgery may worsen the outcome (Sitarz et al., 1983). The only role for surgery appears to be the removal of residual primary tumor after a good response to radiation and chemotherapy.

Radiation Therapy. Radiation therapy has its primary role in the palliation of painful or unsightly metastases. Relatively short treatment to produce doses in the range of 1000 to 2000 rads generally suffices, although higher doses can be useful if the patient is anticipated to have a longer period of time remaining before death from the tumor. A more aggressive approach to Stage IV disease, attempting to achieve a "total cell kill" of tumor by using multiagent chemotherapy, surgical removal of the primary tumor, and irradiation of the tumor bed and areas of metastatic spread, resulted in a 3-year survival rate of 9 per cent, very similar to historical controls for Stage IV disease (Evans, 1982).

Chemotherapy. Chemotherapy for disseminated neuroblastoma has been reported to produce a demonstrable response in up to 70 per cent of patients (Finklestein et al., 1979). The agents that have been demonstrated to be effective include vincristine, cyclophosphamide,

DTIC, VM-26, *cis*-platinum, nitrogen mustard, and doxorubicin (Adriamycin). While various institutions have combined these drugs in many different ways, there does not appear to be any clear advantage to one drug or program. The current protocol being followed by CCSG adds melphalan to the foregoing drugs. Combination chemotherapy does appear to be more effective than any agent used alone. Unfortunately, the use of chemotherapy has done little, if anything, to increase the long-term cure rate for neuroblastoma. The 3-year survival rate is slightly improved and provides some encouragement to those who continue to be aggressive in the treatment of disseminated neuroblastoma.

One exception to these rather depressing results is the use of bone marrow transplant for salvage following lethal combinations of chemotherapy. A combination of doxorubicin, VM-26, and very high-dose melphalan together with total-body irradiation and followed by allogeneic marrow transplantation or autologous marrow infusion has led to a 40 per cent 2-year actuarial survival in ten patients with recurrent Stage IV neuroblastoma (August et al., 1984). Although more than half the children experience recurrence or succumb to the effects of the transplant, to have any survivors following recurrent metastatic neuroblastoma is a significant advance. The role of bone marrow transplantation in the treatment of patients with newly diagnosed Stage IV disease is being explored in a larger multi-institutional study within CCSG.

Treatment of Metastatic Disease—IV-S

Patients with IV-S neuroblastoma confined to the liver, skin, and bone marrow usually are infants. Because the likelihood of spontaneous tumor regression is high, it is usually recommended that these children be observed for a period of time before any form of therapy is initiated (Evans, 1980). Occasionally, infants with massive hepatic involvement develop respiratory difficulty or vascular compression from increasing hepatomegaly. In this situation, low-dose radiation therapy may halt the growth and initiate tumor regression. Radiotherapy administered as 150 rad daily for 3 days through lateral portals angled 15 degrees above the horizontal to avoid the ovaries and spine is recommended by Evans et al. (1980). If there is inadequate reversal of the process, low-dose chemotherapy may be instituted. Cyclophosphamide or vincristine may be used; however, vincristine may be the wiser choice because of the known mu-

tagenic potential of alkalizing agents such as cyclophosphamide. Chemotherapy must be administered in reduced doses because of the increased toxicity in the very young. If radiation therapy and chemotherapy are unsuccessful, a ventral hernia with a Silastic pouch may be effective to temporarily relieve the problem until spontaneous tumor regression ensues (Schnaufer and Koop, 1975).

Future Treatment Expectations

Several promising areas of treatment for neuroblastomas are under investigation. The role of bone marrow transplantation has already been mentioned.

Other approaches are based on numerous observations that suggest that the patient's immune response may play a major part in the cure of neuroblastoma. Lauder and Aherne (1972) reported a better prognosis for patients whose tumors were infiltrated with lymphocytes. It has been proposed (Altman and Baehner, 1976) that opsoclonus may be associated with a good prognosis because the symptom is due to an antibody formed to the neuroblastoma that cross reacts with cerebellar cells to produce the neurologic symptom. Helstrom and Helstrom (1972) demonstrated that lymphocytes from children with neuroblastoma are capable of specific inhibition of neuroblastoma cells. These data suggest that immunotherapy may be useful in the treatment of neuroblastoma (Bernstein, 1980). Sawada et al. (1981) have reported on early work using interferon as an immune enhancer. If neuroblastoma can indeed be treated by immune means, it may be possible to design conjugated monoclonal antibodies against a specific neuroblastoma (Miller et al., 1982).

Further research into the treatment of neuroblastoma experimentally using the C-1300 mouse model (Finklestein et al., 1975) or the nude mouse with transplanted human neuroblastoma (Harlow et al., 1980) may permit the development of more effective treatments for this tumor than are currently available.

RHABDOMYOSARCOMA AND OTHER PELVIC TUMORS OF CHILDHOOD

Incidence

Sarcomas arising in soft tissues are the third most common solid tumor of childhood after central nervous system tumors and neuroblastoma. Rhabdomyosarcoma, a malignancy originating from the same embryonal mesenchyme that gives rise to striated skeletal muscle, is the most common soft tissue sarcoma, representing about 50 per cent of all soft tissue sarcomas of childhood. It constitutes 5 to 15 per cent of all solid malignant tumors and 4 to 8 per cent of all malignant disease in children under 15 years of age (Young and Miller, 1975). In the United States, the incidence is approximately 4.4 per million white children and 1.3 per million black children per year. The ratio of males to females is 1.4:1 (Maurer et al., 1977). There are two age peaks, the first between 2 and 6 years, and the second between 15 and 19 years (Maurer et al., 1977; Sutow et al., 1970). About 70 per cent of cases occur before the age of 10 years.

There appears to be a genetic component to rhabdomyosarcoma. Familial aggregations of rhabdomyosarcoma with other sarcomas, breast carcinomas, and brain tumors have been reported (Li and Fraumeni, 1969). There is an increased incidence of rhabdomyosarcoma in patients with neurofibromatosis (McKeen et al., 1978). Associated congenital anomalies are otherwise not common with rhabdomyosarcoma. Of seven associated congenital anomalies detected in 43 autopsies carried out as part of the Intergroup Rhabdomyosarcoma Study (IRS), there were four malformations of the central nervous system (Ruymann et al., 1977).

Rhabdomyosarcomas may arise from any part of the body that contains embryonal mesenchyme, whether striated muscle tissue is present or not. In the collected experience of the first Intergroup Rhabdomyosarcoma Study (Maurer et al., 1981), tumors arising in the genitourinary region made up approximately 20 per cent of the total. Only head and neck rhabdomyosarcomas occur more commonly. The most common genitourinary sites are the prostate, the bladder (most frequently in the area of the trigone), and the vagina, where tumors tend most frequently to involve the anterior vaginal wall contiguous to the bladder (Fig. 57–15). Paratesticular rhabdomyosarcomas, which arise in the mesenchyme of the spermatic cord, will be discussed with other testis tumors. Rhabdomyosarcomas arising in the pelvis outside the bladder or prostate often come to urologic consideration. These tumors may reach a large size before becoming symptomatic and have a worse prognosis than their counterparts in the bladder, prostate, vagina, or paratesticular region (Raney et al., 1981; Crist et al., 1984).

The natural history of rhabdomyosarcoma includes rapid growth with invasion of adjacent tissue. The tumor tends to be unencapsulated and infiltrative, making total surgical excision often difficult. The tumor may both spread into the regional lymphatic areas of drainage and invade the blood stream. When metastases occur, three quarters will manifest themselves within 6 months of diagnosis and over 80 per cent by 1 year (Heyn et al., 1974). Prior to the development of effective chemotherapy, 70 to 80 per cent of patients with rhabdomyosarcoma died with widespread metastases in spite of local surgical removal and radiotherapy (Mahour et al., 1967; Sutow et al., 1970).

Figure 57–15. Rhabdomyosarcoma: Embryonal tumor—sarcoma botryoides—of wall of bladder appearing like a cluster of grapes in the lumen.

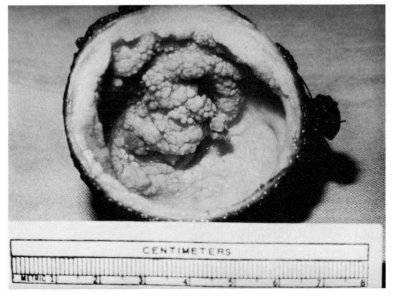

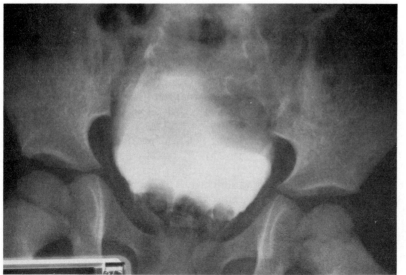

Figure 57–16. Rhabdomyosarcoma: Embryonal tumor—sarcoma botryoides—of bladder base showing characteristic polypoid configuration on cystogram.

Pathology

On gross examination, rhabdomyosarcomas tend to be nodular and firm. When viewed at operation, they are often deceptively well circumscribed while actually infiltrating extensively into adjacent tissue. There are no remarkable gross features of rhabdomyosarcoma excepting *sarcoma botryoides* (Fig. 57–16), which looks like a cluster of grapes and tends to arise in a hollow organ, such as the bladder or vagina.

The histologic classification of rhabdomyosarcoma reflects the wide range of mesenchymal differentiation that may be seen. *Embryonal* rhabdomyosarcoma is the most common type seen in childhood. Morphologically, it resembles developing skeletal muscle as seen in the 7- to 10-week fetus (Patton and Horn, 1962). This type is composed mainly of spindle-shaped cells with a central nucleus and abundant eosinophilic cytoplasm. About 30 per cent demonstrate cross striations. This type accounts for approximately two thirds of the rhabdomyosarcomas of the genitourinary tract and for 50 to 60 per cent of all rhabdomyosarcomas in children (Maurer et al., 1977). Sarcoma botryoides is a polypoid form of embryonal rhabdomyosarcoma.

The *alveolar* form of rhabdomyosarcoma histologically resembles skeletal muscle in the 10- to 21-week fetus. The tumor is often more firm and less myxoid than the embryonal type. Histologically, there are clusters of smaller round cells with scanty eosinophilic cytoplasm. Cross striations are rarely present. This type is more frequent in adolescents and young adults and is more commonly associated with tumors occurring in the extremities and trunk than in the genitourinary tract.

The *pleomorphic* type of rhabdomyosarcoma makes up only about 1 per cent of all childhood cases and is the form usually found in adults. As for the alveolar type, it is more common in the extremities and trunk than in the genitourinary tract. As its name implies, the histologic appearance of the tumor cells varies from racket-shaped to large round cells with giant or multiple nuclei to strap-shaped cells with multiple nuclei in tandem.

One can also encounter histologically *mixed* rhabdomyosarcoma. In addition, there is a group of 10 to 20 per cent of cases that are so undifferentiated that they do not fit into the standard classification. Histologically, they are primitive small round cell tumors, approximately half of which strongly resemble Ewing's sarcoma. The primary difference is that, unlike Ewing's sarcoma, they arise from soft tissue rather than from bone. Thus, many histologic patterns are possible with rhabdomyosarcoma. Mierau and Favara (1980) have suggested that all childhood rhabdomyosarcomas are basically embryonal tumors that vary only in the degree to which they have differentiated or responded to microenvironmental factors.

Presentation

The signs and symptoms of nonparatesticular rhabdomyosarcoma of the genitourinary

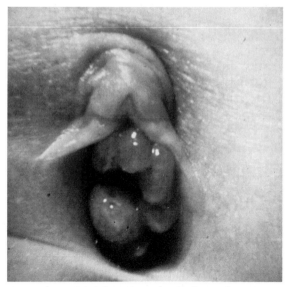

Figure 57–17. Rhabdomyosarcoma: Embryonal tumor prolapsing through urethra in female infant.

tract depend on the site of origin and the size of the tumor (Hays, 1980). If the bladder or prostate is involved, the child may present with strangury due to lower urinary tract obstruction. This may lead to urinary retention and secondary incontinence or infection. Hematuria may occur if tumor breaks through the lining of the genitourinary tract. If the tumor arises in the vagina, a bloody, foul-smelling discharge may be present. In the child with sarcoma botryoides, the tumor may prolapse through the urethra (Fig. 57–17) or be seen in the vagina. Occasionally, a child may void a fragment of tumor tissue. Pelvic rhabdomyosarcomas may grow to a large size before they impinge sufficiently upon the rectum or genitourinary tract to produce symptoms. Indeed, a large palpable mass is the single most common presentation of rhabdomyosarcoma.

Diagnostic Evaluation

Although these children may present with a large abdominal mass whose primary site is difficult to determine, this effort is important because of the different prognoses (see further on) of tumors arising in different sites. These tumors may undergo both hematogenous and lymphatic dissemination, and a careful search for metastatic deposits is important in order to stage the disease accurately.

Diagnostic imaging is usually satisfactorily accomplished using the intravenous urogram,

computerized axial tomography (CAT scans), and/or ultrasound examinations. Filling the bladder or rectum with water may permit better ultrasound imaging. If the tumor has a botryoid configuration, these imaging techniques may strongly suggest the diagnosis. A combination of cystoscopy and vaginoscopy is often useful in delineating the site of the tumor. If the mucosa of the bladder or prostatic urethra is clearly abnormal and an endoscopic biopsy confirms the presence of tumor, the site of origin is most probably in the bladder wall or prostate. Similarly, biopsy performed at vaginoscopy confirms the probable origin of the tumor from that structure. Often, however, these children present with a large pelvic mass that, while displacing the bladder and urethra or vagina, does not appear to involve the mucosal surfaces of these structures. In this case, establishing the site of the primary tumor is much more difficult. Careful bimanual examination with a cystoscope or catheter in the urethra may be useful. A large tumor may so completely fill the pelvis that its exact site of origin may not become evident until significant tumor shrinkage has been produced by chemotherapy or radiotherapy, or both.

The histologic diagnosis of rhabdomyosarcoma is established by biopsy. In obtaining an endoscopic biopsy with the pediatric resectoscope, it is important to be aware that the use of a resectoscope loop electrode may result in sufficient coagulation of the specimen to make it uninterpretable. The cold-cup biopsy forceps are generally more satisfactory These may be passed through a 13 F resectoscope. The 10 F resectoscope can be used with a Collings knife electrode to remove a polypoid specimen by cutting through its base and thus avoiding coagulation artifact in the rest of the specimen.

If, as is often the case, the child presents with a large abdominal mass displacing the bladder, prostate, or vagina but without evidence of mucosal abnormality, a needle biopsy may be useful. Perineal or extraperitoneal suprapubic biopsies may be obtained with needles of the Vim-Silverman type. We have found that the Tru-Cut needle usually produces an excellent core of tissue adequate for diagnosis. If a percutaneous approach to the tumor is not feasible, a laparotomy is required. A careful effort should be made to establish the origin of the tumor. As approximately 20 per cent of genitourinary rhabdomyosarcomas will have spread to the retroperitoneal lymph nodes by the time of diagnosis (Lawrence et al., 1977), a careful inspection and appropriate sampling of these nodes are important to accurately stage the tumor. Extensive deposits may also be evident on CAT scan examination of the chest, which is more successful in detecting metastatic lesions than plain films. Precision of clinical staging is essential because of the prognostic importance of stage and the varying intensity of treatment required.

Clinical Staging

Staging systems for rhabdomyosarcoma have largely depended on the resectability of the primary tumor and the status of the draining lymph nodes. Although there have been a number of different systems, the one most commonly used today is that drawn up by the major collaborative study of rhabdomyosarcoma in the United States—the Intergroup Rhabdomyosarcoma Study (Maurer et al., 1977).

The IRS clinical grouping classification is as follows:

1. Group I. Localized disease; completely removed; regional nodes not involved.
   A. Confined to muscle or organ of origin.
   B. Contiguous involvement with infiltration outside the muscle or organ of origin, as through fascial planes.
      Inclusion in this group includes both gross impression of complete removal and microscopic confirmation of complete removal.
2. Group II.
   A. Grossly removed tumor with microscopic residual disease; no evidence of gross residual tumor; no evidence of regional node involvement.
   B. Regional disease; completely removed (regional nodes involved or extension of tumor into an adjacent organ; no microscopic residual disease).
   C. Regional disease with involved nodes; grossly removed, but with evidence of microscopic residual disease.
3. Group III. Incomplete removal or biopsy with gross residual disease.
4. Group IV. Distant metastatic disease present at onset.

One problem with this staging system is that the stage is dependent on the type of surgical resection carried out prior to initiation of chemotherapy. This may produce a situation where equivalent pathologic stages are considered as different clinical stages. In the report of the first Intergroup Rhabdomyosarcoma Study,

the 118 genitourinary tumors were staged as follows: Group I, 36 patients; Group II, 28 patients; Group III, 27 patients; Group IV, 27 patients (Maurer et al., 1977). As can be seen, almost half of patients have disseminated (Groups III and IV) disease when diagnosed.

Treatment

Historical Approach. Surgical excision of the primary tumor was the first successful form of treatment of rhabdomyosarcoma. Often this required a radical excision, which for genitourinary rhabdomyosarcoma meant an anterior or total pelvic exenteration. Long-term survival with vaginal tumors treated by surgery alone was 40 per cent and for bladder/prostate rhabdomyosarcoma, 73 per cent (Green and Jaffe, 1978). These surgical results were considerably better than those achieved for rhabdomyosarcoma elsewhere in the body. The improved prognosis for bladder/prostate versus vaginal rhabdomyosarcoma may be related to the fact that the former tumors become symptomatic sooner and thus have less opportunity to become disseminated. Ghazali (1973) found that botryoid-type embryonal tumors of the bladder had a better outlook compared with solid embryonal tumors.

Ancillary treatment of rhabdomyosarcoma with radiation therapy began to emerge following the 1950 report by Stobbe and Dargeon that at least some rhabdomyosarcomas are radiosensitive. Experience indicated that persistent local control of tumor often required a high dose of radiation therapy, in excess of 4500 rad (Edland, 1965; Sagerman et al., 1972). D'Angio et al. (1959) recognized the favorable synergism that actinomycin D had with radiation therapy for rhabdomyosarcoma.

Chemotherapy for rhabdomyosarcoma developed with single agents used for the treatment of metastatic disease. The following drugs have been recognized to be effective: vincristine, actinomycin D, cyclophosphamide, mitomycin C, doxorubicin, imidazole carboxamide, *cis*-platinum, and VP-16 (Baum et al., 1981; Green and Jaffe, 1978). Later, these drugs were combined in various protocols for the treatment of metastatic disease.

In 1961, Pinkel and Pickren suggested coordinating aggressive initial surgery with postoperative radiotherapy and "prophylactic" chemotherapy following what appeared to be grossly complete tumor removal, in order to try to eliminate microscopic residual disease. The effectiveness of this approach was confirmed by

Heyn et al. in 1974. These authors reported the results in children with localized rhabdomyosarcoma who were rendered grossly free of tumor by radical surgery. They were then treated with postoperative radiation therapy with or without actinomycin D and vincristine administered for 1 year. Twenty-four of 28 (85.8 per cent) survived relapse-free for 2 years after initial treatment if chemotherapy had been administered, compared with only 7 of 15 (47 per cent) children who received no chemotherapy. The difference was statistically significant. This finding indicated the importance of administration of multiple-agent chemotherapy to all children with rhabdomyosarcoma. An extension of the role of chemotherapy was suggested by Wilbur (1974) in order to make even advanced lesions amenable to surgical treatment.

As more therapeutic alternatives began to open in the treatment of rhabdomyosarcoma, it became evident that the limited clinical experience of individual institutions would not permit an evaluation of the various available options. Thus was born in 1972 the Intergroup Rhabdomyosarcoma Study (IRS). This group has carried out prospective multidisciplinary studies of rhabdomyosarcoma.

The first IRS trial, which ran from 1972 to 1978, adhered to the prevailing approach to management at that time. An effort was made surgically to resect the tumor primarily, with follow-up treatment by radiation therapy and chemotherapy (Hays et al., 1981; 1982a). Of the 62 patients with sarcoma arising in the bladder, prostate, or vagina, 34 (55 per cent) had all gross tumor removed at the primary operation. Chemotherapy consisted of vincristine, actinomycin D, and cyclophosphamide (VAC) for 2 years in most cases. Of the 54 patients with bladder/prostate rhabdomyosarcoma, 47 (87 per cent) were treated with radiation therapy in doses varying from 2000 to 5500 rad. Forty-one of these 54 patients (76 per cent) are alive and relapse-free at a median of 4.5 years. Sixteen of 41 (39 per cent) have avoided exenterative surgery and retain their bladder. There were eight girls with vaginal rhabdomyosarcoma, half of whom were treated with radiation therapy as well as chemotherapy. Seven of the eight (88 per cent) are alive and relapse-free for 4 or more years, and six of the seven (86 per cent) have retained their bladder. The overall survival rate for IRS-I was 50 of 62 patients, or 81 per cent. This is a substantial improvement over the historical series of patients treated by surgery alone.

Recurrence of tumor in IRS-I, whether localized or distant, occurred within 2 years of initiation of treatment in all but two children. These two late recurrences were successfully treated and represent the only survival in recurrent rhabdomyosarcoma. Thus, relapse is particularly ominous with this tumor, with only 2 of 13 patients (15 per cent) being long-term survivors. One patient died of treatment-related causes.

Current Therapeutic Approach. After the demonstration that chemotherapy and radiation therapy were effective, a widespread interest developed in the primary use of these modalities in order to avoid the exenterative surgery so often previously required for genitourinary rhabdomyosarcoma (Maurer, 1980; Ortega, 1979; Rivard et al., 1975). This approach is being studied currently in IRS-II (Hays et al., 1982b; Raney et al., 1983). Primary surgical treatment has been restricted to tumor biopsy only. Subsequent management is as presented in Figure 57–18.

Intense chemotherapy with repetitive monthly courses of VAC (pulse-VAC) is begun. After 8 weeks of treatment, the patient undergoes clinical and radiologic re-evaluation. If there has been a complete or partial response, chemotherapy is continued until week 16. At this time, a similar re-evaluation is followed by surgical exploration, in order to determine the extent of residual disease. If there is gross or microscopic residual disease after surgical resection, the patient has radiotherapy added to the program and then continues on pulse-VAC therapy for a total of 2 years. If there is no residual tumor present after surgery, the radiotherapy is omitted but the patient is maintained on pulse-VAC chemotherapy for 2 years. Some tentative conclusions can be drawn from the information thus far accrued (Raney et al., 1983). The hope that primary chemotherapy would avoid the need for radiation therapy and radical surgery has not been realized. Only about 10 per cent of patients have achieved relapse-free survival with chemotherapy alone. Three quarters of the bladder/prostate tumors required radiotherapy. Approximately two thirds of these patients are alive and relapse-free, with a median follow-up of 2.7 years. Two thirds retain their bladder—somewhat better results than achieved in IRS-I with primary surgical treatment. Of the vaginal rhabdomyosarcomas, all patients are surviving but two thirds have required partial vaginectomy to remove residual tumor. The overall survival rate for IRS-II thus far is 80 per cent, virtually identical to the survival rate in IRS-I.

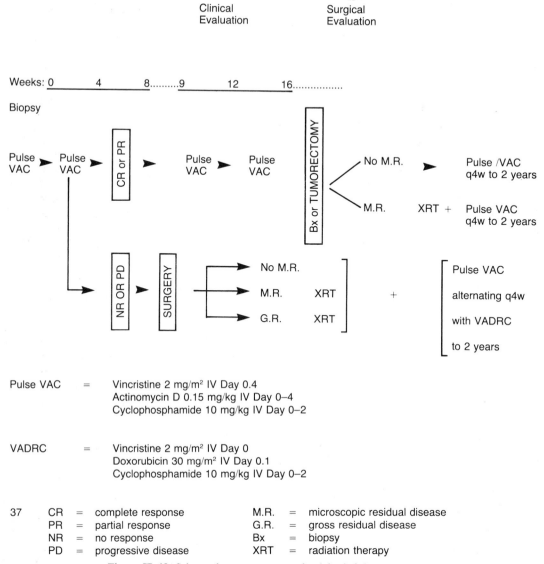

Pulse VAC = Vincristine 2 mg/m² IV Day 0.4
Actinomycin D 0.15 mg/kg IV Day 0–4
Cyclophosphamide 10 mg/kg IV Day 0–2

VADRC = Vincristine 2 mg/m² IV Day 0
Doxorubicin 30 mg/m² IV Day 0.1
Cyclophosphamide 10 mg/kg IV Day 0–2

37	CR	=	complete response		M.R.	=	microscopic residual disease
	PR	=	partial response		G.R.	=	gross residual disease
	NR	=	no response		Bx	=	biopsy
	PD	=	progressive disease		XRT	=	radiation therapy

Figure 57–18. Scheme for management of pelvic rhabdomyosarcoma.

It is clear that optimal therapy for rhabdomyosarcoma has yet to be completely defined. Perhaps a more intense chemotherapy program as advocated by Voute (Voute and Vos, 1977; Voute et al., 1984) will be more effective. With respect to radiotherapy, it has now been recognized that moderately high doses of radiation, in the range of 4000 to 5500 rad, are required to prevent an increased incidence of local recurrence (Tefft, 1981). It may be that altering the timing of radiotherapy will improve results. The timing and nature of surgical intervention may be altered to improve survival. It seems clear that procedures that include total cystectomy will still be necessary in a significant number of cases. It is to be hoped that, in the future, a combination of treatments will be evolved that will permit a high rate of survival without requiring the extensive use of mutilating surgical procedures.

OTHER PELVIC TUMORS

Transitional cell carcinoma of the bladder is very rare prior to puberty (Benson et al., 1983; Ray et al., 1973). Most such tumors in children are of low grade and stage. Almost all can be managed by endoscopic resection or fulguration, or both. Random bladder biopsies rarely detect any further abnormality. When the bladder appears to be free from tumor at the initial follow-up cytoscopy a few months later, it is rare to see a recurrence. It appears likely that transitional cell carcinomas in children are not part of a field defect, as is more likely in adults. When the cancer is invasive in children, it is managed in a fashion similar to that in adults.

Leiomyosarcoma of the bladder is a very rare soft tissue sarcoma in children (Mackenzie et al., 1968). Biologically, the tumor is less aggressive than rhabdomyosarcoma and local excision usually provides adequate therapy.

Adenocarcinoma of the exstrophied bladder or arising from the urachus tends to be seen in adults rather than children (Engel and Wilkinson, 1970). Although endoscopic surveillance of adults with a closed bladder exstrophy appears to be warranted, the risk of cancer is not sufficiently high to discourage attempts at functional reconstruction of bladder exstrophy.

Neurofibroma of the bladder may occur in patients with neurofibromatosis. A case has been reported in which neurofibroma caused such bilateral ureteral obstruction that local excision required bladder augmentation by ileocecal cystoplasty (Schoenberg and Murphy, 1961).

Lymphohemangioma may occur in the pelvis and invade the bladder and ureters. Although it is a benign hamartomatous tumor, we have seen a case causing incontinence through invasion and compression of the bladder. It was satisfactorily treated with restoration of continence by bladder augmentation by ileocecal cystoplasty.

Clear cell adenocarcinoma may occur in either the vagina or the cervix. Maternal use of diethylstilbestrol (DES) during pregnancy has been strongly implicated in the etiology of this tumor (Herbst et al., 1976; Ulfelder, 1976). DES-related adenocarcinoma is very rare before the age of 14 years. The peak incidence is at age 19 years, and the tumor rarely develops after age 24 years. Although much emphasized by the lay press, the actual risk is quite low (1 in 1000) (Herbst et al., 1977). *Benign adenosis*, also caused by diethylstilbestrol, is more common than clear cell carcinoma. Adenosis appears as ridges or folds in the vagina or cervix and, as it contains no glycogen, does not stain with Schiller's iodine. Adenosis, which may be the precursor of adenocarcinoma, appears to heal with time, probably accounting for the incidence of this tumor mainly in young women. These tumors are equally divided between the cervix and the vagina, and survival for clear cell adenocarcinoma is directly related to the size of the primary tumor and the depth of invasion. The larger the tumor, the more likely it is to be symptomatic, and thus, patients with symptoms tend to have a worse prognosis. Radical surgical excision is still advocated, although radiotherapy may also produce a good outcome. Overall 5-year survival is about 80 per cent (Herbst, 1980).

Adenocarcinoma of the infant vagina is a rare, highly malignant tumor that histologically resembles the embryonal cell carcinoma seen in the infant testis (Norris et al., 1970; Chu et al., 1978). Hinman and Perez-Mesa (1958) speculated that this tumor may arise in mesonephric remnants, although an endodermal diverticulum of the yolk sac or extraembryonic membranes could also be a source. The mesonephric papilloma, a form of hamartoma, is occasionally found in the infant vagina and may be the benign form of this tumor.

Squamous cell carcinoma of the cervix (Pollack and Taylor, 1979) and *adenocarcinoma of the uterus* (Lockhart, 1935) are both exceedingly rare tumors in childhood.

TESTIS TUMORS IN CHILDHOOD

Testicular tumors in childhood are common, accounting for about 1 to 2 per cent of all pediatric solid tumors (Ise et al., 1976). Pediatric testicular tumors represent roughly 2 per cent of all testicular tumors (Manger, 1973). The peak incidence occurs at about 2 years of age (Li and Fraumeni, 1972).

In contradistinction to adults, in whom germ cell tumors compose about 95 per cent of all testis tumors, germ cell tumors represent only 60 to 75 per cent of testis tumors occurring in childhood. Another distinction between adults and children is the higher incidence of benign tumors in the pediatric population when compared with the adult (Hopkins et al., 1978). Whereas only a small number of adult testis tumors are benign, between one fourth and one third of pediatric testis tumors are. However, there is no doubt that some testis tumors in children do result in death. From 1960 to 1967, the death rate from testis tumors for children in the United States was calculated at just under 1 death per 10,000,000 population per year, with roughly half of these deaths occurring in patients with yolk sac tumors (Li and Fraumeni, 1972).

TABLE 57–9. CLASSIFICATION OF PREPUBERTAL
TESTIS TUMORS

I. Germ Cell Tumors
  1. Yolk sac tumor   *most common*
  2. Teratoma
  3. Teratocarcinoma
  4. Seminoma
II. Gonadal Stromal Tumors
  1. Leydig cell
  2. Sertoli cell
  3. Intermediate forms
III. Gonadoblastoma
IV. Tumors of Supporting Tissues
  1. Fibroma
  2. Leiomyoma
  3. Hemangioma
V. Lymphomas and Leukemias
VI. Tumor-like Lesions
  1. Epidermoid cyst
  2. Hyperplastic nodule secondary to congenital adrenal hyperplasia
VII. Secondary Tumors
  I. Tumors of Adnexa

From Kaplan, G. W.: Testicular Tumors in Children.
AUA Update Series, 1983.

Classification of Prepubertal Testis Tumors

There has been no universally accepted system for classification of prepubertal testis tumors. As such tumors as seminomas and choriocarcinomas are extremely rare in children, adult classifications are not entirely appropriate. With this in mind, the Section on Urology of the American Academy of Pediatrics has proposed the classification shown in Table 57–9.

The distribution of tumor types is seen in Table 57–10.

TABLE 57–10. DISTRIBUTION OF TUMOR TYPES

Type	Incidence (Per Cent)
Yolk sac	47
Leydig cell	18
Teratoma	14
Sertoli cell	10
Rhabdomyosarcoma	4
Lymphoma	2
Fibrosarcoma	1
Other sarcomas	1
Hemangioma	0.5
Fibroma	0.5
Other	2

Adapted from Hauser, et al. 1965

Presentation

As in adults, the most common presentation is a painless scrotal swelling. Testis tumors may be mistaken for epididymitis, testicular torsion, inguinal hernia, or hydrocele. The last is not surprising, as 10 to 25 per cent of malignant testis tumors are associated with a hydrocele (Karamehmedovic et al., 1975). Aside from an occasionally painful paratesticular rhabdomyosarcoma or hormonally active nongerminal cell tumor, most testis tumors are asymptomatic in children; thus, it is no surprise that there is often a significant delay between notice of a mass and the child's presentation for evaluation.

On physical examination, a hard mass may be readily evident. Conversely, some patients who have hormonally active tumors may have such small lesions that the testis feels normal on palpation. A normal physical examination is not sufficient to exclude a tumor. An ultrasound examination may be particularly useful in this situation (Ilondo et al., 1981). Transillumination of a hydrocele may permit the identification of an enlarged testis; however, ultrasonography is generally more reliable (Leopold et al., 1979). If there has been lymphatic dissemination, an abdominal mass or supraclavicular node may be palpable.

GERM CELL TUMORS

The most common germ cell tumor and, indeed, the most common prepubertal testis tumor overall is the yolk sac carcinoma (Pierce et al., 1970; Weissbach et al., 1984). This tumor has been known by a plethora of terms, including endodermal sinus tumor, orchidoblastoma, embryonal adenocarcinoma, embryonal carcinoma, infantile adenocarcinoma of the testis, and testicular adenocarcinoma with clear cells. Most of these terms reflect confusion as to the exact origin of the tumor. Current opinion supports Teilum's (1959) concept that these tumors originate from yolk sac elements that were present early in the life of the embryo. The histologic hallmark of yolk sac tumors is the presence of eosinophilic, PAS-positive inclusions in the cytoplasm of the clear cells, which by specific staining techniques can be shown to consist of alpha fetoprotein (AFP) (Kurman et al., 1977). AFP is made by yolk sac cells in the embryo but has usually disappeared from the serum by 3 months of age. AFP levels are usually elevated in children with yolk sac carcinoma, and this provides a useful biologic marker for the tumor. The half-life of AFP is 5 days, so that after successful removal of a yolk sac tumor, levels should be normal (less than 20 ng/ml) usually within 1 month.

Although these tumors may bear some histologic resemblance to adult embryonal tumors (Brown, 1976), their clinical behavior is quite different, which has led to controversy concerning management. The tumor tends to occur in infancy (usually under the age of 2 years) and tends to remain localized for a relatively long period of time. When spread occurs, it is predominantly hematogenous to the lungs (20 per cent) and much less commonly by the lymphatics to the retroperitoneal lymph nodes (4 to 5 per cent) (Brosman, 1979). This predeliction for nodal spread is much less common than that seen with embryonal carcinoma in the adult. In the young child, the prognosis is excellent. Brosman (1979) reported a 2-year tumor-free survival rate of 89 per cent in children under 2 years of age; however, survival fell to 23 per cent for those over 2 years. The series of Jeffs (1972), Exelby (1979), and Drago et al. (1978) confirm the favorable prognosis for the young child.

Controversy has centered on management. Although retroperitoneal metastases are not frequent, Staubitz et al. (1965) showed that patients with retroperitoneal disease can be cured by orchiectomy and retroperitoneal node dissection alone. In most series, the retroperitoneal node dissection did not demonstrate tumor; however, microscopic metastases may have been missed. Because of possible long-term morbidity of retroperitoneal node dissection and the presence of a good tumor marker in AFP, the advisability of routine node dissection has been questioned. Additionally, combination chemotherapy with vincristine, actinomycin D, and cyclophosphamide (VAC), with or without doxorubicin, has been effective with this tumor (Colodny and Hopkins, 1977; Exelby, 1979). Kramer (1981) has pointed out the ability of chemotherapy to salvage patients who relapse. Radiotherapy is not indicated unless retroperitoneal nodes are demonstrated to contain tumor (Tefft et al., 1967).

Based upon these facts, our current practice is as follows: A radical inguinal orchiectomy is carried out with initial AFP level determination. Computerized tomography and ultrasound are used to evaluate the retroperitoneum and chest for evidence of dissemination. If a child under 1 year of age has an alpha fetoprotein that rapidly falls to normal and has no evidence of metastatic spread, he is observed for 2 years with chest x-rays and serum AFP levels. If the chest is negative but the retroperitoneum appears suspicious, especially if the AFP value remains elevated after orchiectomy, laparotomy and retroperitoneal node sampling are carried out. All resectable tumor is removed. If the chest is negative but retroperitoneal disease is present, chemotherapy is begun with VAC with or without doxorubicin, as for rhabdomyosarcoma. Radiation therapy is usually not employed. If pulmonary metastases are present, surgical removal may be indicated. If multiple metastases are present, chemotherapy is begun and the child is watched closely for response. If there is not a prompt diminution of tumor, bilateral pulmonary radiotherapy is added. As children over 1 year of age are at increased risk for pulmonary metastases, we generally give a course of vincristine and actinomycin D for a total of six courses over 1 year. Kramer's (1981) report of salvage chemotherapy may call this approach into question. Additionally, vinblastine, bleomycin, and cis-platinum, which have been used in adult testicular carcinoma, may be useful to salvage cases of recurrent yolk-sac carcinoma (Chu et al., 1978; Holbrook et al., 1980). It is apparent that the management of this tumor will continue to evolve.

Other germ cell tumors of childhood are the *teratoma* and *teratocarcinoma*. These tumors contain elements derived from more than one of the three germ tissues: ectoderm, endoderm, and mesoderm. The lesions are often cystic and may transilluminate. They can be bilateral (Carney et al., 1973). On cut section, there may be skin and sebum, hair, neural tissue, bone, and even teeth. Teratomas in infancy and childhood are usually mature, with well-differentiated tissue. Pure immature teratoma with primitive endoderm, neuroectoderm, and mesoderm is extremely rare. About 15 per cent of teratomas contain areas of dedifferentiation with a malignant appearance. In spite of this, testicular teratomas found before 24 months of age are consistently benign. Orchiectomy or the simple removal of the tumor with salvage of the remaining testicular tissue will provide a cure.

Older children with testicular teratocarcinoma are managed similarly to adults with germ cell tumors. Their prognosis has been much improved by chemotherpay regimens employing cis-platinum, bleomycin, and vinblastine. In excess of 80 per cent of patients with disseminated disease can be expected to be long-term survivors (Einhorn and Donohue, 1979).

Seminoma is extremely rare before puberty

(Viprakasit et al., 1977). It is seen in boys in whom puberty and spermatogenesis occur early, and it should in essence be considered a post-pubertal tumor. Management is as in the adult.

NON–GERM CELL TUMORS

Gonadal stromal tumors are the most common nongerminal testicular tumors in children. *Leydig cell tumors* are the most common gonadal stromal tumor both in children and in adults. The peak incidence in children is at about 4 to 5 years of age. Leydig cells, normally producers of testosterone, may continue testosterone synthesis when they undergo neoplastic transformation, and consequently Leydig cell tumors may cause precocious puberty (Pomer et al., 1954). Rapid somatic growth, increased bone age, deepening of the voice, phallic growth, and pubic hair development may precede the appearance of a palpable mass. The hallmark of the diagnosis is the triad of precocious puberty, a testicular mass, and elevated urinary 17-keto steroids. Leydig cell tumors account for about 10 per cent of cases of precocious puberty in boys (Urban et al., 1978). The differentiation from pituitary lesions, which may also cause precocious puberty, is made by finding LH and FSH at prepubertal levels with an elevated serum testosterone value.

Leydig cell tumors may also be associated with gynecomastia. Johnstone (1967) reported gynecomastia in 5 of his 39 reviewed cases of Leydig cell tumor. While estrogen levels are usually increased with these tumors, gynecomastia is more pronounced when the progesterone value is elevated. The estrogen increase is thought to produce an alteration in the normal androgen:estrogen ratio and thus lead to an overproduction of growth hormone. This results in an advancement of bone age, which may not completely regress following removal of the tumor (Ilondo et al., 1981).

Leydig cell tumors must be differentiated from the hyperplastic nodules that often develop in the testis of boys with poorly controlled congenital adrenal hyperplasia (CAH). As CAH is genetically transmitted, a family history may be useful. Moderate elevation of the urinary 17-keto steroid level may occur in both conditions. However, a major elevation is characteristic of the 17-hydroxylase deficiency type of CAH. Urinary pregnanetriol levels are absent with Leydig cell tumors but significantly elevated with the 21-hydroxylase deficiency type of CAH. When CAH is brought under good control by replacement glucocorticoids, the hyperplastic testicular nodules will regress, whereas a Leydig cell tumor remains unchanged.

Treatment for Leydig cell tumors is simple orchiectomy, as they are very rarely malignant (Mostofi and Price, 1973). Simple enucleation of the tumor has been suggested when the diagnosis is made preoperatively (Urban et al., 1978).

Sertoli cell tumors are the next most common gonadal stromal tumors of childhood. They present earlier than Leydig cell tumors, usually as a painless mass in a boy under 6 months of age. Histologically, the tumor resembles the fetal testis (Brosman, 1979). It generally produces no endocrinologic effect on the child. Although several malignant Sertoli cell tumors have been found in adults, only one with documented retroperitoneal metastases has been found in a child (Rosvoll and Woodward, 1968). Orchiectomy alone is sufficient treatment, but careful follow-up for possible retroperitoneal spread is appropriate.

The *gonadoblastoma* is believed to recapitulate gonadal development more completely than any other tumor. It is a neoplasm containing an intimate mixture of germ cells and germinal stromal cells (Scully, 1970). Usually the germ cells overgrow the other elements and the tumor resembles a dysgerminoma (seminoma) and is not hormonally active. In less than 10 per cent of cases, more malignant germ cell tumors may be present. The tumor is bilateral in one third of cases.

The tumor develops almost exclusively in abnormal gonads in children whose karyotype contains a Y chromosome. The most common karyotypes are 46XY and 45XO/46XY. All of these children have sexual abnormalities. Eighty per cent are phenotypic females with intra-abdominal testes (testicular feminization syndrome) or a female phenotype with intra-abdominal streak gonads and a karyotype with a Y (pure gonadal dysgenesis, XY type). Twenty per cent of gonadoblastomas arise in patients whose phenotypes tend more to the male line but often exhibit ambiguity. The gonads may be bilaterally dysgenetic cryptorchid testes or a streak associated with a contralateral testis (mixed gonadal dysgenesis).

The likelihood of gonadoblastoma rises significantly at puberty in these intersex states, all of which have a Y chromosome in the karyotype (Manuel et al., 1976; Mulvihill et al., 1975). Although metastatic spread of gonadoblastoma is not common, appropriate treatment is by gonadectomy before the development of the tumor.

TUMOR-LIKE LESIONS OF THE TESTIS

The hyperplastic testicular nodules associated with congenital adrenal hyperplasia have been discussed under Leydig cell tumors. *Epidermoid cysts* of the testis may present as a painless mass. The cysts are usually single, lined by squamous epithelium, and containing keratinized debris. There are no teratomatous elements. These lesions make up less than 1 per cent of all testis tumors (Price, 1969). These tumors are benign and could be removed with testicular preservation; however, usually an orchiectomy is carried out.

SECONDARY TUMORS

The most common malignancies to secondarily involve the testis are the *lymphomas* and *leukemias*. About 4 per cent of male patients with *Burkitt's lymphoma* have a tumor involving the testis, which may be the main presenting symptom (Lamm and Kaplan, 1974). The testis may also be involved by acute lymphoblastic leukemia (ALL) (Oakhill et al., 1980). Because the testis appears to act as a sanctuary site, perhaps secondary to the blood-testis barrier, it is apparent that as patients with ALL are increasingly controlled by chemotherapy, the testis may come to harbor residual tumor. In many centers, it is now routine to obtain bilateral testicular biopsies before discontinuing treatment in patients who are apparently cured of their leukemia. About 10 per cent will be positive, and about two thirds of these may eventually be salvaged by further chemotherapy and radiation therapy to the testes (Wong et al., 1980; Byrd, 1981). Although enough stromal elements may survive to avoid a need for hormonal replacement, fertility is unlikely.

Rarely, *Wilms' tumor* and *neuroblastoma* may metastasize to the testis.

TUMORS OF THE ADNEXA

Although not actually a testis tumor, *paratesticular rhabdomyosarcoma* must be considered because it arises in the mesenchymal tissue of the spermatic cord and presents as a scrotal mass that is occasionally tender. These tumors may grow rapidly, and a hydrocele may be present.

Most paratesticular rhabdomyosarcomas are of the embryonal type. As with other genitourinary rhabdomyosarcomas, early metastases to lymph nodes or by hematogenous spread are common and long-term survival was less than 50 per cent before the advent of effective chemotherapy and radiotherapy. Recent experience suggests that today close to 90 per cent of these

boys should be long-term survivors (Raney et al., 1978).

Paratesticular rhabdomyosarcoma has a higher incidence of retroperitoneal spread than other genitourinary malignancies. Raney et al. (1978), in their review of the IRS experience, found 40 per cent positive retroperitoneal node dissections and confirmed this percentage by a review of the literature. Although most of these cases can be salvaged by radiotherapy and chemotherapy, this is not without significant morbidity, such as bowel obstruction, intestinal fistula, or myelosuppression (Tefft et al., 1976). A routine retroperitoneal node dissection is indicated to stage the disease (Banowsky and Schultz, 1970; Olney et al., 1979). As there is no convincing evidence that the node dissection itself improves salvage, the dissection is usually a unilateral one on the side of the tumor, with sampling of any suspicious contralateral nodes. By avoiding bilateral node dissection, later problems with ejaculation may be prevented (Bracken and Johnson, 1976).

Our current recommendations for treatment of patients with paratesticular rhabdomyosarcoma are as follows (Cromie et al., 1979): After the diagnosis is confirmed following an inguinal orchiectomy, all patients have retroperitoneal lymph node dissection. If the biopsy results are negative, chemotherapy is carried out as described earlier for rhabdomyosarcoma and radiation therapy is omitted. If the nodes are positive, radiotherapy to the retroperitoneal node area is advised. If a transscrotal procedure to establish the diagnosis has been carried out, then either a hemiscrotectomy or x-ray therapy of the scrotum is indicated. To protect the contralateral testis from radiotherapy, it may be relocated to the thigh (D'Angio et al., 1974).

TUMORS ARISING IN THE UNDESCENDED TESTIS

One clearly identifiable risk factor associated with testicular malignancy is the presence of an undescended testis. About 10 per cent of all germinal tumors of the testis develop in an undescended testis (Fonkalsrud, 1970; Gallagher, 1976). The risk of malignancy in an undescended testis is about 35 times greater than in a descended testis. A testis in the inguinal canal has an approximate 1 per cent risk compared with an approximate 5 per cent risk for the intra-abdominal testis (Campbell, 1942, 1959). The 15 per cent of cryptorchid testis that are intra-abdominal contribute almost 50 per cent of the malignancies. The degree of seminiferous tubule dysgenesis appears to correlate directly with the likelihood of malignant degeneration. Boys with cryptorchidism have a higher incidence of dysgenesis in the contralateral descended testis and, along with that, an increased risk of tumor formation in that testis. Campbell's reviews (1942) indicated that with bilateral cryptorchidism associated with testicular tumors, there is a 25 per cent incidence of bilateral tumors.

The most common tumor that arises in an undescended testis is the seminoma. However, if the testis is brought down into the scrotum, the incidence of embryonal carcinoma rises (Batata et al., 1980). Although it has been always assumed that there would be a higher incidence of inguinal metastases from an undescended testis that had been surgically placed into the scrotum because of disturbance of lymphatic drainage, at least one large review has found this not to be so (Batata et al., 1980). The prognosis for an individual developing a malignancy in a surgically treated undescended testis parallels that of a male with normally descended gonads who develops a malignancy.

Orchiopexy early in life has become common only in recent years. At present, it is rare to see a testis tumor develop in a boy who had an orchiopexy before the age of five years. However, our period of follow-up is not yet adequate to establish this. Since an orchiopexy carried out after puberty does nothing to diminish the risk of malignancy, the current recommendation is for orchiectomy and the placement of a testicular prosthesis if the other testis is satisfactorily in the scrotum (Martin, 1979). Hinman (1979) has suggested the removal of all intra-abdominal testes if the contralateral one appears to be satisfactorily positioned and normal. We continue to carry out orchiopexy for these testes, often by the Fowler-Stephens technique (Gibbons et al., 1979).

As spontaneous testicular descent ceases after 1 year of age, our current recommendation is to carry out orchiopexy as soon after 1 year of age as the diagnosis can be established. As the average age for the development of a tumor in a formerly undescended testis appears to be 40 years, it is clear that prolonged awareness of an increased tumor risk is important. We instruct the families of our patients to see that the boys are taught testicular self-examination beginning after puberty. This seems particularly relevant as testicular tumors are now the leading cause of death from solid tumors in all men between the ages of 15 and 34 years (Grabstald, 1975).

References

Wilms' Tumor

Altman, R. P., Anderson, K. D., Matlak, M. E., et al.: Evolution of surgical treatment of bilateral Wilms' tumor. Surgery, *82*:760, 1977.

Aron, B. S.: Wilms' tumor—a clinical study of eighty-one patients. Cancer, *33*:637, 1974.

Aterman, K., Grantmyre, E., and Gillis, D. A.: Extrarenal Wilms' tumor: a review and case report. Invest. Cell Pathol., *2*:309, 1979.

Banner, M. P., Pollack, H. M., Chatten, J., and Witzleben, C.: Multilocular renal cysts: Radiologic-pathologic correlation. Am. J. Roentgenol., *136*:239, 1981.

Baum, E. S., and Gaynon, P. S.: Phase II trial of cis-dichlorodiammine-platinum II in refractory childhood cancer: Children's Cancer Study Group Report. Cancer Treat. Rep., *65*:815, 1981.

Beckwith, J. B., and Palmar, N. F.: Histopathology and prognosis of Wilm's tumor. Cancer, *41*:1937, 1978.

Belasco, J. B., Chatten, J., and D'Angio, G. J.: Wilms' tumor. *In* Fernbach, D. (Ed.): Clinical Pediatric Oncology. 3rd ed. St. Louis, C. V. Mosby, 1982.

Bennington, J. L., and Beckwith, J. B.: Tumors of the kidney, renal pelvis and ureter. Atlas of Tumor Pathology, Second Series, Fascicle 12. Bethesda, Md., Armed Forces Institute of Pathology, 1975.

Bishop, H. C., Tefft, M., Evans, A. E., and D'Angio, G. J.: Survival in bilateral Wilms' tumor—review of 30 National Wilms' Tumor Study cases. J. Pediatr. Surg., *12*:631, 1977.

Blank, E., Neerhout, R. C., and Burry, K. A.: Congenital mesoblastic nephroma and polyhydramnios. JAMA, *240*:1504, 1978.

Bolande, R. P.: Congenital mesoblastic nephroma of infancy. Perspect. Pediatr. Pathol., *1*:227, 1973.

Bolande, R. P.: Congenital and infantile neoplasia of the kidney. Lancet, *2*:1497, 1974.

Bond, J. V.: Bilateral Wilms' tumour and urinary tract anomalies. Lancet, *2*:721, 1975a.

Bond, J. V.: Bilateral Wilms' tumour. Age at diagnosis, associated congenital anomalies and possible pattern of inheritance. Lancet, *2*:482, 1975b.

Bove, K. E., and McAdams, A. J.: The nephroblastomatosis complex and relationship to Wilms' tumor: a clinico-pathologic treatise. Perspect. Pediatr. Pathol., *3*:185, 1976.

Bracken, R. B., Sutow, W. W., Jaffe, N., et al.: Preoperative chemotherapy for Wilms' tumor. Urology, *19*:55, 1982.

Breslow, N. E., and Beckwith, J. B: Epidemiological features of Wilms' tumor. J. Natl. Cancer Inst., *68*:429, 1982.

Cangir, A., Morgan, S. K., Land, V. J., et al.: Combination chemotherapy with Adriamycin (NSC-123127) and dimethyl triazeno imidazole carboxamide (DTIC) (NSC-45388) in children with metastatic solid tumors. Med. Pediatr. Oncol., *2*:183, 1976.

Carcassone, M., Raybaird, C., and Lebrenil, G.: Clear cell sarcoma of the kidney in children: a distinct entity. J. Pediatr. Surg., *16*:645, 1981.

Cassady, J. R., Tefft, M., Filler, R. M., et al.: Considerations in the radiation therapy of Wilms' tumor. Cancer, *32*:598, 1973.

Castellanos, R. D., Aron, B. S., and Evans A. T.: Renal adenocarcinoma in children: incidence, therapy and prognosis. J. Urol., *111*:534, 1974.

Chatten, J.: Epithelial differentiation in Wilms' tumor: a clinicopathologic appraisal. Perspect. Pediatr. Pathol., 3:225, 1976.

Chatten, J., Cromie, W. J., and Duckett, J. W.: Ossifying tumor of infantile kidney. Report of two cases. Cancer, 45:609, 1980.

Cho, K. J., Thornbury, J. R., Bernstein, J., Heidelberg, K. P., and Walter, J. F.: Localized cystic disease of the kidney: Angiographic-pathologic correlation. Am. J. Roentgenol., 132:891, 1979.

Cochran, W., and Froggatt, P.: Bilateral nephroblastoma in two sisters. J. Urol., 97:216, 1967.

Cohen, A. J., Li, F. P., Berg, S., et al.: Hereditary renal-cell carcinoma associated with a chromosomal translocation. N. Engl. J. Med., 301:592, 1979.

Coleman, M.: Multilocular renal cyst. Case report: ultrastructure and review of the literature. Virchons Arch. Pathol. Anat. Histol., 387:207, 1980.

Colgan, J. R. III, Skaist, L., and Morrow, J. W.: Benign ureteral tumors in childhood: a case report and a plea for conservative management. J. Urol., 109:308, 1973.

D'Angio, G. J.: SIOP and the management of Wilms' tumor (Editorial). J. Clin. Oncol., 1:595, 1983.

D'Angio, G. J., Beckwith, J. B., Breslow, N. E., et al.: Wilms' tumor: an update. Cancer, 45:1791, 1980.

D'Angio, G. J., et al.: Management of children with Wilms' tumor; defining the risk-benefit ratio. In Childhood Cancer: Triumph over Tragedy. Frontiers of Radiation Therapy and Oncology. Vol. 16. Basel, S. Karger, 1982.

D'Angio, G. J., Evans, A. E., Breslow, N., et al.: Results of the Third National Wilms' Tumor Study (NWTS-3): A preliminary report (Abstract #723). Proc. Am. Assoc. Cancer Res., 25:183, 1984.

D'Angio, G. J., Evans, A. E., Breslow, N., et al.: The treatment of Wilms' tumor: results of the Second National Wilms' Tumor Study. Cancer, 47:2302, 1981.

D'Angio, G. J., Evans, A. E., Breslow, N., et al.: The treatment of Wilms' tumor: results of the National Wilms' Tumor Study. Cancer, 38:633, 1976a.

D'Angio, G. J., Meadows, A., Mike, V., et al.: Decreased risk of radiation associated second malignant neoplasms in actinomycin-D treated patients. Cancer, 37(Suppl.):1177, 1976b.

D'Angio, G. J., Tefft, M., Breslow, N., et al.: Radiation therapy of Wilms' tumor: results according to dose, field, post-operative timing and histology. Int. J. Radiat. Oncol. Biol. Phys., 4:769, 1978.

Danis, R. K., Wolverson, M. K., Graviss, E. R., O'Connor, D. M., Joyce, P. F., and Cradock, T. V.: Preoperative embolization of Wilms' tumors. Am. J. Dis. Child., 133:503, 1979.

Dehner, L. P., Leestma, J. E., and Price, E. B., Jr.: Renal cell carcinoma in children—a clinicopathologic study of 15 cases and review of the literature. J. Pediatr., 76:358, 1970.

DeLorimier, A. A.: Surgical treatment of Wilms' tumor. In Pochedly, C., and Miller, D. (Eds.): Wilms' Tumor. New York, John Wiley & Sons, 1976.

DeLorimier, A. A., Belzer, F. O., Kountz, S. L., and Kushner, J. O.: Treatment of bilateral Wilms' tumor. Am. J. Surg., 122:275, 1971.

Donaldson, S. S., Jundt, S., Ricour, C., et al.: Radiation enteritis in children. A retrospective review, clinicopathologic correlation and dietary management. Cancer, 35:1167, 1975.

Donaldson, S. S., Wesley, M. N., Ghavimi, F., et al.: A prospective randomized clinical trial of total parenteral nutrition in children with cancer. Med. Pediatr. Oncol., 10:129, 1982.

Drash, A., Sherman, F., Hartmann, W. H., et al.: A syndrome of pseudohermaphroditism, Wilms' tumor, hypertension and degenerative renal disease. J. Pediatr., 76:585, 1970.

Duckett, J. W., Lifland, J. J., and Peters P. C.: Resection of the inferior vena cava for adjacent malignant disease. Surg. Gynecol. Obstet., 136:711, 1973.

Ehrlich, R. M., Bloomberg, S. D., Gyepes, M. T., Levitt, S. B., Kogan, S., Hanna, M., and Goodwin, W. E.: Wilms' tumor, misdiagnosed preoperatively: a review of 19 National Wilms' Tumor Study I cases. J. Urol., 122:790, 1979.

Ehrlich, R. M., Freedman, A., Goldsobel, A. B., and Stiehn, E. R.: The use of sodium 2-mercaptoethane sulfonate to prevent cyclophosphamide cystitis. J. Urol., 131:960, 1984.

Evans, A. E., Blore, J., Hadley, R., and Tanindi, S.: The LaBrosse spot test: a practical aid in the diagnosis and management of children with neuroblastoma. Pediatrics, 47:913, 1971.

Farber, S.: Chemotherapy in the treatment of leukemia and Wilms' tumor. JAMA, 198:826, 1966.

Farber, S., Toch, R., Sears, E. M., and Pinkel, D.: Advances in chemotherapy of cancer in man. Ad. Cancer Res., 4:1, 1956.

Farewell, V. T., D'Angio, G. J., Breslow, N., and Norkool, P.: Retrospective validation of a new staging system for Wilms' tumor: a report from the National Wilms' Tumor Study. Cancer Clin. Trials, 4:167, 1981.

Filler, R. M., Tefft, M., Vawter, G. F., et al.: Hepatic lobectomy in childhood: effects of x-ray and chemotherapy. J. Pediatr. Surg., 4:31, 1969.

Finklestein, J. Z., Hittle, R. E., and Hammond, G. D.: Evaluation of a high dose cyclophosphamide regimen in childhood tumors. Cancer, 23:1239, 1969.

Ganguly, A., Gribble, J., Tune, B., Kempson, R. L., and Luetscher, J. A.: Renin-secreting Wilms' tumor with severe hypertension. Ann. Intern. Med., 79:835, 1973.

Ganick, D. J., Gilbert, E. F., Beckwith, J. B., and Kiviat, N.: Congenital cystic mesoblastic nephroma. Hum. Pathol., 12:1039, 1981.

Giangiacomo, J., Peachansky, L., Monteleone, P. L., et al.: Bilateral neonatal Wilms' tumor with B-C chromosomal translocation. J. Pediatr., 86:98, 1975.

Green, B., Goldstein, H. M., and Weaver, R. M.: Abdominal pansonography in the evaluation of renal cancer. Radiology, 132:421, 1979.

Green, D. M.: Offspring of patients treated for unilateral Wilms' tumor in childhood. Cancer, 49:2285, 1982.

Gross, R. E., and Neuhauser, E. B. D.: Treatment of mixed tumors of the kidney in childhood. Pediatrics, 6:843, 1950.

Haicken, B. N., and Miller, D. R.: Simultaneous occurrence of congenital aniridia, hamartoma and Wilms' tumor. J. Pediatr., 78:497, 1971.

Harms, D., Gutjahr, P., Hohenfellner, R., and Willke, E.: Fetal rhabdomyomatous nephroblastoma. Pathologic histology and special clinical and biological features. Eur. J. Paediatr., 133:167, 1980.

Hartman, D. S., Lesar, M. S. L., Madewell, J. E., Lichtenstein, J. E., and Davis, C. J., Jr.: Mesoblastic nephroma: radiologic-pathologic correlation of 20 cases. Am. J. Roentgenol., 136:69, 1981.

Heaston, D. K., Libshitz, H. I., and Chan, R. C.: Skeletal effects of megavoltage irradiation in survivors of Wilms' tumor. Am. J. Roentgenol., 133:389, 1979.

Hou, L. T., and Holman, R. L.: Bilateral nephroblastoma in a premature infant. J. Pathol. Bacteriol., *82*:249, 1961.

Howell, C. G., Othersen, H. B., Kiviat, N. E., et al.: Therapy and outcome in 51 children with mesoblastic nephroma: a report of the National Wilms' Tumor Study. J. Pediatr. Surg., *17*:826, 1982.

Hunig, R., and Kinser, J.: Ultrasonic diagnosis of Wilms' tumor. Am. J. Roentgenol., *117*:119, 1973.

Jaffe, N., McNeese, M., Kayfield, J. K., and Riseborough, E. J.: Childhood urologic cancer therapy, related sequelae and their impact on management. Cancer, *45*:1815, 1980.

Janik, J. S., and Seeler, R. A.: Delayed onset of hemihypertrophy in Wilms' tumor. J. Pediatr. Surg., *11*:581, 1976.

Jayabose, S., and Lanzkowsky, P.: Hepatotoxicity of chemotherapy following nephrectomy and radiation therapy for right-sided Wilms' tumor. J. Pediatr., *88*:898, 1976.

Jenkin, R. D. T.: The treatment of Wilms' tumor. Pediatr. Clin. North Am., *23*:147, 1976.

Jereb, B., and Eklund, G.: Factors influencing the cure rate in nephroblastoma. Acta Radiol. Ther., *12*:84, 1973.

Jereb, B., Tournade, M. F., Lemerle, J., et al.: Lymph node invasion and prognosis in nephroblastoma. Cancer, *45*:1632, 1980.

Jones, B.: Metachronous bilateral Wilms' tumor. Am. J. Clin. Oncol. (CCT), *5*:545, 1982.

Kantor, A. F.: Current concepts in the epidemiology and etiology of primary renal carcinoma. J. Urol., *117*:415, 1977.

Katz, A. S., and Landau, S. J.: Pseudotumor of kidney. Urology, *13*:450, 1979.

Katzman, H., Haugh, T., and Berdon, W.: Skeletal changes following irradiation of childhood tumors. J. Bone Joint Surg., *51–A*:825, 1969.

Knudson, A. G., Jr., and Strong, L. C.: Mutation and cancer: a model for Wilms' tumor of the kidney. J. Natl. Cancer Inst., *48*:313, 1972.

Koyanagi, T., Sasaki, K., Arikado, K., et al.: Transitional cell carcinoma of renal pelvis in an infant. J. Urol., *113*:114, 1975.

Kuffer, F., Fortner, J., and Murphy, M. I.: Surgical complications of children undergoing cancer therapy. Ann. Surg., *167*:21, 1968.

Lawler, W., Marsden, H. B., and Palmer, M. K.: Histopathological study of the first Medical Research Council nephroblastoma trial. Cancer, *40*:1519, 1977.

Leape, L. L., Breslow, N. E., and Bishop, H. C.: The surgical management of Wilms' tumor. Ann. Surg., *187*:351, 1978.

Lemerle, J., Voute, P. A., Tournade, M. F., et al.: Preoperative versus postoperative radiotherapy, single versus multiple courses of actinomycin D, in the treatment of Wilms' tumor. Preliminary results of a controlled clinical trial conducted by the International Society of Pediatric Oncology (SIOP). Cancer, *38*:647, 1976.

Lemerle, J., Voute, P. A., Tournade, M. F., et al.: Effectiveness of preoperative chemotherapy in Wilms' tumor: results of an International Society of Pediatric Oncology (SIOP) clinical trial. J. Clin. Oncol., *1*:604, 1983.

Li, F. P., Bishop, Y., and Katsioules, C.: Survival in Wilms' tumour. Lancet, *1*:41, 1975.

Li, F. P., Cassady, J. R., and Jaffe, N.: Risk of second tumors in survivors of childhood cancer. Cancer, *35*:1230, 1975.

Littman, P., Meadows, A. T., Polgar, G., et al.: Pulmonary function in survivors of Wilms' tumor. Cancer, *37*:2773, 1976.

Machin, G. A.: Persistent renal blastema (nephroblastomatosis) as a frequent precursor of Wilms' tumor: a pathological and clinical review. Part 1. Nephroblastomatosis in context of embryology and genetics. Am. J. Pediatr. Hematol. Oncol., *2*:165, 1980.

Machin, G. A.: Persistent renal blastema (nephroblastomatosis) as a frequent precursor of Wilms' tumor: a pathological and clinical review. Part 3: Clinical aspects of nephroblastomatosis. Am. J. Pediatr. Hematol. Oncol., *2*:353, 1980.

Malcolm, A. W., Jaffe, J., Folkman, M. J., and Cassady, J. R.: Bilateral Wilms' tumor. Int. J. Radiat. Oncol. Biol. Phys., *6*:167, 1980.

Marosvari, I., Kontor, F., and Kallay, K.: Renin-secreting Wilms' tumour. Lancet, *1*:1180, 1972.

Marsden, H. B., and Lawler, W.: Bone metastasizing renal tumour of childhood. Histopathological and clinical review of 38 cases. Virchows Arch. Pathol. Anat. Histol., *387*:341, 1980.

Martin, L. W., and Reyes, P. M.: An evaluation of 10 years' experience with retroperitoneal lymph node dissection for Wilms' tumor. J. Pediatr. Surg., *4*:683, 1969.

Martin, L. W., Schaffner, D. P., Cox, J. A., et al.: Retroperitoneal lymph node dissection for Wilms' tumor. J. Pediatr. Surg., *14*:704, 1979.

Mathe, G., and Oldham, R. K.: Complications of cancer chemotherapy, recent results. Cancer Res., *49*:1, 1974.

McBride, G.: Chromosome analysis techniques expanded: new links to cancer. JAMA, *242*:1239, 1979.

McCauley, R. G. K., Safaii, H., Crowley, C. A., and Pinn, V. W.: Extrarenal Wilms' tumor. Am. J. Dis. Med., *133*:1174, 1979.

McVeagh, P., and Ekert, H.: Hepatotoxicity of chemotherapy following nephrectomy and radiation therapy for right-sided Wilms' tumor. J. Pediatr., *87*:627, 1975.

Meadows, A. T., and Jarrett, P.: Pigmented nevi, Wilms' tumor, and second malignant neoplasms. J. Pediatr., *93*:889, 1978.

Mike, V., Meadows, A. T., and D'Angio, G. J.: Incidence of second malignant neoplasms in children: results of an international study. Lancet, *2*:1326, 1982.

Miller, R. W.: Relation between cancer and congenital defects: an epidemiologic evaluation. J. Natl. Cancer Inst., *40*:1079, 1968.

Miller, R. W., Fraumeni, J. F., and Manning, M. D.: Association of Wilms' tumor with aniridia, hemihypertrophy and other congenital malformations. N. Engl. J. Med., *270*:922, 1964.

Mitus, A., Tefft, M., and Fellers, F. X.: Long-term follow up of renal function of 108 children who underwent nephrectomy for malignant disease. Pediatrics, *44*:912, 1969.

Mohammad, A. M., Meyer, J., and Hakami, N.: Long-term survival following brain metastasis of Wilms' tumor. J. Pediatr., *90*:660, 1977.

Morgan, E., and Kidd, J. M.: Undifferentiated sarcoma of the kidney. A tumor of childhood with histopathologic and clinical characteristics distinct from Wilms' tumor. Cancer, *42*:1916, 1978.

Movassaghi, N., Leiken, S., and Chandra, R.: Wilms' tumor metastasis to uncommon sites. J. Pediatr., *84*:416, 1974.

Murphy, D. A., Rabinovitch, H., Chevalier, L., and Virmani, S.: Wilms' tumor in right atrium. Am. J. Dis. Child., *126*:210, 1973.

Neuhauser, R. B. D., Wittenborg, M. H., Berman, C. Z.,

and Cohen, J.: Irradiation effects of roentgen therapy on the growing spine. Radiology, 59:637, 1952.

Novak, R. W., Caces, J. N., and Johnson, W. W.: Sarcomatous renal tumor of childhood: an electron microscopic study. Am. J. Clin. Pathol., 73:622, 1980.

Olsen, B., and Bischoff, A.: Wilms' tumor in adults. Cancer, 25:2, 1970.

Opitz, J. M.: Adenocarcinoma of the colon following Wilms' tumor. J. Pediatr., 96:775, 1980.

Ortega, J. A., Higgins, G. R., Williams, K. O., et al.: Vincristine, dactinomycin and cyclophosphamide (VAC) chemotherapy for recurrent metastatic Wilms' tumor in previously treated children. J. Pediatr., 96:502, 1980.

Palmer, N. F., and Beckwith, J. B.: Multiple primary tumor syndrome in children with rhabdoid tumors of the kidney (RTK). ASCO Abstract C-288, 1981.

Pendergrass, T. W.: Congenital anomalies in children with Wilms' tumor. Cancer, 37:403, 1976.

Penn, I.: Renal transplantation for Wilms' tumor: report of 20 cases. J. Urol., 122:793, 1979.

Pochedly, C.: Two-and-one-half-year survival of patient with ruptured Wilms' tumor. JAMA, 26:334, 1971.

Ramsey, N., Dehner, L., Coccia, P., D'Angio, G. J., and Nesbit, M.: Acute hemorrhage into Wilms' tumor. Pediatrics, 91:763, 1977.

Rance, T. F.: Case of fungus haematodes of the kidneys. Med. Phys. J., 32:19, 1814.

Raney, R. B., Palmer, N., Sutow, W. W., Baum, E., and Ayala, A.: Renal cell carcinoma in children. Med. Pediatr. Oncol., 11:91, 1983.

Riccardi, V. M., Siejansky, E., Smith, A. C., and Francke, U.: Chromosomal imbalance in the aniridia–Wilms' tumor association: 11 p interstitial deletion. Pediatrics, 61:604, 1978.

Riseborough, E. J., Gravias, S. L., Burton, R. I., and Jaffe, N.: Skeletal alterations following irradiation for Wilms' tumor. J. Bone Joint Surg., 5A:526, 1976.

Samuels, L. D., Grosfeld, J. L., and Kartha, M.: Radiation hepatitis in children. J. Pediatr., 78:68, 1971.

Sanyal, S. K., Saldivar, V., Coburn, T. P., et al.: Hyperdynamic heart failure due to A-V fistula associated with Wilms' tumor. Pediatrics, 57:564, 1976.

Scott, J. E. S.: Pubertal development in children treated for nephroblastoma. J. Pediatr. Surg., 16:122, 1981.

Shalet, M. F., Holder, T. M., and Walters, T. R.: Erythropoietin-producing Wilms' tumor. J. Pediatr., 70:615, 1967.

Shalet, S. M.: Abnormalities of growth and gonadal function in children treated for malignant disease: a review. J. R. Soc. Med., 75:641, 1982.

Shalet, S. M., and Beardwell, C. G.: Endocrine consequences of treatment of malignant disease in childhood: a review. J. R. Soc. Med., 72:39, 1979.

Shanklin, D. R., and Sotelo-Avila, C.: In situ tumors in fetuses, newborns and young infants. Biol. Neonate, 14:286, 1969.

Shende, A., Wind, E., and Lanzkowsky, P.: Intrarenal neuroblastoma mimicking Wilms' tumor. N.Y. State J. Med., 79:93, 1979.

Shurin, S. B., Ganderer, M. W. L., et al.: Fatal intraoperative pulmonary embolization of Wilms' tumor. J. Pediatr., 101:559, 1982.

Siegel, S. E., and Moran, R. G.: Problems in the chemotherapy of cancer in the neonate. Am. J. Pediatr. Hematol. Oncol., 3:287, 1981.

Simonowitz, D. A., and Reyes, H. M.: Renal abscess mimicking a Wilms' tumor. J. Pediatr. Surg., 11:269, 1976.

Smith, W. B., Wara, W. M., Margoli, L. W., et al.: Partial hepatectomy in metastatic Wilms' tumor. J. Pediatr., 84:259, 1974.

Snyder, H. S., Lack, E. E., Chetty-Baktavizian, A., Bauer, S. B., Colodny, A. H., and Retik, A. B.: Congenital mesoblastic nephroma: relationship to other renal tumors of infancy. J. Urol., 126:513, 1981.

Sotelo-Avila, C., Gonzalez-Crussi, F., and Fowler, J. W.: Complete and incomplete forms of Beckwith-Weidemann syndrome: their oncogenic potential. J. Pediatr., 96:47, 1980.

Stay, E. J., and Vawter, G.: The relationship between nephroblastoma and neurofibromatosis (von Recklinghausen's disease). Cancer, 39:2550, 1977.

Stevens, P. S., and Eckstein, H. B.: Ureteral metastases from Wilms' tumor. J. Urol., 115:467, 1976.

Sullivan, M. P., Sutow, W. W., Cangir, A., et al.: Vincristine sulfate in the management of Wilms' tumor. Replacement of preoperative irradiation by chemotherapy. JAMA, 202:381, 1967.

Sutow, W. W., and Sullivan, M. P.: Vincristine in primary treatment of Wilms' tumor. Texas State J. Med., 61:794, 1965.

Sutow, W. W., Breslow, N. E., and Palmer, N. F.: Prognosis in children with Wilms' tumor metastases prior to or following primary treatment. Results from the First National Wilms' Tumor Study (NWTS-1). Am. J. Clin. Oncol. (CCT), 5:339, 1982.

Sutow, W. W., Thurman, W. C., and Windmiller, J.: Vincristine (leurocristine) sulfate in the treatment of children with metastatic Wilms' tumor. Pediatrics, 32:880, 1963.

Tan, C., Etcubanas, E., Wollner, N., et al.: Adriamycin: an anti-tumor antibiotic in the treatment of neoplastic disease. Cancer, 32:17, 1973.

Tefft, M.: Radiation related toxicities in National Wilms' Tumor Study Number 1. Int. J. Radiat. Oncol. Biol. Phys., 2:455, 1977.

Tefft, M., D'Angio, G. J., and Grant, W.: Postoperative radiation therapy for residual Wilms' tumor—review of Group III patients in the National Wilms' Tumor Study. Cancer, 37:2768, 1976.

Tefft, M., Mitus, A., and Jaffe, N.: Irradiation of the liver in children: acute effects enhanced by concomitant chemotherapeutic administration? Am. J. Roentgenol. Radium Ther. Nucl. Med., 111:165, 1971.

Thompson, M. R., Emmanuel, I. G., Campbell, M. S., et al.: Extrarenal Wilms' tumors. J. Pediatr. Surg., 8:37, 1973.

Todani, T., Tabucki, K., and Watanabe, Y.: No touch isolation technique for left-sided Wilms' tumor. Z. Kinderchir., 19:93, 1976.

Traggis, D., Jaffe, N., Tefft, M., et al.: Successful treatment of Wilms' tumor with intracranial metastases. Pediatrics, 56:472, 1975.

Waggert, J., and Koop, C. E.: Wilms' tumor: preoperative radiotherapy and chemotherapy in the management of massive tumors. Cancer, 26:338, 1970.

Wang, J. J., Cortes, F., Sinks, L. F., et al.: Therapeutic effect and toxicity of Adriamycin in patients with neoplastic disease. Cancer, 28:837, 1971.

Wara, W. M., Philips, T. L., Margolis, I. W., et al.: Radiation pneumonitis: a new approach to the derivation of time-dose factors. Cancer, 32:547, 1973.

Wasiljew, B. K., Besser, A., and Raffensperger, J.: Treatment of bilateral Wilms' tumors: a 22-year experience. J. Pediatr. Surg., 17:265, 1982.

Wedemeyer, P. P., White, J. G., Nesbit, M. E., et al.: Resection of metastases in Wilms' tumor: a report of three cases cured of pulmonary and hepatic metastases. Pediatrics, *41*:446, 1968.

White, J. C., and Krivit, W.: Surgical excision of pulmonary metastases. Pediatrics, *29*:927, 1962.

Wigger, H. J.: Fetal hamartoma of kidney: a benign symptomatic congenital tumor, not a form of Wilms' tumor. Am. J. Clin. Pathol., *51*:323, 1969.

Williams, D. I., and Martin, J.: Renal tumors. *In* Williams, D. I., and Johnston, J. H. (Eds.): Pediatric Urology. 2nd ed. London, Butterworths, 1982.

Wockel, W., Lagerman, A., and Scheber, K.: Konnatales mesoblastisches nephron und nodulares renales blastem bei einem sangling. Zentralbl. Allg. Pathol., *123*:222, 1979.

Wohl, M. E. B., Griscom, N. T., Traggis, D. G., et al.: Effects of therapeutic irradiation delivered in early childhood upon subsequent lung function. Pediatrics, *55*:507, 1975.

Wolff, J. A., Krivit, W., Newton, W. A., Jr., et al.: Single versus multiple dose Dactinomycin therapy of Wilms' tumor. N. Engl. J. Med., *279*:290, 1968.

Young, J. L. J., Heise, H. W., Silverberg, E., and Myers, M. H.: Cancer incidence, survival and mortality for children under 15 years of age. American Cancer Society Professional Education Publication, September 1978.

Neuroblastoma

Adam, A., and Hochholzer, L.: Ganglioneuroblastoma of the posterior mediastinum: a clinicopathologic review of 80 cases. Cancer, *47*:373, 1981.

Akwari, O. E., Payne, W. S., Onofrio, B. M., et al.: Dumbbell neurogenic tumors of the mediastinum. Diagnosis and management. Mayo Clin. Proc., *54*:353, 1978.

Altman, A. J., and Baehner, R. I.: Favorable prognosis for survival in children with coincident opsomyoclonus and neuroblastoma. Cancer, *37*:846, 1976.

Anders, D., Kindermann, G., and Pfeifer, U.: Metastasizing fetal neuroblastoma with involvement of the placenta simulating fetal erythroblastosis. J. Pediatr., *82*:50, 1973.

Arenson, E. B., Hutter, J. J., Jr., Restuccia, R. D., and Holton, C. P.: Neuroblastoma in father and son. JAMA, *235*:727, 1976.

August, C., et al.: Treatment of advanced neuroblastoma with the supralethal chemotherapy, radiation and allogeneic or autologous marrow reconstitution. J. Clin. Oncol., *2*:609, 1984.

Beckwith, J. B., and Martin, R. F.: Observations on the histopathology of neuroblastomas. J. Pediatr. Surg., *3*:106, 1968.

Beckwith, J. B., and Perrin, E. V.: In situ neuroblastoma: a contribution to the natural history of neural crest tumors. Am. J. Pathol., *43*:1089, 1963.

Bernstein, I. D.: Prospects for immunotherapy of neuroblastoma. *In* Evans, A. E. (Ed.): Advances in Neuroblastoma Research. New York, Raven Press, 1980, p. 243.

Bolande, R. P.: Developmental Pathology. New York, Harper & Row, 1979.

Bond, J. V.: Neuroblastoma metastatic to the liver in infants. Arch. Dis. Child., *51*:879, 1976.

Bray, P. F., Ziter, F. A., Lahey, M. E., et al.: The coincidence of neuroblastoma and acute cerebellar encephalopathy. J. Pediatr., *76*:9833, 1969.

Breslow, N., and McCann, B.: Statistical estimation of prognosis for children with neuroblastoma. Cancer Res., *31*:2098, 1971.

Chatten, J., and Voorhees, M. L.: Familial neuroblastoma. Report of a kindred with multiple disorders, including neuroblastomas in four siblings. N. Engl. J. Med., *277*:1230, 1967.

Coldman, A. J., Fryer, C. J. H., Elwood, J. M., and Sonley, M. J.: Neuroblastoma: influence of age at diagnosis, stage, tumor site and sex on prognosis. Cancer, *46*:1896, 1980.

Cushing, H., and Wolbach, S. B.: The transformation of a malignant paravertebral sympathicoblastoma into a benign ganglioneuroma. Am. J. Pathol., *3*:203, 1927.

D'Angio, G. J., Evans, A. E., and Koop, C. E.: Special pattern of widespread neuroblastoma with a favorable prognosis. Lancet, *1*:1046, 1971.

D'Angio, G. J., Loken, M., and Nesbit, M.: Radionuclear (75 Se) identification of tumor in children with neuroblastoma. Radiology, *93*:615, 1969.

De Gutierrez Moyano, M. B., Bergada, C., and Becu, L.: Significance of catecholamine excretion in the follow up of sympathoblastomas. Cancer, *27*:228, 1971.

Delalieux, C., Ebinger, G., Maurus, R., et al.: Myoclonic encephalopathy and neuroblastoma. N. Engl. J. Med., *292*:46, 1975.

DeLorimier, A. A., Bragg, K. V., and Linden, G.: Neuroblastoma in childhood. Am. J. Dis. Child., *118*:441, 1969.

El Shafie, M., Samuel, D., Klippel, C. H., et al.: Intractable diarrhea in children with VIP-secreting ganglioneuroblastoma. J. Pediatr. Surg., *18*:34, 1983.

Evans, A. E.: Neuroblastoma: diagnosis and management. Curr. Concepts Oncol., *4*:10, 1982.

Evans, A. E.: Staging and treatment of neuroblastoma. Cancer, *65*:1799, 1980.

Evans, A. E., Albo, V., D'Angio, G. J., et al.: Factors influencing survival of children with non-metastatic neuroblastoma. Cancer, *38*:661, 1976.

Evans, A. E., Blore, J., Hadley, R., and Tanindi, S.: The LaBrosse spot test: a practical aid in the diagnosis and management of children with neuroblastoma. Pediatrics, *47*:913, 1971*a*.

Evans, A. E., Chatten, J., D'Angio, G. J., et al.: A review of 17 IV-S neuroblastoma patients at the Children's Hospital of Philadelphia. Cancer, *45*:833, 1980.

Evans, A. E., D'Angio, G. J., and Koop, C. E.: The role of multimodal therapy in patients with local and regional neuroblastoma. J. Pediatr. Surg., *19*:77, 1984.

Evans, A. E., D'Angio, G. J., and Randolph, J.: A proposed staging for children with neuroblastoma. Cancer, *27*:374, 1971*b*.

Everson, I. C., and Cole, W. H.: Spontaneous Regression of Cancer: A Study and Abstract of Reports in the World Medical Literature and of Personal Communications Concerning Spontaneous Regression of Malignant Disease. Philadelphia, W. B. Saunders Co., 1966, p. 88.

Filler, R. M., Traggis, D. G., Jaffe, N., et al.: Favorable outlook for children with mediastinal neuroblastoma. J. Pediatr. Surg., *7*:136, 1972.

Finklestein, J. Z., Eckert, H., Isaacs, H., and Higgens, G.: Bone marrow metastases in children with solid tumors. Am. J. Dis. Child., *119*:49, 1970.

Finklestein, J. Z., Klemperer, M. R., Evans, A., Bernstein, I., Leikin, S., McCreadie, S., Grosfeld, J., Hittle, R., Weiner, J., Sather, H., and Hammond, D.: Multiagent chemotherapy for children with metastatic neuroblastoma: a report from Children's Cancer Study Group. Med. Pediatr. Oncol., *6*:179, 1979.

Finklestein, J. Z., Little, K., Meshnik, R., et al.: Murine neuroblastoma: further evaluation of the C-1300 model with single antitumor agents. Cancer Chemother. Rep., 59:975, 1975.

Fortner, J., Nicastri, A., and Murphy, M. L.: Neuroblastoma: natural history and results of treating 133 cases. Ann. Surg., 167:132, 1968.

Fuks, Z., Strober, S., and Kaplan, H. S.: Interaction between serum factors and T-lymphocytes in Hodgkin's disease. N. Engl. J. Med., 295:1273, 1976.

Gibbons, M. D., and Duckett, J. W.: Neuroblastoma masquerading as congenital ureteropelvic junction obstruction. J. Pediatr. Surg., 14:420, 1979.

Gitlow, S. E., Bertani, L. M., Rausen, A., Gribetz, D., and Dziedzic, S. W.: Diagnosis of neuroblastoma by qualitative and quantitative determination of catecholamine metabolites in urine. Cancer, 25:1377, 1970.

Grosfeld, J. L.: Management of solid tumor in infancy and childhood: The Indiana experience. Jpn. J. Pediatr. Surg., 19:256, 1983.

Grosfeld, J. L., Sitarz, A., Finklestein, J., and Leikin, S.: The effect of primary tumor resection on survival in metastatic neuroblastoma. Proc. Am. Soc. Clin. Oncol., 18:308, 1977.

Gross, R. E., Farber, S., and Martin, L. W.: Neuroblastoma sympatheticum: a study and report of 217 cases. Pediatrics, 23:1179, 1959.

Hann, H. L., Evans, A. E., Cohen, I. J., et al.: Biologic differences between neuroblastoma Stages IV-S and IV. N. Engl. J. Med., 305:425, 1981.

Hann, H. L., Levy, H. M., Evans, A. E., and Drysdale, J. W.: Serum ferritin and neuroblastoma (Abstract 509). Proc. Am. Assoc. Cancer Res. Soc. Clin. Oncol., 20:126, 1979.

Harlow, P. J., Siegel, M. M., Siegel, S. E., et al.: Antitumor activity of chemotherapeutic agents alone or in combination using a human neuroblastoma model system. *In* Evans, A. E. (Ed.).: Advances in Neuroblastoma Research. New York, Raven Press, 1980, p. 319.

Hawthorne, H. C., Nelson, J. S., Witzleben, C. L., et al.: Blanching subcutaneous nodules in neonatal neuroblastoma. J. Pediatr., 77:297, 1970.

Hellstrom, K. E., and Hellstrom, I.: Immunity to neuroblastoma and melanomas. Ann. Rev. Med., 23:19, 1972.

Hepler, A. B.: Presacral sympathicoblastoma in an infant causing urinary obstruction. J. Urol., 39:777, 1976.

Herxheimer, G.: Ueber Tumoren des Nebennierenmarkes, insbesondere das Neuroblastoma sympaticum. Beitr. Pathol. Anat., 57:112, 1914.

Homzie, M. J., and Elkon, D.: Olfactory esthesioneuroblastoma—Variables predictive of tumor control and recurrence. Cancer, 46:2509, 1980.

Hope, J. W., Borns, P. F., and Berg, P. K.: Roentgenologic manifestations of Hirschsprung's disease in infancy. Am. J. Roentgenol. Radium Ther. Nucl. Med., 95:217, 1965.

Imashuku, S., LaBrosse, E. H., Johnson, E. M., Jr., Morgenroth, V. H., and Zenker, N.: Tyrosine hydroxylase in neuroblastoma. Biochem. Med., 5:2229, 1971.

Jaffe, N.: Neuroblastoma: Review of the literature and an examination of factors contributing to its enigmatic character. Cancer Treat. Rev., 3:61, 1976.

Jaffe, N., Cassady, R., Filler, R. M., et al.: Heterochromia and Horner syndrome associated with cervical and mediastinal neuroblastomas. J. Pediatr., 87:75, 1975.

Johnsonbaugh, R. E., and Cahill, R.: Screening procedures for neuroblastoma: false-negative results. Pediatrics, 56:267, 1975.

Knudson, A. G., and Amromin, G. D.: Neuroblastoma and ganglioneuroma in a child with multiple neurofibromatosis. Cancer, 19:1032, 1966.

Knudson, A. G., Jr., and Meadows, A. T.: Developmental genetics of neuroblastoma. J. Natl. Cancer Inst., 57:675, 1976.

Knudson, A. G., Strong, L. C.: Mutation and Cancer. Neuroblastoma and Pheochromocytoma. Am. J. Hum. Genet., 24:514, 1972.

Koop, C. E., and Schnaufer, L.: The management of abdominal neuroblastoma. Cancer, 35:905, 1975.

LaBrosse, E. H.: Biochemical diagnosis of neuroblastoma: use of a urine spot test. Proc. Am. Assoc. Cancer Res., 9:39, 1968.

LaBrosse, E. H., and Karon, M.: Catechol-O-methyltransferase activity in neuroblastoma tumour. Nature, 196:1222, 1962.

LaBrosse, E. H., Comoy, E., Bohmon, C., et al.: Catecholamine metabolism in neuroblastoma. J. Natl. Cancer Inst., 57:633, 1976.

Lauder, I., and Aherne, W.: The significance of lymphocytic infiltration in neuroblastoma. Br. J. Cancer, 26:321, 1972.

Laug, W. E., Siegal, S. E., Shaw, K. N. F., et al.: Initial urinary catecholamine metabolite concentrations and prognosis in neuroblastoma. Pediatrics, 62:77, 1978.

Littman, P., Soper, K., Surti, N., Holmes, J., Shimada, H., O'Neill, J., Chatten, J., and Evans, A.: The role of radiotherapy (RT) in localized neuroblastoma (LNBL). Am. Soc. Clin. Oncol., 3:81, 1984.

Makinen, J.: Microscopic patterns as a guide to prognosis of neuroblastoma in childhood. Cancer, 29:1637, 1972.

Marchand, F.: Beitrage zur Kenntniss der normalen und pathologischen Anatomie der Glandula carotica und der Nebennieren. Festschrift fur Rudolph. Virchows Arch., 5:578, 1891.

Mason, G. H., Hart-Nercer, J., Miller, E. J., et al.: Adrenalin-secreting neuroblastoma in an infant. Lancet, 2:322, 1957.

Miller, R. A., Maloney, D. G., Warnke, R., and Levy, R.: Treatment of B-cell lymphoma with monoclonal anti-idiotype antibody. N. Engl. J. Med., 306:517, 1982.

Miller, R. W., Fraumeni, J. F., and Hill, J. A.: Neuroblastoma: epidemiologic approach to its origin. Am. J. Dis. Child., 115:253, 1968.

Mitchell, C. H., Sinatra, F. R., Crast, F. W., et al.: Intractable watery diarrhea, ganglioneuroblastoma and vasoconstrictive intestinal peptide. J. Pediatr., 89:593, 1976.

Necheles, T. F., Rausen, A. R., King, F. H., and Pochedly, C.: Immunochemotherapy in advanced neuroblastoma. Cancer, 41:1282, 1978.

Odelstad, L., Pahlma, S., Lackgren, E. L., Grotte, G., and Nilsson, K.: Neuron specific enolase: a marker for differential diagnosis of neuroblastoma and Wilms' tumor. J. Pediatr. Surg., 17:381, 1982.

Pearse, A. G. E.: The APUD concept: Embryology, cytochemistry and ultrastructure of the diffuse neuroendocrine system. *In* Friesen, S. R., and Bolinger, R. E. (Eds.): Surgical Endocrinology: Clinical Syndromes. Philadelphia, 1978, J. B. Lippincott, pp. 18–34.

Peterson, D. R., Bill, A. H., Jr., and Kirkland, I. S.: Neuroblastoma trends in time. J. Pediatr. Surg., 4:244, 1969.

Quinn, J. J., and Altman, A. J.: The multiple-hematologic manifestations of neuroblastoma. Am. J. Pediatr. Hematol. Oncol., 1:201, 1979.

Reynolds, C. P., Smith, R. G., and Frenkel, E. P.: The diagnostic dilemma of the "small round cell neoplasm":

Catecholamine fluorescence and tissue culture morphology as markers for neuroblastoma. Cancer, *18*:2088, 1981.

Romansky, S. G., Crocker, D. W., and Shaw, K. N. F.: Ultrastructural studies on neuroblastoma: Evaluation of cytodifferentiation and correlation of morphology and biochemical survival data. Cancer, *42*:2392, 1978.

Sather, H., Siegel, S., Finklestein, J., et al.: The relationship of age at diagnosis to outcome for children with metastatic neuroblastoma (Abstract). Proc. Am. Soc. Clin. Oncol., *22*:409, 1981.

Sawada, T., Takamatsu, T., Tanaka, T., et al.: Effects of intralesional interferon on neuroblastoma: changes in histology and DNA content distribution of tumor masses. Cancer, *48*:2143, 1981.

Schnaufer, L., and Koop, C. E.: Silastic abdominal patch for temporary hepatomegaly in Stage IV-S neuroblastoma. J. Pediatr. Surg., *10*:73, 1975.

Schneider, K. M., Becker, J. M., and Krasna, I. H.: Neonatal neuroblastoma. Pediatrics, *36*:359, 1965.

Senelick, R. C., Bray, P. F., Lahey, M. E., et al.: Neuroblastomas and myoclonic encephalopathy: two cases and a review of the literature. J. Pediatr. Surg., *8*:623, 1973.

Sitarz, A., Finklestein, J., Grosfeld, S., et al.: An evaluation of the role of surgery in disseminated neuroblastoma: a report from the Children's Cancer Study Group. J. Pediatr. Surg., *18*:147, 1983.

Smith, E. I., Krous, H. F., Tunell, W. P., and Hitch, D. C.: The impact of chemotherapy and radiation therapy on secondary operations for neuroblastoma. Ann. Surg., *191*:561, 1980.

Sutow, W. W.: Prognosis in neuroblastoma of childhood. Am. J. Dis. Child., *96*:299, 1958.

Traggis, D. G., Filler, R. M., Druckman, H., et al.: Prognosis for children with neuroblastoma presenting with paralysis. J. Pediatr. Surg., *12*:119, 1977.

Virchow, R.: Hyperplasie der Zirbel und der Nebennieren. *In* Hirschwald, A.: Die krankhaften Geschwulste. Vol. 2. Berlin, 1864–1865.

Voorhees, M. I.: Neuroblastoma with normal urinary catecholamine excretion. J. Pediatr., *78*:680, 1971.

Voute, P. A., Jr., Wadman, S. K., and Van Putten, W. J.: Congenital neuroblastoma: symptoms of the mother during pregnancy. Clin. Pediatr., *9*:206, 1970.

Williams, C., and Greer, M.: Homovanillic acid and vanillylmandelic acid in diagnosis of neuroblastoma. JAMA, *183*:836, 1963.

Wong, K. Y., Hanenson, I. B., and Lampkin, B. C.: Familial neuroblastoma. Am. J. Dis. Child., *121*:415, 1971.

Young, J. L., and Miller, R. W.: Incidence of malignant tumors in U. S. children. J. Pediatr., *86*:254, 1975.

Rhabdomyosarcoma and Other Pelvic Tumors of Childhood

Baum, E. S., Gaynon, P., Greenberg, L., et al.: Phase II trial of cis-dichlorodiammine-platinum II in refractory childhood cancer: Children's Cancer Study Group Report. Cancer Treat. Rep., *65*:815, 1981.

Benson, R. C., Tomera, K. M., and Kelalis, P. P.: Transitional cell carcinoma of the bladder in children and adults. J. Urol., *130*:54, 1983.

Chu, J. Y., O'Connor, D. M., DeMello, D., Razek, A. A., and McElfresh, A. E.: Childhood embryonal carcinoma of testis: report of two unusual cases and the implication on clinical management. Med. Pediatr. Oncol., *4*:175, 1978.

Crist, W., Raney, B., Tefft, M., Heyn, R., Hays, D., Newton, W., Foulkes, M., and Maurer, H.: Soft tissue sarcomas arising in the retroperitoneal space in children: a report from the Intergroup Rhabdomyosarcoma Study Committee (Abstract No. 686). Proc. Am. Assoc. Cancer Res., *25*:173, 1984.

D'Angio, G. J., Farber, S., and Maddock, C. L.: Potentiation of x-ray effects by actinomycin D. Radiology, *73*:175, 1959.

Edland, R. W.: Embryonal rhabdomyosarcoma. Am. J. Roentgenol. Radium Ther. Nucl. Med., *93*:67, 1965.

Engel, R. M., and Wilkinson, H. A.: Bladder exstrophy. J. Urol., *104*:699, 1970.

Ghazali, S.: Embryonic rhabdomyosarcoma of the urogenital tract. Br. J. Surg., *60*:124, 1973.

Green, D. M., and Jaffe, N.: Progress and controversy in the treatment of childhood rhabdomyosarcoma. Cancer Treat. Rev., *5*:7, 1978.

Hays, D. M.: Pelvic rhabdomyosarcoma in childhood: Diagnosis and concepts of management reviewed. Cancer, *45*:1810, 1980.

Hays, D. M., Raney, R. B., Jr., Lawrence, W., Jr., et al.: Rhabdomyosarcoma of female urogenital tract. J. Pediatr. Surg., *16*:828, 1981.

Hays, D. M., Raney, R. B., Jr., Lawrence, W., Jr., et al.: Bladder and prostatic tumors in the Intergroup Rhabdomyosarcoma Study (IRS-I): Result of therapy. Cancer, *50*:1472, 1982a.

Hays, D. M., Raney, R. B., Jr., Lawrence, W., Jr., et al.: Primary chemotherapy in the treatment of children with bladder-prostate tumors in the Intergroup Rhabdomyosarcoma Study (IRS-II). J. Pediatr. Surg., *17*:812, 1982b.

Herbst, A. L.: DES update. Cancer, *30*:326, 1980.

Herbst, A. L., Cole, P., Colton, T., et al.: Age-incidence and risk of diethylstilbestrol related clear cell adenocarcinoma of the vagina and cervix. Am. J. Obstet. Gynecol., *128*:43, 1977.

Herbst, A. L., and Bern, H. A.: Developmental Effects of Diethylstilbestrol (DES) in Pregnancy. New York, Thieme-Stratton, 1981, pp. 1–203.

Heyn, R. M., Holland, R., Newton, W. A., Jr., et al.: The role of combined chemotherapy in the treatment of rhabdomyosarcoma in children. Cancer, *34*:2128, 1974.

Hinman, F., and Perez-Mesa, C.: Infantile carcinoma: a clinicopathological study and classification of 39 cases. Cancer, *11*:181, 1958.

Lawrence, W., Jr., Hays, D. M., and Moon, T. M.: Lymphatic metastases with childhood rhabdomyosarcoma. Cancer, *39*:556, 1977.

Li, F. P., and Fraumeni, J. F.: Soft tissue sarcomas, breast cancer and other neoplasms: a familial syndrome. Ann. Intern. Med., *71*:747, 1969.

Lockhart, H.: Cancer of the uterus in childhood. Am. J. Obstet. Gynecol., *30*:76, 1935.

Mackenzie, A. R., Whitmore, W. F., and Melamed, M. R.: Myosarcomas of the bladder and prostate. Cancer, *22*:833, 1968.

Mahour, G. H., Soule, E. H., Mills, S. D., and Lynn, H. B.: Rhabdomyosarcoma in infants and children: a clinicopathologic study of 75 cases. J. Pediatr. Surg., *2*:402, 1967.

Maurer, H. M.: The Intergroup Rhabdomyosarcoma Study II: objectives and study design. J. Pediatr. Surg., *15*:371, 1980.

Maurer, H. M., Donaldson, M., Gehan, E. A., et al.: The Intergroup Rhabdomyosarcoma Study: Update, November 1978. Natl. Cancer Inst. Monogr., *56*:61, 1981.

Maurer, H. M., Moon, T., Donaldson, M., et al.: The

Intergroup Rhabdomyosarcoma Study: a preliminary report. Cancer, *40*:2015, 1977.

McKeen, E. A., Bodurtha, J., Meadows, A. T., et al.: Rhabdomyosarcoma complicating multiple neurofibromatosis. J. Pediatr., *93*:992, 1978.

Mierau, G. W., and Favara, B. E.: Rhabdomyosarcoma in children: ultrastructural study of 31 cases. Cancer, *46*:2035, 1980.

Norris, H. J., Bagley, G. P., and Taylor, H. B.: Carcinoma of the infant vagina: a distinctive tumor. Arch. Pathol., *90*:473, 1970.

Ortega, J. A.: A therapeutic approach to childhood pelvic rhabdomyosarcoma without pelvic exenteration. J. Pediatr., *94*:205, 1979.

Patton, R. B., and Horn, R. C., Jr.: Rhabdomyosarcoma: clinical and pathological features and comparison with human fetal and embryonal skeletal muscle. Surgery, *52*:572, 1962.

Pinkel, D., and Pickren, J.: Rhabdomyosarcoma in children. JAMA, *175*:293, 1961.

Pollack, R. S., and Taylor, H. C.: Carcinoma of the cervix during the first two decades of life. Am. J. Obstet. Gynecol., *53*:135, 1979.

Raney, R. B., Jr., Donaldson, M. H., Sutow, W. W., Lindberg, R. D., Maurer, H. M., and Tefft, M.: Special considerations related to primary site in rhabdomyosarcoma: experience of the Intergroup Rhabdomyosarcoma Study, 1972–1976. Natl. Cancer Inst. Monogr., *56*:69, 1981.

Raney, B., Hays, D., Maurer, H., et al.: Primary chemotherapy ± radiation therapy (RT) and/or surgery for children with sarcoma of the prostate, bladder or vagina: preliminary results of the Intergroup Rhabdomyosarcoma Study (IRS-II), 1978–1982 (Abstract #C-293). Proc. Am. Soc. Clin. Oncol. 2:75, 1983.

Ransom, J. L., Pratt, C. B., Hustu, H. O., et al.: Retroperitoneal rhabdomyosarcoma in children: results of multimodality therapy. Cancer, *45*:845, 1980.

Ray, B., Grabstald, H., Exelby, P. R., and Whitmore, W. W., Jr.: Bladder tumors in children. Urology, *11*:426, 1973.

Rivard, G., Ortega, J., Hittle, R., et al.: Intensive chemotherapy as primary treatment for rhabdomyosarcoma of the pelvis. Cancer, *36*:1593, 1975.

Ruymann, F. B., Gaiger, A. M., and Newton, W.: Congenital anomalies in rhabdomyosarcoma. Proceedings of Conference on Congenital Birth Defects. Memphis, Tenn., June 9–11, 1977.

Sagerman, R. H., Tretter, P., and Ellsworth, R. M.: The treatment of orbital rhabdomyosarcoma of children with primary radiation therapy. Am. J. Roentgenol. Radium Ther. Nucl. Med., *114*:31, 1972.

Schoenberg, H. S., and Murphy, J. J.: Neurofibroma of the bladder. J. Urol., *85*:899, 1961.

Stobbe, G. C., and Dargeon, H. W.: Embryonal rhabdomyosarcoma of the head and neck in children and adolescents. Cancer, *3*:826, 1950.

Sutow, W. W., Sullivan, M. P., Ried, H. L., et al.: Prognosis in childhood rhabdomyosarcoma. Cancer, *25*:1384, 1970.

Tefft, M.: Radiation of rhabdomyosarcoma in children: local control in patients enrolled into the Intergroup Rhabdomyosarcoma Study. Natl. Cancer Inst. Monogr., *56*:75, 1981.

Ulfelder, H.: The stilbestrol-adenosis-carcinoma syndrome. Cancer, *38*:426, 1976.

Voute, P. A., and Vos, A.: Combination chemotherapy as primary treatment of children with rhabdomyosarcoma to avoid mutilating surgery or radiotherapy Proc. A.A.C.R., *18*:327, 1977.

Voute, P. A., Vos, A., and deKraker, J.: Chemotherapy at initial treatment in rhabdomyosarcoma (Abstract C-341). Proc. Am. Soc. Clin. Oncol., *3*:87, 1984.

Wilbur, J. R.: Combination chemotherapy of embryonal rhabdomyosarcoma. Cancer Chemother. Rep., *58*:281, 1974.

Young, J. L., and Miller, R. W.: Incidence of malignant tumors in U.S. children. J. Pediatr., *86*:254, 1975.

Testis Tumors

Banowsky, L. H., and Shultz, G. N.: Sarcoma of the spermatic cord and tunics: review of the literature, case report and discussion of the role of retroperitoneal lymph node dissection. J. Urol., *103*:628, 1970.

Batata, M. S., Whitmore, W. F., Jr., Chu, F. C. H., et al.: Cryptorchidism and testicular cancer. J. Urol., *124*:382, 1980.

Bracken, R. B., and Johnson, D. E.: Sexual function and fecundity after treatment for testicular tumors. Urology, *7*:35, 1976.

Brosman, S. A.: Testicular tumors in prepubertal children. Urology, *18*:581, 1979.

Brown, N. J.: Teratomas and yolk-sac tumors. J. Clin. Pathol., *29*:1021, 1976.

Byrd, R. L.: Testicular leukemia: incidence and management results. Med. Pediatr. Oncol., *9*:493, 1981.

Campbell, H. E.: Incidence of malignant growth of the undescended testicle. A critical and statistical study. Arch. Surg., *44*:353, 1942.

Campbell, H. E.: The incidence of malignant growth of the undescended testicle: a reply and re-evaluation. J. Urol., *81*:663, 1959.

Carney, J. A., Kelalis, P. P., and Lynn, H. B.: Bilateral teratoma of testis in an infant. J. Pediatr. Surg., *8*:49, 1973.

Chu, J. Y., O'Connor, D. M., DeMello, D., Razek, A. A., and McElfresh, A. E. Childhood embryonal carcinoma of testis: report of two unusual cases and the implication on clinical management. Med. Pediatr. Oncol., *4*:175, 1978.

Colodny, A., and Hopkins, T. B.: Testicular tumors in infants and children. Urol. Clin. North Am., *4*:347, 1977.

Cromie, W. J., Raney, R. B., Jr., and Duckett, J. W.: Paratesticular rhabdomyosarcoma in children. J. Urol., *122*:80, 1979.

D'Angio, G. J., Exelby, P. R., Ghavimi, F., Cham, W. C., and Tefft, M.: Protection of certain structures from high doses of irradiation. Am. J. Roentgenol. Radium Ther. Nucl. Med., *122*:103, 1974.

Drago, J. R., Nelson, R. P., and Palmer, J. M.: Childhood embryonal carcinoma of testes. Urology, *12*:499, 1978.

Einhorn, L. H., and Donohue, J. P.: Combination chemotherapy in disseminated testicular cancer: The Indiana University experience. Semin. Oncol., *6*:87, 1979.

Exelby, P. R.: Testis cancer in children. Semin. Oncol., *6*:116, 1979.

Fonkalsrud, E. W.: Current concepts in the management of the undescended testis. Surg. Clin. North Am., *50*:847, 1970.

Gallagher, H. S.: Pathology of testicular and paratesticular neoplasms. *In* Johnson, D. E. (Ed.): Testicular Tumors. 2nd ed. Flushing, N.Y., Medical Examination Publishing Co., 1976.

Gibbons, M. D., Cromie, W. J., and Duckett, J. W., Jr.: Management of the abdominal undescended testicle. J. Urol., *122*:76, 1979.

Grabstald, H.: Germinal tumors of the testis. CA, *25*:82, 1975.

Hinman, F., Jr.: Unilateral abdominal cryptorchidism. J. Urol., *122*:71, 1979.

Hinman, F., and Perez-Mesa, C.: Infantile carcinoma: a clinicopathological study and classification of 39 cases. Cancer, *11*:181, 1958.

Holbrook, C. T., Crist, W. M., Cain, W., and Bueschen, A.: Successful chemotherapy for childhood metastatic embryonal cell carcinoma of the testicle: a preliminary report. Med. Pediatr. Oncol., *8*:75, 1980.

Hopkins, G. B., Jaffe, N., Colodny, A., Cassady, J. R., and Filler, R. M.: The management of testicular tumors in children. J. Urol., *120*:96, 1978.

Houser, R., Izant, R. J., and Persky, L.: Testicular tumors in children. Am. J. Surg., *110*:876, 1965.

Ilondo, M. M., Van der Mooter, F., Marchal, G., Vereecken, A., Wynants, P., Lauweryns, J. M., Eeckels, R., and Van de Schueren–Looe Weycky, M.: A boy with Leydig cell tumor and precocious puberty: ultrasonography as a diagnostic aid. Eur. J. Pediatr., *137*:221, 1981.

Ise, T., Ohtsuki, H., Matsumoto, K., and Sano, R.: Management of malignant testicular tumors in children. Cancer, *37*:1539, 1976.

Jeffs, R. D.: Management of embryonal adenocarcinoma of the testis in childhood: an analysis of 164 cases. *In* Gooden, J. A. (Ed.): Cancer in Childhood. Toronto, The Ontario Cancer Treatment and Research Foundation, 1972.

Johnstone, G.: Prepubertal gynecomastia in association with an interstitial cell tumor of the testis. Br. J. Urol., *39*:211, 1967.

Kaplan, G. W.: Testicular Tumors in Children. AUA Update Series, Lesson 12, Vol. 2, 1983.

Karamehmedovic, O., Woodtli, W., and Pluss, H. J.: Testicular tumors in childhood. J. Pediatr. Surg., *10*:109, 1975.

Kramer, S. A.: Embryonal cell carcinoma in children. Pediatr Urol. Lett. Club, October 21, 1981.

Kurman, R. J., Scardino, P. T., McIntire, K. R., Waldmann, T. A., and Javadpour, N.: Cellular localization of alpha-feto-protein and human chorionic gonadotrophin in germ cell tumors of the testis using an indirect immunoperoxidase technique: a new approach to classification utilizing tumor markers. Cancer, *40*:2136, 1977.

Lamm, D. L., and Kaplan, G. W.: Urological manifestation of Burkitt's lymphoma. J. Urol., *112*:402, 1974.

Leopold, G. R., Woo, V. L., Scheible, F. W., Nachtsheim, D., and Grosink, B. B.: High-resolution ultrasonography of scrotal pathology. Radiology, *131*:719, 1979.

Li, F. P., and Fraumeni, J. F., Jr.: Testicular cancers in children. Epidemiologic characteristics. J. Natl. Cancer Inst., *48*:1575, 1972.

Manger, D.: Pathology of tumors of the testis in children. *In* Gooden, J. O. (Ed.): Cancer in Childhood. New York: Plenum Press, 1973, p. 60.

Manuel, M., Katayama, K. P., and Jones, H. W., Jr.: The age of occurrence of gonadal tumors in intersex patients with a Y chromosome. Am. J. Obstet. Gynecol., *124*:293, 1976.

Martin, D. C.: Germinal cell tumors of the testis after orchiopexy. J. Urol., *121*:422, 1979.

Mostofi, F. K., and Price, E. B.: Tumors of the Male Genital System. AFIP Fascicle 8, 2nd Series, 1973, p. 99.

Mulvihill, J. J., Wade, W. M., and Miller, R. M.: Gonadoblastoma in dysgenetic gonads with a Y chromosome. Lancet, *1*:863, 1975.

Oakhill, A., Mainwaring, D., Hill, F. G. H., Gornall, P., Cudmore, R. E., Banks, A. J., Brock, J. E. S., Martay, J., and Mann, J. R.: Management of leukemic infiltration of the testis. Arch. Dis. Child., *55*:564, 1980.

Olney, L. E., Narayana, A., Loening, S., et al.: Intrascrotal rhabdomyosarcoma. Urology, *14*:113, 1979.

Pierce, G. B., Bullock, W. K., and Huntington, R. W., Jr.: Yolk-sac tumors of the testis. Cancer, *25*:644, 1970.

Pomer, F. A., Stiles, R. E., and Graham, J. H.: Interstitial cell tumors of the testis in children. Report of a case and review of the literature. N. Engl. J. Med., *250*:233, 1954.

Price, E. B.: Epidermoid cysts of the testis: a clinical and pathologic analysis of 69 cases from the testicular tumor registry. Urology, *102*:708, 1969.

Raney, R. B., Jr., Hays, D. M., Lawrence, W., Jr., Soule, E. H., Tefft, M., and Donaldson, M. H.: Paratesticular rhabdomyosarcoma in childhood. Cancer, *42*:729, 1978.

Rosvoll, R. V., and Woodard, J. R.: Malignant Sertoli cell tumor of the testis. Cancer, *22*:8, 1968.

Scully, R. E.: Gonadoblastoma: a review of 74 cases. Cancer, *25*:1340, 1970.

Staubitz, W. J., Jewett, T. C., Jr., Magoss, I. V., Schenk, W. L., Jr., and Phalakornkulf, S.: Management of testicular tumors in children. J. Urol., *94*:683, 1965.

Tefft, M., Lattin, P. B., Jereb, B., et al.: Acute and late effects on normal tissues following combined chemoand radiotherapy for childhood rhabdomyosarcoma and Ewing's sarcoma. Cancer, *37*:1201, 1976.

Tefft, M., Vawter, G. F., and Mitus, A.: Radiotherapeutic management of testicular neoplasms in children. Radiology, *88*:457, 1967.

Teilum, G.: Endodermal sinus tumors of ovary and testis: comparative morphogenesis of the so-called mesonephroma ovarii (Schiller) and extraembryonic (yolk sac–allantoic) structures of the rat's placenta. Cancer, *23*:1092, 1959.

Urban, M. D., Lee, P. A., Plotnick, L. P., and Migeon, C. J.: The diagnosis of Leydig cell tumors in childhood. Am. J. Dis. Child., *132*:494, 1978.

Viprakasit, D., Navarro, G., Guarin, U. K., and Garnes, H.: Seminoma in children. Urology, *9*:568, 1977.

Weissbach, L., Altwein, J. E., and Stiens, R.: Germinal testicular tumors in childhood. Eur. Urol., *10*:73, 1984.

Wong, K. Y., Ballard, E. T., Strayer, F. H., Kisker, C. T., and Lampkin, B. C.: Clinical and occult testicular leukemia in long-term survivors of acute lymphoblastic leukemia. J. Pediatr. *96*:569, 1980.

INDEX

Note: Page numbers in *italics* refer to illustrations. Page numbers followed by t refer to tables.